INFECTIOUS DISEASE EPIDEMIOLOGY: THEORY AND PRACTICE

Second Edition

Kenrad E. Nelson, MD

*Professor, Departments of Epidemiology, International Health,
and Medicine
Johns Hopkins Medical Institutions
Johns Hopkins University
Baltimore, Maryland*

Carolyn F. Masters Williams, PhD, MPH

*Chief, Epidemiology Branch, Basic Science Program
Division of AIDS
National Institute of Allergy and Infectious Diseases
National Institutes of Health
Bethesda, Maryland*

*Dr. Williams contributed to the book in her personal capacity. The views expressed
are her own and do not necessarily represent the views of the National Institutes of
Health or the United States Government.

JONES AND BARTLETT PUBLISHERS
Sudbury, Massachusetts
BOSTON   TORONTO   LONDON   SINGAPORE

World Headquarters

Jones and Bartlett Publishers
40 Tall Pine Drive
Sudbury, MA 01776
978-443-5000
info@jbpub.com
www.jbpub.com

Jones and Bartlett Publishers
Canada
6339 Ormindale Way
Mississauga, Ontario L5V 1J2
CANADA

Jones and Bartlett Publishers
International
Barb House, Barb Mews
London W6 7PA
UK

Jones and Bartlett's books and products are available through most bookstores and online booksellers. To contact Jones and Bartlett Publishers directly, call 800-832-0034, fax 978-443-8000, or visit our website, www.jbpub.com.

Substantial discounts on bulk quantities of Jones and Bartlett's publications are available to corporations, professional associations, and other qualified organizations. For details and specific discount information, contact the special sales department at Jones and Bartlett via the above contact information or send an email to specialsales@jbpub.com.

Production Credits
Publisher: Michael Brown
Assoc Editor: Kylah Goodfellow McNeill
Production Director: Amy Rose
Associate Production Editor: Daniel Stone
Manufacturing Buyer: Therese Connell
Composition: Best-Set
Cover Design: Kristin E. Ohlin
Cover Image: © Eye of Science/Photo Researchers, Inc.
Printing and Binding: Marketing Manager
Marketing Manager: Sophie Fleck
Cover Printing: Malloy, Inc.

Cover photo is a colored transmission electron micrograph (TEM) of a cluster of coronavirus particles cultured in human cells. Different strains of coronavirus cause diseases such as the common cold, gastroenteritis and SARS (severe acute respiratory syndrome). This is not the specific strain of coronavirus that causes SARS. The coronaviruses derive their name from their crown (corona) of surface proteins (green), which they use to attach and penetrate their host cells. Once inside the cells, the particles use the cells' machinery to make more copies of the virus.

Library of Congress Cataloging-in-Publication Data
Infectious disease epidemiology : theory and practice / [edited by] Kenrad E. Nelson, Carolyn F. Masters Williams.—2nd ed.
    p. ; cm.
Includes bibliographical references and index.
ISBN-13: 978-0-7637-2879-3
ISBN-10: 0-7637-2879-9
1. Communicable diseases—Epidemiology.
    [DNLM: 1. Communicable Diseases—epidemiology. 2. Disease Outbreaks. 3. Epidemiologic Methods. WC 100 I1026 2006] I. Nelson, Kenrad E. II. Williams, Carolyn Masters.
    RA643.I6535 2006
    614.5–dc22

                                             2006005286

6048

The authors, editor, and publisher have made every effort to provide accurate information. However, they are not responsible for errors, omissions, or for any outcomes related to the use of the contents of this book and take no responsibility for the use of the products and procedures described. Treatments and side effects described in this book may not be applicable to all people; likewise, some people may require a dose or experience a side effect that is not described herein. Drugs and medical devices are discussed that may have limited availability controlled by the Food and Drug Adminstration (FDA) for use only in a research study or clinical trial. Research, clinical practice, and government regulations often change the accepted standard in this field. When consideration is being given to use of any drug in the clinical setting, the health care provider or reader is responsible for determining FDA status of the drug, reading the package insert, and reviewing prescribing information for the most up-to-date recommendations on dose, precautions, and contraindications, and determining the appropriate usage for the product. This is especially important in the case of drugs that are new or seldom used.

Printed in the United States of America
10 09 08 07 06 10 9 8 7 6 5 4 3 2

CONTENTS

CONTRIBUTORS

Joan L. Aron, PhD
President
Science Communication Studies
Columbia, Maryland

William R. Bishai, MD, PhD
Professor
Departments of Medicine and Molecular
    Microbiology & Immunology
Johns Hopkins Medical Institutions
Johns Hopkins University
Baltimore, Maryland

Robert E. Black, MD
Professor and Chair
Department of International Health
Bloomberg School of Public Health
Johns Hopkins University
Baltimore, Maryland

Karen C. Carroll, MD
Director, Microbiology Laboratories
Associate Professor
Departments of Pathology and Medicine
School of Medicine
Johns Hopkins University
Baltimore, Maryland

David D. Celentano, ScD
Professor
Departments of Epidemiology, Health
Policy and Management and Human
    Behavior and Health
Johns Hopkins Medical Institutions
Baltimore, Maryland

Richard E. Chaisson, MD
Professor
Departments of Medicine, Epidemiology,
    and International Health
Johns Hopkins Medical Institutions
Johns Hopkins University
Baltimore, Maryland

Rohit Chitale, PhD
Epidemiologist
Department of Epidemiology
Johns Hopkins University
Baltimore, Maryland

Rashid A. Chotani, MD, MPH
Assistant Professor
Department of Emergency Medicine and
    International Health
Johns Hopkins Medical Institutions
Baltimore, Maryland

Jacqueline S. Coberly, PhD
Epidemiologist
The Johns Hopkins Applied Physics
    Laboratory
National Security Technology
    Department
Columbia, Maryland

James Dick, PhD
Associate Professor
Department of Pathology
School of Medicine and W. Harry
    Feinstone
Department of Molecular Microbiology
    and Immunology
Johns Hopkins Medical Institutions
Johns Hopkins University
Baltimore, Maryland

Diane M. Dwyer, MD
Former Maryland State Epidemiologist
  and Director
Epidemiology and Disease Control
  Program
Maryland Department of Health and
  Mental Hygiene
Senior Associate
Department of Epidemiology
Bloomberg School of Public Health
Johns Hopkins University
Baltimore, Maryland

John S. Francis, MD, PhD
Post-Doctoral Fellow
Section of Infectious Diseases
Department of Medicine
School of Medicine
Johns Hopkins University
Baltimore, Maryland

Gregory E. Glass, PhD
Professor
W. Harry Feinstone Department of
  Molecular Microbiology and
  Immunology
Bloomberg School of Public Health
Johns Hopkins University
Baltimore, Maryland

Neil M.H. Graham, MBBS, MD, MPH
Chief Medical Officer
Trimeris Inc
Morrisville, North Carolina

Diane E. Griffin, MD, PhD
Professor and Chair
W. Harry Feinstone Department of
  Molecular Microbiology and Immunol-
  ogy Bloomberg School of Public
  Health
Johns Hopkins University
Baltimore, Maryland

Carmela Groves, RN, MS
Chief, Division of Outbreak
  Investigation
Epidemiology and Disease Control
  Program
Maryland Department of Health and
  Mental Hygiene
Baltimore, Maryland

Susan M. Harrington, MT, MPH, PhD
Department of Laboratory Medicine
Clinical Center
National Institutes of Health
Bethesda, Maryland

Claudio F. Lanata, MD, MPH
Senior Researcher
Instituto de Investigacion Nutricional
Lima, Peru

Anita M. Loughlin, MS, PhD
Assistant Professor
Department of Epidemiology
School of Public Health
Boston University
Boston, Massachusetts

Joseph B. Margolick, MD, PhD
Professor
Department of Molecular
  Microbiology and Immunology,
  Environmental Health Sciences and
  Epidemiology
Bloomberg School of Public Health
Johns Hopkins University
Baltimore, Maryland

Richard B. Markham, MD
Professor
Departments of Molecular Microbiology
  and Immunology and Medicine
Johns Hopkins Medical Institutions
Baltimore, Maryland

Richard H. Morrow, MD, MPH, FACP
Professor of International Health
Bloomberg School of Public Health
Johns Hopkins University
Baltimore, Maryland

William J. Moss, MD, MPH
Assistant Professor
Departments of Epidemiology, Molecular
  Microbiology and Immunology and
  Pediatrics
Johns Hopkins Medical Institutions
Baltimore, Maryland

Kenrad E. Nelson, MD
Professor
Departments of Epidemiology,
  International Health and Medicine
Johns Hopkins Medical Institutions
Johns Hopkins University
Baltimore, Maryland

Martin Ota, MD, FWACP, PhD
Post-Doctoral Fellow
Department of Molecular Microbiology
 and Immunology
Bloomberg School of Public Health
Johns Hopkins University
Baltimore, Maryland

Nikki M. Parrish, PhD
Assistant Professor
Department of Pathology
School of Medicine
Johns Hopkins University
Baltimore, Maryland

Trish M. Perl, MD, MSc
Associate Professor
Director of Hospital Epidemiology and
 Infection Control
Departments of Medicine and
 Epidemiology
Johns Hopkins Medicine Institutions
Johns Hopkins University
Baltimore, Maryland

Mary-Claire Roghmann, MD, MS
Assistant Professor
Hospital Epidemiologist
VA Maryland Health Care System
Departments of Medicine and
 Epidemiology and Preventive
 Medicine
University of Maryland School of
 Medicine
Baltimore, Maryland

Alan L. Scott, PhD
Professor
Department of Molecular Microbiology
 and Immunology
Bloomberg School of Public Health
Johns Hopkins University
Baltimore, Maryland

Richard D. Semba, MD, MPH
Associate Professor
Departments of Ophthalmology and
 International Health
School of Medicine
Johns Hopkins University
Baltimore, Maryland

Clive Shiff, PhD, MSc
Associate Professor
W. Harry Feinstone Department
 of Molecular Microbiology and
 Immunology
Bloomberg School of Public Health
Johns Hopkins University
Baltimore, Maryland

Mark C. Steinhoff, MD
Professor
Departments of International Health,
 Epidemiology and Pediatrics
Johns Hopkins Medical Institutions
Baltimore, Maryland

Frangiscos Sifakis, PhD
Research Scientist
Department of Epidemiology
Bloomberg School of Public Health
Johns Hopkins University
Baltimore, Maryland

Ellen Smit, PhD
Assistant Professor
Department of Social and Preventive
 Medicine
State University of New York at
 Buffalo
Buffalo, New York

Steffanie A. Strathdee, PhD
Professor and Harold Simon
Chair, Chief Division of International
 Health and Cross Cultural Medicine
Department of Family Medicine
University of California at San Diego
San Diego, California

Alice M. Tang, PhD, MS
Assistant Professor
Department of Medicine
School Medicine
Tufts University
Boston, Massachusetts

David L. Thomas, MD, MPH
Professor of Medicine and
 Epidemiology
Johns Hopkins Medical Institutions
Johns Hopkins University
Baltimore, Maryland

Carolyn Masters Williams, PhD, MPH
Chief, Epidemiology Branch, Basic
  Science program
Division of AIDS
National Institute of Allergy and Infec-
  tious Diseases
National Institutes of Health
Bethesda, Maryland

Jonathan M. Zenilman, MD
Professor
Departments of Medicine and
  Epidemiology
Johns Hopkins Medical Institutions
Johns Hopkins University
Baltimore, Maryland

ACKNOWLEDGMENTS

We would like to express our appreciation to all those who assisted us
in putting this book together. The outstanding and steadfast assistance of
Barbara Gray was integral to the completion of the book. We are also
indebted to Mark Kuniholm for his extensive efforts in managing the millions of pieces of paper required to publish a highly illustrated text such as
this one. There are numerous professional contacts who have also helped in
direct and indirect ways as we have shaped the contents of this text book
and developed the emphasis of certain chapters. And lastly, our families who
are incredibly patient when chapters need to be edited, references checked
or emails answered towards a goal of completing the book, we are always
deeply grateful.

Kenrad and Carolyn

PREFACE TO THE SECOND EDITION

Although the first edition of this book is only about four years old, it is apparent that a revision is needed to include the many new developments in infectious diseases since 2001. During this interval we have experienced epidemics of SARS, Monkey Pox, Bioterrorism-related Anthrax, the expansion of West Nile Virus infections in the United States, H5/N1 in birds and humans, and transfusion-transmitted vCJD.

Perhaps more important is the recognition by the world's political leaders of the severity of the continued epidemics of HIV/AIDS, Tuberculosis and Malaria and the need to respond to these neglected crises, especially in Sub-Saharan Africa. The development of the Global Fund, PEPFAR and the support of the Gates Foundation is clearly a much needed step toward controlling these crises. The current level of activity and funding is insufficient, but it is a first step. We have described the current status of these 3 overlapping epidemics and what additional efforts experts believe are urgently needed to reverse these current disasters.

Another long neglected problem is the recurring epidemic of Meningococcal Meningitis in the "Meningitis belt" of Africa. The efforts to eliminate Polio and Measles are important, following on the success with smallpox. This edition covers all of these problems more completely. We have added four new chapters, namely, chapter 1 Meningococcal Disease, chapter 2 Measles, chapter 3 Immunology and chapter 4 Vector borne Emerging Infections.

We believe an effective infectious disease epidemiologist currently needs a basic understanding of molecular biology, immunology, and human behavior in order to design or evaluate programs to control infectious diseases. So the text contains some basic information from these disciplines, as well as classical epidemiology and a description of the epidemiology of the most important infectious diseases.

All of the chapters have been revised and brought up to date. The HIV chapter has been expanded substantially and updated to include issues of Host Genetics in the susceptibility and resistance to HIV, the natural history, viral diversity, risk behaviors, prevention, the global epidemiology and a review of behavioral interventions to control HIV transmission. The recent increase in resources and commitment to control the AIDS pandemic, though insufficient, is nevertheless a very positive development. However, effective control of this pandemic will require that all available prevention efforts be applied and new strategies developed.

We hope the readers of this edition will appreciate our efforts to provide a current and comprehensive but readable text that covers the major issues in infectious disease epidemiology in the early 21st century.

Preparing the second edition, while requiring a great deal of time and effort, was a very important and rewarding experience for the authors and editors. We hope the readers and users of this text will find it useful in understanding the richness and excitement of research and practice in infectious disease epidemiology.

METHODS IN INFECTIOUS DISEASE EPIDEMIOLOGY

CHAPTER ONE

EARLY HISTORY OF INFECTIOUS DISEASE: EPIDEMIOLOGY AND CONTROL OF INFECTIOUS DISEASES

Kenrad E. Nelson and Carolyn F. Masters Williams

Introduction

Epidemics of infectious diseases have been documented throughout history. In ancient Greece and Egypt accounts describe epidemics of smallpox, leprosy, tuberculosis, meningococcal infections, and diphtheria.[1] The morbidity and mortality of infectious diseases profoundly shaped politics, commerce, and culture. In epidemics, none were spared. Smallpox likely disfigured and killed Ramses V in 1157 BCE, although his mummy has a significant head wound as well.[2] At times political upheavals exacerbated the spread of disease. The Spartan wars caused massive dislocation of Greeks into Athens triggering the Athens epidemic of 430–427 BCE that killed up to one half of the population of ancient Athens.[3] Thucydides' vivid descriptions of this epidemic make clear its political and cultural impact, as well as the clinical details of the epidemic.[4] Several modern epidemiologists have speculated about the causative agent. Langmuir et al.[5] favor an influenza and toxin-producing staphylococcus epidemic, while Morrens and Chu suggest Rift Valley fever.[6] A third researcher, Holladay believes the agent no longer exists.[7]

From the earliest times, man has sought to understand the natural forces and risk factors affecting the patterns of illness and death in society. These theories have evolved as our understanding of the natural world has advanced, sometimes slowly, sometimes, when there are profound break-throughs, with incredible speed. Remarkably, advances in knowledge and changes in theory have not always proceeded in synchrony. Although wrong theories or knowledge has hindered advances in understanding, there are also examples of great creativity when scientists have successfully pursued their theories beyond the knowledge of the time.

The Era of Plagues

The sheer magnitude and mortality of early epidemics are difficult to imagine. Medicine and religion both strove to console the sick and dying. However, before advances in the underlying science of health, medicine lacked effective tools, and religious explanations for disease dominated. As early communities consolidated people more closely, severe epidemics of plague, smallpox, and syphilis occurred.

The bubonic plague and its coinfections, measles and smallpox, were the most devastating of the epidemic diseases. In 160 CE plague contributed to the collapse of the Han Empire,[8] and six years later the Roman Empire was ravaged by the Antonine Plague (165–180 CE), which likely killed both coemperors Lucius Verus (130–169 CE) and Marcus Aurelius (121–180 CE) along with 5 million others.[9,10] Plague and other communicable diseases flourished in the cities of the Roman Empire and surely contributed to its final demise.[11] Four centuries later (1104–1110 CE) nearly 90% of Europeans were killed by plague.[8] The plague, or *Black Death* as it was then called, struck again in 1345 and swept across Europe. Starting in the lower Volga, it spread to Italy and Egypt in 1347 on merchant ships carrying rats and fleas infected with the plague bacillus, *Yesinia pestis*.[1] During the next five years (1347–1351), the Black Death killed 3 Europeans out of 10, leaving 24 million Europeans dead with a total of 40 million deaths worldwide.[1,12–14] These waves of bubonic plague fundamentally affected the development of civilizations as well as imposed a genetic bottleneck on those populations exposed. Europeans may be able to attribute their lower susceptibility to leprosy and HIV to the selective pressure of bubonic plague.[15] To survive in an ancient city was no small immunologic feat—and populations that had the immunologic fortitude had an advantage over others when exploration and colonization brought them and their pathogens together.[11]

The first recorded epidemic of smallpox was in 1350 BCE, during the Egyptian–Hittite war.[1] In addition to Ramses V, typical smallpox scars have been seen on the faces of mummies from the time of the 18th and 20th Egyptian dynasties (1570–1085 BCE). Smallpox was disseminated during the Arabian expansion, the Crusades, the discovery of the West Indies, and the colonization of the Americas. Mortality ranged from 10–50% in many epidemics. The disease apparently was unknown in the New World prior to the appearance of the Spanish and Portuguese conquistadors. Cortez was routed in battle in 1520 but was ultimately victorious as smallpox killed more than 25% of the Aztecs over the next year.[8] Mortality rates of 60–90% were described by the Spanish priest Fray Toribio Motolinia. He reported that 1000 persons per day died in Tlaxcala, with ultimately 150,000 total dead.[16] Smallpox then traveled north across the Americas, devastating the previously unexposed American populations.[11]

At that time, there was a reasonable understanding of the epidemiology of smallpox transmission. At the least, it was appreciated that the skin lesions and scabs could transmit the disease. It was known that survivors of the infection were immune to reinfection after further exposure. The practice of inoculation, or variolation, whereby people were intentionally exposed to smallpox was practiced in China, Africa, and India centuries before the practice would be adopted in Europe and the Americas.[17]

Syphilis is another epidemic infectious disease of great historical importance. Syphilis became epidemic in the 1490s as a highly contagious venereal disease in Spain, Italy, and France. By the 1530s, the venereal spread of syphilis was widely recognized in Europe.[18] The name *syphilis* originated from the popular, and extremely long, poem by Girolamo Fracastoro "Syphilis sive morbus Gallicus." Written in 1546, the poem recounts the causes of disease and the origin and treatment of syphilis.[12,18] Fracastoro describes the legend of a handsome young shepherd named Syphilis, who because of an insult to the god Apollo, was punished with a terrible disease, "the French Disease"–or syphilis. The origins of venereal syphilis are debated. One theory proposes that it began as a tropical disease transmitted by direct (nonsexual) contact.[18] In support of this theory, the organism, *Treponema pallidum*, was isolated from patients with endemic (nonvenereal) syphilis (bejel) and yaws. After the first accounts of syphilis, it was reported to spread rapidly through Europe and then North America. In keeping with the hypothesis that syphilis was a recently emerged disease, mortality from syphilis was high in these early epidemics.[11]

Early Epidemiology

In Western medicine, Hippocrates (460–377 BCE) was among the first to record his theories on the occurrence of disease. In his treatise *Airs, Water and Places*, Hippocrates dismissed supernatural explanations of disease and instead attributed illness to characteristics of the climate, soil, water, mode of life, and nutrition surrounding the patient.[2,19-21] It is Hippocrates who coined the terms *endemic* and *epidemic disease* to differentiate those diseases that are always present in a population, endemic, from those that are not always present but sometimes occur in large numbers, epidemic. It was Claudius Galen (131–201 CE), however, who codified the Hippocratic theories in his writings. Galen combined his practical experience caring for gladiators with experiments, including vivisections of animals, to study the anatomy and physiology of man.[22] His voluminous writings carried both his correct and incorrect views into the Middle Ages. It was over a thousand years before Andreas Vesalius (1514–1564), who based his work on dissections of humans, was able to correct Galen's errors in anatomy.[22]

That infectious diseases were contagious was recognized in early epidemics, but because knowledge of the true epidemiology of diseases was lacking, efforts to control the spread of such diseases were flawed. Plague was recognized to be contagious; however, the control measures focused primarily on quarantine and disposal of the bodies and the possessions (presumably contaminated) of the victims. Although it was observed that large numbers of rats appeared during an epidemic of plague, the role of rats and their fleas was not appreciated.

As far back as biblical times, leprosy was believed to be highly contagious. Afflicted patients were treated with fear and stigmatization. Given that leprosy progresses slowly, quarantine of cases late in disease likely had little effect on the epidemic spread. In the Middle Ages lepers were literally stricken from society as leprosy became increasingly equated with sin. Some even required lepers to stand in a dug grave and receive the "Mass of

Separation" from a priest after which they were considered "dead." One example of a Mass of Separation reads as follows:

> I forbid you to ever enter a church, a monastery, a fair, a mill, a market or an assembly of people. I forbid you to leave your house unless dressed in your recognizable garb and also shod. I forbid you to wash your hands or to launder anything or to drink at any stream or fountain, unless using your own barrel or dipper. I forbid you to touch anything you buy or barter for, until it becomes your own. I forbid you to enter any tavern; and if you wish for wine, whether you buy it or it is given to you, have it funneled into your keg. I forbid you to share house with any woman but your wife. I command you, if accosted by anyone while traveling on a road, to set yourself downwind of them before you answer. I forbid you to enter any narrow passage, lest a passerby bump into you. I forbid you, wherever you go, to touch the rim or the rope of a well without donning your gloves. I forbid you to touch any child or give them anything. I forbid you to drink or eat from any vessel but your own.[23]

Persons with leprosy, or suspected leprosy, were forced to carry a bell to warn others that they were coming (see Figure 1-1).

Fracastoro (1478–1553) was much more than just an author of the popular poem on syphilis. As a true Renaissance man, Fracastoro was also an astronomer and doctor. In his book published in 1546, *De contajione, ontagiosis morbis et curatine* (*On Contagion, Contagious Diseases, and Their*

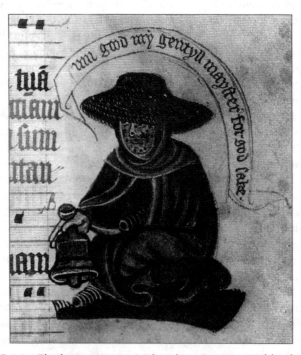

FIGURE 1-1 The leper was required to dress in recognizable clothing and to carry a bell.

Treatment), he proposed the revolutionary theory that infectious diseases were transmitted from person to person by minute invisible particles.[12,24] Fracastoro conceived of the idea that infections were spread from person to person by minute invisible seeds, or *seminaria*, that were specific for individual diseases, were self-replicating, and acted on the humors of the body to create disease. Although revolutionary, Fracastoro did not realize that the seeds of a disease were microbes, and he held to ancient beliefs that they were influenced by planetary conjugation particularly "*nostra trium superiorum, Saturni, Iovis et Martis*" (our three most distant bodies: Saturn, Jupiter, and Mars). He postulated that the environment became polluted with seminaria and that epidemics occurred in association with certain atmospheric and astrologic conditions.[12,24] Fracastoro proposed three modes of transmission of contagious disease: by direct contact from one person to another, through contact with fomites (a term for contaminated articles still used today), and through the air. His theories were respected and certainly far ahead of their time. He was able to persuade Pope Paul III to transfer the Council of Trent to Bologna because of the prevalence of contagious disease in Trent and the risk of contact with contaminated fomites.[1] But it would take the discovery of the microscope 200 years later to prove his theories.

The Observation and Care of Patients

Medical practice was gradually transformed by the introduction of disease-specific treatments during the Renaissance era. Peruvian bark, or cinchona, was imported into Europe for the treatment of malaria around 1630.[25] Its active ingredient, quinine, was the first specific treatment for the disease. Based on the observation that smallpox disease conferred immunity in those who survived, intentional inoculation of healthy people to induce immunity was attempted. This process was known as *variolation* and was advocated by Thomas Jefferson (1743–1826), Benjamin Franklin (1706–1790), and Cotton Mather (1663–1728). Mather learned of it from a man he enslaved, Onesimus, who was innoculated with smallpox in a cut as a child in Africa.[17] In 1796, Edward Jenner (1749–1823), based on the observation that milkmaids were immune to smallpox, greatly improved the process by substituting cowpox in place of the human pathogen. He performed the first vaccine clinical trial by inoculating 8-year-old James Phipps (1788–1853) with lesions containing cowpox (vaccinia virus) and later showed that the boy was immune to variolation, or challenge with variola virus.[26] Thus was born the science of vaccination, which led eventually (180 years later) to the eradication of smallpox.[26] Napoleon (1769–1821) showed his support by vaccinating his army, declaring that "anything Jenner wants shall be granted. He has been my most faithful servant in the European campaigns."[27] It is worthy of mention that other empiric attempts were proposed during the 1700s to induce protection by intentional inoculation, such as for measles (called morbillication) and syphilis. Neither of these efforts were successful.

Changes in the practice of clinical medicine in the 1600s began to differentiate diseases from one another. One of the earliest advocates of careful observation of patients' symptoms and their disease course was the London doctor Thomas Sydenham (1624–1689). He classified different febrile illnesses plaguing London in the 1660s and 1670s in a book entitled *Observations Medicae*. His approach departed from Galen and Hippocrates, who focused on the individual and their illness rather than on trying to differentiate specific diseases. After Sydenham, the Italian physician Giovanni Morgagni (1682–1771) inaugurated the method of clinicopathologic correlation. His book *De sedibus et causis morborum per anatomen indagatis (On the Seats and Causes of Diseases, Investigated by Anatomy)*, based on over 700 autopsies, attributed particular signs and symptoms to pathologic changes in the tissues and organs. The influence of Sydenham and Morgagni on medicine can be seen in Benjamin Rush's (1745–1813) description of dengue among patients afflicted in the 1780 Philadelphia epidemic.[28]

> The pains which accompanied this fever were exquisitely severe in the head, back, and limbs. The pains in the head were sometimes in the back parts of it, and at other times they occupied only the eyeballs. In some people, the pains were so acute in their backs and hips that they could not lie in bed.... A few complained of their flesh being sore to the touch, in every part of the body. From these circumstances, the disease was sometimes believed to be a rheumatism. But its more general name among all classes of people was the Break-bone fever.

This new way of thinking about diseases, requiring careful clinical observation, differentiation, and specific diagnosis, led naturally to the search for specific, as opposed to general, causes of illness.

Expanding on the concept of careful clinical observation of individuals, epidemiologists in the 1800s observed unusual epidemics and performed controlled studies of exposed persons. Epidemiologic theories about the means of transmission of various infectious diseases often preceded the laboratory and clinical studies of the causative organisms. Peter Panum (1820–1885) recorded his observation of an epidemic of measles on the Faroe Islands in 1846.[29] Measles had not occurred on these remote Scandinavian islands for 65 years. Remarkably, the attack rates among those under 65 years old was near 97%, but older persons were completely spared. This demonstrated that immunity after an attack of natural measles persists for a lifetime. Further, Panum described the mean 14-day incubation period between cases.[29] Outbreaks of mumps and other contagious diseases in isolated populations also have contributed to the early understanding of the epidemiology of these diseases.[30,31]

The epidemiology of bacterial diseases also progressed at this time. John Snow (1813–1858) performed classic epidemiology of the transmission of cholera in the mid-1850s, nearly 30 years prior to the identification of the causative organism.[32] William Budd (1868–1953) demonstrated the means of transmission of typhoid fever and the importance of the human carrier in transmission 35 years prior to the isolation of *Salmonella typhi*.[33] Ignatz Semmelweiss (1818–1865) demonstrated with a retrospective record review that an epidemic of puerperal fever, or childbed fever, in 1847 at the Vienna Lying-In hospital was due to transmission of infection on the hands of medical students and physicians who went from the autopsy room to the delivery room without washing their hands. In contrast, the women who were delivered by midwives, who used aseptic techniques (by immersing their hands in antiseptic solution prior to contact with the patient), had much lower rates of puerperal sepsis (Figure 1-2).[34] Unfortunately, while Semmelweiss was correct, bacteria were not yet identified. His theories were not welcomed by the medical profession, and this, combined with his more liberal political views, resulted in his leaving the hospital in 1849.[27] These early epidemiologic theories would have to wait for scientific knowledge to catch up.

The Development of Statistics and Surveillance

Meanwhile, the fields of probability and *political arithmetic*, a term coined by William Petty (1623-1687) to describe vital statistics on morbidity and mortality,[27] were advancing. Gerolamo Cardana (1501-1576) introduced the concept of probability and described that the probability of any roll of the dice was equal so long as the die was fair.[35] Jacques Bernoulli (1654-1705) carried this concept further with the central limit theorem, which states that the observed probability approached the theoretical probability as the number of observations increased.[35] One of the early leaders in the use of statistics to help understand the natural occurrence and epidemiology of infectious diseases was John Graunt (1620-1674), a wealthy haberdasher; he became interested in bills of mortality and published the *Natural and Political Observations—The Bills of Mortality* in 1662.[27,36] Here he detailed the number and causes of deaths in London during the preceding third of a century. He used inductive reasoning to interpret the mortality trends and noted the ratio of male to female births and deaths, mortality by season, and mortality in persons living in rural versus urban locations. He examined several causes of deaths over time and constructed the first life tables.[36] Subsequently, other

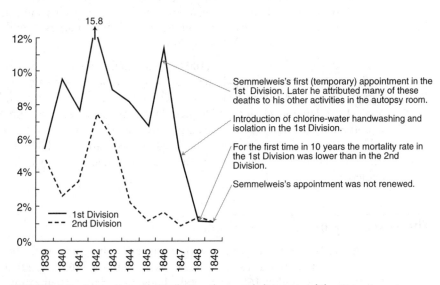

FIGURE 1-2   Mortality rates in first and second divisions of the Department of Obstetrics in the Vienna Lying-In Hospital between 1839 and 1849. Iffy L & Kaminetzky, H, Eds., *Principles of Obstetrics and Perimatology*, Volume 2, © 1981.

observers used public health data for the study of epidemics of infectious diseases. Daniel Bernoulli (1700–1782), the son of Jacques Bernoulli, analyzed smallpox mortality to estimate the risk-benefit ratio of variolation.[12] His calculations determined that the fatality rate of variolation exceeded the benefit in population survival.[37] In England, numerous improvements in public health sanitation and vital registries were made in the 1800s. Edwin Chadwick (1800–1890), an arrogant zealot, managed to institute numerous sanitary reforms when he wasn't annoying his peers.[27] Chadwick used health statistics to effectively change public policy. His 1842 report "to the Poor Law Commission" outlined the cost effectiveness of public health. His report emphasized the understanding that hygiene was closely related to health, but he also linked morality to hygiene and health. He made the following pronouncements:

- ○ That the formation of all habits of cleanliness is obstructed by defective supplies of water.
- ○ That the younger population, bred up under noxious physical agencies, is inferior in physical organization and general health to a population preserved from the presence of such agencies.
- ○ That the population so exposed is less susceptible of moral influences, and the effects of education are more transient than with a healthy population.
- ○ That these adverse circumstances tend to produce an adult population short-lived, improvident, reckless, and intemperate, and with habitual avidity for sensual gratifications.
- ○ That defective town cleansing fosters habits of the most abject degradation and tends to the demoralization of large numbers of human beings, who subsist by means of what they find amidst the noxious filth accumulated in neglected streets and bye-places.
- ○ That the expense of public drainage, of supplies of water laid on in houses, and of means of improved cleansing would be a pecuniary gain, by diminishing the existing charges attendant on sickness and premature mortality.[38]

His countryman William Farr (1807–1883) made important contributions to the improvement and analytical use of public health statistical data. His careful documentation of deaths was used by John Snow to investigate the 1849–1953 London cholera epidemics. Farr initially disagreed with Snow's hypothesis that cholera was transmitted by water. He preferred the miasma theory. However, he was eventually convinced, and his book based on the 1866 epidemic demonstrated that contaminated water was a risk for cholera.[39]

The Discovery of Microorganisms

A significant leap forward in scientific understanding came with the visualization of microorganisms. Anton van Leeuwenhoek (1632–1723) invented the microscope, and in 1683 he described how materials such as rainwater and human excretions had cocci, bacilli, and spirochetes.[8] But he did not evaluate these organisms as agents of disease. Considerable controversy arose over the origin of these minute forms. Because they were often present in decaying or fermenting materials, some people maintained that they were spontaneously generated from inanimate material. However, Leeuwenhoek believed that they were derived from animate life.[27]

Louis Pasteur (1822–1895) demonstrated the dependence of fermentation on microorganisms in 1857 and showed that these organisms came from similar organisms present in the air.[40] Subsequently, Robert Koch (1843–1910) demonstrated in 1876 that he could reproducibly transmit anthrax to mice by inoculating them with blood from sick cattle and that he could then recover the same rodlike bacteria from the sick mice as came from the cattle. Further, he could pass the disease from one mouse to another by inoculating them with these microorganisms.[12] Based on these experiments he proposed the "Henle-Koch postulates" for proof that a microorganism was the cause of an infectious disease. In the subsequent 50 years, numerous microorganisms were identified as the causative agents of important human diseases (Table 1-1) and their epidemiology elucidated. Among these was the causative agent of plague, identified in 1894 by Alexander Yersin (1863–1943) and Shibasaburo Kitasato (1852–1931). They discovered the organism in both rats and humans who had died of plague during an epidemic in Hong Kong.[12,13] Two years later in Bombay, Paul-Louis Simond (1858–1947) of France established that the link between rats and humans was the rat flea, *Xenopsylla cheopis*. Once a rat flea becomes infected with *Yersinia pestis*, the plague bacillus, it cannot digest its food—rat blood. Starving, it looks aggressively for another animal to feed on and, in so doing, passes the organism on to humans. After it is infected, the rat flea can hibernate for up to 50 days in grain, cloth, or other items and spread the disease to humans coming into contact with these items of commerce.[12]

TABLE 1-1   The Scientist Credited with the Discovery of Important Human Pathogens and the Year of That Discovery

Year	Disease or Organism	Scientist
1874	Leprosy	Hansen
1880	Malaria typhoid (organism seen in tissues)	Laveran and Eberth
1882	Tuberculosis glanders	Koch, Loeffler, and Schutz
1883	Cholera streptococcus (erysipelas)	Koch and Fehleisen
1884	Diphtheria Typhoid (bacillia isolate) Staphylococcus Streptococcus Tetanus	Klebs and Loeffler Gaffky Rosenbach Rosenbach Nicolaier
1885	*Escherichia coli*	Escherich
1886	Pneumococcus	Fraenkel
1887	Malta fever, 　Soft chancre	Bruce Ducrey
1892	Gas gangrene	Welch and Nuttall
1894	Plague Botulism	Yersin and Kitasato Van Ermengen
1896	*Hemophilus influenzae*	Pfeiffer
1898	Dysentery bacillus	Shiga

To study disease in a controlled setting, some researchers resorted to self-experimentation. Sometimes with great success, other times not. The first specific published account of human hookworm disease was in 1843 by Angelo Dubini (1813–1902) from Milan.[41] He had found hookworms in the intestines of nearly 20% of autopsies. However, the means of spread was commonly believed to be by the fecal–oral route until the observation of Arthur Looss in Cairo, Egypt, in 1898.[42] Looss was studying *Strongyloides stercoralis* and swallowed several larvae of this organism to infect himself, but, when he examined his stools, he found only hookworm eggs. Then he recalled that he had accidentally spilled a fecal inoculum on his hands that caused a transitory itchy red rash. He then intentionally exposed his skin to another hookworm inoculum and, after a few minutes, was unable to find the organisms on his exposed skin. After several additional careful experiments, he reported the entrance of hookworms into humans by skin penetration of the parasites, rather than by ingestion. One self-experimenter who succumbed was Daniel Carrion (1858–1885), a medical student in Lima, Peru. Carrion injected himself with the material from a chronic skin lesion called *Verraga peruana*. This self-experiment was designed to determine whether the same organism (later identified to be *Bartonella bacilliformis*) could also cause another disease, known as Oroya fever. Oroya fever was a more serious disease, involving the red blood cells. When Carrion developed Oroya fever, he proved that the two diseases were caused by the same infectious organism but the experiment cost him his life.[43]

In the subsequent decades numerous scientists began to focus their investigations on vector-borne disease. The explosive epidemic nature of yellow fever and malaria when they occurred in Europe and the United States, not to mention the military and commercial interests in their control, spurred researchers and their governments to support studies. The first proof that an animal disease was spread by an arthropod was the report in 1893 by Smith and Kilbourne on the transmission of Texas cattle fever by a tick.[44] Another group of landmark studies was organized in Cuba, which led to an understanding of the biology and epidemiology of yellow fever.[45] Although epidemics of yellow fever had been reported as far north as Philadelphia in the 1700s and 1800s, the means of transmission of the disease were unclear. Some believed that the disease was spread directly from person to person. However, Stubbins Firth (1784–1820) in 1804 observed that secondary cases among nurses or doctors caring for patients with the disease were unheard of. To prove that person-to-person transmission wasn't a risk, he undertook a remarkable series of self-experiments, in which he exposed himself orally and parenterally to the hemorrhagic vomitus, other excretions, and blood of patients dying of yellow fever. He was unable to transmit the infection in these experiments, and he concluded that yellow fever wasn't directly transmitted from person to person.[12]

Early in the 1800s, it had been suggested by several physicians that yellow fever might be spread by mosquitoes.[12] The theory was restated by the Cuban physician Carlos Finley (1833–1915) in 1881, but experimental proof was lacking.[12,43] When the United States occupied Cuba during the Spanish-American War, a yellow fever study commission was established and Walter Reed (1851–1902) was dispatched to Cuba in 1899 to study the question further. The commission studied the transmission of yellow fever by *Stegomyia fasciata* mosquitoes, now named *Aedes aegypti*, using human volunteers (because there were no animal models). In the course of the investigation, one of the volunteers, who was a member of the committee, Jesse H. Lazear (1866–1900), contracted yellow fever following a mosquito bite and succumbed to the disease. After several definitive experiments, the commission was able to report that yellow fever was transmitted to humans by the bite of an infected mosquito.[45]

In 1898, Loeffler and Frosh had shown that hoof-and-mouth disease of cattle was caused by an agent small enough to pass through a filter capable of retaining the smallest bacteria.[46] Reed and colleagues demonstrated that the agent of yellow fever was present in filtered blood leading them to conclude that the causative agent of yellow fever was a virus.[45] This conclusion made yellow fever the first identified viral cause of human disease. Furthermore, their studies showed that yellow fever had an obligate insect cycle and was not transmitted directly from person to person.

Mosquitoes were also suspected of transmitting malaria, although early researchers were unsure as to whether they was a marker of poor sanitation or a necessary part of the malaria life cycle. In *De Noxiis Palodum Effloriis* (*On the Noxious Emanations of Swamps*), published in 1717, Giovanni Maria Lancisi (1654–1720) speculated on the manner in which swamps produced malaria epidemics.[12] Lancisi theorized that swamps produced two kinds of emanations capable of producing disease, animate and inanimate. The animate emanations were mosquitoes, and these, he thought, could carry animalcules. Over 150 years later, the microscope was the tool used to wage an intense scientific competition to identify the malaria life cycle. The malaria parasite, *Plasmodium falciparum*, was originally discovered by Alphonse Laveran (1845–1922), a French army surgeon working in Algeria. On November 5, 1880, he "was astonished to observe, [in a soldier's blood specimen] . . . a series of fine, transparent filaments that moved very actively and beyond question were alive."[47] After this discovery, researchers from England and Italy were working around the globe. The Italian research team took a wrong turn and concluded that the parasite might be an amoeba or other spore outside of the human and concentrated on collecting materials from malarious locations, including but not limited to mosquitoes. It was the tireless work of Ronald Ross (1857–1932) in India that finally uncovered the life cycle of avian malaria. Painstakingly dissecting mosquitoes he searched for malaria parasites and finally found the salivary glands packed with the germinal rods of malaria. He described the excitement of his discovery in a letter to Sir Patrick Manson (1844–1922) on July 6, 1898.

> I think that this, after further elaboration, will close at least one cycle of proteosoma, and I feel that I am *almost* entitled to lay down the law by direct observation and tracking the parasite step by step—Malaria is conveyed from a diseased person or bird to a healthy one by the proper species of mosquito and is inoculated by its bite. Remember however that there is virtue in the "almost". I don't announce the law yet. Even when the microscope has done its utmost, healthy birds must be infected with all due precaution. . . . In all probability it is these glands which secrete the stinging fluid which the mosquito injects into the bite. The germinal rods . . . pass into the ducts . . . and are thus poured out in vast numbers under the

skin of the man or bird. Arrived there, numbers of them are probably instantly swept away by the circulation of the blood, in which they immediately begin to develop into malaria parasites, thus completing the cycle. No time to write more.[47]

He was able to demonstrate that birds fed upon by these mosquitoes were infected, and Patrick Manson presented these results to the British Medical Association in Edinburgh at the end of July 1898.[48] Unfortunately for Ross, the British Army required him to work on kala-azar until February of 1899 giving the Italians Amico Bignami, Giovanni Battista Grassi, and Giuseppe Bastianelli the opportunity to finish verifying that anopheline mosquitoes were the vector for malaria and to confirm that the avian life cycle was the same in humans.[49] But the heated rush to decipher the remaining questions in the malaria life cycle pitted the Italians against the near-celebrity Koch who arrived on invitation from the Italian government to "solve the malaria problem."[47] The Italians, bitterly jealous of the German scientific superstar, rushed to publication and failed to give due credit to Ross. The ensuing battle between Ross, Grassi, and Koch was legendary. In fact, when the Nobel committee considered splitting the 1902 Nobel Prize in medicine between Ross and Grassi,[49] Koch's vehement opposition prevented it, allowing Ross the honor alone.[47]

Following the elegant demonstration of yellow fever and malaria transmission, the epidemiology of several other arthropod diseases was described (Table 1-2). Also, many other human diseases caused by viruses were defined in the ensuing decades. The second mosquito-borne human viral infection

TABLE 1-2 The Scientist Credited with the Discovery of Important Vector-Borne Pathogens and the Year of That Discovery

Disease	Disease Vector	Investigator	Year
Babesiosis (Texas cattle fever)	Deer tick	Smith and Kilbourne	1893
Yellow fever	Mosquito	Reed, Carroll, and Lazaer	1900
Dengue	Mosquito	Bancroft, Craig, and Asburn	1906
Rocky Mountain spotted fever	Wood tick	Ricketts, King	1906
Typhus, epidemic	Body louse	Nicolle	1909
Sandfly fever	Sand fly	Doerr, Franz, and Taussig	1909
Murine typhus	Rat louse	Mooser	1931
	Rat flea	Dyer	1931
Colorado tick fever	Wood tick	Topping, Cullyford, and Davis	1940
Rickettsial pox	Mite	Huebner, Jellison, and Pomerantz	1946
Lyme disease	Deer tick	Burgdorfer	1982
Cat scratch fever and bacillary angiomatosis	Cat flea	Koehler	1994
Human monocytic ehrlichiosis	Dog tick and lone star tick	Maedo et al	1986
Human granocytic ehrlichiosis	Deer tick	Chen et al	1994

to be identified was dengue, a reemerging viral infection of increased importance today. Dengue is spread by the same mosquitoes that transmit yellow fever, *A. aegypti*. The means of transmission and the fact that dengue was a filterable virus were discovered by the Australian Thomas Bancroft et al.[12] in the Philippines in 1906.

The Twentieth Century

The identification of the causative microorganisms of specific infections allowed for a much better understanding of their epidemiology, which in turn informed prevention strategies. The disciplines of microbiology, virology, and immunology paralleled and complemented the disciplines of epidemiology, statistics, and public health in the prevention of infectious diseases. Despite advances, epidemic diseases continued to occur in the United States, particularly in the nation's port cities. Cholera, first seen in the Western Hemisphere in 1832,[27] yellow fever, malaria, and plague were constant concerns. Although public health authorities had a better understanding of the diseases, treatments lagged behind, and quarantine remained the staple tool of prevention. Several US congressional acts in 1887, 1901, and 1902 were responsible for creating what would ultimately become the National Institute of Health (NIH). Congress charged the future NIH with the study of "infectious and contagious diseases and matters pertaining to the public health." The first employee was Joseph J. Kinyoun who promoted the science of health and introduced laboratory diagnostics for the confirmation of cholera cases. The Public Health Service was instrumental in addressing sanitation issues during the First World War and also during the influenza epidemic of 1918. In 1930, a financially strapped US government still found funds under the Ransdell Act to further expand the NIH and charged it with investigating basic medical and clinical science. During the Second World War the NIH concentrated on disease of particular importance to the military, including yellow fever and typhus vaccines. After the war, the 1946 Public Health Service Act established the NIH's grant mechanism to fund nonfederal scientists. Finally in 1948, the National Institute of Health was given its last name change and became the National Institutes of Health reflecting the diversity of diseases under study at the NIH.[50]

Greater understanding of the biology of disease pathology also led to better treatments. Treatments for diphtheria with antitoxin and the development of vaccines for rabies, anthrax, diphtheria, and tetanus were developed. However, many of the antisera that were developed and antiseptics that were tried for the therapy of infectious diseases were of only limited effectiveness. Complicating their use was the risk of contamination in the production of these medications. Kinyoun worked hard to establish standards in production of drugs and vaccines. After the death of 13 children in Saint Louis from contaminated diphtheria antitoxin, the US Congress passed the Biologics Control Act.[51] Under this act, standards in biologics were developed and licenses granted to pharmaceutical companies for specific medications or vaccines. In 1924, investigators at the Bayer pharmaceutical company in Germany synthesized a new antimalarial drug, pamaquine (Plasmoquine). Shortly thereafter, they synthesized other antimalarial compounds, including quinacrine (Atabrine).[52] The development of these new drugs gave some hope that specific, effective antimicrobial treatments could be developed for infectious diseases. In 1932, Gerhardt Domagk, experimenting with synthetic dyes, discovered that Prontosil could cure mice challenged with lethal doses of hemolytic streptococci.[52] This led to the development of several sulfa drugs. The sulfonamides were shown during World War II to be quite effective against a number of highly fatal infections, such as meningococcal meningitis. In the 1930s and 1940s, Alexander Fleming, Howard Florey, and Ernst Chain at Oxford University conducted experiments that led to the demonstration that penicillin, a mold product, was effective against many pathogenic organisms.[52] Penicillin was shown to be effective against syphilis, gonorrhea, and pneumococcal infections. For the first time, it was possible to effectively treat a wide range of infections, and this gave birth to the search for new antibiotics produced by organisms in nature or synthesized in the laboratory.

After the conclusion of the Second World War in 1946 the Center for Disease Control (CDC) was established in Atlanta, Georgia.[53] The CDC grew out of an organization known as "Malaria Control in War Areas," which had the mandate to control malaria and other tropical infections, especially scrub typhus and hookworm, in the southern United States. Its founder, Dr. Joseph Mountain, was a visionary public health leader who had high hopes that the CDC would eventually play an important role in public health in the United States. Subsequently, the role of CDC, under the leadership of Dr. Alexander Langmuir, grew dramatically to include surveillance of infectious and noninfectious diseases and the provision of expert scientific advice on health issues to policy makers in the United States as well as to serve as a reference laboratory to the states and inform the public about health issues through the *Morbidity and Mortality Weekly Report*. Today, epidemiologists from the CDC routinely assist state health departments in investigating and controlling outbreaks of infectious and noninfectious diseases. In its role in the field investigation of outbreaks, the CDC is unique among national public health organizations. Since its establishment the CDC has grown to provide leadership, often in partnership with the World Health Organization (WHO), in controlling emerging infectious diseases worldwide.

Although some vaccines were developed earlier, the number and impact of vaccines developed in the 1900s century were monumental. The renamed Centers for Disease Control and Prevention in 1999 published a review of the 10 great public health achievements in the United States during the 1900s.[54] At the top of its list is vaccination. The vaccines developed and licensed to prevent vaccine-preventable diseases are shown in Table 1-3, and an estimate of their effect on reported infectious disease morbidity is shown in Table 1-4.

During the previous century, the average life span of persons in the United States lengthened by about 30 years, and 25 years of this gain has been attributed to advances in public health. The public health actions to control infectious diseases in the 1900s, which included marked improvements in sanitation, chlorination of nearly all public water supplies, and development and use of vaccines to prevent infectious diseases and antibiotics for their treatment, along with improved methods for diagnosis, were reviewed recently by the CDC (Figure 1-3). During the 1900s, infectious disease mortality declined from about 800/100,000 population to under

TABLE 1-3　The Year Effective Vaccines Were Developed Against Different Human Diseases

Smallpox*	1798[†]	Mumps*	1967[†]
Rabies	1885[†]	Rubella*	1969[‡]
Typhoid	1896[†]	Anthrax	1970[‡]
Cholera	1896[†]	Meningitis	1975[‡]
Plague	1897[†]	Pneumonia	1977[‡]
Diphtheria*	1923[†]	Adenovirus	1980[‡]
Pertussis*	1926[†]	Hepatitis B*	1981[‡]
Tetanus*	1927[†]	*Hemophilus influenzae* type b*	1985[‡]
Tuberculosis	1927[†]	Japanese encephalitis	1992[‡]
Influenza	1945[‡]	Hepatitis A	1995[‡]
Yellow fever	1953[‡]	Varicella*	1995[‡]
Poliomyelitis*	1955[‡]	Lyme disease	1998[‡]
Measles*	1963[‡]	Rotavirus*	1998[‡]

* Vaccine recommended for universal use in US children. For smallpox, routine vaccination was ended in 1971.
† Vaccine developed (i.e., first published results of vaccine usage).
‡ Vaccine licensed for use in the United States.

50/100,000 and accounted for most of the improvement in US life expectancy. In 1900, 30.4% of all deaths occurred in children under five years of age. In 1997, the proportion of total mortality in this age group was only 1.4%.[55,56]

What Lies Ahead

The science of health moved forward at breakneck speed in the previous century. The effectiveness of treatments and vaccines coupled with increased financial support fueled spectacular advances as the underlying science of diseases was unraveled. Although many advances are noteworthy, perhaps the discovery of the structure of DNA and ultimately the determination of the entire human genome will have the greatest impact on the future of health research. It was February 28, 1953, when James Watson and Francis Crick first determined the double helix structure of DNA and the mechanism by which it could copy itself and thus serve as the basis for hereditary information. Rosalind Franklin and Maurice Wilkins from King's College in London created images of DNA with X-ray diffraction, and these images, combined with cardboard models, allowed Watson to finally determine the binding of adenine and thymine and guanine and cytosine to form the ladder rungs of the double helix.[57] Franklin died of cancer in 1958, and was unable to share in the Nobel Prize with Watson, Crick, and Wilkins in 1962. Since that time gradual progress in deciphering and manipulating the genetic code of animals and plants had occurred. Dolly the sheep, born July 5, 1996, was the first higher animal to be cloned, and several other animals have followed.[57] In 1990, the US Human Genome Project was undertaken to identify all of the

TABLE 1-4 A Comparison of Morbidity from Infectious Diseases Before and After the Availability of Vaccines

Disease	Baseline 20th-Century Annual Morbidity	1998 Provisional Disease Morbidity	Percent Decrease
Smallpox	48,164*	0	100
Diphtheria	175,885[†]	1	100[‡]
Pertussis	147,271[§]	6,279	95.7
Tetanus	1,314[‖]	34	97.4
Poliomyelitis (paralytic)	16,316[¶]	0[#]	100
Measles	503,282**	89	100[‡]
Mumps	152,209[††]	606	99.6
Rubella	47,745[‡‡]	345	99.3
Congenital rubella syndrome	823[§§]	5	99.4
Hemophilus influenzae type b	20,000[‖‖]	54[¶¶]	99.7

*Average annual number of cases 1900–1904.
[†]Average annual number of reported cases 1920–1922, three years before vaccine development.
[‡]Rounded to nearest tenth.
[§]Average annual number of reported cases 1922–1925, four years before vaccine development.
[‖]Estimated number of cases based on reported number of deaths 1922–1926, assuming a case-fatality rate of 90%.
[¶]Average annual number of reported cases 1951–1954, four years before vaccine licensure.
[#]Excludes one case of vaccine-associated polio reported in 1998.
**Average annual number of reported cases 1958–1962, five years before vaccine licensure.
[††]Number of reported cases in 1968, the first year reporting began and the first year after vaccine licensure.
[‡‡]Average annual number of reported cases 1966–1968, three years before vaccine licensure.
[§§]Estimated number of cases based on seroprevalence data in the population and on the risk that women infected during a childbearing year would have a fetus with congenital rubella syndrome.
[‖‖]Estimated number of cases from population-based surveillance studies before vaccine licensure in 1985.
[¶¶]Excludes 71 cases of *Hemophilus influenzae* disease of unknown serotype.

approximately 25,000 genes in human DNA. The project was completed ahead of schedule and in April 2003 the human genome was published in several articles in *Nature* and *Science*.[58,59] The sequencing project has identified over 10 million locations where single-base DNA polymorphisms (SNPs) occur.[60] Today it is recognized that differences in SNPs between individuals directly affect a person's susceptibility to infection and disease. The fields of genomics and proteomics, the study of protein expression, are rapidly evolving fields that hold great promise for understanding the interaction of humans with infectious pathogens.

Genetics will also play a role in unlikely places. On August 11, 2005, the genome of rice was reported. This was the first of the cereal grains to be deciphered. This genome will be informative for all grains, because rice,

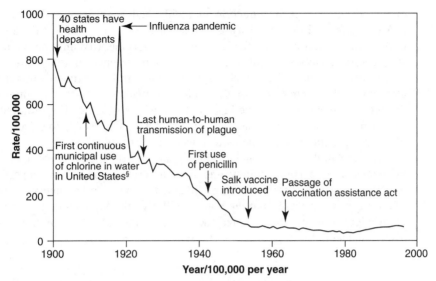

FIGURE 1-3   Crude death rate for infectious disease, United States, 1990–1996.
Source: Achievements in Public Health, 1900–1999: Control of Infectious Diseases.
MMWR, Vol 48, No. 29.

corn, and wheat diverged from a common grass ancestor only 50,000 years ago.[61] Cereals make up the majority of calories in most of the world. Earlier researchers manipulated the rice genome to insert a daffodil gene, which added vitamin A to rice.[62,63] Vitamin A is crucial to immunologic health,[64] and the use of enhanced food products holds promise for improving health. Unfortunately, although genetically modified foods hold great promise, they are also highly controversial. Hardier plants, enhanced with insect repellant genes or drought resistance, threaten to drive out native plants, which could ultimately reduce global genetic diversity. Highly successful seeds are patented, and this elevates the cost of seed beyond the reach of subsistence farmers. The concentration of ownership of seeds is severe, and only a handful of companies own the rights to most of the food seed sold in the world.[65] These controversies, and those surrounding manipulation of the human and other genomes will determine the ethical boundaries and ultimate potential of genomic and proteomic science.

The Infectious Diseases Challenge

In the previous century, such spectacular progress was made in infectious disease control that many health professionals felt that antibiotics and vaccines would soon eliminate infectious disease threats from most developed nations. The confidence of the 1970s was shattered by the 1980s when the AIDS pandemic exploded. The first scientific report of AIDS was June 5, 1981, in the *Morbidity and Mortality Weekly Report*.[66] In this report, cases of *Pneumocystis* pneumonia in previously healthy gay men were described by Dr. Michael Gottlieb. Since that time the magnitude and severity of the HIV/AIDS epidemic has not abated; it is now estimated that more than 5 million people become infected with HIV every year. Because most people infected with HIV acquired it through sexual contact, it is predominately a disease of young adults. The introduction of highly active antiretroviral therapies (HAART) has modified the disease course for those able to afford them, but to date there is neither an effective cure nor a vaccine. HIV and the immune suppression it causes has also allowed for a resurgence of tuberculosis in much of the world. Unfortunately, drug-resistant strains of tuberculosis have also emerged, making control even more difficult. Several other diseases emerged, or reemerged, in the last of the previous century. The unfounded optimism of the mid-1900s has been replaced by greater resolve to solve some of the most intractable problems in infectious diseases.

The remainder of this book will lay out the techniques and tools of infectious disease epidemiology and then describe some of the important infectious diseases. The book is not intended to be a comprehensive study of all infectious diseases, but we hope it will give the fundamental tools and knowledge necessary to advance the reader's understanding of infectious disease epidemiology.

References

1. Watts S. *Epidemics and History: Disease, Power and Imperialism.* New Haven, Conn: Yale University Press; 1997.
2. Ruffer MA, Ferguson AR. Note on an eruption resembling that of variola in the skin of a mummy of the Twentieth Dynasty (1200–1100 BC). *J Pathol Bacteriol.* 1911;15:1–4.
3. Garrett L. *The Coming Plague.* New York, NY: Penguin Books; 1994:236.
4. Poole JCF, Holladay AJ. Thucydides and the plague of Athens. *Classic Q.* 1979;29:282–300.
5. Langmuir AD, Northern TD, Solomon J, Ray CG, Petersen E. The Thucydides syndrome. *N Engl J Med.* 1985;313:1027–1030.
6. Morens DM, Chu MC. The plague of Athens. *N Engl J Med.* 1986;314:855.
7. Holladay AJ. The Thucydides syndrome: another view. *N Engl J Med.* 1986;315:1170–1173.
8. Lee HSJ, ed. *Dates in Infectious Diseases.* Boca Raton, Fla: The Parthenon Publishing Group; 2000.
9. Fears JR. The plague under Marcus Aurelius and the decline and fall of the Roman Empire. *Infect Dis Clin North Am.* 2004;18:65–77.
10. Antonineplague.WikipediaWebpage.Availableat:http://en.wikipedia.org/wiki/Antonine_Plague.AccessedFebruary22,2006.
11. Porter R, ed. *Cambridge Illustrated History of Medicine.* New York, NY: Cambridge University Press; 1996.
12. Rosen G. *A History of Public Health.* Baltimore, Md: Johns Hopkins University Press; 1993.
13. McNeill WH. *Plagues and Peoples.* New York, NY: Doubleday; 1977.
14. Hirst LF. *The Conquest of Plague.* London, England: Oxford University Press; 1953.
15. Duncan SR, Scott S, Duncan CJ. Reappraisal of the historical selective pressures for the CCR5-Delta32 mutation. *J Med Genet.* 2005;42:205–208.
16. Cook ND. *Born to Die, Disease and the New World Conquest, 1492–1650.* Cambridge, England: The Press Syndicate of the Cambridge University Press; 1998.

17. National Library of Medicine. Smallpox and variolation Web page. Available at: http://www.nlm.nih.gov/exhibition/smallpox/sp_variolation.html. Accessed February 22, 2006.
18. Pusey EW. *The History and Epidemiology of Syphilis.* Springfield, Ill: Charles C Thomas; 1933.
19. Temkin O. *Hippocrates in a World of Pagans and Christians.* Baltimore, Md: Johns Hopkins University Press; 1991.
20. Adams F, trans. *The Genuine Works of Hippocrates, Francis Adams Translation.* Baltimore, Md: Williams & Wilkins; 1939.
21. Sigerist HE. *The Great Doctors.* New York, NY: WW Norton & Company; 1933.
22. University of Virginia Health Sciences Library. Antiqua medicina Web page. Available at: http://www.med.virginia.edu/hs-library/historical/antiqua/galen.htm. Accessed February 22, 2006.
23. Mass of Separation. *Cistercian Scholars Quarterly* Web page. Available at: http://www2.kenyon.edu/Projects/margin/lepers.htm. Accessed February 22, 2006.
24. Hall MB. *The Scientific Renaissance, 1450–1630.* Minneola, NY: Dover Publications; 1994.
25. Bruce-Chwatt LJ, de Zulueta J. *The Rise and Fall of Malaria in Europe: A Historico-Epidemiological Study.* London, England: Oxford University Press; 1981.
26. Fenner F, Henderson DA, Anita I, Jezek Z, Ladnyl IR. *Smallpox and Its Eradication.* Geneva, Switzerland: World Health Organization; 1988.
27. Porter R. *The Greatest Benefit to Mankind: A Medical History of Humanity.* New York, NY: WW Norton and Company; 1997.
28. Rosh B. An account of the bilious remitting fever as it appeared in Philadelphia in the summer of 1780. In: *Medical Inquiries and Observations.* Philadelphia, Pa: Richard & Hall; 1789.
29. Panum PL. *Observations Made During the Epidemic of Measles in the Faroe Island in the Year 1846.* [Reprinted by the Delta Omega Society.] New York, NY: FH Newton; 1940.
30. Nelson KE. Invited commentary on observations on a mumps epidemic in a "virgin" population. *Am J Epidemiol.* 1995;142:221–222.
31. Philips RN, Reinhardt R, Lackman DB. Observations on a mumps epidemic in a "virgin" population. *Am J Hyg.* 1959;69:91–111.
32. Snow, J. *On Cholera.* New York, NY: Commonwealth Fund; 1936.
33. William B. *Typhoid Fever: Its Nature, Mode of Spreading and Prevention, London 1873.* New York, NY: Delta Omega; 1931.
34. Semmelweiss IP. The etiology, the concept and the prophylaxis of childbed fever. Murphy FP, trans-ed. *Med Classics.* Jan–Apr 1941:5.
35. Timeweb. Statisticians through history. Available at: http://www.bized.ac.uk/timeweb/reference/statisticians.htm#2 Accessed February 22, 2006.
36. Graunt J. *Natural and Political Observation Made upon the Bills of Mortality.* Wilcox WF, ed. [Reprint of first ed., 1662.] Baltimore, Md: Johns Hopkins University Press; 1937.
37. Shodor Education Foundation. Case studies and project ideas: smallpox Web page. Available at: http://www.shodor.org/succeed/biomed/labs/pox.html.
38. Victorian Web. Edwin Chadwick. Available at: http://www.victorianweb.org/history/chadwick2.html Accessed February 22, 2006.
39. LaborLawTalk.com. William Farr. Available at: http://encyclopedia.laborlawtalk.com/William_Farr. Accessed February 22, 2006.

40. Pasteur L. *The Physiological Theory of Fermentation in Scientific Papers.* Eliot CW, ed. New York, NY: PF Collier and Sons; 1910.

41. Dubini A. Nvove verme intestinalumano (Ancylostoma duodenale) constitutente un sestro gemere dei nematoide: proprii delluomo. *Aanali Universali de Medicina.* 1843:106;5–13. In: Kean B, Mott KE, Russell AJ, trans. *Tropical Medicine and Parasitology.* Vol. 2. Ithaca, NY: Cornell University Press; 1978:287–291.

42. Looss A. Uber das eindringen der ankylostomalarrea in die meatschliche haut. *Zeatral Blatt for Bakteriologic and Parisitenkunde.* 1898;24:441–448,483–488.

43. Altman LK. *Who Goes First? The Story of Self-Experimentation in Medicine.* New York, NY: Random House; 1986:134.

44. Assadian O, Stanek G. Theobald Smith–the discoverer of ticks as vectors of disease. *Wien Klin Wochenschr.* July 31, 2002;114(13–14):479–481.

45. Reed W, Carroll J. The prevention of yellow fever. *Med Rec NY.* 1901;60:641–649.

46. Mahy BW. Introduction and history of foot-and-mouth disease virus. *Curr Top Microbiol Immunol.* 2005;288:1–8.

47. Harrison G. *Mosquitoes, Malaria and Man: A History of the Hostilities Since 1880.* New York, NY: EP Dutton; 1978.

48. Ronald R. *The Prevention of Malaria.* New York, NY: EP Dutton; 1910.

49. Http://www.britannica.com/nobel/micro/369_83.html

50. National Institutes of Health. Office of History Web page. Available at: http://history.nih.gov. Accessed February 22, 2006.

51. Food and Drug Administration. Biologics centennial Web page. Available at: http://www.fda.gov/oc/history/2006centennial/biologics100.html. Accessed February 22, 2006.

52. Dowling HF. *Fighting Infection.* Cambridge, Mass: Harvard University Press; 1977.

53. Etheridge EW. *Sentinel for Health: A History of the Centers for Disease Control.* Berkeley: University of California Press; 1992.

54. Centers for Disease Control and Prevention. Ten great public health achievements–United States, 1900–1999. *MMWR.* 1999;48:241–248.

55. Batelle Medical Technology Assessment and Policy Research Program, Center for Public Health Research and Evaluation. *A Cost Benefit Analysis of the Measles-Mumps-Rubella (MMR) Vaccine.* Arlington, Va: Batelle; 1994.

56. Centers for Disease Control and Prevention. Ten great public health achievements–United States, 1900–1999, control of infectious diseases. *MMWR.* 1999;48:621–629.

57. Davies K. *Cracking the Genome, Inside the Race to Unlock Human DNA.* New York, NY: The Free Press; 2001.

58. Venter JC, Adams MD, Myers EW, et al. The sequence of the human genome. *Science.* 2001;291:1304–1351.

59. The Genome International Sequencing Consortium. Initial sequencing and analysis of the human genome. *Nature.* 2001;409:860–921.

60. NIH. National Human Genome Research Institute Web site. Available at: http://www.genome.gov. Accessed February 22, 2006.

61. International Rice Genome Sequencing Project. The map-based sequence of the rice genome. *Nature.* 2005;436:793–800.

62. Burkhardt PK, Beyer P, Wunn J, et al. Transgenic rice (*Oryza sativa*) endosperm expressing daffodil (*Narcissus pseudonarcissus*) phytoene synthase accumulates phytoene, a key intermediate of provitamin A biosynthesis. *Plant J.* 1997;11:1071–1078.

63. Paine JA, Shipton CA, Chaggar S, et al. Improving the nutritional value of golden rice through increased pro-vitamin A content. *Nat Biotechnol.* 2005;23:482–487.
64. Villamor E, Fawzi WW. Effects of vitamin A supplementation on immune responses and correlation with clinical outcomes. *Clin Microbiol Rev.* 2005;18:446–464.
65. Institute for Science in Society. Monsanto vs. farmers. Available at: http://www.i-sis.org.uk/MonsantovsFarmers.php. Accessed February 22, 2006.
66. Centers for Disease Control and Prevention. Kaposi's sarcoma and prevmocystis prevmonia among homosexual men—New York City and California. *MMWR.* 1981;30:305–308.

EPIDEMIOLOGY OF INFECTIOUS DISEASE: GENERAL PRINCIPLES

Kenrad E. Nelson

Introduction

Studies of the epidemiology of infectious diseases include evaluation of the factors leading to infection by an organism, factors affecting the transmission of an organism, and those associated with clinically recognizable disease among those who are infected. Many epidemiologic concepts were originally developed in studies of infectious diseases. Some of these fundamental concepts were applied later to the study of noninfectious disease. Among these concepts are the following:

- The incubation period—Diseases caused by either an infectious agent or a noninfectious agent, such as a toxin or carcinogen, have an intrinsic incubation period after contact with the agent before disease occurs.
- Resistance—Some individuals may have immunity or resistance to infection on a biologic basis, such as from previous infection, immunization, or because of host genetics, and remain uninfected after exposure.

When new epidemics of infectious diseases are described, they are usually first studied and described according to their epidemiologic characteristics. New infectious diseases can be classified according to their epidemiologic, clinical, or microbiologic features. Certainly, knowledge of all of these characteristics is important. However, the epidemiologic features of a disease are of paramount importance for a public health professional or an epidemiologist who is concerned primarily with controlling or preventing the epidemic spread of an infection. On the other hand, a clinician whose primary role is to treat an individual patient may be more concerned with the clinical symptoms or pathophysiology of the disease. For example, an infectious agent that causes secretory diarrhea will be treated empirically with fluid replacement and symptomatic management of the pathophysiology, irrespective of how the infection was acquired or what the organism is. A microbiologist may be primarily interested in the characteristics of the organism and may try to determine the following:

- How the organism can be isolated?
- How infection can be diagnosed or confirmed in the laboratory?
- Is it possible to prepare a vaccine or treat the infection with an antibiotic?
- What are the essential growth requirements of the organism?

The control, treatment, and prevention of an epidemic usually involves the cooperative efforts of all three groups of specialists: clinicians, microbiologists, and epidemiologists. However, each has a unique orientation and contribution. The perspectives from each of these three areas of study can best be appreciated by considering how infectious diseases are classified by each specialist.

The Classification of Infectious Diseases

Clinicians tend to classify infectious diseases according to their most common or most important clinical manifestation or by the organ systems that are primarily affected. An example of a clinical classification is given in Table 2-1.

The second group of specialists, microbiologists, tend to classify infectious diseases according to the characteristics of the causative organism. An example of a typical microbiologic classification of infectious diseases is shown in Table 2-2.

Epidemiologists usually classify infectious diseases according to two important epidemiologic characteristics—their means of transmission and the reservoir of the organism.

When a new disease appears on the scene, the detailed microbiologic characteristics of the organism usually are not known. The full range of symptoms that may occur after infection often is appreciated only later, after detailed clinical studies of many patients have been carried out. For example, the fact that infection with *Borrelia burgdorferii*, the cause of Lyme disease,

TABLE 2-1   Clinical Classification of Infections

Classification	Infection
Diarrheal diseases	Secretory Invasive
Respiratory diseases	Upper respiratory Lower respiratory
Central nervous system infection	Meningitis (bacterial vs. aseptic) Encephalitis Abscess
Cardiovascular infection	Endocarditis Myocarditis Vasculitis
Sepsis	Disseminated

was responsible not only for the classical skin lesion, erythema chronica migrans (ECM), but also for acute and chronic arthritis, vascular and cardiac disease, and neurologic symptoms, including Bell's palsy and encephalitis, was not appreciated initially. In fact, the full range of clinical manifestations of infection with *B. burgdorferii* is still being defined. Infectious diseases can be classified according to their means of transmission into five distinct categories, as shown in Table 2-3.

The second means for the epidemiologic classification of infectious diseases is according to their major reservoirs in nature. If one is aware of the reservoir of the agent in addition to the means of transmission, it is generally possible to develop a strategy to prevent transmission, even when the microbiologic characteristics of the organism are not known. The demonstration of the water reservoir of cholera by John Snow in London in 1853 preceded the identification of the *Vibrio* cholera by Robert Koch in 1884.[1] The epidemiologic information alone was sufficient to develop public health strategies to

TABLE 2-2   Microbiologic Classification of Infectious Diseases

Classification	Organism
Bacterial	Gram-negative Gram-positive
Viral	DNA virus RNA virus Enveloped vs. nonenveloped viruses
Fungal	Disseminated (biphasic) Localized
Parasitic	Protozoa Helminths Trematodes Cestodes
Prion	Protein

TABLE 2-3   Means of Transmission of Infectious Diseases and Their Characteristic Features

Transmission	Characteristics
Contact	Requires direct or indirect contact (indirect = infected fomite, blood, or body fluid; direct = skin or sexual contact)
Food- or water-borne	Ingestion of contaminated food (outbreaks may be large and dispersed, depending on distribution of food)
Airborne	Inhalation of contaminated air
Vector-borne	Dependent on biology of the vector (mosquito, tick, snail, etc), as well as the infectivity of the organism
Perinatal	Similar to contact infection; however, the contact may occur in utero during pregnancy or at the time of delivery

limit exposure to contaminated water and prevent human infections. Similarly, the demonstration of the importance of human carriers of *Salmonella typhi* as the important reservoir in outbreaks of typhoid fever by Budd in 1858 antedated by 22 years the isolation of the organism in the laboratory by Eberth in 1880. Walter Reed succeeded in transmitting yellow fever by the bite of infected *Aedes aegypti* mosquitoes in 1901. It wasn't until 1928 that Stokes and colleagues isolated the causative virus in the laboratory. In more recent times, investigation of the epidemic at the American Legion convention in Philadelphia in 1976 demonstrated that the outbreak of Legionnaires' disease was due to airborne spread of microorganisms from a contaminated reservoir, the air conditioning system in the Bellevue-Stratford Hotel, and suggested that further infections could be prevented by avoiding exposures to the air in the hotel.[2] The implicated organism, *Legionella pneumophila*, wasn't isolated and characterized in the laboratory until 1978 by McDade and Sheppard at the Centers for Disease Control and Prevention (CDC).

When organisms are classified according to their reservoirs in nature, four general categories are often considered:

1. Human
2. Animal (often called *zoonoses*)
3. Soil
4. Water

Some common examples of infectious diseases classified according to their reservoir are shown in Table 2-4.

Knowledge of the reservoir often is essential prior to devising rational and effective means of preventing transmission of infectious diseases. Prior to John Snow's demonstration that contaminated water was the reservoir of *Vibrio cholerae* in the outbreak in London in the 1850s, the predominant theories were that miasma, or exposure to foul or malodorous air, was the critical exposure leading to infection. However, there were no successful efforts to control the outbreak that were based on the miasma theory.

When Snow demonstrated that attack rates of cholera were highest in those receiving their water from one particular water company and subsequently terminated an epidemic by closing down the pump at one water source, the evidence was persuasive.[1]

TABLE 2-4   Classification of Infectious Organisms by Their Reservoir in Nature

Reservoir	Some Typical Organisms
Human	*Treponema pallidum, Neisseria gonorrhoeae*, HIV, hepatitis B and C virus, *Shigella, S. typhi*
Animals (zoonoses)	Rabies, *Yersinia pestis, Leptospira*, nontyphoid *Salmonella, Brucella*
Soil	*Histoplasma capsulatum* (and other systemic fungi), *Clostridium tetani, Clostridium botulinum*
Water	*Legionella, Pseudomonas aeruginosa, Mycobacterium marinum*

In the Philadelphia outbreak of Legionnaires' disease, the critical exposure was to the contaminated air in the hotel. It was especially noteworthy in this epidemic that no secondary cases occurred among the household contacts of ill patients with pneumonia who did not visit or stay in the hotel.[2] Subsequent study of this outbreak and subsequent Legionellosis outbreaks have found that aerosolization of water contaminated with *L. pneumophila*, often from a cooling tower, was the critical exposure leading to infection and disease.[3-5] Studies of water from a variety of sources have found that contamination with various pathogenic species of *Legionella* is quite common, even in the absence of human illness.[6] Human infection usually requires inhalation of a contaminated droplet of a small particle-sized aerosol (less than 5 μ in diameter) so that the organism can reach the lower respiratory system. However, in the case of *Legionella*, procedures to disinfect the reservoir usually are only undertaken when aerosolization is posing a risk of infection and disease to humans. The water can be decontaminated by heating to temperatures above 120°F, and growth of the organism is inhibited below 70°F.[7]

Infectious Diseases Transmitted by More Than One Means

Some organisms may be spread by several different means, depending on the epidemiologic circumstances. Therefore, it is important for an epidemiologist to keep an open mind to detect unusual epidemiologic features of an infection. A few examples of infectious diseases that have been spread by multiple means are described below.

Tularemia

Perhaps a typical example of a disease that can be spread by more than one means is tularemia, which can be acquired by the bite of infected ticks or deer flies,[8] by contact with infected rabbits or other animals during the hunting season,[9,10] or by inhalation of an aerosol.[11,12] Also, nosocomial infection among microbiology laboratory workers has been reported from inhalation of infected aerosols of the causative organism, *Francisella tularensis*.[13] Curiously, none of the investigators who have studied epidemics of tularemia have found evidence that human-to-human transmission has occurred.[14]

Plague

Plague, the disease that has been associated with perhaps the most serious and extensive epidemic in human history is caused by the plague bacillus, *Yersinia pestis*. The disease is a zoonotic disease of rodents that is transmitted to humans and other mammalian hosts from infected rodents by rat fleas. Percutaneous inoculation of the plague bacillus in humans initiates inflammation of lymph nodes draining the inoculation site, resulting in bubonic plague. Bloodstream invasion may lead to septicemic plague or to infection of other organ systems, such as the lung or meninges. Involvement of the lungs may result in pneumonic plague, which can then be transmitted from person to person via the respiratory route.

Historically, many epidemics of plague have spread rapidly through populations, causing very high mortality. The earliest description of plague dates from the sixth century AD in Egypt, when the epidemic spread throughout North Africa and into Europe. Epidemic plague reappeared in the Far East in the 1300s and subsequently spread to Europe. During the "Great Plague" epidemic in London, which peaked in August and September 1665, 7000 deaths per week were reported in a population of an estimated 500,000 persons. For unknown reasons, plague gradually disappeared from Europe in the 1700s, and the entire continent was free of plague by 1840.[15] Zinsser considers the disappearance of epidemics of plague from Europe to be one of the great mysteries of the epidemiology of infectious diseases.[16]

However, epidemics of plague have occurred in Asia in the late 1800s and more recently in Vietnam, during the war between 1962 and 1975.[17] An epidemic of plague was reported in India in 1994.[18] Sporadic cases of plague have occurred throughout the American Southwest for the past several decades, related to epizootics in infected prairie dogs.[19,20] The organism was first isolated by Yersin in Hong Kong in 1894.[21] A vaccine is available, but its efficacy in preventing pneumonic plague is unknown.

Anthrax

Anthrax is an infection with *Bacillus anthracis*, a gram-positive spore-forming organism that is a zoonotic disease in herbivorous animals. It can be transmitted to humans from contact with infected animals and has three clinical forms in humans: cutaneous, gastrointestinal, and inhalation anthrax.

The organisms from infected animals most often infect humans by contact with contaminated animal hides or pelts; this disease has been called *woolsorter's disease.*[22] Infection can occur also by inoculation of organisms into the skin during butchering of an infected animal; this type of exposure usually leads to cutaneous anthrax, consisting of a black eschar on the skin with swelling and inflammation of the draining lymphatics. Consumption of meat from an infected animal leads to gastrointestinal anthrax, which has a much higher mortality than does cutaneous anthrax. Inhalation anthrax occurs when an infectious aerosol of *B. anthracis* spores is inhaled and germinates in the pulmonary lymphatic tissues. This form of anthrax is rare, which is fortunate because it usually is rapidly fatal.

An epidemic of inhalation anthrax occurred in persons living in Sverdlovsk, Union of Soviet Socialist Republics, in April and May 1979. There were at least 96 cases and 66 deaths. The outbreak also affected cattle within 50 km of the city. Interestingly, Sverdlovsk was known to have a military facility that was suspected of manufacturing biologic weapons, including anthrax spores, for potential use in warfare. Initially, the Soviet authorities maintained that this outbreak was from gastrointestinal exposure due to the consumption of contaminated meat from cattle that had died of anthrax. However, in 1992, Meselson and colleagues visited the site of the epidemic and were able to conduct an epidemiologic investigation, together with Russian scientists. Their study found that all of the human cases were living or working in a narrow belt south of the city on the day the outbreak occurred.[23] Furthermore, the animal deaths also occurred in this belt, up to 50 km distant (Figure 2-1). The wind pattern on the day of the outbreak could explain the geographic

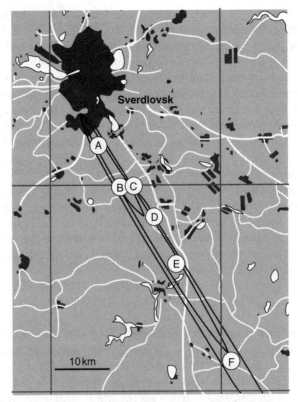

FIGURE 2-1   Russian villages with animal anthrax. Six villages where livestock died of anthrax in April 1979 are shown. Settled areas are shown in gray, roads in white, and calculated contours of constant dosage in black. Reprinted with permission from M. Meselson et al., The Sverdlovsk Anthrax Outbreak of 1979, *Science*, Vol. 266, pp. 1202–1208, Copyright 1994, American Association for the Advancement of Science (AAAS).

distribution of cases. Subsequently, evidence was discovered that many of the human cases had pneumonic anthrax. They concluded that this outbreak, the largest outbreak of human inhalation anthrax ever recorded, was due to an infectious aerosol emanating from the military facility. One very interesting finding in their study was that human cases continued to occur for up to 6 weeks after this point source exposure. Apparently, spores were inhaled and continued to germinate and cause disease for several weeks after they were inhaled. This outbreak has raised considerable concern among scientists and policy makers about the potential for the use of aerosolized *B. anthracis* spores as an agent of biologic terrorism. Indeed, these fears were confirmed in 2001 when an outbreak of 22 cases of anthrax occurred in the United States from intentional contamination of the US mail delivered to a number of persons by the US Postal Service. This outbreak is described in detail in the chapter on emerging infections.

Rabies

Rabies is a nearly uniformly fatal infection of the central nervous system that is almost always transmitted by a bite from an animal infected with the rabies virus. Historically, rabies has nearly always been acquired by a bite from an infected dog, skunk, fox, bat, or other animal. It has been regarded as a typical contact-transmitted infection, in that percutaneous inoculation of rabies virus by a bite is usually required. Nevertheless, a few persons have developed rabies from exposure to infected aerosols in caves harbored by many infected bats.[24] Also, rabies has occurred in a laboratory worker who was exposed to an infectious aerosol[25] and in persons who have received corneal transplants from a donor who died of undiagnosed rabies.[26] In recent years, in the United States, only 2–3 cases have occurred annually; however, reported bite exposures in these cases has been unusual. Of the 32 cases of rabies that were diagnosed in the United States between 1980 and 1996, 25 (78%) had no history of a bite exposure.[27] Some of these non-bite-transmitted cases in the United States have been in persons exposed in the same room (or closed space) to an infected bat; presumably, the transmission in these cases was by aerosol. Genetic analysis of the viruses has shown that 17 (53%) of these cases in the United States were related to rabies viruses found in insectivorous bats.

Brucellosis

Brucellosis is an infectious disease of humans acquired through contact with an infected animal (i.e., a zoonosis). Four species of *Brucellae* have infected humans: *B. abortus* (from cattle), *B. melitensis* (from goats or sheep), *B. suis* (from pigs), and *B. canis* (from dogs). Human infections with the two other known species, *B. ovis* (from sheep) and *B. neotomae* (from desert wood rats), have not been reported. Clinically, the most serious human infections are seen with *B. melitensis*. However, in the early decades of the 1900s infections with *B. abortus* were common, and these infections often were acquired by the consumption of contaminated milk from infected cows. However, after World War II, the US Department of Agriculture (USDA) undertook a campaign to eliminate milk-borne brucellosis as a human health problem in the United States. The program included testing of cattle for *B. abortus* and slaughtering of infected animals or animals from infected herds, and pasteurization of all milk and dairy products.[28] This program was quite successful. More than 6000 cases of human brucellosis were reported each year at the start of this program; the rate was 4.5 cases per 100,000 population in 1948. In the 1990s, only about 100 cases per year were reported; 0.05 cases per 100,000 population were reported in 1993. Furthermore, in recent years, the cases usually had an occupation that directly exposed them to infected animals, such as slaughterhouse workers, farmers, or veterinarians. Brucellosis in these workers was acquired by direct contact with infected animals, not through consumption of infected milk. Also, *B. suis* infections from infected pigs have become proportionally more common, because the brucellosis control program was directed at eliminating the disease in cattle.

Transmission of Microbial Agents by Transfusions

There is evidence that several microbial agents can be transmitted by blood transfusion or contaminated injection if exposure occurs during a time when the organisms are present in the blood stream. Hepatitis B virus, hepatitis

C virus, and HIV are commonly transmitted by the transfusion of blood or blood products. *Trypanosoma cruzii*, a protozoan parasite that causes Chagas' disease, is usually transmitted to humans by the bite of a reduviid bug but can be transmitted by blood transfusion from a carrier.[29] Malaria usually is caused by the transmission of one of four species of *Plasmodium* parasites by the bite of an infected female anopheline mosquito, but it can also be transmitted by blood transfusion or to an infant by perinatal transmission. Hepatitis A virus is generally transmitted by ingestion of contaminated food or water but can be transmitted by blood transfusion during the brief viremic stage early in the infection.

Perinatal Infections

Infections of an infant may be acquired from the mother in utero via placental transfer, during passage through the birth canal, or in the postpartum period.

Rubella

The dramatic effect of rubella infections during the first trimester of pregnancy in producing congenital anomalies in the infant was first reported by Sir Norman Gregg following an outbreak of rubella in Australia in 1940.[30] Gregg noted ocular defects and cardiac lesions in the affected infants. Subsequently, these findings were confirmed by studies during rubella outbreaks in Australia, the United States, and the United Kingdom. These studies further defined the congenital rubella syndrome (CRS) from intrauterine exposure to rubella during the first trimester of pregnancy to include cataracts and other ocular abnormalities, cardiac defects, deafness, microcephaly, and mental retardation. Infants exposed during the first trimester of pregnancy have a 90% risk of developing congenital rubella syndrome; during the early second trimester, the risk of congenital abnormalities declines to 20–40% and often involves only deafness.

In 1962, the rubella virus was isolated by investigators at Harvard University[31] and independently by scientists at the Walter Reed Army Institute of Research.[32] Shortly thereafter, in 1964, a major epidemic of rubella and CRS occurred in the United States.[33] An attenuated live rubella virus vaccine was developed and licensed in the United States in 1969.[34] Subsequently, congenital rubella infections have become rare in the United States, due to routine immunization of infants and screening and selective immunization of susceptible women of childbearing age.

Cytomegalovirus

Cytomegalovirus (CMV) infections during the first trimester of pregnancy are known to lead to congenital malformation, especially of the central nervous system. Cytomegalovirus was first isolated in human fibroblast cultures in 1956.[35-37] It is possible to screen pregnant women for susceptibility to infection during pregnancy. Epidemiologic studies suggest that CMV infection may occur in about 1% of all US births, or about 40,000 infants annually.[38] However, in most instances, these infections are asymptomatic. A national surveillance registry was established in the United States in 1990 by the CDC to monitor congenital CMV infections.[39] The most common clinical manifestation reported was petechiae, observed in 50% of cases, which was often accompanied by hepatosplenomegaly, intracranial calcification, and thrombocytopenia.

Herpes Simplex Virus

In contrast to CMV and rubella, in utero infection with herpes simplex virus (HSV) is rare, and when it does occur, it is most likely to lead to a miscarriage, rather than a congenital malformation. However, infants can be infected when passing through the birth canal if the mother has an active infection, especially with HSV type 2 (HSV-2), which causes recurrent genital tract infection. When the mother has an active HSV infection at the time of delivery, the infant can develop a generalized infection, which is quite serious. The risk to the newborn is higher when the mother has a primary HSV infection than when the HSV is a recurrence; the risk to the newborn is about 40% when exposed to a mother with primary infection, compared with 2–5% when the mother has a recurrent infection. In the latter situation, the infant's risk is modified by maternal passive transfer of antibodies to HSV-2 and by lower maternal viral load. Cesarean section is recommended to prevent neonatal herpes in children born to women with active HSV at the time of delivery. However, most cases of neonatal HSV occur where the mother was not identified as having active HSV infection. For example, during an 18-month hospital-based surveillance study, the CDC identified 184 cases of neonatal herpes but only 22% of the mothers had a history of genital HSV infection, and only 9% had lesions at the time of delivery.[40]

Toxoplasmosis

Congenital infection with *Toxoplasma gondii* occurs when a pregnant woman develops infection, especially early in pregnancy. Clinical manifestations in the infant at birth include a maculopapular rash, generalized lymphade-nopathy, hepatomegaly, splenomegaly, jaundice, or thrombocytopenia. Also, the infant can develop meningoencephalitis with cerebrospinal fluid abnormalities, hydrocephalus, microcephaly, chorioretinitis, and/or convulsions. However, congenital infection is usually asymptomatic at birth, although sequelae can become apparent several years later. Sequelae of congenital toxoplasma infection include mental retardation and learning disability. Also, ocular toxoplasmosis most often results from reactivation of a congenital infection, but it can occur from an acquired infection, as well. Ocular toxoplasmosis usually occurs among adults.

Syphilis

Syphilis is caused by infection with the spirochete *Treponema pallidum.* Syphilis is usually transmitted sexually but can be transmitted by the peri-natal (congenital) route by infection through the placenta, especially in the second and third trimesters, or, more rarely, transmission can occur during delivery by contact of an infant with the mucosa of a woman with primary or secondary syphilis during the birth process. Congenital syphilis can be asymptomatic or it may manifest as multisystem involvement, including osteitis, hepatitis, lymphadenopathy, pneumonitis, mucocutaneous lesions, anemia, and hemorrhage. Late manifestation may involve the central nervous system, bones, teeth, and/or eyes. Rates of congenital syphilis parallel the rates of primary and secondary syphilis in women and can be prevented by treatment of infected pregnant women with penicillin, to which the organism is uniformly sensitive. Rates of congenital syphilis have increased in the late 1980s and early 1990s, in part related to the epidemic of crack cocaine use in the United States.[41]

Because newborns infected with each of these agents have similar clinical symptoms, pediatricians often consider all of them in the differential diagnosis of perinatal infections. The syndrome of congenital infection is often referred to by the abbreviation *TORCHS* to signify the most common etiologies: toxoplasmosis, rubella, CMV, HSV, and syphilis.

Hepatitis B Virus

Women who are carriers of hepatitis B virus (HBV) may transmit the virus to their infants in utero or at the time of birth (peripartum). Infection of a newborn with HBV carries a very high risk of chronic infection, with the possibility of subsequent chronic active hepatitis, cirrhosis, or liver cancer when carriage persists for decades. Most perinatal transmission of HBV can be prevented by screening pregnant women for HBsAg and administering hepatitis B immunoglobulin and a course of HBV vaccine to the infants of HBsAg carriers, beginning immediately after birth.

Human Immunodeficiency Virus

Human immunodeficiency virus (HIV) is an important viral infection that can be transmitted perinatally from an infected woman to her newborn infant. Worldwide, the number of infected infants born each year in the 1990s was estimated to be about 500,000.

Although the risk of the prenatal transmission of HIV can be reduced to 5–10% or less by screening pregnant women and treating them with antiviral drugs, perinatal transmission still commonly occurs in sub-Saharan Africa. The various reported studies and research strategies to reduce perinatal HIV transmission are discussed in detail in the chapter on HIV.

Other Infectious Agents

The most important infectious diseases that are transmitted by the perinatal route are discussed above; however, there is some evidence of transmission of several other agents, such as parvovirus B-19, varicella-zoster virus, and others. The most common agents incriminated in perinatal infection and the effects of perinatal infection with these agents on the fetus and newborn infant are listed in Table 2-5.

TABLE 2-5   Effects of Transplacental Fetal Infection

Organism or Disease	Effect of Infection on the Fetus and Newborn Infant				
	Prematurity	Intrauterine Growth Retardation and Low Birth Weight	Developmental Anomalies	Congenital Disease	Persistent Postnatal Infection
Viruses					
Rubella	−	+	−	+	+
Cytomegalovirus	+	+	+	+	−
Herpes simplex	+	−	−	+	+
Varicella-zoster	−	(+)	−	+	−
Mumps	−	−	−	(+)	−
Rubeola	+	−	−	+	−
Vaccinia	−	−	−	+	−
Smallpox	+	−	−	+	−
Coxsackieviruses B	−	−	(−)	−	−
Echoviruses	−	−	−	−	−
Polioviruses	−	−	−	−	−
Influenza	−	−	−	−	−
Hepatitis B	+	−	−	+	+
Human immuno-deficiency virus	(+)	(+)	(−)	+	+
Lymphocytic chorio-meningitis virus	−	−	−	+	−
Parvovirus	−	−	−	(+)	−

Notes: +, evidence for effect; −, no evidence for effect; (−), association of effect with infection has been suggested and is under consideration.
Source: Reprinted with permission from Epidemiologic Concepts and Methods, in *Viral Infections of Humans*, 4th Ed., A.S. Evans & R.A. Kaslow, eds., p. 30, Copyright © 1997, Plenum Publishing Corporation.

Epidemiologic Characteristics of Infectious Diseases

Incubation Period

The incubation period of an infectious disease is the time between exposure to an infectious agent and the onset of symptoms or signs of infection. Each infectious disease has a typical incubation period that requires multiplication of the infectious agent to a threshold necessary to produce symptoms or laboratory evidence of infection, such as antibodies, viral isolation, and nucleic acids in the host. The incubation period for infectious diseases shows some variation, which occurs for a variety of reasons, including the dose or inoculum of the infectious agent, the route of inoculation, and the rate of replication of the organism. Even when numerous persons are exposed at the same time to a similar inoculum of the same strain of an infectious agent, such as consumption of food contaminated with *Salmonella* at a picnic, the length of the incubation period varies between individuals. A plot of the incubation period for persons exposed at the same time usually follows a log normal distribution. The antilogarithm of 1 standard deviation from the mean log incubation period has been referred to by Sartwell as the *dispersion factor*.[42] The dispersion factor multiplied by the mean log of the incubation period will define an interval above which 16% of the periods will fall, and the mean divided by the dispersion factor will define the period below which 16% will occur. Even diseases with very long incubation periods have been shown to follow similar patterns of distribution of their incubation periods. A recent study of the incubation periods of AIDS found that a log normal distribution reasonably described the incubation period of this disease as well.[43]

The usual ranges of the incubation periods for a number of infectious diseases are shown in Figure 2-2. These incubation periods range from 6 to 12 hours for *B. cereus* and staphylococcal food poisoning to 5–10 years for AIDS and leprosy. The extrinsic incubation period applies to vector-borne infections; it is the time that a vector-borne agent requires for maturation to infectivity in the vector before it becomes infectious to humans. The extrinsic incubation period also has a medium and range that are unique to each organism. Also, the extrinsic incubation period can be affected by environmental conditions. For example, when *A. aegypti* mosquitoes were infected with dengue type 2 virus and held at 30°C, the mean extrinsic incubation period before they become infectious was 12 days, whereas between 32° and 35°C, they became infectious after only 7 days.[44] The extrinsic incubation periods for various species of *Plasmodium* are discussed in more detail in the chapter on malaria.

Biologic Characteristics of the Organism

Infectivity

Infectivity is defined as the ability of an agent to cause infection in a susceptible host. The basic measure of infectivity is the minimum number of infectious particles required to establish infection. In diseases spread from person to person, the proportion of susceptible individuals who develop infection after exposure—the secondary attack rate—is a measure of the infectivity of an organism (see Table 2-6 below).

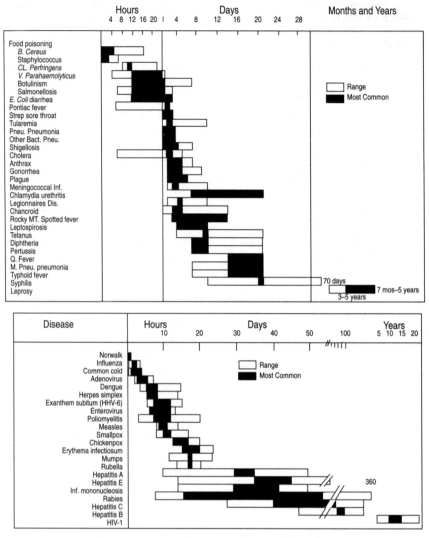

FIGURE 2-2 Incubation periods of common bacterial diseases (*top panel*) and viral diseases (*bottom panel*). Reprinted with permission from *Viral Infections of Humans*, 4th Edition, A.S. Evans and R.A. Kaslow, eds., p. 20, Copyright © 1997, Plenum Publishing Corporation.

Pathogenicity

Pathogenicity refers to the ability of a microbial agent to induce disease. Diseases such as rabies, smallpox, measles, chicken pox, and rhinovirus colds have high pathogenicity. Others, such as polio and arbovirus (mosquito-borne) infections, have low pathogenicity.

Virulence

Some dictionaries use the terms *virulence* and *pathogenicity* interchangeably. However, it is useful to consider them to be separate properties of an infectious agent. *Virulence* can be defined as the severity of the disease

TABLE 2-6   Ranking of Infection by Infectivity, Pathogenicity, and Virulence

Severity*	Infectivity (Secondary Attack Rate = Ill/Number Exposed)	Pathogenicity (Illness Rate = Ill/Number Infected)	Virulence (Severe/Fatal Cases) Total Cases
High	Smallpox Measles Chicken pox	Smallpox Rabies Measles Chicken pox Common cold	Rabies Smallpox Tuberculosis Leprosy
Intermediate	Rubella Mumps Common cold	Rubella Mumps	Poliomyelitis Measles
Low	Tuberculosis	Poliomyelitis Tuberculosis	Measles Chicken pox
Very low	Leprosy	Leprosy	Rubella Common cold

*The "severity" of an infection varies by how it is being measured.
Source: Reprinted with the permission of Simon & Schuster from Epidemiology: Man and Disease by John P. Fox, Carrie Hall & Lila R. Elveback. Copyright © 1970 Macmillan Publishing Company.

after infection occurs. Although smallpox and rhinoviruses both usually cause symptoms (both are pathogenic), smallpox infections are much more virulent. Virulence can best be measured by the case fatality rate or as the proportion of clinical cases that develop severe disease. It is possible to classify organisms based on their infectivity, pathogenicity, and virulence. Only a few diseases, such as smallpox, airborne anthrax, and Ebola virus, will be classified as ranking high in all three characteristics. Several diseases are ranked by these characteristics in Table 2-6.

It is important to recognize that these properties of an infection may change over time under different circumstances. At one time, syphilis and streptococcal infections were highly virulent infections with high mortality rates, but these diseases are now much less virulent. Changes in the epidemiologic characteristics of infectious diseases will be discussed in greater detail later in this chapter and elsewhere in this book.

Immunogenicity

Immunogenicity is the ability of an organism to produce an immune response after an infection that is capable of providing protection against reinfection with the same or a similar organism. Some organisms, such as measles, polio, HBV, or rubella, lead to solid, lifelong immunity after an infection. Others, such as *Neisseria gonorrhoeae* or *Plasmodium falciparum*, are weakly immunogenic, and reinfection commonly occurs. Studies of the antigens that produce protective immunity after natural infections often have led to the development of effective vaccines. It should be noted that some microorganisms may provoke an immune response that is not protective from future infections. In a sense, they are immunogenic. However, sometimes these immune responses even may be deleterious to the host.

Several types of group A streptococci can provoke an immune response that leads to glomerulonephritis or acute rheumatic fever because of cross-reactive antibodies elicited in response to the streptococcal infection that react with endocardial or glomerular basement membrane antigens. In other instances, antibodies may occur that are markers of a previous or current infection but do not provide immunity to the organism or terminate an ongoing infection. These antibodies are often called *binding antibodies*, and they react to nonneutralizing antigens (or epitopes) of the organism. Examples of antibodies of this type are found in patients with hepatitis C virus infection, HIV infection, and HSV-2 infection. Persons with these antibodies have been or are infected with the virus and have antibodies but are not immune.

Inapparent Infections

An inapparent infection is an infection that can be documented by isolation of an organism by culture, demonstration of nucleic acid by polymerase chain reaction (PCR) amplification, or by demonstrating a specific immune response in a person who remains asymptomatic. The proportion of individuals with asymptomatic or clinically inapparent infections is a measure of the pathogenicity of the organism, as defined above. Inapparent infections are quite common in many infections and may play an important role in the propagation of an epidemic in some circumstances. The proportion of infected individuals who do not develop symptoms varies with different organisms. For example, most polio infections are inapparent. Also, inapparent nasopharyngeal carriage of meningococci is quite common, during an epidemic especially. Identification and treatment of carriers of meningococci or *Staphylococcus aureus* have been shown to help control epidemic transmission, because healthy carriers may play an important role in transmission. In the United States, persons who convert their tuberculin skin test and are infected but asymptomatic carriers of *Mycobacterium tuberculosis* are often treated to prevent clinically active tuberculosis from developing later in their life and subsequent spread of infection to their contacts. On the other hand, inapparent infections with some organisms are quite rare. Most persons with measles, varicella, smallpox, or hanta virus infection are symptomatic. The proportion of infections that are symptomatic is of considerable importance in understanding the transmission during an epidemic and in designing methods to control epidemic or endemic transmission. The proportion of infections that are clinically inapparent among individuals infected with some important organisms is shown in Table 2-7.

The Carrier State

The epidemiologic importance of the asymptomatic carrier in the transmission of infectious diseases has been recognized for some time. An early classic example was an Irish cook in New York City in the early 1900s, Mary Mallon, who became known as "Typhoid Mary." She was quite healthy but had worked as a cook in many homes where the residents developed typhoid fever after she was hired. Eventually, 53 cases of typhoid fever were

TABLE 2-7   Subclinical/Clinical Ratio in Selected Viral Infections (Inapparent/Apparent Ratio)

Virus	Clinical Feature	Age at Infection (Years)	Estimated Subclinical/Clinical Ratio	Percentage of Infection with Clinical Features
Poliomyelitis	Paralysis	Child	±1000:1	0.1–1
Epstein-Barr	Heterophil-positive	1–5	>100:1	1
	infectious	6–15	10–100:1	1–10
	mononucleosis	16–25	2–3:1	35–50
Hepatitis A	Jaundice	<5	20:1	5
		5–9	11:1	10
		10–15	7:1	14
		Adult	2–3:1	35–50
Rubella	Rash	5–20	2:1	50
Influenza	Fever, cough	Young adult	1.5:1	60
Measles	Rash, fever	5–20	1:99	95
Rabies	CNS symptoms	Any age	0:100	100

Source: Reprinted with permission from Viral Infections of Humans, 4th Ed., A.S. Evans & R.A. Kaslow, eds., p. 25, Copyright © 1997, Plenum Publishing Corporation.

traced to her. After she was located and cultures of her stool consistently grew *S. typhi*, she was confined and not allowed to work in food service between 1907 and 1910. After her release, she disappeared and changed her name. Two years later, outbreaks of typhoid fever involving over 200 persons were detected in hospitals in New York and New Jersey that were traced to her.[45] This remarkable story illustrates the potential importance of the carrier state in the transmission of typhoid fever. Patients infected with *S. typhi* may carry the organism in their gall bladders and excrete the organism in their stool for many years. Generally, antibiotic therapy is ineffective in curing their infections, but many chronic carriers can be cured by cholecystectomy.[46]

Another, more modern example is that of "patient 0," who was at the center of a large cluster of men who developed Kaposi's sarcoma (KS), with or without *Pneumocystis carinii* pneumonia (PCP), in 1980–1981. This patient was a male homosexual flight attendant who had visited several large US cities. He had sexual contact with all of the men who later became ill. This cluster of cases of KS and PCP was one of the early outbreaks of AIDS in the United States.[47] The carrier state may be of epidemiologic importance in any infectious disease that is transmitted from person to person. However, the average length of the carrier state, the site of replication and infectivity of the organism, and the usual means of spread determine the epidemiologic importance of asymptomatic carriers.

Outbreaks have been documented from chronic carriers in the respiratory tract, stool, genital tract, or blood. Nosocomial transmission from hospital workers to patients, from one patient to another, or from patients to health care workers is common. Currently, transmission of antibiotic-resistant staphylococci by healthy carriers of these organisms is of major concern in hospitals in the United States. Patients who are chronic carriers of hepatitis B virus pose a significant risk to health care workers. As a result, use of HBV vaccine is routinely recommended for health care professionals who are likely to be exposed. These issues are covered in more detail in the chapter on nosocomial infection.

Transfusion-Transmitted Infection

The transmission of infections by transfusion has received increasing attention in the last 20 years. Although transfusion-transmitted HBV was recognized for several decades, the introduction of screening of donors for HBsAg in 1973 reduced this risk. Subsequently, it became apparent that after screening of blood donors for hepatitis virus was introduced, posttransfusion hepatitis declined to about half of the previous rate but was not eliminated. The hepatitis C virus was identified and screening implemented in 1990. Also, the occurrence of HIV infection and AIDS among transfusion recipients and hemophiliacs has highlighted the risks of the transmission of infection by transfusion of blood or blood products from healthy carriers.

Currently, blood donors undergo extensive questioning about their risks to a variety of infectious agents, and they are screened for the presence of several pathogens. Pooled plasma products also undergo several viral inactivation steps and are heat-treated prior to their use. Nevertheless, the list of agents that may possibly be transmitted by the transfusion of blood or blood products continues to expand (Exhibit 2-1).

Exhibit 2-1   Infections Transmitted by Transfusion

- Viruses
  - HIV, HTLVI/II
  - HBV, HCV, HAV (rare)
  - Parvovirus B-19
  - CMV
  - KSHV (HHV-8)
  - Others
- Bacteria
  - *T. pallidum* (rare)
  - *Y. enterocolitica*
  - Various gram-positive organisms by platelet transfusion (especially)
  - *Ehrlichea* (rare)
- Parasites
  - *Trypanosoma cruzii*
  - *Plasmodium* species
  - *Babesia necrotica*
- Other agents
  - New variant Creutzfeldt-Jakob disease prion

The Host–Parasite Relationship

Patterns of Natural History

After infection occurs, the subsequent course or natural history of an infection can be quite variable. Many infections are characterized by acute symptoms, some of which may be severe and even terminate fatally. In some infections, the proportion of patients with asymptomatic or clinically inapparent infections varies, but once the acute phase is over, the patient is immune to reinfection with the same agent. The common childhood contagious diseases, such as measles, mumps, and rubella, are characterized by this type of natural history.

In other infections, some patients may develop chronic or recurring infection, and others may recover and develop lasting immunity. Hepatitis B virus and herpes virus types 1 and 2 typify this type of natural history. Infection with some agents may lead to chronic sequelae, due to an autoimmune reaction or chronic tissue damage that occurs after the acute infection has subsided and without persistence of the organism or chronic infection. Poststreptococcal glomerulonephritis or rheumatic fever are typical of this type of natural history.

Some infectious agents may recur or relapse, even after the acute infection has resolved without sequelae. Typical of this pattern is HSV-1 and HSV-2, varicella-zoster virus, and cytomegalovirus infections. Some infections may become chronic, with a variable proportion leading to progressive tissue damage at the primary site of the infection. Typical of this pattern is hepatitis C virus, HBV, and HIV.

Finally, some infections may become chronic and eventually lead to cancer in the target organ of the infection. Typical of this type of infection are human papillomavirus, HBV, and *Helicobacter pylori* infections. Infections that often exhibit each of these various natural history patterns are listed in Table 2-8.

It has been estimated by the World Health Organization (WHO) that greater than 15% of human cancers worldwide are caused by chronic infections. The proportion and types of human cancers associated with infectious agents are shown in Table 2-9.

The Immune Response to Infection

A detailed discussion of the immune responses to infection is well beyond the scope of this chapter. The topic is covered in the chapter on immunology. However, it might be useful to provide a very brief overview to introduce some concepts and nomenclature relative to the immune responses to infection.

Protection against infection consists of both specific immune responses against particular pathogens and nonspecific defenses directed against organisms or foreign antigens. Several compounds present in the normal intact skin, including lipids, lipoproteins, and peptides, are toxic to many organisms. Lysozyme in the tears and several proteins in the oral cavity have bactericidal activity. The acidic pH of the stomach is lethal to moderate doses of many enteric pathogens. The normal ciliary activity of the respiratory tract and the mucous layer coating the bronchus and bronchioles are

TABLE 2-8   Natural History Patterns of Some Important Infectious Diseases

Natural History	Disease
Acute with recovery and long-term immunity	Measles, mumps, rubella, polio, diphtheria
Acute with some chronic carriers	HBV, HSV-1 and HSV-2, VZV, *Chlamydia trachomatis* infections
Acute disease, chronic sequelae without carrier state	Group A streptococcal (ARF, AGN), syphilis, Lyme disease
Chronic carriers common (or usual)	HIV, HBV, HSV-2, HPV, HCV, *H. pylori* infections, *Opisthorchis viverrini, Schistosoma* infections
Chronic carriers may develop cancer	HBV—Hepatocellular CA HCV—Hepatocellular CA HPV—Cervical or laryngeal CA *H. pylori*—Gastric CA HTLV-1—T-cell leukemia EBV—Nasopharyngeal carcinoma HHV-8—Kaposi's sarcoma Opisthorchis—Cholangiocarcinoma

TABLE 2-9   Infection and the Burden of Cancer Worldwide (1990)

Cancer	No. of Cases	Agent	% of Total Cancers
Stomach	504,928	*H. pylori*	5.3
Cervix, vulva	447,400	HPV	4.8
Liver	398,600	HBV, HCV	4.3
Lymphoma	46,779	EBV	0.5
Kaposi's sarcoma	43,525	HIV, HHV-8	0.5
Bladder	10,249	*Schistosoma hematobium*	0.1
Leukemia	2,662	HTLV-1	0.1
Cholangiocarcinoma	808	Liver flukes (microns)	0.1
Total infection-related cancers	1,454,951		15.6
Total no. of cancers	9,327,165		

Data from the World Health Organization.

an important first line of defense against respiratory organisms. The low pH of the vagina serves as a first line of defense against many sexually transmitted pathogens. Furthermore, natural killer (NK) cells and cells of the monocyte-macrophage lineage can provide some nonspecific defense against a pathogen. However, the immune responses generated by cells and antibodies that have been stimulated to respond to a specific pathogen usually are more effective.

The immune system consists of a few main classes of cells and a large variety of cell subsets. Lymphocytes provide direction for the main activities of the immune system and govern the nature of the immune response.

Those that originate in the bone marrow are called *B lymphocytes*; those that originate in or traffic through the thymus are called *T lymphocytes*. Other cells of the immune system include circulating monocytes or macrophages, tissue macrophages, dendritic cells, Langerhans cells, NK cells, mast cells, eosinophils, and basophils. Granulocytes are involved in phagocytosis of bacterial pathogens, and eosinophils are involved in the reaction to parasitic pathogens and in allergic and autoimmune reactions.

B Lymphocytes and Humoral Immunity

The B lymphocytes are responsible for humoral immunity. These cells produce antibodies in the form of immunoglobulins that are reactive with foreign antigens. Five different isotypes of antibody are produced by B cells, namely, IgM, IgD, IgG, IgE, and IgA. Generally, the acute response to infection is characterized by a predominance of IgM antibodies that switch later to an IgG predominance. This pattern is useful in differentiating a recent, as in within the past 3–6 months, from a more remote infection. For example, persons with IgM antibodies to hepatitis A virus (HAV) or the core antigen of HBV have had their primary HAV or HBV infections in the past 6 months. Persons with only IgG antibodies to HAV or HBV but no IgM antibodies were infected longer than 6 months ago. Antibodies of the IgA class may provide neutralization of pathogens on mucosal surfaces. IgE antibodies are often involved in the immune responses to parasites and in allergic reactions to foreign protein antigens.

Local Immunity—The Mucosal Secretory IgA System

B lymphocytes secrete IgA antibodies, both in the blood and at the mucosal surfaces. These antibodies may be critical for resistance to infection in the respiratory, intestinal, and urogenital tracts. They are secreted after natural infection or following the administration of some whole virus vaccines. Vaccines given parenterally are less effective in inducing mucosal IgA. Therefore, some live virus vaccines, such as oral polio virus vaccines, may be more effective in preventing infection than killed vaccines because they provide resistance to mucosal infection, as well as resistance to invasive infection.

T Lymphocytes and Cell-Mediated Immunity

T lymphocytes are important regulatory cells of the immune system. They interact with antigen-presenting cells and secrete numerous cytokines that activate effector cells and interact with cells through the major histocompatibility complex (MHC) proteins at the cell surface. T lymphocytes can be classified as helper cells if they have CD4$^+$ markers on their surface. The CD4$^+$ helper cells activate B cells, monocytes-macrophages, and other T helper cells by binding directly to these cells or by secreting specific cytokines that stimulate cell proliferation. The cells that have CD8$^+$ markers on their surface are cytotoxic T cells that lyse other cells that contain foreign proteins or viruses. Also, CD8$^+$ T cells can help modulate the immune response by suppressing the activation of effector cells, such as macrophages.

Granuloma reactions to an infection with a mycobacteria consists of an organized cellular immune response with phagocytic effector cells, surrounded by CD4$^+$ cells and CD8$^+$ T suppressor cells on the periphery to provide a localized and controlled immune response to the organism. Natural killer cells resemble lymphocytes but have some distinctive properties, such as expression of a specific receptor for the Fc portion of IgG. In some circumstances, these NK cells can kill virus-infected or neoplastic cells by secretion of interferon gamma (IFN-G), especially when induced to do so by tumor necrosis factor (TNF) and other cytokines produced by macrophages. Macrophages and monocytes function to process and deliver antigens for recognition by lymphocytes. Macrophages also can destroy intracellular virus-infected cells. These cells can respond to IFN-G secreted by the T cell, which activates the toxic oxygen and enzymatic pathways of the macrophage.

Granulocytes and Complement

Granulocytes are phagocytic cells that are involved in the protection against bacterial infections by ingesting and killing extracellular bacteria. The complement system is a set of enzymes and other proteins that attach to bacteria or foreign proteins and promote their destruction by phagocytosis. Persons who are deficient in some components of the complement system (especially C6, C7, or C8) have markedly increased susceptibility to recurrent infection with meningococci.[48]

Innate Immunity

In addition to acquired immunity it has long been recognized that animals are protected from invasion by pathogenic organisms by a system of innate or native immunity. A few years ago transmembrane receptor named Toll was identified in Drosophila insects that was responsible for establishing dorso-ventral polarity during embryogenesis. Subsequently it was found that Toll was also responsible for protecting insects against fungal infections. More recently it was discovered that humans and all animals have Toll-like receptors (humans have 10TLRS) that recognize patterns of non-self molecules, such as bacterial lipopolysaccharides or viral DNA or RNA, which then sets off an intracellular defense reaction involving cytokines and enzymes, to destroy the foreign material. Innate immunity has been recognized recently as a critical component of the defense against infection.

Quantitation of Infectious Diseases

Epidemiologists use a variety of measurements to quantify the occurrence of disease. Fundamentally, these measurements are intended to estimate the burden of disease in a population or the incidence of disease—the rate at which the disease is spread among persons in the population. The prevalence of disease in a population is the number of people who are infected divided by the number of people in the population. The numerator is those who are ill, those who have specific symptoms of the illness, or those who have microbiologic evidence of infection but do not exhibit symptoms. Each of these definitions yields different information, and each is a valid measure of the prevalence. However, it is critical that the definition of what constitutes infection be defined. The denominator in the prevalence equation is also defined by the epidemiologist. It may be the number of persons in the population, regardless of known exposure status, or it may be persons who were exposed. In the former case, the measurement of prevalence defines the burden of disease in the population overall; in the latter case, the definition gives the prevalence of disease among those exposed. Where exposure is common, age-specific population prevalence is commonly measured. Where exposure is rare, prevalence rates by exposure group are more frequently used.

The other commonly used measure is the incidence of disease. The incidence is the rate at which persons acquire the disease or the rate at which the infectious agent is being transmitted throughout the population. The incidence of disease always includes a unit of time—the number of cases of influenza in a given year, month, or week, for example.

The incidence and prevalence of disease are related to each other by the duration of disease. In cases where the duration of disease is short, the prevalence of disease will be approximately equal to the incidence of disease because most infections will be relatively recent. If, in contrast, the duration of the disease is long, the prevalence of disease will include both new and former cases of disease and will be larger than the incidence of disease. This relationship can be described by the equation:

$$Prevalence = Incidence \times Duration$$

At times, the incidence may be decreasing at the same time that prevalence is rising. Such may be the case with HIV infections in the United States and Western Europe at present, because combined antiretroviral therapy has prolonged survival and thereby increased the prevalence, but because of the effect of the drugs in reducing viral load, the transmission, or incidence of new cases, may be decreasing.

In other infectious diseases that have short duration but infected persons remain susceptible to reinfection, the incidence may exceed the point prevalence. Persons may have several episodes of diarrheal disease or rhinovirus respiratory infections per year that last only a few days. In these diseases, the point prevalence may be low but the annual incidence may be quite high. It may be preferable to measure the impact of these diseases with annual incidence rates. In contrast, in malaria hyperendemic areas, young children may receive hundreds of bites from infected mosquitoes every year. In this situation, the annual incidence of malaria is so high that it is difficult to measure. However, a blood film will allow determination of the point prevalence of infection, because the parasites persist in the blood for some time. Malaria prevalence data are more useful to differentiate populations at very high risk or of hyperendemic foci in an endemic area. These issues are discussed further in the chapters on malaria, diarrheal infections, and respiratory infections.

Surveillance of Infectious Diseases

Surveillance of infectious diseases is essential to understand their epidemiology. *Surveillance* can be defined as the ongoing and systematic collection, collation, and analysis of data, and the dissemination of the results to those who need to know to avoid or prevent infections or epidemics.

In the United States, surveillance of infectious diseases is done by physicians and other health care workers, laboratories, clinics, and public health departments. Cases or outbreaks of selected infectious diseases are reported to the local health department by health care providers, laboratories, or hospitals. These reports are analyzed and forwarded to each state's health department, which reports the data to the CDC in Atlanta. Additional details of infectious disease surveillance are covered in Chapter 4.

Temporal Trends of Infectious Diseases

Many infectious diseases undergo temporal variation in incidence. This temporal variability is sometimes easy to explain by changes in the exposure to the agent over time, such as in different seasons of the year or in different years.

Seasonal Variation

Vector-transmitted diseases, such as malaria, dengue, or St. Louis encephalitis (SLE), depend on exposure to infected mosquito vectors for their transmission. Therefore, these diseases are present only during the warm months of the year in temperate climates when the appropriate mosquito vectors are present. The seasonal distribution of SLE virus infections of the central nervous system in the United States that were reported to the CDC between 1988 and 1997 is shown in Figure 2-3. The marked and consistent seasonality of SLE is readily apparent and easily understood, because the transmission depends on bites of susceptible humans by infected *Culex pipiens* or other related mosquitoes. These mosquitoes breed only in the summer in temperate climates and must reach a certain density and level of infection with SLE virus before human infections occur.

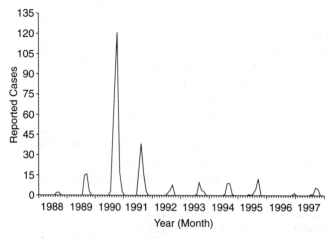

FIGURE 2-3 Arboviral infections (of the central nervous system)—reported laboratory-confirmed cases caused by St. Louis encephalitis virus, by month of onset, United States, 1988–1997. Reprinted from *MMWR*, Summary of Notifiable Disease, 1997, Centers for Disease Control and Prevention.

A description of the epidemiologic cycle of SLE in nature is shown in Figure 2-4.

The important reservoir hosts for SLE are infected birds, both wild and domestic, that carry the virus without illness and develop high-level, persistent viremia with SLE virus after infection. These birds serve as the reservoir to infect mosquitoes. Because humans and other animals that may be bitten by SLE-infected mosquitoes have low levels of virus in the blood that is very transient, they are not effective as reservoir hosts to infect additional mosquitoes and maintain the epidemic. For this reason, they are termed *dead-end hosts*. In other mosquito-borne arboviral infections, such as Eastern equine encephalitis, Western equine encephalitis, or Venezuelan encephalitis, horses may commonly be infected when bitten by infected mosquitoes and develop

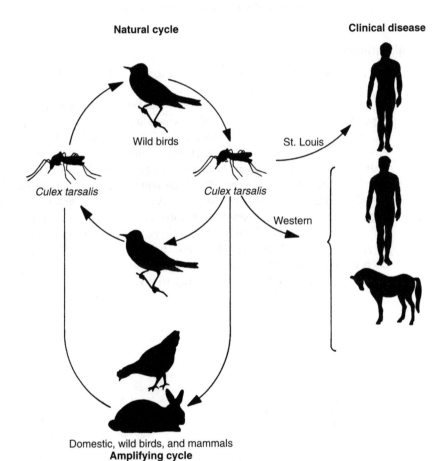

FIGURE 2-4   The sylvatic cycles of Western and St. Louis encephalitis viruses. The natural inapparent cycle is between *Culex tarsalis* and nestling and juvenile birds, but this cycle may be amplified by infection of domestic birds and wild and domestic mammals. Western encephalitis virus can replicate in mosquitoes at cooler temperatures, so epidemic disease in horses and humans may occur earlier in the summer and farther north into Canada. St. Louis encephalitis virus in the eastern United States involves *Culex pipiens* and other urban mosquitoes and causes urban epidemics. Reprinted with permission from R.T. Johnson, *Viral Infections of the Nervous System,* © 1998. Lippincott Williams & Wilkins.

symptomatic, even fatal, illness after infection. The rate of inapparent infections in humans may be 1000 to 1 or higher; whereas, a much higher proportion of infected horses is symptomatic. Therefore, severe or fatal encephalitis in horses may serve as a harbinger that a subsequent human epidemic may follow. Substantial variations in the number of reported SLE infections by year are seen in the CDC data. Beyond the seasonal pattern, the year-to-year variation in the number of cases is not readily predictable. These mosquito-borne viral infections vary in relation to the number of mosquitoes, which may vary in density due to rainfall and temperature patterns; the number of reservoir hosts (especially wild birds) that are infected; and contact patterns between mosquitoes and birds and between infected mosquitoes and susceptible humans. Because of the interaction of these variables, it is difficult to predict from one year to the next whether an epidemic will occur. The important arthropod-borne virus infections of humans are discussed further in the chapter on emerging vector-borne infections.

Annual Variation

Prior to the development of effective vaccines for the prevention of many of the common childhood infections (measles, mumps, rubella, and varicella), these infections exhibited marked and repetitive cyclical trends, which depended largely on an epidemic exhausting the susceptible population and another birth cohort replenishing it. For measles, the cycle for a major epidemic in an urban population in the United States repeated every other year, at which time, the number of cases roughly doubled, compared with the preceding and following years. With the widespread routine use of effective measles vaccine, the rates of measles have decreased dramatically, and the cyclical occurrence of cases has changed. However, cycles at 3- to 4-year intervals have persisted for reported cases of pertussis between 1967 and 1997 (Figure 2-5). This cyclical pattern indicates that persistent transmission of pertussis related to contact between an infected case and a susceptible host still occurs, despite the availability of a vaccine that has been used quite

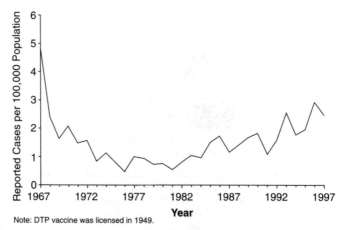

Note: DTP vaccine was licensed in 1949.

FIGURE 2-5   Pertussis (whooping cough) by year, United States, 1967–1997. Reprinted from *MMWR*, Summary of Notifiable Disease, 1997, Centers for Disease Control and Prevention.

widely. In part, this persistence may relate to waning of the immunity induced by the whole-cell pertussis vaccine over time, the role of older children and adults in maintaining the transmission cycle of pertussis, and the periodic replenishment of the susceptible population. Most of the childhood infections are more common in the winter and early spring seasons. This seasonality has been postulated to be related to greater transmissability when populations spend more time indoors during the winter. Also, the low humidity of indoor air and the presence of other respiratory infections, which cause coughing and sneezing, may be critical factors in promoting the transmission during the winter.

Herd Immunity

Prior to the epidemiologic theories proposed by Kermack and McKendrick and by Reed and Frost from Johns Hopkins, the predominant theory was that epidemics occurred due to variation in the infectivity of the organism. Instead, these investigations showed that patterns of epidemics could be explained by the proportion and distribution of susceptible persons. In certain diseases that are spread from person to person, the level of immunity of the population may be critical in determining whether an epidemic will occur and, therefore, the risk of infection for a susceptible individual in the population. Because transmission is based on contact between an infected person and a susceptible person, if the number of immune persons is high enough that it is unlikely that a susceptible will have contact with an infected person, the population is said to have *herd immunity*. Even though some susceptible persons remain in the population, epidemics are not sustained because the day-to-day contacts between persons do not result in contact between infected persons during the period that they are contagious and others who are still susceptible. The level of immunity required to attain herd immunity is dependent on the characteristics of the infectious disease. Those that are spread more readily will require a higher level of immunity in the population than will those that are less infectious. The levels of herd immunity and individual susceptibility to infections are major epidemiologic factors that have influenced the periodicity and secular trends observed in many diseases, such as measles, rubella, varicella, and polio. A new epidemic of measles, prior to the era of widespread immunization, was dependent on the existence of a large cohort of susceptible individuals. A large enough pool of susceptibles to sustain an epidemic occurred every other year as new children were born. After an effective measles vaccine became available, epidemics were less common, less predictable, and often involved older individuals. Epidemics occurred even in immunized populations when clusters of susceptibles were exposed to an infectious case, such as on college campuses. The theoretical modeling of epidemics is covered more thoroughly in the chapter on modeling.

Variations of Infectious Diseases Over Decades

Tuberculosis

Many classic infectious diseases, such as tuberculosis, have decreased in incidence and mortality in the United States and Europe during the past century.

Tuberculosis is still one of the most important infectious diseases globally. However, in the United States, the mortality rates from tuberculosis began to decline in the late 1800s. Between 1950 and 1985, tuberculosis morbidity declined at a rate of about 5% per year. Tuberculosis mortality by age in the United States is highest in older age groups.[49] However, the age-specific tuberculosis mortality data were studied in another way by Wade Hampton Frost. He examined the risk of tuberculosis death by birth cohort, rather than as cross-sectional age-specific mortality.[50] When the data are studied in this way (as the risk of mortality from tuberculosis in a cohort of persons born in the same year), different conclusions are reached about the age-specific risk of mortality. In Figure 2-6, the mortality rates are depicted as age-specific mortality by birth cohort. The cohort analysis shows tuberculosis mortality. The reason for the higher mortality among older persons is that they were born at a time when the risk of tuberculosis was higher than it is at present. Their higher mortality reflects their elevated risk of infection due to subsequent activation of an infection that originally occurred when the incidence of tuberculosis was higher than more recent cohorts.[50,51]

Changes in Infectious Disease Morbidity and Mortality During the 1800s and 1900s

During the 1700s, 1800s, and early 1900s, infectious diseases were the major cause of morbidity and mortality. Reliable mortality data are available from the United Kingdom from the 1800s because early leaders, such as John Graunt and William Farr, recognized the importance of surveillance data to evaluate improvements in public health and promoted routine reporting of infectious disease mortality. The mortality rates from whooping cough, enteric fevers, and tuberculosis decreased over 100-fold between 1900 and 1960 in persons living in the United Kingdom. The mortality rates from these diseases decreased in the United States and other developed countries in Europe in a parallel fashion to those reported from the United Kingdom. In 1900, the death ratio from 10 of the most common infectious diseases varied from 202.2 per 100,000 population for influenza and pneumonia to 6.8 per 100,000 population for meningococcal infections. By 1970, only influenza and pneumonia infections were associated with mortality rates above 3 per 100,000 (Table 2-10).

A recent analysis of the trends in infectious disease mortality in the United States during the 1900s documented the effect of the control of infectious diseases. The overall mortality from infectious diseases, which was 797 deaths per 100,000 in 1900, declined to 36 deaths per 100,000 in 1980.[52] However, the decline in mortality was reversed between 1980 and 1995, when the death rate increased to 63 deaths per 100,000 persons.[53] The trend of a steady decline was interrupted by a sharp spike of increased mortality during the 1918 influenza epidemic. Between 1938 and 1952, the decline was particularly rapid, with mortality decreasing by 8.2% per year. Pneumonia and influenza were responsible for the largest number of infectious disease deaths throughout the century. Tuberculosis caused a large number of deaths early in the century, but tuberculosis mortality declined sharply after 1945. Although the crude mortality rate for infectious diseases was dramatically reduced during the first eight decades of the 1900s, the mortality from all noninfectious diseases has not shown a similar change (Figure 2-7). In fact,

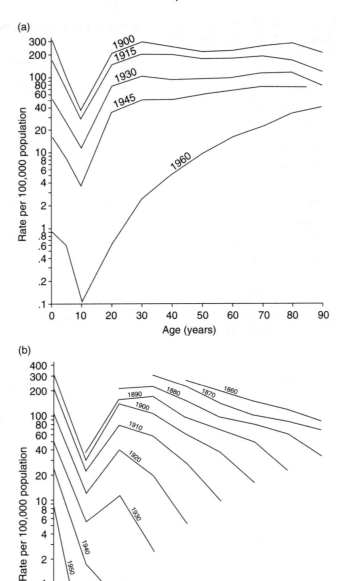

FIGURE 2-6a & b (a) Death rates from tuberculosis by age group for selected years; (b) Cohort analysis of death rates from tuberculosis by age group, 1860–1960. The line associated with each year indicates death rates by age group for persons born in that year. Reprinted with permission from T.G. Doege, Tuberculosis Mortality in the United States, 1900 to 1960, *JAMA*, Vol. 192, pp. 1045–1048, © 1965, American Medical Association.

TABLE 2-10   Death Rates for Common Infectious Diseases in the United States in 1900, 1935, and 1970

Infectious Disease	Mortality Rate per 100,000 Population		
	1900	1935	1970
Influenza and pneumonia	202.2	103.9	30.9
Tuberculosis	194.4	55.1	2.6
Gastroenteritis	142.7	14.1	1.3
Diphtheria	40.3	3.1	0.0
Typhoid fever	31.3	2.7	0.0
Measles	13.3	3.1	0.0
Dysentery	12.0	1.9	0.0
Whooping cough	12.0	3.7	0.0
Scarlet fever (including streptococcal sore throat)	9.6	2.1	0.0
Meningococcal infections	6.8	2.1	0.3

Source: Reprinted from National Office of Vital Statistics, USPHS and Centers for Disease Control and Prevention.

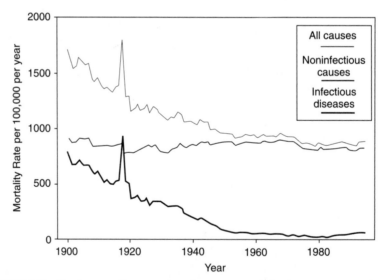

FIGURE 2-7   Crude mortality rates for all causes, noninfectious causes, and infectious diseases. Reprinted from G.L. Armstrong, L.A. Conn, and R.W. Pinner, Trends in Infectious Disease Mortality in the United States during the 20th Century, *JAMA*, Vol. 281, pp. 61–66, 1999.

most of the decline in mortality during the 1900s can be attributed to the dramatic reduction in infectious disease mortality. In the last two decades of the 1900s, the mortality from coronary heart disease has declined substantially; however, this has been offset by increasing mortality for lung cancer and other diseases. Clearly, the decline in mortality from infectious diseases during the 1900s stands as a tribute to the advances in public health and safer lifestyles, compared with that in previous centuries.

What caused these remarkable reductions in the mortality from common infectious diseases? One might surmise that the development of modern microbiology with the understanding the discipline provided about the pathogenesis of specific infections led to the development of vaccines and effective antibiotics to prevent or treat infections. However, for most of these infections, the evidence suggests a more complex scenario. The decline in the annual death rates for tuberculosis in England and Wales antedated the identification of the tuberculosis bacillus; however, the slope of the declining mortality increased after 1948, with the availability of streptomycin, isoniazide, and other chemotherapeutic agents (Figure 2-8).

Similarly, death rates from scarlet fever, diphtheria, and whooping cough (pertussis) in children under age 15 in England and Wales began to decline well before these organisms were identified in the laboratory, and the availability of effective antibiotics had a small effect on the overall mortality decline (Figure 2-9).[54]

Also, dramatic declines in the death rates from measles and pertussis were seen among children in England and Wales decades prior to the identification of these organisms and the availability of vaccines or antibiotics to treat infected persons. What, then, can account for these declines in mortality? Recent experience with some of these diseases in poor and often malnourished children from developing countries in Africa has shown that some of these diseases still have high mortality in certain populations. For example, measles, which is rarely fatal when it occurs in children in the United States, is still associated with a 15–20% mortality in infants and children in sub-Saharan Africa. Hypotheses to explain this difference have included poorer nutritional status, earlier ages at exposure, other concomitant infections, higher infectious dose, and greater crowding during epidemic spread among infants in Africa.[55,56] All of these factors may play a role, but it is difficult to

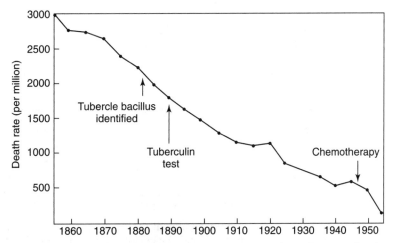

FIGURE 2-8 Mean annual death rate from respiratory tuberculosis, England and Wales. E. Kass, Infectious Diseases and Social Change, *Journal of Infectious Diseases*, Vol. 23, No. 1, p. 111, © 1971, University of Chicago Press.

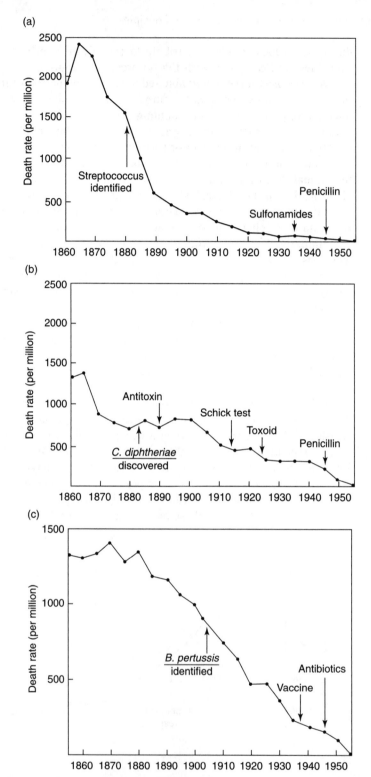

FIGURE 2-9 a, b, & c. (a) Mean annual death rate from scarlet fever in children under 15 years of age, England and Wales; (b) Mean annual death rate from diphtheria in children under 15 years of age, England and Wales; and (c) Mean annual death rate from whooping cough in children under 15 years of age, England and Wales.

Source: E. Kass, Infectious Diseases and Social Change, *Journal of Infectious Diseases*, Vol. 23, No. 1, p. 111, © 1971, University of Chicago Press.

evaluate their independent contribution. Clearly, the complex changes that have occurred in society, hygiene, and lifestyle in the United States and in Europe during the late 1800s and early 1900s have had a profound effect on these diseases.

Recent Trends in Infectious Disease Morbidity and Mortality in the United States

Although the mortality from the classical infectious diseases declined dramatically in the late 1800s and the first 80 years of the 1900s, several cultural and environmental changes occurred that fostered the emergence of a number of new infections and the reemergence of older, well-recognized infections. Indeed, it has been estimated that a larger number of new infections have emerged in the last decade or so than in the hundred years previously.

The most heralded, of course, is the HIV/AIDS epidemic, which probably originated as a mutant or recombinant primate retrovirus that was spread to humans from chimpanzees in Africa in the 1950s or 1960s. The ensuing pandemic of AIDS has led to the emergence of many new and previously recognized but rare human pathogens, such as *P. carinii*, *Mycobacteria avium*, *Cryptosporidia parvum*, *Microsporidia*, *Bartonella rochelimea*, and *Penicillium marneffei*. The epidemic of AIDS is covered in more detail in the chapter on AIDS. In addition to HIV and AIDS, modern chemotherapy of neoplasms, aging of the population, increased invasive therapeutic procedures in hospitalized patients, crowding of elderly patients in nursing homes and infants and children in day care centers, widespread use of broad spectrum antibiotics, environmental pollution, and other factors have led to the emergence of infectious diseases. These issues are covered in detail in Chapter 12.

An analysis was done by investigators for the CDC of all deaths in the United States between 1980 and 1992.[53] In this interval, the death rate due to infectious diseases as the underlying cause of death increased 58%, from 41 to 65 deaths per 100,000 population in the United States. Age-adjusted mortality from infectious diseases increased 39% during the same period. Infectious disease mortality increased 25% among those aged 65 years or older, from 271 to 338 per 100,000 population, and 5.5 times among 25- to 44-year-olds, from 6.9 to 38 deaths per 100,000 population. Mortality due to respiratory tract infections increased 20%, the death rate from septicemia increased 83%, and AIDS emerged as a major cause of death. These national data are quite sobering because they clearly demonstrate that an increased infectious disease mortality has occurred recently in the US population, which is not limited to newly emerging diseases, such as AIDS. The 10 leading underlying causes of mortality caused by infectious diseases in the United States in 1980 and 1992 are listed in Table 2-11.

Recent Worldwide Trends in Infectious Disease Morbidity and Mortality

Infectious diseases play a leading role in mortality and morbidity globally, due in large part to the continued importance of infectious diseases in

TABLE 2-11 Leading Underlying Causes of Mortality Caused by Infectious Diseases in the United States, 1980 and 1992

Rank	1980 Infectious Disease Group	No. of Deaths	Mortality per 100,000	1992 Infectious Disease Group	No. of Deaths	Mortality per 100,000
1	Respiratory tract infections	56,966	25.1	Respiratory tract infections	77,336	30.3
2	Septicemia	9,438	4.2	HIV/AIDS	33,581	13.2
3	Infections of kidney/urinary tract	8,006	3.5	Septicemia	19,667	7.7
4	Infections of the heart	2,486	1.1	Infections of kidney/urinary tract	12,399	4.9
5	Tuberculosis	2,333	1.0	Infections of the heart	3,950	1.5
6	Bacterial meningitis	1,402	0.6	Hepatobiliary disease	2,494	1.0
7	Gastrointestinal tract infections	1,377	0.6	Mycoses	2,298	0.9
8	Hepatobiliary disease	1,227	0.5	Tuberculosis	1,851	0.7
9	Perinatal infections	1,035	0.5	Gastrointestinal tract infections	985	0.4
10	Mycoses	680	0.3	Perinatal infections	965	0.4
Total infectious diseases		93,407	41.1		166,047	65.1
All deaths		1,989,841	878.0		2,175,613	852.7

Source: Reprinted with permission from Pinner RW et al., Trends in infectious diseases mortality in the United States, JAMA, Vol. 275, No. 3, pp. 189–193, Copyright 1996, The American Medical Association.

sub-Saharan Africa, Asia, and Latin America. Data were published recently from the Global Burden of Disease Study, which was initiated in 1992 in collaboration with the World Bank and the WHO. The goals of this study were to make reasonable estimates from the available data of the impact of various diseases as causes of disability, to develop unbiased assessments for major disorders, and to quantify the burden of disease with a measure that could be used for cost-effectiveness analysis. This study found that 98% of all deaths in children younger than 15 years of age are in the developing world, and 50% of deaths between ages 15 and 59 years of age were in the developing world.[57] The probability of death between birth and 15 years of age ranges from 22% in sub-Saharan Africa to 1.1% in the established market economics. Probabilities of death between 15 and 50 years of age range from 7.2% for women in established market economies to 39.1% in sub-Saharan Africa. Worldwide in 1990, communicable, maternal, perinatal, and nutritional disorders accounted for 17.2 million deaths, noncommunicable diseases for 28.1 million deaths, and injuries for 5.1 million deaths. The leading causes of death in 1990 were ischemic heart disease (6.3 million deaths), cerebrovascular accidents (4.4 million deaths), lower respiratory infections (4.3 million deaths), diarrheal diseases (2.9 million), perinatal disorders (2.4 million), chronic obstructive pulmonary disease (2.2 million), tuberculosis (2.0 million), measles (1.1 million), road traffic accidents (1.0 million), and lung cancer (0.9 million).

This WHO–World Bank study also concluded that effective treatment of tuberculosis is the most cost-effective health measure that could be implemented in developing countries in terms of prevention of mortality and increasing disability-adjusted life years (DALY).[58] The analysis of tuberculosis programs in Malawi, Mozambique, and Tanzania has shown that treating smear-positive tuberculosis costs $20–52 per death averted. The cost per discounted year of life saved, therefore, is $1–3. There are few other interventions that are as cost-effective as is tuberculosis case treatment. This WHO analysis estimated that $150 million would be needed to treat 65% of smear-positive cases in low-income countries and 85% of middle-income countries with short-course chemotherapy. Clearly, the interaction between HIV and tuberculosis has made the tuberculosis problem more acute and intractable. The rapid and extensive spread of AIDS in countries in the developing world, where a high proportion of the population has latent tuberculosis, indicates that a public health strategy that is limited to treating active cases is unlikely to control the emerging tuberculosis epidemic effectively. However, recent research has shown that active tuberculosis generally is treatable with current chemotherapeutic regimens, even in the face of HIV infection. This issue is reviewed in greater detail in the chapter on tuberculosis.

Other health interventions are cost-effective for the prevention of infectious disease morbidity and mortality, including effective sexually transmitted disease (STD) treatment; oral rehydration therapy for diarrhea; immunization for childhood diseases, including HBV; ivermectin for the treatment and prevention of onchocerchiasis and schistosomiasis; and zidovudine for the prevention of the perinatal transmission of HIV. The chemotherapy and chemoprophylaxis of malaria and antibiotic prophylaxis for the prevention of postsurgical infections are also cost-effective; these issues are reviewed in the chapters on malaria and nosocomial infections.

Currently, the world's population is in a very delicate balance with respect to infectious diseases. The continual emergence of new infectious diseases and the reemergence of old infections, together with the potential for their global spread, underline the need for accurate surveillance and the development of newer strategies for their control and prevention. However, the successes of the last century should provide hope that infectious diseases can be controlled with the proper understanding and effort.

References

1. Snow J. *On Cholera.* New York, NY: Commonwealth Fund; 1996.
2. Fraser DW, Tsai TR, Orenstein W, et al. Legionnaire's disease. Description of an epidemic of pneumonia. *N Engl J Med.* 1977;297:1189–1197.
3. Dondero TJ, Rentdorff RL, Mallison GF, et al. An outbreak of Legionnaire's disease associated with a contaminated air-conditioning cooling tower. *N Engl J Med.* 1980;302:365–370.
4. Cords LG, Fraser DW, Skailly P, et al. Legionnaire's disease outbreak at an Atlanta, Georgia, country club: evidence for spread from an evaporative condenser. *Am J Epidemiol.* 1980;111:425–431.
5. Garbe PL, Davis BJ, Weisfeld JS, et al. Nosocomial Legionnaire's disease: epidemiologic demonstration of cooling towers as a source. *JAMA.* 1985;254:521–524.
6. Morris GK, Patton CM, Feeley JC, et al. Isolation of the Legionnaire's disease bacterium from environmental samples. *Ann Intern Med.* 1979;90:664–666.
7. Moraca E, Yu VC, Goetz A. Disinfection of water distribution system for Legionnella: a review of applicator procedures and methodologies. *Infect Control Hosp Epidemiol.* 1990;11:79–88.
8. Francis E. Deer-fly fever: a disease of man of hitherto unknown etiology. *Public Health Rep.* 1991;34:2061–2062.
9. Waring WB, Ruffin JJ. A tick-borne epidemic of tularemia. *N Engl J Med.* 1946;234:137.
10. Young LS, Bickewell DS, Archer BG, et al. Tularemia epidemic: Vermont 1968: forty-seven cases linked to contact with muskrats. *N Engl J Med.* 1969;280:1253–1260.
11. Teutsch SM, Martone WJ, Brink EW, et al. Pneumonic tularemia on Martha's Vineyard. *N Engl J Med.* 1979;301:826–828.
12. Dahlstrand S, Ringertz O, Zetterberg B. Airborne tularemia in Sweden. *J Infect Dis.* 1971;3:7–16.
13. Barbeito MS, Alg RL, Wedum AG. Infectious bacterial aerosol from dropped Petri disk cultures. *Am J Med Technol.* 1961;27:318–322.
14. Hornick RB. Tularemia. In: Evans A, Brachman PS, eds. *Bacterial Infections of Humans: Epidemiology and Control.* 3rd ed. New York, NY: Plenum Publishing; 1998:823–837.
15. Hirst CF. *The Conquest of Plague.* London, England: Oxford University Press; 1953.
16. Zinsser H. *Rats, Lice and History.* Boston, Mass: Little, Brown; 1934.
17. Marshall JD Jr, Joy RJT, Ai NY, et al. Plague in Vietnam 1965–1966. *Am J Epidemiol.* 1967;86:603–616.
18. Campbell GL, Hughes JM. Plague in India: a new warning from an old nemesis. *Am Int Med.* 1995;122:151–153.

19. Eskey CR, Haas V. Plague in the western part of the United States. *Public Health Bull.* 1940;254:1–82.
20. Mann JM, Martone WJ, Myoce JM, et al. Endemic human plague in New Mexico: risk factors associated with infections. *J Infect Dis.* 1979;140:397–401.
21. Butler T. *Plague and Other Yersinia Infections.* New York, NY: Plenum Publishing; 1983.
22. Laforce FM. Woolsorter's disease. *Acad Med.* 1978;54:956–963.
23. Meselson M, Guillemin J, Hugh-Jones M, et al. The Sverdlousk anthrax outbreak of 1979. *Science.* 1994;266:1202–1208.
24. Constantine DG. Rabies transmission by non-bite route. *Public Health Rep.* 1963;77:287–289.
25. Winkler WG, Fashinell TR, Leffingwell C, Howard P, Conomy JP. Airborne rabies transmission in a laboratory worker. *JAMA.* 1973;226: 1219–1221.
26. Hooff SA, Burton RC, Wilson RW, et al. Human-to-human transmission of rabies by a corneal transplant. *N Engl J Med.* 1979;300:603–604.
27. Noah DC, Drenzik CL, Smith JS, et al. Epidemiology of human rabies in the United States, 1980 to 1996. *Ann Intern Med.* 1998;128:922–930.
28. Brown GM. The history of the brucellosis eradication program in the United States. *Ann Selavo.* 1977;19:20–34.
29. Grant IH, Gold JW, Witner M, et al. Transfusion-associated Chagas' disease acquired in the United States. *Ann Intern Med.* 1989;111:849–851.
30. Gregg NM. Congenital cataract following German measles in the mother. *Trans Ophthalmol Soc.* 1941;3:35–46.
31. Weller TH, Neva FA. Propagation in tissue culture of cytopathic agents from patients with rubella-like illness. *Proc Soc Exp Biol Med.* 1962;11:215–225.
32. Parkman PD, Bueschler EL, Artenstein MS. Recovery of rubella virus from army recruits. *Proc Soc Exp Biol Med.* 1962;111:225–230.
33. Krugman S, ed. Rubella symposium. *Am J Dis Child.* 1965;110:345–476.
34. Krugman S, ed. International conference on rubella immunization. *Am J Dis Child.* 1969;118:2–410.
35. Smith MG. Propagation in tissue culture of a cytopathic virus from human salivary gland virus (SGV) disease. *Proc Soc Exp Biol Med.* 1956;92:424–430.
36. Rowe WP, Hartley JW, Waterman S, Turnan HC, Huebner RJ. Cytopathic agent resembling human salivary gland virus recovered from tissue culture of human adenoids. *Proc Soc Exp Biol Med.* 1956;92:418–424.
37. Weller TH, MaCaulay JC, Craig JM, Wirth P. Isolation of intranuclear inclusion producing agents from infants with illness resembling cytomegalic inclusion disease. *Pro Soc Exp Biol Med.* 1957;94:4–12.
38. Gershon AH, Gold E, Nankervis GA. Cytomegalovirus. In: Evans AS, Kaslow RA, eds. *Viral Infections of Humans, Epidemiology and Control.* New York, NY: Plenum Publishing; 1997:229–251.
39. Dobbins JG, Stewart JAS. Surveillance of congenital cytomegalovirus disease 1990–1991. *MMWR.* 1992;41:SS-2.
40. Stone KM, Brooks CA, Guinan ME, Alexander ER. National surveillance for neonatal herpes virus infections. *Sex Transm Dis.* 1989;16:152–156.
41. Mcllinger AK, Goldberg M, Wade A, et al. Alternative case-finding in a crack-related syphilis epidemic–Philadelphia. *MMWR.* 1991;40:77–80.

42. Sartwell PE. The distribution of incubation of disease. *Am J Epidemiol.* 1950;51:310–318.
43. Muñoz A, Kirby AJ, He DY, et al. Long-term survivors with HIV-1 longitudinal patterns of CD4⁺ lymphocytes. *J Acquir Immunodeficiency Syndr.* 1995;8:496–505.
44. Watts DM, Burke DS, Harrison BA, et al. Effect of temperature on the vector efficiency of *Aedes aegypti* for dengue 2 virus. *Am J Trop Med Hyg.* 1987;36:143–152.
45. Soper GA. The curious case of typhoid Mary. *Acad Med.* 1939;15:698–712.
46. Anders W, Conde F, Stephen W. Surgical treatment of the chronic typhoid carrier: report of 102 operated cases. *Dtsch Med Wochenschr.* 1955;89:1637–1648.
47. Shilts R. *And the Band Played On.* New York, NY: St. Mortons Press; 1987.
48. Peterson BH, Lee TJ, Snyderman R, Brooks GF. *Neisseria meningitidis* and *Neisseria gonorrhoeae* bacteremia associated with C6, C7, C8 deficiency. *Ann Intern Med.* 1979;90:917–920.
49. Rieder HL, Cauthen GM, Kelly GD, et al. Tuberculosis in the United States. *JAMA.* 1989;262:385–389.
50. Frost WH. The age selection of mortality from tuberculosis in successive decades. *Am J Hyg.* 1939 (Section A);30:91–96.
51. Doege TG. Tuberculosis mortality in the United States, 1900 to 1960. *JAMA.* 1965;192:1045–1048.
52. Armstrong GL, Conn LA, Pinner RW. Trends in infectious disease mortality in the United States during the 20th century. *JAMA.* 1999;281:61–66.
53. Pinner RW, Teutsch SM, Simonsen L, et al. Trends in infectious diseases mortality in the United States. *JAMA.* 1996;225:189–193.
54. Kass EM. Infectious disease and social change. *J Infect Dis.* 1971;123:110–114.
55. Aaby P, Bakh J, Lisse IM, Snits AJ. Measles mortality, state of nutrition, and family structure: a community study on Guinea-Bissau. *J Infect Dis.* 1983;147:693–701.
56. Aaby P. Malnutrition and overcrowding-exposure in severe measles infection: a review of community studies. *Rev Infect Dis.* 1988;10:478–491.
57. Murray CJ, Lopez AD. Alternative projections of mortality and disability by course, 1990–2020: global burden of disease study. *Lancet.* 1997;349:1498–1504.
58. Murray CJ, Lopez AD. Mortality by cause for eight regions of the world: global burden of disease study. *Lancet.* 1997;349:1269–1276.

CHAPTER THREE

STUDY DESIGN

Carolyn F. Masters Williams and Kenrad E. Nelson

Introduction

Epidemiology is based on two fundamental tenets. The first is the observation that human disease does not occur at random. The second is that there are causal, and possibly preventable, factors that influence the development of disease. Epidemiologic studies of infectious diseases try to evaluate the contribution of different factors in the transmission and acquisition of infections and those factors favoring endemic transmission and epidemics. Epidemiologic studies can also be used to evaluate the effects of interventions, such as HIV protease inhibitors on AIDS mortality or the protective effect of bed nets in malaria prevention. How to structure the processes of observing, or study design, is a critical step. The study design must optimize the researcher's ability to evaluate and measure the relationship between risk factors and disease in the study population, which can then be applied to the population as a whole.

Epidemiologic studies of an infectious disease can be designed to explore landmarks along the entire temporal process during which an individual is at risk, acquires infection, develops an infectious disease, or succumbs to it. Several chronic infectious diseases, such as tuberculosis or AIDS, may have different risk factors that are important for acquiring infection and the development of disease. In addition to understanding disease among individuals, epidemiologists attempt to understand the burden of disease at a population level and the factors leading to epidemics. From these studies, measurements of the prevalence and incidence of disease and correlates and risk factors for infection are evaluated.

Goals of Epidemiologic Research

The epidemiologic triangle is used to describe the relationship between the host (i.e., the diseased person), the agent (i.e., the infecting virus, bacteria, parasite, or fungi), and the environment (i.e., the setting in which transmission occurs) (Figure 3-1). This conceptual framework is useful in modeling the transmission dynamics of an infectious disease. Human hosts differ in susceptibility to infections because of genetic, environmental, behavioral, and other characteristics. Infections differ in some respects from other diseases of humans in that genetic and phenotypic variability of both the agent and the host can affect the microorganism's ability to cause disease and its epidemiology. Humans have interacted with infectious agents throughout evolutionary history, and changes in both the host and the agent have resulted from this selective interaction. Major epidemic diseases, such as malaria, tuberculosis, smallpox, and plague, have led to selective genetic changes in human populations. The evolution of several mutations among Africans and Asians has resulted primarily from the selective pressure of hyperendemic malaria. Sickle hemoglobin, glucose-6-phosphate dehydrogenase deficiency, thalassemia, hemoglobin C, and hemoglobin E may be disadvantageous in homozygous individuals, but they have evolved in certain populations because they confer significant protection from malaria in heterozygous individuals.[1] In fact, it is possible to estimate the mortality rates from malaria that would have been necessary in previous generations to account for the current sickle cell hemoglobin gene frequency using the Hardy-Weinburg equation. On the agent side, escape mechanisms—techniques used by parasites to evade the host's immune system—may require a large portion of the parasite's genome but are effective enough that they are retained in the genome.

The environment also plays a significant role in infectious disease epidemiology. It is important to understand and characterize the environment in which transmission occurs and to be aware of environmental factors that facilitate the agent's survival or infectivity. It is straightforward to envision the role of environment for agents that have an extrinsic cycle, such as hookworm. For example, soil humidity, temperature, and other soil characteristics can influence the development of infectious *Ancylostoma duodenalae* larvae. However, the environment is also important in the transmission of airborne viruses, such as influenza and varicella, because it affects the length of time that the viral particles remain infectious as an aerosol. The winter

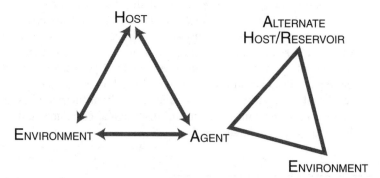

FIGURE 3-1   The epidemiologic triangle. For some diseases, the interaction may be described by the interaction between the host, environment, and agent. For other diseases, the interaction must include a second triangle to describe the extrinsic life cycle of the agent outside of the human host.

environment in temperate climates also facilitates transmission of influenza by bringing people indoors. However, influenza epidemics have been interrupted by extreme cold weather that has forced schools to close, thereby interrupting transmission among children and introduction of the virus into the home.[2]

Epidemiologic studies are used to evaluate these relationships and efforts to alter them to our advantage, be they preventive or therapeutic in nature. Several designs have been used, including ecologic and surveillance studies, cohort studies (parallel and pre- and postintervention designs), and traditional randomized clinical trials. Increasingly, meta-analysis, in which data from many studies is systematically combined to study a research question, is being used. In this chapter, we review several important and frequently used epidemiologic study designs and illustrate their use in evaluating infectious diseases.

Choosing a Study Design

The optimal study design for a research question is a function of the hypothesis under investigation and the information that is available at the time of analysis. Prior to initiating an epidemiologic study, it is useful to consider these questions:

- Who is to be studied (sampling)?
- What data are going to be collected (data collection)?
- How are these data going to be analyzed (analysis)?

These issues may influence the design of an epidemiologic study.

Sampling

The design of epidemiologic studies requires the successful translation of an idea to a hypothesis that can be tested by measurable observations in a relevant study population. It is rarely possible to study the entire population at risk for a disease. Therefore, an epidemiologic study must first define the study sample—those persons who will be included in the study. Epidemiologists must "sample" from the population to have a manageable study. The study sample must be at risk for the disease and representative of the populations to which the study results will be applied. Also, the sample size must be large enough to ensure sufficient statistical power to evaluate the study hypothesis. Finally, the researchers must take into account other considerations of the sampling protocol. Issues such as cost, quality of data, degree of cooperation that can be expected from a given population, and the accessibility of the population for enrollment and follow-up can influence sampling protocols. Practical issues, such as the reliability and validity of data obtained by questionnaire or other means, confidentiality of the data, and effects of the study process on data gathering, may influence the study results.

Data Collection

Infectious disease epidemiology shares many of the considerations common to epidemiologic studies of other diseases. Data collection must ensure meaningful, reliable data. Data collection itself may involve the use of employment or medical record review, personal interviews, medical exams, environmental measurements, and other relevant information. Interviews may be conducted in person, by phone, by mail, or by computer. The participant may complete the questionnaire or may be asked the questions by a trained interviewer. Each of these methods has its advantages and disadvantages in reliability, reduction in response bias, and expense.

To conduct an epidemiologic study of an infectious disease, it must be possible to measure the occurrence of infection or disease. Although this may seem obvious, in practice, the occurrence of disease may be difficult or costly to determine (Figure 3-2). The study design must take into account what methods are available to ascertain whether an infection is present or has occurred, as well as the methods' reliability and appropriateness in answering the research question. Depending on the study question, data may be collected as self-reports, abstracted from medical charts or laboratory reports, or the study may do the testing. Despite the expense, conducting testing within the study protocol can have a number of advantages, including standardized specimen collection and assay and the development of a specimen archive for future studies.

Analysis

Evaluation of the study results includes evaluation of the conduct of the study as well as the data. Was the study performed in the manner in which it was designed? Did any deviations from the design alter the quality of the results? Evaluation of the success of sampling procedures should be conducted. Who was ultimately studied? Also, the study should be evaluated with respect to any potential biases. Were biases introduced into the study by the manner

---

Many infectious diseases result in the formation of antibodies. Antibodies are generally long lasting and indicate that a person has been exposed to a disease. However, using antibodies as a marker of disease is more complicated than it first appears:

1. **When was the person exposed?** Antibodies to mumps are long lasting and could indicate infection in the distant past or a recent infection. Immunoglobulin type M (IgM) antibodies are the first to form, and high levels of these antibodies indicate that the infection is recent. IgG antibodies form later in the course of infection. Variation in the timing (but not the sequence) of the different antibody classes is seen among individuals and for different infections.
2. **Has immunity waned or never formed?** Antibodies are not long lasting for some infectious agents. Antibodies form several months after exposure to *B. burgdorferi* (the agent of Lyme disease) and may either wane or not form at all in persons who are treated early.
3. **Was the person exposed or vaccinated?** It may not be possible to differentiate those who are vaccinated from those who had disease. Vaccination against polio with the inactivated injection and oral inoculation will generate immunity that cannot be diffientiated from immunity from polo infection. th In contrast, the hepatitis B vaccine results in antibodies against only one viral protein (HBsAg). An infected individual will have antibodies to other viral proteins not included in the vaccine.
4. **Did the person have the disease or just infection?** Antibody formation can occur in those who suffered severe disease and in those with subclinical symptoms. The presence of antibodies only demonstrates infection, not disease status. Cholera has low rates of clinical disease, and the prevalence of antibodies to cholera are not a measure of the mortality and morbidity of a cholera epidemic.

FIGURE 3-2 Issues in determining the occurrence of an infectious disease.

in which it was conducted? Comparisons should be made between the actual study sample and the population targeted for study, the response rate of subgroups, and the composition of the population from which the sample was drawn. Data should be compared with studies of the research question in other populations by other investigators. Researchers may then determine whether the observed data are valid. Key questions that an epidemiologist should address are: How much of the measured effect may be explained by bias? Is there a dose-response effect? How do the results compare with other data available on this subject?

Specific study designs and the analysis of the data are reviewed here briefly, and examples of their application to infectious diseases are described below. The reader should consult other sources for a more detailed description. Recommended references include Rothman and Greenland[3] and Diggle, Liang, and Zeger.[4]

Types of Epidemiologic Study Design

Descriptive Studies

Epidemiologic studies of infectious diseases are designed for several purposes. When a new disease is recognized, the main purpose may be to describe the nature of the disease and to evaluate the probable means of transmission, reservoir, and natural history. Sometimes, a new disease is known to be caused by a specific organism, such as staphylococcal toxic shock syndrome; often, it is not, such as Hanta virus pulmonary syndrome, Legionnaires' disease, and AIDS. Early studies may consist of descriptions of cases or groups of cases that sometimes can be linked by a possible transmission route or exposure to a reservoir. These studies do not necessarily compare cases of an infectious disease with controls but only describe the disease and the exposures in the cases. At times, case reports or case series provide considerable understanding about the epidemiology of an infectious disease.

Case Reports

Case reports are a careful evaluation of a single case of disease in which the epidemiologist may describe the transmission, natural history, and/or treatment. Although case reports are based on an infection in a single patient, they may yield important new epidemiologic information regarding the disease. Examples of illustrative case reports follow.

Rabies

Rabies is a zoonotic viral infection that is spread to humans by contact with body fluids, most commonly, saliva, from an infected animal. Prior to rabies vaccination of domestic animals, most US transmissions were associated with domestic animal bites.[5] Rabies transmission was believed to require direct inoculation via a bite or other invasive contact with the infected animal. Infection is initially confined to the site of exposure without systemic viremia. Because of this, the rabies vaccine can be given after exposure to prevent infection of the central nervous system (CNS). Such postexposure prophylaxis is usually successful. However, if not given, rabies was believed to be universally fatal once the virus infected the CNS and signs and symptoms of CNS infection occurred. Two case reports of rabies overturned these long-held beliefs about the means of transmission of the virus and its natural history. Aerosol transmission of rabies was described in a cave explorer, a spelunker, who developed rabies after exploring a cave inhabited by large numbers of bats in Frio, Texas.[6] In this case, there was no history of a bite. This case was followed by a series of experiments in which animals were placed in the cave and protected from bites and even insect transmission but were exposed to the air in the infected cave. After several animals developed rabies during this exposure, the classic concepts of rabies transmission were challenged.[6] This was confirmed in additional laboratory studies which showed that rodents could be infected by aerosol inoculation.[7,8] The importance of this route of infection was confirmed by a review of case reports of rabies in the United States in the last 20 years; it was found that the majority of human cases were acquired after nonbite exposures to bats.[9] The control of rabies in domestic animals in the United States has resulted in fewer human cases, but a higher proportion of cases are due to wild animal nonbite exposures (Table 3-1). These exposures are not as readily recognized as rabies risks, and preventive vaccination may not be initiated (Figure 3-3).

The uniform fatality of rabies has also been challenged. In October 1970, a 6-year-old boy was bitten by a rabid bat. He was given 14 doses of duck embryo rabies vaccine but developed rabies 21 days later. He eventually recovered completely after treatment with intensive care for nearly 2 months.[10] A second report of survival from clinical rabies was reported in October 2004 in a previously healthy 15-year-old Wisconsin female who was bitten on the left finger by a bat while at church.[11,12] About 1 month later she complained of fatigue and tingling and numbness of her left hand.

TABLE 3-1 Sources of Human Exposure to Rabies in the United States

Year	Domestic Animal*	Wildlife	Other Sources[†]	Unknown[‡]	Total No. of Cases
		number of cases (percent)			
1946–1955	86 (72)	8 (7)	0	26 (22)	120
1956–1965	21 (55)	7 (18)	0	10 (26)	38
1966–1975	6 (38)	7 (44)	1 (6)	2 (12)	16
1976–1985	6 (30)	1 (5)	2 (10)	11 (55)	20
1986–1995	2 (12)	1 (6)	0	14 (82)	17
1996–2003	4 (19)	2 (10)	0	15 (71)	21

*After 1979, there were no cases involving documented exposure to a domestic animal known to be rabid or probably rabid. Thereafter, all cases originated in countries where canine rabies was endemic.
[†]Other sources of exposure include laboratory aerosol (in 1972 and 1977) and corneal transplantation (in 1978).
[‡]If a definitive source of exposure was not identified in the patient's history, the source of exposure was considered to be unknown, regardless of the source suspected on the basis of antigenic or genetic characterization.
Source: Rupprecht, C.E., Gibbons, RV Prophylaxis against Rabies *The New England Journal of Medicine*, Vol. 351; 25 pp. 2626–2635. Copyright 2004 Massachusetts Medical Society.

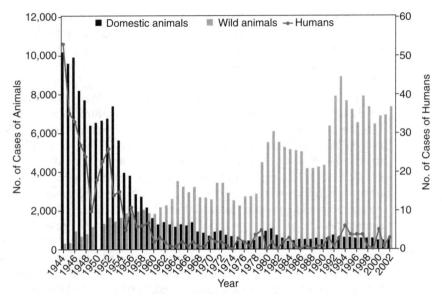

FIGURE 3-3   Temporal trends in the diagnosis of rabies in the Untied States, 1994 to 2002. Rupprecht, C.E., Gibbons, RV Prophylaxis against Rabies *The New England Journal of Medicine*, Vol. 351; 25 pp. 2626–2635. Copyright 2004 Massachusetts Medical Society.

Within 3 days she developed diplopia and subsequently slurred speech, blurred vision, and unsteady gait. On day 6 of her illness the diagnosis of rabies was considered when the history of a bat bite was obtained. She was transferred to a tertiary care hospital and treated aggressively with ketamine, midazolam, ribavirin, and amantadine. Ketamine is a dissociative anesthetic agent and a noncompetitive antagonist of the N-methyl-D-aspartate (NMDA) receptor. It had been shown in laboratory studies to inhibit rabies viral transcription.[13] The use of gamma-aminobutyric acid (GABA) receptor agonists with benzodiazepines and barbiturates was to reduce excitotoxicity, brain metabolism, and autonomic reactivity. Clinical reports of rabies cases had suggested that death resulted from the secondary complications of infections, primarily "neurotransmitter imbalance" and autonomic failure, rather than direct cytolysis from rabies virus. This was the first case of human rabies reported to have survived without the use of rabies vaccine or rabies immunoglobulin. However, at five months posttreatment she still had significant neurologic sequelae including choreoathetosis, dysarthria, and an unsteady gait. Although rabies still has the highest case fatality rate, this case and its successful treatment provides important insight into the pathophysiology of human rabies and offers promise for advances in its treatment.

Spontaneous Cure of HIV

HIV is unique among infectious diseases in that clearance of disease was not believed to ever occur. Bryceson and her colleagues from the University of California at Los Angeles reported a case of an infant who was born after 36 weeks' gestation to an asymptomatic HIV-positive woman.[14] She reported a history of sex with a former injection drug user. The pregnancy was uncomplicated, and the mother had a CD4+ T-cell count of over 1000 cells/mm³ at the time of delivery. The infant was normal at birth but required hospitalization for 8 days because of mild respiratory distress syndrome. Laboratory studies on the infant found a negative culture of cord blood for HIV. However, the infant's blood culture was positive at 19 and 51 days of age, and the PCR was positive at 33 days of life. Subsequently, HIV antibodies disappeared by 12 months of age. Multiple cultures of peripheral blood lymphocytes and plasma for HIV were negative between 3 months and 5 years of age. The child was asymptomatic and had no laboratory evidence of HIV infection at 5 years of age. The authors believed that the infant was infected but cleared the HIV infection by immunologic or other mechanisms. This case report was followed up by a search for similar cases of spontaneous resolution of perinatal HIV infection in infants by other investigators; however, no similar cases have been reported. In adults there have been extremely small numbers of persons who may have cleared an established HIV infection. Dr. Miles Cloyd has reported on several highly exposed patients who he believes to have been transiently infected. This work is being explored further, and it is not yet clear if these cases can be confirmed in other laboratories.[15]

Case reports have shed light on the immune response to HIV. Infection with one strain of HIV was believed to prevent infection with a subsequent strain. Natural infection is commonly the greatest stimulator of an immune response. Persons who are HIV positive have high antibody titers and often robust cellular immune responses. Superinfection in the face of this immunity was felt to be unlikely, particularly in persons who were not substantially immunologically impaired. Unfortunately, this was disproven by a case of superinfection reported in 2002.[16] A long-term nonprogressor, who had controlled his HIV infection without therapy for several years, became infected with a second strain of HIV. He was unable to control the second strain of HIV and had a rapid decline in his immune status. Subsequent to this case, several cases of superinfection have been documented, and it is now clear that HIV-positive persons are at risk for superinfection. However, whether they might have partial protection from superinfection is unclear. Nevertheless, HIV recombinant viruses are quite common, so superinfection or coinfection with two strains occurs more commonly than was appreciated.

Case Series

A second type of descriptive epidemiologic study is a case series. In this type of study, data from a cluster or series of cases are reported. No comparison is made with controls; instead, the exposures of the cases are often described. These case series may be reported in sufficient epidemiologic detail that it is possible to infer the means of transmission and the risk factors for infection. A case series of AIDS patients, which was reported early in the epidemic and prior to the identification of HIV, is described below.

AIDS Cluster

A cluster of homosexual men with Kaposi's sarcoma (KS) and/or *Pneumocystis carinii* pneumonia (PCP) was reported in 1984, prior to the identification of HIV.[17] The investigators enumerated the sexual contacts of the first 19 homosexual male AIDS patients reported from Southern California. One of the men had sexual contacts with 12 of the AIDS patients within 5 years of the onset of their symptoms. Four of the patients from Southern California had contact with a non-California AIDS patient, who was also the sex partner of four AIDS patients from New York City. Ultimately, 40 AIDS patients in 10 cities were linked by sexual contact in this extensive sexual network (Figure 3-4). This remarkable study led the investigators to conclude that AIDS was caused by a sexually transmitted agent. The sexual network linking these patients with the new disease was remarkably similar to the networks of patients with syphilis that were described four decades earlier. At the epicenter of this cluster was "patient 0," who estimated that he had had about 250 different male sexual partners each year from 1979 through 1981 and was able to name 72 of his 750 partners during this 3-year period; 8 of these partners had developed AIDS.

Ecologic Studies

Ecologic studies are another type of epidemiologic study. Ecologic studies measure the exposure and rates of disease at a population level, rather than at an individual level, which is to say, they compare the prevalence of risk

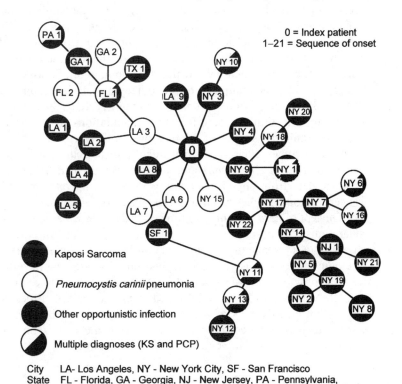

FIGURE 3-4 Sexual contacts among homosexual men with AIDS. Each circle represents an AIDS patient. Lines connecting the circles represent sexual exposures. Indicated city or state is place of residence of a patient at the time of diagnosis. "0" indicates Patient 0 (described in text). D. Auerbach et al., *American Journal of Medicine*, Cluster of Cases of the Acquired Immune Deficiency Sundrome, Patients Linked by Sexual Contact, Vol. 76, pp. 487–492, Copyright 1984. Excerpta Medica Inc.

or beneficial factor(s) and disease rates across different populations. In an ecologic study, whether an individual member of a population is exposed and has disease or whether there is an association between a risk factor and a disease at the individual level is unknown. Furthermore, it is not possible to assess whether there are confounding factors at the individual level in the relationship between the exposure and disease. Despite the inability to make conclusions at the individual level, because ecologic studies are based on the population level and not the individual level, individual factors that may confound an analysis of individual data can be ignored in an ecologic analysis. For example, commonly the most ill patients are the ones most likely to initiate therapy. This "selection by indication" can bias a measured treatment response as those who use therapy appear sicker than those who do not use therapies. The ecologic study avoids this bias by comparing populations with different access to treatment without regard to individual therapy choices. Ecologic studies may be useful to explore hypothesized associations and to test hypotheses that may not be easily tested by other types of studies. Ecologic studies also may be conducted with relatively less financial or other resources than other epidemiologic studies. Data may be available from national or community-wide surveys of exposures and disease rates, which can be accessed inexpensively. Ecologic studies also allow for comparisons between populations that are too geographically dispersed for individual-based study designs. In some populations, the range of exposure may be too narrow to allow easy analysis of the association with a disease outcome at an individual level within that population. Studies of host nutrition status, such as vitamin A, on the outcome of an infection might best be evaluated in a population containing vitamin A-deficient individuals or by comparing infection outcome in several populations with different vitamin A levels. Similarly, studies of the relationship between infectious agents and unusual outcomes, such as the liver fluke *Ophisthorcus viverini* and bile duct cancer or *Helicobacter pylori* and stomach cancer, can be strengthened by ecologic data from populations with widely varying rates of infections and cancer. Ecologic studies can also be applied to the study of protective factors. The concept of *herd immunity* to infectious diseases is based on ecologic considerations. The proportion of a population that is immune to an infectious disease can influence the risk of infection in an individual in the population. Ecologic studies are also extremely important for assessing the effect of intervention programs on the targeted population. For example, the efficacy of measles vaccination is well established from randomized clinical studies, but population effectiveness of a vaccination program can be assessed only by surveillance using an ecologic design. Two ecologic studies, one of rheumatic fever and one of HIV infection, are described below.

Crowding and Rheumatic Fever

Early studies led to the hypothesis that household crowding was an important environmental factor in the transmission of group A streptococci and high rates of acute rheumatic fever. Conversely, it has been hypothesized that the reduction in household crowding may be one of the factors in the decreased rates of acute rheumatic fever in the last half of the 1900s in comparison with earlier periods.[18] The data in Figure 3-5 show the

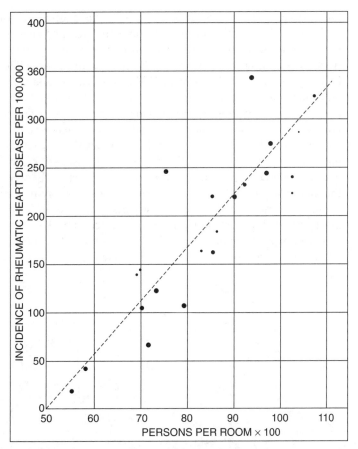

FIGURE 3-5   The correlation between the incidence of rheumatic heart disease per 100,000 and the number of persons per room (×100), as found by Perry and Roberts in various districts of the city of Bristol, England, in 1927–1930. (The size of the dots indicates roughly the comparative population size of the districts.) E. Kass, Infectious Diseases and Social Change, *Journal of Infectious Diseases*, Vol. 23, No. 1, p. 113, copyright 1971. Chicago Press.

association between the incidence of rheumatic heart disease per 100,000 and the number of persons per room in various districts in the city of Bristol, England, in 1927–1930.

Circumcision and HIV Transmission

Male circumcision is a surgical procedure in which the foreskin, or prepuce, of the male penis is removed so that the end of the penis, the glans, is exposed. After circumcision the penile shaft skin becomes keratinized over time resulting in a thicker stronger outer layer. In contrast, the foreskin has characteristics that increase its susceptibility to HIV. The foreskin is rich in immune cells, which may be infected by HIV; it is delicate and may develop microtears that may serve as an entry point for HIV, and the foreskin may trap HIV in a warm moist environment allowing more time for infection to occur. Because of these physical differences, it has been hypothesized that uncircumcised males might be at higher risk for HIV infection. Circumcised men have been found to have lower rates of other sexually transmitted diseases (STDs).[19] An ecologic study of circumcision rates and HIV seroprevalence was conducted in several African countries.[20] Data on circumcision practices were extracted from an ethnographic database, the Human Relations Area File in New Haven, Connecticut, and combined with HIV seroprevalence data from a variety of published scientific literature sources and governmental data. These data were mapped to demonstrate geographical overlap between cultures that do not practice male circumcision and a high seroprevalence rate of HIV infection among males (Figure 3-6). This study introduced the hypothesis that a lack of male circumcision increased the risk of HIV transmission. However, there are obvious behavioral, cultural, and religious differences between ethnic groups that may alter the risk of HIV acquisition. Most notably that circumcised men are more likely to be Muslim in most parts of the world. Differences in sexual practices, alcohol use, and hygiene may reduce the risk of HIV among Muslim men. Because an ecologic study design does not collect individual-level data, it cannot control for these confounding factors.

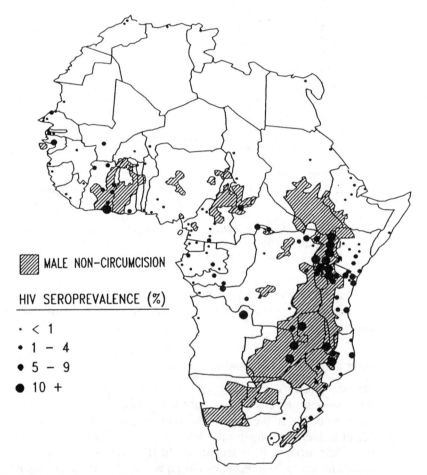

FIGURE 3-6   Map of Africa showing political boundaries and usual male circumcision practice, with point estimates of general adult population HIV seroprevalence superimposed. S. Moses et al., Geographical Patterns of Male Circumcision Practices in Africa: Association with HIV Seroprevalence, *International Journal of Epidemiology*, Vol. 19, pp. 693–697, copyright 1990, Oxford University Press.

Based on the strength of these ecologic data and several cross-sectional studies, three randomized clinical trials of male circumcision, in Kenya, South Africa, and Uganda, were initiated in 2001. Male circumcision is a controversial procedure. Although circumcision is common in the United States, it is significantly less common in other parts of the world and is equated with genital mutilation by some. Before such a controversial surgical intervention can be endorsed for the prevention of HIV it will be necessary to definitively demonstrate its efficacy with multiple trials in different populations.

Analytic Studies

Several different types of analytic studies have been used to study the natural history or risk factors for an infection. Among these are cross-sectional, cohort, case-control and nested case-control studies, and clinical trials. In these types of studies, the epidemiologist measures exposures and disease status in individuals to evaluate associations (Table 3-2). These study designs differ in the following ways:

- Their temporal nature, whether they are conducted at a given point in time or are conducted over an interval of time
- The characterization of subjects, whether they define individuals according to their risk factors for disease or according to their disease status
- The measures of association between risk factors and disease

Temporal Differences in Study Designs

Epidemiologists may be able to measure the occurrence of disease and other characteristics in a population at a given point in time—a cross-sectional study. A cross-sectional study can measure the prevalence of disease in a population. Cross-sectional and case-control studies measure the association between a disease and possible risk factors. Although correlates of disease are not always causes of the disease, a causal association is more likely if the association is strong, consistent in several studies, and biologically plausible. These study designs may collect exposure data at the time that cases and controls are selected or they may use previously collected data to add temporal depth to their study. Later in the chapter, case-control studies that are "nested" in cohort studies are discussed.

In contrast, cohort studies are longitudinal studies in which participants are followed over time. In cohort studies, a researcher identifies and enrolls a population (cohort) that does not have the disease at baseline and measures various factors to identify those that precede the development of disease and those that may be causal factors. When such associations are confirmed in multiple studies, when other factors which may be confounders of the relationship are controlled for, and when the factors can be shown to have a biologic association with disease, it can fulfill the epidemiologic criteria to be considered a cause or cofactor in the disease.

Exposure Status Versus Disease Status

All of the study designs measure the strength of the association between disease and a characteristic or exposure of a population. However, the

TABLE 3-2 Summary of Basic Analytic Study Designs

Study Design	Temporal Nature	Characterization of Subjects at Enrollment	Measures of Association
Cross-sectional	Point in time May collect retrospective data	Exposure and disease status measured simultaneously	Prevalence = $\dfrac{\text{N with disease}}{\text{N in total population}}$ Odds ratio = $\dfrac{\dfrac{\text{N exposed with disease}}{\text{N exposed without disease}}}{\dfrac{\text{N unexposed with disease}}{\text{N unexposed without disease}}}$
Case-control	Point in time May collect retrospective data	Diseased and nondiseased	Odds ratio = $\dfrac{\dfrac{\text{N exposed with disease}}{\text{N exposed without disease}}}{\dfrac{\text{N unexposed with disease}}{\text{N unexposed without disease}}}$
Cohort	Follow participants over time	Exposed and nonexposed	Incidence of disease = $\dfrac{\text{N with new disease}}{\text{N in total cohort}}$ Relative risk = $\dfrac{\dfrac{\text{N exposed with new disease}}{\text{Total N exposed}}}{\dfrac{\text{N unexposed with new disease}}{\text{Total N unexposed}}}$ Odds ratio = $\dfrac{\dfrac{\text{N exposed with disease}}{\text{N exposed without disease}}}{\dfrac{\text{N unexposed with disease}}{\text{N unexposed without disease}}}$
Clinical trial	Follow participants over time	Similar with respect to disease status, randomly assigned an exposure status (treatment)	Incidence of disease = $\dfrac{\text{N with new disease}}{\text{N in total cohort}}$ Relative risk = $\dfrac{\dfrac{\text{N exposed with new disease}}{\text{Total N exposed}}}{\dfrac{\text{N unexposed with new disease}}{\text{Total N unexposed}}}$ Odds ratio = $\dfrac{\dfrac{\text{N exposed with disease}}{\text{N exposed without disease}}}{\dfrac{\text{N unexposed with disease}}{\text{N unexposed without disease}}}$

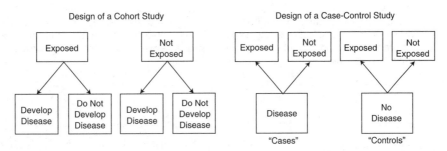

FIGURE 3-7   Cohort and case-control study designs. L. Gordis, Epidemiology, p. 163, copyright 1996 with permission from Elsevier.

approaches are based on different definitions of the study population. The study population can be defined according to disease or exposure status, or both (Figure 3-7). In a cross-sectional design, the study population is defined simultaneously by exposure characteristics and disease status. Patients with the disease are compared to nondiseased controls, and risk factors, or exposures, are measured in the two groups.

Prospective cohort studies enroll persons who are at risk of developing a disease but who are disease free at baseline. Possible risk factors, or exposures (i.e., interview data and/or biologic specimens) are measured, as is the incidence of new cases of the disease. Multiple biologic specimens, such as serum, cells, and tissues, can be collected and stored in a repository for subsequent testing when new hypotheses are developed.

Disease status is used for enrollment in case-control and cross-sectional studies. In a case-control study, the researcher defines cases based on a specific definition of disease status and compares the prevalence of exposure between those with and without disease. In a case-control study, it is usually possible to specify multiple rigorous criteria for the enrollment of a case, so that the case definition is not arguable. However, to be sure that controls are disease free, cases and controls should have the same level of scrutiny. Because controls are by definition not cases, they may not have received the same level of medical diagnostic tests to rule out disease. A rigorous case definition may make selection of a suitable control population more difficult.

Measures of Association

Regardless of the study design, the goal is to measure the association between exposure to a risk factor and the occurrence of a disease. Both cross-sectional and prospective studies can express the data obtained in a 2 × 2 table or a 2 × N (several categories) table. In these tables, the number of study participants who are exposed are stratified according to their disease status. In a 2 × N table, there may be multiple levels of exposure (Figure 3-8).

The calculation of the association between exposure and disease differs, based on the design of the study. In a cross-sectional study, in which the proportion of diseased individuals from a defined reference population is not

Epidemiologic data can be presented according to the disease and exposure status of the study participants. In the simplest case, the data may be presented as a 2 × 2 table. In instances where there are multiple exposures, the 2 × 2 table may be generalized to include as many exposure categories as necessary.

	2 × 2 Table			2 x _N_ Table		
		Disease Status			Disease Status	
		+	-		+	-
Exposure	Yes	A	B		High	A	B
Status	No	C	D	Exposure	Medium	C	D
				Status	Low	E	F
					None	G	H

FIGURE 3-8   Epidemiologic data presentation.

fixed by the study design, the association between exposure and disease is termed the relative risk (RR) and is expressed as follows:

$$RR = \frac{\dfrac{A}{(A+B)}}{\dfrac{C}{(C+D)}} = \frac{\text{Prevalence of disease in exposed}}{\text{Prevalence of disease in nonexposed}}$$

The above equation shows that if the prevalence of disease among those exposed is greater than the prevalence in the unexposed, the RR will be greater than 1, meaning the exposed are more likely to have the disease (a risk factor). Conversely, if the prevalence in the exposed is significantly less than the prevalence in the unexposed, the RR will be less than 1, and the exposed are less likely to have disease (protective). The greater the difference from 1, the stronger the effect of the exposure is on the disease. Statistical tests are used to determine whether the measured RR is likely to be a true effect or different due to chance. It is important to remember that the size of the effect and the level of statistical significance are not one and the same thing. For instance, a very small effect size, where the relative risk is not very different from 1, that is highly significant should be interpreted as an exposure that has a small, but real, impact on the risk of disease. When reporting the results of epidemiology studies, the size of the effect (e.g., the RR) should always be reported because that describes the strength and importance of the association. The level of statistical significance describes the likelihood that the association is real but does not describe its impact on the disease process. Data from a cross-sectional study may be analyzed to determine the ratio of odds of exposure in cases and controls, or the odds ratio (OR), as described below.

In a prospective cohort study, the incidence rate, expressed as the number of cases of disease per unit of time or per person-years of observation may be used instead of the prevalence:

$$RR = \frac{\text{Incidence/person-years in exposed}}{\text{Incidence/person-years in nonexposed}}$$

Statistical Significance

To determine whether the association is statistically significant, the epidemiologist must be able to demonstrate that the results are unlikely to be explained by chance alone. Epidemiologists commonly use the 95% confidence interval to illustrate the possible range of values that the RR could take, given the distribution of the data. In other words, the researcher is confident that, 95% of the time, the measured RR will be between the upper and lower limits of the confidence interval if the experiment were repeated. If the confidence interval does not include 1, then the researcher can report that there is a statistically significant association, within the 95% confidence limits, between the exposure and the disease. The use of the 95% confidence limits as indicating "statistical significance," though standard, is arbitrary. Other confidence limits could be used in some circumstances and sometimes are. One could also calculate the p-value, or the probability of a chance association, instead of the 95% confidence limits. The p-value, in contrast to the 95% confidence limits, gives only the probability of a chance association and not the strength, or importance, of the association. Weak associations can have a significant p-value if the sample size is very large. Therefore, the odds ratio or relative risk with the 95% confidence limit is preferable, because it more clearly depicts the magnitude of the association, as well as demonstrating its statistical significance.

The method usually used to calculate the 95% confidence limit of the RR is shown below:[17]

$$\text{Variance of natural log (RR)} = \frac{\dfrac{B}{A}}{(A+B)} + \frac{\dfrac{D}{C}}{(C+D)}$$

$$\text{Standard error of the natural log(RR)} = (\text{Variance lnRR})^{1/2}$$

$$\text{95\% Confidence Interval lnRR} = \text{lnRR} \pm z_{\alpha=0.05} * \text{SE (lnRR)}$$

$$\text{upper limit lnRR} = \text{lnRR} + 1.96 * \text{SE (lnRR)}$$

$$\text{lower limit lnRR} = \text{lnRR} - 1.96 * \text{SE (lnRR)}$$

$$\text{upper limit RR} = e^{\text{upper limit lnRR}}$$

$$\text{lower limit RR} = e^{\text{lower limit lnRR}}$$

In contrast, case-control studies, which have a predetermined proportion of diseased and disease-free participants (i.e., a given number of controls are chosen per case), compare the RR of exposure among those with and without disease. The formula is shown below:

$$\text{RR of exposure} = \frac{A/A+C}{B/B+D}$$

However, although the RR of exposure can evaluate the strength of the association between a risk factor and disease, it is not an intuitively easy measurement to evaluate. Instead, the odds of disease among exposed, or OR, is more commonly calculated from case-control data:

$$\text{Odds Ratio} = \frac{AD}{BC}$$

The 95% confidence interval for the OR is calculated in a similar manner to the method used for calculating the confidence interval of RR in a cohort study:[17]

$$\text{Variance of lnOR} = \frac{1}{A} + \frac{1}{B} + \frac{1}{C} + \frac{1}{D}$$

$$\text{Standard error of the lnOR} = (\text{Variance lnOR})^{1/2}$$

$$\text{95\% Confidence Interval lnOR} = \text{lnOR} \pm z_\alpha = 0.05 \ * \ \text{SE (lnOR)}$$

$$\text{upper limit lnOR} = \text{lnOR} + 1.96 \ * \ \text{SE (lnOR)}$$

$$\text{lower limit lnOR} = \text{lnOR} - 1.96 \ * \ \text{SE (lnOR)}$$

$$\text{upper limit OR} = e^{\text{upper limit lnOR}}$$

$$\text{lower limit OR} = e^{\text{lower limit lnOR}}$$

In a case-control study, the OR of disease may be a close approximation of the RR of disease when the prevalence of the disease in the population is low. As a rule of thumb, when the prevalence of disease is less than 5%, the RR and OR are nearly equal:

$$\text{RR} = \frac{A / A + B}{C / C + D} = \frac{AD}{BC} = \text{OR}$$

When the disease is rare, A and C are very small, A + B is approximately equal to B, and C + D is approximately equal to D:

$$\frac{A / B}{C / D} = \frac{AD}{BC}$$

In addition to these simple measures of exposure and disease associations, a variety of other statistical methods are available to the infectious disease epidemiologist. Powerful computer programs for exploratory analysis, graphing, and statistical software for simultaneous control of the effect of multiple variables in disease outcome are now available. A clear understanding of the statistical tools used in analysis is vital to achieving accurate results in the analysis of data, because statistical programs will give results even when inappropriately applied! A description of these methods is beyond the scope of this chapter. The reader is advised to consult other references for a detailed description of these methods: Breslow and Day,[21] Rothman and Greenland,[3] Diggle, Liang, and Zeger,[4] and Brookmeyer and Gail.[22]

Some Specific Details of Analytic Study Designs

Cross-Sectional Studies

Cross-sectional studies measure the occurrence of disease in a population at a single point in time; this measurement is called the prevalence. Case-control studies collect data on participants that are used to evaluate the prevalence of disease with respect to exposures of interest. The prevalence is a measure that is very useful to public health professionals in assessing the current burden of disease in a community. This "snapshot" of a disease is inherently static, but if multiple cross-sectional studies are conducted in a population, changes over time may be evaluated. Because cross-sectional studies may not be able to define the temporal relationship between factors, they cannot determine whether the exposure or disease came first. Thus, these studies are limited in their ability to draw conclusions about cause and effect. However, in some studies determining the temporal relationship is possible. Cross-sectional studies also can be done several times within a defined cohort, which can yield valuable information. Some examples are described below.

Cross-Sectional Studies of HIV Prevalence in Young Men in Northern Thailand

Multiple cross-sectional studies of HIV prevalence in male military conscripts in Thailand have been used to evaluate the national HIV control program. Serial cross-sectional studies of HIV prevalence and behavioral risk factors among 21-year-old men conscripted into the Royal Thai Army (RTA) were conducted between 1991 and 1998.[23] The HIV/AIDS epidemic began in Thailand in 1988 and spread rapidly among urban and rural populations, especially in northern Thailand. The predominant means of spread was by heterosexual sex, although transmission by injecting drug use, homosexual sex, and perinatal transmission also occurred.

The government responded to this widespread, rapidly evolving epidemic with a program called the 100% condom program. This program included intensive health education about the risk of HIV transmission, especially during commercial sex, the provision of free condoms, and the promotion of their use wherever commercial sex occurred.

The serial cross-sectional studies were used to document temporal trends in HIV prevalence, changes in the frequency of commercial sex, condom use, and the prevalence of STDs in these young men. These data were an unbiased estimate of the prevalence of HIV and associated risk factors because selection of the conscripts was by a random lottery system. Approximately 9% of all eligible 21-year-old men were conscripted by lottery each year. Men were not excluded based on their HIV status, a history of male-to-male sexual behavior, or injecting drug use. Furthermore, because the average age of sexual debut was 17 years, HIV prevalence in 21-year-old males represented recently acquired infection and could be used to evaluate the success of the Thai control program. The prevalence of HIV declined from 11.9% in 1991–1993 to 4.7% in 1997, whereas the lifetime history of an STD declined from 42% to 4.2% during this period. A history of paying for sex in the past year declined from 60% in 1991 to 18% in 1997, and condom use during commercial sex increased from 67% in 1991 to 95% in 1997 (Figure 3-9). These cross-sectional data documented the effectiveness of the HIV prevention program in Thailand.

HIV Cross-Sectional Studies Within a Cohort: Multicenter AIDS Cohort Study

Any particular visit of the individuals enrolled in a cohort study is an opportunity to conduct a cross-sectional analysis. In many cohort studies, the study population is characterized initially at baseline. Such cross-sectional studies allow for description of the cohort being followed and a preliminary assessment of the association of risk factors with disease outcome. The Multicenter AIDS Cohort Study (MACS) enrolled more than 6000 homosexual men in 1984 from four urban areas (Los Angeles, Chicago, Baltimore-Washington, and Pittsburgh) in a prospective study to evaluate the risk factors and natural

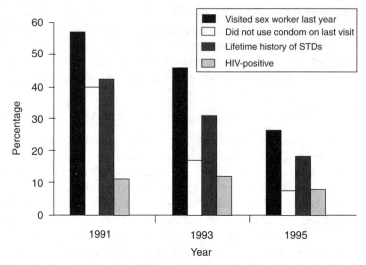

FIGURE 3-9   Sexual behavior, STDs and HIV in 21-year-old men in Northern Thailand, 1991–1995. Nelson, et al., Changes in sexual behavior and a decline in HIV infection among young men in Thailand. *The New England Journal of Medicine*, Vol. 335, pp. 297–303. Copyright 1996. The Massachusetts Medical Society.

history of HIV/AIDS. Enrollment criteria were men who had sex with men, over 18 years of age, and willing to be followed with repeated interviews and physical exams (Table 3-3). After the HIV antibody test became available nearly three years after the study began, the research team was able to test specimens stored in the national repository to measure the HIV seroprevalence among study participants at the baseline visit, even though they had been enrolled prior to the availability of an HIV antibody test (Table 3-3).[24] HIV seroprevalence rates were reported according to the participants' demographic characteristics, including city of residence, age, race, educational level, and occupational group. These data give a "snapshot" of the HIV prevalence and risk factors for HIV infection in the MACS population. They demonstrated that men who were 25–34 years old, nonwhite, with no more than a high school education, and who were service, craft, or repair workers had a higher prevalence of HIV infection early in the study. The HIV prevalence at baseline varied in the men from the participating cities; HIV prevalence was 11% in subjects from Pittsburgh, 29% in Baltimore-Washington, 30% in Chicago, and 42% in Los Angeles. The number of partners and sexual practices were similar in men from the different sites. However, men from Los Angeles were more likely to have had sex with a partner who developed AIDS, reflecting the fact that the epidemic was older in Los Angeles. Prevalence of HIV infection at baseline was also associated with having had receptive anal intercourse with a larger number of partners and reporting a history of an STD (Table 3-4).

HIV Cross-Sectional Studies Within a Cohort: Women's Interagency HIV Study

Another HIV cohort study is the Women's Interagency HIV Study (WIHS), which was initiated to study the effect of HIV-related immune suppression on gynecologic pathology and the natural history of HIV in women (Table 3-3).[25] A cross-sectional study was done in this cohort to evaluate the association

TABLE 3-3   Enrollment Criteria for the Multicenter AIDS Clinical Study (MACS), the AIDS Link to the Intravenous Experience (ALIVE), and the Women's Interagency HIV Study (WIHS). www.statepi.jhsph.edu

Characteristics	MACS (N = 4955)	ALIVE (N = 2960)	WIHS (N = 2058)
Risk group	Men who have sex with men	Injected drugs at least once after 1978	Women with and without HIV infection
Age group	18–70 years	18 years or more	13 years or more
Gender	Males	Males and females	Females
Recruitment method	Existing HBV study, word of mouth referrals, community outreach, media outreach, clinic referral	Street recruitment, word of mouth, clinic/hospital/ treatment center referral	Community outreach, hospital-based and research programs, women's support groups, drug treatment, word of mouth, HIV testing sites, clinic referral
HIV serostatus	Unknown	Tested at first visit	Tested at first visit
AIDS	AIDS-free	AIDS-free	AIDS and AIDS-free
Study visit schedule	6-month visits	6-month visits	6-month visits
Physical exam	All	All HIV-seropositives, subset HIV-seronegatives	All
Routine specimens	Serum, plasma, lymphocytes, throat washings/saliva, urine, feces, semen	Serum, plasma, lymphocytes	Serum, plasma, lymphocytes, cervical lavage, urine, throat washings/saliva
Risk exposure data	1-hour interviewer-administered questionnaire	1-hour interviewer-administered questionnaire	1-hour interviewer-administered questionnaire

between HIV and human papillomavirus (HPV) infection among more than 2500 subjects, composed of both HIV-negative and HIV-positive women who were enrolled at six clinical sites throughout the United States. Data collected included physical exams, medical history, behavioral and demographic factors, as well as CD4$^+$ cell count and quantitative RT-PCR measurement of HIV RNA and prevalence of HPV infection using hybrid capture and PCR amplification. This allowed the investigators to examine the association between HIV and HPV prevalence.[26]

In this study, HIV-positive women with a CD4$^+$ T-cell count of less than 200 cells/mm^3 were at the highest risk of HPV infection, regardless of HIV RNA load (OR = 10.13; 95% confidence interval [CI] = 7.32, 10.34). A lower risk was seen among women with a CD4$^+$ T-cell count greater than 200 cells/mm^3 but who had a high viral load, HIV RNA greater than 20,000 copies/ml (OR = 5.78, 95% CI: 4.17–8.08). The lowest risk was for women

TABLE 3-4 Cross-Sectional Analysis of Data from the Multicenter AIDS Cohort
Study (MACS)

	% Seropositive*			
	Baltimore/ Washington, DC	Chicago	Los Angeles	Pittsburgh/ Tristate area
Age (years)				
18–24	29	30	42	11
25–34	35	49	53	26
35–44	31	42	52	19
45+	18	33	38	11
Race				
White	30	42	51	20
Black	47	60	52	35
Other	46	50	41	27
Educational level				
≤12th grade	35	60	65	26
Some college	34	46	51	21
Some graduate work	27	33	46	17
Occupation				
Management/professional	29	39	47	21
Technical/sales	32	39	51	18
Service	36	57	62	23
Craft/repair	38	71	52	21
Operator/laborer	30	41	50	24

*Prevalence of ELISA antibody to human immunodeficiency virus and relationship to
demographic features among homosexual men, by center of the MACS, at entry, April 1984–
April 1985.
Source: R. Kaslow et al., The Multicenter AIDS Cohort study: Rationale, Organization, and
Selected Characteristics of the Participants, *American Journal of Epidemiology*, Vol. 126, p. 317,
Copyright 1987 Oxford University Press.

with a $CD4^+$ T-cell count greater than 200 cells/mm^3 and a low viral load, less
than 20,000 HIV RNA copies/ml. This study suggested there was a correlation
between HIV-related immune suppression and HPV infection. The next step
would be to evaluate the association in a prospective study design so that a
causal link could be evaluated.

Case-Control and Nested Case-Control Studies

Case-control studies are the natural extension of a descriptive case series
study. They are also related to a cohort study when the cases and controls
are drawn from or can be related back to a defined or similar population, or a
population "set." In a case-control study, a group of persons with a disease—
the cases—is compared with a group of persons without the disease—the
controls. Because the proportion of those with disease in the study is fixed
by the study design, the analysis is based on comparing the rate of exposure
in those with and without the disease. In a case-control study, the researcher
concentrates on assembling a group of persons with and without disease. This
fundamental characteristic of the study design has several advantages. It is
possible to study rare diseases because resources can be efficiently used to

evaluate known or readily available cases of a disease. More than one exposure can be evaluated because the original study population was not restricted with respect to exposure. Typically, case-control studies have smaller sample sizes than cohort studies, allowing for greater resources to be expended per participant and for lower costs to the study overall. Resources can be used to define disease status and the absence of disease with greater certainty, reducing the risk of misclassification bias.

Case-control studies are especially useful for evaluating potential risk factors in an outbreak of an infectious disease, because they can be done quickly and efficiently. However, the determination of exposure data may be difficult. Sometimes, the exposure may have occurred many years prior to the onset of the disease, so recall bias may be a problem. However, in acute outbreaks of infectious diseases, such as with toxic shock syndrome or food-borne outbreaks, the exposures are recent, so recall bias may be less important than when the time from exposure to disease is long. Recall often can be differential; persons who have developed a disease that is putatively linked to an exposure may recall exposure more readily than will those in whom no disease occurred. Also, case-control studies of chronic infectious diseases may be affected by survival bias: the cases must live long enough to be diagnosed and enrolled, and this may mean they lived longer than other cases. Case-control studies are sensitive to biases because the study population is highly selected (Table 3-5). However, it would be incorrect to assume that other study designs are not also susceptible to some of these same biases.

TABLE 3-5   Biases of Epidemiologic Studies

Response bias occurs when persons who have a disease or their medical care providers examine their past behaviors and exposures so carefully that they are more likely to report behaviors or risk that they feel are associated with a disease. Conversely, they may also be more likely to suppress information that they feel would incriminate them as the cause of their own illness.

Ibrahim-Spitzer bias is when the selection of cases and controls results in a distorted measure of association between the exposure and disease.

Prevalence-incidence bias, or Neyman bias, may occur if the duration of disease is affected by exposure. Prevalence-incidence bias can raise or lower the observed association between an exposure and a disease. If persons who are exposed to a factor have a more rapid course of disease, they may die before they can be identified by researchers. This will spuriously reduce the relative risk. Conversely, if exposure increases survival, the relative risk measured by the study will be higher than the true association.

Latency bias occurs if the analysis is begun prior to the development of disease among exposed cases. For example, liver cancer cases would not be manifested if a study of the role of hepatitis C infection in cancer was initiated only a few months after exposure.

Berksonian bias occurs if there is referral bias of exposed persons to study personnel.

Detection bias occurs when persons who are known to be exposed to a hypothesized etiologic exposure undergo more rigorous screening. Thus, exposed persons are more likely to be cases because the sensitivity of screening is higher among exposed than unexposed.

Nonresponse bias cases may be either too sick to participate or have died prior to the study. Researchers may have to rely on exposure ascertainment data from surrogate respondents. Thus, data may be collected differently from cases and controls.

In analytical case-control studies, the researcher attempts to determine the exposures among the cases and controls. Because the analysis is based on comparisons within the study sample, generalizability of the results to the overall population is less important than the appropriate selection of the control population. The overriding consideration in the selection of controls is to select them in such a way that they are representative of the same population from which the cases arose. Studies have sought controls from other patients in hospitals or clinics, friends of the cases, family members of cases, neighborhood or geographic controls, or other accessible populations. Whereas the risk of disease may differ between cases and controls, controls should be similar enough to cases that they too have a risk of developing disease. If the controls were completely immune to developing a disease, the risk factor of importance in the case group may not be different between the groups. For instance, a study of genetic traits and ovarian cancer should not have men as the control group. A less extreme example is that HIV seronegative persons are not suitable controls for a study of Kaposi sarcoma (KS) in AIDS patients; the researcher should instead choose individuals with a similar level of immune suppression but who are KS free. Researchers must also decide whether controls should be chosen from populations with other diseases or from nondiseased persons. Frequently, data are available on persons diagnosed with another disease as a result of diagnosis or treatment that can be used to compare risk factors between cases and controls. When controls with other diseases are selected, it is important to ensure that the exposure being evaluated is not also related to the control's disease. Sometimes, it may be difficult to rule out the presence of disease in persons who have not received certain diagnostic procedures. However, if a study requires that the controls have had extensive diagnostic tests, it may compromise generalizability or external validity because only a select group of people will have undergone the testing requirements.

To maximize the study's ability to analyze a given risk factor, the study design should minimize differences between cases and controls with respect to other known risk factors. Controls may be matched with cases to varying degrees. Controls may be simply drawn from homogeneous populations, such as clinics that serve only specific types of patients. More closely matched controls may be chosen from subpopulations that closely conform to the demographic characteristics of the cases. Individual matching may also be used. Individual matching can reduce the variability between the cases and controls with respect to confounding factors, known and unknown, but there are several potential drawbacks. The inability to find a matched control for a particular case could result in exclusion of the case. This would be a particular problem if cases were rare. Matching increases the complexity of enrollment of participants, and this complexity could result in errors in enrollment. Because cases and controls have been chosen so that they are similar with respect to the matching variables, the distribution of the matched variables will be the same in the cases and controls. Future analysis of these matched variables cannot be assessed. In most instances, statistical adjustment of the data during analysis can account for differences in the distribution of known risk factors. Given its drawbacks, matching should only be done when the matching variables are likely to confound the data even after statistical adjustment and are of no research interest in and of themselves. In a matched analysis, the data may be expressed in a 2 × 2 table. Instead of each study participant being counted in the table, data are entered by pairs. For example, a pair where both the case and control are exposed would be recorded as one data point in the A cell of the table. When a matched design is used in a case-control study, the OR is expressed as the ratio of the discordant pairs.

Controls

		Exposed	Not exposed
	Exposed	A	B
Case	Not exposed	C	D

$$\text{Odds ratio (matched pair)} = \frac{B}{C}$$

Nested Case-Control Studies

One of the major problems with case-control studies is the reliability and validity of the measurement of the exposure. Also, it may not be possible to determine whether the exposure occurred prior to the onset of disease. One type of study design that can be used to avoid these issues is a nested case-control study. Cases are selected from a cohort after the onset of illness, and they are matched with controls from the same cohort on whom similar exposure information is available and who have had the same opportunity to be diagnosed with disease. Controls should have been followed for a similar length of time as the cases, and they should have received the same diagnostic procedures. Many of the biases that can arise in reconstructing retrospective exposure data are reduced or eliminated when previously collected data from a cohort study are used. Furthermore, nested case-control study designs have the advantage that the researcher can know the temporal relationship between the exposure and disease. Analysis of stored specimens from the cohort study also ensures that changes in laboratory methods or artifacts due to specimen storage do not affect the study results differentially between cases and controls.

There are two commonly used methods for selecting controls in the nested case-control study. When controls are matched to cases by selecting participants from the cohort who are disease free at the time the case becomes ill, the procedure is referred to as incidence density sampling. A second method is to select controls from the cohort at baseline—a case-cohort design. In the case-cohort study, all or some known proportion of the original cohort is sampled for the analysis. When the case-cohort design is used, it is possible to estimate the prevalence of disease in the cohort and to calculate the population-attributable risk.[21] Examples of case-control and nested case-control study designs are given below.

Examples of Case-Control Studies

Kaposi's Sarcoma and Pneumocystis carinii Pneumonia in Homosexual Men

After the recognition of the cluster of homosexual/bisexual men with KS and PCP in 1981, the Centers for Disease Control and Prevention (CDC) did a case-control study to determine the factors that placed these men at increased risk of AIDS.[27] For this study, 50 men with KS or PCP were matched by age and geographic area with 120 controls, who were homosexual men without AIDS. The rates of different exposures were compared between the cases and controls. The variable most strongly associated with illness was a greater number of male sex partners per year. Compared with controls, cases were also more likely to have been exposed to feces during sex, have had syphilis or hepatitis B virus infection, have been treated for enteric parasites, and had a higher reported lifetime use of various illicit substances, especially amyl nitrite (Table 3-6). These results led the investigators to hypothesize that the illness was spread sexually and was associated with certain aspects of the homosexual lifestyle. When a similar disease appeared in injection drug users, transfusion recipients, and hemophiliacs, the hypothesis was strengthened that AIDS was caused by a specific infection.[28] The hypothesis that the agent was sexually transmitted was strengthened further when studies of the wives of men with hemophilia and AIDS or lymphadenopathy found that the wives also had low CD4+ lymphocyte counts.[29]

Reye's Syndrome and Aspirin Exposure

Reye's syndrome was also studied using a case-control design. The first case-control study of Reye's syndrome was conducted in Phoenix, Arizona, in 1976. This study showed a significant association between the use of aspirin during influenza illness and Reye's syndrome.[30] Also those with Reyes syndrome used more salicylates than the controls. However, the controls with influenza were more likely to use other antipyretics, such as acetaminophen. Subsequently, the incidence of Reye's syndrome in the United States increased significantly between 1972 and 1983. A number of case-control studies were done, and all of them showed a significant association with a similar OR.[30-32] Because of some lingering concerns about the representativeness of controls in these studies, the CDC did a case-control study in which controls were selected from four different populations for each case.[33] This case-control study agreed with the results of the other studies and showed

TABLE 3-6 Rates of Risk Behaviors Measured in a Case-Control Study

	Patients	Controls	
	Cases (N = 50)	Clinic (N = 78)	Private Practice (N = 42)
Median male sexual partners per year	61	27	25
Mean feces exposure scale	2.3	1.9	1.9
History of syphilis (%)	68	36	36
History of non-B hepatitis (%)	48	30	33
History of drugs for enteric parasites (%)	44	19	50
Use of ethyl chloride (%)	50	35	38
Lifetime nitrite use (days)	336	168	264

Source: H. Jaffe et al., National Case-Cntrol Study of Kaposi's Sarcoma and *Pneumocystis carinii* Pneumonia in Homosexual men. *Annals of Internal Medicine.* Vol. 99, pp. 145–151, Copyright 1983 American College of Physicians—American Society of Internal Medicine

a significant association between aspirin use for influenza and Reye's syndrome. Because of these findings, the CDC[34] and the American Academy of Pediatrics recommended that physicians warn parents of the risk of Reye's syndrome. The Food and Drug Administration mandated warning labels about this hazard on aspirin bottles. In the last decade, Reye's syndrome has virtually disappeared as aspirin use during influenza season declined (Figure 3-10).[35]

Examples of Nested Case-Control Studies

Epstein-Barr Virus Infection and Hodgkin's Disease

For several years, epidemiologists have questioned whether Hodgkin's disease (HD) might be caused by an infectious agent, especially in those with onset at an earlier age. Some investigators have found evidence of an increased prevalence of Epstein-Barr virus (EBV) antibodies in patients with HD. Also, EBV is known to cause other tumors, especially nasopharyngeal carcinoma, and to persist after the initial infection. However, EBV infection is not uncommon. To show a causal association, it was necessary to demonstrate that EBV infection preceded the development of HD.

A community-based public health epidemiologic study in Washington County, Maryland, afforded the opportunity to test the hypothesis that EBV might be etiologically related to HD.[36] In this study, a sera repository was collected in 1963. Over two decades later, specimens from persons who had developed HD in the interim were selected, matched with controls, and tested for serologic evidence of EBV. The data showed a significant association between EBV antibodies prior to the onset of HD in cases, compared with matched controls (RR = 2.6–4.0 for various serologic markers of infection). This evidence strengthened the argument that EBV infection might be in the causal pathway for the development of HD because EBV infections were more common in the cases and preceded the onset of HD.

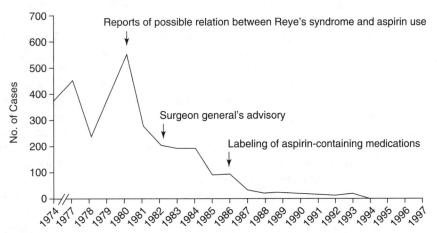

FIGURE 3-10 Number of reported cases of Reye's syndrome in relation to the timing of public announcements of the epidemiologic association of Reye's syndrome with aspirin ingestion and the labeling of aspirin-containing medications. Belay et al., Reye's Syndrome in the United States from 1981 through 1997, *New England Journal of Medicine*, Vol. 340, pp. 1377–1382. Copyright 1999 Massachusetts Medical Society.

Kaposi's Sarcoma and HHV-8 (KSHV)

The presence of nucleic acid sequences of a new herpes virus (HHV-8) were detected in the lesions of AIDS patients with KS by Chang et al.[37] It then became important to determine whether infection with HHV-8 preceded the occurrence of KS in patients with HIV-1 infection. The availability of specimen repositories from several large cohorts of homosexual men allowed investigators to perform nested case-control studies. The sera were examined at baseline for antibodies to HHV-8 to estimate the RR of subsequent KS in men with and without HHV-8 antibodies. Also, Kaplan-Meier survival analysis was done to estimate the rate of new KS cases in HIV-positive men after HHV-8 infection. Nested case-control studies showing an association between HHV-8 infection and KS have been published from several cohorts, including a Danish homosexual cohort, an Australian cohort, and the Multicenter AIDS Cohort Study (MACS).[38–40]

Case-Cohort Study of HIV Seroconversion Among Health Care Workers

A nested case-cohort study of the risk of HIV seroconversion among health care workers (HCWs) in France, the United Kingdom, and the United States was published in 1995.[41] This study was done to determine whether treatment with zidovudine (or other antiretroviral drugs) after parenteral exposure in HCWs reduced the rate of HIV transmission. Several animal studies suggested that postexposure prophylaxis conferred protection after challenge with simian immunodeficiency virus (SIV). Furthermore, at the time of the study, zidovudine had been shown to be effective in preventing vertical transmission of HIV. Prospective studies suggested that the risk of HIV transmission after parenteral exposure was only 0.35%.[42] Therefore a prospective study, or clinical trial, would need to be extraordinarily large to have sufficient statistical power to evaluate the benefit of therapy. Also, recruitment of participants for a randomized clinical trial would be difficult because zidovudine was generally felt to be effective in preventing HIV transmission, and participants who were randomized to the control arm might insist on receiving the unproven antiretroviral therapy. In this study, available data from the United States and France were analyzed in which the exposure and treatment history of all known cases of HIV transmission to HCWs ($n = 31$ cases) was compared with that of all reported uninfected exposed HCWs ($n = 679$, cohort). Exposure was defined as those who had a documented penetrating injury with an instrument contaminated by blood from an HIV-positive patient. Cases and cohort members had received either zidovudine or no antiretroviral prophylaxis and had been followed at least 6 months, as of August 1994. The risk factors for HIV infection and protective effect of zidovudine are shown in Table 3-7.

Based on this study, it was recommended by the CDC that all HCWs receive zidovudine after percutaneous exposure to HIV-infected blood. However, it is clear that there are some potential biases in this study. For example, if there was significant underreporting of HCWs in whom transmission failed to occur and who had not received prophylaxis, the transmission rate in the control group could be inflated. This referral (or enrollment) bias would decrease the measured OR and increase the apparent protective efficacy of zidovudine

TABLE 3-7 Risk Factors for HIV Infection Among Health Care Workers After Percutaneous Exposure to HIV-Infected Blood

Risk Factors	Adjusted OR	(95% CI)
Deep injury	16.1	(6.1–44.6)
Visible blood on device	5.2	(1.8–17.7)
Procedure involving needle placed directly in vein or artery	5.1	(1.9–14.8)
Terminal illness in source patient	6.4	(2.2–18.9)
Postexposure use of zidovudine	0.2	(0.1–0.6)

Notes: OR, odds ratio; CI, confidence interval.
Source: Morbidity and Mortality Weekly Report, Vol. 44, pp. 929–931, Centers for Disease Control and Prevention.

postexposure prophylaxis above the actual efficacy. Certainly, data from a randomized controlled clinical trial could provide more valid data. However, clinical trials are not always feasible (as in this case) or ethical to conduct, and other study designs must often be used to answer important policy questions.

Cohort Studies

Enrollment

The word *cohort* was originally used to describe a unit of 300–600 men in the ancient Roman army. In epidemiology, a cohort is a group of persons with similar characteristics who are followed over time. The characteristic used to define the cohort may be an exposure, an occupation, a genetic trait, a geographic location, or another population characteristic determined by the epidemiologist. To conduct a prospective cohort study, participants who are disease free at baseline but at risk for disease are enrolled and followed over time to measure the occurrence of disease.

A cohort study is best suited for diseases with high incidence rates among exposed persons and frequent exposures to the variable of interest. The study needs to have adequate numbers of individuals who are exposed and who develop disease after enrollment for the statistical analysis to have sufficient power to detect associations. If a disease were rare, even among exposed people, an unrealistically large cohort would have to be assembled. If exposures were uncommon, this could also affect the size of the population needed in the cohort. Cohorts can be assembled for which there are special resources available for follow-up. For example, members of HMOs or occupational groups with employment records can be selected. Occupational cohorts may also represent persons with high exposure to an agent. For example, HCWs were an ideal group from which to draw a cohort to study the risk of HBV, cytomegalovirus and HIV transmission.[42] Unfortunately, although the high levels of exposure and the ensuing high numbers of cases may make demonstrating a link between an exposure and an outcome easier, the unusual exposure levels may make results of such cohorts more difficult to generalize to the population. Nevertheless, internal validity, or whether an exposure and disease are truly related in the study population, is more important than generalizability to populations outside the study. Cohort studies can be very expensive and often require a large staff and great motivation on the part of the study subjects to remain in follow-up. Cohort studies with large losses to follow-up may not yield data that are interpretable, because the risks for disease may be different in those lost to follow-up than in the subjects who were successfully followed. The enrollment criteria for three HIV/AIDS cohorts—the Multicenter AIDS Cohort Study (MACS), the AIDS Link to the Intravenous Experience (ALIVE), and the Women's Interagency HIV Study (WIHS) are shown in Table 3-3.

Although most cohort studies enroll and follow subjects prospectively, cohorts may also be assembled retrospectively, after disease has occurred. Such a study could bring together previously collected medical or exposure records or incorporate previously collected data with current and future assessment of disease among those exposed. A retrospective cohort, or histori-cal cohort design, takes advantage of records and specimens collected in the past and can generate results more rapidly than a truly prospective design, which must wait for the development of disease. Within existing cohorts, subgroups can evaluate hypotheses prospectively that were not proposed at the outset of the original cohort. These studies, nested cohorts, are able to study participants enrolled in the parent cohort and take advantage of the infrastructure, data, and even specimens collected by the original cohort.

Data Collection

Cohort studies collect information on exposure and on the development of disease. Simplistically, a cohort is assembled from a group of exposed individuals, and the study measures the incidence of disease in the group. Practically, however, cohorts assemble persons with a range of risk expo-sures and measure the incidence of disease across the range of risk levels. Often, it is possible in cohort studies to measure a dose-response effect of increasing disease incidence (because of higher attack rates or shorter incubation periods) with higher levels of exposure. Furthermore, in cohort studies, the subjects can develop infection or disease of varying severity. Thus, defining the appropriate end point is critical. In some cohort studies, several end points may be measured. For example, a study of influenza could measure serologically or virologically confirmed infection, clinical illness, illness with a physician visit or time away from work, hospital-ization, or death. A cohort study of influenza vaccine in the elderly has found the vaccine to be more efficacious in preventing death than it is in preventing infection.[43]

An interviewer-administered questionnaire can collect more detailed and complex information, can allow for more flexibility in collecting infor-mation, and often results in more complete and standardized information being collected. Interviewer-administered questionnaires can also create a stronger bond with the study participants, so they are more likely to share information and are more likely to continue their participation in the study. In some populations, literacy levels may be low, necessitating an interviewer-administered design. Other cohort studies have relied on less expensive data collection techniques, such as mail or telephone inter-views. These data collection techniques commonly have lower response rates than do interviewer-administered questionnaires but are significantly less expensive. Repeated interviews of ongoing cohorts may encounter problems with "socially desirable responding" particularly on questions to assess risk behaviors. In this situation, participants respond to questions according to what they believe the interviewer might view as desirable behavior. This is not always intentional misreporting or "lying" about behavior by the subject. Sometimes, the subject's memory is influenced by the social situation of the interview. Care must be taken to ensure that interviewers are well trained and that the questionnaire is carefully conducted to minimize these potential biases. One recent technique that has been evaluated to reduce socially desirable responses is to replace the interviewer with a computer response system. The interview is administered by an audio-adapted computer assisted interview (ACASI). Another advantage of ACASI data collection over self-completed questionnaires is that ACASI questions are more readily understood by persons with low literacy levels, because the questions are printed on the computer screen but also spoken through the audio connection. Although some participants prefer the personal interaction with the interviewer, the use of ACASI to measure risk behavior generally results in higher levels of reported risk behaviors. For example, more adolescents reported unprotected sex and injection drug on ACASI than was reported in a standard interview.[44]

Analysis

Unlike other epidemiologic study designs, cohort studies are able to measure the rate at which participants develop disease per unit of time—the incidence rate. The incidence rate is the number of people who develop disease divided by the cumulative time in the study for all participants up until the time that they develop disease.

To measure associations, cohort studies compare the incidence rate of disease among persons with different exposures or other characteristics at baseline or during the follow-up period. The ratio of the incidence rates according to exposures is expressed as the relative risk, risk ratio, or relative hazard of disease (Table 3-2). Analysis may be extended to include Kaplan-Meier types of survival curves and Cox proportional hazard analysis, in which data are stratified according to exposure characteristics and survival curves are compared. Cohort studies can also use data obtained by testing multiple biologic specimens collected from subjects during the course of the study.

In addition to methods that define exposure at an arbitrary baseline time point, there are analytical methods that take into account changes in exposure among individuals over time. Because cohort studies follow participants over time, the level of exposure to different risk factors may fluctuate for an individual over time. For example, an individual who uses illicit drugs may have times of abstinence and episodes of heavy drug use. Exposures that fluctuate over time, either qualitatively (e.g., present/absent) or quantitatively (e.g., heavy/light), are termed *time-dependent covariates*. Those covariates that don't change, such as sex, histocompatibility locus antigen (HLA) type, ethnicity, age at baseline, are termed *fixed covariates*. Note that while participants contribute data to the study at each visit, how those data are distributed in the analysis depends on their risk behaviors at that point in time. A single individual may contribute data to both the exposed and the unexposed categories over the course of the cohort study. The fluctuation in personal behaviors is accounted for in the person time analysis and gives cohort analysis considerable statistical power, as each data point from each participant is used.

The ability to assess time-dependent covariates is useful when assessing the effects of long-term therapy on chronic disease outcomes. The patients may have periods when they go off treatment (e.g., due to side effects) or may even change therapy, so that a baseline assessment of exposure would lead to misclassification of such patients. In studies of nutrition, for example, calorie intake can fluctuate with seasonal food supplies and may need to be assessed several times over a year.

The analysis of longitudinal data requires attention to some of the assumptions of the statistical models. Longitudinal data contain repeated measurements on risk behaviors for a single individual over time. The distribution of these risk behaviors is not normal, nor is it independent. For example, a person who injects illicit drugs frequently will probably continue to inject at a high frequency. A plot of a hundred measurements of injection frequency on a single participant would differ from single measurements on a hundred participants. The variation in data from the single person would be much less than the variability in data from a hundred individuals. Many statistical programs assume that the data are normally distributed and that the values are independent of each other. An analysis of longitudinal data that does not take into account the smaller variance of repeated measures will give estimates of the variance that are too small and will construct confidence intervals for the estimates that are too small. In other words, the model will report that the data are better than they really are. Numerous programs are able to perform analysis on repeated measurement data and should be used for longitudinal data analysis when appropriate.

One such generalized approach, the Generalized Estimating Equations (GEE), was developed by Zieger and Liang. GEE adjusts for within-person correlation of multiple observations from the same individual[45] and allows analyses that can model changes in exposure status over time. These methods were used to assess the effects of zidovudine therapy and antibiotics for PCP on HIV disease progression and death at the population level.[46,47] An extension of the Cox proportional hazards model that allows for time-dependent covariates also gives the epidemiologist the ability to assess the effects of changes in exposure over time. This approach has been used to assess the effectiveness of switching therapy among HIV-infected patients who were taking nucleoside reverse transcriptase inhibitor therapy at baseline.[47]

Examples of Cohort Studies

The use of cohort studies to evaluate the incidence of HIV, natural history of HIV, and the effectiveness of drug therapies is shown in the following four examples, two from the ALIVE cohort and two from the MACS cohort.

HIV Infection and Risk Behaviors in the ALIVE Study

A cohort of 2960 participants was recruited and screened for HIV infection in Baltimore between February 1988 and March 1989. Criteria for enrollment were age of 18 years or more, a history of injection of illicit drugs in the past 10 years, AIDS-free status at baseline, and willingness to be followed prospectively. Those who were HIV-seropositive were enrolled in a study of the natural history of HIV infection in injection drug users. A sample of HIV-negative injecting drug users (IDUs) was followed to determine the incidence of HIV infection. Among the HIV-negative participants at baseline 1532 were followed, and 188 (12.3%) had seroconverted by December 1992. The incidence of HIV over time was analyzed. Risk factors of interest in this study were active drug use within the past 6 months (a time-dependent covariate), age <35 years versus ≥35 years, and gender (a fixed covariate).[48]

The analysis showed that the incidence of HIV was highest in young females who continued using drugs (3.17/100 person-semesters, or 6.34/100 person-years) and was lowest in both males and females who had stopped injecting drugs (1.37/100 person-semester) (Table 3-8). The higher incidence continued among younger drug users and was stable between 1988 and 1992 (Table 3-8). The incidence rates were higher in female than in male drug users during the early years of the study but declined between 1990 and 1992; whereas the incidence rates among males who continued injection were stable at about 2.0/100 person-semesters (i.e., 4.0/100 person-years) between 1988 and 1992 (Figure 3-11).

HIV Viral Load and Progression to AIDS

As new laboratory methods were developed to evaluate the natural history of HIV, the existence of sample repositories accelerated the rate at which hypotheses could be tested. After a reliable methodology to quantitate HIV RNA in plasma was developed, stored samples from cohort studies were tested to determine how viral load might predict the risk of progression. In the MACS cohort, Mellors et al. were able to describe the viral load with respect to the natural history of HIV infection.[49] They found an early viral burst with high levels of HIV RNA in the plasma that was followed after a few months by a relatively stable lower plateau in the viral load until shortly prior to the onset of clinical AIDS, when viral load again rose.[49] These studies found that infected individuals generally developed different steady states, or set

TABLE 3-8   Incidence of HIV-1 Infection per Person-Semester by Gender and Age Among a Cohort of Injecting Drug Users, Baltimore, MD, 1988–1992

Age (years)	PSs at Risk	Number of Seroconverters	Incidence per PS (%)	95% CI
		Male		
≥35	3864.74	53	1.37	1.05–1.80
<35	3846.17	86	2.24	1.81–2.76
		Female		
≥35	727.52	10	1.37	0.74–2.50
<35	1168.75	37	3.17	2.29–4.37

Notes: HIV-1 indicates human immunodeficiency virus type 1; CI, confidence interval; PS, person semester.
Source: K. Nelson et al., *Archives of Internal medicine*, No. 155, pp. 1305–1311. Copyright 1995. American Medical Association.

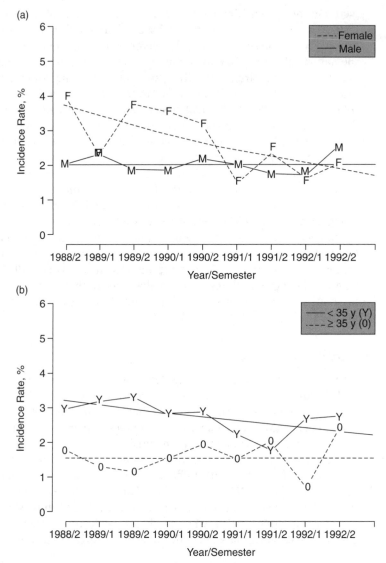

FIGURE 3-11a & b   HIV seroincidence rates decreased over time. (a) Trend of human immunodeficiency virus seroconversion among current drug users by semester between July 1988 and December 1992 by gender. The line was fitted to the data by Poisson regression, which was given by: exp [−388 + 0.60 (female) − 0.087 (female) × semester]. (b) Trend of human immunodeficiency virus seroconversion among current drug users by semester between July 1988 and December 1992 by age. The line was fitted to the data by Poisson regression, which was given by: exp [−4.15 + (age < 35 y) × 0.72 + (semester × age < 35 y) × 0.043]. K. Nelson et al., *Archives of Internal Medicine*, Vol. 155, p. 1310, Copyright 1995, American Medical Association.

points, of viral load during their periods of clinical latency. The level of the viral load set point was strongly predictive of the duration of the period of clinical latency. Some individuals with high viral load progressed to AIDS in 2–3 years, but others with low viral load remained free of AIDS for more than 12 years. Moreover, the viral load data could be combined with the CD4+ T-cell count to predict more accurately the time to development of AIDS.

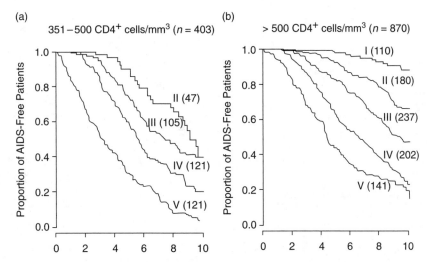

FIGURE 3-12a & b   Time to AIDS for participants with (a) 351–500 and (b) >500 CD4+ T cells/mm³. The five categories of HIV-1 RNA are defined as follows: I, 500 copies/mm³ or less; II, 501 to 3000 copies/mm³; III, 3001 to 10,000 copies/mm³; IV, 10,001 to 30,000 copies/mm³; and V, more than 30,000 copies/mm³. Mellors et al., Plasma Viral Load and CD4+ Lymphocytes as Prognostic Markers of HIV-1 Infection, *Annals of Internal Medicine*, Vol. 126, pp. 946–954, © 1997, American College of Physicians–American Society of Internal Medicine.

Figure 3-12 shows the Kaplan-Meier curves of time to AIDS for participants who had 351–500 CD4+ T-cells/mm³ and those with greater than 500 CD4+ T-cells/mm³.

Examples of Nested Cohorts

Effect of Therapy on HIV/AIDS Survival

A second type of ecologic study utilizes the cohort study structure to analyze longitudinal data to evaluate disease outcomes in different eras. For example, changes in disease outcomes can be compared across periods of time when different therapies were available. As with all ecologic designs, the individual's therapy exposure and outcome are not compared. Instead, calendar periods can be characterized by the dominant therapies used during that time, and therapeutic effectiveness can be examined at the population level. A publication from the MACS and WIHS cohorts assessed the effectiveness of highly active antiretroviral therapy (HAART) in a nested cohort study of those select participants who had a known date of their first AIDS illness. Because the date of AIDS or death was known (within a six-month window); the researchers could evaluate differences in the time from AIDS to death over different calendar periods. Five periods were defined based on therapy use patterns: the no or monotherapy era (July 1984–December 1989); the monotherapy/combination therapy era (January 1990–December 1994); HAART introduction era (January 1995–June 1998); short-term stable HAART use era (July 1998–June 2001); and moderate-term stable HAART use era (July 2001–December 2003). In a Weibull regression, the researchers showed that in the monotherapy era 25% of patients died 6 months after an AIDS diagnosis; it was 4 and 5 years, respectively, before 25% of patients

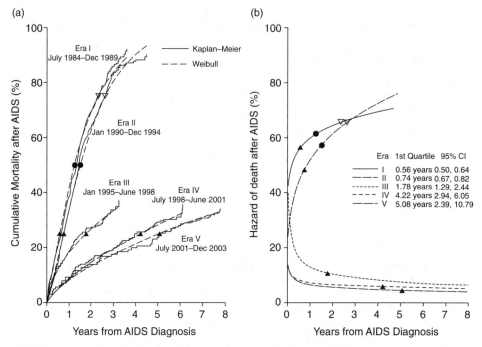

FIGURE 3-13a & b   Time from AIDS to death for MACS and WIHS participants in different therapy eras. Schneider MF, Gange SJ, Williams CF, Anastos K, Greenblatt R, Kingsley L, Detels R, Munoz A. Patterns of the Hazard of Death after Acquired Immunodeficiency Syndrome through the Evolution of Antiretroviral Therapy: 1984–2004. *AIDS*. 19(7), pp. 2009–2018.

died in the two stable HAART eras. If the conditions of the latest era were to remain, the model predicts that 50% of persons with AIDS will survive more than 16 years after their initial AIDS diagnosis. This would be greater than a 10-fold improvement from the observed median survival of 1.2 years in the no/monotherapy eras. These findings demonstrate that even among patients who have already had an AIDS diagnosis, HAART remains highly effective (Figure 3-13).[50]

Human Papillomavirus and Cervical Intraepithelial Neoplasia

A nested cohort design was used to test the hypothesis that HIV infection facilitates and enhances the persistence of HPV and that such persistence was correlated with an increased incidence of cervical intraepithelial neoplasia (CIN).[51] This nested cohort study relied on stored samples from the biannual collection of cervicovaginal washings to test for HPV DNA among HIV-seropositive and HIV-seronegative female participants in the ALIVE study. The proportion of HPV-positive women and the persistence of HPV positivity in individual women were measured. Persistence of HPV was evaluated according to the participants' HIV status and CD4 cell count. Immune-suppressed HIV-seropositive participants were found to have greater persistence of HPV infection. To evaluate the risk of CIN among participants according to the persistence of HPV, all female ALIVE participants were invited to participate in the nested cohort by receiving a colposcopic examination and biopsies when indicated. The independent effect of HPV persistence and HIV infection among women who had biopsy-confirmed CIN was evaluated. This study found that HPV persistence was a risk factor for CIN among HIV-seropositive women.

Clinical Trials

Clinical trials evaluate the effect of planned interventions. In contrast with cohort or case-control studies, clinical trials are experimental, rather than observational. The investigator assigns certain subjects to receive one treatment—the experimental group—and other subjects to receive another treatment—the control or comparison group. Clinical trials of interventions to prevent or treat infectious diseases are commonly used to evaluate the efficacy of vaccines; antimicrobial agents; and behavioral, immunologic, or other interventions to prevent or treat infectious disease. For a more detailed discussion of the design and analytical and ethical issues involved in clinical trials in infectious diseases the reader is referred to several excellent resources.[52,53]

In a clinical trial, a control or comparison group is usually necessary to determine whether and to what extent the treatment was efficacious or, in some instances, harmful. Although some studies are done in which a new intervention is compared with data from historical controls, this type of study is subject to many potential temporal biases and, for that reason, is not often used.

In the classic double-masked (or double-blinded) trial, subjects are assigned by a random procedure to receive an experimental treatment or placebo, and neither the subject nor the investigator knows which treatment the subject is receiving. Under some circumstances, this type of trial is not possible, for a variety of reasons. It may not always be possible to conceal the treatment group from the trial participants or the investigators. For instance, trials of medical procedures may be obvious, or medications may have certain side effects. Also, there may be times when a suitable placebo is not available. Another method of randomization is to allocate treatment or interventions at a community level. One community receives the experimental treatment or intervention while another serves as the control community. Whatever the details of conducting a trial, it is critical to utilize a comparison or control population where the intervention was not applied and that is as similar to the experimental group as possible, with regard to both factors affecting the risk of disease and the measurement of the outcome. Trial study populations are often less representative of the population affected by a disease than cohort studies for two reasons. First, because the study is designed to maximize the observable differences between the treated and untreated groups, subject selection may result in a less generalizable population. Second, because the study is an intervention, the researchers must take every step to maximize the safety of the study participants. This may require that the study team choose participants who have more mild disease, or who have few other conditions. Intervention trials in infectious diseases can use various outcome measures, such as infection rates, disease rates, and progression of disease or death.

Determining the size of the trial is crucial for its ultimate success. The factors that are important in the determination of the sample size are:

- The difference in infection or disease outcome to be detected
- An estimate of the likely disease incidence in the placebo group
- Level of significance desired (the alpha or p value)
- Power of the study required (1-beta)
- Whether the significance test should be one- or two-sided

Estimating these parameters is not always easy. Infection or disease incidence in a population may not always be known. When estimates are available, they are often obtained under different conditions than will be present during a clinical trial. However, during a clinical trial, persons at lower risk may be more likely to enroll, and the incidence might be lower than predicted. Also, study subjects may not be compliant with the intervention, and the loss to follow-up may be higher than anticipated. Some trials can even be affected by competing mortality from other diseases. Furthermore, ethical considerations often mandate interventions other than the one under study, and the effects of this intervention may obscure the role of the experimental intervention.

Ethical issues have had extensive discussion and controversy in many large clinical trials of HIV/AIDS and other serious chronic infectious diseases. Nevertheless, the enormously important role played by clinical trials in evaluating treatments or preventive strategies for improving the prognosis of HIV/AIDS is acknowledged, even by those critical of the trials, though often in retrospect. Ethical questions that have arisen include the following:

- Is it ethical to use a placebo for an illness known to be serious or fatal, such as HIV/AIDS?
- To what extent should other interventions known to be effective be promoted in the subjects in a trial when the use of this intervention in the population from whom the subjects are recruited is not available, except during the trial? For example, in trials of HIV transmission in Africa, do researchers need to compare interventions that are economically feasible in the country to expensive protocols used in the United States (i.e., ACTG 076) or offer procedures not generally available in the country (i.e., advanced cancer screening or care)?
- How much promotion of condoms and safe sex counseling is required in a trial of microbicides or other interventions in countries where these services are not available outside the study protocol?
- Is it coercive and unethical to offer the "best available treatment" to trial participants when they cannot receive these treatments without participating?

Issues such as these have been considered by the World Health Organization/United Nations AIDS (UNAIDS) program, National Institutes of Health, CDC, and other organizations that fund or supervise AIDS research. Some examples of recent illustrative clinical trials are summarized below.

Perinatal HIV Transmission: Intrapartum and Single-Dose Nevirapine (HIVNET 012 Trial)

A landmark clinical trial was reported in 1994 on the use of zidovudine therapy of HIV-infected pregnant women during their last two trimesters, during labor and delivery, and in the newborn for the first 6 weeks of life to prevent maternal-fetal transmission of the virus.[54] From April 1991 through December 20, 1993, the study enrolled women from numerous clinics in the United States and France. The transmission rates from the infected mothers to their infants among the first 363 births were 8.3% (95% CI = 3.9–12.8) in the zidovudine group and 25.5% (95% CI = 18.4–32.5) in those who did not receive zidovudine, a 67.5% reduction in transmission (Figure 3-14).

Although the Adult AIDS Clinical Trial Group (ACTG) 076 regimen and a subsequently tested short-course zidovudine study were effective,[55] these regimens were beyond the economic means of many African countries, where HIV seropositivity rates in pregnant women were very high, often 30% and higher. Furthermore, HIV infection was often not identified until delivery, which is too late to start either AZT preventive strategy. Because it was not ethical to use a placebo in the study, a revised short-course AZT therapy was used in the trial.

The HIV Prevention Network initiated the HIVNET 012 trial in Kampala, Uganda.[56] Nevirapine is a nonnucleoside reverse transcriptase inhibitor that passes rapidly through the placenta. It acts more quickly than zidovudine to reduce HIV viral load and has a long half-life (median 61–64 hours in pregnant women after a single dose during labor and 45–54 hours in infants). The trial consisted of randomly assigning women to receive a single oral dose of 200 mg of nevirapine at the onset of labor and 2 mg/kg to babies within 72 hours of birth, or zidovudine 600 mg orally to mother at onset of labor and 300 mg every 3 hours until delivery and 4 mg/kg orally to babies for 7 days after birth. Nearly all infants were breast-fed. The infection rates in the infants by age 14–16 weeks was 25.1% in the zidovudine group and 13.1% in the nevirapine group, an efficacy of 47% (95% CI = 20–64) for the nevirapine regimen.

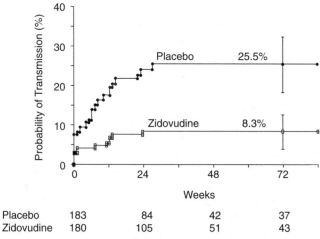

FIGURE 3-14 Kaplan Meier plots of the probability of HIV transmission according to treatment group. The estimated percentages of infants infected at 72 weeks are shown. Connor et al., Reduction of Maternal-Infant Transmission of Human Immunodeficiency Virus Type 1 with Zidovudine Treatment, *The New England Journal of Medicine*, Vol. 331, pp. 1173–1180, Copyright © 1994, Massachusetts Medical Society.

This simple, low-cost, easy-to-administer regimen of a single dose of oral nevirapine to mother and infant has revolutionized the prevention of HIV infection around the world. Its ease of use, low toxicity, and acceptability has lead to massive reductions in HIV transmission to infants even in those communities with few resources and high HIV prevalence. A cost-effectiveness analysis of this nevirapine regimen found universal treatment ratios of $138 per infant HIV infection averted and $5.25 per disability-adjusted life-year (DALY) in populations where the HIV prevalence was 30% in pregnant women (as in many countries in East and South Africa). The researchers concluded that the HIVNET 012 regimen was likely to be as cost-effective as other public health interventions, such as immunization, in developing countries.[57]

Nonoxynol 9 Film to Prevent Sexual Transmission of HIV in Cameroon

Worldwide, the most frequent means of transmission of HIV is through sexual intercourse. Although condoms are known to be highly effective in preventing the sexual transmission of HIV when used consistently and correctly, they are often not used in populations at high risk of infection. Therefore, additional means of preventing HIV transmission, especially those methods initiated and controlled by women, are needed. Vaginal microbicides, are being developed that are both virucidal for HIV and HSV, as well as bactericidal for other STD pathogens and may or may not be contraceptive. One product already in use for its contraceptive properties was the detergent Nonoxynol 9 (N-9). N-9 had been shown to be moderately effective in vivo as prophylaxis against infection by *Neisseria gonorrhoeae* and *Chlamydia trachomatis*, and vaginal infection with *Trichomonas vaginalis*.[58] However, the compound also had adverse effects; when applied to mucosal surfaces, it disrupts normal mucosa, and this could lead to increased HIV transmission. A double-blind placebo-controlled clinical trial of a film containing N-9 was done among female sex workers in Cameroon.[59] The film dissolves in 2–5 minutes, requires no applicator, is easy to use, and is not messy or affected by heat. For ethical reasons, the study made condoms available without charge to the women, and they were counseled to use them with each partner and not to assume that the film would protect them. At baseline, condoms had been used with the last client by about only 50% of the women.

The study found no difference in the rates of HIV, gonorrhea, or *C. trachomatis* infection between the N-9 and placebo groups (Table 3-9). However, one unanticipated problem emerged in the analysis of the data. Although the film was used by women in about 88% of episodes of sex with clients and 82% of sex with nonclients, the reported use of condoms also increased dramatically. Condoms were reportedly used by the women in 95% of coital episodes with clients and 83% of episodes with nonclients. Therefore, the numbers of coital events in which N-9 or placebo film only was reported to be used were quite small (Table 3-10).

This study illustrates the difficulty of doing a clinical trial of an intervention predicted to be modestly effective when the use of a more effective prevention (condoms) increases during the trial. In fact, it is not uncommon to find that the incidence of HIV or other STDs is lower due to behavior change among participants who are enrolled in a trial than was seen in the same population prior to a trial.

TABLE 3-9   Rates of HIV, Gonorrhea, and Chlamydia Infection in the Placebo and Nonoxynol 9 Group

Infection and Treatment Group	No. of Women	Woman-years	No. of Events	Event Rate*	Rate Ratio (95% CI)[†]
HIV					
Placebo	575	698	46	6.6	
Nonoxynol 9	595	720	48	6.7	1.0 (0.7–1.5)
Gonorrhea					
Placebo	435	357	111	31.1	
Nonoxynol 9	441	342	114	33.3	1.1 (0.8–1.4)
Chlamydia					
Placebo	420	365	81	22.2	
Nonoxynol 9	451	384	79	20.6	0.9 (0.7–1.3)

*The event rate is the rate per 100 woman-years.
[†]The placebo group served as the reference category. CI denotes confidence interval.
Source: Roddy et al., A Controlled Trial of Nonoxynol 9 Film to Reduce Male-to-Female Transmission. *The New England Journal of Medicine*, Vol. 339, pp. 504–510. Copyright © 1998, Massachusetts Medical Society.

TABLE 3-10   Reported Use of Condoms and Films for Vaginal Sexual Acts During the Study, According to Type of Sexual Partner

Variable	Placebo Group		Nonoxynol 9 Group	
	Client	Nonclient	Client	Nonclient
	Number (percentage)			
Use of film only	3,465 (4)	9,270 (18)	2,792 (3)	7,446 (15)
Use of condom only	11,530 (12)	6,891 (13)	9,967 (10)	5,808 (11)
Use of film and condom	77,830 (83)	33,442 (63)	83,146 (86)	35,305 (69)
Use of neither film nor condom	1,267 (1)	3,247 (6)	956 (1)	2,576 (5)
Total no. of coital acts	94,092	52,850	96,861	51,135

Source: Roddy et al., A Controlled Trial of Nonoxynol 9 Film to Reduce Male-to-Female Transmission, *The New England Journal of Medicine*, Vol. 339, pp. 504–510. Copyright © 1998, Massachusetts Medical Society.

Subsequent pathogenesis research has found that the detergent properties of N-9 are excessively disruptive to the mucosal epithelium.[60] Research is moving forward with other types of microbicides. As these are tested, the trials must be powered to accommodate unexpected problems such as differential compliance with the intervention, poor follow-up rates, and, in this example, compliance with another, more effective intervention at higher rates than were predicted.

Reduction of Malaria Transmission: Insecticide-Treated Bed Nets

In some situations, clinical trials are done in which it is more appropriate to randomize communities, rather than individuals. This is the case when the intervention is ecologic and is applied at the community level, rather than at the individual level. Clinical trials of health education using mass media are an example of such an intervention. Also, in infectious diseases with a human reservoir where transmission is person to person, an intervention targeted at decreasing the prevalence of infected persons or the duration of their infectivity would be expected to decrease the risk of new infection among individuals in the community.

A community-based randomized trial of insecticide-treated bed nets (ITN) was initiated in 1996.[61] The trial was conducted in Asembo and Gem, two rural areas of western Kenya that sit on the shores of Lake Victoria. For this trial, villages were randomized by public lottery to receive ITN or not, and then mortality and morbidity due to malaria were assessed in children up to 5 years of age. Every 6–11 months study personnel returned to the houses to re-treat the bed nets. Adherence with using the ITN was assessed by unannounced visits to the homes in the early morning, 4:30–6:30 am. To be fully adherent, children under the age of 5 years had to have their body completely covered by the hanging net. Prior to the start of the study a cross-sectional survey of the communities was conducted to assess malaria-specific morbidity and mortality. Because of the substantial burden malaria has on the health of young children, the study team included broad measures of health such as weight and diarrheal disease as well as specific markers of malaria morbidity such as anemia and parasitemia. At 14 and 22 months after deployment of the ITNs study personnel returned to the villages to conduct additional cross-sectional surveys of morbidity and mortality.

In the baseline survey 70% of children had parasitemia; however, only 4% were symptomatic with a fever. *Plamodium falciparum* accounted for the majority of cases (86.1%). A majority of the children had hemoglobin levels less than 11.0 g/dl (90%) and nearly one third (30%) had severe anemia with hemoglobin levels less than 7.0 mg/dl. The follow-up surveys found a reduction in all-cause morbidity by 14.6%, an increase in anemia by 0.5 mg/dl overall, with a corresponding decrease in severe anemia (39%) in ITN villages as compared to control villages. The prevalence of malaria parasitemia was reduced by 19% and clinical cases of malaria decreased by 44% in ITN villages when compared to control villages. Subsequent research on this population has found that ITN benefits are sustained for up to 6 years of follow-up.[62]

HIV Prevention: Reducing HIV Sexual Risk Behavior

Because sexually transmitted HIV infection occurs due to high-risk sexual behavior, interventions to reduce this risk are very important. However, designing, implementing, and evaluating behavioral intervention trials are quite difficult. Problems arise in designing an intervention to be applied to a group of high-risk people. Also, valid measurement of the reduction in risk behavior is difficult because the behavior is private and cannot be observed. Some social scientists have relied on risk behavior change reported by study subjects as an end point. However, after subjects have received extensive counseling, it may be difficult to differentiate socially desirable reporting from true reductions in high-risk behavior.

Clinical trials of behavioral change with HIV infection as an outcome have not been done frequently because of these difficulties and the large number of subjects required for such a trial. One alternative to a trial requiring HIV incidence as an end point is to measure the incidence of other STDs as a surrogate marker for HIV risk behavior because those who develop other STDs are engaged in behaviors that can result in HIV transmission if the partners are discordant for HIV infection.

Two randomized controlled clinical trials have been done recently in the United States to study the efficacy of a standardized behavioral intervention to prevent sexually transmitted HIV; incident STDs and reported high-risk behaviors were the end points. These are the NIMH Multisite HIV Prevention Trial[63] and Project Respect, a CDC multisite trial.[64] The results of the NIMH trial are described here.

In the NIMH trial, 3706 sexually active adults were recruited from 37 clinics in the United States.[65] Participants were HIV-negative persons who had recently engaged in high-risk sexual behavior, as evidenced by unprotected high-risk vaginal or anal sex in the past 90 days with a new partner, more than one partner, an injection drug user, or a person infected with HIV. Participants were then assigned randomly to the control counseling group ($N = 1855$) or the intensive behavioral counseling group ($N = 1851$). Controls received a single 1-hour AIDS education session. Those in the intervention group received seven 90- to 120-minute HIV risk-reduction counseling sessions. Reported condom use increased above baseline in both the intervention and control groups at 3 months. However, there was a 47% greater increase in reported condom use in the intervention group, which persisted for 12 months. Overall, the rates of reported STDs were not different in the two groups. However, in the participants recruited from an STD clinic, the rates of newly diagnosed gonorrhea in the intervention group was half that of the rate in the control group. Incident HIV was not studied in this population.

Special Issues

Agent and Host Factors in Infectious Diseases

Infectious diseases differ somewhat from those with noninfectious etiologies, in that there is biologic variation in either the host or the agent—or both—that can influence the natural history of and susceptibility to infection. Furthermore, it is often of importance to detect less virulent or avirulent infectious agents that share characteristics of the virulent wild-type agent, because this information could lead to the development of a preventive vaccine. The classic example of this was Jenner's discovery that immunity to vaccinia (the cowpox virus) was protective against human smallpox. Some examples of infectious disease studies designed to differentiate host and agent factors that influence the natural history of infectious diseases are reviewed here: first, a study of HIV/AIDS that illustrates how research can be targeted specifically to evaluate the role of the infecting organism in the natural history of a disease, and second, twin studies and other genetic studies that demonstrate the role of host susceptibility in the natural history of a disease.

Transfusion-Transmitted HIV Infection

One situation in which the natural history of an infection can be studied in two or more persons infected with the same agent is transfusion-transmitted HIV infection. When more than one person has been transfused with blood from the same donor, the recipients have been challenged with the same inoculum. Furthermore, because the exact date of the infection is known in the transfused patients, the rate of progression can be accurately determined. The CDC studied 694 recipients of transfused blood from 112 donors who later developed AIDS and from 31 donors later found to be positive for the HIV antibody.[66] These donors had given blood prior to the availability of an HIV antibody test to screen donors.

The rate of disease progression in the transfusion recipients was compared with the donor's rate of progression. Among the recipients of blood from donors who developed AIDS within 29 months of their donations (group 1), 49% developed AIDS within 4 years, compared with 4% of those receiving blood from donors who had not developed AIDS by 29 months after their donations (group 2). Furthermore, among those who developed AIDS, progression was more rapid in group 1, compared with group 2 recipients (Figure 3-15). These data suggested that viral characteristics (possibly visal load) may be important in the rate of HIV progression after infection, because the

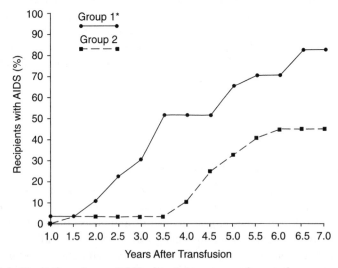

FIGURE 3-15 Progression to AIDS of recipients, according to donor group. AIDS developed in Group 1 donors within 29 months of donation and in Group 2 donors 29 months or more after donation. The asterisk denotes a significant difference between groups (P = 0.005). J.W. Ward et al., The Natural History of Transfusion-Associated Infection with Human Immunodeficiency Virus-Factors Influencing the Rate of Progression to Disease, *The New England Journal of Medicine.* Vol. 321, pp. 947–952. Copyright © 1989, Massachusetts Medical Society.

recipients of blood from rapidly progressing donors also progressed rapidly, and vice versa.[65]

Twin Studies

Several studies have been reported of the natural history of infectious diseases in twins. By comparing monozygotic with dizygotic twins to other control populations, it is possible to evaluate the role of host genetics in the immune response and natural history of an infection. The differences in the natural history of infection between monozygotic twin pairs and dizygotic twin pairs could reflect the role of the genetically controlled immune response of the host because environmental and agent differences would be minimized between same-age siblings. Susceptibility of humans to tuberculosis and leprosy have both been studied among monozygotic and dizygotic twins. One of the most extensive twin studies of tuberculosis was done by Dr. Barbara Simmons in London.[65] This study evaluated 202 twins of patients with tuberculosis in whom the zygosity could be determined. The concordance for tuberculosis infection was over twofold higher in monozygotic twins compared with dizygotic twins, indicating that there was important host genetic susceptibility. A similar study of leprosy was done by Chakravarti and Vogel.[67] This study enrolled 62 monozygotic and 40 dizygotic twin pairs. These investigators found a significantly increased rate of leprosy in the opposite twin when the twins were monozygotic, compared with those who were dizygotic. Also, in cases where both twins had leprosy, the type of leprosy, tuberculoid or lepromatous, was more likely to be concordant if the pair was monozygotic. Again, the similar risk of disease and similarities in the type of disease indicated that there was a genetic component that was important in determining susceptibility to leprosy.

Other Genetic Studies

The sequence of the human genome was completed ahead of schedule in 2003.[68] This achievement has burst open new opportunities in genetic evaluations. The technical advances of the field of genetics now allow for rapid and relatively inexpensive evaluations of multiple genes in many persons. This has expanded our capacity to explore differences in genetics and the expression genes between people. Research has moved forward in evaluating differences in the sequence of genes between people. These different gene alleles have varying risk of disease. In addition to the 30,000 genes now believed to be coded by the human genome, there are large stretches of DNA that do not code for specific gene products but which are crucial in determining the expression of genes near them. Variations in these regulatory regions have also been found to be important in determining disease risk. Fundamentally, genes code for proteins and the expression of genes is the phenotype of an individual. Many genes are not present in a single copy but may have multiple copies in a genome. Copy number has recently been correlated with the risk of progression with HIV. And lastly, the field of proteomics is studying the phenotypic expression of genes—what proteins are actually produced and when. These studies are rapidly widening our understanding of immunology and genetic variation in susceptibility to disease.

HLA Studies

Several studies have been done of the association of HLA markers with infectious diseases. HLA genetic diversity is the basis of the adaptive immune system and is the most highly polymorphic biologic system known. The polymorphism is driven by the underlying HLA type, and there are biologic and ethnic variations in the distribution of HLA frequencies. These differential distributions arose from the evolutionary pressure of previous epidemics that selected resistant genotypes. Some HLA types are strongly associated with several diseases, such as B27 with ankylosing spondylitis, DR4 with rheumatoid arthritis, and DR3 with chronic hepatitis.[69] HIV progression has also been associated with several HLA polymorphisms.[70-73]

Research has also been done on genetic variability in important genes that interact with pathogens. Notably, the gene mutation that causes sickle cell anemia also makes red cells resistant to *P. falciparum* malaria. Despite the detrimental effect of sickle cell on survival, this gene has persisted in populations that are also under evolutionary pressure from *P. falciparum* malaria because of the malaria protection it affords to those who are heterozygous.[74]

Genetic Mutation in HIV Receptors

The primary receptor for HIV-1 is the CD4 surface molecule expressed on the surface of T helper cells. However, fusion and cell entry is mediated by a second receptor. It was found recently that several chemokines, MIP-1 alpha, MIP-1 beta, and RANTES, suppressed infection by macrophage tropic isolates of HIV-1.[75] Subsequently, it was discovered that the cell receptor for these chemokines, CCR5, was the second receptor for fusion and entry of macrophage-tropic isolates of HIV-1 into cells.[76] Several investigators discovered that individuals who were homozygous for a 32 base pair deletion in the CCR5 molecule were resistant to infection with macrophage-tropic isolates.[77,78] Furthermore, individuals who were heterozygous for this deletion, although they were susceptible to infection, had slower progression of HIV disease after they were infected.[79,80] Subsequent to this it has been shown that the number of copies of some genes alters an individual's risk of disease. Gonzalez et al. measured the impact of the number of copies of the gene that codes for MIP-1alphaP on HIV progression.[81] This protein can block HIV-1 from entering the cell by engaging with the CCR5 receptor and directly interfering with HIV binding. They found that the lower the copy number of the CCL3L1 gene the greater the risk of disease progression. In this study, the impact of the copy number of CCL3L1 was at least as strong as the CCR5 gene itself, and the disease-accelerating influence of CCR5 variation was dependent upon CCL3L1. The research on CCR5 and its ligands depended on having populations of participants in whom the natural history of HIV disease was well documented. To evaluate differences in infectivity and survival, it was necessary to have populations of HIV-negative persons who were at risk and to follow them to know which genetic profiles were associated with susceptibility or resistance, and then to measure the length of time from HIV seroconversion to the development of AIDS or death. Furthermore, these cohort studies needed to have a wide diversity of genetics to ensure that genetic polymorphisms could be adequately studied.

Meta-Analysis

A meta-analysis is a statistical analysis of a collection of studies, especially an analysis in which studies are the primary units of analysis. Meta-analysis has been used commonly by epidemiologists to synthesize data for which there is controversy between various studies or sometimes to arrive at an overall summary estimate of a relationship when individual studies are under-powered. Some of the problems with meta-analysis include the effects of publication bias that can occur when negative studies aren't published. Also the combined analysis of data from studies in which the exposure measurements or outcomes are significantly different may not clarify an association but lead to erroneous conclusions.

A Meta-Analysis of Mortality Associated with Vancomycin-Resistant and Vancomycin-Sensitive Enterococcal (VSE) Blood Streams Infections

Enterococcal infections have emerged as the third or fourth most frequent cause of nosocomial blood stream infections in hospitalized patients in the United States.[82] Also the prevalence of vancomycin-resistance has increased to 14–25% of all nosocomial enterococcal bacteremic strains. In 1995, the CDC published guidelines to prevent transmission of vancomycin-resistant enterococci (VRE), and several pharmaceutical firms are developing anti-biotics to use against VRE. However, some clinicians have argued that VRE strains are not commonly virulent and have questioned whether they should be given special attention. Therefore, a meta-analysis of the mortality rates associated with vancomycin-resistant (VR) compared to vancomycin-sensitive (VS) enterococcal nosocomial bacteremia was done (Figure 3-16). All articles listed in the MEDLINE database from January 1988 through March 2003 were identified, as well as those in the Cochrane Library through March 2003. Studies were included if they assessed mortality after enterococcal blood stream infection (BSI), compared mortality after VRE BSI with VSE BSI, and adjusted for underlying severity of illness. Individual study validity was assessed, with attention to selection bias and misclassification bias.

Of 114 studies, 9 met the inclusion criteria. All of the 9 studies found a significant increased OR for mortality associated with VRE BSI compared to VSE BSI; however, the 95% confidence interval of 3 studies overlapped (Figure 3-16).[82]

Efficacy of BCG Vaccine in the Prevention of Tuberculosis—A Meta-Analysis of the Published Literature

BCG vaccine is one of the oldest and most frequently used vaccines through-out the world. It is included as one of the routine vaccines in the expanded program on immunization (EPI) in most developing countries. However, the efficacy of BCG in the prevention of tuberculosis has been uncertain and quite variable; efficacy has varied from 80% to 0%. Therefore, a meta-analysis of reported studies was published in 1994.[83] In this study MEDLINE was reviewed for published papers on BCG vaccine efficacy. Also tuberculosis experts at WHO and CDC were consulted to find unpublished studies. A total of 1264 articles or abstracts were reviewed, and 14 prospective trials and 12

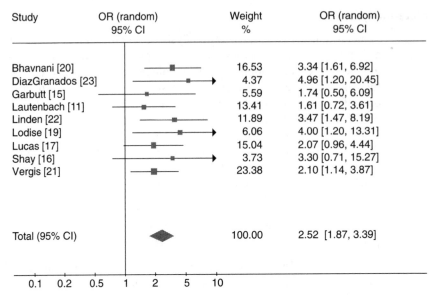

Study	OR (random) 95% CI	Weight %	OR (random) 95% CI
Bhavnani [20]		16.53	3.34 [1.61, 6.92]
DiazGranados [23]		4.37	4.96 [1.20, 20.45]
Garbutt [15]		5.59	1.74 [0.50, 6.09]
Lautenbach [11]		13.41	1.61 [0.72, 3.61]
Linden [22]		11.89	3.47 [1.47, 8.19]
Lodise [19]		6.06	4.00 [1.20, 13.31]
Lucas [17]		15.04	2.07 [0.96, 4.44]
Shay [16]		3.73	3.30 [0.71, 15.27]
Vergis [21]		23.38	2.10 [1.14, 3.87]
Total (95% CI)		100.00	2.52 [1.87, 3.39]

0.1 0.2 0.5 1 2 5 10

FIGURE 3-16 Meta-analysis plot using a random effects model. The dots represent the point estimates for the measure of effect of each study. The horizontal lines represent the 95% CIs for each study. The rhomboidal figure represents the summary measure and 95% CI. The right column shows the numeric values for each study and summary measure.
Source: Diaz Grandos CA, Zimmer SM, Klein M and Jernigan JA. Comparison of mortality associated with Vancomycin-resistant and Vancomycin-susceptible enterococcal bloodstream infections: A meta-analysis. *Clin Infect Dis* 2005; 41:327–333. Copyright University of Chicago Press.

case-control studies were included in the analysis. In the clinical trials the RR for tuberculosis was 0.44 (95% CI, 0.34–0.70), and in the case-control studies the OR for tuberculosis was 0.50 (95% CI, 0.39–0.64). Seven trials reporting tuberculosis deaths showed a protective efficacy of BCG vaccine of 71% (RR = 0.29; 95% CI, 0.16–0.53) and five studies showed a protective effect for meningitis of 64% (RR = 0.36; 95% CI, 0.18–0.70). Geographic latitude of the study site and study validity explained 66% of the heterogeneity among trials in a random effects regression model.

The conclusions from this meta-analysis are debated by some experts. The trials of BCG have produced highly variable results in different populations and times. Generally, BCG vaccine has been found to be less protective in tropical populations, such as Puerto Rico and Madras, India, than in temperate areas. One hypothesis to explain this variability is that nontuberculous mycobacteria may be more common in the tropics and either interfere with BCG vaccine immune protection or confer some immunity among controls in tropical populations. Second, and more important, is that the BCG vaccines used in these trials all were different from each other. Therefore, the same BCG strain was not used in each of the studies included in the meta-analysis. The initial BCG vaccine was developed in 1921 by Calmette and Guiren after 230 in vitro passages. However, no stock BCG culture was established. Instead, the vaccine has undergone over 1000 subsequent passages. Behr and Small have shown a reduction in BCG efficacy over time.[84] Also, they have shown the *M. bovis* BCG organism has lost important genes, which may have conferred

TABLE 3-11 Vaccine Efficacy and Vaccine Attributable Incidence

Efficacy	$= \dfrac{\text{Ic} - \text{Iv}}{\text{Ic}}$	= **(relative difference)**
		= % of cases prevented
	$= \dfrac{120 - 10}{120}$	= 92%
"Probe study"	= **Ic − Iv**	= **(absolute difference)** = vaccine-preventable disease incidence
	= 120 − 10	= 110/100,000

Notes: Ic = incidence/10^5 control group; Iv = incidence/10^5 vaccine group.

efficacy in earlier vaccines that no longer exist in the current BCG vaccines.[85] Finally, the effect of the HIV pandemic on increasing the risk of tuberculosis has probably overwhelmed any protective efficacy of BCG.

Vaccines Used as Probes to Assess Infectious Diseases*

A standard vaccine efficacy trial measures disease to learn about the vaccine efficacy. A vaccine probe study uses a vaccine of known efficacy to estimate disease incidence. In summary, the intent of the two types of studies is reversed, but the methods are similar.

A vaccine probe study must be done with a proven well-characterized vaccine with known efficacy in the prevention of standard clinical outcomes. Like a vaccine efficacy trial, the probe trial needs careful randomization between vaccinees and controls, blinding or masking of participants to the intervention, high-quality nondifferential surveillance in both study groups, standard disease definitions with well-characterized specificity, and of course, an adequate sample size.

Vaccine efficacy is usually expressed as a *relative difference* or percentage reduction between the placebo group and the vaccine group. In a probe study to determine disease burden, one can calculate both the relative and *absolute difference* in incidence between the two groups.

The study incidence difference is the measurement of the incidence of vaccine-prevented cases or *vaccine-prevented incidence (VPI)* and is a pragmatic direct measure of the effect of vaccine, in the local setting, without concern for variable and often insensitive microbiological estimates. VPI also incorporates all the local effects of immune response, vaccine storage and handling, the actual age of immunization, and other local variations. It has an understandable direct application for local policy. In the example in Table 3-11, the VPI would be 110/100,000, or approximately 1 case prevented for every 1000 immunized children.

One of the oldest examples of this kind of assessment was a reanalysis of a cholera vaccine trial in Bangladesh. The original trial evaluated a cholera vaccine with a tetanus toxoid vaccine as a control. The reanalysis evaluated mortality in children of women who received tetanus toxoid vaccine

---

*This section contributed by Mark C. Steinhoff

compared with the children of women who received the cholera vaccine. Deaths in the 0 to 28 day neonatal period were reduced by 50%. Earlier surveillance had not revealed that tetanus was responsible for so high a proportion of infant deaths.[86]

For example, influenza vaccine is 60% to 90% effective in reducing culture-proven influenza illness. A series of recent influenza vaccine trials has shown a relatively high proportion of clinical illnesses are prevented by influenza vaccine (in addition to confirming the high level of efficacy against lab-proven influenza). For example clinically diagnosed otitis media in children in day care was reduced by 84%.[87] Similar flu vaccine studies in adults have shown an approximately 20% reduction in all febrile respiratory illness and a ~36% reduction of absenteeism from work.[88] A study among health care workers showed that use of influenza vaccine averted 11 days of sick leave during the winter season for every 100 persons immunized, another version of VPI.[89]

Several recent studies of *Haemophilus influenza* type B (Hib) vaccine has shown its effectiveness in reduction of laboratory-confirmed Hib meningitis and blood culture-positive Hib pneumonia. The new data related to analyses of the reduction of clinical syndromes suggest that use of Hib vaccine reduces hospitalized severe pneumonia by approximately 20% in the Gambia and approximately 4% in Indonesia.[90,91] In contrast, when analyzed for the absolute reduction of illness, the incidence per 100,000 of vaccine-preventable clinically severe pneumonia was estimated at 83 in children under 5 years in the Gambia and 264 in children under 2 years in Indonesia. These rates of Hib vaccine-preventable severe pneumonia are far higher than rates previously estimated by standard blood culture studies and are likely a better measure of disease burden. Similarly in a prospective trial the incidence of laboratory-proven Hib meningitis in control group children younger than 2 years in Indonesia was 19/100,000. However, the use of Hib vaccine prevented 67/100,000 meningitis cases in children admitted to hospital with lumbar puncture. These data on Hib vaccine-prevented meningitis cases suggest that only 28% of all Hib meningitis cases were detected through routine hospital surveillance and standard culture techniques, again showing the true burden of vaccine-preventable illness.

The use of vaccines with careful analysis of their effect can provide substantial new information regarding the full spectrum of morbidity associated with specific vaccine-preventable agents.[92,93]

References

1. Miller L. Impact of malaria on genetic polymorphism and genetic disease in Africans and African Americans. In: Roisman B, ed. *Infectious Disease in an Age of Change. The Impact of Human Ecology and Behavior on Disease Transmission.* Washington, DC: National Academies Press; 1995:99–111.
2. Glezen WP, Couch RB, Taber LH. Epidemiologic observations on influenza B virus infections in Houston, Texas, 1976–1977. *Am J Epidemiol* January 1980; 111(1):13–22.
3. Rothman G, Greenland S. *Modern Epidemiology.* New York, NY: Lippincott-Raven; 1998.

4. Diggle P, Liang K-Y, Zeger S. *Analysis of Longitudinal Data*. Oxford, England: Clareden Press; 1994.

5. Rupprecht CE, Gibbons RU, Prophylaxis against rabies. *NEJM*. 2004;351:2626–2635.

6. Constantine D. Rabies transmission by non-bite route. *Public Health Rep*. 1962;77:287–291.

7. Hronovsky V, Benda R. Development of inhalation rabies infection in suckling guinea pigs. *Acta Virol*. 1969;13:198–202.

8. Hronovsky G, Benda R. Experimental inhalation of infection of laboratory rodents with rabies virus. *Acta Virol*. 1969;13:193–197.

9. Noah D, Drezik C, Smith J, et al. Epidemiology of human rabies in the United States. *Ann Intern Med*. 1998;128:922–930.

10. Hattwick M, Weis T, Stechschulte J, Baer GM, Gregg M. Recovery from rabies, a case report. *Ann Intern Med*. 1972;76:931–942.

11. Centers for Disease Control and Prevention. Recovery of a patient from clinical rabies—Wisconsin, 2004. *MMWR*. 2004;53:1171–1173.

12. Willoughly RE Jr, Tieves KS, Hoffman GM, et al. Survival after treatment of rabies with induction of coma. *N Engl J Med*. 2005;352:2508–2514.

13. Luckhart BP, Tordo N, Tsiang H. Inhibition of rabies virus transcription in rat cortical neurons with the dissociative anesthetic ketamine. *Antimicrob Agents Chemother*. 1992;36:1750–1755.

14. Bryceson Y, Pang S, Wei L, et al. Clearance of HIV infection in a perinatally infected infant. *N Engl J Med*. 1995;332:833–838.

15. Sahu GK, McNearney T, Evans A, et al. Transient or occult HIV infections may occur more frequently than progressive infections: changing the paradigm about HIV persistence. *Arch Virol*. 2005;19 (Suppl):131–145.

16. Altfeld M, Allen TM, Yu XG, et al. HIV-1 superinfection despite broad CD8 T-cell responses containing replication of the primary virus. *Nature*. 2002;420:434–439.

17. Auerbach D, Darrow W, Jaffe H, et al. Cluster of cases of the acquired immune deficiency syndrome. Patients linked by sexual contact. *Am J Med*. 1984;76:487–492.

18. Kass E. Infectious disease and social change. *J Infect Dis*. 1971;123:110–114.

19. Cook L, Koutsky L, Holmes K. Circumcision and sexually transmitted diseases. *Am J Public Health*. 1994;84:197–201.

20. Moses S, Bradley J, Hagelkerke N, et al. Geographical patterns of male circumcision practices in Africa: association with HIV seroprevalence. *Int J Epidemiol*. 1990;19:693–697.

21. Breslow NE, Day NE. *Statistical Methods in Cancer Research: The Analysis of Case-Control Studies*. Lyon, France: International Agency for Research on Cancer; 1980:1.

22. Brookmeyer R, Gail MH. *AIDS Epidemiology: A Quantitative Approach*. New York, NY: Oxford University Press; 1994.

23. Nelson K, Celentano D, Eiumtrakol S, et al. Changes in sexual behavior and a decline in HIV infection among young men in Thailand. *N Engl J Med*. 1996;335:297–303.

24. Kaslow R, Ostrow D, Detels R, et al. The Multicenter AIDS Cohort Study: rationale, organization, and selected characteristics of the participants. *Am J Epidemiol*. 1987;126:310–318.

25. Barkan S, Melnick S, Preston-Martin S, et al. The Women's Interagency HIV Study. WIHS Collaborative Study Group. *Epidemiology*. 1998;9:117–125.

26. Palefsky J, Minkoff H, Kalish L. Cervicovaginal human papillomavirus infection in human immunodeficiency virus-1 (HIV)-positive and high risk HIV-negative women. *J Natl Cancer Inst.* 1999;91:226–236.

27. Jaffe H, Choi K, Thomas P, et al. National case-control study of Kaposi's sarcoma and *Pneumocystis carinii* pneumonia in homosexual men. 1. Epidemiologic results. *Ann Intern Med.* 1983;99:145–151.

28. Curren JW. The epidemiology and prevention of the acquired immunodeficiency syndrome. *Ann Intern Med.* 1985;103:657–662.

29. deShazo R, Andes W, Nordberg J, et al. An immunologic evaluation of hemophiliac patients and their wives. *Ann Intern Med.* 1983;99:159–164.

30. Starko K, Ray C, Domingues L, et al. Reye's syndrome and salicylate use. *Pediatrics.* 1980;66:859–864.

31. Waldman R, Hall W, McGeeh H, et al. Aspirin as a risk factor in Reye's syndrome. *JAMA.* 1982;247:3089–3094.

32. Halpin T, Holtzhauer F, Campbell R, et al. Reye's syndrome and medication use. *JAMA.* 1982;248:687–691.

33. Pinsky P, Hurwitz E, Schonberger L, et al. Reye's syndrome and aspirin. Evidence for a dose-response effect. *JAMA* 1988;260:657–661.

34. Centers for Disease Control and Prevention. Surgeon General's advisory on the use of salicylates and Reye's syndrome. *MMWR.* 31(22):289–290.

35. Belay E, Bresee J, Holman R, et al. Reye's syndrome in the United States from 1981–1987. *N Engl J Med.* 1999;340:1377–1382.

36. Mueller N, Evans A, Harris N, et al. Hodgkin's disease and Epstein-Barr virus. Altered antibody pattern before diagnosis. *N Engl J Med.* 1989;320:689–695.

37. Chang Y, Cesarman E, Pessin M, et al. Identification of herpesvirus-like DNA sequences in AIDS-associated Kaposi's sarcoma. *Science.* 1994;266:1865–1969.

38. O'Brien T, Kedes D, Ganem D, et al. Evidence for concurrent epidemics of human herpesvirus 8 and human immunodeficiency virus type 1 in US homosexual men: rates, risk factors, and relationship to Kaposi's sarcoma. *J Infect Dis.* 1999;180:1010–1017.

39. Jacobson L, Yamashita T, Detels R, et al. Impact of potent antiretroviral therapy on the incidence of Kaposi's sarcoma and non-Hodgkin's lymphomas among HIV-1-infected individuals. Multicenter AIDS Cohort Study. *J AIDS.* 1999(suppl 1):S34–S41.

40. Dore G, Li Y, Grulich A, et al. Declining incidence and later occurrence of Kaposi's sarcoma among persons with AIDS in Australia: the Australian AIDS cohort. *AIDS.* 1996;10:1401–1406.

41. Centers for Disease Control and Prevention. Case-control study of HIV seroconversion in health care workers after percutaneous exposure to HIV-infected blood—France, United Kingdom, and United States, January 1988-August 1994. *MMWR.* 1995;44:929–931.

42. Gerberding J. Incidence and prevalence of human immunodeficiency virus, hepatitis B virus, hepatitis C virus, and cytomeglovirus among healthcare personnel at risk for blood exposure and final report studies. *J Infect Dis.* 1994;170:1410–1417.

43. Glezen W. Serious morbidity and mortality associated with influenza. *Epidemiol Rev.* 1982;4:25–44.

44. Turner C, Ku L, Riogers S, et al. Adolescent sexual behavior, drug use, and violence: increased reporting with computer survey technology. *Science.* 1998;280:867–873.

45. Zieger SL, Liang KY. Longitudinal data analysis for discrete and continous outcomes. *Biometrics.* 1986;42:121–130.

46. Graham N, Zeger S, Park L, et al. The effects on survival of early treatment of human immunodeficiency virus infection. *N Engl J Med.* 1992;326:1037–1042.
47. Graham N, Hoover D, Park L, et al. Survival in HIV-infected patients who have received zidovudine: comparison of combination therapy with sequential monotherapy and continued zidovudine monotherapy. Multicenter AIDS Cohort Study Group. *Ann Intern Med.* 1996;124:1031–1038.
48. Nelson K, Vlahov D, Solomon L, et al. Temporal trends of incident human immunodeficiency virus infection of injecting drug users in Baltimore, MD. *Arch Intern Med.* 1995;155:1305–1311.
49. Mellors J, Munoz A, Giorgi J, et al. Plasma viral load and CD4$^+$ lymphocytes as prognostic markers of HIV-1 infection. *Ann Intern Med.* 1997;126:946–954.
50. Schnieder MF, Gange SJ, Williams CF, et al. Patterns of the hazard of death after acquired immunodeficiency syndrome through the evolution of antiretroviral therapy: 1984–2004. *AIDS.* Nov 18 2005;19(17):2009–2018.
51. Ahdieh L, Munoz A, Vlahov D, et al. Cervical neoplasia and repeated positivity of HPV infection in HIV seropositive and HIV seronegative women. *Am J Epidemiol.* Jun 2000;151:1148–1157.
52. Piantadosis S. *Clinical Trials, a Methodologic Perspective.* New York, NY: John Wiley & Sons; 1997.
53. Meinert CL. *Clinical Trials: Design, Conduct, and Analysis.* New York, NY: Oxford University Press; 1986.
54. Connor E, Sperling R, Gelber R, et al. Reduction of maternal-infant transmission of human immunodeficiency virus type 1 with zidovudine treatment. Pediatric AIDS Clinical Trials Group Protocol 076 Study Group. *N Engl J Med.* 1994;331:1173–1180.
55. Shaffer N, Chuachoowong R, Mock P, et al. Short-course zidovudine for perinatal HIV-1 transmission in Bangkok, Thailand: a randomised controlled trial. Bangkok Collaborative Perinatal HIV Transmission Study Group. *Lancet.* 1999;353:773–780.
56. Guay L, Musoke P, Fleming T, et al. Intrapartum and neonatal single-dose nevirapine compared with zidovudine for prevention of mother-to-child transmission of HIV-1 in Kampala, Uganda: HIVNET 012 randomized trial. *Lancet.* 1999;354:795–802.
57. Marseille E, Kahn J, Mmiro F, et al. Cost effectiveness of single-dose nevirapine regimen for mothers and babies to decrease vertical HIV-1 transmission in sub-Saharan Africa. *Lancet.* 1999;354:803–809.
58. Louv W, Austin H, Alexander W, et al. A clinical trial of nonoxynol-9 for preventing gonococcal and chlamydial infections. *J Infect Dis.* 1988;158:518–523.
59. Roddy R, Zeking L, Ryan K, et al. A controlled trial of nonoxynol-9 film to reduce male-to-female transmission of sexually transmitted diseases. *N Engl J Med.* 1998;339:504–510.
60. Hillier SL, Moench T, Shattock R, Black R, Reichelderfer P, Veronese F. In vivo: the story of nonoxynol 9. *J Acquir Immune Defic Syndr.* 2005;39:1–8.
61. Lindblade KA, Eisele TP, Gimnig JE, et al. Impact of permethrin-treated bed nets on malaria and all-cause morbidity in young children in an area of intense perennial malaria transmission in western Kenya: cross-sectional survey. *Am J Trop Med Hyg.* 2003;68(4 suppl): 100–107.

62. Linblade K, Eisele TP, Gimnig JE, et al. All sustainability of reductions in malaria transmission and infant mortality in western Kenya with use of insecticide-treated bednets: 4 to 6 years of follow-up. *JAMA*. 2004;291:2571–2580.

63. The NIMH Multisite HIV Prevention Trial: reducing HIV sexual risk behavior. *Science*. 1998;280:1889–1894.

64. Kamb M, Fishbein M, Douglas J Jr, et al. Efficacy of risk-reduction counseling to prevent human immunodeficiency virus and sexually transmitted diseases: a randomized controlled trial. Project RESPECT Study Group. *JAMA*. 1998;280:1161–1167.

65. Comstock G. Tuberculosis in twins: a re-analysis of the Prophit survey. *Am Rev Respir Dis*. 1978;117:621–624.

66. Ward J, Bush T, Perkins H, et al. The natural history of transfusion-associated infection with human immunodeficiency virus. Factors influencing the rate of progression to disease. *N Engl J Med*. 1989;321:947–952.

67. Fine P. Leprosy: the epidemiology of a slow bacterium. *Epidemiol Rev*. 1982;4:161–188.

68 The genome international sequencing consortium: initial sequencing and analysis of the human genome. *Nature*. 2001;409:860–921.

69. Leffell MS, Donnenberg AD, Rose NR. *Handbook of Human Immunology*. Boca Raton, FL: CRC Press; 1997.

70. Kaslow R, Carrington M, Apple R, et al. Influence of combinations of human major histocompatibility complex genes on the course of HIV-1 infection. *Nature Med*. 1996;2:405–411.

71. Just J. Genetic predisposition of HIV-1 infection and acquired immune deficiency virus syndrome. A review of the literature examining associations with HLA. *Hum Immunol*. 1995;44:156–169.

72. Tang J, Costello C, Keet I, et al. HLA class I homozygosity accelerates disease progression in human immunodeficiency virus type 1 infection. *AIDS Res Hum Retrovirus*. 1999;15:317–324.

73. Carrington M, Nelson G, Martin M, et al. HLA and HIV-1: heterozygote advantage and B*35-Cw*04 disadvantage. *Science*. 1999;283: 1748–1752.

74. Miller LH. Impact of malaria on genetic polymorphism and genetic diseases in Africans and African Americans. *Proc Nat/Acad Sci*. 1994;91:2415–2419.

75. Cocchi F, DeVico A, Garzino-Demo A, et al. Identification of RANTES, MIP-1 alpha, and MIP-1 beta as the major HIV-suppressive factors produced by CD8+ T cells. *Science*. 1995;270:1811–1815.

76. Alkhatib G, Combadiere C, Broder C, et al. CC CKR5: a RANTES MIP-1-alpha, MIP-1-beta receptor as a fusion cofactor for macrophage-trophic HIV-1. *Science*. 1996;272:1955–1958.

77. Huang Y, Paxton W, Wolinsky S, et al. The role of a mutant CCR5 allele in HIV-1 transmission and disease progression. *Nature Med*. 1996;2:1240–1243.

78. Michael NL, Chang G, Louie LG, et al. The role of viral phenotype and CCR-5 gene defects in HIV-1 transmission and disease progression. *Nat Med*. 1997 March;3(3):338–340.

79. Dean M, Carrington M, Winkler C, et al. Genetic restriction of HIV-1 infection and progression to AIDS by a deletion allele of the CKR5 structural gene. Hemophilia Growth and Development Study, Multicenter AIDS Cohort Study, Multicenter Hemophilia Cohort Study, San Francisco City Cohort, ALIVE Study. *Science*. 1996;273:1856–1862.

80. Zimmerman PA, Buckler-White A, Alkhatib G, et al. Inherited resistance to HIV-1 conferred by an inactivating mutation in CC chemoking receptor 5: studies in populations with contrasting clinical phenotypes, defined racial backdground, and quantified risk. *Mol Med.* 1997 January;3(1):23–36.

81. Gonzalez G, Kulkarni H, Bolivar H, et al. The influence of CCL3L1 gene-containing segmental duplications on HIV-1/AIDS susceptibility. *Science.* 2005;307:1434–1440.

82. DiazGrandos CA, Zimmer SM, Klein M, Jernigan JA. Comparison of mortality associated with vancomycin-resistant and vancomycin-susceptible enterococcal bloodstream infections: a meta-analysis. *Clin Infect Dis.* 2005;41:327–333.

83. Colditz GA, Brewer TF, Berkey CS, et al. Efficacy of BCG vaccine in the prevention of tuberculosis: meta-analysis of the published literature. *JAMA.* 1994;271:698–702.

84. Behr MA, Wilson MA, Gill WP, et al. Comparative genomics of BCG vaccines by whole-genome DNA microarray. *Science.* 1999;284:1520–1523.

85. Behr MA, Wilson MA, Gill WP, et al. Comparative genomics of BCG vaccines by whole-genome DNA microarray. *Science.* 1999;284: 1520–1523.

86. Black RE, Huber DH, Curlin GT. Reduction of neonatal tetanus by mass immunization of non-pregnant women: duration of protection provided by 1 or 2 doses of alumi-num-absorbed tetanus toxoid. *Bull WHO.* 1980;58:927–930.

87. Clements DA, Langdon L, Bland C, et al. Influenza A vaccine decreases the incidence of otitis media in 6- to 30-month-old children in day care. *Arch Pediatr Adolesc Med.* 1995;149:1113–1117.

88. Nichol KL, Lind A, Margolis KL, et al. The effectiveness of vaccination against influenzae in healthy, working adults. *N Engl J Med.* 1995;333:889–893.

89. Wilde JA, McMillan J, Serwint J, et al. Effectiveness of influenza vaccine in health care professionals: a randomized controlled trial. *JAMA.* 1999;281:908–913.

90. Mulholland K, Hilton S, Adegbola R, et al. Randomised trial of *Haemophilus influenzae* type-b tetanus protein conjugate vaccine [corrected] for prevention of pneumonia and meningitis in Gambian infants. *Lancet.* 1997;349:1191–1197.

91. Gessner BD, Sutanto A, Linehan M, et al. Incidence of vaccine-preventable *Haemophilus influenzae* type b pneumonia and meningitis in Indonesian children: hamlet-randomized vaccine-probe trial. *Lancet.* 2005;365:43–52.

92. Orenstein WA, Bernier RH, Hinman AR. Assessing vaccine efficacy in the field: further observations. *Epidemiol Rev.* 1988;10:212–241.

93. Clemens J, Brenner R, Rao M, Tafari N, Lowe C. Evaluating new vaccines for developing countries. Efficacy or effectiveness? *JAMA.* 1996;275:390–397.

CHAPTER FOUR

SURVEILLANCE

Kenrad E. Nelson and Frangiscos Sifakis

Introduction

Surveillance of infectious diseases is the continuous systematic collection of data on illness or infections in a defined population to monitor the incidence or prevalence of a disease or a behavior that is placing people at risk of disease or ill health. Although surveillance originally focused on infectious diseases, especially the major epidemic conditions, the activity has been broadened to include noninfectious diseases, such as cancer, heart disease, renal disease, and strokes. More recently, routine surveillance data have been collected on risk factors, disability, behavior, and health practices.

The Centers for Disease Control and Prevention (CDC) in 1986 defined *epidemiologic surveillance* as follows:[1,2]

> Epidemiologic surveillance is the ongoing systematic collection, analysis, and interpretation of health data essential to the planning, implementation, and evaluation of public health practice, closely integrated with the timely dissemination of these data to those who need to know. The final link in the surveillance chain is the application of these data to prevention and control. A surveillance system includes a functional capacity for data collection, analysis, and dissemination linked to public health programs.

This concept of surveillance differentiates surveillance from occasional surveys and from planned comprehensive research programs. Also, a surveillance program involves analysis, interpretation, and dissemination of the data for the purpose of improving the health of the population and preventing disease. Therefore, surveillance needs to be selective, planned, and tailored to meet a specific goal in the prevention of disease.

This chapter reviews the history of the development of surveillance systems and their applications to the recognition, control, and prevention of infectious disease. Several current surveillance programs are described, along with their application to the prevention of infectious disease.

History of Surveillance

The responsibility of local governments to control and prevent disease in the population dates back to early times. Governments assumed responsibility for disease control by identifying possible sources of disease and quarantining infectious cases to prevent further spread.[3] Illness was monitored, regulations were enacted to prevent pollution of streets and public water supplies, and instructions were specified for burial and food handling. Unfortunately, this was not always based on a sound understanding of disease transmission as when the Mayor of London ordered the slaughter of cats and dogs to slow the bubonic plague epidemic of 1665. Cases continued to rise as rat populations were unchecked over the summer and only slowed when flea populations died off in the fall. The epidemic was finally ended when the crowded houses of London, which sustained the epidemic, burned in the Great Fire of London on September 2, 1666.[4]

In the 1600s, John Graunt published the bills of mortality for the surveillance of disease in London.[5] In Germany, Johann Peter Frank advocated that public health surveillance include maternal and child health, injuries, occupational illnesses, and school health.[6]

The modern concepts of surveillance were developed by William Farr in Great Britain. He was the superintendent of the Statistical Department of the Registrar General's Office of England and Wales from 1839 to 1879. Farr collected, analyzed, and published mortality and morbidity statistics for England and Wales and reported the data to responsible public health authorities and the general public.[7]

Surveillance in the United States

Infectious disease surveillance in the United States began soon after the colonies were established. In 1741, Rhode Island passed legislation requiring tavern keepers to report contagious disease among their patrons. Two years later, a law was passed requiring the reporting of smallpox, yellow fever, and cholera.[2]

National disease surveillance began in 1850, when mortality statistics were first published by the federal government, based on the decennial census. The legal requirement to collect national morbidity data in the United States was initiated in 1878, when Congress authorized the US Public Health Service (USPHS) to collect reports of the occurrence of the quarantineable diseases, cholera, plague, smallpox, and yellow fever. In 1902, the Surgeon General of the USPHS was directed by Congress to provide forms for collecting data on these infectious diseases and officially reporting the surveillance data. Each state and municipality had laws requiring reporting of selected communicable diseases, such as smallpox, tuberculosis, and cholera.[2] In 1913, the state and territorial health authorities recommended that every state send weekly telegraphic summaries reporting infectious diseases to the PHS.[8] In 1949, the National Office of Vital Statistics (NOVS) was established, and this office received, analyzed, and published infectious disease surveillance reports. These data were published in the official PHS journal, *Public Health Reports*. When this became a monthly journal, the NOVS issued a separate weekly bulletin, the *Morbidity and Mortality Weekly Reports* (*MMWR*), which was distributed to epidemiologists and others interested in health data. In July 1960, the responsibility for receiving morbidity reports on infectious diseases and publishing the *MMWR* was transferred from the NOVS to the Centers for Disease Control (CDC) in Atlanta.

The CDC was established in Atlanta after World War II. Its initial mission was to evaluate the health threat of malaria in the southeastern United States at a time when many World War II veterans were returning from malaria-endemic areas in the Pacific and Mediterranean. Although reports of indigenous malaria were common in the 1940s and 1950s, when CDC established routine surveillance and evaluated the reported cases, it was determined that few of these reported cases could be confirmed and that malaria had already ceased to be an important endemic disease in the United States. Despite its negative finding, the rigorous malaria surveillance system convinced government and public health officials of the value of surveillance.

Alexander Langmuir, who became director of the epidemiology program at CDC in the early 1950s, emphasized the value of surveillance as a critical public health activity.[9] In 1951, the Epidemic Intelligence Service (EIS) was established at CDC, which trained a cadre of field epidemiologists to investigate unusual epidemics anywhere in the United States upon invitation from the states.[9] Subsequently, the value of systematic surveillance was demonstrated for other diseases. In 1955, inactivated polio vaccine, shown to be efficacious in a clinical trial, was used on a wide scale to control a polio epidemic.[10] Tragically, several cases of polio appeared among those vaccinated in the previous 30 days. A review of reported cases implicated specific lots of vaccine that were incompletely inactivated and thus contained residual infectious polio virus.[11] This outbreak of vaccine-associated illness established the value of national surveillance of poliomyelitis, which continues to the present.

In 1957, a major pandemic of influenza occurred when a new genetic strain of influenza (Asian influenza, an H2/N2 recombinant virus) appeared, resulting in the establishment of influenza surveillance by the CDC. The CDC also included broader surveillance for deaths from pneumonia or influenza in 121 major US cities to enhance their ability to track influenza epidemics.[12] The CDC placed an emphasis on the development of novel methods for displaying surveillance data to ensure its ultimate value. Serfling and colleagues at CDC devised a clear and straightforward method for analyzing large surveillance databases.[13] They plotted influenza case rates as an average over specific time periods that were compared with the same time period in the previous years when an influenza epidemic was known to be absent (Figure 4-1). Whenever two or three consecutive weeks exceeded the 95% confidence limits of mortality in a nonepidemic year, the excess mortality warned of a possible influenza epidemic. Subsequently, many other infectious diseases were targeted for surveillance, due either to the development of new vaccines (e.g., measles, rubella, or pertussis) and the need to monitor their effectiveness at a population level or to the emergence of new diseases (e.g., toxic shock syndrome, Reye's syndrome, Legionnaires' disease, Hanta virus pulmonary syndrome) that required ongoing epidemiologic investigation and control (Figure 4-2).

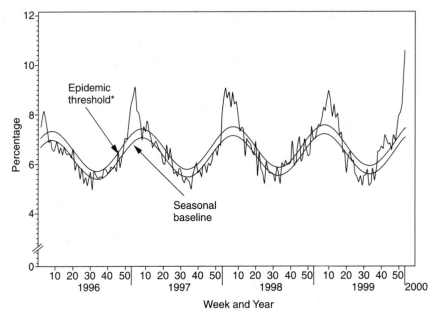

*The epidemic threshold is 1.645 standard deviations above the seasonal baseline. The expected seasonal baseline is projected using a robust regression procedure in which a periodic regression model is applied to observed percentages of deaths from P&I since 1983.

FIGURE 4-1   Percentage of mortality attributable to pneumonia and influenza (P&I) in 122 cities, by week of report United States, 1996–2000. Reprinted from *MMWR*, Vol. 39, p. 30, 1990, Centers for Disease Control and Prevention.

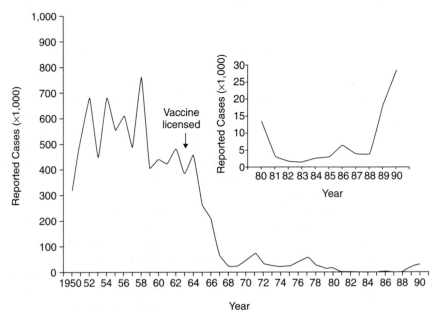

FIGURE 4-2   Measles (rubeola): by year, United States, 1950–1990. [Inset: Measles by year, United States, 1980–1990.] Reprinted from *MMWR*, 39:30, 1991, the Centers for Disease Control and Prevention.

Reportable Diseases

Currently, a total of 52 infectious diseases is officially reportable in the United States. These are listed in Table 5-1 in Chapter 5. The list of nationally reportable infectious diseases changes periodically. Diseases may be added to the list as new pathogens emerge or when a previously recognized pathogen becomes more important. Also, some diseases may be deleted from the list as their incidence or importance declines.

To standardize the cases reported to the CDC, official definitions of what constitutes a case have been published by CDC for all reportable and many of the nonreportable diseases.[14] Some diseases require laboratory confirmation for diagnosis, regardless of clinical symptoms; whereas, others are diagnosed solely on clinical criteria. Examples of those requiring laboratory confirmation are infections from *Salmonella* species, *Shigella* species, *Escherichia coli* 0157:H7, and hepatitis A (HAV) or B (HBV) viruses; whereas, botulism, tetanus, varicella, and toxic shock syndrome are diagnosed solely by clinical criteria.

The official case definition of some diseases may be changed in some instances as new scientific information is accumulated. For example, as the HIV/AIDS epidemic has evolved, the official case definition of acquired immune deficiency syndrome (AIDS) has changed. Prior to the identification of the human immunodeficiency virus (HIV), the case definition of AIDS included the most characteristic, yet unique, clinical symptoms associated with the new disease, such as Kaposi's sarcoma, *Pneumocystis carinii* pneumonia, cytomegalovirus retinitis, or another opportunistic infection, plus signs of otherwise unexplained immune suppression as measured by CD4$^+$ T-cell count. In 1987, a commercial test for the virus became available. However, it was not known what proportion of those infected with HIV would progress to severe disease. The case definition of AIDS was modified to require clinical symptoms, several of which were newly added in 1987, as well as being positive for the HIV virus.[15] In 1993, research demonstrated that those with CD4 T-cell counts below 200/μL were at high risk for developing AIDS clinical symptoms. Based on this, the definition was changed to include those with clinical symptoms, *or* a CD4 T-cell count below 200/μL and HIV infection. Because a patient's risk of developing an opportunistic infection was affected by their immune state, their exposure to specific pathogens, and their level of prophylactic care, the low CD4 T-cell count case definition was felt to be a more consistent measure of HIV progression. Furthermore, the effective prophylactic care for HIV-positive patients was lowering the occurrence of opportunistic infections that suppressed the number of cases reported to CDC. The 1993 case definition sought to correct for this underreporting of AIDS cases by removing the previous requirement that an immune-suppressed HIV-infected patient also have a documented opportunistic infection.[16] Because many cases were reported solely on the basis of T-cell counts, there was a substantial increase in the number of officially reported AIDS cases in 1993 and 1994. However, the number of AIDS cases declined from this peak level in the subsequent years as the bolus of immune-suppressed, yet asymptomatic, cases was reported earlier than would have happened with the 1987 definition. To facilitate comparisons across time, data in research and surveillance reports must clearly state which AIDS definition is being used. In fact, data are often reported using both the 1987 and 1993 definitions.

The case definition for tuberculosis has also changed several times during the past decades. The official case definition for tuberculosis raises some interesting issues. Patients with tuberculosis may respond to therapy and their disease resolve, only to reactivate at a later date. Should such a patient be reported twice? The current official practice for the CDC statistics is that such a patient should not be reported twice if the relapse occurs in the same year. However, if a patient responds and is released from therapy but relapses at a later date, both episodes should be reported as separate events. These examples are described in some detail to illustrate why it is important for epidemiologists to be familiar with the details of the case definition in order to understand and properly interpret the official statistics on reportable diseases and, especially, to evaluate temporal trends in infectious disease morbidity.

Types of Reports

Some diseases are reported to health departments as individual case reports, such as tuberculosis. Others are reported as the aggregate number of cases seen at a facility, such as varicella. For some diseases, the level of certainty of the diagnosis may vary from case to case. Sometimes, the appropriate laboratory specimens are not obtained or the patient is seen too late in the illness or after treatment, so that microbiologic confirmation of the disease is not possible. This level of certainty is reported on the case report, as in laboratory-confirmed case, clinically compatible case, or epidemiologically linked case.

Many diseases are reported *passively*, meaning that the health care providers report cases to health departments as a matter of routine. Other diseases are under *active surveillance* because of their potential public health importance. When active reporting is being done, health department personnel contact selected health care providers at regular intervals to solicit case reports. Active surveillance is particularly useful when an epidemic is suspected or in progress. For example, during an influenza-associated outbreak of Reye's syndrome, an epidemiologist might establish active surveillance for potential cases of Reye's syndrome by calling all of the neurologists in the area on a weekly basis. During an influenza outbreak, special surveillance methods are often instituted, such as monitoring school or workforce absenteeism, emergency room visits, or visits to select sentinel physicians' offices with compatible respiratory symptoms. These data are analyzed in concert with the pneumonia-influenza mortality statistics and published weekly in the *MMWR* during the influenza season or whenever the epidemic threshold is exceeded for several consecutive weeks.

Official CDC case definitions of three reportable diseases are shown in Table 4-1.[14] The reader is referred to the CDC Web site (www.cdc.gov) for a comprehensive list of criteria for the 52 officially reportable diseases.

Guidelines for Evaluating a Surveillance System

Surveillance data are collected and analyzed to provide useful and current information on important infectious diseases to epidemiologists, health officials, clinicians, laboratory scientists, and the public to develop and evaluate

TABLE 4-1   Case Definitions for Infectious Disease Surveillance—Examples

Cases of infectious diseases are reported to health officials by health care providers, laboratories, and other public health personnel. Included below are case definitions for a few reportable infectious diseases.

- *Botulism:* Ingestion of botulinum toxin results in an illness of variable severity. Common symptoms are diplopia, blurred vision, and bulbar weakness. Symmetric paralysis may progress rapidly.
    - ○ *Laboratory criteria for diagnosis:*
        - ■ Detection of botulinum toxin in serum; stool on patients' food
    - ○ *Case classification:*
        - ■ *Probable case:* A clinically compatible case with an epidemiologic link (e.g., ingestion of a home-canned food within the previous 48 hours)
        - ■ *Confirmed case:* A clinically compatible case that is laboratory confirmed or that occurs among persons who ate the same food as persons who have laboratory-confirmed botulism
- *Chlamydia trachomatis:* Infection with *C. trachomatis* may result in urethritis, epididymitis, cervicitis, acute salpingitis, or other syndromes when sexually transmitted; however, the infection is often asymptomatic in women. Perinatal infections may result in inclusion conjunctivitis and pneumonia in newborns. Other syndromes caused by *C. trachomatis* include lymphogranuloma venereum and trachoma.
    - ○ *Laboratory criteria for diagnosis:*
        - ■ Isolation of *C. trachomatis* by culture or
        - ■ Demonstration of *C. trachomatis* in a clinical specimen by detection of antigen or nucleic acid
    - ○ *Case classification:*
        - ■ *Confirmed case:* A case that is laboratory confirmed
- *Varicella (chickenpox):* An illness with acute onset of diffuse (generalized) papulovesicular rash without other apparent cause
    - ○ *Laboratory criteria for diagnosis:*
        - ■ Isolation of varicella virus from a clinical specimen or
        - ■ Significant rise in serum varicella immunoglobulin G antibody level by any standard serologic assay
    - ○ *Case classification:*
        - ■ *Probable case:* A case that meets the clinical case definition, is not laboratory confirmed, and is not epidemiologically linked to another probable or confirmed case
        - ■ *Confirmed case:* A case that is laboratory confirmed or that meets the clinical case definition and is epidemiologically linked to a confirmed or probable case

Source: Reprinted from *MMWR*, Vol. 46 (RR10): pp. 1–55, 1997, Centers for Disease Control and Prevention.

methods for their prevention. Table 4-2 shows some sources of surveillance data on infectious diseases. To be useful for this purpose, surveillance systems need to have several qualities that promote efficiency and reliability of the data. The CDC has published a set of attributes and criteria by which to evaluate a surveillance system.[17] These criteria can be used to evaluate an existing surveillance system or to establish a new system. The judgment of which criteria are most important depends on the primary purposes for which the surveillance data will be used. For example, surveillance systems that are designed to track an eradication campaign or to control an epidemic of a serious disease need to be comprehensive, rapid, and sensitive. The efforts and funding allocated to such a system will be much higher than surveillance for a less severe endemic disease. In this case, the surveillance system

TABLE 4-2   Sources of Surveillance Data on Infectious Diseases

Source	Description/Examples
1. Mortality registration	Primary and underlying causes of death
2. Morbidity reporting	52 reportable diseases
3. Epidemic/outbreak reports	Acute outbreaks reported to health department
4. Laboratory	Laboratory reports are required for several reportable diseases, e.g., syphilis and salmonella. Blinded surveys of HIV
5. Case investigations	Individual cases of certain diseases are investigated, e.g., rabies, polio, plague.
6. Nosocomial infection surveillance	NNIS;* all hospitals are required to do nosocomial infection surveillance to maintain licensure (Joint Commission).
7. Animal disease surveillance	Done by veterinary section of health department
8. Adverse reactions to vaccines	VAERs, VSD*
9. Food-borne illness	FoodNet, PulseNet
10. Vector populations	Targeted to specific vector-borne diseases
11. Behavioral risk factors	DAWN* behavior risk factor survey
12. Targeted disease surveillance	
• Hepatitis	Sentinel Counties Study
• Influenza	Pneumonia/Influenza Mortality in 121 US cities
• Tuberculosis	Contact investigations of active cases
• Syphilis	Contact investigation and "epidemiologic treatment" of exposed contacts

*NNIS: National Noscomial Infection Surveillance Programs. VAERS: Vaccine Adverse Events Reporting System. VSD: Vaccine Safety Data Link. DAWN: Drug Abuse Warning Network.

may not count every case that occurs as long as those it does receive are representative of the populations at risk, and it can detect fluctuations in the disease incidence. A passive reporting system is the most cost-effective here, in which the criteria for a case are quite specific but less sensitive. This system is sufficient to detect major fluctuations in incidence, even when many cases go undetected or unreported.

The CDC recommended attributes of a surveillance system are as follows:

- *Sensitivity*: To what extent does the system identify all or most cases in a target population? As described above, good sensitivity may be more important for a surveillance system designed to control an outbreak or to evaluate an intervention than for monitoring disease trends.
- *Timeliness*: This refers to how rapidly reports are received, evaluated, and analyzed and the information provided to those in a position to intervene. This may be critical to control an outbreak of an acute disease.
- *Representativeness*: This refers to whether the likelihood of reporting a disease is the same within subgroups of the population or in different populations. If surveillance reports are not representative, this could affect the application of control efforts.

- *Predictive Value Positive*: This refers to the specificity of the case report. To what extent are the reported cases really cases? This is an important attribute of surveillance systems in most situations.
- *Simplicity*: This refers to both the system's structure and ease of operation. Surveillance systems should be as simple as possible, while still meeting their objectives. It is costly and burdensome to collect data that will not be used. A system that is too costly risks having its funds cut while a burdensome system may have poor compliance.
- *Acceptability*: This refers to the willingness of individuals and organizations to participate in the surveillance system. Obviously, this is a critical characteristic of all surveillance systems.
- *Flexibility*: This refers to a system's ability to adapt to changing information needs or operating conditions with little additional costs in time, personnel, or funding. Some disease-reporting systems are quite flexible and can accommodate the need to monitor new diseases. Generally, simple systems are more flexible. The system that reports the 52 diseases that are officially reported by all the states to the CDC is generally quite flexible. A newly recognized or emerging infectious disease usually can be added to the list. The decisions as to what diseases are to be reported are made regularly by the Council of State and Territorial Epidemiologists, and the definitions to be used to report cases are developed in consultation with the CDC.

Communication and Presentation of Data

The primary purposes of a surveillance system are to collect data on the health status and/or risk factors for disease in a population and to analyze, interpret, and utilize the data in a manner that will lead to prevention and control of disease. Therefore, a critical component of this activity is the interpretation and communication of the data in an ongoing fashion, so that health care providers or officials can take appropriate action when necessary. Investigations of epidemics of infectious diseases should occur promptly in a journal with a wide distribution to health professionals, the public, and the news media, such as *MMWR*, and should include (1) the results of the investigation, (2) the control measures instituted, and (3) interpretive comments to put the epidemic in context. Such reports have been successful in informing policies or procedures to prevent future epidemics.

Presentations of data on endemic infectious diseases are also important to assess progress or lack of progress toward a healthier society. The CDC issues annual reports on the epidemiology of several diseases, where longer-term trends are analyzed. Also, CDC regularly presents the weekly reports of infectious diseases in a graphic form, in which the number or rates of reported cases of several infectious diseases are compared with the number reported in recent weeks or in a comparable period in a previous year (Figure 4-3). Another method of data presentation is to show the temporal trends of disease incidence in reference to a targeted prevalence or incidence rate of the disease in the future, such as 2010. This type of graph allows the reader to determine whether a predetermined goal is likely to be met. These PHS goals were specified and published in the PHS publication *Healthy People 2000* (Figure 4-4).

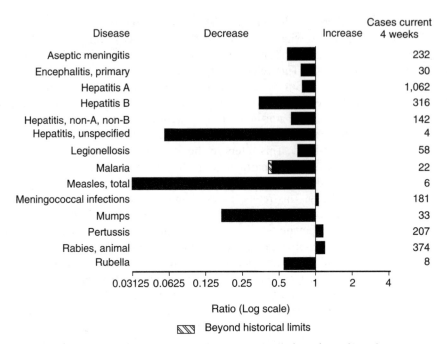

FIGURE 4-3   Notifiable disease reports, comparison of week totals ending February 4, 1995, with historical data—United States. Reprinted from Centers for Disease Control and Prevention, National Center for Infectious Diseases.

Not Just Counting Cases

Surveillance as a Tool to Describe Risk Groups

One important purpose of routine, ongoing surveillance of infectious diseases is to gather descriptive data about important health problems. The data reported usually contain demographic data on the cases, such as gender, age, geographic location, and occupation. These data sometimes allow public health programs to be implemented or altered. For example, several decades ago, the case reports of tetanus appeared more often among adult women than in men, especially in female illicit drug users. The data supported the hypothesis that lower-class men were more often immunized upon entry to military service or the workforce or as a result of occupational injuries than were women. These surveillance data led to an effort to immunize women who had previously gone unimmunized.

Prior to the AIDS epidemic, syphilis was most common among men who have sex with men (MSMs); however, a reduction in high-risk sex among MSMs and an increase in risky sex among cocaine users changed the demographics of the disease.[18] In 2005, an increase in syphilis and rectal gonorrhea in men in several cities has signaled a dangerous resumption of high-risk sex among MSMs.

The data available from the routinely reported cases with simple demographic characteristics have often triggered more detailed epidemiologic studies that have led to the design and implementation of prevention strategies. A critical feature of these routine reports is that they are published in the *MMWR* and widely distributed to public health authorities, government

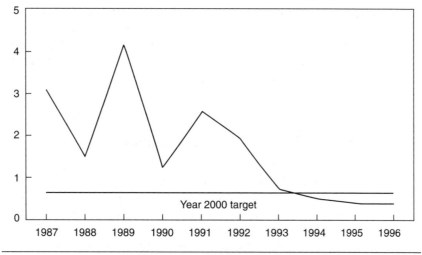

(a)

Number of new cases
(thousands)

	1987	1988	1989	1990	1991	1992	1993	1994	1995	1996	Year 2000 target
Occupationally exposed workers. . . .	3090	1520	4189	1258	2576	1923	727	506	407	391	623

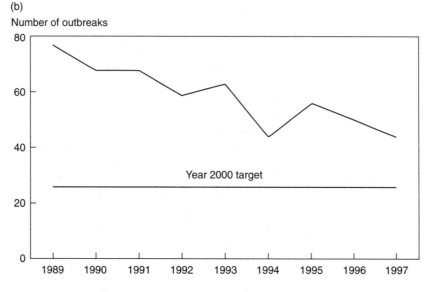

(b)

Number of outbreaks

	1989	1990	1991	1992	1993	1994	1995	1996	1997	Year 2000 target
All persons	77	68	68	59	63	44	56	50	44	25

FIGURE 4-4 (a) Number of new cases of hepatitis B infections among occupationally exposed workers: United States, 1987–1996, and year 2000 target for objective 10.5. (b) Outbreaks of infections due to *Salmonella enteriditis*: United States, 1989–1997, and year 2000 target for objective 12.2. Reprinted from the Centers for Disease Control and Prevention, National Center for Infectious Diseases, Salmonella Surveillance System.

officials, news media, and public interest groups. In addition to the nationally distributed *MMWR*, many state and local health departments analyze and publish data about local health problems on a regular basis. For example, in response to the increase in syphilis among MSMs, behavioral researchers studied whether this is due to a decrease in concern about HIV as effective therapies have changed the disease's prognosis or if it is due to exhaustion with practicing safe sex behaviors.[19]

Surveillance as a Tool to Evaluate Vaccines

Routine surveillance is often a critical component of the evaluation of vaccines and other public health prevention programs. After a vaccine is licensed, it is important to continue surveillance to measure its effectiveness in controlling the disease in the population and the extent of its use. Prelicensure clinical trials of vaccines cannot take into account the great variety of conditions under which a vaccine might be used or inappropriately used in the field. Outside of the tightly controlled setting of a clinical trial, differences in the disease strain, patient characteristics, vaccine administration, and concomitant medications may all interfere with vaccine efficacy. Several examples of changes in vaccine practices after analysis of postlicensure surveillance data follow.

Modification of Dosing Schedule

The measles vaccine is highly effective for the prevention of measles. Its efficacy is estimated to be 95–97% or higher, when given at 12–15 months of age, after the disappearance of maternal antibodies. However, postlicensure surveillance of children vaccinated at 12 months found somewhat lower vaccine efficacy than when the vaccine was given at 15 months.[20] Based on these surveillance data the vaccine recommendations were changed to encourage vaccination at 15 months instead of at 12 months.[21] After the original licensure of live attenuated measles vaccine in 1963, reported cases of measles declined by over 95%.[22] However, reported cases of measles increased in 1979–1980, 1984–1986, and 1989–1991.[22] Many of these cases occurred in children who had been appropriately vaccinated. Because measles is highly infectious, it is not possible to establish herd immunity, thus the 2% to 5% of the population who do not respond to the initial measles vaccine are at risk for endemic transmission. The occurrence of measles epidemics in highly vaccinated populations led to the recommendation that a second dose of measles, mumps, and rubella (MMR) vaccine be given at 4–6 years of age.[23,24] This strategy has further reduced measles incidence. However, imported cases continue to be reported, and indigenous cases, especially among persons who refuse vaccine for religious reasons, are not uncommon.

Modification of Vaccine Components

The importance of postlicensure surveillance to determine vaccine effectiveness in a diverse situation occurred in Brazil when an outbreak of type 3 polio occurred among vaccinees.[25] Investigation of this outbreak disclosed that the ratio of types 1, 2, and 3 of 10 : 1 : 3 in the vaccine proved to be inadequately immunogenic for type 3 polio. The trivalent vaccine was then changed to a 10 : 1 : 6 mixture, which provided improved immunogenicity for type 3 polio.[25]

Monitoring Vaccine Administration

During the trial, storage of vaccines usually is optimal. Some live attenuated vaccines require refrigeration and a "cold chain" from the manufacturer to the care setting must be maintained to prevent loss of immunogenicity. However, it is not uncommon for problems with maintenance of a cold chain to impair vaccine effectiveness, especially in tropical, developing country settings. The mode of vaccine delivery can also affect immunogenicity, which may not be realized until postlicensure surveillance. Postlicensure studies of HBV vaccine found unexpected low immunogenicity of the vaccine among those who received the vaccine subcutaneously, rather than by the intramuscular route.[26] The trial for intradermally administered rabies vaccine showed sufficient immunogenicity among veterinary medicine students. Based on this, the vaccine was given to Peace Corps volunteers intradermally. The postlicensure evaluation of a rabies death in a vaccinated Peace Corps volunteer in Africa showed that chloroquine, used for malaria prophylaxis, inhibited the immune response to intradermal vaccine.[27]

Calculating Vaccine Effectiveness

Vaccine effectiveness can be measured epidemiologically by comparing the rates of disease in vaccinees and nonvaccinees. The standard formula for calculating vaccine efficacy (VE) compares the attack rates for disease in the unvaccinated (ARU) with those in the vaccinated (ARV), as follows:

$$VE(\%) = \frac{(ARU - ARV)}{ARU} \times 100$$

The problems in ascertaining cases and assigning vaccine status in a postlicensure study are substantial. Disease manifestation may be altered in vaccinated patients, and care must be taken when developing the case definition to ensure equal ascertainment of cases in the two groups. Even with a highly effective vaccine, cases can occur among vaccinated individuals. If 90% of a population were vaccinated with a vaccine that was 90% effective, only 81% of the population would be immune. Of those not immune, half would have a history of having received vaccine and half would be nonvaccinees. Also, difficulties may exist in determining whether the exposure and risk of disease are comparable in the vaccinated and unvaccinated populations. Variation in the sensitivity and specificity of the case definition and biased case ascertainment that is linked to vaccination status can falsely increase or decrease vaccine efficacy. For example, vaccinated patients may have greater access to health care and may be more likely to be diagnosed as a case than those without access to care, thus falsely decreasing the apparent vaccine efficacy (Table 4-3). The details of measurement of vaccine effectiveness after licensure are covered in greater detail in Chapter 10.

TABLE 4-3 Effects of Different Methodological Problems on Estimation of Vaccine Efficiency

Problem	Likely Effects On		
	ARU	ARV	VE
a. Lack of sensitive definition; equal sensitivity in vaccinees and nonvaccinees; 100% specificity	↓	↓	No change
b. Low-sensitivity definition but more sensitive in nonvaccinees than vaccinees; 100% specificity	↓	↓↓	↑
c. Nonspecific definition; background illnesses are classified as cases; 100% sensitivity	↑↑	↑↑↑	↓
d. Nonspecific definition; low sensitivity	↑	↑↑↑	↓↓
e. Cases are classified with knowledge of vaccination status; bias toward detecting cases in unvaccinated and toward failing to detect cases in vaccinated	No change	↓	↑
f. Cases are classified with knowledge of vaccination status; bias toward detecting cases in vaccinated and toward failing to detect cases in unvaccinated	↓	No change	↓

Note: ARU, attack rate in the unvaccinated; ARV, attack rate in the vaccinated; VE, vaccine efficacy.
Source: Reprinted with permission from WA Orenstein, RH Bernier and RR Hinman. Assessing vaccine efficacy in the field: further observation. *Epidemiology Rev.* 1988;10:212–241.
Source: Reprinted with permission from W.A. Orenstein, R. Bernier, A.R. Hinman, Assessing Vaccine Efficacy in the Field Further Observation, *Epidemiologic Reviews*, Vol. 10, pp. 212–241, © 1988, Oxford University Press.

Surveillance as a Tool to Eradicate Disease

Smallpox Eradication

After the successful program for the eradication of smallpox, several other infectious diseases were targeted for eradication, including polio, guinea worm, and measles. The smallpox campaign showed that an active and aggressive surveillance program is required. The smallpox eradication program not only relied on reports of smallpox cases to health authorities but actively sought cases by having regular contacts with health care providers, intensive surveillance of villages where cases had occurred, and providing monetary rewards to citizens for reporting confirmed cases.[28] This highly active surveillance system was coupled with vaccination of case contacts and preventing their contact with additional susceptible persons during the infectious period. The method became known as the *surveillance and containment strategy*. It replaced the older, ineffective method of attempting to vaccinate 100% of the population.[28] Fenner and Henderson detail the smallpox control and eradication campaign in their book *Smallpox and Its Eradication*.[29]

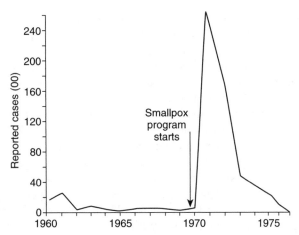

FIGURE 4-5 Evidence of the underreporting of variola minor. Increase in the number of reported cases in Ethiopia following the initiation of intensified surveillance in 1971. Reprinted with permission from F. Fenner, D.A. Henderson, C. Arita, et al., *Smallpox and Its Eradication*, 1st ed., © World Health Organization.

The implementation of active surveillance to supplant the passive reporting of cases of smallpox resulted in an apparent large increase in the incidence of cases. This is shown by the surveillance data from the smallpox eradication program in Ethiopia in the 1970s (Figure 4-5). Another issue associated with concerted efforts to increase surveillance is that patients with other diseases having similar clinical manifestations may be reported. That is, efforts to increase sensitivity of reporting may lead to decreased specificity, or at least some nonspecificity, of the case reports. In the smallpox eradication program, cases of atypical varicella with clinical features similar to smallpox were commonly reported as possible cases of smallpox.[29] In addition, human cases of monkey pox, a newly recognized human infection, were reported, especially in Africans having close contact with monkeys.[30] Conversely, cases of monkey pox were underreported, and this disease is more frequently recognized since the eradication of smallpox.[30]

Poliomyelitis Eradication

Following the successful eradication of smallpox, the Pan American Health Organization (PAHO) in May 1985 proposed a plan to eradicate poliomyelitis from the Western Hemisphere within the next five years.[31] The proposal was accepted by all PAHO member countries, and a major initiative was launched within months. The program aimed to interrupt the indigenous transmission of wild poliovirus. It relied on the use of trivalent oral polio vaccine given to every child under 5 years of age on national vaccination days, held twice yearly in each country, and on active surveillance for polio cases, especially patients with acute flaccid paralysis. Efforts were made to document each reported case virologically to confirm whether or not the case was due to acute infection with wild poliovirus. A standard benchmark definition of "adequate surveillance" was established that included a very sensitive marker of disease: identification of acute flaccid paralysis (AFP) at a rate of $\geq 1:100,000$ population of children under 5 years old and a very specific marker of disease: two stool cultures for polio virus isolation from AFP cases taken within 14 days of onset in $\geq 80\%$ of AFP cases. Confirmation of viral etiology was necessary as polio cases declined because other viral infections, especially enterovirus, cause AFP in at least 1 per 100,000 children child under age 1.

Similar to the smallpox eradication program, extensive active surveillance for cases involving not only health professionals but the general public as well was a central component of the program. However, in the polio eradication program, in contrast to the smallpox eradication program, surveillance was also directed at detecting wild poliovirus in humans and in the environment. In August 1991, the last case of indigenous polio in the Western Hemisphere occurred in a 2-year-old boy in Peru. Three years later, after no additional indigenous cases were detected, despite intensive surveillance, an independent international commission certified to PAHO that polio had been eradicated from the Western Hemisphere.[32] While there is considerable hope that polio could be eradicated globally, setbacks in polio control in Nigeria have substantially undermined this campaign.

Surveillance as a Tool to Prevent Disease Spread

Surveillance may also be used to prevent spread of the disease to others. When a patient with active tuberculosis is identified, the report is usually followed by an investigation of the contacts. Any contacts who are infected are given prophylactic therapy. Contact investigation and prophylactic treatment of all contacts are recommended for infectious syphilis, meaning primary or secondary syphilis and meningococcal disease. Surveillance and prevention of nosocomial infections in hospitals and other health care institutions have become integral and critical components of modern health care. These issues are reviewed in detail in Chapter 13.

Specialized Surveillance Programs

There are numerous specialized surveillance programs operating in the United States and globally. These programs address identified needs and are an important part of the public health infrastructure. They also provide useful data for epidemiologic research beyond their primary mission. These are described in greater detail below.

The National Nosocomial Infection Surveillance System

The National Nosocomial Infection Surveillance System (NNIS) began in 1970 when selected US hospitals agreed to report their nosocomial infection surveillance data routinely to a national database maintained by the hospital infection program at CDC. In the 30 years since NNIS was begun, the program has been expanded to include 231 acute care hospitals. Also, considerable attention has been directed to standardization of the definitions for each site of nosocomial infection and requirements for adequate personnel and laboratory resources for the diagnosis of nosocomial infections to ensure that the data are reasonably accurate and comparable among different hospitals.

The objectives of NNIS are the following:

1. Estimate the extent and nature of nosocomial infections in the United States.
2. Identify changes in the incidence of nosocomial infections and the pathogens that cause them.
3. Provide hospitals with comparative data on nosocomial infection rates.
4. Develop efficient and effective data collection management and analysis methods.
5. Conduct collaborative research studies of nosocomial infections.

Epidemiologists from the hospital infection program at CDC frequently assist hospitals, both those participating in NNIS and others, in the investigation and control of nosocomial outbreaks.

Nosocomial infections are a very important health problem in the United States, and antibiotic-resistant organisms often may be selected for and transmitted in this setting. It has been estimated that over 2 million patients develop a nosocomial infection in the United States each year, at a cost of approximately $3.5 billion. The NNIS is the only ongoing surveillance program of nosocomial infections in acute care hospitals in the United States. Data from the NNIS program are described in detail in Chapter 14.

Emerging Infections

Recently, considerable attention has been directed at emerging and reemerging infections. This topic is covered in detail in Chapter 13 of this book. A sensitive system of surveillance for the early detection of emerging infections is a critically important component of the public health response to this problem.

The Institute of Medicine of the National Academy of Sciences reviewed the problem of emerging infectious diseases in 1991.[33] This expert committee recommended that the CDC develop a strategy for improved early detection and response to the threat of emerging infections. The CDC established an emerging infections program (EIP) in seven states: California, Connecticut, Georgia, New York, Maryland, Minnesota, and Oregon. The goals of the EIP are to improve national surveillance for new and emerging infectious diseases, conduct applied epidemiologic and laboratory research, develop prevention and control measures, and strengthen the national public health infrastructure.

To further these goals, the CDC granted a Cooperative Agreement Program Award to the Infectious Diseases Society of America (IDSA) in 1995. The main objective of the award was for IDSA to establish a provider-based emerging infections sentinel network. The Emerging Infections Network (EIN) currently includes over 900 infectious disease (ID) member specialists worldwide. The EIN members serve as field officers to identify new and unusual clinical events. Because of their professional experiences, EIN members can link to the broader community of ID specialists—local, national, and global public health practitioners—to tap into their collective resources and research knowledge. The EIN members communicate electronically via a listserv. The listserv acts as an informal mechanism for the flow of information, as well as a venue for administration of formal, either urgent or periodic, surveys. Outbreak investigations merit urgent queries; whereas, periodic surveys of the membership evaluate ongoing public health needs in the field. The EIN contributes annually to tracking of influenza and availability of vaccines and has participated in information gathering relating to diseases such as West Nile virus encephalitis, smallpox vaccination, *Clostridium difficile*-associated disease, and severe acute respiratory syndrome (SARS).

Syndromic Surveillance

The terrorist attacks of September 11, 2001, and the subsequent anthrax outbreak emphasized the need for the development of a system that would enhance the US terrorism preparedness. The main goal of such a surveillance system is the early detection of outbreaks caused by intentional emergence of biologic and chemical agents.[34] Clusters of human illness need to be quickly identified and described in an accelerated fashion due to the nature and scope of the threat and the imperative to limit human casualties.

The resulted innovation is the development of *syndromic surveillance.* The CDC defines syndromic surveillance as "an investigational approach where health department staff, assisted by automated data acquisition and generation of statistical alerts, monitor disease indicators in real-time or near real-time to detect outbreaks of disease earlier than would otherwise be possible with traditional public health methods."[35] The fundamental premise of syndromic surveillance is that in order to identify disease clusters early, potential cases of a biological or chemical outbreak are defined by virtue of their symptoms and before their clinical or laboratory confirmation and reporting via traditional surveillance channels. Figure 4-6 provides a graphic representation[36] of the lead time allowed by detection of early symptoms, as opposed to clinical disease manifestation, thus allowing public health officials time for a rapid response in limiting the outbreak.

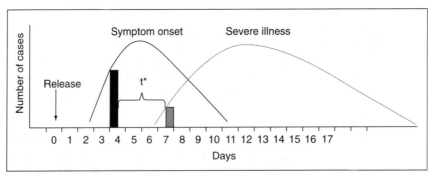

* t = time between detection by syndromic (prediagnostic) surveillance and detection by traditional (diagnosis-based) surveillance.

FIGURE 4-6   Syndromic surveillance—rationale for early detection.
Source: Henning KJ; Centers for Disease Control and Prevention (CDC). What is syndromic surveillance? MMWR Morb Mortal Wkly Rep. 2004 Sep 24;53 Suppl:5–11.

Standardization of syndromic surveillance protocols remains a complex and unresolved issue. Despite deployment of different systems by numerous local and regional jurisdictions following the anthrax outbreaks of 2001, implementation challenges remain. Statistical signaling of an unexpected disease cluster is very difficult because of limitations on the knowledge of strong correlations between nonspecific symptoms and disease, the relative inexperience of clinical and public health respondents with biologic and chemical agents, and the wide array of data sources, such as emergency department patient volume aberrations, poison control center calls, medical examiner data, medication sales, and Internet-based health-related inquiries by the public. Further research is needed to define optimal data sources, evaluate syndromic definitions, standardize signal-detection methods, incorporate information from existing surveillance systems, and develop response protocols.[36]

In addition to syndromic surveillance, the CDC already had in place several specific programs to monitor intentional and unintentional epidemics. These include the FoodNet, PulseNet, ArboNET, and tuberculosis programs.

FoodNet and PulseNet

The Food-Borne Diseases Active Surveillance Network (FoodNet) is the food-borne disease component of CDC's EIP. FoodNet is a collaborative project among CDC, the seven EIP sites, the US Department of Agriculture (USDA), and the US Food and Drug Administration (FDA). It consists of active surveillance for food-borne diseases and related epidemiologic studies designed to help improve public health officials' understanding of the epidemiology of food-borne disease in the United States. The total population included in the special surveillance efforts of the FoodNet catchment areas is 20.3 million people, or 8% of the population of the United States. FoodNet provides a network for responding to new and emerging food-borne diseases of national importance, monitoring the burden of food-borne diseases, and identifying the source of specific food-borne diseases.

The program includes surveillance of several populations, including the following:

- Active laboratory-based surveillance
- Survey of clinical laboratories
- Survey of physicians
- Survey of the population
- Case-control studies

Closely linked to FoodNet is another laboratory-based program called PulseNet. PulseNet is a national network of public health laboratories that performs DNA fingerprinting of bacteria that might be the cause of food-borne illnesses. The network permits rapid comparison of the DNA fingerprint patterns through an electronic database at the CDC. The DNA fingerprinting method used is pulsed-field gel electrophoresis (PFGE). The PFGE methods are described in some detail in Chapter 8. The data from FoodNet and PulseNet allow a better understanding of the epidemiology of food-borne diseases of national significance.

ArboNET

The first domestically acquired cases of West Nile virus (WNV) encephalitis were described in the United States in the summer of 1999.[37-42] By 2002, the WNV epidemic had spread to 44 states, the District of Columbia, and Canada, making it the largest documented WNV epidemic in the Western Hemisphere. To assist in the development of WNV surveillance and response, the CDC implemented an electronic-based surveillance and reporting system, ArboNET, to track WNV infection. Although state jurisdictions may employ varied surveillance systems, the CDC is coordinating the reporting of WNV infection data in humans, other mammals, birds, and mosquitoes to the national ArboNET system in a standardized format and schedule.

The objectives of this system are to monitor the geographic and temporal spread of WNV in the United States; to develop national public health strategies for WNV surveillance, prevention, and control; to develop a more complete regional picture of the distribution and incidence of the other clinically important arboviruses (e.g., eastern and western equine encephalitides, St. Louis encephalitis, La Crosse, Powassan) in the United States; to provide national and regional information to public health and government officials and the general public; and to evaluate the need for additional resources.[43]

ArboNET reporting incorporates data from sentinel surveillance of avian, equine, and mosquito morbidity and mortality as indicators for epizoonotic activity and human risk, as well as surveillance of human syndromes (i.e., encephalitis cases), diagnostic tests of antibody specimens, physician surveys, and specific research projects, such as case-control studies. Information technology advancements allow for ArboNET to be readily accessible by local jurisdictions for data entry and verification in real time, thus facilitating WNV monitoring. This electronic-based system enables a multidisciplinary team of public health and agriculture officials to assess WNV epidemic implications and coordinate the local and national WNV response with effective allocation of resources.

Tuberculosis Surveillance

Enhanced tuberculosis surveillance was established as part of the CDC's EIP in response to the reemergence of tuberculosis in the United States caused by the neglect of tuberculosis in the decades prior to the AIDS epidemic and then the resurgence of TB in populations with or at risk for HIV/AIDS. The reinvigorated programs have included increased funding to health departments for more active case detection, directly observed therapy (termed *DOTS*) of active cases with effective drug combinations and molecular characterization of all isolates from patients in the seven EIP states. These molecular epidemiologic studies of isolates from patients with recent tuberculosis have led to a reassessment of the proportion of cases in adults that are due to reactivation versus recent tuberculosis. Studies from several locations have suggested that recent infections in adults are more common than had been previously believed, accounting for about 35% of active cases in some areas.[44] Also, several clusters of tuberculosis cases acquired by casual contact and unusual exposures, such as bronchoscopy, have been documented.[45] These issues are reviewed in greater detail in Chapter 18.

Influenza Surveillance

Influenza has probably received more systematic global surveillance than any other disease in the last several decades. Active surveillance of influenza is necessary to monitor the emergence of new influenza viruses that arise by genetic drift or reassortment (genetic shift). The detection of new influenza viruses on a global basis is required to have sufficient lead time to produce and distribute new influenza vaccines. Because of the great genetic variability of influenza viruses, the vaccine must be reformulated on an annual basis. The World Health Organization (WHO) has established a global network of influenza surveillance laboratories, where isolates from infected persons are characterized serologically and genetically. Each year, a panel of experts meets and makes a prediction as to which of the circulating viruses is most likely to be responsible for an epidemic during the ensuing influenza season. Vaccine preparation for the next year is based on this recommendation (see Chapter 11).

In addition to this program of global influenza surveillance, the CDC maintains an influenza surveillance program in the United States. This program, which is described in more detail in Chapter 17, monitors influenza and pneumonia deaths in adults in 121 US cities. Also, special influenza surveillance programs include monitoring visits to sentinel physicians and hospital emergency rooms, as well as obtaining data concerning hospital admissions and school absenteeism in selected populations. For several years, Baylor University in Houston, Texas, has maintained comprehensive community-wide surveillance of influenza in Harris County, Texas, with funding from the National Institutes of Health (NIH) to evaluate the influenza morbidity and mortality at the population level.[46]

Hepatitis Surveillance

The hepatitis program at CDC has established the Sentinel County Study, a collaborative network of county health departments for the purpose of monitoring the epidemiology of viral hepatitis. This program has been in operation since 1982. The counties involved in this surveillance program are provided with personnel to do active surveillance of hepatitis occurring in residents of these sentinel counties. This surveillance includes maintaining regular active contact with physicians, other health care providers, and laboratories to detect all cases of hepatitis. Each hepatitis case is interviewed to determine risk factors, and laboratory evaluation is done to establish the hepatitis virus type. The data from the Sentinel County Study have been of considerable value in monitoring the incidence, temporal trends, and risk factors for infection with the different hepatitis viruses in the United States. Although viral hepatitis is one of the reportable diseases in the United States, the reporting is incomplete, and the passively reported data do not provide reliable estimates of the type of hepatitis or the risk factors for infection. The epidemiology of viral hepatitis and the data from the Sentinel County Study are reviewed in more detail in the chapter on hepatitis (Chapter 22).

Vaccine Adverse Event Reporting System

The National Childhood Vaccine Injury Act of 1986 mandated the reporting of certain adverse events following vaccination to help ensure the safety of vaccines distributed in the United States. This act led to the establishment of the Vaccine Adverse Event Reporting System (VAERS) in November 1990. The program is operated jointly by the CDC and FDA. VAERS receives about 800–1000 reports each month from health care providers, vaccine manufacturers, and vaccine recipients or their parents or guardians. One of the dilemmas in public health is the imbalance between the tremendous benefits from vaccines during the 1900s in reducing morbidity and mortality and the high degree of suspicion that the public has about the dangers of new vaccines or vaccines in general. This has led to reluctance to develop, test, and license new vaccines among some pharmaceutical firms, due to concerns about litigation, as vaccines are blamed for health events that are merely coincidental. This situation, which is inimical to further advances in public health, has been addressed in part by the VAERS surveillance program. Although VAERS is a passive reporting system and does not include denominator data, it identified an uncommon complication of the rotavirus vaccine. On further study, intussusception was attributed to 1 in 5000–10,000 vaccine recipients.[47]

In 1991, the CDC, in collaboration with several large health maintenance organizations (HMOs), established another surveillance system to monitor adverse reaction to vaccines. This program is called the Vaccine Safety Datalink Project (VSD).[48] The VSD project contains a large database of vaccinated children and adults where adverse events can be linked to denominator data on the number of vaccines administered.

Because the HMO populations included in the VSD project are relatively stable and receive all of their health care through the HMO, these data are less subject to bias than the VAERS passive reporting systems.

Other Surveillance Data

There are several surveillance systems in the United States that have been established to obtain data for other purposes that could be utilized to evaluate infectious diseases issues. Among these are the Surveillance, Epidemiology, and End Results (SEER) project of the National Cancer Institute and the National Health and Nutrition Assessment Study (NHANES) of the National Center for Health Statistics.

SEER Study

The SEER project of the National Cancer Institute of NIH includes cancer registries in 11 geographic areas, including 6 states, 1 territory, and 4 metropolitan areas. Through contacts with hospitals and pathologists, the occurrence of incident cases of cancer are monitored, and ascertainment is believed to be very complete. Data collected on cancer patients include demographic characteristics; exposures, such as industrial or occupational histories; characteristics of the cancer (site, morphology, stage); treatment; and outcomes. These patients have been enrolled in a number of studies. They are a useful population for the study of infectious causes of cancer, such as hepatitis B virus (HBV), hepatitis C virus (HCV), *Helicobacter pylori*, human papillomavirus (HPV), Epstein-Barr virus, and other infections.

National Health and Nutrition Survey

The NHANES involves a random sample of the US population, which is done about every 10 years to evaluate the prevalence of health conditions and the nutritional status of the US population. Randomly selected subjects are asked to participate in a survey that includes a detailed assessment of health conditions and disabilities, a physical examination, and collection of blood specimens. The blood specimens are evaluated for several biochemical and nutritional components, and a repository is created. Several studies of infectious diseases have been evaluated using the repository and questionnaire data, including the prevalence of infection with HBV, HCV, and herpes simplex viruses types 1 and 2. These data are discussed in Chapters 22 and 23.

Behavioral Surveillance

The Behavioral Risk Factor Surveillance System is an ongoing telephone survey that is conducted by over 40 state health departments in the United States. The survey includes standardized questions on various risk factors for disease, including cigarette smoking, alcohol use, seat belt use, and exercise. These data are analyzed and published by the CDC and are very useful in evaluating temporal trends in health risk behaviors. Additional questions are added periodically.

Another example of an active behavioral surveillance effort is the national HIV Behavioral Surveillance (NHBS), which began in 2004 and is funded by CDC. NHBS is an anonymous, community-based survey of populations, such as men who have sex with men (MSM), injection drug users (IDU), and high-risk heterosexuals, who are at an elevated risk for the acquisition of the HIV virus. A standardized behavioral questionnaire is administered in 25 metropolitan areas around the United States on an annual basis to individuals of the aforementioned HIV-risk groups. These individuals are actively recruited using generalizable sampling methods. Data from NHBS are used to assess the prevalence of HIV-related risk behaviors, ascertain changes over time in the prevalence of these behaviors, and enlighten city and state health departments as to the local needs for HIV prevention resource allocation.

Drug Abuse Warning Network

The Drug Abuse Warning Network (DAWN) collects data on morbidity and mortality related to illicit drug use from hospital emergency departments and medical examiners or coroners' offices in 27 metropolitan areas. It is a useful source of data on the types of illicit drugs in common use in a geographic area and the associated health problems associated with their use. The DAWN data have been useful in detecting changing types of drug use that have adverse health consequences. The DAWN study is especially useful for detecting changes in the rates of drug overdose.

International Surveillance Systems

In addition to the numerous sources of data on health events in the United States listed above, there are various sources of international surveillance data. Most national governments have established surveillance programs on cancer and infectious diseases. Some of those data are published in the *Weekly Epidemiologic Record* of the WHO. Also, the International Union Against Tuberculosis and the International Cancer Control Organization in Lyon, France, collect and publish data on tuberculosis and cancer, respectively.

The importance and effectiveness of international surveillance of infectious diseases coordinated by the World Health Organization was demonstrated during the global SARS outbreak in 2003. Reports of SARS cases were made to the WHO Global Outbreak Alert & Response Network (GOARN), and the response to the disease was coordinated through the Global Public Health Intelligence Network (GPHIN) of WHO. This coordinated response permitted the identification of a novel coronavirus (SARS-Co-V) as the etiologic agent. This in turn informed control strategies within a few weeks of the recognition of the epidemic. The WHO is building on their successful response to the global SARS epidemic with improved surveillance and response using an available field team of epidemiologists and coordinating with other international health agencies, such as CDC and Medicine Sans Frontieres (MSF).

Other Surveillance Issues

Confidentiality of Data

For many diseases, it is of critical importance to maintain the confidentiality of surveillance data. For some conditions, such as HIV/AIDS, the issues of confidentiality are critical and must be considered in order to obtain valid data and to prevent harm to the persons surveyed. The issue of confidentiality arose over a plan to test sera from NHANES participants for HIV antibodies. After the plan was proposed initially, it was dropped because of fears that testing the sera for HIV would substantially reduce the participation rate and the representativeness of the sampled population if counseling and informed consent were required of the subjects studied. If only persons at low risk to HIV participated in NHANES, it would not only compromise the validity of the HIV prevalence estimate but of other health conditions measured in NHANES, as well. Eventually an anonymous, random survey of HIV prevalence in the general population was done by the NCHS.[49]

One method of dealing with this ethical and scientific dilemma is to use blinded, anonymous serologic surveys to estimate the prevalence of disease in critical populations. In blinded surveys, serologic testing can be performed on sera remaining after a clinically indicated test is completed and patient identifiers have been removed. Because the specimens are not linked to any personal identifiers, informed consent is not required. Ideally, the sera are available from an unbiased sample of a population. Examples of unbiased specimens include mandated programs such as infant screening programs for lead, pheylketonuria (PKU), hypothyroidism, and glucose-6-phosphate deficiency, or syphilis screening of persons attending sexually transmitted disease clinics. In hospitals, it is also possible to sample from the many clinical specimens collected to generate unbiased samples of the patient population. This method was used, originally in Massachusetts but later across the entire United States, to determine the prevalence of HIV in pregnant women.[50] Maternal antibodies are passively transferred to the infant during pregnancy so that HIV serology tests of blood collected from the infant at birth are a reflection of the maternal HIV status, not the infant's. The results from the infant blinded screening surveys provided valid and valuable public health data on the prevalence of HIV early in the US epidemic. These surveys receive considerable negative political attention as concerns were raised that all pregnant women should be required to have an HIV test to protect the infant from HIV. Rather than transform the program from blinded serosurveys to mandatory testing, which many public health officials feared would destroy the unbiased nature of the surveys and drive at-risk mothers away from health care, the CDC ended the maternal surveys. Despite the end of the maternal surveys, blinded anonymous surveillance of HIV seroprevalence in other populations continued and has been extremely important in tracking the US epidemic.[51]

Particularly, HIV testing is voluntary, making it inherently biased, and it was not a reportable disease early in the epidemic. Blinded serosurveys are not only used for diseases with confidentiality issues such as HIV but may also be applied to any infection where laboratory identification is possible.

Conclusion

Whether it is to define the burden of disease in a population to inform policy makers and caregivers, to evaluate the success of vaccine or other prevention programs, to monitor intentional or unintentional emerging diseases, or to provide insight into underlying health and risk behaviors in a population, surveillance is one of the cornerstones of public health.

References

1. Centers for Disease Control and Prevention (CDC). *Comprehensive Plan for Epidemiologic Surveillance.* Atlanta, GA: CDC; 1986.
2. Thacker SD, Berkelman RL. Public health surveillance in the United States. *Epidemiol Rev.* 1988;10:164–190.
3. Hartgerink MJ. Health surveillance and planning for healthcare in the Netherlands. *Int J Epidemiol.* 1976;5:87–91.
4. Politzer R. Plague. *World Health Organ Monogr Series.* 1954;22:1–198.
5. Wilcox WF, ed. *Natural and Political Observation Made upon the Bills of Mortality.* John Graunt (reprint of first edition, 1662). Baltimore, Md: Johns Hopkins University Press; 1937.
6. Frank JP. The people's misery: mother of disease. An address delivered in 1790. Sigerist H, trans. *Bull History Med.* 1941;9:81–100.
7. Langmuir AD. William Farr: Founder of modern concepts of surveillance. *Int J Epidemiol.* 1976;5:13–18.
8. Chapin CV. State health organization. *JAMA.* 1916;66:699–703.

9. Langmuir AD. The surveillance of communicable diseases of national importance. *N Engl J Med.* 1963;268:182–192.

10. Francis T Jr, Korus RF, Voight RB, et al. An evaluation of the 1954 poliomyelitis vaccine trials. Summary report. *Am J Public Health.* 1955; 45 (5,2):1–63.

11. Nathanson N, Langmuir AD. The Cutter incident: poliomyelitis following formaldehyde inactivated poliovirus vaccine in the United States in the spring of 1955. *Am J Hyg.* 1963;78:16–28.

12. Luik J, Kendal AP. Impact of influenza epidemics on mortality in the United States from October 1972 to May 1985. *Am J Public Health.* 1987;77:712–716.

13. Serfling RE. Methods for the current statistical analysis of excess pneumonia: influenza deaths. *Public Health Rep.* 1963;78:494–566.

14. Centers for Disease Control and Prevention. Case definitions for surveillance purposes. *MMWR.* 1997;46(RR19):1–15.

15. Centers for Disease Control and Prevention. Revision of the surveillance case definition for acquired immunodeficiency syndrome. *MMWR.* 1987;36:35–55.

16. Centers for Disease Control and Prevention. 1993 revised classification system for HIV infection and expanded surveillance case definition for AIDS for adolescents and adults. *MMWR.* 1992;41:1–19.

17. Centers for Disease Control and Prevention. CDC guidelines for evaluating surveillance systems. *MMWR.* 1988;37:1–18.

18. Minkoff HL, McCalla S, Delike I, et al. The relationship of cocaine use to syphilis and human immunodeficiency virus infection among inner city parturient women. *Am J Obstet Gynecol.* 1990;163:521–526.

19. Centers for Disease Control and Prevention. Gonorrhea among men who have sex with men selected sexually transmitted disease clinics, 1993–1996. *MMWR.* 1997;46:889–892.

20. Marks JS, Hayden GF, Orenstein WA. Measles vaccine efficacy in children previously vaccinated at 12 months of age. *Pediatrics.* 1978;62:955–960.

21. Orenstein WA, Markowitz L, Preblod SR, et al. Appropriate age for measles vaccination in the United States. *Dew Biol Stand.* 1985;65:13–21.

22. Centers for Disease Control and Prevention. Summary of notifiable diseases, United States, 1990. *MMWR.* 1991;39:30.

23. Shasby DM, Shope TC, Dowas K, et al. Epidemic measles in a highly vaccinated population. *N Engl J Med.* 1977;296:585–589.

24. The National Vaccine Advisory Committee. The measles epidemic: the problems, barriers and recommendation. *JAMA.* 1991;266:1547–1552.

25. Patriarca PA, Laender F, Palmeira E, et al. A randomized trial of alternative formulations of oral polio vaccine in Brazil. *Lancet.* 1988;1:429–433.

26. Ukena T, Esber H, Bessette R, et al. Site of injection and response to hepatitis B virus vaccine. *N Engl J Med.* 1985;313:579–580.

27. Pappaioanou M, Fishbein DR, Dreesen DW, et al. Antibody response to pre-exposure human diploid-cell rabies vaccine given concurrently with chloroquine. *N Engl J Med.* 1986;314:280–284.

28. Foege W. The eradication of vaccine-preventable diseases. In: Levine MM, Woodrow GC, Kapes JB, Cobon GS, eds. *New Generation Vaccines.* New York, NY: Marcel Dekker; 1997.

29. Fenner F, Henderson DA, Arita C, et al. *Smallpox and Its Eradication* Geneva, Switzerland: World Health Organization; 1988.

30. Mukinda VBK, Mwema G, Kilanda M, et al. Reemergence of human, monkey pox in Zaire. *Lancet.* 1997;349:1449–1450.
31. Pan American Health Organization. Director announces campaign to eradicate poliomyelitis from the Americas by 1990. *Bull Pan Am Health Org.* 1985;19:213–215.
32. Robbins FL, de Quadros LA. Certification of the eradication of indigenous transmission of wild poliovirus in the Americas. *J Infect Dis.* 1997;175(suppl. 1):S281–S285.
33. Lederberg J, Shope RE, Oaks SC Jr, eds. *Institute of Medicine, Committee on Emerging Microbial Threats to Health: Emerging Infections.* Washington, DC: National Academies Press; 1992.
34. Buehler JW, Hopkins RS, Overhage JM, Sosin DM, Tong V. Framework for evaluating public health surveillance systems for early detection of outbreaks: recommendations from the CDC Working Group. *MMWR Recomm Rep.* 2004;53:1–11.
35. Henning KJ. What is syndromic surveillance? *MMWR.* 2004;53 (suppl):5–11.
36. Duchin JS. Epidemiological response to syndromic surveillance signals. *J Urban Health.* 2003;80:i115–i116.
37. Centers for Disease Control and Prevention. Update: West Nile-like viral encephalitis—New York, 1999. *MMWR.* 1999;48:890–892.
38. Nash D, Mostashari F, Fine A, et al. The outbreak of West Nile virus infection in the New York City area in 1999. *N Engl J Med.* 2001;344:1807–1814.
39. Anderson JF, Andreadis TG, Vossbrinck CR, et al. Isolation of West Nile virus from mosquitoes, crows, and a Cooper's hawk in Connecticut. *Science.* 1999;286:2331–2333.
40. Briese T, Jia XY, Huang C, Grady LJ, Lipkin WI. Identification of a Kunjin/West Nile-like flavivirus in brains of patients with New York encephalitis. *Lancet.* 1999;354:1261–1262.
4l. Jia XY, Briese T, Jordan I, et al. Genetic analysis of West Nile New York 1999 encephalitis virus. *Lancet.* 1999;354:1971–1972.
42. Lanciotti RS, Roehrig JT, Deubel V, et al. Origin of the West Nile virus responsible for an outbreak of encephalitis in the northeastern United States. *Science.* 1999;286:2333–2337.
43. Centers for Disease Control and Prevention. *Epidemic/Epizootic West Nile Virus in the United States: Guidelines for Surveillance, Prevention, and Control.* Atlanta, Ga: Centers for Disease Control and Prevention; 2003.
44. Small P, Hopewell P, Singh S, et al. The epidemiology of tuberculosis in San Francisco. *N Engl J Med.* 1994;330:1703–1709.
45. Michele T, Cronin W, Graham NMH, et al. Transmission of mycobacterium tuberculosis by a fiber-optic bronchoscope. *JAMA.* 1997;278:1093–1095.
46. Perrotta DM, Decker M, Glezen WP. Acute respiratory disease hospital patterns as a measure of impact of epidemic influenza. *Am J Epidemiol.* 1985;122:468–476.
47. Centers for Disease Control and Prevention. Intussusception among recipients of rotavirus vaccine, United States, 1998–1999. *MMWR.* 1999;48:577–581.
48. Chen RT, Glasser JW, Rhodes PH, et al. Vaccine Safety Datalink project: a new tool for improving vaccine safety monitoring in the United States. *Pediatrics.* 1997;99:765–773.

49. McQuillan GM, Ezzati-Rice TM, Siller DB, Visschev N, Morley P. Risk behavior and correlates of risk for HIV infection in the Dallas County Household Survey. *Am J Public Health.* 1994;84:747–753.

50. Gwinn M, Pappaianou M, George JR, et al. Prevalence of HIV infection in childbearing women in the United States: surveillance using newborn blood samples. *JAMA.* 1991;265:1704–1708.

51. Centers for Disease Control and Prevention. *National HIV Serosurveillance Summary: Results Through 1992.* Atlanta, Ga: Department of Health and Human Services; 1994.

OUTBREAK EPIDEMIOLOGY

Diane M. Dwyer and Carmela Groves

Introduction

Outbreak epidemiology is the study of a disease cluster or epidemic in order to control or prevent further spread of disease in a population. The word *epidemic*, defined as an increase in the number of cases of a disease above what is expected, is derived from the Greek (epi-demos), meaning "that which is upon the people." This meaning enriches our understanding of epidemics by emphasizing the burdensome toll they have on a population or "a people." This definition also allows us to realize that epidemics are not always caused by infectious agents. Many other hazards, such as chemicals or physical conditions, can cause unusually high numbers of cases of disease in a given population. Nevertheless, the techniques used to investigate and control outbreaks are generally similar, regardless of the etiology of the disease.

Accounts of outbreaks have been recorded throughout the centuries. Cholera, influenza, malaria, smallpox, and the plague are extensively documented as causes of epidemics and pandemics that have altered the outcome of wars, disrupted political structures, killed millions of people, and affected the lives of countless others.[1] The prevention of disease through improved sanitation was recognized even before the causes of these diseases had been identified.

Today, there are new challenges in the control of infectious diseases. Public health officials and health care providers face the emergence of new diseases and the re-emergence of diseases that were no longer thought to be a threat to the public's health.[2] The intentional use of biologic agents or their toxins (e.g., anthrax, plague, botulism, and smallpox) as weapons of bioterrorism has occurred recently in the United States and has resulted in increased attention on outbreaks potentially caused by intentionally released agents. Changes in the environment; in industrial practices; in agriculture and food processing; in international transportation of people, foods, and goods; and changes in human behaviors have increased the risk of disease and the speed at which communicable disease can spread. Concurrently, the number of people at high risk and the density of human populations have increased. People with immunosuppression (e.g., those infected with human immunodeficiency virus), the elderly, or people with medical therapy for cancer, kidney failure, etc. are more susceptible to infectious diseases, including ones that may not have been medical concerns in the past. These compromised individuals may present with unusual symptoms that complicate the diagnosis, and their infections may be more difficult to treat. Immunosuppression may also increase the infectiousness of the individual, either by increasing the number of infectious organisms that the individual sheds or by increasing the length of time that the individual is infectious. The increasing density of the human population, especially in some developing nations, creates situations that foster the spread of new and old infectious diseases. However, the advantage is not all to the microbes. Advances in laboratory techniques and medical interventions, such as antibiotics, sanitation, and epidemiology, have increased our ability to identify and control infectious diseases.

In recent years, the news media have enhanced outbreak awareness. The names of organisms such as *Escherichia coli* O157:H7, Ebola virus, *Cryptosporidium*, Group A *Streptococcus* ("the flesh-eating bacteria"), and antibiotic-resistant *Streptococcus pneumoniae* conjure up reports of outbreaks that have been sensationalized in the press. Although some may take issue with the manner in which these reports have been presented, the reports have brought the results of outbreak investigations to the attention of the public. That *E. coli* O157:H7 can cause fatal hemolytic uremic syndrome, especially in children, was demonstrated in the US outbreaks caused by contaminated ground beef and in the Japanese outbreak caused by contaminated radish sprouts.[3,4] The speed at which international diseases could become threats to US citizens was underscored by the reports of Ebola virus isolated in monkeys in Reston, Virginia.[5] Reports of outbreaks of strains of *Mycobacterium tuberculosis* and *S. pneumoniae* that are resistant to antibiotics have raised the public awareness of the danger of inappropriate or excessive antibiotic use. Investigation of outbreaks such as these allows epidemiologists to identify risk factors and to determine preventive measures that will limit and control the spread of disease.

Today there may be a variety of reasons that an outbreak occurs, ranging from poor food handling practices to intentional acts of terrorism. An epidemiologist must investigate cases of disease with an awareness of all these possibilities. However, the basic techniques in investigation remain the same. This chapter will review the methods used to investigate and control outbreaks of infectious disease.

Surveillance and Outbreak Detection

Outbreaks may come to the attention of health professionals through a report from a doctor's office, a hospital, a nursing home, a laboratory, or even a patient's call to the health department. Alternatively, outbreaks may be recognized through analysis of reports of individual cases of disease.

In the United States, individual cases of certain diseases are "nationally notifiable" (Table 5-1), meaning the Council of State and Territorial

TABLE 5-1   Nationally Notifiable Diseases

Acquired immunodeficiency syndrome	Hemophilus influenzae (Invasive Disease)	Psittacosis Rabies, animal
Anthrax	Hansen disease (leprosy)	Rabies, human
Botulism*	Hantavirus pulmonary syndrome	Rocky Mountain spotted fever
Brucellosis		Rubella
Chancroid*	Hemolytic uremic syndrome	Salmonellosis*
Chlamydia trachomatis genital infection	post-diarrheal Hepatitis A	Shigellosis* Streptococcal disease,
Cholera	Hepatitis B	invasive, group A
Coccidioidomycosis* Congenital rubella syndrome	Hepatitis C/non-A, non-B HIV infection, pediatric	Streptococcus pneumoniae, drug-resistant*
Congenital syphilis Cryptosporidiosis	Legionellosis Lyme disease	Streptococcal toxic-shock syndrome
Diphtheria	Malaria	Syphilis
Encephalitis, California	Measles (Rubeola)	Tetanus
Encephalitis, Eastern Equine	Meningococcal disease	Toxic-shock syndrome
Encephalitis, St. Louis	Mumps	Trichinosis
Encephalitis, Western Equine	Pertussis	Tuberculosis
Escherichia coli O157:H7	Plague	Typhoid fever
Gonorrhea	Poliomyelitis, paralytic	Yellow fever

Note: Although varicella is not a nationally notifiable disease, the Council of State and Territorial Epidemiologists recommends reporting of cases of this disease to CDC.
* Not currently published in the *MMWR* weekly tables.
Source: Centers for Disease Control and Prevention.

Epidemiologists (CSTE) and the federal Centers for Disease Control and Prevention (CDC) recommend that 52 notifiable diseases be included in national surveillance.[6] States have individual laws, regulations, or both that govern which diseases and conditions are reportable and the method and timing of reporting, thus there are some variations across states. Reporting of outbreaks is generally included in a state's disease reporting system.

In routine passive surveillance in public health, reporting occurs from multiple sources. Physicians, laboratories, hospitals, prisons, schools, child-care centers, other facilities, and vital records departments (e.g., using death records) may generate reports (Figure 5-1). Cases are generally reported to state or local health departments with information such as diagnosis, name, age, gender, address, and date of onset. Reports may also include additional information, such as laboratory results, treatment, occupation, setting of occurrence, and risk factors (Figure 5-2 and Figure 5-3). Case reports, usually without personal identifiers, are then transmitted weekly from states to the CDC for inclusion in national summary data published in the *Morbidity and Mortality Weekly Report*.

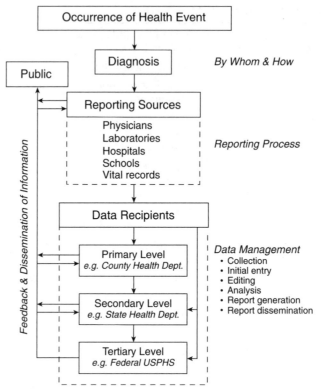

FIGURE 5-1   The flow of surveillance information.
Source: Public Health Surveillance, W. Halperin and E. Baker, eds., p. 30,
Copyright © 1992, Van Nostrand Reinhold.

Information collected as part of the disease reporting system is compiled
and evaluated at the local, state, and federal levels. The information collected
as part of the surveillance network is available for additional epidemiologic
evaluation. These data represent years of continuous data collection that can
be used to examine disease trends in a community. However, these data are
not collected for the conduct of epidemiologic studies. Rather, surveillance
data are collected to detect disease and to describe cases found in a community. Epidemiologic research data ideally would be collected to address
specific hypotheses. Surveillance data are collected according to those procedures that maximize consistency and minimize the barriers to reporting.
Surveillance databases often include data collected by passive reporting and
have only minimal information on cases. Research data may, instead, require
more detailed data collection to examine specific hypotheses and may require
employees dedicated to managing complex data collection systems. Because
of these differences, surveillance data may be inadequate to answer some
epidemiologic questions. However, surveillance data are an excellent source
of information to establish baseline rates and detect outbreaks, to identify
new problems or trends in a community, to evaluate programs, to assist
health professionals in estimating the magnitude of a health problem, and to

MARYLAND CONFIDENTIAL MORBIDITY REPORT
SEND TO LOCAL HEALTH DEPARTMENT

NAME OF PATIENT – LAST	FIRST	M	DATE OF BIRTH OR AGE			M □	W □ B □ Asian □ Am.Ind. □ Unk. □
			MO	DAY	YR	F □	Hispanic: Yes □ No □ Unk. □

ADDRESS	CITY OR TOWN		ZIP CODE	COUNTY

TELEPHONE NO.	OCCUPATION	WORKPLACE. SCHOOL. CHILD-CARE FACILITY. ETC (NAME. ADDRESS)

DISEASE OR CONDITION (IF STD OR TS COMPLETE REVERSE SIDE ALSO)	DATE OF ONSET			ADMITTED	DATE ADMITTED			HOSPITAL
	MO	DAY	YR	NO □ YES □	MO	DAY	YR	

PERTINENT CLINICAL INFORMATION:	LABORATORY TEST(S) IF VIRAL HEPATITIS			(SPECIMEN. TEST. RESULT. DATE)	SURVIVED □	IMPORTED
		pos	neg	date		DIED □	YES INTERSTATE □ INTERNATIONAL □
	HAV IgM	□	□	_____		DATE ____	NO □
	HBsAg	□	□	_____			UNK □
	HBcAb	□	□	_____			
	HBcIgM	□	□	_____		SUSPECTED SOURCE	
	HBsAb	□	□	_____			
	HCV AB	□	□	_____			

ACQUIRED IMMUNODEFICIENCY SYNDROME (AIDS) AND SYMPTOMATIC HIV INFECTION		LABORATORY TEST(S)
FEVER. WEIGHT LOSS. OR DIARRHEA □	SECONDARY CANCERS (KS, ETC.) □	CD4 + T-CELLS < 200/μL □
MYELOPATHY. OR PERIPHERAL NEUROPATHY □	OTHER CONDITIONS ATTRIBUTED TO	ELISA □
SECONDARY INFECTIONS (PCP. ETC) □	HIV INFECTION □	WESYERN BLOT □
		OTHER ____ □

REPORTED BY:	ADDRESS	TELEPHONE NO.	DATE OF REPORT		
			MO	DAY	YR

□ CHECK HERE IF YOU NEED ADDITIONAL MORBIDITY REPORT CARDS   DHMH-1140   5/94

SEXUALLY TRANSMITTED DISEASE (STD) (SEE INSTRUCTIONS)
STAGE OF SYPHILIS

PRIMARY □	SECONDARY □	EARLY LATENT (LESS THAN 1 YR) □	CONGENITAL □	OTHER STAGES □ SPECIFY ____

GONORRHEA | OTHER STD (SPECIFY)

UNCOMPLICATED □   PID □   RECTAL □   PHARY-NGEAL □   OPHTHALMIA NEONATORUM □   OTHER □ (SPECIFY) ____

Specify Lab Test (RPR or VDRL, FTA-ABS. FTA-IgM. Darkfield, Smear, Culture. Other)				TREATMENT GIVEN		
DATE	TEST	RESULTS	DATE	DRUG	DOSAGE	

TUBERCULOSIS DISEASE (SEE INSTRUCTIONS)
MAJOR SITE OF DISEASE | FOREIGN BORN: YES □

Pulmonary □ Ploural □ Lymphatic □ G/U □ Military □ Bone Joint □ Moningeal □ Periloneal □ Other □ ____	COUNTRY
Additional Sites: ____	DATE ENTERED USA ____

SUPPORTING BACT./HISTOLOGICAL EVIDENCE	CHEMOTHERAPY	NO □ UNK □
SPUTUM SPCEIMEN: DATE ____	CURRENT RX. DATE STARTED ____	TUBERCULIN TEST
POS NEQ PENDING NOT DONE	INH □ RIF □ PZA □ EMB □	PPD ____ mm
SMEAR □ □ □ □	SM □ OTHER □ ____	DATE ____
CULTURE □ □ □ □	NONE □	NOT DONE □
OTHER SPCEIMEN: TYPE ____ DATE ____	DIRECTLY OBSERVED THERAPY YES □ NO □ UNK □	X-RAY
POS NEG PENDING NOT DONE	PREVIOUS RX FOR TB DISEASE	NORMAL □
SMEAR □ □ □ □	YES □ YEAR ____ NO □ UNK □	ABNORMAL NON-CAVITARY □
CULTURE □ □ □ □	PREVIOUS INH PROPHYLAXIS	CAVITARY □
HISTOLOGY □ □ □ □	YES □ YEAR ____ NO □ UNK □	NOT DONE □
DATE ____		

5/94

FIGURE 5-2 Morbidity Case Report Form for transmission to the state or local health department.
Source: Maryland Department of Health and Mental Hygiene.

identify possible hypotheses that can be explored by enhancing surveillance or by a research study.

Because outbreak epidemiology is concerned primarily with the control of disease, the sensitivity of the surveillance or reporting network is of

Gastroenteritis Case Report Form
Maryland Department of Health & Mental Hygiene
Epidemiology & Disease Control Program

Source of Case Report _____

Date of Case Report _____

| Disease | ☐ Campylobacteriosis ☐ Shigellosis ☐ Unknown ☐ Salmonellosis ☐ Other _____ |
| Status | ☐ Sporadic Case ☐ Outbreak |

Patient Data

Name	Last	First
Telephone	Home	Work
Address	Street	
	County	City	State	Zip
Age	Date of Birth	/ /
Race	☐ White ☐ Hispanic ☐ Other ☐ Black ☐ Asian ☐ Unknown

Occupation, Student, or Situation

Name of Employer, School or Day Care

Clinical and Lab Data

Data of Onset ___/___/___ Time _____ am or pm

☐ Diarrhea ☐ Bloody Stool ☐ Cramps

☐ Fever ☐ Vomiting ☐ Other _____

Duration of Symptoms ___ days

| Outcome | ☐ Survived ☐ Died |
| Hospitalized | ☐ Yes ☐ No |

Name of Hospital

Date Admitted ___/___ Date Discharged ___/___/___

Date of Death ___/___/___

Name of Lab confirming diagnosis

Was the culture of specimen sent to the State Lab for serotyping or confirmation? ☐ Yes ☐ No ☐ Unknown

Agent (Check one)
☐ Campylobacter   Serotype _____
☐ Giardia
☐ Salmonella Group ___   Serotype _____
☐ Shigella   Serotype _____
☐ Other _____

Type of Specimen
☐ Bacterial ☐ Viral ☐ Ova and Parasite ☐ Serological

Source of Specimen
☐ Stool ☐ Urine
☐ Blood ☐ Other _____

Travel

Did patient travel to another state or country in the 2 weeks prior to symptom's onset? ☐ Yes ☐ No

Where _____ When _____

Animal Contact

Did patient have contact with the following animals [ ] hours/days* prior to symptom's onset?

☐ Dogs ☐ Parakeets ☐ Cows
☐ Cats ☐ Chickens ☐ Turtles
☐ Ducks ☐ Other _____

Food History

Did patient eat any of the following within [ ] hours/days* prior to onset of illness?

	Yes	No	Unknown
1. Eggs			
a. Cooked eggs: scrambled, hard fried, other _____	☐	☐	☐
b. Undercooked eggs: poached, soft, scrambled, sunny side up, other _____	☐	☐	☐
c. Raw eggs: egg nog, Caesar salad, hollandaise sauce, meringue, bearnaise, other _____	☐	☐	☐
2. Raw or undercooked poultry (chicken, turkey)	☐	☐	☐
3. Raw or undercooked red meat	☐	☐	☐
4. Raw (unpasteurized) milk	☐	☐	☐
5. Homemade/unpasteurized cheese	☐	☐	☐
6. Raw or undercooked fish/shellfish	☐	☐	☐

Other Exposure

Within [ ] hours/days* prior to onset of symptom(s) did patient:

	Yes	No	Unknown
1. Handle raw poultry?	☐	☐	☐
2. Have exposure to a day care or nursery?	☐	☐	☐
3. Have household member or sexual partner with similar symptoms?	☐	☐	☐
4. Hike, camp, fish, swim?	☐	☐	☐
5. Drink from a spring, stream or lake?	☐	☐	☐
6. Take antibiotics in month prior to onset of illness?	☐	☐	☐

Disposition

Work or school restrictions? ☐ Yes ☐ No

Is yes, specify _____

Was patient advised of appropriate precautions? ☐ Yes ☐ No

Is yes, how?
☐ Telephone ☐ Fact Sheet ☐ In Person ☐ In Writing

DHMH 4458 (June 1992)

FIGURE 5-3 Maryland Gastroenteritis Case Report Form.
Source: Maryland Department of Health and Mental Hygiene.

paramount importance. If cases of disease are not reported, an outbreak may not be detected or may continue unabated.

Most commonly, outbreak investigations are conducted by facilities (e.g., hospitals, nursing homes) or at the local or state public health level. Generally, the CDC is consulted in multistate outbreaks or in outbreaks of diseases that

Food History for Food-borne Diseases. List the foods eaten within [   ] hours/days* prior to onset:

[12 hours]   [24 hours]   [48 hours]   [72 hours]

Breakfast _____

_____

_____

Lunch _____

_____

_____

Dinner _____

_____

_____

_____

Household Members. List household contacts, even if asymptomatic; give onset if symptomatic:

Name	Age	Relationship to Case	Symptoms Y/N?	Onset of Symptoms	lab Testing (Date Collected, Result)	Occupation/Employer School/Grade, Day Care

Summary of Investigation - action taken on patients and contacts - outcome:

_____

_____

_____

_____

_____

_____

_____

Name of person completing form   Date of Interview

* Use the incubation period which applies to the agent/disease under investigation: e.g., bacillus cereus (1–24 hours), Campylobacter (1–10 days), Clostridium (6–24 hours), E. coli (9–60 hours), Giardia (5–25 days), Listeria (3–70 days), Salmonella (6–72 hours), Shigella (12–96 hours), Staphylococcus (30 min.–7 hours), Typhoid fever (1–3 weeks), Vibrio (4–96 hours), Viral agent (24–72 hours).

FIGURE 5-3   Continued

require resources or skills that state and local agencies are unable to provide. The laboratory and epidemiologic capabilities of the CDC are used to assist with domestic and international disease outbreaks of unusual etiology or of major public health significance.

Local and state health departments make the decision to conduct an outbreak investigation based on health regulations and on their professional judgment regarding the outbreak and its public health impact or implications.

Regardless of the etiologic agent, the setting in which the disease may have been transmitted, or the population at risk, it is possible to summarize the basic steps and goals of the investigation. The primary motivation of any outbreak investigation is to control the spread of disease within the initial population at risk or to prevent the spread to additional populations. Many outbreaks occur in confined populations, groups, or settings, such as a food-borne outbreak at a wedding banquet or a potluck dinner. Fortunately, these outbreaks generally have a single exposure, where the contaminated vehicle may have been consumed or eliminated before the first cases are apparent. In other outbreaks, where transmission is ongoing, such as legionellosis among hospitalized patients, the epidemiologic investigation must be initiated quickly and control measures implemented to halt transmission. Regardless of the current transmission status, prevention of disease requires that the investigation seek to identify the etiologic agent, its source, the mode of transmission, and the vehicle. Information learned is important in preventing and controlling outbreaks of the same disease in the future and may be useful in linking sporadic cases to the same source.

Outbreak Investigation

Based on experience with outbreak investigations, there is a series of steps that can be used to guide any epidemiologic field investigation.[7-10] The outbreak epidemiologist is the "Sherlock Holmes" or disease detective of public health. Outbreak investigation is a systematic process of evaluating data to form hypotheses, then collecting additional data to test the hypotheses. An understanding of the basic steps of outbreak epidemiology can guide the type of data to collect and how to collect them; however, each outbreak is unique, and it is equally important to be aware of how the current outbreak differs from previous outbreaks.

The steps for conducting an outbreak investigation are outlined in Figure 5-4. A hallmark of outbreak epidemiology is that these steps do not necessarily proceed in a specified sequence. In actuality, several steps in the investigation usually occur simultaneously. These steps are tailored to the situation and depend on factors such as the urgency to implement control measures; the availability of staff, resources, and time; and the difficulty in obtaining the data. Multiple persons may perform activities concurrently. Action and reaction proceed, based on new and cumulative information. Most obviously, implementation of control measures is central to the goal of any outbreak investigation. Measures to control the spread of disease must be implemented early in the investigation and may be altered as data are collected and analyzed.

Prepare for Field Work

Preparing for the outbreak investigation and planning the investigation are critical to a successful outcome. It is imperative to identify the investigation team members, to assign responsibilities, to begin the investigation as soon as possible, and to conduct progress meetings at regular intervals. The multidisciplinary investigative team may be composed of epidemiologists,

Prepare for field work
Confirm the existence of an outbreak—verify
    the diagnosis
Identify and count cases and exposed persons
    Select a case definition
    Identify cases, population at risk, and
        controls
Choose a study design
Collect risk information
Tabulate the data in terms of time, place, and
    person
Collect specimens for laboratory analysis
Conduct an environmental investigation
Institute control measures
Formulate and test hypotheses
Conduct additional systematic studies
Communicate the findings

FIGURE 5-4   Steps in an outbreak investigation.

health care professionals, laboratorians, sanitarians, etc. Often, the personnel who initiate an outbreak investigation are predetermined: health departments, hospitals, schools, or nursing homes commonly have personnel responsible for disease control who are dedicated to outbreak activities when the need arises. For many small-scale epidemiologic investigations, the initial outbreak "team" will be a single epidemiologist or other professional who will assess the situation and determine what needs to be done. As the investigation proceeds, personnel may need to be added or reassigned to carry out the investigation.

Successful investigations require effective communication at all levels of authority. Summaries or specific findings need to be shared on an ongoing basis (as appropriate and as allowed by confidentiality laws) with critical individuals and parties, such as facilities or businesses where the outbreak occurred, colleagues, health care providers, other regulatory agencies, the media, or the public. In the United States, communication among the local health department, state health department, and federal agencies such as the CDC, the Food and Drug Administration (FDA), and the US Department of Agriculture (USDA) is routine.

Confirm the Existence of an Outbreak—Verify the Diagnosis

An early step of any outbreak investigation is to confirm the existence of an outbreak. Important questions to ask are: Are there cases in excess of the expected baseline rate for that disease and setting? Is the reported case actually a case of the disease or a misdiagnosis? Do all (or most) of the "suspect cases" have the same infection or similar manifestations? For some diseases, a single case is sufficient to warrant an outbreak investigation. For example, anthrax, human rabies, food-borne botulism, polio, or bubonic plague are so rare in the United States and so serious that an investigation would be initiated with a single suspected case. As was the case with the single case of anthrax reported in October 2001 (CDC ongoing investigation of anthrax–Florida October 2001. *MMWR* 2001, 50;877), which initiated the full-scale investigation of the intentional release of anthrax in multiple locations across the eastern United States. Those investigating an epidemic must be aware of the background level of disease in a population under surveillance. For example, malaria infection acquired in the United States would be treated quite differently than a case of malaria acquired in sub-Saharan Africa. A review of existing state, local, or facility baseline rates of disease can be compared with the current case number. It is important to take into account the population in which the cases are occurring. Cases of diarrhea in a nursing home may be a common occurrence, whereas the same number would represent an outbreak if they occurred clustered in time among healthy adults after a picnic. It is also important to consider seasonal variations in disease rates. Influenza outbreaks can be expected to occur in the winter, whereas bacterial enteric diseases are more common in the summer.

As an outbreak investigation is initiated, it is important that the diagnosis be confirmed–and that the specificity of the case definition be good. This involves a review of available clinical and laboratory findings that support the diagnosis and often involves obtaining more clinical or laboratory information than is initially reported. For example, before deciding that *Neisseria meningitidis* is the organism causing disease, the investigator must confirm that the specimen was taken from a sterile body site (e.g., blood or cerebrospinal fluid), rather than from a body site where the organism may be a part of the normal flora (e.g., throat). Several cases of rash illness in a school may signal a scabies outbreak if the diagnosis is confirmed, or they may simply represent a cluster in time of rashes of different etiologies and, therefore, not an outbreak.

Identify and Count Cases and Exposed Persons—Select a Case Definition

A case definition is needed to identify and count cases in order to determine who may be affected by the outbreak. Components of the case definition may include information about time and place of exposure, laboratory findings, and clinical symptoms. For example, an early definition in a food-borne outbreak may read: "A case of illness is defined as any diarrhea, vomiting, abdominal cramps, headache, or fever that developed after attending the implicated event." This broad definition neither assumes that all cases will have the same symptoms, nor does it make any assumptions about the risk factors for illness (e.g., those who ate a particular food or had contact with specific people). This initial case definition has greater emphasis on sensitivity than on specificity. As additional information is gathered about the cases, the nature of exposure, and the symptoms, the case definition can be refined as appropriate to improve the specificity. A subsequent case definition may state: "A case of illness is defined as diarrhea or vomiting with onset within 96 hours of consuming food served at the implicated meal." This refined definition is more specific and will serve to exclude unrelated cases of gastroenteritis or other illnesses.

In outbreak investigations, as in routine surveillance, cases of disease are commonly separated into those that are confirmed and those that are probable cases. Confirmed cases are generally those with laboratory findings (such as a positive culture or antigen test, antibody titer rise, or a positive polymerase chain reaction [PCR]) for the organism, and probable cases are those who have certain symptoms meeting a clinical case definition but without laboratory confirmation.[11] For some diseases (e.g., pertussis), a case can be confirmed if there is a compatible clinical illness and the case is epidemiologically linked to a laboratory-confirmed case. Frequently, laboratory confirmation is complicated by a number of factors: People may test positive for the organism for a short time around the acute phase of illness; some pathogens produce toxins for which there is no laboratory test; the organism may be shed only transiently or intermittently; antibody tests may be difficult to interpret if individuals have been exposed to the pathogen in the past; persons with mild disease may not seek medical attention and, thus, will not have laboratory tests completed; and persons may be treated at different medical facilities with different laboratory procedures. If laboratory confirmation is important and the outbreak is identified rapidly enough, the outbreak investigation team may want to collect samples promptly or obtain multiple specimens to confirm the initial cases in order to establish the agent responsible for the outbreak. However, this commitment of resources may not be necessary to confirm every case during the investigation. If the case definition can be made sufficiently specific without the use of laboratory tests, collecting and testing specimens may only represent an additional burden and expense to the exposed population and the research team.

Identify Cases, Population at Risk, and Controls

During the outbreak investigation, the investigator should seek to identify additional cases not known or reported at the time of the initial report. Case-finding techniques used to enhance surveillance for additional cases include reviewing existing surveillance data (e.g., morbidity reports received by a health department or monthly summaries of illness); reviewing outbreak–complaint logs kept by the local health department; reviewing past laboratory data; and surveying hospitals, emergency rooms, or physicians. In certain outbreaks, such as those occurring in a restaurant where there is no list of attendees, a useful technique for finding additional cases and controls is questioning known cases to identify others who were in attendance. (See section on case-control studies.)

The investigator should identify the population at risk or the exposed group in which to conduct expanded surveillance for cases. The exposed group or cohort will vary, depending on the setting, and it may not always be possible to identify or enumerate the entire population at risk. Examples of exposed groups include a group of persons who attended a wedding banquet; all people who dined in a food establishment on one particular day; children who attend a day-care center, their household members, and the employees of the center; or all persons who were exposed to an implicated manufactured lot or shipment of a commercial product. The exposed population, therefore, can range from as few as one person to as many as thousands of individuals in multiple locations. Records maintained by the establishments involved can facilitate identification of persons at risk. Wedding invitation lists, guest books, credit card receipts, and customer lists are often available and are very helpful to investigators. However, individuals located by use of their credit card receipt may be concerned about how the investigators got their names! Explaining the purpose of the investigation and how information will be handled may be vital to securing their cooperation in the investigation. State and federal public information laws vary in what information is to be held confidential in outbreak situations.

Choose a Study Design

During an outbreak investigation, the study design is chosen based on factors such as the size and availability of the exposed population, the speed with which results are needed, and the available resources. The characteristics of the exposed population are generally determined after interviewing a few of the initial cases. Exposed populations fall into four broad categories: small enumerable exposed groups, large enumerable exposed groups, large or small groups where the exposure situation can be pinpointed but where the exposed population cannot be enumerated, and finally, cases of disease where the exposed population is not known or identifiable. The study design that is chosen will then dictate the appropriate analysis and hypothesis testing as discussed below.

Cohort Studies

Cohort studies, which include persons based on their exposure status, are appropriate when it is possible to enumerate or assemble a list of persons potentially exposed and to contact the people in a timely manner. Outbreaks that are suspected to have occurred at a specific event, such as a party, or in a specific place, such as a worksite or cruise ship, are often suited to cohort investigations. If the group is small enough, a study can be designed to include all of the people in the exposed cohort. Alternatively, a selection (using a random number table or selecting a random starting point and then choosing, e.g., every fourth name) can be made from a large enumerated exposed population. The demographic statistics, attack rates, and relative risks are calculated when data are collected on the cohort or on a randomly selected fraction of the cohort. (See section on formulating and testing hypotheses.)

Case-Control Studies

For outbreaks associated with large events (such as a convention or a state fair), or for community-wide outbreaks or uncommon diseases reported from a population, especially where the potential exposure is unknown, it may not be possible or economically feasible to obtain or assemble a list of all those exposed or to interview all people in the cohort or exposed population. These outbreak investigations lend themselves to studies that include all or a selected group of cases, and a selected group of not-ill individuals for comparison. A full description of the types of case-control studies, their nomenclature, and their analyses can be found in several references and in Chapter 3.[12-14]

When a list of a large cohort of potentially exposed people is available (i.e., the cohort can be enumerated) but a cohort study is not desirable or feasible, information on identified cases can be included and compared with information from a random sample of not-ill persons chosen from the baseline cohort, such as the list of those exposed (called a case-control study within a specific cohort, a case cohort study,[14] or a cumulative ["epidemic"] case-control study[13]). The number of not-ill people for comparison, and the manner in which the not-ill participants are chosen, differentiates these studies from traditional case-control studies. These studies maximize the number of cases included, and include a manageable number of not-ill people for comparison. The analysis of data is based on odds ratios, but attack rates and relative risks can also be calculated if the study group is a known fraction of the total cases and not-ill people.

Another common outbreak situation arises when cases are occurring within a known exposed population (e.g., attendees at a state fair or a specific restaurant) but the exposed population cannot be enumerated and there is no list of attendees from which to identify cases and controls. In this situation, it is important to secure data on a representative sample of people who were potentially exposed. Cases can be identified from reports of illness. Both cases and controls can be identified from the exposed group through friends of cases or through media reports, credit card receipts, lists of hospital patients, etc. Publicizing through a press release in local print or on television and radio may be necessary to secure a sufficient number of not-ill participants. People who know someone who became ill are more likely to know about the outbreak investigation and volunteer to participate. The volunteers, however, may share characteristics with those who are cases and may not represent all of those who attended the event. Small groups may be identified who attended a larger event, such as a church group who attended a national convention or a state fair, and the group members may serve as a source of investigation participants. The use of such identified groups can aid recruitment because they may have a list of participants for inclusion. For outbreaks such as these, analysis of the data would necessarily proceed using odds ratios as in a case-control study because data are neither available on the entire cohort nor from a known fraction of the group of exposed persons.

For situations in which an exposed cohort or population is not known or identifiable, a case-control study design is appropriate to determine risk factors for disease. Examples of this situation include increases in the number of community-wide cases of an unusual *Salmonella* serotype, or the need to identify risk factors for sporadic cases of *Campylobacter* infection. In these situations, cases are selected based on their disease status rather than their exposure status. All known cases are included in the study along with a group of controls, selected, for example, by random digit dialing, or from friends or neighbors of cases. For increased statistical power, up to four controls per case are selected. A further refinement of the case-control study is the matched case-control design. In these studies, controls are matched to cases with respect to potentially confounding variables. In matched case-control studies the effect of these matched variables is removed from the analysis so that the effect of other factors can be more readily observed. For example, to determine the risk factors for a cluster of cases of a rare *Salmonella* serotype, all known cases would be interviewed. Controls may be identified by randomly calling homes with incrementally higher or lower telephone numbers from the case's telephone number. If a household is found in which a member matches the case within a certain age grouping, that person is included as a control in the study and is interviewed.

Because outbreak investigations are primarily concerned with the prevention of the spread of disease, the speed at which case-control studies can be assembled makes them an attractive alternative to cohort studies. The case-control design is also efficient with respect to collection of data and the expense of conducting the study. The toxic shock syndrome epidemic of 1980 was alarming for the speed at which cases occurred and the severity of the illness.[15,16] Investigation was needed as rapidly as possible. Using a case-control study design, investigators assembled study populations using cases and selecting as controls their friends of the same sex. Controls were matched to cases within 3 years of age. Lives were saved because of the speed at which these investigations were completed and the subsequent speed at which health interventions were initiated (Figure 5-5).

Collect Risk Information

As the case investigation continues, the investigator assimilates information regarding the affected population to answer questions regarding person, place, and time (also referred to as who, what, when, and where). As part of the investigation, the investigator may use a questionnaire or survey instrument to collect pertinent data (Figure 5-6). Questionnaires should be administered as soon as possible. The ability to recall one-time exposures after an event is poor, even in the best of circumstances, and will diminish rapidly with time. Initially, questionnaires may need to be broad and capture as much information as possible regarding suspected exposures, such as in widely distributed or geographically clustered outbreaks like the large cryptosporidiosis outbreak in Milwaukee.[17]

The questionnaire instrument collects pertinent information about the exposed population or the cases and controls, and about the situation under investigation. Questionnaires usually include variables sufficient to define cases and to identify exposures. Each survey must be tailored to the outbreak and the possible routes of exposure for the agent involved. Demographic information allows the investigator to answer the *who* question and usually includes personal identifiers, such as the person's name, home address, telephone number, age, gender, race/ethnicity, occupation/school, and work address.

These variables are used to characterize both the ill and well populations. Clinical information helps the investigator with the *what* and *when* questions and includes symptoms of illness, date and time of onset and length of symptoms, specimen collection dates and results, severity of illness, medical care sought, and outcome information, such as hospitalization or death. These variables allow the characterization of identified cases and assist with hypothesis generation. Exposure information helps the investigator to answer the *where* and *when* questions and helps detail the suspected event or situation that put the individuals at risk. The questionnaire should consider exposures other than the most obvious exposure. For example, if ill individuals all attended a wedding, they should be asked not only about the

Identified as a severe systemic illness in children, toxic-shock syndrome (TSS) burst on the national scene when cases suddenly appeared, first in Wisconsin and Minnesota and then nationwide, among young adult women during their menstrual periods. The disease was serious and caused substantial mortality. Recovery was complete among survivors; however, recurrences were common during a subsequent menses unless the *S. aureusvaginal* infection was effectively treated with antibiotics. Eventually, 941 cases were reported from every state in the United States. However, 247 (26%) of the cases occurred in Minnesota and Wisconsin.

In the interest of speed and because the number of cases was small, a case-control study design was chosen. To control for unknown confounders and to assemble a study population rapidly, the investigators chose to use friends of cases for the initial investigation. Controls were the same gender as the cases (female) and matched to cases within 3 years of age. In the initial investigations, conducted June 13–19, 1980, one control was matched to each case. These studies implicated tampons and hormonal contraception as risk factors for TSS during menstruation. However, women had been

using tampons and hormonal contraception for years. Why an outbreak now? And why were the cases concentrated in Wisconsin and Minnesota? The epidemiologic team was aware that a new brand of tampons had been marketed in these states, and they suspected that these super-absorbent tampons might be associated with the outbreak. Although a few brands of tampons were common among women with TSS, these tampon brands were found to be popular with women in general (as measured by market share). A third case control outbreak investigation was conducted September 5–8, 1980. In this study, cases were matched to three age- and gender-matched controls. To reduce misclassification bias, participants were asked to get any boxes of tampons they had in the house and to read the brand information to the telephone interviewer. In this investigation, one brand of super-absorbent tampons was identified and subsequently recalled on September 22, 1980. The incidence of TSS declined dramatically and fell even further when polyacrylate tampons (super-absorbent tampons) were withdrawn altogether, although some cases are still reported.

FIGURE 5-5 Investigation of toxic shock syndrome.

wedding but also about events related to the wedding, such as a common hotel swimming pool exposure, or attendance at other events, such as the rehearsal dinner.

Errors in recall can result in "baseline noise" or misclassification bias. Misclassification bias occurs when persons are randomly incorrectly classified with respect to exposure or illness. Misclassification bias results in the measured risk of disease for persons exposed being lower than the actual risk. Thus, a study could underestimate or miss a significant exposure. Figure 5-7 shows an example of how a 20% misclassification of exposure among all attendees at a dinner underestimates the true relative risk by half. One technique used to aid respondents is to ask directed questions of what they "usually" would eat. Using these questions in combination with more traditional food survey questions may help to reduce misclassification bias. For example: "If given a choice between chicken salad and roast beef, which would you usually take?" In addition to improving the quality of data collected, timely collection of data allows for a faster public health response, such as closure of a facility or a product recall or embargo. The Tennessee Department of Health and Environment conducted a planned study to

The Health Department is investigating some reports of illness that occurred after the _____ (event) _____ on __ day, _____.
It is important that anyone who attended fill out a questionnaire, even if you did not get sick.

Last name _____ First name _____ Age _____

Home phone number: (__ __ __) __ __ __ -__ __ __ __   Sex: M F (circle one)

Did you eat at this event?   Yes   No

Please circle YES for any food item you ate at the event and circle NO for each item that you did not eat.
All items should be marked.

Ate item?   Ate item?

Food 1 .... Yes   No   Food 7 .... Yes   No
Food 2 .... Yes   No   Food 8 .... Yes   No
Food 3 .... Yes   No   Food 9 .... Yes   No
Food 4 .... Yes   No   Food 10 .... Yes   No
Food 5 .... Yes   No   Food 11 .... Yes   No
Food 6 .... Yes   No   Food 12 .... Yes   No

Did you have any drinks on ice?   Yes   No
Did you have any soft drinks on ice?   Yes   No
Did you have any alcoholic drinks on ice?   Yes   No   (Number_____)
Did you have any non-iced alcoholic drinks?   Yes   No   (Number_____)

Was anyone in your household ill with diarrhea or vomiting in the week preceding the event?
Yes   No   (If yes, Who? & When?_____)

Have you become ill **since** attending the event?   Yes   No

If yes, please circle   YES   or   NO   for **each** of the following symptoms:

Diarrhea   Yes No   If yes, total number of stools on worst day _____
                                 Was there any blood in your stool? Yes   No
Stomach cramps   Yes No
Nausea   Yes No
Vomiting   Yes No
Fever   Yes No   If yes, what was your highest temperature?_____
Headache   Yes No
Body aches   Yes No
Chills   Yes No

Date illness began: _____   Time illness began: ___:___ AM? or PM? (circle answer)

Still having symptoms? Yes No
  (If no, symptoms ended: Date: ___ Time: ___:___ AM? or PM?)
Did you take any medicines for this illness?   Yes No   If yes, what medicines? _____
Did you go to your doctor or an emergency room for this illness?   Yes No
  If yes, did they collect specimens?   Yes No   If yes, name of doctor: _____
Were you admitted to the hospital for this illness?   Yes No   If yes, name of hospital:_____

FIGURE 5-6 Sample questionnaire for a food-borne illness outbreak.

Ate Birthday Cake	Ill	Not Ill	Attack Rate	Relative Risk
Yes	30	30	30/60 = 50%	50%/10% = 5.0
No	15	135	15/150 = 10%	

Now, assume that, on the questionnaire, 20% of all attendees made an error in whether or not they ate birthday cake. The table below shows the resulting calculation with the relative risk underestimated at 2.5.

Ate Birthday Cake	Ill	Not Ill	Attack Rate	Relative Risk
Yes	30 − 6 + 3* = 27	30 − 6 + 27 = 51	27/78 = 34.6%	34.6%/13.6% = 2.5
No	15 − 3 + 6 = 18	135 − 27 + 6 = 114	18/132 = 13.6%	

Note: 30 people ate birthday cake, minus 20% (or 6) who make an error and say they did not eat cake, plus 20% of the 15 (or 3) people who did not eat cake but in error say that they did.

FIGURE 5-7   Example of the effect that misclassification bias has on the relative risk calculation.

determine the degree of misclassification of food consumption after a luncheon.[18] By comparing videotapes of the luncheon to participants' answers on a subsequent food survey, investigators found that 32 attendees failed to report 58 food items actually selected and reported selecting 24 items not actually selected, or a total of 82 errors. Only 12.5% of participants made no errors.

Figure 5-7 shows the true exposures to birthday cake and true illness in a cohort of 210 people who attended a banquet: 50% of those who ate cake became ill, compared with only 10% of those who did not eat the cake. The true relative risk of illness is 5.0, or "Those who ate birthday cake were five times as likely to become ill, compared with those who did not eat cake."

The design of the survey instrument is determined by how much the investigative team already knows. In cases where some of the epidemiologic questions have been answered, the questionnaire can be more specific. Questions can be in a closed format with "yes" or "no" answers, or they can be quantitative (e.g., maximum number of stools per day or amount of food consumed). This assures consistency in response and facilitates analysis of the data. In cases where less is known, investigators must keep an open survey instrument to collect any information that may be of use. In such instances, the initial interview or survey instrument should include open-ended questions to encourage people to recall how, where, and over what period they may have been exposed. The questionnaire must be flexible enough to take into account the variable incubation periods for different diseases. For example, two diseases that might initially be reported as diarrheal diseases, salmonellosis and giardiasis, have incubation periods of 1–3 days and 7–10 days, respectively. Until the agent is known through laboratory results, the questionnaire would need to be broad enough to cover exposures during both periods of risk. The epidemiologist must evaluate all the questionnaires to see whether any common links can be found. This sort of evaluation will require knowledge about the clinical syndrome, incubation period, duration, possible etiologies, and possible routes of transmission. This detailed initial process may be conducted even verbally, with as few participants as necessary to define the outbreak better. Once the questionnaire can be simplified, a new, more specific questionnaire without open-ended questions can be administered to a larger group of participants to complete the investigation.

More than one questionnaire can be used during an investigation to capture the necessary information. The initial questionnaire may not be specific enough to answer all of the epidemiologic questions of interest, such as the qualitative and quantitative details of exposure. Furthermore, different populations affected by the epidemic may have different roles in its transmission. For example, a survey of patrons of a food establishment might be administered to the exposed group to find cases and to record clinical and risk information. A different questionnaire would be administered to food service workers that would collect information on illnesses prior to the event, food preparation and handling, hygiene practices, food intake at the event, and any illnesses after the event. Similarly, in a hospital nursery outbreak, the questionnaires completed on newborn cases and controls would be very different from the questionnaires for hospital personnel.

Tabulate and Orient the Data in Terms of Time, Place, and Person

The organization of data is critical to the timely and successful analysis of the outbreak data. A useful tool to organize data is the line listing. An example of a line listing is provided in Figure 5-8. Using a spreadsheet-style format, key variables on each ill person are listed, either on paper or computerized. Information on well persons can also be included. A line listing allows the investigator to visualize and summarize pertinent variables quickly, including the total number of cases, the number of individuals with specific symptoms, their ages, gender, hospitalization, date and time of onset, exposures, and rates of illness. Another traditional method for organizing outbreak data is to use cards, where each person's characteristics are recorded on a single index card. Sorting the cards in different ways allows investigators to determine risk factors for cases. Obviously, card and paper methods were devised prior to the use of computers, and any of the spreadsheet or database programs available today can be used for data management and analysis. The CDC has developed the EpiInfo computer software program, in which questionnaires can be created, data entered and analyzed, and line listings produced. This program is currently in worldwide use because it is free, easy to use, has modest computer requirements, is designed specifically for surveillance systems and outbreak epidemiology, and is sufficiently powerful for most investigations. Information on EpiInfo can be obtained from the CDC home page on the Internet (www.cdc.gov).

Visual representations of data can be helpful in understanding an epidemic. Spot maps of cases by residence, site of care, or location in a facility can help explain the occurrence of cases. More complex methods of combining outbreak data with other sources of data are explained in the chapter on Geographical Information Systems (GIS). Graphs, such as an epidemic curve, or epi-curve, provide a visual summary of data (Figure 5-9). The epidemic curve depicts the frequency of cases over time by plotting the number of cases by date or time of onset. This provides information regarding the nature

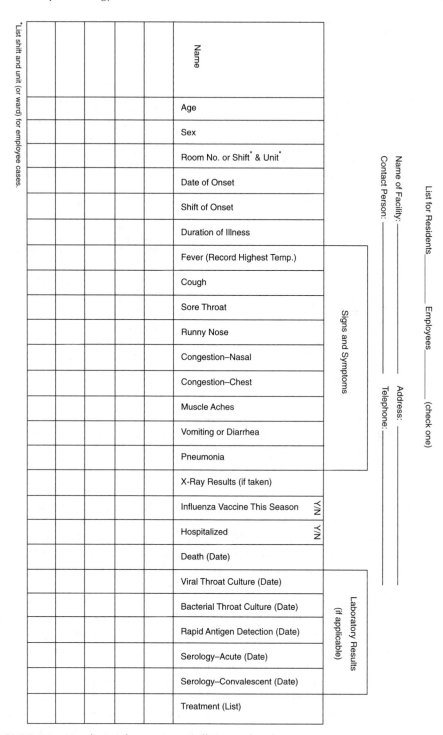

FIGURE 5-8 Line listing for respiratory illness outbreaks.

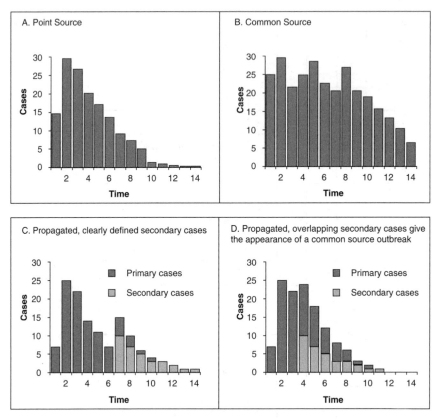

FIGURE 5-9 Examples of epidemic curves illustrating that the shape of the curve gives clues to the mode of transmission and incubation period.

and time course of the outbreak. The epi-curve can allow an estimate of the incubation time of the infection, which may help in the identification of the organism. The time from the presumed exposure to the peak of the epidemic curve is the hypothesized median incubation time. The epi-curve can also give an indication of whether transmission is continuing or has ended. This information is vital to knowing whether control measures may be needed because the current outbreak is continuing and whether control measures are containing the outbreak. Epidemics in which the number of cases rises abruptly and falls again in a log linear fashion are possible point source epidemics: The population at risk was exposed at one point in time. Cases occur suddenly after the minimum incubation time and continue for a brief period of time related to the variability in the incubation time in infected individuals. Unless there is secondary spread of the pathogen to others not exposed originally, the epidemic ends.

Second, in cases where there is continued exposure of individuals, a common source epidemic, cases rise suddenly after the minimum incubation time but do not disappear completely because more individuals continue to be exposed to the source.

Third, a propagated outbreak will show an increase in cases after exposure, then a fall in the number of cases after the epidemic has exhausted those susceptible from the initial exposure. Later, there is a second increase in cases one incubation period after the peak of the first cases, due to secondary cases infected by person-to-person spread. Because an incubation period may be shorter than the rate at which case rates decline after the initial exposure, propagated outbreaks and common source outbreaks can be difficult to distinguish on the basis of their epi-curves alone.

Perform Laboratory Analysis

The laboratory investigation consists of collecting and testing appropriate specimens. To identify the etiologic agent, the collection of laboratory specimens needs to be appropriately timed. Examples of specimens include food and water samples, other environmental samples (e.g., air settling plates), and clinical specimens (e.g., stool, blood, sputum, or wound specimens) from cases and controls. Hypotheses about the suspected agent and source should guide the laboratory tests that are performed. Further description of organisms through speciation and other specialized laboratory testing, such as pulsed field gel electrophoresis (PFGE),[19] plasmid analysis,[20] PCR,[21-23] or DNA fingerprinting (restriction fragment length polymorphism [RFLP]),[24] is useful to link cases with each other and with the hypothesized source(s). For example, to confirm the source in a legionellosis investigation, it is important to obtain an isolate of *Legionella* from the patient and from the epidemiologically implicated water source to determine whether the isolates are identical. Chapter 8 covers the methods and use of laboratory techniques in more detail.

Conduct an Environmental Investigation

An assessment of the environment where the exposure occurred should be performed when appropriate. The environmental investigation assists in answering How? and Why? questions. This includes an inspection of the facility, a review of practices and procedures for the operation, and an assessment of employee illness. Staff members (including paid employees and volunteers) at facilities such as day-care centers, restaurants, and health care facilities may play a key role in outbreaks and may be either the source of the problem or cases in the outbreak. Their evaluation as potential sources and cases, as well as the information they provide in the environmental investigation, may be critical.

The facility assessment may include an inspection by an environmental specialist or other investigator to review procedures and compliance with existing regulations and to identify breakdown of preventive measures. Timely inspection of facilities is of utmost importance to the control of an outbreak. When violations are noted, corrective actions are recommended and compliance monitored. In a food-borne outbreak, an inspection should focus on the kitchen and food preparation areas, whereas in a legionellosis outbreak, inspection should focus on water sources, such as the cooling tower, heating and ventilation systems, potable hot water and plumbing systems, and other areas of water aerosolization, such as showers, decorative fountains, and respiratory equipment. In a nursing home outbreak with person-to-person spread, inspection and interviews should focus on adherence to appropriate infection control procedures, including hand washing and exclusion of ill employees.

While conducting the physical inspection of the facility, the investigator must pay careful attention to the details of the suspected procedure, such as food preparation, administration of medications, hand washing, or endoscope cleaning. Investigating each step in a procedure with observations of their use and open-ended questions enables the epidemiologist to identify potential problem areas or violations. A review of existing standard operating procedure manuals or materials is helpful in the process. In the United States, food providers are recommended (or, in some states, required) to have a hazard analysis, critical control point (HACCP) procedure outlined for each food product they serve.[25] The HACCP plan outlines the ingredients, food preparation techniques, storage until serving, serving conditions, and handling of leftover food (Figure 5-10). However, the investigator must assess how the procedure was done at the time of the outbreak, instead of how the procedure should be done or how it is usually done. For example, in an outbreak of egg-associated *Salmonella* serotype *Enteritidis* in Maryland, pasteurized eggs were always used in the preparation of crab cakes, and the crab cakes were reportedly cooked to an adequate internal temperature according to their procedure. On one occasion when no pasteurized eggs were available and the facility was exceptionally busy, the facility used fresh shell eggs in the mixture and the crab cakes were not cooked to an internal temperature necessary to kill *Salmonella*. Thus, *Salmonella* in the raw shell eggs and breaks in the usual operating procedures were responsible for the outbreak.[26]

The investigator may need to replicate the process described to determine where the break in food handling procedures occurred. A Maryland outbreak of cholera was found to be associated with a coconut dessert prepared in an individual's home.[27] The cook explained that the commercial, fresh-frozen coconut milk had been brought to a boil. After replicating the recipe and cooking procedures, investigators found that coconut milk brought to a low boil reached only 160° F. After "boiling," the coconut milk had been allowed to sit on the counter for several hours at room temperature in the summer before being eaten, offering an excellent opportunity for the *Vibrio cholerae* organisms to multiply.

Implement Control Measures

As soon as preliminary data indicate the magnitude and severity of the outbreak, a hypothesis should be made regarding the time, place, and person; the suspected etiologic agent(s); and the mode of transmission. Steps should be taken to contain the outbreak. Additional recommendations for control may be developed as the investigation progresses and new information is gathered. Appropriate control measures depend on knowledge of the etiologic agent, the mode of transmission, and other contributing factors. Public health law gives health officials substantial authority to take action to prevent the spread of disease to others. Some examples of control measures include:

- Recalling or destroying remaining contaminated food products[27,28]
- Restricting infected workers from high-risk occupations[29]
- Closing affected facilities to prevent continued exposure
- Correcting procedural practices identified as inadequate or improper (such as food handling in a salmonellosis outbreak[30] or patient care practices in a methicillin-resistant *Staphylococcus aureus* outbreak[31])

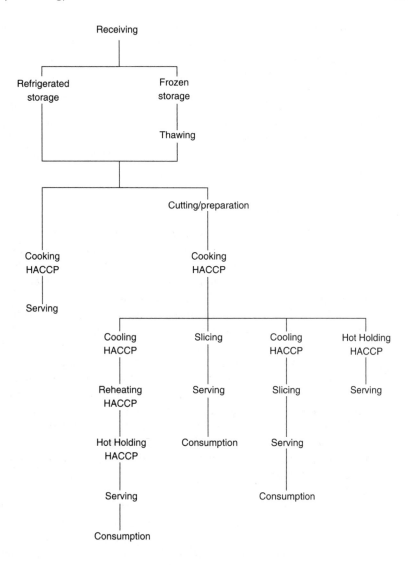

FIGURE 5-10   Sample hazard analysis, critical control point chart that follows an item (e.g., raw meat) from the point of receiving the raw product through storage and cooking to the point of consumption.
Source: Maryland Department of Health and Mental Hygiene.

- Recommending a prophylactic therapeutic agent and/or vaccine (e.g., use of rifampin in an outbreak of meningococcal disease)[32]
- Enforcing hand washing (e.g., in an outbreak of nosocomial gastroenteritis)
- Educating the public about risk and prevention (e.g., recall of beef contaminated with *E. coli* O157:H7, coupled with the message to cook hamburger to greater than or equal to 160° F)[28]

Surveillance for additional cases will allow the investigator to evaluate how the control measures are working. Depending on the disease and the incubation period, additional reports of cases may be expected, even after control measures have been implemented and control achieved. For example, successful control of an outbreak of hepatitis A (with an incubation period of 2–6 weeks) does not prevent additional cases from occurring that were exposed in the past and incubating at the time that control measures were implemented.

Recommendations or control measures from an outbreak investigation may lead to the development of procedural changes, guidelines, regulations, or laws that will be applied more broadly as public health policy and are intended to prevent additional cases or outbreaks in similar settings in the future.

Formulate and Test Hypotheses

As the outbreak is investigated, data are assessed informally so that control measures can be implemented and hypotheses can be developed that may lead to further data collection or data analysis. Data are also assessed formally, using standard descriptive and analytic epidemiologic techniques to determine the specific cause(s) of the epidemic.

A primary goal of data analysis is to determine means of transmission and the source and the vehicle of the agent, so that the most effective preventive measures can be initiated. Laboratory data can be conclusive but may not be available, especially at the beginning of an outbreak. An evaluation of symptoms, including their description, frequency, and severity, is a first step in determining the probability of the causal agent. Also, the mean, median, mode, and range of the incubation period can be determined from the epi-curve or by direct calculation. As mentioned above, it is important to separate primary and secondary cases of disease, when possible, to avoid errors in estimating the incubation period. The epi-curve and interviews can be used to determine whether the epidemic is most likely a point source, a common source, or a propagated epidemic.

Another goal of data analysis is to determine the risk factors for disease. As has been done throughout the investigation, analysis starts by answering global questions and works toward answering more specific questions—nesting more specific questions within the context of having answered the broader ones. Initially, analysis will be directed toward determining what population is at risk for disease. Initial hypotheses will be questions such as, "Are people who attended the wedding at greater risk of disease than the general public (was there an outbreak)?" Subsequently, the question will be, "Among those who participated in the wedding party events are people who ate at the wedding buffet, or swam in the pool, or attended the rehearsal dinner at greater risk of disease than those without these exposures?" More specifically, the hypotheses will be in the form, "Among those who ate at the buffet, are people who ate the Caesar salad (or other specific food item) at greater risk than those who did not?" To answer these questions, measures of risk will be calculated.

The measure of risk used in outbreaks investigated using cohort design is the risk-specific attack rate (e.g., food-specific attack rate for food-borne outbreaks), which is the number of persons who became ill who reported the risk behavior divided by the total number of people who reported that risk behavior. Commonly, the risk-specific attack rate is expressed as a percentage.

Figures 5-11, 5-12, and 5-13 illustrate the nested hypothesis testing in a typical outbreak of diarrheal disease associated with a picnic. In Figure 5-11, 42.9% (30 of 70) of attendees who ate hors d'oeuvres were ill (that is, the risk-specific attack rate for hors d'oeuvres was 42.9%, higher than the attack rates for other risk factors examined).

The second step of analysis is to compare the attack rates for different groups. In this way, it can be determined whether persons reporting a particular behavior are at higher risk of illness than those who do not report the risk behavior. The relative risk (RR) is the attack rate among those exposed to the risk factor divided by the attack rate in those who were not exposed. If those who ate hors d'oeuvres were no more likely to become ill than those who did not, the attack rates would be equal, and the RR would be 1. If those who ate hors d'oeuvres were more likely to become ill than those who did not, this ratio would be greater than 1, and hors d'oeuvres would be a risk factor for illness. Conversely, if the ratio is less than 1, having that factor would be protective against illness. In Figure 5-11, the attack rate in those who ate hors d'oeuvres is divided by the attack rate in those who did not,

Risk Factor Present	Cases $N = 35$	Not Cases $N = 100$	Risk-Specific Attack Rate (AR)
Swimming	15	39	$\frac{15}{54} = 27.7\%$
Volleyball	5	20	$\frac{5}{25} = 20.0\%$
Ate box lunch	20	95	$\frac{20}{115} = 17.3\%$
Ate evening hors d'oeuvres	30	40	$\frac{30}{70} = 42.9\%$

Figure 5-11 Example of the attack rate and relative risk calculations in a typical outbreak.

		Case	Not Case	AR	
Swimming	Yes	15	39	$\frac{15}{54} = 27.7\%$	Relative Risk $= \frac{27.7\%}{24.7\%} = 1.1$
	No	20	61	$\frac{20}{81} = 24.7\%$	

		Case	Not Case	AR	
Ate hors d'oeuvres	Yes	30	40	$\frac{30}{70} = 42.9\%$	Relative Risk $= \frac{42.9\%}{7.7\%} = 5.6$
	No	5	60	$\frac{5}{65} = 7.7\%$	

Figure 5-12 Follow-up analysis using a case-control study to determine the odds of disease according to consumption of specific hors d'oeuvres.

The investigators were concerned that one of the ingredients used in the preparation of the stuffed mushrooms was also used in a dipping sauce for chips. In particular, they were concerned about a prepared meat product used to stuff the mushrooms and to flavor the dipping sauce. To determine whether the two hors d'oeuvres were independent risk factors for illness, the investigators first reviewed the risk of disease for participants who ate the mushrooms and for those who ate the dipping sauce. They then conducted a cohort study because they were using data from the entire cohort who ate the evening hors d'oeuvres ($N = 70$), and they were able to calculate relative risks.

		Case	Not Case	AR	
Ate	Yes	15	9	$\frac{15}{24} = 62.5\%$	
Stuffed					Relative Risk = 1.9
Mushrooms	No	15	31	$\frac{15}{46} = 32.6\%$	

		Case	Not Case	AR	
Ate	Yes	16	14	$\frac{16}{30} = 53.3\%$	
Dipping					Relative Risk = 1.5
Sauce	No	14	26	$\frac{14}{40} = 35.0\%$	

Next, they conducted a stratified analysis to determine the risk-specific attack rates of people who ate both of the hors d'oeuvres, dipping sauce only, stuffed mushrooms only, and neither item.

Ate Dipping Sauce

	Yes					No		
	Case	Not Case	AR			Case	Not Case	AR
Ate	Yes	4	1	$\frac{4}{5} = 80.0\%$	Ate	Yes	11	8	$\frac{11}{19} = 57.9\%$
Stuffed					Stuffed			
Mushrooms	No	12	13	$\frac{12}{25} = 48.0\%$	Mushrooms	No	3	18	$\frac{3}{21} = 14.3\%$

Based on these results, investigators concluded that both stuffed mushrooms and dipping sauce were risk factors for illness, without evidence of additive interaction between them. An investigation was initiated into the common ingredient—prepared meat. Further laboratory tests confirmed that packages of prepared meat were contaminated, and appropriate control measures instituted.

Figure 5-13 Additional analysis to determine whether there was interaction between foodstuffs consumed at the picnic.

or 42.9% divided by 7.7%, for an RR of 5.6. In this example, the statement could be made that those who ate hors d'oeuvres were more than five times as likely to become ill than those who did not eat hors d'oeuvres. Usually, additional statistical calculations are made, including the confidence interval around this point estimate of risk and the probability that this result occurred by chance.

In a case-control study, the total population exposed to the risk factor is not available; the ratio of cases to controls is determined by the investigator. Therefore, in the case-control study design (or, frequently, in the case cohort design, unless the cases and not-ill individuals are a known fraction of the cohort of ill and not-ill individuals), it is not possible to measure the risk-specific attack rates. However, it is possible to measure the number of cases who reported the risk behavior and compare this to the number of controls who report the same risk behavior. In the example in Figure 5-12, a small case-control study was done within the picnic cohort in order to determine which hors d'oeuvre was the culprit. Fifteen cases and 30 controls were asked additional questions. In this case-control study, the question was, "How many cases ate stuffed mushrooms?" rather than, "How many of those who ate stuffed mushrooms became cases?" as would be asked in a cohort study. The odds ratio (OR) is used to compare the odds of risk behaviors between cases and controls. The odds of eating stuffed mushrooms in cases (9/6, or 3:2) is divided by the odds in controls (6/24, or 1:4). Thus the OR or relative odds is 6.0. The OR is interpreted in the same manner as the relative risk: Values greater than 1 indicate that the risk behavior is associated with being a case (a risk factor), values less than 1 indicate that the risk behavior is associated with being a control (a protective factor). An OR greater than 1 would be stated as "the relative odds of eating stuffed mushrooms among cases compared to controls was 6.0." Confidence intervals and probabilities can be calculated for the OR as well.

In an outbreak investigation, it is important to consider the possibility that there may be relationships between the variables that influence their association with the risk of disease. Three commonly seen relationships are: interaction, effect modification, and confounding of the data. Variables are said to interact if the presence of one changes the risk of disease for another. In an additive model, the effect of a variable increases the risk of the other as though the risks were being added. If the risk of disease in those people exposed to both risk factors exceeds the sum of the two individual risks, the two factors are said to show positive additive interaction or synergism. Similarly, the presence of a multiplicative interaction is evaluated against a multiplicative model for disease risk where the baseline risk is multiplied in the presence of one or more factors.[12]

In the example provided in Figure 5-13, a third analysis of the picnic data was conducted to examine additive interactions. All of the guests who had eaten the evening hors d'oeuvres were further queried about whether they had eaten specific items including stuffed mushrooms and dipping sauce. First, a two-by-two table was constructed for each item and it was found that the relative risk of disease was 1.9 for those who had eaten the stuffed mushrooms and 1.5 for those who had eaten the dipping sauce. Second, a stratified analysis was performed, where the risk of disease after eating stuffed mushrooms was stratified according to whether or not the guest also ate the dipping sauce. In this analysis, it was found that those who ate both the mushrooms and the dipping sauce were over five times more likely to be cases than those who ate neither (80% vs 14.3%; the risk attributable to consuming both items above the baseline rate of disease is 80% minus 14.3%, or 65.7%). The risk of disease after consuming both is slightly lower than the sum of the risks of only eating stuffed mushrooms and the risk of only eating the dipping sauce (i.e., 65.7% is slightly lower than 77.3%), the sum of the individual risks (57.9% − 14.3%) + (48.0% − 14.3%). An additive risk model makes biological sense in this example: If both items were equally contaminated and people ate equal amounts of both items, then those who ate both items would get twice the dose of the pathogenic agent. Although the number of people in the example is small, the combined risk is approximately the sum of the risk of the two items alone—or no evidence of additive interaction.

Another type of relationship is effect modification. Effect modification is when the value of one variable affects the relative risk or odds ratio of another variable. For example, age is often an effect modifier: The risk of disease is higher among infants and the elderly who consume a particular food. Confounding occurs when the causal effect of one variable is modified by the value of another variable. For example, it may initially appear that gender is a risk factor for a particular disease until it is determined that a second factor is differentially distributed by gender. A preliminary review of the data might show that male participants at an event were more likely to be cases than were female participants. After additional investigation, it was found that the water fountain near the men's restrooms was contaminated; thus, more men were exposed than were women. The variable gender was confounded by whether the participant drank from a contaminated water fountain. When investigating an outbreak, it is important to consider the possibility of interaction or confounding and to continue to explore the relationships between variables to ensure that any of these effects in the data have been evaluated.

The OR and RR are similar measures of risk that can be used and interpreted interchangeably when the attack rate in the population being studied is less than 5%. This is done because many find it simpler to describe or to conceptualize the risk and relative rate of disease than the odds and relative odds of disease. The assumption that the OR approximates the RR is known as the rare disease assumption; mathematically, the OR estimates the RR at low attack rates. Although the rare disease assumption is usually valid in epidemiologic research on diseases of low prevalence, it is commonly not valid in outbreak investigations. Attack rates of 30% or more are common in outbreak studies—clearly much higher than the 5% cutoff used by convention. It is important to realize that the OR and RR are both valid measures of the association between disease and the risk factor at any level of attack rate. However, when the disease is common, the investigator may often not be able to use the OR to estimate the RR. For example, the OR in Figure 5-12 for stuffed mushrooms is 6.0; whereas the RR in Figure 5-13 is 1.9. Both measures point to an association between the mushrooms and illness.

It is possible for associations to be found that are due to chance, rather than because of any true association between the risk factor and disease. Statistical tests (e.g., p-value and confidence interval) are used to evaluate the possibility that the findings are due to chance alone. These statistical tests assess the possibility that the distribution of cases by risk group could have happened by chance alone. In other words, how likely is it that, by chance alone, 30 of the 70 people who ate hors d'oeuvres became ill, versus 5 of the 65 who did not eat them? If the possibility that this distribution of data would occur by chance is less than 5% ($P < .05$), the distribution of the data is attributed to an association between the factors, meaning the exposure is associated with disease. In outbreak studies, it is common for multiple comparisons to be made, such as the risk of disease is compared for exposure to 20 different foods. If the cutoff value for statistical significance is set at 5% ($P < .05$), it would be expected that one of 20 comparisons would appear to be a significant association by chance alone. To correct for multiple comparisons, the most conservative approach is to lower the p value, according to the number of comparisons being made. To assess the possibility that the distribution is by chance alone, the statistical test will make some assumptions about the distribution of data. For instance, the test will commonly assume that the data are "normally distributed." This means that the test is comparing the distribution of data found in the study to a hypothetical data set, where the distribution of data would fit a normal curve. If there are very few people (less than 40) in the study, the assumption of normally distributed data may be false. Some corrections have been devised to overcome the assumption of normality, such as Cornfield or Fisher's exact test. These alterations to the basic statistical equations are available in most software packages, including EpiInfo.

In some outbreak investigations, the data are sufficiently complex that analysis using 2×2 tables is difficult or insufficient. Stratifying the data may be necessary to remove confounding factors. Logistic regression may also be used to control for certain variables. However, the basic goal remains the same: to determine the important risk factors for disease and to prevent its spread or recurrence.

Outbreak investigations should look beyond the current circumstances to determine how to prevent future outbreaks. In food-borne outbreaks, determination that a particular food was responsible for the disease is only the first step. It may be possible to follow the flow diagram of the food production to determine how the food became contaminated with the pathogen or how the food was improperly handled so that a pathogen could persist or multiply. Corrections to the handling of the food should be made to prevent problems in the future. This step may take the investigation across state or national boundaries. In Figure 5-13, once the prepared meat in the stuffed mushrooms is determined as the most likely cause of illness, the investigators can further query the food handlers who prepared the item by developing an HACCP chart, detailing food preparation, storage, and serving. Laboratory data, if available, will be used to support the epidemiology.

In the case of the cholera outbreak in Maryland, epidemiology and laboratory results pointed to the coconut milk as the vehicle for *Vibrio cholera*.[27] It was determined that raw coconut was washed in stream water in the country of origin. Subsequently, the coconut milk was not pasteurized but, instead, frozen and shipped to the United States. The contamination from the stream water exposed US residents to pathogens from thousands of miles away. Changes in US import laws may be required to reduce the risk of future outbreaks.

Plan Additional Studies

The data derived from the outbreak investigation may lead to questions that can be answered only with further planned studies, including epidemiologic research or laboratory investigation at academic, private, or governmental agencies. Outbreaks of *E. coli* O157:H7 have identified undercooked hamburger and apple cider as vehicles. In follow-up, institutional review board–approved case-control studies of sporadic cases of diarrhea in numerous states caused by this pathogen are under way to determine additional specific risk factors. Similarly, nationwide outbreaks of *Salmonella serotype enteritidis* linked to grade A shell eggs led to studies of chickens, the hen house environment, the heat lability of the pathogen, the transport and storage requirements of eggs, etc., with the goal of preventing future cases.

Communicate Findings

Investigators communicate interim findings and recommendations verbally and in writing during the investigation to those needing to know, such as the facility or public health agencies. At the conclusion of the investigation, the investigators should write a summary report to document the investigation, the actions taken, and the outcome. If the investigation was conducted by a local, state, or federal health agency, the report becomes a document that will provide feedback to the personnel at the facility or site where the outbreak occurred. Final reports may, in some instances, lead to recommendations, publications, or regulatory changes that will prevent disease and improve outbreak response in the future (see Figure 5-14).[33]

Background: In November 1993, we investigated an outbreak of gastroenteritis associated with eating raw oysters.

Methods: We interviewed 14 groups of two or more ill persons who had eaten raw oysters together. Source beds for oysters were identified using oyster sack tags and dealer records. Oyster harvesters were interviewed. Stool samples from ill persons were tested by electron microscopy (EM) and reverse transcription-polymerase chain reaction (RT-PCR) for Norwalk-like virus (NLV); viral genome was also sequenced.

Results: Of 78 raw oyster eaters, 65 (83%) became ill, compared with 2 (5%) of 41 associated persons who did not eat raw oysters (Risk Ratio [RR] = 17.1, 95% Confidence Interval [CI] 4.4–66.3). The 67 persons had vomiting (71%) or diarrhea (92%) 5–60 hours after eating (median 31 hours). Nine stool samples from persons in

three of the groups were tested for NLV; six were positive by EM, and nine were positive by RT-PCR. Viruses sequenced to date are identical. In the 13 outbreaks where tracing information was available, implicated oysters were harvested November 9–13 from a single area of beds remote from sewage contamination and ship traffic. Four harvesters who did not eat oysters were ill with vomiting and diarrhea while working in the implicated beds on November 7–9 and disposed of their feces and vomitus overboard.

Conclusions: Because the infectious dose for NLV is small (1–10 virus particles) and because oysters concentrate enteric pathogens, virus-containing stool from four ill harvesters may have contaminated a sufficient number of oysters to cause this outbreak. Enforcement of regulations governing waste disposal by fishing boats might prevent similar outbreaks from occurring.

Figure 5-14 An outbreak of oyster-related Norwalk-like virus gastroenteritis traced to fecal contamination from fishing boats.
Source: M.A. Kohn et al., An Outbreak of Oyster-Related Norwalk-Like Virus Gastroenteritis Traced to Fecal Contamination from Fishing Boats, presented at the Epidemic Intelligence Service 43rd Annual Conference, 1994, Centers for Disease Control and Prevention.

Conclusion

Outbreaks afford opportunities to gain information about diseases, pathogens, and changing risk factors for disease. Epidemiologic field investigations or outbreak investigations involve a series of methodical, well-planned steps for the collection and analysis of data. Armed with the knowledge of how to investigate an outbreak, the epidemiologist is able to execute a timely and thorough study of the cause and contributing factors of an outbreak while quickly taking measures to control the outbreak. Cooperation and communication are key elements in the smooth operation of this process. Issues of confidentiality and the release of information should be taken into account, with the operating procedure of the jurisdiction guiding the action to release information. Public health officials in local, state, and federal agencies can provide expert advice and assistance in the investigation of outbreaks.

References

1. Zinsser H. *Lice and History—The Biography of a Bacillus: A Bacteriologist's Classic Study of a World Scourge*. Boston, Mass: Atlantic, Little, Brown; 1963.
2. Institute of Medicine. Lederberg J, Shope RE, Oaks SC Jr, eds. *Emerging Infections: Microbial Threats to Health in the United States*. Washington, DC: National Academies Press; 1992.
3. Bell BP, Goldoft M, Griffin PM, et al. A multistate outbreak of *Escherichia coli* O157:H7-associated bloody diarrhea and hemolytic uremic syndrome from hamburgers: the Washington experience. *JAMA*. 1994;272:1349–1353.
4. Yukioka HK. *Escherichia coli* O157 infection disaster in Japan 1996. *S Eur J Emerg Med*. 1997;4:165.
5. Centers for Disease Control. Ebola virus infection in imported primates—Virginia, 1989. *MMWR*. 1989;48:831–838.
6. Centers for Disease Control and Prevention. Summary of notifiable diseases, United States, 1997. *MMWR*. 1998;54:iii–iv.
7. Goodman RA, Buehler JW, Koplan JP. The epidemiologic field investigation: science and judgment in public health practice. *Am J Epidemiol*. 1990;132:9–16.
8. Dwyer DM, Strickler H, Goodman RA, Armenian HK. Use of case-control studies in outbreak investigations. *Epidemiol Rev*. 1994;16:109–123.
9. Reingold AL. Outbreak investigations—a perspective. *Emerg Infect Dis*. 1998;4:21–27.
10. El-Gazzar RE, Marth EH. Foodborne disease: investigative procedures and economic assessment. *Environ Health*. 1992;55:24–26.
11. Centers for Disease Control and Prevention. Case definitions for infectious conditions under public health surveillance. *MMWR*. 1997;46 (RR-10):1–5.
12. Schlesselman JJ. *Case-Control Studies: Design, Conduct, Analysis*. New York, NY: Oxford University Press; 1982.
13. Rothman KS, Greenland S. *Modern Epidemiology*. 2nd ed. Philadelphia, Pa: Lippincott-Williams & Wilkins; 1998:108–111.
14. Szklo M, Nieto FJ. *Epidemiology: Beyond the Basics*. Gaithersburg, Md: Aspen Publishers; 1999:1–51.

15. Langmuir AD. Toxic-shock syndrome—an epidemiologist's view. *J Infect Dis.* 1982;145:588–591.
16. Centers for Disease Control. Toxic-shock syndrome, United States, 1970–1982. *MMWR.* 1982;31:201–204.
17. MacKenzie WR, Hoxie NJ, Proctor ME, et al. A massive outbreak in Milwaukee of cryptosporidium infection transmitted through the public water supply. *N Engl J Med.* 1994;331:161–167.
18. Decker MD, Booth AS, Dewey MJ, et al. Validity of food consumption histories in a foodborne outbreak investigation. *Am J Epidemiol.* 1986;124:859–863.
19. Centers for Disease Control and Prevention. Multistate outbreak of Salmonella serotype Agona infections linked to toasted oats cereal—United States, April-May 1998. *MMWR.* 1998;47:462–464.
20. Morris JG, Jr, Dwyer DM, Hoge CW, et al. Changing clonal patterns of Salmonella enteritidis in Maryland: evaluation of strains isolated between 1985 and 1990. *J Clin Microbiol.* 1992;30:1301–1303.
21. Kohn MA, Farley TA, Ando T, et al. An outbreak of Norwalk virus gastroenteritis associated with eating raw oysters: implications for maintaining safe oyster beds. *JAMA.* 1995;273:466–471.
22. Dowell SF, Groves C, Kirkland KB, et al. A multistate outbreak of oyster-associated gastroenteritis: implications for interstate tracing of contaminated shellfish. *J Infect Dis.* 1995;171:497–503.
23. Moe CL, Gentsch J, Ando T, et al. Application of PCR to detect Norwalk virus in fecal specimens from outbreaks of gastroenteritis. *Clin Microbiol.* 1994;32:642–648.
24. Braden CR, Templeton GL, Cave MD, et al. Interpretation of restriction fragment length polymorphism analysis of *Mycobacterium* tuberculosis isolates from a state with a large rural population. *J Infect Dis.* 1997;175:1446–1452.
25. US Public Health Service. Food Code. *1998 Recommendations of the United States Public Health Service, Food and Drug Administration.* National Technical Information Service Publication, Bethesda, MD.
26. Maryland Department of Health and Mental Hygiene, Epidemiology and Disease Control Program, Division of Outbreak Investigation. Unpublished data.
27. Taylor JL, Tuttle J, Pramukul T, et al. An outbreak of cholera in Maryland associated with imported commercial frozen fresh coconut milk. *J Infect Dis.* 1993;167:1330–1335.
28. Centers for Disease Control and Prevention. *Escherichia coli* O157:H7 infections associated with eating a nationally distributed commercial brand of frozen ground beef patties and burgers—Colorado. *MMWR.* 1997;46:777–778.
29. Rodriguez E, Parrott C, Rolka H, et al. An outbreak of viral gastroenteritis in a nursing home: importance of excluding ill employees. *Infect Control Hosp Epidemiol.* 1996;17:587–592.
30. Meehan PJ, Atkeson T, Kepner DE, Melton M. A food-borne outbreak of gastroenteritis involving two different pathogens. *Am J Epidemiol.* 1992;136:611–616.
31. Boyce JM, Jackson MM, Pugliese G, et al. The AHA Technical Panel on Infections within Hospitals. Methicillin-resistant *Staphylococcus aureus* (MRSA): a briefing for acute care hospitals and nursing facilities. *Infect Control Hosp Epidemiol.* 1994;15:105–115.
32. Jackson LA, Schuchat A, Reeves MW, Wenger JD. Serogroup C meningococcal outbreaks in the United States: an emerging threat. *JAMA.* 1995;273:383–389.

33. Kohn MA, Farley T, Curtis M, et al. An outbreak of oyster-related Norwalk-like virus gastroenteritis traced to fecal contamination from fishing boats. Abstract presented at: Epidemic Intelligence Service 43rd Annual Conference; April 18–22, 1994.

CHAPTER SIX

MATHEMATICAL MODELING: THE DYNAMICS OF INFECTION

Joan L. Aron

Introduction

Mathematical models are important for understanding the population dynamics of the transmission of infectious agents and the potential impact of infectious disease control programs. As an example, consider the information available for a decision to introduce an immunization program to control an infectious agent circulating in a population of 50 million people. Studies of the biology of the agent could identify its basic biochemical and genetic characteristics and possibly even its entire genome. Studies of the clinical effects of the agent could describe the natural history of disease, including the likelihood of permanent damage or death. Studies of the epidemiology of the agent could estimate its prevalence and incidence in various demographic subgroups and identify likely modes of transmission and various risk factors. Studies of the vaccine itself could determine its level of efficacy in protecting an individual from infection or disease. Nevertheless, an enormous extrapolation is required to contemplate the effect of an immunization program on 50 million people and the populations of the infectious agent they harbor. Therein lies the role of the mathematical model.

Still, personal common sense, a so-called mental model, might seem to be more reliable than extensive computer calculations based on a mathematical model whose details are comprehended fully by only a few individuals. After all, the quality of a mathematical model of complex phenomena depends on the accuracy of its underlying assumptions, which cannot always be verified. However, mental models for making decisions are often ambiguous, difficult for others to comprehend, or just plain wrong.[1] The way out of this quandary is an approach to analyze and understand the differences between mental models and mathematical models, where the term *mathematical model* is used here interchangeably with *computer model* because computer software is often used to construct mathematical models. Insights about the role of mathematical models in evaluating social and economic policies also apply to infectious disease control policies:

> Computer modeling is thus an essential part of the educational process rather than a technology for producing answers. The success of this dialectic depends on our ability to create and learn from shared understandings of our models, both mental and computer. Properly used, computer models can improve the mental models upon which decisions are actually based and contribute to the solution of the pressing problems we face.[1]

Public health professionals can gain a better understanding of infectious disease epidemiology by becoming intelligent "consumers" of the literature on mathematical models. Furthermore, public health professionals frame the questions to be addressed, thereby playing a major role in guiding the development of applications of mathematical models.

As a first step in introducing mathematical models to public health professionals, it is necessary to define what a mathematical model is (and, by implication, what it is not). A mathematical model is an explicit mathematical description of the simplified dynamics of a system. The use of the word *simplified* is essential because the art and science of modeling require the appropriate selection of information in order to achieve a specific purpose. A model is therefore always "wrong," but may be a useful approximation, permitting conceptual experiments that would otherwise be difficult or impossible. The results of mathematical models can help determine the plausibility of epidemiologic explanations, improve understanding by a demonstration of unexpected interrelationships among empirical observations, and predict the impact of changes on the dynamics of a system. An extensive literature on mathematical models of the epidemiology of infectious diseases is closely linked to the field of population biology, which incorporates aspects of ecology, demography, and genetics, as well as mathematics and statistics.[2–8]

The transition from a clinical and biologic understanding of the course of an infectious disease to a mathematical model of the dynamics of transmission requires selection of features of the disease to represent in the model. For example, the population size of an infectious agent that replicates inside a host may grow from a small inoculum and later decline and disappear altogether (Figure 6-1). It is common to represent this process as a series of stages of infection, starting with a susceptible host who becomes infected. The level of infection must grow for the infected host to be able to transmit the infection to others, that is, to become infective. The *latent period* refers to the period of time that elapses before an infected host becomes infective. When the host is no longer able to transmit infection, the host is removed from the cycle of transmission in the population. Removal might involve death caused by the infection or the acquisition of natural immunity that clears infection and prevents reinfection. (Mortality unrelated to the infection may occur at any stage and is not part of the natural history of infection per se.) Removal might also involve curative treatment that leaves the host free of infection and disease, and prevents the host from reinfection. For some diseases, removal does not occur because a host becomes susceptible to reinfection after recovery. The relative length and importance of different stages vary with the host population and the agent.

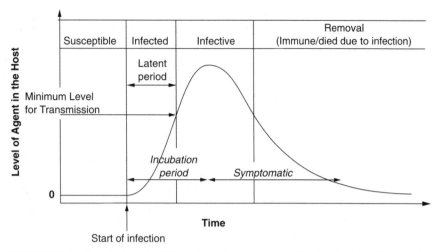

FIGURE 6-1 Population size of an infectious agent replicating inside a host and classification of stages of infection.

The distinction between infection and disease is essential. Figure 6-1 shows stages of infection relevant to the dynamics of transmission. In general, symptoms of disease might occur before or after the host becomes infective. The period of time from infection until the onset of symptoms is the incubation period, which is not to be confused with the latent period. Hypothetical incubation and symptomatic periods appear in italics in Figure 6-1. In cases of asymptomatic infection, symptoms never appear. In some situations, acute symptoms that occur close in time to the period of infectivity could be followed by damage that persists long after the infection is cleared from the body. The appearance of symptoms is important for case diagnosis and treatment, case definition in a disease surveillance program, and estimation of the harm caused by disease as the justification for a disease control program. However, the fundamental process represented in mathematical models of the epidemiology of infectious diseases is the transmission of infectious agents.

Transmission occurs when a susceptible host contacts an infective host and the infectious agent initiates an infection in the susceptible host. Contact is defined according to the appropriate mode of transmission for a specified agent, such as direct person-to-person transmission of measles via coughs or indirect vector-borne transmission of malaria via mosquito bites. The ability of the agent to infect people is dependent on inherent characteristics of the agent; some infectious agents are more readily transmitted than are other infectious agents under similar conditions. Mathematical models characterize transmission in terms of infection rates related to the frequency of contact between individuals and the likelihood of transmission given a contact between a susceptible host and an infective host.

If the chain of transmission from infective host to susceptible host is maintained in a population, the infection is considered to be endemic. In other words, one would expect to find the infectious agent somewhere in the population at any time. However, the chain of transmission may be interrupted for many reasons. Environmental and social conditions may no longer support transmission of the infectious agent (in effect, reducing contact), treatment may interfere with the infectious stage, or most of the host population may be immune. The last situation is called *herd immunity*, to suggest the analogy between the immune status of a population preventing spread of infection, and the immune status of an individual host preventing internal replication of an infectious agent. The term *herd* is used instead of *population* because of a history of related work on infections in large herds of animals. Mathematical models provide a theoretical framework for understanding how transmission is maintained and can be interrupted.

This chapter will focus on infections that are directly transmitted and confer lifelong immunity. The prototypical example of this class of infections is the measles virus, which causes a respiratory infection transmitted from person to person. If a person survives a case of measles, that person cannot be infected again. The basic model structure also provides a framework for adding structural details to address other epidemiologic problems. An important theme is that different models, characterized by type and degree of complexity, are appropriate for different kinds of questions.

The class of infections represented by the measles virus has several advantages that make it especially useful as an introduction to mathematical models of the epidemiology of infectious disease. The model needs to account for relatively simple characteristics of transmission. The infectious agent is transmitted from one human host to another without a disease vector. An individual who is not infected can be clearly defined as either susceptible or immune without intermediate stages of immunity. Immunity is acquired after a single infection. Although these model assumptions may seem restrictive, several childhood immunizable diseases have these characteristics.

The application of mathematical models to childhood immunizable diseases has contributed to the development of important concepts that are used widely in the field of public health. These concepts illustrate basic features of the epidemiology and control of infectious disease that might not be readily understood in personal mental models. Analysis according to the age of the host is particularly critical. Immunization of a percentage of the population does not necessarily result in a proportionate drop in incidence across all age groups and, indeed, may even increase incidence in some age groups. Further, even if the only laws affecting immunization apply to school entry, it does matter whether children are immunized at school entry or well before school entry. Another problem is that extrapolating the conditions for interrupting transmission from one population to another is often invalid. If a small town is able to interrupt transmission of a respiratory infectious disease by immunizing 70% of its population, the same target is unlikely to have the same effect in a metropolitan area. It is also risky to assume that immunization can be delivered as a single time-limited campaign, even if such a campaign is followed in one instance by a few years free of infection and disease. Careful comparison of the results of mathematical modeling with erroneous ideas demonstrates the utility of modeling.

Basic Theory for SIR Model

The basic theory for the dynamics of transmission of directly transmitted infections that confer lifelong immunity describes a population divided into three classes or states. The classes are taken from the depiction of the natural history of infection in Figure 6-1. The first class is susceptibles (S) who can acquire infection. The second class is infectives (I) who can transmit infection to susceptibles. The third class is removals (R) who are immune or dead as a consequence of infection. Because many conclusions from the basic model are not affected by the class of individuals shown in Figure 6-1 with latent infection, that is, those who are infected but not yet infective, discussion of this class is deferred until later in this chapter. The initial letters of the names of the three classes (S, I, R) are used to name the SIR model. Throughout this chapter, the last class always refers to immune individuals. The immune individuals are often called *recovered*, and the process of removal from infective to immune is often called *recovery*.

The development of the basic theory is structured around three important concepts—endemicity, age at infection, and mass immunization/herd immunity. *Endemicity* refers to an endemic infection, that is, an infection that is always present in a population. *Age at infection* refers to the age of a susceptible host when infection occurs. The distribution of ages at which infection occurs is characteristic of a particular infection that is endemic in a particular population. The average age at infection is an indirect indicator of the underlying dynamics of transmission whose components may be difficult to measure directly. *Mass immunization* is a strategy to control disease by administering a vaccine to a large segment of a population. It may even be possible to create *herd immunity* so that transmission is completely interrupted because of a high percentage of immune individuals. The theory of mass immunization and herd immunity is based on the concepts of endemicity and age at infection.

Endemicity

Empirical Example

Infectious agents can have very different patterns of endemicity in populations. An epidemiologic comparison of poliovirus and hepatitis B virus demonstrates how differences in natural history affect endemicity. Both kinds of viruses have been studied in seroprevalence surveys that use the presence of antibodies as an indicator of prior exposure to virus. A prevaccine poliovirus study in an isolated Eskimo village in Greenland examined the prevalence of antibodies to the three different types of poliovirus according to the age of the host (Figure 6-2a).[9] For each type of poliovirus, there appeared to be an age cutoff that split the population into an older group previously exposed to the poliovirus and a younger group who had not been previously exposed. This pattern is consistent with the introduction and extensive spread of the virus in the population, followed by rapid disappearance of the virus from the population in a short period of time. Poliovirus disappears in an isolated population because those infected with poliovirus develop immunity to the infection, and too few susceptibles remain to maintain transmission. In contrast, another study of Eskimos in Greenland showed that the prevalence of antibodies to hepatitis B virus rose slowly with age (Figure 6-2b).[9] This pattern is consistent with some risk of exposure present all of the time. The

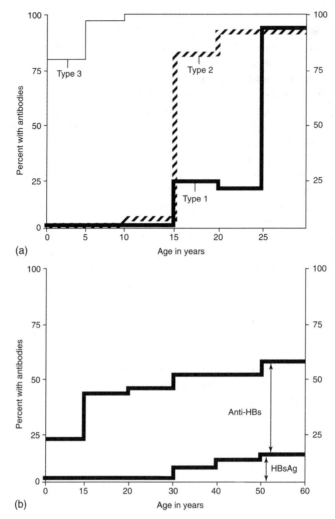

(a)

(b)

FIGURE 6-2 a & b (a) Age distribution of poliomyelitis antibodies in an isolated Eskimo village, Narrsak, Greenland; and (b) age distribution of hepatitis B surface antigen (HbsAg) and antibody to HbsAg (anti-HBs) in Eskimos of southwest Greenland.
Source: J.A. Yorke et al., American Journal of Epidemiology, Vol. 109, p. 106, © 1979, The Johns Hopkins University School of Hygrene and Pubilc Health.

key to understanding the difference between hepatitis B and polio is the hepatitis B carrier state, which is a chronic infection in an individual host, indicated by the presence of the hepatitis B surface antigen. In the hepatitis B study population, the prevalence of the hepatitis B surface antigen rose with the age of the host (see Figure 6-2b). The establishment of the hepatitis B carrier state in some individuals allows hepatitis B virus to remain endemic in a population where poliovirus transmission cannot be maintained.

The dynamics of poliovirus display the characteristics of an infection obeying the basic assumptions of the SIR model. The presence of the carrier state in hepatitis B infection is not part of the assumptions of the SIR model. Analysis of the SIR model helps to develop a deeper understanding of the phenomenon of epidemic spread and disappearance.

Assumptions in the Threshold Theorem

The formulation of the SIR model is based on the Kermack–McKendrick Threshold Theorem.[6] The Kermack–McKendrick Threshold Theorem considers population size in relation to area, that is, population density. The variables X, Y, and Z denote the population densities of the three classes in a SIR model (Figure 6-3). The population is closed, which means that no one enters or leaves the population. Although the assumption that the population is closed appears to ignore births, deaths, and migrations that happen in every human population, a population can be effectively closed during an epidemic if the epidemic moves quickly through the population before the processes of demographic change have a significant effect. (For other applications in which the removals are not immunes but, rather, deaths from the disease, the removals are counted as part of the population during the course of the epidemic.) Short-term travel movements in and out of the defined population may also violate the assumption of a closed population. However, in many settings, travel may not contribute very much to transmission during the time scale of an epidemic, especially for children, who typically travel less than do adults. Under the assumption of a closed population, the three classes add up to a fixed total population density, N.

Transmission of the infectious agent is characterized by a mass-action term (βXY) for the rate of transfer of individuals from the susceptible class X to the infective class Y. The contact parameter β incorporates an area of movement per person per day and a probability that a contact between an infective and a susceptible results in transmission of the infectious agent. The multiplication of X and Y corresponds to mass-action mixing, the simplest assumption for random mixing. The removal of infectives is characterized by a term (γY) for the rate of transfer of individuals from the infective class Y to the immune class Z. The recovery parameter γ is a rate, but it is easier to think about the transition from the infective state to the immune state in terms of $1/\gamma$, the average duration of infectivity. A rapid rate of recovery results in a short duration of infectivity. The model is written as a system of differential equations showing the rates of change of the population densities of X, Y, and Z with respect to time t (see also Figure 6-3).

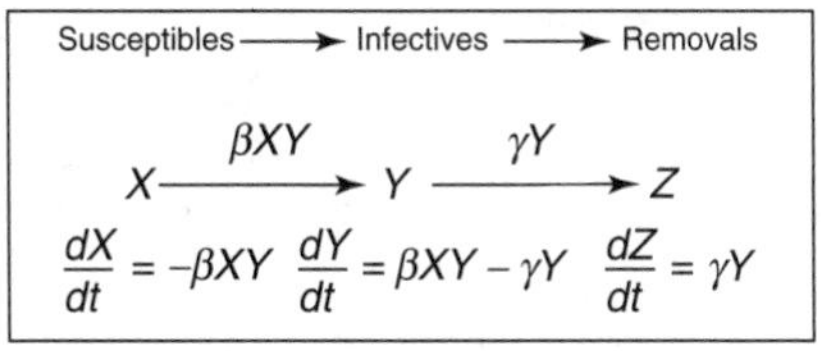

FIGURE 6-3 SIR model for a closed population.

$$\frac{dX}{dt} = -\beta XY$$

$$\frac{dY}{dt} = \beta XY - \gamma Y$$

$$\frac{dZ}{dt} = \gamma y$$

$$X + Y + Z = N \qquad\qquad (1)$$

Results from the Threshold Theorem

The conditions for transmission in an epidemic model are usually analyzed in terms of a scenario in which a single infective is introduced into an otherwise susceptible population. For the Kermack–McKendrick Threshold Theorem using population density, the introduction of an infective corresponds to a very small density of infectives. In the system described in Equation (1), an epidemic will start only if the density of susceptibles X exceeds a threshold γ/β.

The threshold condition is derived from an analysis of the growth in the density (or number) of infectives, Y, at $t = 0$, which is the conventional starting time. An epidemic means that the number of infections grows beyond the number initially introduced.

$$\text{At } t = 0, \frac{dY}{dt} = (\beta X - \gamma)Y > 0 \text{ if } X > \frac{\gamma}{\beta} \qquad\qquad (2)$$

If the density of susceptibles exceeds the threshold γ/β, the rate at which susceptibles become infectives (βXY) exceeds the rate at which infectives are removed (γY). That is, the net rate of growth of the population density of infectives is positive. Because it is assumed that almost everyone is susceptible at the outset ($X \cong N$), the statements about the density of susceptibles, in effect, refer to the population as a whole. In other words, the initiation of an epidemic requires that the population density exceed the threshold γ/β. If there is an epidemic, it eventually terminates. At the end of the epidemic, the population consists of susceptibles below the threshold density and removals (immunes). A more detailed mathematical analysis of the system in Equation (1) may be found elsewhere.[10]

Hypothetical SIR Epidemic in Baltimore City

A hypothetical infection in Baltimore City provides an example to demonstrate calculations of the variables and the parameters of the SIR model, as well as the progress of the epidemic. The threshold condition is stated in terms of the density of susceptibles required for an epidemic to spread and an alternative formulation of secondary cases per introduced case. Evidence of the great power and generality of this restatement of the threshold condition will be seen later in this chapter.

Baltimore City has a population density, N, of 8700 people per square mile. The epidemic is assumed to start with $X = 8699$, $Y = 1$, and $Z = 0$.

The contact term β incorporates an area of movement per person per day of .001 square miles. Thus, a typical infective would encounter an average of 8.7 (8700 × .001) people per day, virtually all of whom are susceptible at the start of the epidemic. The parameter β is reduced from .001 to .0004 because it is further assumed that only 40% of contacts between susceptibles and infectives result in transmission. So the number of people infected per day by a single infective at the start of the epidemic would be only 3.48 (βN). The recovery parameter γ of .5 per day means that a person is infective, on average, for 2 days before becoming immune. Under these assumptions, the threshold condition in Equation (2) for the density of susceptibles becomes 1250 people per square mile (.5/.0004). In this example, the population density of 8700 people per square mile clearly exceeds the threshold, and so the epidemic spreads. The SIR epidemic for the system in Equation (1) demonstrates the classic rise and fall in the population density of infectives, Y, over time as the epidemic progresses (Figure 6-4).

The assumptions about the contact parameter β can be subtle. The key assumption is that everyone in the population has a typical pattern of contact, characterized by the population density and a typical area of movement. However, it is sometimes erroneously stated that everyone in the population must have an equal chance of contacting everyone else in the population. Because this pattern of contact is obviously impossible for large populations in cities or countries, it would be easy to reject the model for failure to meet this assumption. This misinterpretation is encouraged when population size is used to define population density. For example, one could achieve the same numerical results for Baltimore City by constructing a new unit of area to be 80.8 square miles and using the total city population of 702,979 instead of 8700 people per square mile.

An alternative expression of the threshold condition is in terms of secondary cases per introduced case instead of population density. Simply put, the epidemic will spread if a single case introduced into a susceptible population generates more than one new case. Therefore, the threshold density of 1250 people per square mile becomes a threshold of one secondary case. The number of secondary cases generated by a single introduced case is the product of the number of new cases generated per day and the number of days of infectivity. As discussed earlier, the values for the Baltimore City example

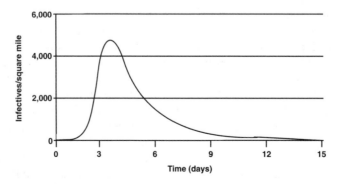

FIGURE 6-4   Population density of infectives during a SIR epidemic.

are 3.48/day (βN) and 2 days ($1/\gamma$), respectively. Because there are, on average, 6.96 secondary cases per introduced case, the epidemic will spread.

There are other ways of describing the progress of an epidemic. The ratio of the population density of infectives, Y, to the total population density, N, yields the prevalence, that is, the proportion of the population that is infective. For example, the value in Figure 6-4 of 5000 infectives per square mile corresponds to roughly 57% of the population. In addition, the ratios of population density and proportion of infectives to the average duration of infectivity provide approximate measures of incidence (see relationships among prevalence, incidence, and the duration of infectivity in Chapter 2). For example, the value in Figure 6-4 of 5000 infectives per square mile corresponds to an incidence of 2500 people per square mile per day, or roughly 29% of the population per day at that point in the progress of the epidemic. These numbers translate to about 202,000 cases per day for the city as a whole. The true incidence of infection may actually be shifted in time because, technically, this approximation estimates the rate at which infective cases become immune rather than the rate at which susceptible individuals become infective. Epidemic statistics are often cited in terms of incident cases for entire populations in political jurisdictions. Although such reporting is useful for public health services, it may generate confusion among population density, population size, and assumed patterns of contact in the underlying model of transmission. It should be noted that the shape of the epidemic curve remains the same for all of these alternative measurements, except that the delays in the appearance of symptoms and reporting may shift the observed timing.

Epidemiologic Insights from the Threshold Theorem

The development of the SIR epidemic theory and the Kermack–McKendrick Threshold Theorem have led to important epidemiologic insights about endemicity for directly transmitted infections that confer lifelong immunity. The central result has been a better understanding of the dynamics of the susceptible population.

Epidemics cannot spread in a population of susceptibles whose density is very low. If the density of susceptibles is sufficient for the initial spread of epidemics, infection in the population cannot be sustained (i.e., become endemic) without an influx of susceptibles. If new susceptibles do not arrive quickly enough, the population is effectively "closed," and the infection dies out. The episodic appearances and disappearances of poliovirus in remote Eskimo villages demonstrate the consequences of an inadequate supply of susceptibles (Figure 6-2a). Endemicity of infection generated by a steady influx of susceptibles is discussed in the section on age at infection.

Epidemics can wax and wane as a function of the supply of susceptibles. Although the role of the susceptible population may seem obvious in retrospect, the study of the causation of epidemics has been characterized by vigorous debate. An old epidemic theory postulated the need for increases and decreases in the transmissibility of the agent.[11]

Finally, the eradication of an infection by mass immunization can be understood in terms of reducing the density of susceptibles below a threshold required for the spread of infection. Thus, herd immunity is theoretically possible because eradication can, in principle, be achieved with less than

100% effective immunization. The section on mass immunization and herd immunity provides more details.

Age at Infection

Empirical Example

Infections that obey the basic assumptions of the SIR model remain endemic in open populations with a steady influx of susceptibles. For these endemic infections, the distribution of age of the susceptible host at time of infection may vary by disease and location. For example, the average ages of measles and whooping cough (pertussis) cases reported in Maryland from 1908 to 1917 demonstrate differences between urban and rural areas and differences between the two diseases (Table 6-1). The average age of measles cases is lower in urban areas (6.9 years) than in rural areas (10 years). Similarly, the average age of pertussis cases is lower in urban areas (4.9 years) than in rural areas (6.5 years). A comparison within urban and rural areas shows that pertussis tends to strike at younger ages than does measles. Analysis of the SIR theory of endemic infection helps to develop a deeper understanding of the underlying population dynamics of infection reflected in the relationships observed in Table 6-1.

SIR Model of Endemic Infection

An influx of susceptibles is required to maintain transmission of an infection characterized by the basic assumptions of the SIR model. An influx of susceptible hosts changes a closed population to an open population (see Figure 6-5). The simplest formulation of a SIR model of an endemic infection permits the derivation of new concepts about endemicity. Three basic elements characterize the turnover of population. First, the steady influx of susceptibles is assumed to be the births in the host population. The short period of passive immunity provided by maternal antibodies is ignored. Second, mortality unrelated to the infection acts equally on all epidemiologic classes in the model. Third, the total population size remains fixed because the influx of births exactly balances the loss due to mortality. The influx of births is represented by B, and the deaths are represented by $\mu X + \mu Y + \mu Z$, where μ is the mortality rate. When the parameters for birth and death are added to the system in Equation (1), the result is the system in Equation (3).

TABLE 6-1   Average Age at Infection in Maryland, 1908–1917

	Age at Infection (yrs)	
Disease	**Urban**	**Rural**
Measles	6.9	10.0
Whooping Cough	4.9	6.5

Note: Age at infection is measured as age of the cases.
Source: Data from R.M. Anderson, Directly Transmitted Viral and Bacterial Infectious of Man. In: Anderson R.M., ed., Population Dynamics of Infectious Diseases, London, Chapman and Hall © 1982

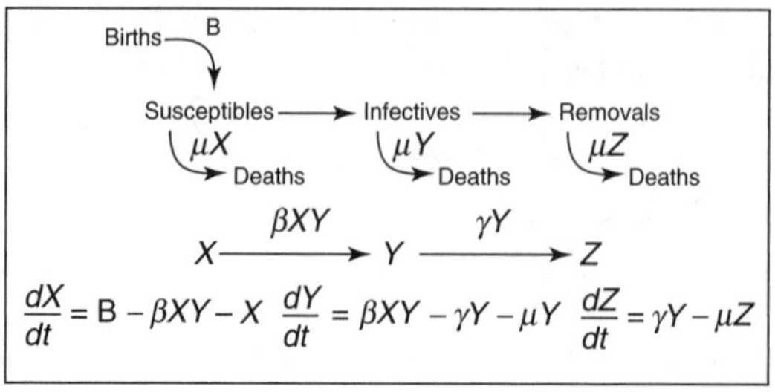

FIGURE 6-5 SIR model for a population with births and deaths.

$$\frac{dX}{dt} = -\beta XY + B - \mu X$$

$$\frac{dY}{dt} = \beta XY - \gamma Y - \mu Y$$

$$\frac{dZ}{dt} = \gamma Y - \mu Z$$

$$B = \mu N, \ X + Y + Z = N \tag{3}$$

Basic Reproduction Ratio

The basic reproduction ratio, R, is the number of secondary cases generated from a single infective case introduced into a susceptible population. (R is sometimes called R_0, and the basic reproduction ratio is sometimes called the *basic reproductive rate*.) If R is greater than 1 and there is a steady influx of births of susceptibles, as shown in Equation (3), an infection obeying the basic assumptions of the SIR model becomes endemic. The threshold condition for the basic reproduction ratio is the generalization of the alternative formulation of the threshold condition in terms of secondary cases per introduced case. R is the product of an effective contact rate and the average duration of infectivity. In terms of the notation for the hypothetical Baltimore City example, these values are 3.48/day (βN) and 2 days ($1/\gamma$). (Technically, the effect of mortality can alter the duration of infectivity because of the chance of dying during the period of infectivity. This effect can be ignored for practical purposes if this chance of dying is small.) It may be useful to re-express the effective contact rate in terms of new parameters for the contact rate c and the probability of transmission per contact q.

$$R \cong (\beta N)(1/\gamma) = cq(1/\gamma) \tag{4}$$

With c of 8.7 people per day, q of .4, and ($1/\gamma$) of 2 days, the basic reproduction ratio has a value of 6.96 that exceeds the threshold of a single secondary case. By focusing on the contacts instead of just population density, attention is directed to the underlying social and biologic determinants of transmission. For example, if regional schools in rural districts bring children together from large areas, the contact rate is not as small as would be expected on the basis of residential population density alone.

Equation (4) shows that larger R is associated with a greater contact rate, a greater duration of infectivity, and a greater probability of transmission per contact. In turn, a greater contact rate is often associated with a greater population density, especially for respiratory infections. Therefore, R would be expected to be higher in urban areas than in rural areas in regional comparisons of a particular infection. (As noted above, social mixing patterns may make the differences less pronounced than the differences in residential population density.) Also, a greater duration of infectivity and a greater probability of transmission per contact are associated with greater infectivity of infectious agents and reflect intrinsic differences between different infectious agents. In comparisons of different infections within the same population, one would expect R to be consistently higher for some infections.

The great contribution of the SIR theory is that the value of R can be used to analyze the dynamics of transmission, both when infection has just been introduced into a population and when infection has long been endemic. When R is greater than 1, the dynamics of infection in the system of equations in (3) tend toward an equilibrium with infection present (i.e., an endemic equilibrium). At the equilibrium (denoted with the bar over the variable), the fraction susceptible, $\bar{X}/N$, is equal to the inverse of the basic reproduction ratio:

$$\frac{\bar{X}}{N} = \frac{1}{R} \qquad (5)$$

The intuitive explanation is that a single case will generate, on average, R new cases if everyone else is susceptible but only a single new case at the endemic equilibrium. (If the number of cases is growing, the dynamics of infection cannot be at an equilibrium.) That means that only a fraction, *1/R*, of the possible contacts is susceptible at the endemic equilibrium. From Equation (5), it is clear that the susceptible fraction at equilibrium decreases with larger R.

The susceptible fraction is also related to the mean life expectancy *L* and the average age at infection *A*:

$$\frac{\bar{X}}{N} \cong \frac{A}{L} \qquad (6)$$

A more detailed explanation of the reasoning based on following the experience of a birth cohort may be found elsewhere.[12] However, an intuitive explanation is that the earlier a birth cohort experiences infection (smaller *A*), the fewer will be the people remaining susceptible at equilibrium (smaller $\bar{X}$). Combining Equation (5) and Equation (6) yields a relationship between the basic reproduction ratio and the average age at infection:

$$R \cong \frac{L}{A} \qquad (7)$$

The larger basic reproduction ratio R is associated with lower average age at infection *A*. (A variation on the formula in Equation [7] shows the value 1 added to the right-hand side. This variation is related to technical differences in the definition of the average age at infection,[13] but the effects are minor in most situations.)

The relationship in Equation (7) provides a basic understanding of the average ages of measles and pertussis cases in Maryland shown in Table 6-1. Urban areas have higher population density, which is associated with greater contact rates for respiratory infections. Therefore, measles and pertussis should have higher basic reproduction ratios in urban areas. In turn, these higher basic reproduction ratios in urban areas are associated with lower average ages at infection reflected in the average age of reported cases. It is important to focus on the contact pattern and not on urban living per se. For example, a study of hepatitis A found lower ages at infection in rural areas, a reversal of the urban–rural pattern described for measles and pertussis.[14] Apparently, poor sanitation is more important than population density in determining contact rates for hepatitis A, whose mode of transmission is fecal–oral.

Equation (7) also helps elucidate the differences between measles and pertussis. If pertussis tends to occur at younger ages than measles in the same populations, pertussis should have a larger basic reproduction ratio than measles. Pertussis could be more infective than measles because of a longer duration of infectivity or a greater probability of transmission per contact, or both.

Admittedly, this reasoning about infectivity of different infectious agents is indirect. However, this indirect reasoning was bolstered by empirical evidence of an inverse relationship between infectivity and the average age at infection. A study of measles, varicella, and mumps in England compared the (infection) attack rates of susceptibles within households[15] of an index case with the average age of cases in the community (Table 6-2). The attack rate is an indicator of infectivity because it measures the percentage of susceptible people in the household who become ill from an initial case in the household. (The usage of the term *rate* is for a proportion of a population at risk.) In the English study, the attack rate was highest for measles and lowest for mumps, whereas the average age of the reported cases was lowest for measles and highest for mumps. Such studies are more difficult to perform after diseases are controlled by immunization programs. However, a study of pertussis[16] in unvaccinated household contacts demonstrated a very high attack rate that is consistent with an infection even more contagious than measles (Table 6-3).

Mass Immunization and Herd Immunity

Immunization and the Basic Reproduction Ratio

Immunization, when effective, transfers an individual directly from the susceptible class to the immune class without experiencing disease. Mass immunization is a program to control disease by vaccinating large segments of the population; mass immunization policy often aims for universal coverage. When many people are immunized, the dynamics of transmission are altered. Potentially infectious contacts that would have been made with susceptible individuals are made instead with immune individuals. From the perspective of an infectious agent that requires a steady supply of susceptible hosts to

TABLE 6-2   Empirical Evidence for Inverse Relationship Between Infectivity of Agent and Average Age at Infection

Factor	Disease		
	Measles	Varicella	Mumps
Exposures	266	282	264
Transmissions	201	172	82
Exposure Attack Rate	75.6%	61.0%	31.1%
Average Age at Infection (yrs)	5.6	6.7	11.5

Note: Medical records were used to determine which household members were susceptible to the infection. All susceptibles in the household of an index case were considered as possible exposures.
Source: Data from R.E. Simpson, Infectiousness of Communicable Diseases in the Household (Measles, Chickenpox and Mumps), Lancet, 2(12):549–54, © 1952.

TABLE 6-3   Pertussis Secondary Attack Rates in Unvaccinated Household Contacts

Statistic	<1 Year Old	1–5 Years Old
Total Contacts	9	5
Illnesses	8	5
Attack Rate	89%	100%

Source: Data from C.V. Broome et al., Epidemiology of Pertussis, Journal of Pediatrics, Vol. 98, pp. 362–367, © 1981.

maintain propagation, mass immunization transforms a high-density population into a low-density population.

The effect of mass immunization is to reduce the basic reproduction ratio. A change in the basic reproduction ratio refers to permanent changes in the conditions of transmission as a result of an ongoing immunization program. If, for any reason, the immunization program does not continue, the original conditions for transmission will eventually return as new susceptibles enter the population. Defining R′ to be the basic reproduction ratio after immunization and v to be the proportion vaccinated and effectively immunized,

$$R' = R(1 - v) \qquad (8)$$

A higher proportion immunized means a lower basic reproduction ratio after immunization. The theoretical proportion immunized does not include the administration of vaccine to individuals who are already immune as a result of natural infection. Consequently, because older individuals are more likely to have been exposed to infection, careful assessment of the effectiveness of immunization programs should consider the age of the recipient of vaccine. If, for example, substantial transmission occurs before the typical age at which a child enters school, immunization at time of school entry is less likely to reach susceptible individuals than is immunization at younger ages.

Eradication

When the basic reproduction ratio is reduced below 1, transmission is, in theory, eradicated, and herd immunity is achieved.

$$R' < 1 \tag{9}$$

The magnitude of the basic reproduction ratio before the start of an immunization program is an indicator of the difficulty of disease eradication because the proportion that should be immunized to achieve eradication increases with the magnitude of the basic reproduction ratio. Figure 6-6 illustrates how the target immunization level for eradication increases if the preimmunization basic reproduction ratio increases from 2 to 5. More generally, the target level of immunization to achieve herd immunity may be expressed by combining Equation (8) and Equation (9):

$$v > 1 - \frac{1}{R} \tag{10}$$

Selected values of the target level of immunization are shown in Table 6-4. It should be noted that many estimates of the basic reproduction ratio for SIR-type diseases are at least 10, meaning that at least 90% of the population must be effectively immunized. Eradication by mass immunization still requires a large effort, even with the help of the herd immunity principles.[17]

The theory also demonstrates that it is generally invalid to use a target level of immunization simply because it was effective in another location. If there are important differences in the dynamics of transmission, as reflected in the value of the basic reproduction ratio, the target levels must differ also. For example, one would expect the target levels for eradication of a respiratory infection to be higher in an urban setting than in an otherwise comparable rural setting because the basic reproduction ratio is probably higher.

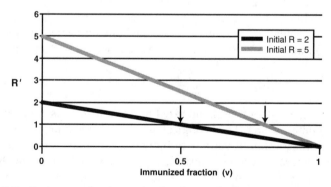

FIGURE 6-6 Basic reproduction ratio after immunization.

TABLE 6-4   Immunization Percentage to Achieve Herd Immunity

Preimmunization Basic Reproduction Ratio	Target Immunization Percentage
2	50%
5	80%
10	90%
20	95%

Increased Average Age at Infection

If mass immunization reduces transmission without interrupting it, then $1 <$ $R' < R$. Total incidence is reduced but, because a lower basic reproduction ratio is associated with a higher average age at infection, the average age at infection is increased. That is, the population that remains unimmunized indirectly experiences the effect of mass immunization by a delay in the age at which infection occurs. Despite the drop in the total number of cases, older age groups may actually experience an increase in the number of cases.

The impact of measles immunization provides an excellent example of this phenomenon. After the measles immunization program was introduced in the United States in 1963, the overall risk of measles infection was dramatically reduced. During the program, however, measles became a new risk on college campuses as measles cases appeared at ages older than was typical before the immunization program began.[18] The risk of measles on college campuses has subsequently been reduced through the introduction in 1989 of a second dose of vaccine to compensate for primary vaccine failure, in combination with campus policies to require proof of immunization.

Developing Applications

Extensions of the SIR Model

The basic SIR model provides useful insights about the persistence of infection in populations, factors determining the average age at infection, the response to mass immunizations, and the possibilities of interrupting transmission. However, the development of applications usually requires the incorporation of considerably more epidemiologic detail than shown earlier. The challenge is identifying specific questions and the level of information needed to address them. Several examples of extensions of the SIR model will be used to illustrate the issues.[13]

Age Differences in Contact Rates

The simple SIR model makes a strong general prediction that mass immunization raises the average age at infection. However, the simple SIR model assumes that everyone in the population has the same contact rate, regardless of age. The limitations of the simple SIR model can be seen in an explicit description of how the average age at infection should change in response to immunization. If A is the average age before immunization, A_I is the average age after immunization, and v is the fraction effectively immunized,

$$A_I(1 - v) = A \tag{11}$$

For example, if $v = .5$, then the average age of the cases should double after the immunization program is in place. However, a study of the impact of immunization in Britain shows that the results of the simple SIR model do not make reliable quantitative predictions about the magnitude of the increase in the average age of measles cases.[19,20] During the period from 1970 to 1980, when measles vaccine uptake in children was around 50%, the effect of immunization was to raise the average age of the cases from 4.5 to 5.5 years, much smaller than the doubling predicted by the simple model. The reason for the discrepancy is thought to be the enhanced contact rates among school-aged children that accelerated the rate of exposure at around the age of 5 years. Therefore, the results of the simple SIR model applied to the study of the average age at infection are only semiquantitative, in that the model can reliably identify the direction of change but not the magnitude of change.

Other models of the impact of immunization in Britain have estimated the percentage of the population that needed to be effectively immunized in order to eradicate measles.[21-23] Three different models yielded 96%, 89%, and 76%. The differences among the three predictions correspond to different assumptions about disease contact rates for adults—low for 76%, intermediate for 89%, and high for 96%. The adult contact rates are important because the average age at infection increases as an immunization program is implemented. The degree of difficulty of eradication is related to transmission patterns among adults. Projections of the eradication of disease based on studies of children may be misleading when extrapolated to adults.

Enhanced contact among school-aged children could also lead to a policy of immunizing those children in order to reduce the spread of influenza to the unvaccinated population. This approach is quite different from the current policy of reducing influenza mortality by directly vaccinating those at greatest risk of complications, who are primarily older adults and people with chronic illnesses. The idea of targeting children is not novel (e.g., see references 24 and 25), but a new, nasally administered influenza vaccine and a growing body of evidence from community-based studies are generating more interest in a policy of immunizing children against influenza.[26]

Latent Period

Infectious diseases typically have a latent period between the time that a host becomes infected and a host is able to transmit infection to others. For an analysis of latency, an exposed but latent class E transforms the model from SIR to SEIR. The importance of the latent period depends on the epidemiologic problem under investigation. For example, the values of the immunization thresholds needed to eradicate infection and the reservoirs of infection when systems are at an endemic equilibrium depend on the basic reproduction ratio but not usually on latency. Latency does not affect the basic reproduction ratio unless there is a probability of dying during the period of latency. For the diseases presented in this chapter, the probability of dying during the period of latency is usually small enough to have a negligible effect on the basic reproduction ratio. However, latency always affects time-dependent phenomena, such as the speed of the epidemiologic response to changes in immunization or the speed of an epidemic. For example, in following a chain of measles transmission, the generation time from case to case is approximately 14 days. Because the latent period accounts for the majority of the generation time, the elimination of the latent period would significantly accelerate the spread of disease.

Demographic Effects

Epidemiologic models usually assume a fixed population size for diseases affecting human populations. This simplifying assumption is justified on the basis that the dynamics of infectious agents operate on a much faster time scale than do changes affecting human populations. However, the difference between crude birth rates and crude death rates in many developing countries is large enough to affect the population dynamics of infection and, in particular, contribute to the reduction of the average age at infection.[2]

Spatial Effects

The fact that populations are geographically dispersed has important implications for the spread of disease and the design of disease control programs. Measles is one of many diseases whose geographic aspects have been studied in detail.[27] Explicit representation of a collection of populations (a metapopulation) permits joint analysis of characteristics for individual populations, such as birth rate and population size, and contacts between populations in a region (geographic coupling).[28] Before a measles immunization program was introduced in England and Wales, the pattern of maintenance or interruption of transmission at a local level was strongly influenced by geographic coupling. New technologies for geographic information systems have expanded opportunities for studying spatial characteristics of disease (see Chapter 7).

Stochastic Effects

Deterministic models, which are the focus of this chapter, have fixed rules for change. Given the same initial conditions, a deterministic model will produce the same result. However, there is also an extensive literature on stochastic, or probabilistic, models in which chance plays a role. Deterministic models tend to be more appropriate when many infectives are circulating and immunization levels are moderate. Stochastic effects tend to be more important when few infectives are circulating, immunization levels are high, and cases tend to occur in clusters. In some settings, the differences between deterministic formulations and stochastic formulations may be quite substantial.[2,29,30]

Other Epidemiologic Models

Modes of Transmission

Vector-borne transmission is indirect transmission, in that one person can infect another person only by transmitting the infectious agent through an invertebrate animal, that is, the disease vector, which is typically an insect, tick, or snail (see discussion of vector-borne disease in Chapter 24). The specific details of transmission cycles are as varied as the diseases and vectors involved, but the example of malaria can be used to demonstrate the basic concepts. The cycle of transmission starts when a person harboring the infectious stage of malaria in the blood is bitten by an anopheline mosquito that ingests the infectious stage. The malaria parasite develops and migrates to the salivary glands of the mosquito vector, and the cycle of transmission continues when the mosquito transfers the parasite while biting another human host. A standard model for this process counts both the human and the mosquito population, dividing each population into those who are susceptible and those who are infected.[31] The only contacts are mosquito bites that transmit infections from people to mosquitoes and from mosquitoes to people. As with infections that are transmitted directly from person to person, the basic reproduction ratio of the number of new human cases generated from an initial human case in a susceptible population is a fundamental concept. However, the basic reproduction ratio must be generalized as the product of two quantities:

1. The number of mosquitoes that become infective by biting an infective person
2. The number of people who become infective due to the bites of an infective mosquito

Models of transmission of infection by sexual contact share some features with both direct transmission and vector-borne transmission. Homosexual contact is structured as direct transmission, and heterosexual contact is structured as vector-borne transmission, in which females and males are counted as separate populations. That is, the basic reproduction ratio of transmission considers how many new cases among females are generated from a single infected female (or how many new cases among males are generated from a single infected male). It may also be useful to construct separate subpopulations within a homosexual population (i.e., use the structure of a heterosexual transmission model) if specific sexual practices result in asymmetric patterns of risk between partners. The sharing of needles for injecting drugs, resulting in the spread of blood-borne diseases, can be considered a form of direct transmission. Although all contact patterns display some heterogeneity within populations, the effects are perhaps the most extreme for sexual contacts. The existence of a subset of the population with very high contact rates, called *superspreaders* or the *core population*, is central to models of sexually transmitted infections.[2,32] Such social heterogeneity renders population averages very misleading; an understanding of the spread of sexually transmitted disease in a population depends on detailed studies of personal sexual behavior.

In zoonotic diseases, the reservoir of infection is maintained in a vertebrate animal population, and humans are infected only occasionally.[33] The model structures that have been applied to the human population are used for the animal host population; the framework may be applied to animal infections whether or not they present a problem to humans.[34]

Another mode of transmission is vertical transmission, in which a parent transmits infection to unborn offspring. This may be of importance in maintaining transmission in the reservoir of infection in some circumstances, such as transovarial transmission by ticks[35] and hepatitis B transmission in humans.[2] For populations of ticks, a full ecologic model of the growth of the affected population is required. A model of hepatitis B transmission can incorporate population turnover of births and deaths in a manner similar to that shown in Figure 6-5, except that there are two types of birth—infected and uninfected. In contrast, the transmission of HIV from mother to fetus is a tragic consequence of other modes of transmission, but it is not a major contributor to the reservoir of infection.

Natural Histories

The most fundamental distinction in the natural history of infection is whether or not immunity is acquired after infection. For epidemiologic purposes, the key consideration is whether a person is subject to repeated infection and not whether there is some evidence of an immunologic response. (For some diseases, an immunologic response may not be effective, at least not at first.) Hethcote[10] provides a comparative analysis of the SIR model in which a person acquires immunity and the SIS model in which a person reverts to the susceptible state after infection. For either natural history, an infection will spread initially if the basic reproduction ratio exceeds 1. However, in a closed population, infection will become endemic in the SIS model and will disappear in the SIR model. The maintenance of transmission in a SIR model with births and deaths is also discussed.

An elaboration of the SIS model of infection and reinfection counts the number of parasites in a host. This structure has been used extensively for diseases caused by worms, such as schistosomiasis, and is considered a model for macroparasites.[2] In contrast, the models used in this chapter are considered models for microparasites that typically are smaller and replicate inside their hosts. Analysis of the replication of macroparasites is in terms of the number of parasites generated per parasite.

Persistent infection, which is characterized as SI, is also important for facilitating transmission of infection. This kind of infection is often asymptomatic and may be referred to as a *carrier state,* as with hepatitis B virus.[2] A carrier state of an infection helps it to establish and maintain endemicity (see the discussion of Figure 6-2b).

Host Genetic Factors

Genetic factors of the host that affect susceptibility to infection can be incorporated into models by dividing the host population into subgroups based on genotypes. Although this type of heterogeneity has played a relatively small role in epidemiologic models, it has been explored for a subset of the population that develops an asymptomatic carrier state of hepatitis B infection.[2] The genetics of host–parasite interactions are being investigated in diverse ways,[36,37] and more is being learned about the importance of host genetic factors in a variety of infectious diseases, including Puumala hantavirus infection, tuberculosis, Lyme disease, and HIV/AIDS.[38] The emerging picture is that infectious diseases are typically polygenic, meaning they are influenced by several genetic loci for susceptibility and resistance, each of which produces small effects.[39] With advances in understanding the genetic basis of disease, it is expected that models of the epidemiology of infectious diseases will incorporate more genetic information.

Pathogen Genetic Factors

Key epidemiological characteristics, such as transmissibility, pathogenicity, and immunogenicity, may vary greatly between strains of pathogens. The genetic structure of infectious agents provides clues about their origin, evolution, and spread, as shown in studies of mosquito-borne flaviviruses, which include yellow fever, Japanese encephalitis, West Nile, and dengue.[40] The general approach to modeling multiple strains of an infection is to treat them as distinct infections that interact in a host population.[41,42] Much more remains to be learned about the evolution of these systems.

Earth System Science and Remote Sensing

Growing awareness of global ecosystem change has stimulated interest in the effects such change has on public health.[43] Ecosystem change and its impact on public health is an example of the application of earth system science, a rich characterization of the dynamic interactions of air, water, land, and life that is enhanced by remote sensing data from space-based platforms.[44] One prominent application of earth system science is the study of the impact of climate on infectious disease transmission.[45,46] Malaria, a mosquito-borne illness with global impacts, serves to illustrate key issues of ecosystem change and climate.[47] Planning for malaria control is starting to take advantage of climate forecasts on seasonal to interannual timescales, as shown in reports about southern Africa and Colombia.[48,49] Although malaria is traditionally a rural disease, it is also a growing urban public health problem in developing countries, many of which are undergoing rapid urbanization with poor economies that have difficulty providing resources for disease control.[50] The increasing urbanization of malaria is motivating greater use of remote sensing for public health in urban areas. Sensors, such as the US Air Force Defense Meteorological Satellite Program's (DMSP) Operational Linescan System (OLS), provide data on nighttime lights used to infer the density of human settlements.[50,51]

Bioterrorism

Bioterrorism is terrorism that utilizes biological agents as the mechanism of attack. Although, from a social science perspective, *terrorism* is a term with great rhetorical power but limited scientific precision, *terrorism* does have a useful working definition with three elements: the illegal use, actual or threatened, of force or violence; the intent to coerce societies or governments by inducing fear in their populations; and an extra-societal aspect, be it domestic or foreign.[52] Combating terrorism is now a central policy concern in the United States and around the world as a consequence of the attacks of September 11, 2001, and the release of anthrax spores in subsequent months.

In the context of bioterrorism, the Centers for Disease Control and Prevention (CDC) have classified biological agents in terms of their risk to national security.[53] The greatest attention is paid to the highest priority agents, which are designated Category A: anthrax, botulism, plague, small-pox, tularemia, and viral hemorrhagic fevers (filoviruses and arenaviruses). Category A agents are deemed high risk because they satisfy one or more of the following criteria: ease of dissemination from person to person; high mortality rates and the capacity for major public health impact; potential of causing public panic and social disruption; and the need for special action for public health preparedness.

Epidemiological modeling applied to bioterrorism has a distinctive focus on scenarios of intentional release of biological agents, especially Category A agents. One central area of debate is the role of preparations in advance of an identified outbreak. For example, an analysis of public health vaccination policies for containing an anthrax outbreak concludes that mass pre-exposure vaccination would require very high coverage in order to have outcomes superior to those of a strategy of targeted and rapid post-exposure antibiotic prophylaxis.[54] On the other hand, the analysis of a model of the potential consequences of the introduction of 100 people infected with smallpox into a city subway system supports mass vaccination as the best strategy.[55] Scenarios of terrorist attacks also require the analysis of the capability of sensors to detect hazardous biological and chemical substances in air and water.[56]

Although traditional public health approaches are at the heart of strategies for countering bioterrorism, they must allow a broader scope for two major reasons. First, impacts to both human health and agricultural health are important.[57] The destruction of livestock and crops can cause enormous economic damage even if the organisms involved are not pathogenic to humans directly. Second, advances in technology for designing drugs and vaccines are a two-edged sword. The very tools that offer such promise to protect public health can also be misused to create new agents that pose even greater threats.[57]

Health Impacts

An analysis of the dynamics of transmission alone is not sufficient to inform policy makers. Measures of the impact of infectious diseases and other health problems are used to identify priorities for action. Measures of the burden of disease based on estimates of mortality and disability have become more widespread,[58] although such estimates are not without controversy. Translating a disease burden into economic impacts is another step that takes into account the cost of treatment and the cost of morbidity and mortality. For example, the global AIDS epidemic has been analyzed in terms of the cost of treating an AIDS patient, the effect on the health care sector, and the effect on poverty due to the loss of adults in a household.[59] Another important area of application is planning for economic development projects in terms of an economic analysis of environmental impacts, including possible adverse health impacts.[60,61] For example, water development projects in Africa have long demonstrated the capacity to increase the incidence of malaria or schistosomiasis.[62]

Social Processes and the Use of Model Predictions

Model predictions of disease transmission are highly dependent on time and place. For example, an infectious agent will not spread in exactly the same way in different populations (comparing either two geographic settings in the same time period or one geographic setting in two different time periods). These processes are different from the invariant "laws of nature" for which the term *prediction* really means explanation and inference.[63] Traditional natural science that constructs invariant "laws" is reductionist in that it breaks down nature into component parts and studies those parts. Complex systems for disease transmission and other problems characterize the interaction of the component parts. Efforts to predict the behavior of complex systems to aid in making decisions face a distinct set of challenges.

The use of predictions from complex systems in a policy context involves social processes in (at least) four important ways. First, individuals and societies may respond to the announcements of predictions, altering the outcomes.[64] Indeed, that may be the purpose of making such announcements, which should be linked to a growing body of knowledge about constructing messages for public health.[65] Second, when the political stakes of a controversy are high, political and scientific scrutiny of the problem will increase. Sources of uncertainty will increase because competing interests will bring different perspectives to strategies and solutions.[66] Third, different disciplinary approaches and different societal groups often make different value judgments about important outcomes. The selection of analytical tools in valuing outcomes, such as cost-benefit analysis, may appear to be straightforward but in fact involve implicit assumptions that may not be acceptable to all parties.[67] Fourth, when the aim is to use a model to examine the consequences of alternative policies, decisions are incorporated into the model so that forecasts are conditional upon the selection of a policy. Such forecasts cannot be assessed in terms of accuracy because real-world policies are never identical to idealized policies; rather, evaluation of the model should instead focus on the exposition of theory and method.[64,68]

The projections of the potential impact of HIV/AIDS in Asia illustrate the interplay of social processes and uncertainties in using model predictions in infectious disease epidemiology. A 2004 report reviewed outlooks for the HIV/AIDS epidemic in Asia amid concerns that the HIV/AIDS epidemic in Asia could end up on the same scale as the HIV/AIDS epidemic in Africa.[69] At the time of the report, the HIV/AIDS epidemic had appeared in high-risk groups of Asian intravenous drug users, sex workers, and gay men and had reached at least 5% prevalence in some subnational Asian populations. The forecasts addressed the risk of a "generalized epidemic" in Asia spread by heterosexual sex. A relatively reassuring forecast for an Asian epidemic limited primarily to sex workers and injecting drug users projected that HIV prevalence in the total sexually active population would never reach 0.5%. In contrast, a forecast for a "generalized epidemic" projected 15 million HIV cases in China and 25 million HIV cases in India (corresponding to an adult prevalence in India of 4%) by the year 2010. The discrepancies between forecasts were due primarily to differing assumptions about the potential for HIV to spread in relation to sexual practices, sexual partners, and circumcision. The issue of timing was a more subtle problem. The Asian HIV/AIDS had been progressing more slowly than the African HIV/AIDS epidemic, but a slow speed could nevertheless be consistent with a high ultimate prevalence of HIV. Predicting the speed of an epidemic is notoriously difficult in general, as illustrated by the slower-than-expected spread of a strain of dengue virus introduced into Puerto Rico, which was well known to have the right conditions for high levels of transmission—a large mosquito vector population, a large susceptible human population, and a suitable climate.[70]

The divergence in forecasts of the AIDS epidemic in Asia, an indicator of gaps in data and real uncertainties, elicited different responses from health researchers and program managers about how to guide public communications. The report[69] identified concerns about both overestimating and underestimating the impact of the AIDS epidemic, which are related to the importance of maintaining the credibility of public warnings.[65] How to galvanize support for interventions to limit the impact of the HIV/AIDS epidemic in Asia was a central focus. A model about high-risk groups in the Asian HIV/AIDS epidemic demonstrated the potential benefit of targeted early interventions by concluding that prevention of the HIV/AIDS epidemic among intravenous drug users in Jakarta, Indonesia, would have prevented the spread of the epidemic through sex workers and their clients in that city. This model also indicated that the number of female sex workers and their clients was a powerful determinant of Asian HIV/AIDS epidemics. A suggested communications strategy was to promulgate the most pessimistic model with the argument that the worst outcomes could not be ruled out. However, another worry was that the announcement of a scenario of widespread HIV transmission could cause people to become fatalistic and do nothing. A distinct but related issue put forth in the discussion was that the framing of the forecasting controversy in terms of the potential for a "generalized" HIV/AIDS epidemic could suggest that preventing a "generalized" epidemic was the only valued outcome for disease control. Public health workers stressed the importance of preventing spread in high-risk groups whereas most HIV/AIDS prevention campaigns in Asia had been addressing the general population and not high-risk groups.

To more effectively use science and technology to address complex societal problems, the US National Research Council has recommended the development of knowledge-action systems.[71] Generalizing from their study of the applications of seasonal to interannual climate forecasting, they have identified six components of effective knowledge-action systems.

1. Problem definition that is collaborative but user-driven
2. Complete inclusion on the continuum of decision maker to knowledge produced ("end-to-end systems")
3. Boundary organizations that act as intermediaries between nodes in the system—most notably between scientists and decision makers
4. Design for learning rather than knowing (featuring flexible processes and institutions)

5. Funding strategies tailored to the dual private–public character of such systems and with sufficient continuity to foster long-term relationships between users and producers
6. Long-term investments in people who can work across disciplines, issue areas, and the knowledge–action interface

The development of knowledge–action systems therefore stresses the importance of understanding and managing the social processes that influence the use of model predictions. Such an approach is consistent with calls in the science policy community to view science not as a predictive oracle but rather as a tool to facilitate consensus and action with an iterative and incremental approach to making decisions.[66] This process must grapple with questions of values up front, seeking agreement on the questions to be asked and the social uses of the answers.[64,72]

Conclusion and Prospects

This chapter has focused primarily on mathematical models of directly transmitted infections that confer lifelong immunity, such as measles and many other childhood immunizable diseases. The model and its extensions are usually referred to as SIR, for epidemiologic states corresponding to people who are susceptible, infective, or recovered/removed. A central concept is the basic reproduction ratio, which is the number of secondary cases generated from a single case in an otherwise susceptible population. The basic reproduction ratio affects patterns of endemicity, the age at which a host becomes infected, and the epidemiologic response to mass immunization. Mathematical analysis demonstrates how the basic reproduction ratio depends on the structure of the host population and the characteristics of the infectious agent.

This chapter has also provided a brief overview of issues in developing applications beyond the basic SIR model. Common extensions of the SIR model involve the age structure of contact patterns and latent periods, as well as demographic, spatial, and stochastic effects. An understanding of the SIR model forms the basis for understanding applications to infectious diseases with different modes of transmission, different natural histories, a strong dependence on host or pathogen genetic factors, linkages to earth system science, or a context of bioterrorism. For any disease, links between the dynamics of transmission and health impacts are needed for the analysis of policies for disease control and prevention. To use model predictions effectively in making decisions, attention must be paid to the social processes shaping the knowledge–action system relevant to the problem of interest.

Mathematical models of the epidemiology of infectious diseases provide numerous examples of the exchange of ideas among disciplines, demonstrating a benefit of interdisciplinary communication that is gaining greater appreciation throughout the scientific world. The origin of the mass-action mixing term used in epidemiological models for contact between susceptibles and infectives lies in chemistry mass-action kinetics, which in turn is similar to that derived from scattering theory based on spherical geometry in physics. The formal similarities between the SIR model in epidemiology and the basic model for the intensity of light produced by lasers contribute to more cross-fertilization between biology and physics.[73,74] And in the modern world of the Internet, the epidemiological perspective provides insights about the transmission and control of computer viruses.[75,76]

Trends in research reveal two apparently contradictory directions. On the one hand, adverse effects of global environmental change on public health are a growing concern.[77] Models of the dynamics of transmission of infectious diseases should be linked to models of environmental phenomena on a global scale.[43] On the other hand, microbial change is a major cause of the emergence and re-emergence of infectious diseases.[78] Models should examine the dynamics of infection at the level of replication of the infectious agent, taking into account genetic changes[79,80] and the dynamics of the immune response,[81] for an overall evolutionary perspective.[82] Both macro and micro factors must be considered in practical applications to public health, such as the development of an immunization program to combat a large epidemic of diphtheria in the former Soviet Union or the threat of pandemic influenza.[83,84]

The complexity of the dynamics of transmission can easily overwhelm any attempt to develop mathematical models of multiple factors operating at radically different scales. Quantitative predictions will require highly detailed models. However, it is important to remember that the development of applications has an inherent tension between simple and complex models. As stated in the introduction, mathematical models are supposed to aid the educational process and not simply be "black boxes" that produce answers. For conceptual understanding, a limited number of assumptions are an advantage.

The trade-off between simplicity and complexity arises again and again in different contexts. Experiences in other fields are useful in gaining insight about this issue in the epidemiology of infectious diseases. An evaluation of a global model of population and resources led to the comment below on the problem of losing conceptual understanding of a complex model:

> Although the model suppresses a great deal of detail, it is complicated enough to make understanding difficult. When you discover some new aspect of its behavior, it can be difficult to track down the mechanism responsible. Thus, adding more structure in the cause of realism would not necessarily teach us much. We might well reach a point where we could not understand the model any better than we understand the real world.[85]

A report on the use of geographic information systems emphasizes the problem of making decisions using highly detailed data:

> Realistic modeling of spatial and temporal phenomena generally demands disaggregation (i.e., large detailed models and/or databases)—but in terms of decision making, such levels of disaggregation are usually counterproductive. Decision making demands aggregation, and therein lays the dilemma. From a scientific viewpoint, we must disaggregate "to be real"—from a decision-making viewpoint, we must aggregate "to be real."[86]

In selecting an appropriate degree of complexity during the process of model development, it is essential to focus on specific questions to be addressed.[13] Variations of a model with different levels of structure may be useful in different phases of development.

The challenge of developing and utilizing mathematical models to aid in understanding and controlling the spread of infectious diseases continues to evolve. It is hoped that researchers and practitioners in public health can use the concepts and approaches presented in this chapter as a starting point in meeting the challenge.

Acknowledgments

I thank Martin Ruzek and Ira Schwartz for suggestions and comments.

References

1. Sterman JD. A skeptic's guide to computer models. In: Barney GO, Kreutzer WB, Garrett MJ, eds. *Managing a Nation: The Microcomputer Software Catalog*. Boulder, Col: Westview Press; 1991:209–229.
2. Anderson RM, May RM. *Infectious Diseases of Humans*. London: Oxford University Press; 1991.
3. Scott ME, Smith G. *Parasitic and Infectious Diseases: Epidemiology and Ecology*. San Diego, CA: Academic Press; 1994.
4. Mollison D, ed. *Epidemic Models: Their Structure and Relation to Data*. Cambridge, UK: Cambridge University Press; 1995.
5. Grenfell BT, Dobson A, eds. *Ecology of Infectious Diseases in Natural Populations*. Cambridge, UK: Cambridge University Press; 1995.
6. Bailey NTJ. *The Mathematical Theory of Infectious Diseases and Its Applications*. New York, NY: Oxford University Press; 1975.
7. Levin SA, Hallam TG, Gross LJ, eds. *Applied Mathematical Ecology*. Biomathematics. Vol. 18. Berlin, Germany: Springer-Verlag; 1989.
8. Hastings A. *Population Biology: Concepts and Models*. New York, NY: Springer-Verlag; 1997.
9. Yorke JA, Nathanson N, Pianigiani G, Martin J. Seasonality and the requirements for perpetuation and eradication of viruses in populations. *Am J Epidemiol*. 1979;109:103–123.
10. Hethcote HW. Three basic epidemiological models. In: Levin SA, Hallam TG, Gross LJ, eds. *Applied Mathematical Ecology*. Berlin, Germany: Springer-Verlag; 1989:119–144.
11. Fine PEM. John Brownlee and the measurement of infectiousness: an historical study in epidemic theory. *J R Stat Soc* [A]. 1979;42:347–362.
12. Anderson RM. Directly transmitted viral and bacterial infections of man. In: Anderson RM, ed. *Population Dynamics of Infectious Diseases*. London, UK: Chapman and Hall; 1982.
13. Aron JL. Simple versus complex epidemiological models. In: Levin SA, Hallam TG, Gross JJ, eds. *Applied Mathematical Ecology*. Berlin, Germany: Springer-Verlag; 1989:176–192.
14. Lobel HO, McCollum RW. Some observations on the ecology of infectious hepatitis. *Bull WHO*. 1965;32:675–682.
15. Hope Simpson RE. Infectiousness of communicable diseases in the household (measles, chickenpox, and mumps). *Lancet*. 1952;2:549–554.
16. Broome CV, Preblud SR, Bruner B, et al. Epidemiology of pertussis, Atlanta, 1977. *J Pediatr*. 1981;98:362–367.

17. Fine PEM. Herd immunity: history, theory, practice. *Epidemiol Rev.* 1993;15:265–302.
18. Centers for Disease Control. Current trends. Practices in college immunization–United States. *MMWR.* 1987;36:209–212.
19. Fine PEM, Clarkson JA. Measles in England and Wales. I. An analysis of factors underlying seasonal patterns. *Int J Epidemiol.* 1982;11:5–14.
20. Fine PEM, Clarkson JA. Measles in England and Wales. II. The impact of the measles vaccination programme on the distribution of immunity in the population. *Int J Epidemiol.* 1982;11:15–25.
21. Anderson RM, May RM. Directly transmitted infectious diseases: control by vaccination. *Science.* 1982;215:1053–1060.
22. Anderson RM, May RM. Age-related changes in the rate of disease transmission: implications for the design of vaccination programmes. *J Hyg* (Camb). 1985;94:365–436.
23. Schenzle D. An age-structured model of pre- and postvaccination measles transmission. *IMA J Math Appl Med Biol.* 1984;1: 169–191.
24. Longini IM, Halloran ME, Nizam A, Wolff M, Mendelman PM, Fast PE, Belshe RB. Estimation of the efficacy of live, attenuated influenza vaccine from a two-year, multi-center vaccine trial: implications for influenza epidemic control. *Vaccine* 2000;18:1902–1909.
25. Monto AS, Maassab HF. Use of influenza vaccine in non-high risk populations. *Dev Biol Stand.* 1977;39:329–335.
26. Cohen J. Vaccine policy. Immunizing kids against flu may prevent deaths among the elderly. *Science.* 2004;306:1123.
27. Cliff A, Haggett P, Smallman-Raynor M. *Measles: An Historical Geography of a Major Human Viral Disease from Global Expansion to Local Retreat, 1840–1990.* Oxford, UK: Blackwell Reference; 1993.
28. Finkenstadt B, Grenfell B. Empirical determinants of measles metapopulation dynamics in England and Wales. *Proc R Soc Lond B Biol Sci.* 1998;265:211–220.
29. Nasell I. The threshold concept in stochastic epidemic and endemic models. In: Mollison D, ed. *Epidemic Models: Their Structure and Relation to Data.* Cambridge, UK: Cambridge University Press; 1995: 71–83.
30. Diekmann O, Heesterbeek H, Metz H. The legacy of Kermack and McKendrick. In: Mollison D, ed. *Epidemic Models: Their Structure and Relation to Data.* Cambridge, UK: Cambridge University Press; 1995: 95–115.
31. Aron JL, May RM. The population dynamics of malaria. In: Anderson RM, ed. *Population Dynamics of Infectious Diseases.* London: Chapman and Hall; 1982:139–179.
32. Hethcote HW, Yorke JA. Gonorrhea: transmission dynamics and control. *Lect Notes Biomath.* 1984;56:1–105.
33. Wilson ML. Ecology and infectious disease. In: Aron JL, Patz JA, eds. *Ecosystem Change and Public Health: A Global Perspective.* Baltimore, Md: Johns Hopkins University Press; 2001:283–324.
34. Barlow ND. Critical evaluation of wildlife disease models. In: Grenfell BT, Dobson AP, eds. *Ecology of Infectious Diseases in Natural Populations.* Cambridge, UK: Cambridge University Press; 1995: 230–259.
35. Smith G, Basanez M-G, Dietz K, et al. Macroparasite group report: problems in modelling the dynamics of macroparasitic systems. In:

Grenfell BT, Dobson AP, eds. *Ecology of Infectious Diseases in Natural Populations.* Cambridge, UK: Cambridge University Press; 1995: 209–229.

36. Wakelin D. Host populations: genetics and immunity. In: Scott ME, Smith G, eds. *Parasitic and Infectious Diseases: Epidemiology and Ecology.* San Diego, Calif: Academic Press; 1994:83–100.

37. Lively CM, Apanius V. Genetic diversity in host-parasite interactions. In: Grenfell BT, Dobson AP, eds. *Ecology of Infectious Diseases in Natural Populations.* Cambridge, UK: Cambridge University Press; 1995:421–449.

38. McNicholl J. Host genes and infectious diseases. *Emerg Infect Dis.* 1998;4:423–426.

39. Frodsham AJ, Hill AV. Genetics of infectious diseases. *Hum Mol Genet.* 2004;13:187–194.

40. Mackenzie JS, Gubler DJ, Petersen LR. Emerging flaviviruses: the spread and resurgence of Japanese encephalitis, West Nile and dengue viruses. *Nature Medicine.* 2004;10:S98–S109.

41. Abu-Raddad LJ, Ferguson NM. The impact of cross-immunity, mutation and stochastic extinction on pathogen diversity. *Proc R Soc Lond B Biol Sci.* 2004;271:2431–2438.

42. Rohani P, Green CJ, Mantilla-Beniers NB, Grenfell BT. Ecological interference between fatal diseases. *Nature.* 2003;422:885–888.

43. Aron JL, Patz JA, eds. *Ecosystem Change and Public Health: A Global Perspective.* Baltimore, Md: Johns Hopkins University Press; 2001.

44. Ruzek M. Earth system science in a nutshell. In: *Starting Point Teaching Entry Level Geoscience, Using an Earth System Approach,* Science Education Resource Center, Carleton College; 2004. Available at: http://serc.carleton.edu/introgeo/earthsystem/nutshell/index.html. Accessed 14 Mar 2006.

45. National Research Council. *Under the Weather: Climate, Ecosystems, and Infectious Disease.* Washington, DC: National Academies Press; 2001.

46. Kovats S, Ebi KL, Menne B, eds. *Methods of Assessing Human Health Vulnerability and Public Health Adaptation to Climate Change.* Copenhagen, Denmark: World Health Organization Regional Office for Europe; 2003.

47. Aron JL, Shiff CJ, Buck AA. Malaria and global ecosystem change. In: Aron JL, Patz JA, eds. *Ecosystem Change and Public Health: A Global Perspective.* Baltimore, Md: Johns Hopkins University Press; 2001: 353–378.

48. DaSilva J, Garanganga B, Teveredzi V, Marx SM, Mason SJ, Connor SJ. Improving epidemic malaria planning, preparedness and response in Southern Africa. *Malaria J.* 2004;3:37.

49. National Research Council. *Knowledge-Action Systems for Seasonal to Interannual Climate Forecasting: Summary of a Workshop.* Washington, DC: National Academies Press; 2005.

50. Keiser J, Utzinger J, de Castro MC, Smith TA, Tanner M, Singer BH. Urbanization in sub-Saharan Africa and implication for malaria control. *Am J Trop Med Hyg.* 2004;71(Suppl 2):118–127.

51. Tatem AJ, Hay SI. Measuring urbanization pattern and extent for malaria research: a review of remote sensing approaches. *J Urban Health; Bull NY Acad Med.* 2004;81:363–376.

52. National Research Council. *Terrorism: Perspectives from the Behavioral and Social Sciences.* Washington, DC: National Academies Press; 2002.

53. Centers for Disease Control and Prevention. Emergency Preparedness and Response. Agents, Disease and Other Threats. Bioterrorism Agents; 2005. Available at: http://www.bt.cdc.gov. Accessed 14 Mar 2006.

54. Brookmeyer R, Johnson E, Bollinger R. Public health vaccination policies for containing an anthrax outbreak. *Nature.* 2004;432: 901–904.

55. Castillo-Chavez C, Song B, Zhang J. An epidemic model with virtual mass transportation: the case of smallpox in a large city. In: Banks HT, Castillo-Chavez C, eds. *Bioterrorism: Mathematical Modeling Applications in Homeland Security.* Philadelphia, Pa: Society for Industrial and Applied Mathematics; 2003:173–197.

56. Schwartz IB, Billings L, Holt D, Kusterbeck AW, Triandaf I. Chemical and biological sensing: modeling and analysis from the real world. In: Banks HT, Castillo-Chavez C, eds. *Bioterrorism: Mathematical Modeling Applications in Homeland Security.* Philadelphia, Pa: Society for Industrial and Applied Mathematics; 2003:55–86.

57. Institute of Medicine. *Countering Bioterrorism: The Role of Science and Technology.* Washington, DC: National Academies Press; 2002.

58. Murray CJL, Lopez AD. The *Global Burden of Disease: A Comprehensive Assessment of Mortality and Disability from Diseases, Injuries and Risk Factors in 1990 and Projected to 2020.* Cambridge, Mass: Harvard University Press; 1996.

59. World Bank. *Confronting AIDS: Public Priorities in a Global Epidemic.* New York, NY: Oxford University Press; 1997.

60. World Bank. *Economic Analysis and Environmental Assessment. Environmental Assessment Sourcebook Update, no. 23, Environment Department.* Washington, DC: World Bank; 1998.

61. World Bank. *Health Aspects of Environmental Assessment. Environmental Assessment Sourcebook Update, no. 18, Environment Department.* Washington, DC: World Bank; 1997.

62. Hunter JM, Rey L, Scott D. Man-made lakes and man-made diseases: towards a policy resolution. *Soc Sci Med.* 1982;16:1127–1145.

63. Sarewitz D, Pielke RA Jr. Prediction in science and policy. In: Sarewitz D, Pielke RA Jr, Byerly R Jr, eds. *Prediction: Science, Decision Making, and the Future of Nature.* Washington, DC: Island Press; 2000: 11–22.

64. Aron JL, Ellis JH, Hobbs BF. Integrated assessment. In: Aron JL, Patz JA, eds. *Ecosystem Change and Public Health: A Global Perspective.* Baltimore, Md: Johns Hopkins University Press; 2001:116–162.

65. Institute of Medicine and National Research Council. *Public Health Risks of Disasters: Communication, Infrastructure, and Preparedness.* Washington, DC: National Academies Press; 2005.

66. Sarewitz D. How science makes environmental controversies worse. *Environmental Science & Policy.* 2004;7:385–403.

67. Aron JL, Zimmerman RH. Cross-disciplinary communication needed to promote the effective use of indicators in making decisions. *Canadian Journal of Public Health.* 2002;93(suppl 1):S24–S28.

68. Ascher W. Beyond accuracy. *Int J Forecasting.* 1989;5:469–484.

69. Cohen J. HIV/AIDS in Asia. News. Asia and Africa: on different trajectories? *Science.* 2004;304:1932–1938.

70. Rigau-Pérez JG, Ayala-López A, García-Rivera EJ, Hudson SM, Vorndam V, Reiter P, Cano MP, Clark GG. The reappearance of dengue-3 and a subsequent dengue-4 and dengue-1 epidemic in Puerto Rico in 1998. *Am J Trop Med Hyg.* 2002;67:355–362.

71. National Research Council. *Knowledge-Action Systems for Seasonal to Interannual Climate Forecasting: Summary of a Workshop.* Washington, DC: National Academies Press; 2005.

72. Herrick C, Jamieson D. The social construction of acid rain: some implications for science/policy assessment. *Global Environ Change.* 1995;5:105–112.

73. Billings L, Bollt E, Morgan D, Schwartz IB. Stochastic global bifurcation in perturbed Hamiltonian system. *Discrete and Continuous Dynamical Systems,* supplemental volume entitled *Fourth International Conference on Dynamical Systems and Differential Equations, May 24–27, 2002. Journal of Discrete and Continuous Dynamical Systems.* 2003:123–132.

74. Kim M-Y, Roy R, Aron JL, Carr TW, Schwartz IB. Scaling behavior of laser population dynamics with time-delayed coupling: theory and experiment. *Physical Review Letters.* 2005;94:Art. No. 088101.

75. Aron JL, O'Leary M, Gove RA, Azadegan S, Schneider MC. The benefits of a notification process in addressing the worsening computer virus problem: results of a survey and a simulation model. *Computers & Security.* 2002;21:142–163.

76. Liebovitch LS, Schwartz IB. Information flow dynamics and timing patterns in the arrival of email viruses. *Physical Review E.* 2003;68:Art. No. 017101.

77. WRI/UNEP/UNDP/World Bank. *World Resources 1998–99.* New York, NY: Oxford University Press; 1998.

78. Institute of Medicine. *Microbial Threats to Health: Emergence, Detection, and Response,* Washington, DC: National Academies Press; 2003.

79. Burke DS. Evolvability of emerging viruses. In: Nelson AM, Horsburgh CR, eds. *Pathology of Emerging Infections.* Washington, DC: American Society of Microbiology Press; 1998.

80. Burke DS, Grefenstette JJ, Ramsey CL, De Jong KA, Wu AS. Putting more genetics into genetic algorithms. *Evolutionary Computation.* 1998;6:387–410.

81. Perelson AS, Nelson PW. Mathematical analysis of HIV-1 dynamics in vivo. *SIAM Rev.* 1999;41:3–44.

82. Levin BR, Lipsitch M, Bonhoeffer S. Population biology, evolution, and infectious disease: convergence and synthesis. *Science.* 1999;283:806–809.

83. Vitek CR, Wharton M. Diphtheria in the former Soviet Union: reemergence of a pandemic disease. *Emerg Infect Dis.* 1998;4:539–550.

84. Institute of Medicine. *The Threat of Pandemic Influenza: Are We Ready? Workshop Summary.* Washington, DC: National Academies Press; 2005.

85. Hayes B. Balanced on a pencil point. *Am Scientist.* 1993;81:510–516.

86. Glass GE, Aron JL, Ellis JH, Yoon SS. *Applications of GIS Technology to Disease Control.* Baltimore, Md: Dept. of Population Dynamics, Johns Hopkins School of Hygiene and Public Health; 1993.

CHAPTER SEVEN

GEOGRAPHIC INFORMATION SYSTEMS

Gregory E. Glass

Introduction

A common definition of geographic information systems (GIS) is that they are procedures to input, store, retrieve, manipulate, analyze, and output data that have spatial attributes associated with them.[1] Typically, the results are presented as maps or images that summarize the data or analyses performed on the data. Infectious disease epidemiology, almost by the very nature of the interaction of hosts and the pathogens within the environment (as well as vector and reservoir populations with vector-borne and zoonotic diseases), lends itself to GIS, at least as a way to summarize the sometimes complex relationships associated with disease transmission.

Snow's classic study of cholera transmission around Broad Street in London in the mid-1850s is often summarized by the map of deaths he plotted in relation to the Broad Street pump, as well as the pump's spatial relationship to other features such as workhouses, residences, and factories (Figure 7-1). As such, the manual construction of a map to present these data conforms to the definition of a GIS. Despite the convincing nature of the data when presented in this way, it is critical to keep in mind an important feature of Snow's analysis that has characterized the limited application of GIS in epidemiology: The map that he created did not lead him to conclude that (1) cholera was a water-borne illness and (2) the pump was the source of contagion (contrary to popular lore); rather, the map was a method that he used to summarize his data to his audience and a tool he used to try to convince others of his conclusions. As Vandenbroucke[2] noted, "As an historical example, it remains important to remember that Snow's theory on the communication of cholera was not derived from his epidemiologic observations, but preceded them." Although Snow may have applied GIS well, it was a relatively restricted application. The restriction has been due, historically, to technical limitations rather than to conceptual ones.

213

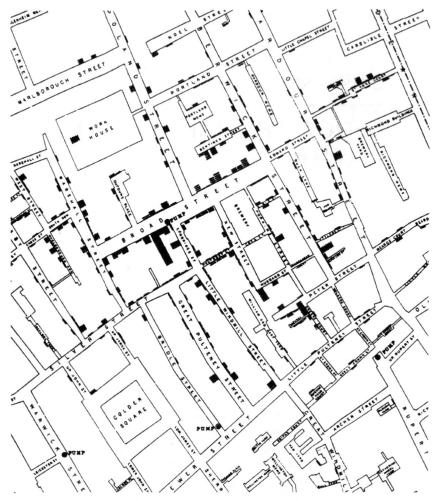

FIGURE 7-1 Map of the cholera outbreak in London around Golden Square and the Broad Street pump, indicating deaths, the pumps in the vicinity, and various land use features as drafted by John Snow.
Source: Historical Collection, Institute of the History of Medicine, The Johns Hopkins University.

However, even today GIS still often remains a tool to represent complex spatial relationships rather than being used to explore epidemiologic patterns and identify risk factors. Although the spatial distribution of cases is recognized as important in understanding infectious disease transmission, the statistical and geographic tools have not been generally available to make the examination of spatial distributions of infectious diseases an important analytical method for epidemiologic investigations. The increased development of GIS as an analytical approach in epidemiology results from improved access to automated computer systems and their associated software. To date, most of the progress in spatial epidemiology has been made where point exposures to a single factor (e.g., a pollutant or radiation) are responsible for human disease. An analogous situation occurs during outbreak investigations from a single source of infection. The graphical presentation of these data is little removed from Snow's early representations, demonstrating that the spatial consequences of epidemiologic processes deduced from more traditional means can be compelling. For example, in 1979 an outbreak of anthrax was reported from the Sverdlovsk region in Russia involving deaths of both humans and domestic animals. Occasional anthrax outbreaks had been known from that region since at least the early 1900s. Anthrax is a disease caused by infection with *Bacillus anthracis*, and the severity of the disease caused by infection varies with the route of exposure. Cutaneous infection is least likely to cause mortality, whereas ingesting contaminated meat has a higher rate of mortality and inhalation of the agent is commonly fatal. Official reports indicated the outbreak was associated with contact with naturally infected animals. However, rumors persisted that the outbreak was related to an accidental release of bacteria from a military facility. Subsequent epidemiologic investigations, summarized by Meselson et al.[3] with the mapping of human and animal cases, indicated both the locations and timing (based on meteorologic conditions) were immediately downwind of the military facility (see Chapter 2). Examination of autopsy materials confirmed the human cases resulted from inhalation rather than ingestion of the bacteria.

Probably one of the most striking early examples that moved beyond simple graphic representation and demonstrated the power of examining spatial patterns in developing hypotheses for infectious disease epidemiology was Maxcy's[4] implication of rodent arthropod vectors in the transmission of murine typhus. Comparison of the spatial distributions of typhus cases in Montgomery, Alabama, from 1922 to 1925, by places of residence and places of occupation, showed substantial aggregation by place of occupation rather than residence. Thus, the differences in the spatial distributions of cases by alternate, possible places of exposure were used to generate inferences about modes of transmission. Maxcy hypothesized that if human lice served as vectors of typhus (as was assumed by many at that time), then multiple cases should occur in and around the same household because of close human contact. However, spatial clustering of cases was more evident when place of occupation was examined (Figure 7-2); typhus was especially common among workers associated with food services, leading Maxcy to propose that an arthropod vector associated with food services was responsible. Subsequent work[5] showed the vector of murine typhus to be the rat flea, whose hosts infested many of the food facilities at that time.

Clearly, one factor that historically limited the use of spatial data was the methodological difficulties associated with manipulating spatial data. The problem with manually plotting information, such as Maxcy's, multiplies significantly with each environmental factor examined, the spatial (and temporal) relationships of these factors, and the epidemiologic associations to be evaluated. These difficulties have been greatly reduced by the accessibility of relatively powerful computing systems in epidemiologic research and the development of dedicated GIS software that is designed to perform functions associated with mapping spatial data. When coupled with spatial analytic methods that have developed during the past two decades, it seems that we may be able to use the spatial patterns of infectious diseases in an analytical fashion, rather than intuitively, to provide important clues to the epidemiology of infectious diseases. This is true even when multiple

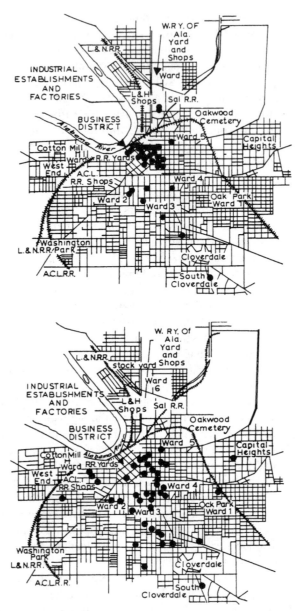

FIGURE 7-2   The distribution of cases of typhus fever in Montgomery, Alabama, plotted by K.F. Maxcy in 1926. Top shows distribution of cases by place of work (or residence if unemployed); bottom by place of residence. The more focal distribution of cases by place of work (top) was used by Maxcy to infer that endemic typhus was not transmitted by lice.
Source: Historical Collection, Institute of the History of Medicine, The Johns Hopkins University.

environmental factors interact to influence disease rates. The most intriguing possibility of these systems is that they will allow us to develop and test hypotheses about infectious disease epidemiology in ways that have previously been impossible.

This chapter provides an overview of GIS with its structure discussed in functional terms. The influence of computer systems on the field means that many software systems have been developed to apply to spatial data, each with its own limitations. The field of GIS has rapidly grown during the past decade and various textbooks exist as introductions to the methods and approaches of the technology especially as they relate to public health.[6,7] Thus, after the brief overview of GIS, the rest of the chapter contains discussion of each of the major applications of GIS as they apply to infectious disease epidemiology. A series of case studies, from simple situations involving data storage through analysis and decision making, is provided. These examples represent studies that will provide some ideas of the broad scope of the technology's application. The chapter is completed with a brief overview of remotely sensed (satellite) data as a way of gathering updated information on the environment, as well as some of the major analytical issues with spatial analyses.

Overview

Geographic information systems can be used for a variety of purposes in infectious disease epidemiology and these functions are fairly general to any field using spatial data. GIS can be used to help collect and store data, manage data, query data, model the processes generating the data, and make programmatic decisions. It is important to realize that these latter tasks, especially modeling and decision making, are not independent of the earlier functions; the quality of modeling, for example, is critically influenced by how well data have been collected and managed.

An excellent recent synopsis of GIS can be found in Vine et al.[8] Briefly, a major feature that distinguishes GIS from other computer-based systems is that a GIS contains within the stored data information concerning the spatial relationships among geographic features, and provides methods to study the relationships among selected, relevant features. Two major formats are used to represent these features. Software systems tend to be predominantly one or the other, but more recent versions usually provide algorithms for alternating between formats. GIS tend to present data in either vector or raster formats.

Vector Format

Vector format GIS represent features in two-dimensional space as points, lines, or polygons. Raster format GIS represent features in two-dimensional space in (usually) a uniform grid. Other data formats, such as quadtrees, which are something of a hybrid format, also exist but they are generally less common in their current usage. The major conceptual difference between vector- and raster-based systems is in how the data are represented. In vector format, points are located by specific x,y coordinates that typically represent a specific place on the earth's surface. Lines are interconnected points, linked one to another, whereas polygons represent features with areas and are joined line segments in which the first and last point have the same coordinates.

These three types of features are used to represent objects on a map. For example, points might be used to indicate the location of health care facilities, lines might be used to represent transportation networks (e.g., roads), and polygons may be used to indicate the geographic extent of service areas for the clinics. In vector formats, the points, lines, and polygons are usually thought of as being fairly precisely located and, in the case of polygons, the area to the inside of the polygon's boundary is assumed to be homogeneous. This is only approximately true for most environmental features and this raises an issue of data quality that must be assessed in any analysis.

How objects are represented in vector format depends on the scale at which the data are gathered. For example, a clinic might be presented as a point at one scale but as one moves to a larger scale (zooms in), such as floor plans, the outside walls of the buildings making up the clinic may be best represented by polygons. Issues related to choice of scale for GIS application are critical to the study design and outcome. The choice of scale, to some extent, is often determined by the initial resolution of the epidemiologic data. Consider, for example, that Lyme disease, a tick-borne bacterial infection, is a nationally reportable disease in the United States. However, the summary data may only be available at state or, at best, county level. Consequently, the scale for the GIS applications of the problem may be no better than county resolution, with cases known to occur somewhere within the county boundary. This indicates that a fairly small scale is most appropriate for presentation of these data and this scale places limits on the types of questions that can be addressed. In properly maintained databases, the minimal mapping unit (or the extent of smallest feature identified) is indicated, which is an important consideration in the selection of databases for study.

Raster Format

By contrast, raster formats are typically represented as grids of a study area, and locations are determined by the row and column locations much like a Cartesian coordinate system so that each x,y coordinate represents the location of a cell. Probably the most obvious example of raster-based data is satellite imagery in which reflected light from the earth is recorded by sensors on the satellite. The brightness of the reflected light is recorded for an area of the earth's surface. This area represents the spatial resolution of the image. No points or lines are used in raster formats, as all features have some minimal area assigned to them. Additionally, polygons, as used in vector formats, do not exist but are represented by large numbers of adjacent cells with the same data value. This data format has two consequences in GIS. First, the locations of points, lines, and boundaries of areas are approximate in that they are located somewhere within the specified cells, although their precise locations are not specified. This means that the locations of features are somewhat "fuzzy"—which may be more realistic for natural features, such as habitat edges. Spatial accuracy of raster features is determined by the spatial resolution of the grid. The raster format sometimes provides a more detailed characterization of features in the inside of regions than vector formats, which assume features are uniform within a polygon. Second, because the spatial resolution is determined by the interval distances between the rows and columns, the shorter the intervals, the finer the resolution. This produces a computational trade-off between improved spatial resolution, made by increasing the numbers of rows and columns, and the size of the database. This is because, unlike vector formats, the data value for each cell has to be recorded. To minimize the size of files and the time needed to process data, various methods of data encoding have been developed to try to reduce the computational loads associated with raster formats.

Data Structure

The development of relational databases in which different databases can be linked by a common, key field was a major contribution for integrating GIS within infectious disease epidemiology. Relational database structures make it possible to use GIS as a tool within a larger, investigative analysis rather than forcing studies within specified data frameworks. Data for GIS can be derived from a variety of sources, both specifically for study (e.g., survey data) and as part of the regular duties of agencies (administrative data). As long as at least one of the variables in the gathered data can be linked to a geographic location (e.g., postal codes, addresses, census tracts, states, provinces, countries), the information can be incorporated in a GIS.

More typically, studies derive information from both administrative and specific study design sources. Information on environmental conditions (e.g., land use or land cover patterns, property ownership patterns, soils, watersheds) can all be accessed from appropriate governmental agencies that gather the data as part of their administrative responsibilities. These data can form a portion of the analysis, whereas specific survey data to study disease incidence, morbidity patterns, and so forth can be gathered as part of a specific study by investigators who then attempt to link observed disease patterns with the spatial distribution of environmental covariates.

Data quality, especially when not gathered by the investigators, is a substantial, often ignored, issue. Epidemiologists are often used to considering misclassification errors associated with attribution (false-positive and false-negative findings); however, four additional sources of error can be overlooked in GIS analyses: spatial, resolution, interpretive, and temporal errors.

Spatial errors involve misplacement of mapped features to their locations in the coordinate system. These errors can occur from simple data entry mistakes or from the methods used to locate the mapped features. An example of spatial errors introduced by methodologies concerns address-matching algorithms using digitized street maps. Digitized street map databases in vector formats often use an "arc–node" design to code information where street intersections are nodes and the streets are the arcs. The numbering of the buildings is rarely done by actually locating each property boundary. Rather, the "even" and "odd" sides of the streets are indicated in the file and the possible range of addresses is given. The geographic location of a residence is then determined by the linear interpolation of the building number relative to the range of numbers for the street. Introduced errors by this coding method can be striking in some areas where block numbers have specific local meaning. In Baltimore, Maryland, blocks north and south of Baltimore Street are numbered in 100s north or south (e.g., 600 block of North Wolfe Street). At the intersection the block changes in units of 100. Even if only 10 buildings, numbered 600 through 618 occupy one side of a block, on the next block the first building is numbered 700. Thus, with the arc–node format all the buildings will be mapped within the lower one fifth of each block even though they cover its entire length. If the spatial resolution of the study is not too fine, this error can be relatively insignificant; however, if exposures need to be specified with a high degree of spatial accuracy, the error could be substantial. Regardless, such errors need to be identified and empirically evaluated for each study.

Resolution errors can occur because when the databases that make up the GIS are created tbey are made at some level of spatial resolution, or detail. This is sometimes known as a minimal mapping unit. That is, because of limitations of resources or space, the databases are abstractions of the real world they represent. For example, a database of forest boundaries rarely, if ever, shows the exact location of each tree in the forest. Rather, the edge of the forest is approximated to some level of resolution. In addition, open spaces in the forest that support small meadows or grasslands may not be shown if these open spaces are too small (i.e., they are smaller than the minimal mapping unit). This abstraction is necessary but can limit the usefulness of a particular database for a specific study. Information on the level of resolution when the data layer was created should exist within the metadata that are generated as part of the database. Even if every environmental feature, such as each tree, could be located, epidemiologic investigations of infectious diseases rarely have sufficient accuracy themselves to make such detail meaningful. An example of this is Lyme disease, a bacterial infection transmitted by small, hard-bodied ticks. Clearly, an epidemiologic investigation that attempts to identify environmental risk factors of the disease requires identifying places of exposures for cases. However, the ticks associated with most disease transmission in the eastern United States are so small that only a few individuals can accurately identify where or when exposure occurred to any useful level of accuracy. Many people do not even recall getting tick bites.

The epidemiologic issue related to place of exposure is often a critical one with the application of GIS. Placing a "case" on a map has significant implications for any viewer of the data, but such conclusions may be incorrect. This is especially true when the place of exposure is unknown. The example of Maxcy's study[4] of murine typhus is a classic example of such a phenomenon. But such situations occur frequently. Recently, for example, Kitron et al. examined the risk of LaCrosse encephalitis (LAC) in Illinois.[9] This California group encephalitis virus is transmitted by mosquitoes and can produce severe disease, primarily in children. However, most cases are clinically not apparent and the symptoms vary widely, making diagnosis difficult. Consequently, it is difficult to identify where and when cases of LAC are likely to occur. Therefore, they selected the epidemiologically best characterized subset of cases and used a GIS with spatial analyses to identify clusters of LAC cases, specifically to determine if regions existed where cases occurred at higher than expected frequencies. Their results showed significant spatial clustering in the state within three counties surrounding Peoria. Demonstration of this clustering then allowed them to investigate what environmental factors occurred within the regions around these sites. Identifying these conditions would permit targeted interventions that would minimize environmental impacts associated with controlling mosquito vectors and to reduce most cases of LAC in the region.

Another condition in which the place of exposure is subject to significant error is when the time between exposure and onset of disease is relatively long, such as with human immunodeficiency virus (HIV), acquired immunodeficiency syndrome (AIDS), or tuberculosis. In this situation, use of current place of residence or place of work, for example, could give misleading results. This is especially critical during the occurrence of syndromes whose causes are unknown. Thus, workers using a GIS need to take special care in selecting what data are to be presented and how they are to be shown.

Interpretive errors are misclassification errors in the databases. In many cases when databases are obtained from other sources such errors are difficult to estimate unless "ground truthing," in the case of environmental data, is conducted. Epidemiologists often fail to appreciate the level of error in these databases, especially when they are presented as maps. For example, remotely sensed data (e.g., those collected by satellites) can be used to interpret land cover patterns. Land cover is classified based on the reflectance patterns from regions of the electromagnetic spectrum using various classification algorithms. However, when sites are "ground truthed" and compared with their predicted land cover, error rates of 15% to 20% are common, especially in complex environments, such as residential or rural environments.[10] Improvements in the classification algorithms remain a major research focus. For example, Gong[11] demonstrated that the use of evidential reasoning and artificial neural networks substantially improved classification rates of environmental data from multiple sources compared with the more traditional approaches.

Temporal errors are another source of error that is often overlooked. All of the developed databases have a temporal aspect associated with their collection. This is evident for epidemiologic data gathered during an outbreak investigation, for example. However, it is easy to forget that spatial databases gathered for a GIS also have temporal components that can change rather dramatically over various time scales. For example, soil databases may be relatively time invariant, whereas land cover, especially in rapidly developing areas, can change within a few years and precipitation patterns can vary in a matter of hours. Consequently, using databases in GIS as part of infectious disease studies can produce classification errors if the environmental conditions during the time of the study differ substantially from those when the database was created. In many areas of the world recently updated databases simply do not exist, hence the interest and application of remote sensing in these GIS.

Application Examples

Data Collection and Storage

A major feature of computerized systems is their capacity to input and store large quantities of data with relative ease. When data are being collected to answer a specific focused research question, the data gathered are often limited to those variables needed to test the hypotheses associated with the question. In these cases, the data collection and storage needs may be relatively small and a GIS primarily serves to present the data visually.

By contrast, some agencies are required to gather certain data as part of their administrative responsibilities. These data files can be extensive, both in the numbers of records included and in the number of data fields incorporated into each record. If spatial attributes are associated with these data, especially if they are combined from multiple sources, a GIS can prove a useful system for organizing and updating the data. Schistosomiasis is a disease caused by infection with various species of parasitic worms of the genus *Schistosoma*. The disease causes substantial morbidity worldwide and is often associated with large-scale agro-ecosystem developments. Infection in humans requires contamination of water sources by infectious individuals, subsequent development in snail hosts, and then infection of susceptible people who contact contaminated water.

This complex interplay of hosts and environmental variables creates significant data storage issues when detailed epidemiologic studies of transmission patterns are undertaken. However, GIS can be exceptionally useful for such storage. For example, the Schistosomiasis Research Program (SRP) was a joint effort of the Egyptian Ministry of Health and the United States Agency for International Development (USAID) that was undertaken as part of its research program into detailed ecological conditions of factors associated with schistosome transmission at six sites in Egypt. Irrigation canals at these sites represented the primary source of environmental exposure. The sites were sampled once a month for more than a year. The issues related to data storage involved the large number of environmental variables being recorded at a very fine spatial scale over the extended period of the project. Every 50 meters 84 variables were recorded including factors related to the type of canal, the abundance and size of host snails, whether the snails were infectious, the abundance of other species of snails, water chemistry, aquatic vegetation, and temperature. Because irrigation systems in these villages typically were 50 to 70 km long, it was usual to have 1400 collecting locations at each of the six sites. This resulted in the production of large volumes of data. Nearly 50,000 sheets of data were generated for each study site. This longitudinal sampling of many data variables at many collecting locations for multiple sites presented a substantial data storage problem. Because collections were performed repeatedly at fixed collecting locations along the canals, a GIS represented a simple way of storing and organizing the data (Figure 7-3). Each collection location served as a key field in the data record and those places were geocoded to their locations along the canals. Figure 7-3, a simple schematic of the study area, shows major features of one site, such as roads, canals, and collecting sites. The primary difference from many such hand-drawn schematics is that the locations of all the features are spatially accurate and are referenced to particular locations on the earth's surface. As a result, querying the data (see below) to identify where snail hosts were located and when transmission could occur became a simple process that examined the spatial relationships among various features of interest.

Data Management

Once data are entered, validated, and stored in the GIS, managing, updating, and editing them can be straightforward. GIS, in this sense, serves as a system

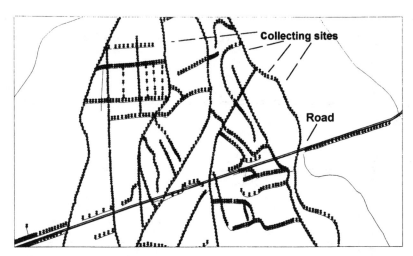

FIGURE 7-3 Collecting locations and selected features at one site in Egypt used to sample for snails that serve as host for schistosome parasites. Collecting sites are densely located along canals (thin lines). A major road (thick line) bisected the region. More than 1400 collecting locations were sampled each month during the study, but the same collecting locations were revisited each time, making data storage within a geographic information system feasible.

to integrate data from various sources (e.g., paper maps, reports, administrative and test data) into a coherent system. Thus, GIS can be especially helpful in quality control issues, both those related to geographic locations and those used in evaluating consistency among different data sources.

In Baltimore, Maryland, the Baltimore City Health Department (BCHD) has as one of its responsibilities monitoring the number of cases of several reportable sexually transmitted infections (STIs). The city has an area of approximately 240 square kilometers and a population of approximately 700,000 people; however, even in this small region, substantial ethnic, racial, and socioeconomic diversity exists. The administrative data are derived from several sources, including several public health care clinics where patients can be treated and offices of private physicians who diagnose their patients and take samples for laboratory workups; a network of public and private health care systems conduct laboratory diagnoses and report the results to either the city or state health departments (depending on the source of the specimen). The data include a required array of demographic and personal information. To coordinate all the information obtained from these various sources, the BCHD developed a data management scheme[12] that allows the information from laboratory tests and clinic records to be integrated and merged into a single large database (Figure 7-4). A GIS was incorporated into the data management scheme using place of residence as the geographic identifier.

The GIS provided an additional level of quality control for the database and health care delivery. For example, examination of the data showed substantial differences in the quality of data reporting by public and private providers for several important demographic variables. Public clinics reported racial data for 99% of cases compared with 72% of cases for private providers. It is thought that STIs occur at substantially different rates in different

Collection Site	Date	Depth of Canal (Meters)	Site	Sampling Technique N = Canal Bed S = Surface	Non-Vector Snail Species			Schistosomiasis Vector Snail Species	
					Paspal	Phrag	Planor	Biomm9	Biom+ Bioml 13
321.0000	6/29/93	0.10	1	N		1	0	0	0 0
321.0000	6/29/93	0.10	1	S		1	0	0	0 0
322.0000	6/29/93	0.10	2	N		1	0	0	0 0
322.0000	6/29/93	0.10	2	S		1	0	0	0 0
323.0000	6/29/93	0.10	3	N		2	0	0	0 0
323.0000	6/29/93	0.10	3	S		2	0	0	0 0
324.0000	6/29/93	0.10	4	N	2		0	0	0 2
324.0000	6/29/93	0.10	4	S	2		0	1	1 2
325.0000	6/29/93	0.10	5	N	1	1	0	1	0 0
325.0000	6/29/93	0.10	5	S	1	1	0	0	0 0
326.0000	6/29/93	0.10	6	N		1	0	0	0 1
326.0000	6/29/93	0.10	6	S		1	0	0	0 0
327.0000	6/29/93	0.10	7	N	1	1	0	0	0 0
327.0000	6/29/93	0.10	7	S	1	1	0	0	0 1
328.0000	6/29/93	0.20	8	N		1	0	0	0 0
328.0000	6/29/93	0.10	8	S		1	0	0	0 1
329.0000	6/29/93	0.10	9	N	1		0	0	0 0
329.0000	6/29/93	0.10	9	S	1		0	0	0 0
330.0000	6/29/93	0.10	10	N	1		0	0	0 0
330.0000	6/29/93	0.10	10	S	1		0	0	0 0
331.0000	6/29/93	0.10	11	N	1		0	0	0 0
331.0000	6/29/93	0.10	11	S			0	0	0 0

FIGURE 7-3 Continued

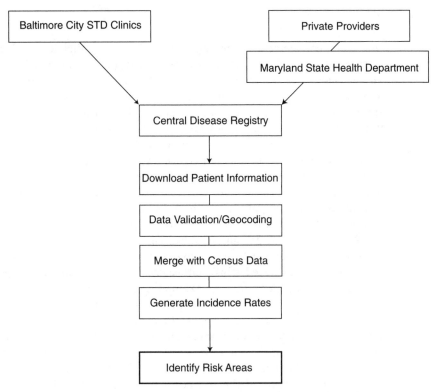

FIGURE 7-4   Data management of clinical information with the Baltimore City Health Department (BCHD) for sexually transmitted diseases. Cases could be seen initially at clinics run by BCHD or at private providers such as hospitals. If patients were seen by private providers, the information first was reported to the Maryland State Health Department before integration in the Central Disease Registry. The information then was downloaded to the geographic information system for validation, cleaning, and geocoding. Subsequently, the information could be merged with census information, as shown here, to generate rate maps of selected sexually transmitted diseases (STDs) and identify high-risk areas.

portions of the population, but the extent to which reporting bias affects this interpretation is uncertain. In general, if such administrative data were used to make programmatic decisions such conclusions could be significantly in error.

Management of the data files using GIS also showed several places in the actual implementation of both services and the data management where problems had arisen. For example, a small subsample of patients with an STI were seen at private health care systems and the public clinics for the same disease within a single day. This was not identified in the previously used system because private and public clinics used different identification numbers for the same individuals. However, the GIS identified cases with identical demographic information at the same locality. Subsequent examination of confidential information by appropriate staff identified individuals who had been sent from the private facilities to the public clinics for treatment rather than receiving care at the initial facility.

Querying

Once data management is ongoing within a GIS, its application in identifying disease patterns becomes of interest. Data querying in GIS, which represents an approach to examine past or current infectious disease patterns, is probably the most frequent use of a GIS. Querying uses many of the features specific to GIS, especially the spatial relationships of features to one another (topology). These include issues such as how far cases of disease are from a potential site of transmission, or how close they are to one another. This is often referred to as a "problem of adjacency." Querying often relies on taking survey and administrative data that are collected and using the GIS to summarize and categorize the data. Such questions usually involve determining the numbers and geographic distributions of cases of disease within a region and their relationship to various features of interest.

Adjacency problems can be addressed by several methods in GIS. Typically, fairly "low-end" GIS technology can deal with many querying tasks; when fairly sophisticated relational aspects are investigated, more powerful systems are needed. Consider the example of schistosomiasis discussed above (Figure 7-3). An obvious question arises: Where are the snails found that serve as hosts for the schistosomes? Remembering how large the database was and how many sites were sampled, the utility of GIS queries is immediately obvious. When the database is queried for a simple tally of captures of *Biomphalaria*, the genus of snail host, throughout the year (Figure 7-5) and this is compared with all the collecting sites (Figure 7-3), it is evident that the snails are very restricted in their distribution within the canals. If only sites with large numbers of snails (e.g., 14–42 snails) are considered, these sites are extremely limited. This raises several questions that then can be further queried. What is there about these nine sites (out of 1450 sampled) that differs from the others? Is it related to vegetation cover, water chemistry, other species of snails, where people conduct certain activities? From a programmatic perspective, it also suggests that focused snail control in a very limited number of locations could have a substantial impact on the total abundance of the host snail population.

Other querying functions include extracting information from the databases for specific geographic regions. This process of overlaying features is an often-used feature of GIS that has benefited from the development of relational database formats. The value of relational databases is that they permit the linking of data from multiple sources to obtain information that is not uniquely available in any one source. The STI data obtained by the city of Baltimore provide a useful example. An important concern is whether the rates of selected STIs differ substantially within the city. Estimation of rates requires a denominator of the estimated population at risk. The STI database (Figure 7-4), however, does not include such information. It is possible to acquire from the US Census Bureau data on the census information gathered in the city of Baltimore (Figure 7-6). A portion of the database is shown, along with a map of the census tracts in the city. Note that one of the data fields is the census tract number.

The distribution of gonorrhea cases in Baltimore can be mapped on a similar base map to Figure 7-6 using place of residence (Figure 7-7). The geographic locations of these residences were determined by geocoding the

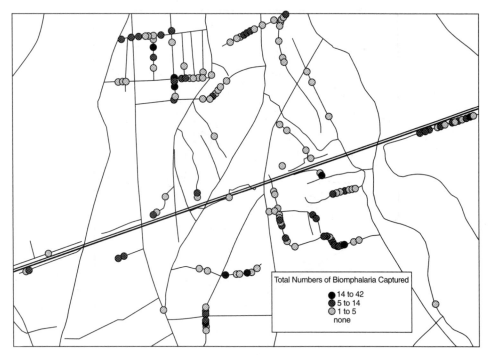

FIGURE 7-5 A data query of the schistosomiasis database for the map shown in Figure 7-3. This query involved locating all sites that captured *Biomphalaria*, one of the genera of snail that serves as a host for schistosoma in the region, for the entire collecting interval. Intensity of captures is shown by increasing darkness of the circles. Collecting localities that captured no snails are not indicated. Comparison with Figure 7-3 shows very few sites had any snails captured and only a few of these had significant numbers.

addresses to another database of street addresses for the city. Rates of gonorrhea were estimated by overlaying the census tract data on the locations of gonorrhea cases. The GIS was used first to count the numbers of cases in specific age–ethnicity–gender categories contained in the STI database, and then the appropriate categories from the census data were used as denominators to estimate rates. A large-scale portion of the data (Figure 7-7) shows that even in an area of intense transmission, substantial local variation in rates of disease is seen.[13] These data then might be used to identify and target regions where rates of disease are above some threshold for action.

Another important feature of GIS that involves data querying is the ability of the system to measure distances from one feature of interest to another feature. If only two points are involved, this can be done manually. However, in the situation of multiple cases or irregular features this task becomes quite difficult, if not impossible. For example, Lyme disease is transmitted by hard-bodied ticks (genus *Ixodes*) that live in forests (see Chapter 25). To assess the importance of peridomestic exposure, it would be of interest to know how far the residences of cases of human Lyme disease are from the nearest forest (Figure 7-8). Forests have irregular boundaries, multiple cases of Lyme disease occur, and, practically, it would be impossible to measure the

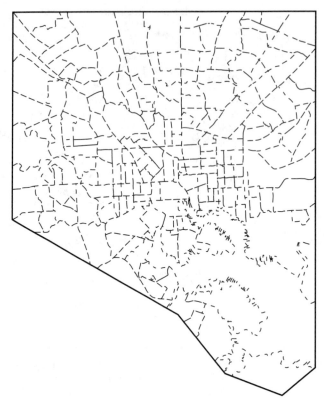

Tract90	Totalper	Perusamp	Per100	Pctinsam	Males	Females
010100	3508	477	3,508	13.6	1646	1862
010200	3435	494	3,431	14.4	1613	1822
010300	2414	344	2,418	14.2	1135	1279
010400	2244	292	2,218	13.2	1158	1086
010500	1942	285	1,968	14.5	962	980
020100	2078	260	2,148	12.1	1012	1066
020200	1863	264	1,916	13.8	987	876
020300	2088	240	1,965	12.2	1154	934
030100	1685	225	1,660	13.6	748	937
030200	2763	326	2,714	12.0	1461	1302
040100	1632	163	1,683	9.7	938	694
040200	1474	159	1,497	10.6	744	730
050100	3828	439	3,828	11.5	1568	2260
060100	3246	430	3,246	13.2	1530	1716
060200	4094	559	4,094	13.7	1910	2184

FIGURE 7-6 One database of census data for the city of Baltimore showing the geographic boundaries of census tracts within the city. Shown below the map is the database linked to the map indicating census tract number and population data.

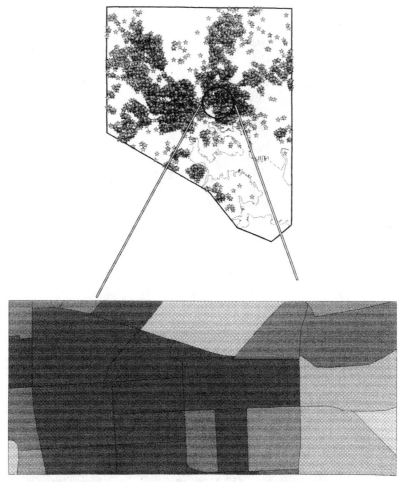

FIGURE 7-7 The geographic distribution of cases of gonorrhea for the city of Baltimore (top figure; cases have been randomly shifted to protect confidentiality). Using overlay procedures and census data (Figure 7-6), it is possible to link two unrelated databases to estimate disease rates for any portion of the city. An enlarged area is shown below. Rates of disease increase are shown with darker shading.

distance from the site of each Lyme disease case to the nearest forest edge. With aerial photographs and knowledge of where cases of disease occurred, it would be possible to estimate the distances with a ruler and a conversion method. This supposes that a procedure exists for identifying which forest edge is nearest to the site of each case. However, GIS can be used to measure the distances from the edges of all forests to each case by overlaying one data layer, the distribution of forests, with the distribution of Lyme disease cases in another layer, and calculating the distances between each case and the nearest forest edge. In the county of Baltimore, the distribution of the residences of Lyme disease cases appears to be clustered along the edge of forested areas (Figure 7-8), an observation confirmed by the histogram of cases relative to the distance from the edge of the forest. None of the persons

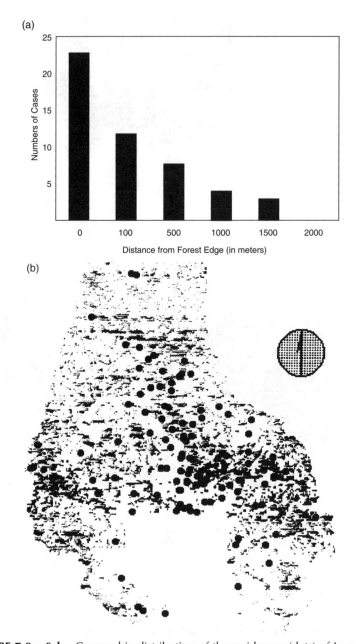

FIGURE 7-8 a & b Geographic distribution of the residences (dots) of Lyme disease in Baltimore County in relationship to forested areas (gray areas). (Places of residences have been randomly shifted to protect confidentiality.) Using a buffer procedure it is possible to determine distances between the nearest forest edges and the residences of Lyme disease cases and summarize the results (graph above map). Results suggest nearness to forest edge may be a risk factor for disease.

infected resided more than 2000 m from the edge of the forest and most lived within 100 m of the forest edge. Before confirming such a relationship, however, the distribution of a representative sample of all residences from the forest edges would need to be determined, as residence in or near forests can be a culturally preferred behavior.

Modeling

One obvious feature of GIS database development is that a large number of potential environmental risk factors for a selected infectious disease can be evaluated. Any feature that can be given a geographic location can be considered in the epidemiologic investigation. Consequently, the investigator is faced with the task of selecting from among these features the most appropriate ones to examine and analyze. In some cases of infectious diseases this can be straightforward. The basic epidemiology is well understood and the environmental factors, both proximate and ultimate, are fairly clear. For many vector-borne diseases, for example, only one or a few vectors transmit the pathogen and the environmental conditions that favor the vector have been characterized. These conditions are so well defined that all that needs to be done is to overlay the distributions of the appropriate conditions to identify the predicted distribution of disease. For example, Beck et al.[13] used information on the breeding, feeding, and flight habits of *Anopheles albimanus*, a major vector of malaria in the Americas, and the locations of villages to model the predicted risk of malaria in a region of coastal Mexico using satellite imagery to identify key environmental features. It is not often appreciated, however, that the variables selected in the analysis and the way the biological information is used by the researcher represent a model of the disease process. The model is developed outside the GIS and the GIS then is used to identify where the stated conditions exist. With such models, the GIS simply serves its query function. For many infectious diseases with alternate hosts or vectors, however, such simple models cannot be developed. In addition, for many infectious diseases the conditions that cause disease outbreaks are not clearly understood, in which case the GIS can be used as an exploratory data analysis tool to develop and test hypotheses about the potential importance of environmental factors. In this situation, statistical methods are used to identify "important" factors associated with disease. The GIS can be used to query the environmental data (Figure 7-8) associated with disease. This information can be exported and analyzed by various statistical procedures. Then, the GIS can graphically represent the results.

Many infectious diseases with arthropod vectors are influenced by environmental conditions affecting the survival of the vector and any other hosts or reservoirs of the pathogen. Lyme disease (see Chapter 25) is common along the coastal regions of northern and central North America (as well as elsewhere). It is the most common vector-borne disease in the United States, and it is associated with substantial morbidity. In some areas, Lyme disease has a dramatic impact on outdoor activities of residents. Although exposure can be associated with recreational activities, a significant problem with Lyme disease in the northeastern United States is that much of the exposure appears to occur as part of daily activities around the place of residence.

Baltimore County, Maryland, is located along the western shore of the Chesapeake Bay, and surrounds Baltimore City on three sides. The county is a mixture of industrial, fairly high-density residential, and rural environments. Since Lyme disease was recognized in Maryland, Baltimore County has had the largest number of cases reported annually; its population in 1990 was approximately 700,000. In 1991, 38 cases of Lyme disease were reported.

To better understand the epidemiology of the disease, the areas within the county at high risk for the disease need to be identified. A number of environmental factors have been thought to influence the survival of the tick vector, the rodent reservoir of the Lyme disease spirochete, and the white-tailed deer, the host for the adult tick. Presumably, how these factors interact influences where and how intense Lyme disease transmission would occur.

To model Lyme disease risk, a case-control design was developed using confirmed cases of Lyme disease. Place of residence was selected as the likely site of exposure. This was based on interviews conducted with patients, few of whom indicated any other likely site. Because residential site was used for exposure, control sites were a randomly selected sample of all residential addresses within the county. A GIS was used to extract environmental variables (e.g., land use characteristics, soil types, distance to forests, elevation, aquatic drainage systems) that were thought to influence Lyme disease risk from the areas around case residences, as well as randomly selected residential sites.[14] These data were analyzed by logistic regression analysis. The environmental variables, weighted by their appropriate regression coefficients, then were mapped throughout the region (Figure 7-9) as a measure of Lyme disease risk. The results of the risk map were evaluated on follow-up by comparing the numbers of cases of Lyme disease the following year, relative to a new set of randomly selected control sites. Cases were 16 times more likely to occur in high-risk than in low-risk areas the following year. A number of statistical approaches are unique to modeling data with spatial components and those are discussed more, below. However, a few more general comments are discussed here. A significant risk of statistical modeling with GIS once the databases are developed is that in many situations the number of potential environmental variables is as great or greater than the numbers of cases of disease. As such, the potential exists for the model to be unstable and dependent on idiosyncrasies of the data. This is not unique to GIS modeling and is always a risk in exploratory data analysis; however, because it is relatively easy to incorporate many variables once the databases are constructed, it is an important aspect to remember with GIS. Another potential problem with statistical modeling of spatial data is rarely explicitly considered in traditional epidemiologic analyses. In general, most traditional analyses assume that observations are independent of one another. However, this is unlikely to be true, especially when considering the spatial distribution of infectious diseases. This is fairly obvious for contagious diseases. However, even when diseases, such as Lyme disease, are not contagious, significant spatial structure is generated by the underlying spatial correlation of environmental factors that influence the risk of disease. The major consequence for statistical models appears to be that the spatial structure creates a false sense of precision in the statistics.[15] A basic introduction to the measures and effects of spatial correlation on data can be found in Griffith.[16]

One approach using statistical modeling to identify risk factors is to explicitly incorporate spatial aspects of the data, as well as the other environmental data, and any information of the known biological processes. For example, Das et al.[17] used hierarchical linear modeling to develop a spatially explicit model of tick vector abundance for adult *Ixodes* found on its principal host, white-tailed deer, that incorporated both spatial correlation of the data and overdispersion in the outcome variable, tick abundance. This hierarchical model had the advantage in both identifying environmental covariates

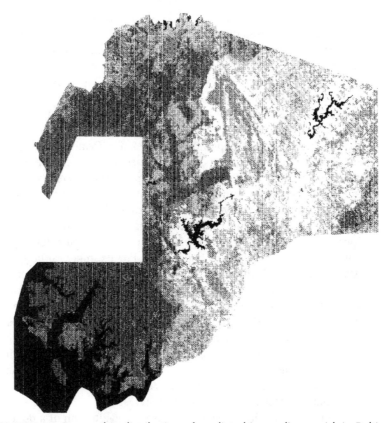

FIGURE 7-9   Geographic distribution of predicted Lyme disease risk in Baltimore County using a geographic information system to create an environmental database of potential risk factors for a case-control study design. Risk is mapped as four quartiles using the results of logistic regression analysis. Risk increases with increasing lightness.
Source: G.E. Glass et al., Environmental Risk Factors of Lyme Disease Identified with Geographic Information Systems, American Journal of Public Health, Vol. 85, No. 7, p. 946, © 1995, American Public Health Association.

of vector abundance, as well as factors influencing the overdispersion in the abundance of the tick vectors.

Decision Making

A major application of GIS technology that has been recognized, but little used in infectious disease epidemiology, is in decision making and targeted public health interventions. Throughout this chapter the policy implications of the data collected for the various examples, such as targeting schistoso-miasis control programs or developing STD interventions, have been mentioned. In principle, this use of a GIS would allow policy makers a better method of identifying areas at risk for the outcome of an infectious disease process and then direct resources toward preventing disease or targeting the at-risk population for screening and treatment while minimizing collateral (and potentially undesirable) impacts. In fact, development of accurate spatial models that incorporated the dynamics of infectious diseases might allow the testing of alternative strategies to identify the best strategy or combination of strategies for disease control. As noted, however, this goal requires substantial, accurate databases that have been incorporated into a GIS, as well as a detailed understanding of disease processes. Given the lack of development of GIS in infectious disease epidemiology, it is not too surprising that few examples of this application exist. However, GIS should be extremely useful in targeting such interventions. The example discussed below demonstrates its application in evaluation of vaccine trials by identifying target populations at risk for Lyme disease. Until recently, public health interventions for Lyme disease primarily involved education and encouraging individuals to take appropriate personal protective measures to reduce exposure to vectors. However, recently several recombinant vaccines have been developed and tested. Although Lyme disease represents the most common vector-borne disease in North America and may be locally common, the numbers of individuals infected often represent a very small portion of the entire population. For example, although the state of Maryland ranks fifth nationally in numbers of cases, the crude incidence in 1995 was approximately 9 per 100,000. A major problem in conducting population-based vaccine trials for diseases, such as Lyme disease, that lack a well-defined at-risk group is the large number of individuals who would need to be recruited to demonstrate efficacy of a vaccine if individuals were recruited at random. Given the tremendous costs associated with recruiting patients for vaccine trials, testing them, and following up the population for evaluation, it would be nearly impossible to conduct vaccine trials by such a population-based recruitment strategy.

Maryland was included as a site for the evaluation of a double-blind trial for one candidate vaccine. Power estimates indicated that, assuming a vaccine efficacy of 80% and 4000 people in each of two arms of the study, it would be necessary to recruit from areas where the seasonal incidence was 500 per 100,000.[18] To identify an appropriate population, therefore, the GIS and the model of Lyme disease risk described above were used to recruit individuals into the study. The map of Lyme disease risk (Figure 7-9) was overlaid with street maps of the region. Streets that overlaid high-risk areas were identified, and individuals who lived in these high-risk areas were contacted and asked to participate in the trial until 200 individuals were enrolled, the population size needed for the Maryland portion of the study (Figure 7-10). This approach reiterates the points made earlier that each use of GIS relies on the earlier ones: using databases that have been developed and checked, linking them with epidemiologic data, modeling the factors associated with disease, and then querying the results for specific conditions (residence in high-risk areas).

If this strategy was successful, we would expect to see a significant increase of Lyme disease cases, compared with the crude population rate, making it possible to conduct the trial with substantially fewer participants and more power than would be possible otherwise. If the vaccine were successful, the cases should be (nearly) confined to the control group. As part of the 2-year surveillance, Lyme disease diagnostics were performed twice a year. By the end of the study Lyme disease incidence in the control group was 2% per year. This was substantially above both the crude population

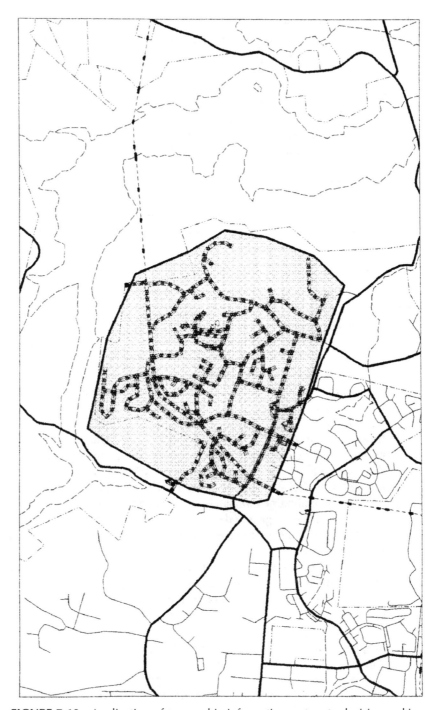

FIGURE 7-10 Application of geographic information system to decision making showing the high-risk area for Lyme disease shown in outlined region overlaid on street map. Street addresses falling in high-risk areas were selected to recruit individuals for vaccine trial based on the assumption that peridomestic risk was an indicator of individuals likely to be at high risk of disease.

level and the targeted incidence rate, and was sufficient to demonstrate the effectiveness of the vaccine with a limited sample size.

More recently, the use of GIS in decision making has been formalized by its integration into decision support systems. These systems develop explicit rule-making processes for monitoring, planning, and health care delivery—often relying on expert systems for planning purposes. GIS may represent the backbone for data reporting and planning in these systems. An excellent example of this use is a malaria control decision support system that is part of the malaria control program instituted by the Medical Research Council of South Africa. This system uses GIS to integrate clinical surveillance, epidemiologic data, surveillance of mosquito vector populations and demographic information to monitor and plan interventions for malaria control in South Africa and southern Mozambique. Since its inception, the decision support system has made substantial inroads into disease burden while allowing careful use of limited resources.

Remote Sensing and GIS

A substantial challenge for GIS in infectious disease epidemiology is obtaining up-to-date information on environmental conditions that could act as risk factors of disease at the appropriate spatial and temporal scales. Remotely sensed data can serve as such a source. Remotely sensed data from commercially available sources typically measure the strength of reflected electromagnetic (EM) energy from the earth's surface. By combining the data on the reflected energy from different parts of the EM spectrum, the data are interpreted to convey information about various aspects of the environment, such as land cover, soil moisture, and temperature. Such information can be gathered from various sources, such as airplanes, for survey studies, but most current sources of remotely sensed data rely on instruments maintained on satellites. Weather satellites are easy examples of these systems. A large number of satellite platforms are currently gathering data and many more sensor systems are planned by governments and private agencies.

The satellite systems vary in their spatial resolution, temporal resolution, duration of data gathering, and the portions of the electromagnetic spectrum that are monitored. For example, one of the longest active systems is the Landsat Thematic Mapper platform. It surveys each part of the earth every 16 days. It scans in seven regions (bands) of the electromagnetic spectrum—three in the visible portion and four in the infrared region, with a spatial resolution of approximately 30 m. This is considered a moderate spatial and temporal resolution system. By contrast, the Advanced Very High Resolution Radiometer (AVHRR) system surveys each region twice daily, scanning in five bands of the electromagnetic spectrum, with a spatial resolution of 1.1 km—a spatially coarse but temporally fine resolution system. Some current, and other planned high-resolution systems record spatial details at a meter or less. The very high resolution imagery provides nearly photographic level detail and is useful for characterizing details such as the enumeration of households in areas where such census information is lacking. However, even fairly coarse-resolution data can be used to characterize environmental conditions associated with disease risk.[19]

Analysis of archived satellite imagery is a useful method to examine changes in environmental conditions over time or to review environmental conditions at the times of previous disease outbreaks. The choice of satellite data is influenced then by both the time when the epidemiologic data were gathered and the spatial and temporal resolution needed for the environmental data. Interpretation of the satellite imagery, or any remotely sensed data, can be a difficult task and requires substantial training. In some cases the interpreted results can be used in epidemiologic studies, especially when the relationship between environmental risk factors and satellite data are already known. In other situations the data from the sensors, themselves, can be used to generate new interpretations of the environment. Thus, in GIS, the remotely sensed data serve as an updated data source on environmental conditions, but the quality of the interpretation involves skills and techniques outside of GIS.[20]

Data Analysis

A unique aspect of data analysis for mapped epidemiologic data is that correlations among health outcomes are expected. This is in contrast to many basic analytical methods where a primary assumption is that the observations are independent of one another. Positive spatial correlation (outcomes that are nearer to one another are more similar) is probably the most anticipated outcome with spatial data. A site that has a case of disease may be geographically closer to another site with disease than expected, and similarly, the absence of disease in a location may also be associated with fewer cases nearby than expected. The mechanism by which contagious diseases induce this effect is obvious, but even for diseases that are not contagious, the spatial structure of common environmental risk factors is likely to produce positive spatial correlation. The methods associated with detecting and characterizing clusters of disease cases are a major focus of research itself. But in addition there are a number of other public health problems that rely on spatial statistics. An excellent recent textbook discussing the field is by Waller and Gotway.[21]

One way of structuring problems in spatial analysis is to consider the types of data available and question being considered. For some problems we sample the environment at a number of locations and want to obtain the best estimate of environmental conditions at sites that are not sampled. For example, estimating the elevation of a particular point given the elevation at other points is a typical problem of spatial correlation that is analogous to the problem of estimating the risk of disease at a particular location from which there is no data. These types of analyses have been most thoroughly developed in geostatistics. Methods such as kriging use information about variation in the internal spatial structure of the data to interpolate a "best" answer. Ordinary kriging does not make use of information concerning the underlying pattern of other environmental conditions that may influence the distribution of the outcome in question. Instead, universal kriging has been developed as an approach for incorporating the spatial patterns of other covariates into estimates of interest.

A second, common type of problem arises when we have locations of health outcomes (e.g., cases or controls) that can be represented as points on a map. This differs from the data described above in that the outcome is measured as the (non)occurrence of an event, rather than being quantified (e.g., risk, elevation). With these problems we often are interested, initially, in whether events cluster, either globally or locally. From the answers to these questions we focus on whether the risk of disease varies in space and if so, what the environmental risk factors are and how strong their effects are with the associated disease.

There are many methods for cluster detection and these range from establishing the occurrence of clustering in relationship to a common feature (such as a source of contamination), to clustering compared to the general population as a whole. The occurrence of clustering per se may be a relatively uninteresting problem because most populations are spatially clustered naturally. Thus, finding that cases of disease are clustered without considering the underlying distribution of the population at risk leaves open far too many questions to be of much utility. A number of techniques for comparing the pattern of interest to the underlying population distribution have been investigated.

A final common type of data problem arises as data are aggregated to some area or region. In GIS we often make chloropleth maps with counts or rates of disease cases by arbitrary regions, such as countries, postal codes, or census tracts. These problems of discrete spatial variation provide a statistical evaluation of the patterns observed on the maps and include a wide variety of methods to detect significant patterns of local and global spatial correlation. More recent efforts have focused on adding a temporal component to analyses so that clusters in space and time can be identified with the goal of improving the sensitivity of analyses. Regardless of the methods, statistical analyses have as their overarching goal allowing us to establish the certainty of our interpretation of results generated from manipulating data within a GIS.

Conclusion

The applications of GIS to infectious disease epidemiology are extremely diverse, ranging from data storage and management to modeling and programmatic decision making. As a tool for the field, GIS remains highly underutilized, but this is beginning to change. The opportunities to apply the technology are only limited by the users' abilities to apply the technology. For much of the practical infectious disease epidemiology, low-end data querying systems are perfectly adequate. These systems are fairly easily mastered in a short period of time. Most important, many services are being developed in which critical data layers are professionally constructed, which minimizes the time and resources needed to create and update needed data layers. Along with this, however, will be the risk that data are used inappropriately or beyond the level of their quality. Unlike many other investigative tools in epidemiology, because GIS produces derivative products, such as maps, these errors will be more difficult to detect. The parallel development in the field of spatial statistics provides an important adjunct for improving the interpretation of results generated from GIS approaches and is an area that will deserve better integration within the GIS framework in the future. Despite these concerns, the opportunities for a better understanding of infectious diseases using GIS outweigh the risks.

References

1. Aronoff S. *Geographic Information Systems: A Management Perspective.* Ottawa, Can: WDL Publications; 1989.
2. Vandenbroucke JP. Re: "A new perspective on John Snow's communicable disease theory." *Am J Epidemiol.* 1997;146:363–364.
3. Meselson M, Guillemin J, Hugh-Jones M, et al. The Sverdlovsk anthrax outbreak of 1979. *Science.* 1994;266:1202–1208.
4. Maxcy KF. An epidemiological study of endemic typhus (Brill's disease) in the southeastern United States with special reference to its mode of transmission. *Public Health Rep.* 1926;41:2967–2995.
5. Woodward TE. President's address: typhus verdict in American history. *Trans Am Clin Climatology Assoc.* 1970;82:1–8.
6. Cromley EK, McLafferty SL. *GIS and Public Health.* New York, NY: Guilford Press; 2002.
7. Antenucci JC, Brown K, Croswell PL, Kevany MJ. *Geographic Information Systems: A Guide to the Technology.* New York, NY: Van Nostrand Reinhold; 1991.
8. Vine MF, Degnan D, Hanchette C. Geographic information systems: their use in environmental epidemiologic research. *Environ Health Perspect.* 1997;105:598–605.
9. Kitron U, Michael J, Swanson J, Haramis L. Spatial analysis of LaCrosse encephalitis in Illinois. *Am J Trop Med Hyg.* 1997;57:469–475.
10. Harris R. *Satellite Remote Sensing: An Introduction.* London: Routledge and Kegan Paul; 1987.
11. Gong P. Integrated analysis of spatial data from multiple sources: using evidential reasoning and artificial neural network techniques for geological mapping. *Photo Eng Remote Sens.* 1996;62:513–523.
12. Becker KM, Glass GE, Brathwaite W, Zenilman JM. Geographic epidemiology of gonorrhea in Baltimore, Maryland, using a geographic information system. *Am J Epidemiol.* 1998;147:709–716.
13. Beck LR, Rodriguez MH, Dister SW, et al. Assessment of a remote sensing-based model for predicting malaria transmission risk in villages of Chiapas, Mexico. *Am J Trop Med Hyg.* 1997;56:99–106.
14. Glass GE, Schwartz BS, Morgan JM, Johnson DT, Noy PM, Israel E. Environmental risk factors for Lyme disease identified with geographic information systems. *Am J Public Health.* 1995;85:944–948.
15. Breslow NE. Extra-poisson variation in log-linear models. *Applied Statistics.* 1984;33:38–44.
16. Griffith DA. *Spatial Autocorrelation: A Primer.* Washington, DC: Association of American Geographers; 1987.
17. Das A, SR Lele, GE Glass, T Shields, JA Patz. Modeling a discrete spatial response using generalized linear mixed models: application to Lyme disease vectors. *Intl J GIS.* 2002;16:151–166.
18. Steere AC, Sikand VK, Meurice F, et al. Vaccination against Lyme disease with recombinant *Borrelia burgdorferi* outer-surface lipoprotein A with adjuvant. *N Engl J Med.* 1998;339:209–215.

19. Ostfeld RS, Glass GE, Keesing F. Landscape epidemiology: an emerging (or re-emerging) discipline. *Trends in Ecology and Evolution.* 2005;20: 328–336.

20. Lillesand TM, Kieffer RW, Chipman JW. *Remote Sensing and Image Interpretation.* 5th ed. Hoboken, NJ: John Wiley and Sons; 2004.

21. Waller LA, Gotway GA. *Applied Spatial Statistics for Public Health Data.* Hoboken, NJ: Wiley Interscience; 2004.

MICROBIOLOGY TOOLS FOR THE EPIDEMIOLOGIST

James Dick and Nikki M. Parrish

Introduction

Medical microbiology is the study of interactions between organisms that result in infectious disease. Despite our concentration on microoganisms that cause disease, the vast majority of microorganisms we continuously interact with do not result in disease. In fact, many are beneficial and essential for our health and well-being. Pathogenic viruses, bacteria, fungi, and parasites have cellular structures, products, or toxins that result in disease in a specific host. These are termed virulence factors and can be classified into those factors that permit the microorganism to:

1. Colonize
2. Evade host defense mechanisms
3. Invade and disseminate

The resulting host response, combined with virulence factors, results in toxicity or tissue damage to the host. Alternatively, some microorganisms produce toxins that cause the pathology to the host. Of equal importance in understanding the interactive nature of infection and disease is an understanding of the host mechanisms that continually operate to prevent infection. Despite the vast numbers of bacteria that inhabit our mouth, teeth, gastrointestinal tract, urogenital tract, and skin, only a small number of microorganisms associated with man and animals cause disease. The prevention of infection and disease is in large part due to an array of defense mechanisms that we have developed to deal with these continuous intimate interactions. *Mechanical barriers* are typically the first line of defense. Examples include: skin and mucous membranes as a physical barrier, ciliated cells and mucus in the respiratory tract, and the washing action of tears and urine. *Chemical barriers* are produced at these sites, many by resident normal flora, such as fatty acids and propionic acid, which prevent colonization by pathogens. Other compounds produced by the host that are inhibitory include lysozyme in tears, blood, urine, and sweat; acid in the stomach, vagina, and skin; basic polyamines and complement in plasma; and acute-phase proteins, such as β-antitrypsin, fibrinogen, C-reactive protein, and β2-micro-globulin. In addition to mechanical and chemical mediators, *defensive cells* such as phagocytic cells including macrophages, polymorphonuclear neutrophils, monocytes, and eosinophils are all components of nonspecific host resistance or innate immunity. The fourth type of defense in man and other vertebrates is our *specific immunity*, which is comprised of both the humoral immune system, involving antibody-mediated B-cell functions, and the cellular immune system, involving T-lymphocyte-mediated functions. A compromise in any of these defense mechanisms can lead to infection and disease in the host. Pathogens of low virulence or pathogenicity, as well as true pathogens, can cause infection in these situations and are termed opportunistic pathogens.

In this chapter, a basic broad overview of the classification, taxonomy, structure, and methods of diagnosis of infectious agents is presented. Although by no means comprehensive, it is hoped that the information will provide a basis of understanding for further in-depth study of microbiology as it relates to infectious disease epidemiology.

Taxonomy, Classification, and Structure of Infectious Agents

Early biologists realized that microorganisms such as algae, protozoa, fungi, and bacteria did not readily fit into the already-established plant and animal kingdoms. This led to the proposal by Haechel in 1886 of a third kingdom, the Protista. As viruses were still unknown, they were not included in this classification system. Subsequent advances in the biologic sciences, specifically microscopy, led to a further subdivision of the Protista into eukaryotic cells, which included the algae, fungi, and protozoa, as well as members of the plant and animal kingdoms and prokaryotic cells that represent the bacteria. The terms *eukaryotic* and *prokaryotic* reflect only the presence of a true nucleus, eukaryotic, or the absence of a well-delineated nucleus, prokaryotic. Significant structural and other biologic differences are described in Table 8-1, although the presence of transition forms can result in a blending of some of the listed characteristics.

A variety of characteristics has been used to name and identify microorganisms. Initially these included phenotypic properties and morphology, such as size and shape, staining characteristics, biochemical properties, physiology, metabolism, ecologic niche, etc. Currently, taxonomy is moving toward a genetic basis for differentiation among microorganisms. Genetic methods use DNA and RNA homology and nucleic acid base sequence similarity to evaluate relatedness. Highly conserved genes with variable regions, such as bacterial 16s and 23s ribosomal RNA genes, are commonly used to differentiate bacteria. Microorganisms are taxonomically organized into orders, families, genera, and species.

The naming of microorganisms, with the exception of the viruses, is binomial and includes the genus and species name, as in *Staphylococcus aureus*. Microorganisms can be further subdivided on characteristics that do not warrant a separate species designation but do differentiate a specific member of a species or strain from other members or strains of a particular species.

TABLE 8-1　Comparison of Eukaryotic and Prokaryotic Cells

Form	Multicellular	Single cells
Nucleus	Nuclear membrane	DNA in contact with cytoplasm
Organelles	Membrane-bound organelles present	No organelles
Sterols	Always	Only in Mycoplasma
Ribosomes	80s = 40s + 60s	70s = 30s + 50s
Cell wall	Absent or cellulose	Peptidoglycan
Mitosis	Yes	No

Differences or similarities used for subspecies or strain designation within a species can include a variety of parameters, such as structural or functional differences, phenotypic differences, antigenic differences in surface or sub-surface structures, and genomic polymorphism. Strain differentiation is an important component of epidemiologic studies, as the significant diversity within species may result in different clinical manifestations or may be useful in defining a cluster of cases.

Viruses

Viruses are the smallest of the infectious agents, with the exception of prions or agents of spongiform encephalopathies, such as scrapie and Creutzfeldt–Jakob disease. Viruses range in size from 20 to 200 nm and, as such, are not readily visible by light microscopy. They contain a single form or type of nucleic acid, either DNA or RNA, which functions as their genome. In addition to a single form of nucleic acid, viruses compositionally may contain proteins, lipids, and glycoproteins as structural components, depending on their level of complexity. Viruses are obligate intracellular parasites, and their replication is host-cell dependent, directed by their DNA or RNA. Viral subversion of the host's cellular machinery favors the synthesis of viral nucleic acid and structural proteins. Viral infection is host-cell specific and depends on the presence of specific surface receptors (attachment molecules) for successful entry. There are viruses specific for almost every organism. Even bacteria may be infected by the phage viruses, an interaction which has been useful in the laboratory for introducing genes into bacteria. The ultimate outcome of virus-infected cells varies for different viruses and includes a spectrum from rapid lysis (influenza) to continued growth of the cell and continued release of new virus particles (adenovirus). Some viruses are capable of integrating their nucleic acid into the host cell genome, establishing a latent (herpes viruses) or quiescent state. Latency can continue for long periods of time before reactivation with initiation of viral replication and subsequent lysis of the host cell (herpes viruses).

Classification

Viruses are classified into families, genera, and species, as are other microorganisms, but are not named in a generally binomial classification, as in genus and species (Figure 8-1). Commonly, viruses are referred to by their single names. The viral classification system is based on the nature of the following:

1. Viral genome: DNA or RNA; single- or double-stranded, linear or circular, segmented or nonsegmented; and genome capping with a protein or polynucleotide
2. Size and shape of the capsid and whether it is enveloped or nonenveloped
3. Method of replication
4. Pathophysiology of the virus such as host range, antigenic composition, vectors, and tissue tropism
5. Physical/chemical features, such as susceptibility to acid or lipid solvents

The medically important virus families are shown in Table 8-2. Various elements of a virus are used to categorize them into families. The type of genetic material, the size, and whether the virus has an envelope surrounding the capsid are all used. Viruses are either RNA or DNA viruses. Among the DNA viruses they are further subdivided into those genomes that are single- or double-stranded, linear or circular. Although the criteria

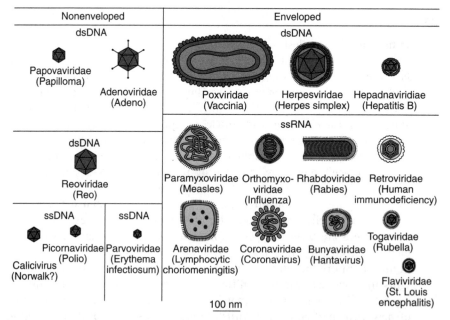

FIGURE 8-1 The 18 families of animal viruses pathogenic for humans. Filoviridae is not included because human infection by this family of viruses has not been documented in the United States.
Source: E.J. Baron et al., *Medical Microbiology: A Short Course*, p. 606, Copyright © 1994. Reprinted by permission of Wiley-Liss, Inc., a subsidiary of John Wiley & Sons, Inc.

TABLE 8-2 Classification of Viruses

Family	Example	Genome Size, Kilobases of Kilobase Pairs	Envelope
RNA Viruses			
Single-stranded			
Picornaviridae	Poliovirus	7.2–8.4	No
Togaviridae	Rubella virus	12	Yes
Flaviviridae	Yellow fever virus	10	Yes
Coronaviridae	Coronaviruses	16–21	Yes
Rhabdoviridae	Rabies virus	13–16	Yes
Paramyxoviridae	Measles virus	16–20	Yes
Orthomyxoviridae	Influenza viruses	14	Yes
Bunyaviridae	California encephalitis virus	13–21	Yes
Arenaviridae	Lymphocytic choriomeningitis virus	10–14	Yes
Retroviridae	HIV	3–9	Yes
Double-stranded			
Reoviridae	Rotaviruses	16–27	No
DNA Viruses			
Single-stranded			
Parvoviridae	Human parvovirus B-19	5	No
Mixed strandedness			
Hepadnaviridae	Hepatitis B	3	Yes
Double-stranded			
Papovaviridae	JC virus	8	No
Adenoviridae	Human adenoviruses	36–38	No
Herpesviridae	Herpes simplex virus	120–220	Yes
Poxviridae	Vaccinia	130–280	Yes

are similar to those used to categorize DNA viruses, RNA viruses are categorized by the mechanism they use to produce viral proteins. One category of viruses that possess polycistronic RNA use messenger RNA (mRNA) to produce a large single protein that is subsequently cleaved to yield several smaller proteins. These include the Coronaviridae, Paramyxoviridae, Picornaviridae, Togaviridae, and Rhabdoviridae. Alternatively, viruses with segmented genomes without polycistronic RNA, requiring cleavage of nested genes, include Arenavirus, Bunyavirus, Orthomyxoviridae, Reovirus, Rotavirus, and the Retroviridae. The RNA viruses are further subdivided on the basis of transcription requirements for their RNA. Positive-strand viruses use their RNA as messenger RNA (mRNA) for translation for required protein. In contrast, negative-stranded RNA viruses require their own RNA-dependent RNA polymerase with production of mRNA and subsequent translation of essential proteins.

Structure

The complete infectious virus is termed a *virion*. It is composed of its specific nucleic acid, DNA or RNA, surrounded by a protein coat known as the capsid. The capsid is further subdivided into capsomers, repeating identical morphologic protein subunits. Each capsomer subunit is composed of one or more polypeptides. Viruses construct several different capsid shapes, according to how these proteins combine. Arrangement of capsomers in the shape of an icosahedron (polygon with 20 faces) results in cubic symmetry. In a cubically symmetrical virus, some capsomers are surrounded by five (penton) capsomers, whereas others are surrounded by six (hexon) capsomers. In helical viruses, the capsid proteins are arranged around a helical nucleic acid core. In addition to icosahedral and helical viruses, the complex viruses have more intricate structural elements. The viral genome can have an associated protein complex that is referred to as the nucleocapsid and forms the viral core. Enveloped viruses possess a lipoprotein coat that surrounds the virion and is acquired from infected host cell membrane. Nonenveloped viruses are termed naked viruses. Finally, viruses may possess glycoprotein spikes, known as peplomers, which protrude from the envelope and function in the attachment of the virus to target host cells.

Bacteria

Classification

As they were discovered earlier, bacteria have been subjected to human classification schemes for longer than the viruses. As with other organisms, prokaryotic bacteria are named using the binomial system of genus and species (Table 8-3). Further subdivision can occur among species, such as subspecies, serotype, etc. Taxonomic classification for bacteria was based on morphologic and biochemical characteristics. More recently, genetic methods indicative of the phylogenetic or evolutionary relationships among the various genera have been applied for classification. Morphologic classification of bacteria has developed on the basis of staining characteristics, shape, and size of the microorganism when visualized by light microscopy. The gram stain reaction, which is a reflection of cell wall structure of bacteria, has been used extensively for classification. The gram stain procedure is a relatively simple staining method that utilizes gentian or crystal violet (purple dye) as the initial stain, followed by fixation with iodine, decolorization with 95% ethanol or acetone–alcohol, and final counterstaining with safranin (a red dye). Crystal violet and iodine form large aggregates within the cell, which, depending on the nature of the cell wall, will be retained or washed out by the action of alcohol. Cells that retain the crystal violet–iodine complex will appear blue/purple, whereas those with thinner cell wells will stain red/pink with the safranin counterstain. Bacteria that retain the dye and stain blue/purple are referred to as gram-positive bacteria, whereas those that do not retain the dye and stain red/pink are referred to as gram-negative bacteria. Another widely used stain for differentiation of bacteria is the acid-fast stain, also known as the Ziehl–Nielsen stain. The

TABLE 8-3   Examples of Bacteria of Medical Importance

Family, Genus, and Species	Disease
Gram-positive cocci	
Staphylococcus	
S. aureus	Abscess, toxic shock, food poisoning
S. epidermidis	Nosocomial infections
Streptococcus	
S. pyogenes (Group A)	Pharyngitis, rheumatic fever, glomerulonephritis, toxic shock
S. agalactiae (Group B)	Neonatal meningitis
S. pneumoniae	Lobar pneumonia, meningitis
Enterococcus	
E. faecalis	Nosocomial infections
Gram-positive bacilli	
Bacillus (spore-forms)	
B. anthracis	Anthrax
Clostridium (spore-forms)	
C. botulinum	Botulism
C. tetani	Tetanus
C. perfringens	Gas gangrene, food poisoning
C. difficile	Pseudomembranous colitis
Listeria	
L. monocytogenes	Meningitis
Corynebacterium	
C. diphtheriae	Diphtheria
Actinomyces	
A. israelii	Actinomycosis
Nocardia	
N. asteroides	Pulmonary disease, brain abscess
Gram-negative spirochetes	
Borrelia burgdorferi	Lyme disease
Treponema pallidum	Syphilis
Leptospira interrogans	Leptospirosis
Acid-fast gram-positive bacilli	
Mycobacterium	
M. tuberculosis	Tuberculosis
M. leprae	Leprosy
M. avium complex	Disseminated infection in immunocompromised hosts
Gram-negative bacilli	
Enterobacteriaceae	Urinary tract infection, diarrhea
Escherichia coli	Meningitis, bacteremia

continued

TABLE 8-3   continued

Family, Genus, and Species	Disease
Klebsiella pneumoniae	Pneumonia, urinary tract infection
Salmonella typhi	Typhoid fever
Salmonella species	Diarrhea, food poisoning
Shigella species	Diarrhea, gastrointestinal disease
Yersinia enterocolitica	Gastroenteritis
Yersinia pestis	Bubonic plague
Pasteurella multocida	Cat bite infections
Hemophilus influenzae	Meningitis, pneumonia, otitis media, and epiglottiditis
Bordetella pertussis	Whooping cough
Brucella species	Brucellosis
Francisella tularensis	Tularemia
Legionella pneumophila	Legionnaires' disease
Pseudomonas aeruginosa	Opportunistic infections
Bacterioides fragilis	Anaerobic abscesses
Fusobacterium nucleatum	Abscesses, oral infections
Gram-negative curved or helical bacilli	
Campylobacter jejuni	Gastroenteritis
Helicobacter pylori	Gastritis, peptic ulcers
Vibrio cholerae	Cholera
Vibrio parahaemolyticus	Gastroenteritis
Gram-negative cocci	
Neisseria	
N. gonorrhoeae	Gonorrhea
N. meningitidis	Meningitis
Gram-negative, obligate intracellular bacteria	
Rickettsia	
R. prowazekii	Epidemic typhus
R. rickettsii	Rocky Mountain spotted fever
Coxiella burnetii	Q fever
Chlamydia	
C. trachomatis	Lymphogranuloma venereum
C. pneumoniae	Pneumonia
Trachoma	
C. psittaci	Psittacosis
Ehrlichia	
E. chaffiensis	Ehrlichiosis
Mycoplasma (lacking a cell wall)	
Mycoplasma pneumoniae	Pneumonia
Ureaplasma urealyticum	Urethritis

acid-fast stain differentiates members of the genus *Mycobacterium*, which includes *M. tuberculosis* and *M. leprae*, the etiologic agents of tuberculosis and leprosy. The differentiation is based on the ability of mycobacteria to retain a primary carbolfuchsin stain when decolorized with 95% alcohol containing 3% hydrochloride (HCl). All other bacteria will decolorize during the acid wash. In addition to differential staining characteristics, bacteria are also morphologically classified on the basis of their shape and arrangement. Three general shapes have been identified:

1. Cocci—round or spherical cells
2. Bacilli—rod-shaped cells
3. Curved, spiral forms

Further descriptive terms include coccobacilli, which are short, rod-shaped cells, and pleomorphic cells, which demonstrate variable morphologies. Morphologically, bacteria are also categorized based on their arrangement when grown in cell culture. For example, *Streptococcus pneumoniae* is frequently described as gram-positive diplococci (pairs of cocci) because it grows in characteristic pairs. Whereas *Staphylococcus aureus*, translated from Greek and Latin as "golden grapes arranged in bunches," is most often described as gram-positive cocci in clusters.

The ability of most bacteria to grow in vitro has allowed for their biochemical and morphologic classification. These taxonomic characteristics are based on the metabolic and physiologic differences between different groups of organisms and are most commonly referred to as phenotypic characteristics. A variety of methods has been developed to test for the presence or absence of particular enzymes. Commonly used taxonomic classification tests by this method include determining whether a bacteria can use specific nutrients for growth or whether it metabolizes particular substrates, such as carbohydrates. Other phenotypic methodologies directly test for the presence of an enzyme, such as catalase. Catalase is an enzyme that breaks down H_2O_2 to water and oxygen and can be readily tested by applying hydrogen peroxide to a growing colony. The solution will bubble, due to the release of oxygen, if the organism possesses the catalase enzyme. The presence of particular enzyme systems is most commonly detected by colorimetric assays wherein, if the enzyme is present, there will be a pH change or production of a colored product in the culture medium. Similarly, antigen–antibody reactions have been utilized to distinguish between species, subspecies, or serotypes within a genus. In these tests, antibodies that bind to specific bacterial surface antigens can be used to identify bacteria that produce these proteins. Advances in genetics have resulted in classifications that reflect evolutionary and phylogenetic relationships. These methods have reclassified many bacteria at the genus level. Genetic methods have gone through an evolution with earlier tests, utilizing the measurement of DNA homology of the *entire* chromosome as the determinant of genetic relatedness. Although still used as a tool for genetic classification, hybridization techniques using cloned or amplified *portions* of the genome have also been developed that look for the presence of a specific DNA sequence. These methods have been used extensively in diagnostic microbiology. Current genetic taxonomy has evolved to the use of sequence analysis of highly conserved genes for determination of phylogenetic relationships. The most commonly used genes are the ribosomal RNA genes, which include the 16s, 23s, and 5s genes. These genes are found in all prokaryotes and contain both highly conserved and variable regions. Sequence, or base, changes in these genes reflect evolutionary and phylogenetic relationships among bacteria.

Bacterial Structure

Figure 8-2 illustrates the basic structure of a bacterial cell. Although all of the structures shown in Figure 8-2 are involved in the life and survival of these versatile cells, many are important virulence factors and are briefly described with emphasis on their roles in pathogenesis. Figure 8-2 shows bacterial cell structure. Moving from the outermost structures inward, the flagella are long, complex structures that are responsible for motility or movement. They are nonessential (not all bacteria have them) and are composed of protein, which is an important antigen (H antigen) for identification and classification among those bacteria that possess them. Fimbriae or pili are short, nonflexible structures that surround the surface of the cell. As with flagella, they are nonessential but function in adherence. In bacterial pathogens, these structures are responsible for adherence to host cell membranes through a very specific interaction, which frequently determines the organotropism of a particular pathogen. A type of pili known as sex or F pili permits attachment and DNA transfer between similar species through a process known as conjugation. This process is the most common method for acquisition of antibiotic resistance determinants by bacteria. Capsules are secreted polysaccharides and, in some cases, proteins that surround some bacterial cells. In general, they are nonessential. In the environment, their primary function is to prevent dehydration of the cell, but in pathogens they are a major virulence factor through interference of phagocytosis by the host.

The cell wall is an essential component of all bacteria, with the exception of the mycoplasma. In addition to determining the size and shape of the cell, it serves as an exoskeleton, preventing lysis of the cell. As discussed earlier, the differences in cell wall structure form the basis for taxonomic differences or groupings of bacteria through the gram-stain reaction. As shown in Figure 8-3, an essential component all of bacterial cell walls is peptidoglycan. Peptidoglycan is a complex polymer composed of alternating units of N-acetyl-glucosamine and N-acetyl muramic acid in a β-1, 4 linkage. The polysaccharide chains are cross-linked through peptide bonds between a pentapeptide chain (typically, four amino acids ending in D-alanine) and the muramic acid residue of N-acetyl muramic acid. This interlinked polymer forms the strong backbone for all other cell wall components. The gram-positive cell wall is composed of a very thick layer of peptidoglycan. Despite its thickness, the gram-positive cell wall is not a permeability barrier for the bacteria's cytoplasmic membrane. A unique component of the gram-positive cell wall is teichoic acid. This polymer is composed of either glycerol or ribitol with phosphate linkages. It is frequently attached to the cytoplasmic membrane and can activate host macrophages with the release of interleukin-1 and tumor necrosis factor alpha (TNF-α). In contrast to the gram-positive cell wall structure, gram-negative bacteria have a significantly more complex

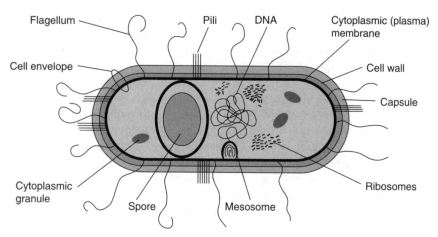

FIGURE 8-2 Schematic diagram illustrating bacterial cell structure.
Source: E.J. Baron et al., Medical Microbiology: A Short Course, p. 8, Copyright
© 1994. Reprinted by permission of Wiley-Liss, Inc., a subsidiary of John Wiley &
Sons, Inc.

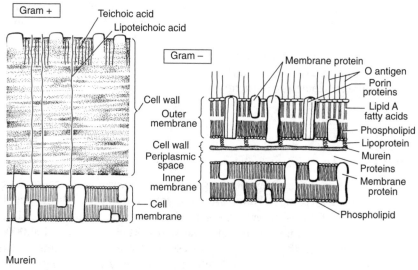

FIGURE 8-3 The envelope structure of a gram-positive (left) and a gram-negative
(right). Capsules and appendages are not shown, nor are surface proteins such
as the M protein of streptococci indicated. Note the 20-fold greater amount of
peptidoglycan in the gram-positive. The outer membrane of the gram-negative
envelopes show O antigen polysaccharide molecules covering the outer layer.
Source: M. Schaechter, G. Medoff and B.I. Esenstein, Mechanisms of Microbial
Disease, p. 31, © 1993, Lippincott Williams & Wilkins.

cell envelope. The outermost portion of the gram-negative cell wall is a lipid
bilayer referred to as the outer membrane. Under the outer membrane is
an area called the periplasmic space, which contains a variety of metabolic
and transport enzymes. The peptidoglycan layer of gram-negative bacteria
is significantly thinner than that of gram-positive bacteria. The outer leaflet

of the outer membrane contains lipopolysaccharide (LPS) or endotoxin, a major virulence factor of gram-negative bacteria. Lipopolysaccharide is a three-component molecule. Lipid A is the toxic component of LPS and is located innermost in the lipid bilayer. Extending from lipid A is the core, an oligosaccharide composed of some unusual sugars. The composition of the core oligosaccharide is similar among all gram-negative bacteria. The outermost portion of LPS is a series of repeating oligosaccharides, the somatic antigen, which is a primary antigenic determinant of the cell. In addition to LPS, the outer membrane of gram-negative bacteria has a variety of proteins associated with it. A group of these outer membrane proteins are porins. These proteins are frequently trimers (three identical proteins bound together) and have a central channel that provides for the passage of hydrophilic compounds through the hydrophobic outer membrane. Unlike gram-positive bacteria, the cell wall of gram-negative bacteria is a permeability barrier to the cell, due to the presence of the hydrophobic outer membrane. Hydrophilic compounds with a molecular weight greater than approximately 800 cannot pass through the porin protein channels. Beneath the cell wall, all bacteria are surrounded by a cytoplasmic membrane, which is the primary osmotic barrier for the cell. The cytoplasmic membrane is a lipid bilayer composed of phospholipids and protein. Unlike eukaryotic cells, bacteria do not have sterols, such as cholesterol, in their membranes. Within the cytoplasm, ribosomes for protein synthesis and the bacterial chromosome are the essential structural components. In addition, many bacteria possess granules that can be visualized within the cytoplasm. These granules are most commonly storage depots for nutrients.

Fungi

The study of pathogenic fungi and the diseases they cause is known as medical mycology. Fungi are eukaryotic organisms, which include a wide variety of forms, from single-cell microscopic yeasts to the multicellular and macroscopic mushrooms and toadstools. There are over 100,000 different species of fungi, which play an essential role in degrading organic waste in nature. Despite their ubiquitous nature, only a few fungi are of medical importance (Table 8-4). As eukaryotes, the fungi have a defined nucleus, surrounded by a nuclear membrane, a plasma membrane that contains sterols, mitochondria, golgi apparatus, 80S ribosomes, and a cytoskeleton, as well as a cell wall or exoskeleton.

Characteristics of Pathogenic Fungi

The pathogenic fungi have two forms: yeasts, which are unicellular and reproduce by extension of buds from the mother cell; and molds, which are multicellular, with a division of function among the individual cellular components. Molds grow as a filamentous, branching strand of connected cells, which form what is called a hypha. Hyphae may have intracellular divisions or septa, or may lack them entirely. The majority of fungi can be grown

TABLE 8-4   Selected Fungi of Medical Importance

Fungus	Classification	Disease
Malassezia furfur	Yeast	Superficial mycoses
Trichophyton rubrum	Filamentous	Tinea, cutaneous mycoses
Microsporum audouinii	Filamentous	Tinea, cutaneous mycoses
Epidermophyton floccosum	Filamentous	Tinea, cutaneous mycoses
Candida albicans	Yeast	Mucocutaneous and systemic mycoses
Sporothrix schenckii	Dimorphic	Subcutaneous mycoses
Histoplasma capsulatum	Dimorphic	Systemic mycoses, histoplasmosis
Blastomyces dermatitidis	Dimorphic	Systemic mycoses, blastomycosis
Coccidioides immitis	Dimorphic	Systemic mycoses, coccidioidomycosis
Paracoccidioides brasiliensis	Dimorphic	Systemic mycoses, paracoccidioidomycosis
Penicillium marneffei	Dimorphic	Systemic mycoses, penicilliosis
Cryptococcus neoformans	Yeast	Systemic mycoses, opportunistic cryptococcosis
Candida species	Yeast	Opportunistic infections
Aspergillus fumigatus	Filamentous	Opportunistic infections
Aspergillus flavus	Filamentous	Opportunistic infections
Rhizopus species	Filamentous	Opportunistic infections
Mucor species	Filamentous	Opportunistic infections
Absidia species	Filamentous	Opportunistic infections
Pneumocystis carinii	Dimorphic, cysts, and trophozoites	Opportunistic infections, pneumonia

in vitro and form colonies that are either cottony or velvety in appearance. In contrast, yeast grows as moist, smooth colonies similar to bacteria. Fungi are classified by the type and method of sexual reproduction. Fungi not known to reproduce sexually have been classified together and produce spores that are called conidia. Fungi with sexual reproduction must reduce the DNA content to half that of the normal cell and fuse the gametes to make the next generation. The hemigenetic cells are known as spores, with a prefix that describes the origin of the spore. Examples include: arthrospores, which are formed within a septate hypha; chlamydospores, which also develop within a hyphal strand; blastospores, which are the sexual spores of yeasts and are the daughter buds from yeast cells; and sporangiospores, which develop within a saclike structure known as a sporangium (Figures 8-4 and 8-5). These terms are frequently prefixed with *micro* or *macro*, which refer to the size of the spore.

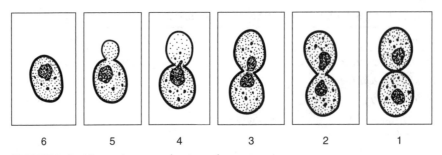

6   5   4   3   2   1

FIGURE 8-4   Vegetative reproduction of yeast.
Source: M. Schaechter, G. Medoff and B.I. Esenstein, Mechanisms of Microbial Disease, p. 563, © 1993, Lippincott Williams & Wilkins.

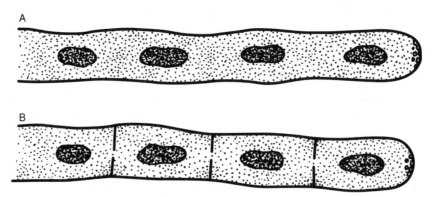

FIGURE 8-5   Somatic hyphae. A. Apical portion of nonseptate (coenocytic) hypha; the protoplasm is continuous and multinucleated. B. Apical portion of septate hyphae; protoplasm is interrupted by cross walls.
Source: M. Schaechter, G. Medoff and B.I. Esenstein, Mechanisms of Microbial Disease, p. 563, © 1993, Lippincott Williams & Wilkins.

Many of the truly pathogenic fungi have two growth forms and can exist as either molds or yeasts, depending on environmental conditions. This phenomenon is known as dimorphism. This yeast–filamentous or filamentous–yeast transition is most commonly associated with environment or functional roles, such as free-living versus parasite or pathogen. In most cases, the infectious or pathogenic form of the dimorphic fungi is the yeast form, with the filamentous or mycelial form being found in the environment. An exception to this exists with *Candida*, in which the pathogenic form is most commonly associated with the filamentous or pseudohyphal form (aggregates of newly budded cells that remain attached and become elongated), whereas the yeast form is associated with colonization or noninvasive behavior.

Classification

Historically, the fungi have been classified on the basis of morphologic characteristics and type or lack of sexual reproduction. As a group, the fungi are included in a separate biologic kingdom called Fungi. Within the kingdom are five phyla: Zygomycota, Ascomycota, Basidiomycota, Deuteromycota, and Mycophycophyta. Pathogenic fungi are found in the first four phyla, with the majority belonging to the Ascomycota and Deuteromycota. Members of the various phyla, genera, and species are frequently referred to or grouped by replacing the suffix *ota* with *etes*.

Fungi of medical importance can be grouped according to the type or location of infection that they cause. These groupings include:

1. Superficial mycoses or infections that involve only the outermost layers of the skin and hair
2. Cutaneous mycoses that involve primarily the epidermis
3. Subcutaneous mycoses that cause infections of the dermis and subcutaneous tissue
4. Systemic mycoses, which are infections of internal organ systems

The systemic mycoses can be further subdivided into those caused by true or primary pathogens, which are capable of causing disease in healthy individuals, and opportunistic pathogens, which are marginally pathogenic and cause disseminated or deep-tissue infection in compromised or debilitated hosts.

There are four fungi associated with superficial mycoses. *Malassezia furfur* is a lipophilic yeast that causes a mild, asymptomatic infection of the stratum corneum known as pityriasis or tinea versicolor. *Phaeoannellomyces wenckii* is the etiologic agent of tinea negra palmaris, an asymptomatic infection, usually of the palms of the hands, which produces flat areas of pigmentation. *Piedraia hortae* and *Trichosporon beigelii* are the etiologic agents of black piedra and white piedra, respectively. The piedras are diseases of the hair shaft. Cutaneous mycoses can be caused by a variety of fungi and include such diseases as ringworm and athlete's foot, etc. Although yeasts such as *Candida* species and some other miscellaneous fungi can cause infections of the skin, the most common etiologic agents of cutaneous infections include members of the genera *Microsporum*, *Trichophyton*, and *Epidermophyton*. As a group, these agents are referred to as dermatophytes, and the diseases they cause are termed tineas, which are further described by the specific area of the body infected. For example, infection of the head is termed tinea capitis; infection of the body is termed tinea corporis, and so on.

Subcutaneous mycoses are caused by a variety of fungi, which are found in soil and other environmental sources. Infection occurs by direct inoculation through broken skin, with the subsequent development of a localized infection, which rarely disseminates beyond the regional lymphatics. The most common cause of subcutaneous mycoses is *Sporothrix schenckii*, a dimorphic fungus on plant surfaces and in the soil. Infection occurs through implantation of microconidia of the filamentous stage into tissue through a puncture or abrasion, with subsequent conversion to the yeast form, resulting in an ulcer and potential spread to the lymphatic system. Two other subcutaneous infections include mycetoma and chromoblastomycosis. Mycetoma is a subcutaneous infection, usually of the foot or ankle, as a result of inoculation. Mycetomas are rare in the United States and are caused by a variety of relatively unusual fungi. Similar to mycetoma, chromoblastomycosis is most commonly a disease of the tropics. The disease manifests as a warty or cauliflower-like growth on the foot or ankle as a result of subcutaneous fungal growth. There are multiple etiologic agents of chromoblastomycosis, with the majority producing dark brown, pigmented hyphae in tissue and culture.

The primary etiologic agents of systemic mycoses include *Histoplasma capsulatum*, *Blastomyces dermatitidis*, *Coccidioides immitis*, *Para-coccidioides brasiliensis*, and *Cryptococcus neoformans*. All except *Cryptococcus neoformans*, a yeast only, are dimorphic fungi, existing as yeasts in vivo during infection and in the filamentous hyphal form in the soil. The infective stage is the microconidium of the hyphal form. The route of entry for all of the primary systemic mycoses is the respiratory tract with potential dissemination, if not controlled by the host, to other organ systems. Person-to-person transmission does not occur. The epidemiology of the systemic mycoses varies geographically.

H. capsulatum and *B. dermatitidi*s are found predominantly in the Mississippi, Missouri, and Ohio river valleys and, for *B. dermatitidis*, Canada. In contrast, *C. immitis* is found primarily in the soil of North, Central, and South America, as well as the southwestern United States; *P. brasiliensis* is found only in South and Central America.

The opportunistic systemic mycoses include a spectrum of fungi, from the primary system fungi described above to the usually nonpathogenic, saprophytic *Aspergillus* or *Rhizopus* species. Opportunistic fungi cause disease in hosts that have a depressed immune system, such as infants, diabetics, the elderly, patients with AIDS, or patients receiving cytotoxic drug therapy. As a group, they are ubiquitous and are frequently found as part of the normal flora. Initial infection can progress to serious system diseases, depending on the degree and duration of immunosuppression of the host. The most common opportunistic fungi are members of the genus *Candida*, particularly *C. albicans*, *Aspergillus fumagatus*, and *A. flavus*; members of any of the three genera of the *Zygomycetes*, *Rhizopus*, *Mucor*, *Absidia*; and *Pneumocystis carinii*. Also, one species of the genus *Penicillium*, *P. marheffei*, is a frequent opportunistic pathogen causing disseminated mycotic infections in AIDS patients in Southeast Asia.

Medical Parasitology

The study of protozoan and animal parasites that infect humans is known as medical parasitology. Organisms considered in this field fall into two major categories: the protozoa and the helminths, in which the adult stage is a worm. A few parasites of medical importance from each of these categories are discussed in the following section. Diagnosis of parasitic infections often involves direct examination of stool specimens for the presence of ova and parasites using standard light microscopy, which is mentioned in greater detail in the next section.

Parasitic diseases are spread in conditions of poverty. Substandard housing, poor water treatment, and crowding facilitate their transmission. Table 8-5 shows the burden of these diseases globally.

TABLE 8-5 Burden of Parasitic Diseases

	TDR Disease Category	Disease Burden DALYs* (thousands)			Deaths (thousands)		
		Total	Male	Female	Total	Male	Female
African trypanosomiasis	1	1,598	1,029	568	50	32	18
Leishmaniasis	1	2,357	1,410	946	59	35	24
Malaria	2	42,280	20,024	22,256	1,124	532	592
Schistosomiasis	2	1,760	1,081	678	15	11	5
Chagas disease	3	649	333	316	13	7	6
Lymphatic filariasis	3	5,644	4,317	1,327	0	0	0
Onchocerciasis	3	987	571	416	0	0	0

*DALYs: Disability Adjusted Life Years (the number of healthy years of life lost due to premature death and disability).
Source: World Health Report, 2004. World Health Organization.

Protozoa

The protozoa belong to a subkingdom, Protozoa, because they are neither plant nor animal. The morphology of protozoa varies widely and includes oval, spherical, and elongated cells that can range in size from 5–10 to 1–2 mm. Structurally, the protozoa resemble other eukaryotic cells in possessing a cytoplasmic membrane that encloses cytoplasm containing membrane-bound nuclei, mitochondria, 80S ribosomes, and a variety of specialized organelles associated with higher life forms. The majority of protozoa are aquatic, living in soil water, rivers, oceans, etc. However, there is a relatively small subset which are obligate parasites of animals which are capable of producing both acute and chronic disease (Table 8-6).

Like fungi, many protozoa are capable of both asexual and sexual reproduction. Asexual reproduction usually involves division of a cell into two daughter cells of equal size and composition through transverse (crosswise) or longitudinal (lengthwise) fission. Some species are capable of unequal fission or division through budding or multiple fission. In contrast, the method of sexual reproduction involves the fusion of two morphologically disparate cells (conjugation) with exchange of nuclear material and segregation of two daughter cells. Reproductive cycles of some protozoa are complex, in that a part of the life cycle is required in one host, such as a human or other vertebrate, and another stage is required in an invertebrate host. In instances where two different hosts are required in the life cycle, the host in which sexual reproduction occurs is known as the definitive host, whereas the host in which only asexual multiplication occurs is termed the intermediate host. Not unlike spore-forming bacteria, some protozoa are capable of forming cysts that can survive in unfavorable environmental conditions. During conversion to the cyst form, protozoa become morphologically round or oval and secrete a protective coating around themselves that is resistant

TABLE 8-6 Major Disease-Causing Protozoa in Humans

Disease	Causative Agent	Transmission to Humans	Reservoir/Hosts	Geographic Distribution
Amoebiasis	*Entamoebae histolytica*	Ingestion of cysts	Humans	More prevalent in tropical/subtropical regions
Balantidiasis	*Balantidium coli*	Ingestion of cysts	Hogs, humans	Worldwide
Giardiasis	*Giardia lamblia*	Ingestion of cysts	Humans	Worldwide
Trichomoniasis vaginitis	*Trichomonas vaginalis*	Contact	Humans	Worldwide
West African sleeping sickness	*Trypanosoma gambiense*	Inoculation (bite of tsetse fly, *Glossina* species)	Humans, animals including cattle	West Africa
East African sleeping sickness	*Trypanosoma rhodesiense*	Inoculation (bite of tsetse fly, *Glossina* species)	Humans, animals including cattle	Eastern and Central Africa
Chagas disease	*Trypanosoma cruzi*	Reduviid bugs (contamination from feces). Vertically from mother to child	Humans, armadillos, opossums	Mexico, Central and South America, more rarely southern United States
Leishmaniasis (visceral)	*Leishmania donovani*	Inoculation (bite of sand fly, *Phlebotomus* species)	Humans, dogs	Middle and Far East Africa
Leishmaniasis (cutaneous)	*Leishmania tropica*	Inoculation (bite of sand fly, *Phlebotomus* species)	Humans, dogs	Near East, Mediterranean, Africa, southern Russia, and southern Asia
Leishmaniasis (mucocutaneous)	*Leishmania braziliensis*	Inoculation (bite of sand fly, *Phlebotomus* species)	Humans, possibly dogs	South America
Malaria	*Plasmodium falciparum*	Inoculation (Anopheline mosquitoes)	Humans	Tropics and subtropics
	Plasmodium vivax			Central and South America, India, Southeast Asia
	Plasmodium ovale			Sub-Saharan Africa
	Plasmodium malariae			Tropics and subtropics

to temperature changes, toxic chemicals, and drying. Encysted protozoa are capable of survival outside of their specific host until they gain access to a new host, with resumption of growth and infection.

Classification

As with bacteria and fungi, only a limited number of the ~40,000 species of protozoa cause disease in humans. Pathogenic protozoa are found throughout the phylogeny of the subkingdom Protozoa. In the following sections, members of three phyla are discussed: Sarcomastigophora, Ciliophora, and Apicomplexa.

In the phylum Sarcomastigophora, amoebae comprise a subphylum known as Sarcodina. Amoebic infections of humans are generally confined to the intestine but can occasionally be carried in the blood to other organs of the body, such as the liver, lungs, spleen, pericardium, and brain. Amoebae do not possess complex organelles and do not undergo sexual reproduction, but rather multiply by binary fission. They are known for their ability to acquire food through the use of fingerlike projections known as pseudopodia, meaning "false feet." These projections are also used for motility. Under adverse conditions, many species are capable of forming cysts that can change into actively feeding trophozoites when conditions are more favorable.

Of the Sarcodina, *Entamoeba* is the most prevalent genus found associated with humans. In most instances, species of this genus exist as normal flora of the human intestinal tract. However, one species in particular, *Entamoebae histolytica*, is a potential pathogen in humans. Infections with *E. histolytica* are referred to as amebiasis and can be the cause of amebic dysentery. In such cases, actively growing organisms (trophozoites) invade the intestinal mucosa, resulting in lesions that can cause a range of symptoms from a few daily loose stools with small amounts of blood and mucus to acute cases with numerous intestinal ulcers causing severe diarrhea and substantial amounts of blood and mucus. In a small proportion of individuals, these intestinal ulcers may erode into adjoining blood vessels, allowing spread to other organs, especially the liver and lungs, and eventually leading to abscess formation.

Amebiasis is more prevalent in tropical and subtropical regions than in temperate zones and is often associated with poor sanitary conditions. In most instances, transmission is the result of ingestion of cysts from chronic carriers who shed the cyst form of the organism in their feces. Unlike acute cases, which tend to shed the trophozoite forms in feces, cysts are relatively resistant to harsh environmental conditions and, therefore, survive long enough to establish new infections.

Also in the phylum Sarcomastigophora, the subphylum Mastigophora comprises a group of flagellated protozoa commonly divided into two groups: those causing disease in the intestinal or genital tracts of humans (intestinal flagellates) and those transmitted by blood-sucking insects (hemoflagellates). Intestinal flagellates can produce a spectrum of disease, ranging from asymptomatic to severe, whereas the hemoflagellates may produce severe disease that is often fatal.

Of the intestinal flagellates, *Giardia lamblia* is the only one that produces specific intestinal disease. The actively growing form of this organism is bilaterally symmetric, with two nuclei and four pairs of flagella that provide its motility. It also produces cysts. Infections in adults range from asymptomatic to mild, including abdominal cramps and diarrhea. However, in severe cases, malabsorptive deficiencies may result in the small intestine. This organism is ubiquitous throughout the world and in the United States and may contaminate surface water. Furthermore, as it is resistant to chlorine, even treated water supplies can become contaminated if the water is not properly filtered.

Another flagellated protozoan, *Trichomonas vaginalis*, is the causative agent of trichomoniasis, a relatively common sexually transmitted disease infecting both men and women. Infection in both men and women can be asymptomatic or in women can cause a thin, watery, vaginal discharge, accompanied by burning and itching. This parasite does not form cysts and has four anterior flagella with one posterior flagellum that forms the outer edge of an undulating membrane.

Hemoflagellates are those flagellated protozoa that are transmitted to humans by the bites of infected, blood-sucking insects. Two genera are of importance in this particular category: *Trypanosoma* and *Leishmania*. In both cases, cells of each of these genera pass through similar stages in their life cycles. This involves development in both vertebrate and invertebrate hosts. Four principal stages are typically involved in the life cycles of these parasites and are characterized by the presence or absence of an undulating membrane and flagella: trypomastigotes, which characteristically possess an undulating membrane running the entire length of the organism, the outer edge of which is formed by a single flagellum that extends anterior to the cell; the epimastigotes, in which the undulating membrane originates in the central part of the cell; the promastigotes, which lack an undulating membrane but have a single anterior flagellum; and amastigotes, which are rounded, nonmotile forms. It is important to remember that for each species of parasite, some forms develop in the vertebrate host and others develop in the invertebrate host.

Trypanosomes are the causative agents of West and East African sleeping sickness. Specifically, *Trypanosoma gambiense* is the etiologic agent of West African sleeping sickness, and *T. rhodesiense* is the etiologic agent of East African sleeping sickness (also known as Rhodesian trypanosomiasis). Transmission occurs as the result of a bite from an infected tsetse fly, and the organisms migrate through the blood, eventually invading the lymph nodes, which results in attacks of fever. These attacks can be intermittent and recur over a period of weeks to months, often resulting in heart damage. As the disease progresses, trypanosomes invade the central nervous system, causing a meningoencephalitis, resulting in slurred speech and difficulty walking. Later stages are characterized by convulsions, paralysis, mental deterioration, and increasing sleepiness that ultimately progresses to coma and death. This process may take several months to reach its ultimate conclusion. Although West and East African sleeping sickness are similar in clinical presentation, the East African form of the disease typically progresses much more rapidly, with death occurring well before the onset of the meningoencephalitis. Frequently, myocarditis is the cause of death.

Another disease caused by a trypanosome is American trypanosomiasis, also known as Chagas' disease. This disease is found in the southern United States and Central and South America and the burden of Chagas is high in several South American countries. The causative agent of this disease is *T. cruzi*, which is transmitted to humans by reduviid bugs also called kissing or assassin bugs. Reduviid adults can be over two inches in length. They emerge from the walls and ceilings of substandard tropical housing to feed on humans at night. Their bite is painless and can occur on any exposed skin—commonly the face. They shed trypanosomes in their feces. As the bugs feed, they continually defecate, contaminating the bite site and, thus, infecting the host. Chagas may also be transmitted by blood transfusion and vertically from mother to child. This particular species of trypanosome is unable to multiply outside the cell in its vertebrate host; thus, it undergoes a morphologic change to the amastigote form and is found multiplying in virtually every cell in every organ of the body. The organ most often affected is the heart, and growth of the parasite in this organ induces an inflammatory reaction that enlarges the heart. The chronic phase of the disease is long and mostly asymptomatic; untreated death occurs in approximately 30% of patients usually from disturbances in heart rhythm or congestive heart failure.

The genus *Leishmania* is another hemoflagellate that infects humans. All species of this parasite are transmitted from one animal to another by the bite of an infected sand fly of the genus *Phlebotomus*. In general, the form of the parasite introduced by the bite of the sand fly is the flagellated promastigotes (the form present in the insect's gut), which transform into nonmotile amastigotes that then proliferate in cells of the reticuloendothelial system, specifically, macrophages and endothelial cells. Three species of this genus are of particular medical importance in humans: *Leishmania tropica*, the causative agent of cutaneous leishmaniasis; *L. braziliensis*, the causative agent of mucocutaneous leishmaniasis; and *L. donovani*, the causative agent of visceral leishmaniasis. These diseases vary in regions of the world in which they are found and in severity of disease. Cutaneous leishmaniasis occurs primarily in the Near East, Mediterranean countries, Africa, southern Russia, and southern Asia. It is characterized by a papule that appears at the bite site and eventually develops into an ulcer. Secondary bacterial infection can be a problem but, in general, the ulcer heals within a year, leaving a depigmented scar. Mucocutaneous leishmaniasis is a variant of the cutaneous form, involving the mucous membranes of the nasopharyngeal area. If untreated, the nasal septum, lips, and the soft palate may be destroyed, resulting in asphyxiation due to airway collapse or secondary bacterial infection. This form of leishmaniasis is typically found in South America. Visceral leishmaniasis, also known as kala-azar, is a form of the disease in which the parasites are able to invade the reticuloendothelial system throughout the body, especially the liver and spleen. As a result, these organs become enlarged, causing abdominal swelling, and often culminate in death an average of two years after onset of initial symptoms.

In the phylum Ciliophora, only one of these free-living species, *Balantidium coli*, causes disease in humans. Actively growing trophozoites are covered in tiny, hairlike projections called cilia, which provide motility in aqueous environments. This organism has both a macronucleus that controls the metabolic activities of the cell and a micronucleus involved in sexual reproduction of the cell, which divides by transverse fission. In addition, this parasite is capable of forming cysts that provide a means of transmission upon ingestion of contaminated food or water. *B. coli* typically resides in the lumen of the intestine, obtaining food by ingesting bacteria. Occasionally, this organism can cause symptoms not unlike those seen in amebic dysentery.

The phylum Apicomplexa contains one class, the Sporozoa, which is of relevance to human disease. Members of this particular class are obligate parasites of animal hosts. Among the diseases caused by these organisms are malaria and toxoplasmosis, as well as intestinal infections. Because the life cycles of the Sporozoa are much more varied than those of the other protozoa, only a few of them are covered in this chapter.

Malaria is caused by one of four parasites belonging to the class Sporozoa: *Plasmodium vivax, P. ovale, P. malariae,* and *P. falciparum.* Although the clinical signs and symptoms can vary with each species of malaria, in general, these include chills and fever at intermittent, regular intervals, followed by profuse sweating. Because the life cycle of the malarial parasite is complex and varies by species, only a brief description is presented here. Transmission occurs when an individual is bitten by an infected female mosquito of the genus *Anopheles.* Sporozoites are released into the bloodstream of the host from the salivary glands of the mosquito as it feeds. Subsequently, the sporozoites migrate to the hepatocytes of the liver and undergo one or more rounds of asexual reproduction before returning to the bloodstream as merozoites, where they invade red blood cells. Two species of parasite, *P. ovale* and *P. vivax,* are associated with relapsing malaria. This particular form of disease is caused by dormant parasites in the liver, which may erupt weeks, months, or years after the initial episode. Merozoites undergo several developmental stages and asexual reproduction within the red blood cells, eventually causing rupture of the cells and release to the bloodstream, where other red blood cells can then be infected and the process started again. It is during the time of red blood cell rupture and parasite release that the symptoms of the disease are present. In addition, after asexual reproduction has occurred in the red blood cells, some of the merozoites do not divide, but rather undergo a transition to male and female gametocytes. These, in turn, are ingested by a feeding mosquito, and the gametocytes are converted into male and female gametes that fuse, producing a zygote during sexual reproduction in the gut of the mosquito. The zygote undergoes several developmental transitions within the mosquito before once again reaching the sporozoite stage and repeating the infectious cycle.

In endemic areas, significant morbidity and mortality are the result of anemia, due to the high level of parasitized red blood cells. *P. falciparum,* the most dangerous of the malarial parasites, is adept at invading red blood cells and, in addition, can induce conformational changes in these cells that result in blocked capillaries, leading to hemorrhages in the brain, lungs, and kidneys. For this reason, severe infection with this species of parasite is often fatal.

Toxoplasmosis is caused by another member of the class Sporozoa, *Toxoplasma gondii.* This parasite is one of the most widespread in the world, infecting vertebrate hosts. Very often, the disease is mild to asymptomatic in humans; however, it can present a particular threat in neonates and immuno-compromised individuals. This parasite is widespread throughout the animal kingdom and, thus, a common source of infection for humans is ingestion of undercooked or raw meat containing either the trophozoite or cyst forms. In particular, these parasites undergo their sexual reproduction in the intestinal cells of members of the cat family and are shed as oocysts in the feces of these animals. Infection can also result from ingestion of these oocysts, which release enclosed sporozoites that then travel to infect epithelial cells, leukocytes, the reticuloendothelial system, and the central nervous system. The parasites then multiply within these cells.

Cryptosporidium, the causative agent of cryptosporidiosis, is also included in the class Sporozoa. Both the sexual and asexual reproductive cycles occur in one host. Infectious oocysts are shed in the feces, which can then infect another susceptible host. Clinically, the disease is characterized by mild to severe diarrhea and nausea that spontaneously resolve in an average of 1–10 days. Although infection with *Cryptosporidium* produces asymptomatic to mild, self-limiting illness in most individuals, it can cause a persistent diarrhea in immunocompromised patients and may even be fatal.

Helminths

The numbers of invertebrates that parasitize humans are seemingly endless. Helminths are typically classified into two phyla: Platyhelminthes, or flatworms, and Aschelminthes, or roundworms. Generally speaking, many live only in the intestinal tract of a parasitized host, whereas others invade organs such as the liver, lungs, blood, brain, and subcutaneous tissue. Most of these parasites are large, macroscopic organisms.

The flatworms are the most primitive of the Platyhelminthes and characteristically have no digestive tract or only a rudimentary one. They are typically flat, and most contain both male and female reproductive organs (hermaphroditic). Although many require an alternation of hosts to complete their life cycles, humans are often the definitive host for the adult worms, and other animals are the hosts for the intermediate stages.

Intestinal cestodes, or tapeworms, of humans inhabit the intestinal tract. Adult tapeworms are long and ribbonlike, and are divided into segments with a head, which has either suckers or hooks that provide for attachment to the intestinal wall. In general, the animal in which the larval stage develops into an adult worm is the definitive host, and the animal in which the eggs develop into the larval stage is the intermediate host. Humans are the only definitive host for the beef and pork tapeworms, *Taenia saginata* and *T. solium*, respectively. *Taenia saginata* is acquired by ingestion of beef infected with the larval stage of the parasite. Once the larvae reach the small intestine, the worm head emerges and attaches itself to the intestinal mucosa. Mature worms can reach a length of 8–12 meters. Eggs are passed in the feces and can infect other animals, such as cattle. The eggs subsequently hatch, and the embryos disseminate throughout the body, particularly the muscles. There, they develop into the larval stage, or cysticercus, which will die in about 9 months if not ingested by the definitive host, humans. Most infections are asymptomatic, although malnutrition, anemia, and weight loss can result. The adult pork tapeworm develops similarly to that of the beef tapeworm and can attain a length of 2–3 meters. However, pigs can ingest eggs on fecally contaminated food. The larvae that develop can survive for several years in the musculature of the animal. If the larvae are ingested, very often no symptoms are present. Unlike infection with the beef tapeworm, humans can serve as an intermediate host. This arises when an individual ingests food or water contaminated with fecal material containing eggs from another human carrier. These eggs hatch, and the resulting larvae disseminate throughout the body, forming cysticerci. The resulting condition, cysticercosis, can cause an asymptomatic infection if either the subcutaneous tissues or muscles are involved. However, more severe complications and death can occur if vital organs become infected, such as the central nervous system. Another tapeworm infection of humans is acquired by eating raw or undercooked fish infected with *Diphyllobothrium latum*, the fish tapeworm.

Other Platyhelminthes of human medical importance are the trematodes, also known as flukes. Adult worms are typically smaller than the cestodes, ranging in size from 1 mm to several centimeters and use suckers to attach themselves to host tissue. These parasites are found worldwide, although most human infections occur in the Far and Near East. Trematodes require snails as their intermediate host. In general, parasite eggs hatch in fresh water and undergo several larval stages, one of which involves the snail, until the infective-stage larvae are formed. Humans become infected by ingestion of infective-stage larvae or, as in the case of the schistosomes, the larvae burrow directly through the skin of an individual standing in contaminated water. These parasites are typically classified as intestinal, liver, lung, or blood flukes. Intestinal flukes, such as *Fasciolopsis buski*, involve humans only accidentally. Liver flukes, such as *Fasciola hepatica*, mature into adult worms in the bile ducts of the liver. Lung flukes, such as *Paragonimus westermani*, cause a major disease of the lungs, paragonimiasis, and are found only in the Far East. Blood flukes of the genus Schistosoma cause schistosomiasis and vary by anatomic region in which the adult worms reside. For example, adult worms may reside in the inferior mesenteric veins of the large intestine (*S. mansoni*), the superior mesenteric veins of the small intestine (*S. japonicum*), or the rectal vessels and veins surrounding the bladder (*S. haematobium*). In the latter case, ulceration of the bladder is common, thus leading to the presence of blood in the urine.

Aschelminthes

Nematodes, or roundworms, are small and possess functional digestive systems, including an anus. Human infections caused by these worms are largely divided into intestinal roundworms and blood and tissue roundworms. Of the intestinal roundworms, *Trichinella spiralis* is the cause of trichinosis in carnivorous animals. Human infection usually is the result of ingestion of the encysted larvae in undercooked or raw pork. After ingestion, the cysts reach the intestine, where the larvae are liberated and develop into adult worms. Adult female worms penetrate the intestinal mucosa, producing larvae that then migrate via the lymphatics to the muscles, etc., and become encysted.

The severity of symptoms varies with the magnitude of the initial infection. Thus, infection can be asymptomatic or severe, with initial symptoms including fever, diarrhea, and malaise, due to the activities of the adult worms in the intestines. In severe cases, muscle pain throughout the entire body can also occur, due to migration of the larvae into the skeletal muscles. However, this is most commonly seen in cases of moderate to heavy infection. In addition, although encystment occurs only in muscle, larvae can infect other organs of the body, such as the lungs, heart, meninges, and brain. In particular, myocarditis, the most common cardiac lesion caused by the larvae, can lead to arrhythmias and congestive heart failure. The invasion of any of these organs during the early weeks of infection can be fatal.

Ascaris lumbricoides is the largest nematode infecting humans and often attains a length of 20–30 cm. It is most frequently found in the tropics and some areas of the southern United States. Humans become infected by ingesting infectious eggs containing second-stage larvae. Once in the intestine, the larvae hatch, penetrate the intestinal mucosa, and eventually reach the lungs after the portal circulation picks them up. Once in the lung, the parasites undergo differentiation, are coughed up and swallowed, and eventually return to the small intestine, where adult worms remain attached. Only in cases of heavy infection are symptoms such as abdominal pain or complications arising from invasion of the liver, etc., seen.

Whipworm disease, caused by *Trichuris trichiura*, is found primarily in the tropics and occasionally in the southern United States. The adult worm lives in the human cecum and is attached to the intestinal mucosa. Eggs are passed in feces, and, as a result, transmission occurs via ingestion of contaminated food or water. Heavy infections are associated with chronic diarrhea, abdominal pain, vomiting, constipation, headache, and, in some cases, anemia.

Pinworms, *Enterobius vermicularis*, are strictly human parasites. Humans become infected by ingestion of fertilized eggs. As in the preceding example, adult worms live in the cecum. Female worms migrate to and lay their eggs in the perianal area, which produces an intense itching. Most infections are asymptomatic and resolve after all of the female worms have died. Human hookworm disease is caused by *Necator americanus* and *Ancylostoma duodenale*. Both species are widely distributed in tropical regions; however, *A. duodenale* is also present in Europe. The eggs of both species are passed in the feces and develop into rhabditiform, or first-stage larvae, which are generally noninfectious. These larvae feed on vegetation and bacteria in the soil and subsequently develop into infectious, filariform larvae. Filariform larvae infect a host by direct penetration of the skin, usually of the foot, and migrate to the lungs, where they are coughed up and swallowed. Adult worms reside in the small intestine, attached to the mucosa. Although the life cycles of these two species are similar, only *N. americanus* has an obligatory requirement for development in the lungs, whereas *A. duodenale* can bypass this particular stage. In addition, *A. duodenale* can also infect a host orally, as well as by direct skin penetration.

Symptoms of hookworm disease range from mild to severe and include headache, fever, nausea, and hemoptysis due to the migration of the larvae in the lungs, intestinal symptoms such as diarrhea and vomiting, and, in extreme cases, anemia, due to the feeding activity of the worms in the intestines.

Creeping eruption, also known as cutaneous larva migrans, can also result from the migration of the larvae beneath the skin.

Blood and tissue nematodes, unlike their intestinal counterparts, are not spread by fecal–oral transmission. Most are carried from one host to another by the bite of an arthropod vector. In general, most worms in this category belong to the superfamily Filarioidea, and the human infection they cause is called filariasis. Adult worms generally range in size from 2 to 30 cm in length, and females are ordinarily twice the size of males. Unlike other nematodes, females do not lay eggs, but rather give birth to prelarval forms known as microfilariae. Microfilariae are subsequently picked up by a blood-sucking vector, which then transmits the filariae from one host to another. These parasites are divided largely into two groups, based on the habitat of the adult worms: the lymphatic group (*Wuchereria bancrofti* and *Brugia malayi*) and the cutaneous group (*Loa loa* and *Onchocerca volvulus*). *Wuchereria bancrofti* is the etiologic agent of elephantiasis. This mosquito-borne disease is found in the Pacific Islands and Africa, and occurs sporadically in the Near and Far East and Central and South America. Within the human host, the larvae enter the lymphatic vessels and nodes and eventually develop into adult worms. Because the adult worms tend to prefer the lymphatics of the lower extremities, in extreme cases, especially in endemic areas, fibrous tissue can develop around the worms, leading to an obstruction of lymphatic flow and the characteristic massive edema of the legs, scrotum, breasts, or female genitalia known as elephantiasis. However, this particular complication is relatively rare, and more often, light infections cause only slightly enlarged lymph nodes. *Brugia malayi*, the causative agent of Malayan filariasis, is similar in life cycle to *W. bancrofti*. It is endemic on the Malay Peninsula, although it is also present in India, Indonesia, Thailand, Sri Lanka, and Vietnam.

Loa loa, often referred to as the African eye worm, is transmitted by mango or deer flies and found only in Africa. Unlike other filarial parasites, adult worms of this particular species migrate through the subcutaneous tissue throughout the body and, in some cases, can affect the facial area. There they can be seen as they migrate across the bridge of the nose or the subconjunctival tissue of the eye.

River blindness is caused by *Onchocerca volvulus*, which is typically found in Central Africa and in some areas of Central and Northern South America. Infection is transmitted to humans by the bite of infected sand flies carrying infectious larvae. Adult worms reside in subcutaneous tissue and routinely become encased in a fibrous capsule that can often be seen beneath the skin. Microfilariae migrate from the capsules and move throughout the dermis and connective tissue and can cause ocular lesions, which may ultimately result in blindness.

Diagnostic Microbiology

Since the study of microorganisms began with their initial observation in 1683 by Antony van Leeuwenhoek, using the first microscope, continuous progress has resulted in the discovery and development of methods to detect and identify members of this previously unseen universe. Historically, this initially involved improvements in microscopy and methods to cultivate microorganisms outside of their normal hosts. The subsequent development of immunology and the sensitivity and specificity of antigen–antibody reactions led to a rapid expansion of noncultural techniques for the detection and identification of microorganisms. The incorporation of these extraordinarily sensitive and specific molecular methods for detection of microbial pathogens with older visualization methods has lead to ever greater specificity and accuracy. In the following section, the four major categories of microbial detection–microscopy, culture, immunology, and those utilizing molecular/nucleic acid methods–are briefly reviewed.

Microscopy

Light Microscopy

The current light microscope contains a built-in light source and a compound lens system, which means that at least two separate lenses are used. Specimens are visualized by transillumination, with light being focused on the object, which is then seen against a bright background. The major components of the microscope can be divided into lens systems and mechanical parts. The purposes of microscopy include:

1. Magnification of an image
2. Maximization of resolution
3. Optimization of the contrast between structures, organisms, cells, and background

The lens system utilized today in microscopes offers a variety of magnifications through a number of objective lenses in conjunction with a fixed (usually 10×) ocular lens. Light microscopes should be equipped with objective lenses of low-power (10×), high-dry (40×), and oil immersion (100×), which will result in final magnifications, in conjunction with the ocular lens, of 100×, 400×, and 1000×, respectively. As important as magnification, resolving power is an essential component of microscopy. Resolving power is the ability of the lens system of the microscope to distinguish two objects as separate, rather than one. Resolving power is dependent on the wave length (L) of light used to illuminate the specimen or object and the numerical aperture of the microscopic system. Numerical aperture is a measure of the angle of the maximum cone of light that can enter the objective lens of the microscope. Resolving power of the microscope can be optimized through proper use of the condenser, which focuses light into the plane of the specimen. The most commonly used condensers can produce a numerical aperture of 1.25. Resolving power can also be increased by adjusting the medium through which the light passes between the specimen or object and the objective lens. Special oils, termed immersion oil, have a refractive index similar to glass, permitting more light to be incorporated in the image, thus improving resolving power. Visualization of bacteria usually requires the use of the 100× objective and immersion oil. This combination will result in resolution of approximately 0.2 microns.

Optimization of resolving power and magnification may require further adjustment of contrast and must be incorporated into microscopic systems to differentiate or distinguish various elements within a microscopic field. This is due to the similar refractive indices of many microorganisms and the matrices in which they are being observed. Although some adjustment can be made through a decrease or increase in admitted light, the majority of biologic structures cannot be visualized without the use or application of differential stains. Biologic stains are basically dyes that are used to improve contrast between structures in specimens and objects. The contrast is improved through a color differentiation—an attraction of a particular dye molecule, based on charge, pH, or other physiochemical interaction between a specific structural component and the dye. Due to the relative nonspecific staining characteristics of dyes, most staining techniques involve a stepwise application of chemicals for differentiation. These usually include a primary stain, which is amphoteric and can act either as an acid or a base, depending on the predominance of anionic (acidic) or cationic (basic) moieties in the dye. In general, basic dyes stain structures that are acidic, such as nuclear chromatin, whereas acid dyes react with basic structures, such as cytoplasm and cell walls. The second step involves the application of mordant, which fixes the primary stain to its target, followed by decolorization, which removes unbound dye/stain from the structure in the microorganism. Finally, a secondary or counterstain is added to provide color to nontargeted structures or microorganisms. This process is best explained by the gram-stain and acid-fast stain of bacteria, described earlier.

Variations on bright-field microscopy are employed in the diagnosis of infectious disease. Dark-field microscopy is utilized to increase apparent resolving power of light microscopy below 0.2 microns. In dark-field microscopy, the condenser, which focuses light directly onto a plane, is replaced by a special dark-field condenser, which permits entry of light only from the periphery or circumference of the object or structure. As a result, objects within the field or specimen appear to glow. Although there is no real increase in resolution, this technique does permit the visualization of microorganisms with diameters between 0.1 and 0.2 microns. This technique has been limited in application to visualization of spirochetes, such as *Treponema pallidum*, the causative agent of syphilis, in secondary syphilitic lesions; *Borrelia burgdorferi*, the agent of Lyme disease in spinal fluid; and *Leptospira* species in urine or blood.

Fluorescence Microscopy

Fluorescence is a phenomenon that occurs when a molecule is impacted by a given wavelength of light and emits light at a wavelength longer than the one to which it was exposed. In fluorescent microscopy, specimens are labeled with a fluorescent dye (molecule) and exposed to ultraviolet (UV) light of a specific wavelength, which results in emission of longer-wavelength visible light. Specificity or selectivity is dependent on the nature of the fluorescent dye and the staining process. Examples of this direct fluorescence staining technique are auramine–rhodamine dye staining of mycobacteria and acridine orange staining of bacteria. The specificity of the mycobacterial fluorescent system is the staining technique, which utilizes the acid-fast nature of this group of bacteria. In contrast, acridine orange at low pH can intercalate into nucleic acid with bacterial nucleic acid fluorescing green when the appropriate UV wavelength light is utilized. Fluorescent microscopy is significantly more sensitive than light microscopy because organisms that bind and retain dye are visualized as brightly glowing objects in a dark background.

Another powerful adaptation of this technique is direct florescent antibody detection, which combines the sensitivity of fluorescent microscopy with the specificity of antigen–antibody reactions. In this technique, a fluorescent dye is linked to a specific antibody that binds only to a specific antigen. It is then possible to detect the presence and cellular location of any antigen because they literally "light up." Different antigens within a single specimen can be detected by using antibodies labeled with different florescent dye, also known as a flurochrome. More commonly, indirect fluorescent antibody (IFA) methods are used to determine the presence of specific antigens. IFA uses a "second antibody," tagged with a flurochrome, which binds to the antigen-specific antibody. The second antibody is derived from another species and is directed against multiple epitopes on the antibody class of the antigen specific antibody. In this way, IFA may be more sensitive than the direct method.

Electron Microscopy

The resolving power of any microscope is directly related to the wavelength of light, which is used for visualization. The use of an electron beam decreases the resolution from the 0.2 microns possible with a light microscope to 0.0005 microns in the electron microscope. Although the substantial increase in resolution of electron microscopy has led to significant scientific discoveries in the ultrastructure of microorganisms, a major disadvantage is the inability to examine living cells. In addition, the preparation process can result in the creation of artifacts. Two types of electron microscopy are available that include transmission and scanning. Transmission electron microscopy uses an electron beam that travels directly through the specimen with a resulting two-dimensional image. Scanning electron microscopy produces a three-dimensional image of the specimen or object through the use of modified electron beams. In electron microscopy, contrast is achieved through differences in electron density. As a result, specimens are treated with chemicals to accentuate the electron density differential. To optimize this electron density differential, three methods of preparation have been developed: negative staining, which utilizes a heavy metal, such as uranium or gold, to stain the background, leaving the target structures lighter; freeze-etching which involves rapid cooling of the specimen with subsequent fractures along planes of the object or specimen; and, finally, osmium tetroxide or glutaraldehyde fixation and embedding in epoxy resins with very thin, fine sectioning of the specimen and, in some cases, enhancement with heavy metal treatment.

Culture

Almost all medically important bacteria and fungi can be cultivated outside of the host on artificial culture media. Due to the growth characteristics of bacteria, a single cell, when placed on appropriate culture medium and environmental conditions, will reproduce to numbers sufficient to be visible to the naked eye (i.e., colony) or other means of detection (Table 8-7). Culture media can be prepared as a fluid, broth medium, or as a solid medium through the addition of a gelling agent—most commonly, agar, a polysaccharide extracted from specific types of seaweed. Agar becomes liquid upon boiling and solidifies when cooled to <50 °C. The advantage of solid or agar medium is that specimens may be "streaked" thin enough across the plate that single organisms may multiply to form visible colonies. Isolated colonies growing on a solid surface represent pure cultures, or a single strain, which may subsequently be identified and tested for susceptibility to therapeutic drugs using standard methodologies.

The medium can also be a diagnostic tool. Pathogenic microorganisms require a source of energy, electrons, carbon, nitrogen, oxygen, sulfur, and phosphorus. In addition, trace elements, such as potassium, calcium, magnesium, and iron, are required as are very low concentrations of zinc, copper, manganese, nickel, boron, and cobalt. Many of the more fastidious microorganisms require vitamins, which function as coenzymes or precursors for coenzymes. Media utilized to cultivate microorganisms are known as defined and undefined. Defined media are formulated from chemically known ingredients in known quantities. Undefined media are prepared from ingredients in which not all of the components are known but do contain adequate amounts of essential or growth-promoting ingredients. Examples of ingredients frequently used in undefined culture media include partial digests

TABLE 8-7   Media Used for Growth and Isolation of Pathogenic Bacteria

Medium	Cultivation
Enrichment Media	
Brain–heart infusion broth	Most bacteria
Trypticase soy broth	
Thioglycolate broth	Anaerobes, facultative anaerobes
Blood agar	Most pathogens
Chocolate agar	Most pathogens, including *Hemophilus* and *Neisseria* species
Selective Media	
MacConkey	Nonfastidious gram-negative bacteria-differential for lactose fermentation
Colistin–nalidixic acid	Gram-positive bacteria only
Blood agar	
Hektoen agar	*Salmonella* and *Shigella* species
Specialized Media	
Thayer-Martin medium	Selective for *N. gonorrhoeae* and *N. meningitidis*
Thiosulfate-citrate-bile-sucrose agar	Selective for *Vibrio* species
Bordet–Gengou agar	Selective for *Bordetella pertussis*
Lowenstein–Jensen medium	*Mycobacteria*

of animal or vegetable protein, yeast extract, serum, or blood. The majority of diagnostic media are undefined because of their lower cost and their ability to support the growth of a broad range of pathogenic organisms. The use of complex media components, such as yeast extract, in media formulations for the routine growth and recovery of microbial pathogens obviates the need to add trace minerals and vitamins. Bacteriologic media are usually categorized into three groupings: enrichment, selective, and differential media.

Enrichment media are formulated to encourage the growth of a wide variety of bacteria, although a single medium that will support the growth of all bacteria has not been found. Examples of enrichment media used for the recovery of pathogenic bacteria include blood agar, chocolate agar (a descriptor which is based on the color of the medium, not the ingredients), trypticase soy broth, and brain–heart infusion broth. Selective media are used when specific pathogens are sought from specimens or sites that contain normal flora. In these instances, the pathogen of interest may be overgrown, due to a slower growth rate or smaller numbers being present at the site by the expected resident flora. Selective media usually contain chemicals, dyes, or antibiotics that are inhibitory to contaminating bacteria but not the specific pathogen of interest. Differential media contain indicator systems that permit the differentiation of groups of organisms, based on a selective metabolic or physiologic characteristic. Commonly, this includes the addition of a specific carbohydrate and a pH indicator to the base medium. Fermentation of the carbohydrate results in a reduction of pH and a color change in the colony. Erythrocytes added to base media can also be differential in indicating hemolysin and the presence or absence of a hemolysis, a common virulence factor. Frequently, the properties of enrichment, selective, and differential media are combined in the same medium. Culture media commonly used in the clinical laboratory are listed in Table 8-7.

In addition to the rational requirements for in vitro growth of microorganisms, the optimal physical conditions for successful cultivation must be considered. Most human pathogens are mesophiles, which is to say they grow optimally at human body temperature, 37 °C, and can only tolerate temperatures between 25° and 40 °C. Similarly, the ideal pH range for most bacteria lies between 6.5 and 7.5. The principal gases that affect bacterial growth are oxygen and carbon dioxide. Aerobic organisms require oxygen for growth and can be cultivated in an air atmosphere. In contrast, anaerobic bacteria cannot use oxygen as a terminal electron acceptor; oxygen is toxic and they cannot be cultivated in an air atmosphere. Facultatively anaerobic bacteria do not require oxygen for growth, although if it is available, they are capable of using it as a terminal electron acceptor. Facultative anaerobes are capable of growth in the presence or absence of air. Microaerophilic organisms require low levels of oxygen; they are cultivated at 5–10% CO_2, but cannot tolerate the level of oxygen present in atmospheric air.

In addition to visualization of growth through colony formation on agar media or turbidity in broth media, several methods have been developed that do not depend on visual changes for detection of growth. The techniques include detection of carbon dioxide as a result of bacterial metabolism, bioluminescence, changes in electric impedance, and chromatographic detection of metabolic end products. All of these methods require growth or metabolism by the microorganism for successful detection.

Growth of Other Organisms

Viruses and some other microorganisms are obligate intracellular pathogens and, as such, cannot be cultivated using the techniques described above. Because growth and replication of these pathogens require living cells, three techniques have been used: inoculation of tissue or cell culture, embryonated hens' eggs, and experimental animals. Tissue culture is the most common method of viral culture. Cells are grown as monolayers in the presence of nutrient media until a confluent layer of cells is achieved. Cell culture monolayers are of three basic types: primary cell culture, transformed haploid or heteroploid cell lines, and diploid cell lines or stains. In primary cell culture, the cells have a normal chromosome count (diploid) and are derived from initial cell cultivation from a tissue source such as monkey or human embryonic kidney cells. Continued subculture and regrowth of primary cell lines usually result in one of two events: the cells will eventually die or they will undergo spontaneous transformation. Transformed cell lines have altered growth characteristics; the chromosome count varies (haploid or heteroploid); and their susceptibility to viral infection can be altered. In addition, transformed cell lines are immortal, in that they can be subcultured or regrown through serial passage many times without dying. Transformed cells can also be obtained from malignant cells or tissue, or through mutagenesis in vitro. A common transformed cell line used diagnostically is Hep-2, derived from a human epithelial carcinoma. The third type of tissue culture is composed of diploid cells, usually of fibroblast origin that can be subcultured or regrown through 30–40 passages, prior to dying out or transforming. The ability to cultivate virus in vitro is highly dependent on the specific cell line in which it is placed. As a result, successful cultivation of human viral pathogens requires the use of a number of cell lines for diagnosis unless a specific viral pathogen is being sought.

Microbial growth in cell culture can be visualized or detected through a variety of methods. Most commonly, growth can be detected through cytopathic effect. Lytic or cytopathic viruses produce alterations in cell morphology during replication in susceptible cell lines, which can be observed directly by light microscopy. The morphologic changes observed are usually characteristic of a particular virus growing in a specific cell line. For example, as its name implies, respiratory syncytial viruses cause fusion of cells to produce multinucleated giant cells, termed syncytia.

Some viruses produce proteins that are expressed on the membrane of infected cells. These viral proteins bind erythrocytes and this can be detected by testing for hemadsorption or hemagglutination. Hemadsorption is when erthrocytes added to the infected cell culture adhere to the cell culture monolayer. Hemagglutination is when released virus causes added erthrocytes to clump. Detection and visualization of viruses that produce little or any cytopathic effect (CPE) do not possess hemagglutinins or do not completely replicate in cell culture can be achieved through immunologic or nucleic acid probes. Most commonly IFA is used to detect viruses, although direct florescent antibody techniques are possible. Another commonly utilized immunologic method for viral identification is neutralization. In this technique, viral infectivity is neutralized through mixing of subcultured virus with specific individual antibodies against different viruses and inoculation of cell lines with treated and untreated aliquots of the unknown viral agent. The identity of the virus is indicated by an inability of the virus to grow in the presence of specific antibodies compared to untreated controls. Finally, animal inoculation is used in the recovery of some viruses. Suckling mice in the first 48 hours of life are very susceptible to viral infection. Depending on the virus, the mice can be inoculated intracerebrally, subcutaneously, or intraperitoneally. Evidence of viral replication/infection is manifested by clinical disease. Confirmation and identification of the infecting virus can be achieved through histology, immunofluorescent staining, or detection of specific antibody response. Arboviruses and rabies virus are detected using this system.

Diagnostic Immunology

Previously used techniques for the investigation of infectious diseases included culture, serologic tests, and biochemical assays. Initially, serodiagnosis was achieved through a variety of techniques, including antigen–antibody, agglutination, and complement fixation. However, these techniques were labor intensive and lacked specificity and sensitivity. These drawbacks improved significantly with the development of immunofluorescence, radioimmunoassays, and enzyme immunoassays.

In general, the use of immunoassays for the diagnosis of infectious diseases involves one of two main principles: testing for specific microbial antigens or testing for specific microbial–antigen antibodies. These assays may involve the detection of a microbial antigen directly from a clinical specimen or the detection of a specific antigen, once an organism is cultured in vitro.

Tests for antibodies may be designed to detect any antibody isotype or a particular isotype, such as IgM or IgG. Precautions must be taken in using IgM or IgG due to markers for infection as a result of the temporal expression of each of these isotypes. For example, in many infections IgM appears rapidly following infection, peaks within 7–10 days, and wanes after several weeks. In contrast, detectable IgG requires at least 4–6 weeks to develop and persists longer than IgM. In general, the presence of IgM antibodies is indicative of recent infection. However, because IgM appears on second exposure to most agents and may persist in some individuals for long periods of time, interpretation of results must be carefully evaluated for each infectious agent. Therefore, in most cases, paired sera are required for the measurement of total antibody. This includes both an early sample taken the first week to 10 days after onset of symptoms and a subsequent sample taken during convalescence (3–4 weeks). In general, a fourfold rise or greater in antibody titer indicates a positive test. Other antibody isotypes, such as IgA and IgE, are not routinely used in immunodiagnosis. As IgA is primarily released at mucosal surfaces the levels and persistence in sera are highly variable. IgE plays an important role in parasitic infections but has little role in the control of other infectious agents.

In terms of sensitivity and specificity in immunodiagnostics, several important terms and how they are applied should be remembered. In addition to the traditional meaning of the term, *sensitivity*, in reference to immunodiagnostics, may also refer to the minimum level of antigen or antibody that can be detected by a given test. Specificity may also refer to the ability of a particular assay to distinguish one antigen from another. The following sections contain a brief summary and outline of several of the most commonly used immunodiagnostic methods.

Complement Fixation

Complement refers to series of serum proteins that become activated by a variety of biologic mechanisms. One of the functions of complement includes lysis of red blood cells (RBCs) in the presence of RBC-specific antibody, which has become the basis for the complement fixation test. This assay involves incubation of test serum in the presence of a particular microbial antigen. If antibodies to that antigen are present, indicating infection, complement is activated and depleted from the sample. As a result, reaction mixtures containing RBCs as an indicator of complement activity will not be lysed, due to the depleted complement in the sample. In the event that the test sample does not contain antigen-specific antibody, complement is not depleted, and the RBCs are lysed. This particular type of diagnostic assay has some inherent problems associated with it, including the fact that it is relatively labor intensive and can lack sensitivity. In addition, other factors in the serum can activate complement nonspecifically, producing false-positive results.

Agglutination Assays

Agglutination assays involve the immobilization of a particular antigen or antigen-specific antibody on polystyrene beads or latex particles that are then mixed with a test specimen. This specimen is then examined for evidence of clumping. These reactions are typically performed in a tube or on a slide and often are measured photometrically. In addition, agglutination assays can usually be completed within 30 minutes and the antigen- or antibody-coated beads are relatively stable for long periods of time.

This particular type of assay has been especially useful in the detection of soluble antigens from sterile body fluids, such as cerebrospinal fluid, urine, and serum, especially in the case of infections due to *Haemophilus influenzae*, *Streptococcus pneumoniae*, *Neisseria meningitidis*, *Cryptococcus neoformans*, and both Groups A and B streptococci. However, they have not been developed for rapid diagnosis of viral infections because this method lacks sensitivity for this particular type of agent.

Neutralization and Hemagglutination Inhibition Assays

Both of these assay types are used primarily for viral identification. Hemagglutination inhibition is used to detect viruses containing hemaglutinin, such as the influenza virus. This assay requires a mixture of viral hemaglutinin, RBCs, and a test sample. If virus-specific antibodies are present, they react with the viral hemaglutinin, thus preventing agglutination of the RBCs. The neutralization assay is one of the most important standard techniques for the detection of cultivable viruses. Test samples are mixed with virus and subsequently incubated in the presence of a susceptible cell type. If antibodies to the particular virus are present, adsorption to the cells or another stage of viral replication will usually be blocked, resulting in a decrease in infectivity, which can then be measured.

Enzyme Immunoassay

The discovery that antibodies could be labeled with enzymes that could subsequently be used in histochemical staining procedures led to the development of enzyme immunoassays (EIAs), also known as enzyme-linked immunoabsorbent assays (ELISAs). In general, several types of EIAs are currently in use and can be divided into two broad categories: assays that detect microbial antigens and those that detect antigen-specific antibodies (Figure 8-6). Antigen detection methods are either direct or indirect, versus antibody detection methods, which are either competitive or noncompetitive. Both types of EIAs typically use a solid-phase (e.g., microtiter plates, tubes, beads, or nitrocellulose membranes) to which an antigen or antibody probe is immobilized. In the direct EIA an antibody that is specific against a pathogen's antigen is attached to the solid-phase support. The patient sample is added to the test well. Next, another antigen-specific enzyme-labeled detector antibody is added, followed by a chromogenic enzyme substrate. The amount of color generated is directly proportional to the amount of antigen present in the test specimen. The indirect EIA also uses an antigen-specific antibody that binds antigen, and then the specific, unlabeled detector antibody is added. However, instead of the chromogenic enzyme, another antibody directed against the detector antibody is added. This antiglobulin antibody is enzyme-labeled. Once the chromogenic enzyme substrate is added, a color change will occur if the antigen in question is present in the test sample. Again the amount of color is proportional to the amount of antigen present. As with fluorescent

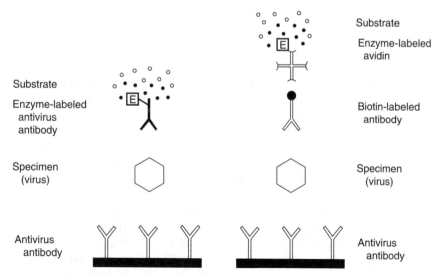

FIGURE 8-6   Enzyme immunoassays (EIA or ELISA) for detection of virus and/or viral antigen. Left: Direct. Right: Avidin–biotin.
Source: D.O. White and F.J. Fenner, Medical Virology, 4th edition, p. 197, © 1994, Academic Press, Inc.

microscopy the antiglobulin antibody, because it binds to multiple epitopes of the detector antibody, amplifies the signal and makes the test more sensitive than the direct methods.

Antibody detection is achieved largely through the use of competitive or noncompetitive EIAs. The noncompetitive EIA uses a solid support onto which the antigen has been fixed. The patient sample is added to the well and antibodies specific to the antigen will bind. The solid support is washed so that only bound antibodies remain. Next, an enzyme-labeled antiglobulin directed against the class of antibody is added, along with a chromogenic enzyme substrate. The amount of color produced is directly proportional to the amount of specific antibody present in the test specimen. The competitive version of this assay differs slightly, in that the test specimen is added simultaneously with an enzyme-labeled antibody specific for the antigen bound to the solid support. This is followed by the addition of a chromogenic enzyme substrate. High levels of antibody in the test specimen will compete for antigen with the enzyme-labeled antibody; thus, the amount of color produced is inversely proportional to the amount of antigen-specific antibody present in the test sample.

Radioimmunoassay

Radioimmunoassay, or RIA, is a technique similar to EIA. However, a radioactive rather than an enzyme label is used, and specific binding is determined using a gamma- or beta-ray counter, depending on the isotope. Therein lie the disadvantages of RIA—adherence to radiation safety protocols and the restrictions that accompany working with radioactive substances. In addition, the immunoreagents used for RIAs are typically not stable for as long a period of time as those used in EIAs.

Fluorescent Antibody Techniques

Fluorescent antibody (FA) techniques have been widely used in the past for the detection of both microbial antigens and antigen-specific antibodies, and still have many applications today. Tests can be either direct or indirect. Antigen detection requires specimens that contain live virus and cannot be used to test patient serum or feces, which rarely contain virus. The microbe is grown, from a patient swab or other specimen, on glass slides and then fixed. In the direct method, a fluorescein-labeled antibody specific for a particular antigen is incubated with a test specimen fixed on a glass microscope slide. If the antigen is present in the specimen, a bright yellow–green fluorescence will be seen under a fluorescent microscope. The indirect method involves the use of a primary, unlabeled, antigen-specific antibody and a fluorescein-labeled anti-immunoglobulin specific for the primary antibody. Both are incubated with the test specimen, and results are interpreted the same as for the direct FA. Indirect fluorescent antibody techniques can also detect patient antibodies. Because antiglobulin antibodies are directed against classes of antibodies, the indirect method allows for the differentiation of IgM and IgG and is more sensitive and specific in identifying viruses, as compared with traditional cell culture. However, FA is commonly used for the detection of antibodies to *Legionella pneumophila* and serodiagnosis of several parasitic diseases, including malaria, leishmaniasis, African trypanosomiasis, pneu-mocystosis, toxoplasmosis, and schistosomiasis. It can also be used for the direct detection of antigen in clinical samples and is used in the diagnosis of respiratory syncytial virus, influenza virus type A, and parainfluenza viruses types 1 through 3.

Molecular Diagnostics

Over the past 10 years, advances in molecular biology have resulted in the application of these techniques in diagnostic microbiology. Although microscopy, culture, and phenotypic characterization remain the mainstay for microbial diagnosis, application of molecular techniques can potentially enhance the speed, sensitivity, and sometimes the specificity of diagnosis and identification of etiologic agents. A variety of molecular techniques has evolved from initial hybridization and nucleic acid probes, including signal amplification, target amplification, and postamplification technologies.

The underlying principle of nucleic acid probe technology is the selec-tion of unique genomic sequences for a particular group of etiologic agents or specific genes with subsequent cloning, synthesis, and utilization. Probes can hybridize with either DNA or RNA with high specificity to complemen-tary sequences of the target nucleic acid. Hybridization is detected by label-ing the probe with radioisotopes, enzymes, antigens, or chemoluminescent compounds that can be measured through instrumentation specific for the label. Three nucleic acid probe hybridization methods have evolved: liquid-phase, solid-phase, and in situ hybridization; for liquid-phase hybridization, a single-stranded probe that does not hybridize to itself is utilized. The most common method used in diagnostics is the hybridization protection assay. A labeled probe is mixed with the potential target and subjected to alkaline hydrolysis. The signal molecule is protected from hydrolysis, if hybridized, and is detected directly in the liquid specimens. In solid-phase hybridization, nucleic acid-bound nylon membranes or nitrocellulose are hybridized with the nucleic acid probe. Unbound probe is washed off, and hybridization can be detected using any of the signal systems mentioned earlier. In situ hybrid-ization utilizes tissue or whole cells fixed to microscope slides. Probes are hybridized targets in the cells, using the same principles employed in solid-phase hybridization. The sensitivity of this method is limited by penetration of the probe into the cell, but does have the advantage of visualization by microscopy of the location and cell type in which hybridization is occurring. Nucleic acid probes have been used successfully for the detection of fastidious, slow-growing, or nonculturable organisms and antibiotic resistance genes, as well as for identification of phenotypically difficult microorganisms.

Signal amplification methods are designed to increase the signaling capac-ity of the hybridization reaction of a probe to its target through an increase in the concentration of the label. Signal amplification methods increase the amount of signal generated by a fixed amount of probe/target hybrid. These methods do not increase the amount of target the way amplification methods do. Therefore, these methods are less susceptible to contamination than target amplification but are comparatively limited in sensitivity. Two examples of signal amplification techniques are a solution hybridization antibody capture assay that uses chemiluminescent detection and the branched DNA (bDNA) probe assay. The former utilizes RNA probes that hybridize with DNA target sequences to form an RNA–DNA hybrid. These hybrids are captured on a solid surface by attached antibodies specific for RNA–DNA hybrids. The immobilized hybrids are then reacted with another enzyme-conjugated antibody specific for the hybrids. Signal amplification occurs through multiple antibody binding to the hybrid, with detection through the addition of a chemiluminescent substrate. The branched DNA probe technique uses a branched multiple probe–enzyme complex. This system utilizes three probes for detection of a primary probe (target-specific), a branched secondary probe, and a short enzyme-labeled tertiary probe. The primary probes are used to capture target on a solid surface. Branched oligonucleotide probes (bDNA amplifiers) specific for the hybridized primary probe are added, followed by the short enzyme-labeled tertiary probes. Chemiluminescent substrate is then added, and the signal can be quantitated.

The polymerase chain reaction (PCR) has in many ways revolutionized diagnostic microbiology. As the first amplification technology, it has been developed for the widest number of applications. Other target amplification systems that have been developed but are not yet as widely used include: transcription-mediated amplification (TMA) and similar methodologies, and strand displacement amplification (SDA). As a target amplification method, PCR is based on the ability of DNA polymerase to copy a strand of DNA when two primers (oligonucleotides) bind to complementary strands of target DNA. The enzyme initiates elongation at the 3′ end of a primer bound to the target strand of DNA. The sequence between the two specific primers is amplified exponentially with each cycle of PCR. A cycle consists of three steps:

1. A DNA denaturation step, in which the double-stranded target DNA is separated into single strands.
2. Primers anneal or bind to their complementary target sequences at a lowered temperature.
3. DNA polymerase synthesizes or extends the target sequences between the primers.

With each cycle, the PCR product or target sequences are doubled. The reaction is performed in a programmable thermal cycler, usually with 30–50 cycles, resulting in amplification of <100 copies of target sequence to a detectable level. There has been a variety of adaptations to PCR, which include:

- RT–PCR, developed to amplify RNA targets through the initial use of the enzyme reverse transcriptase for conversion of the RNA target to cDNA
- Nested PCR, designed primarily to increase sensitivity through the use of two primer sets directed at the same target, one set within the other
- Multiplex PCR, in which two or more sets of primers specific for different targets are utilized in the same reaction

Other technologies for target amplification include transcription-mediated amplification systems and strand-displacement amplification. In addition to target amplification, two systems, QB replicase (QBR) and the DNA ligase reaction, are based on amplification of a probe.

The application of molecular technology to the diagnosis of infectious disease has enhanced the speed, sensitivity, and specificity of microbial diagnosis. Although improving the ability to make some diagnoses, these techniques are currently more research tools than standard clinical diagnostic tools. Although significant strides have been made, false positives from contamination or false negatives from a failure of the process are possible. Unlike culture systems, which are able to detect multiple pathogens, molecular tests are intended to only identify one pathogen. For the detection of more than one pathogen, additional tests have to be performed. The cost of molecular diagnostics is also higher than traditional culture. However, molecular techniques are warranted in situations where currently available culture techniques are unable to recover or grow the organism in vitro, or instances where current methods are too insensitive, too costly, or too time consuming. The reader is referred to Chapter 9 for a more detailed description of molecular techniques and their utility in infectious disease epidemiology.

Suggested Reading

Ajello L, Hay RJ. Medical mycology. In: Collier L, Balows A, Sussman M, eds. *Topley and Wilson's Microbiology and Microbial Infections.* 9th ed. Vol. 4. New York, NY: Oxford University Press; 1998.

Baron EJ, Chang RS, Howard DH, Miller JN, Turner JA. *Medical Microbiology: A Short Course.* New York, NY: Wiley-Liss; 1994.

Barrett JT. *Microbiology and Immunology Concepts.* Philadelphia, Pa: Lippincott-Raven Publishers; 1998.

Flint SJ, Enquist LW, Krug RM, Racaniello VR, Skalka AM. *Virology, Molecular Biology, Pathogenesis, and Control.* Washington, DC: American Society of Microbiology (ASM) Press; 2000.

Garcia LS, Bruckner DA. *Diagnostic Medical Parasitology.* 3rd ed. Washington, DC: ASM Press; 1997.

Mandell GL, Bennett JE, Dolin R. *Principles and Practice of Infectious Diseases.* 5th ed. Philadelphia, Pa: Churchill Livingstone; 2000.

Murray PR, Baron EJ, Pfaller MA, Tenover FC, Yolken RH. *Manual of Clinical Microbiology.* 7th ed. Washington, DC: ASM Press; 1999.

Mims CA. *The Pathogenesis of Infectious Disease.* 3rd ed. Orlando, Fla: Academic Press; 1987.

Nelson KE, Kaufman L, Cooper CR, Merz WG. Penicillium mannettei: biology and infections with this emerging fungal pathogen. *Infect Med.* 1999;16:118–121.

Salyers AA, Whitt DD. *Bacterial Pathogenesis: A Molecular Approach.* Washington, DC: ASM Press; 1994.

Schaechter M, Medoff G, Esenstein BI. *Mechanisms of Microbial Disease.* 2nd ed. Baltimore, Md: Williams & Wilkins; 1993.

Volk WA, Gebhardt BM, Hammarskjold M-L, Kadner RJ. *Essentials of Medical Microbiology.* 5th ed. Philadelphia, Pa: Lippincott-Raven Publishers; 1996.

CHAPTER NINE

MOLECULAR EPIDEMIOLOGY AND INFECTIOUS DISEASES

John S. Francis, Susan M. Harrington, Karen C. Carroll, and William R. Bishai

Introduction

The past 20 years have seen significant advances in the ability of the clinical microbiologist to identify substrains of bacterial pathogens and use this information to track infectious diseases. Most strain typing has focused on bacteria, but fungi and viruses can also be typed. Medical diagnostic evaluations for a particular infectious disease usually end with identification of pathogens to their species; most clinical microbiology laboratories do not routinely identify organisms to the substrain level. For example, strains of *Staphylococcus aureus*, implicated in many hospital-acquired (or nosocomial) infections, are identified to the species level, but are not routinely evaluated for evidence of belonging to a particular type. Similarly, *Haemophilus influenzae* isolates can be identified by serotype, as well as by species. However, the subtyping is not part of a routine microbiology culture result. Serotyping is generally only performed to rule out serotype B infection in children.

Strain typing is used to determine how close isolates of the same species are related to one another. When isolates from different patients are related or identical to one another, it may indicate a common source of the infection. This information is useful to epidemiologists who are responsible for tracking communicable diseases within a health care institution or a community. Such information helps them to identify point sources and transmission patterns of infections so that appropriate interventions may be applied.

Likewise, when isolates are found to differ by subspecies analysis, it suggests a different source of infection. Hence, if two people are diagnosed with tuberculosis in the same community at the same time, differences by strain typing indicate that the individuals are highly unlikely to have passed the infection between them.

In short, the goal of strain typing is to distinguish epidemiologically related isolates from those which are unrelated, based on the premise that related isolates share detectable characteristics that will distinguish them from others. Established criteria for evaluation of typing systems include typeability, reproducibility, ease of both interpretation and performance. As with other kinds of epidemiological investigations, control strains known to be unlinked epidemiologically must be included in a subtyping analysis. A typing system must be able to delineate control strains from those thought to be part of an outbreak or cluster. The ability of a typing method to distinguish epidemiologically related isolates from epidemiologically unrelated isolates is termed "discriminatory power." It is important to mention that, although strain typing is a very powerful tool for the epidemiologist, it should be done with clear goals in mind and should be used to enhance a sound epidemiologic investigation.

Application of Typing Techniques

Strain typing systems are widely used to characterize bacteria, fungi, and, more rarely, viruses. Many applications for typing methods exist. Some example applications include studying the relationships between colonizing and infecting strains, documenting nosocomial transmission, distinguishing relapse from reinfection, establishing clonality of isolates within clusters of patients in the hospital or community, and tracking spread of isolates between hospitals or communities over time.[1]

Often the laboratory is asked to subtype isolates when an epidemiologist notices increased disease associated with a specific pathogen or increased isolation of a microbe on routine surveillance of microbiology culture results. For example, during a 6-year period an increased incidence of pediatric empyema was noted at a Children's Medical Center in Salt Lake City associated with infection due to *Streptococcus pneumoniae*. Each pneumococcal strain was determined to be serotype 1 and pulsed-field gel electrophoresis indicated that the isolates were indistinguishable or closely related, supporting clonal spread.[2] Sometimes a relatively rare organism recovered over a short period of time from patients not obviously linked epidemiologically may be an indication of disease transmission. Three cases of *Listeria monocytogenes* bacteremia, noted in two departments in the same hospital within a 2-week time period, led investigators to suspect a common source of contamination. Molecular typing quickly determined the isolates to be distinct and no further investigation was indicated.[3] As part of a prospective study of tuberculosis transmission in Baltimore, two patients whose only link was the hospital wherein they were treated were found to have the same *Mycobacterium tuberculosis* subtype. Upon further examination, the second patient was thought to have acquired tuberculosis from a contaminated bronchoscope that had been used on the other patient 2 days earlier.[4]

Reports of unusual pathogens (e.g., those with rare antimicrobial resistance patterns or unexpected isolates from environmental sources) alert microbiologists and epidemiologists to potential outbreaks. Molecular analysis of plasmid DNA has been found useful in demonstrating clonality of a relatively rare strain of chloramphenicol-resistant *Salmonella* in California. The Los Angeles County Health Department Laboratory noticed a 4.9 times increase in this species; 87% were chloramphenical-resistant. A case-control study showed the illness to be associated with consumption of ground beef derived from feedlots using antibiotics in cattle. The strain was further linked to contaminated beef, slaughterhouses, and dairy farms.[5] Use of polymerase chain reaction and DNA sequencing was essential in identifying monkeypox (usually isolated in Africa) during an outbreak in the midwestern United States associated with individuals who had contact with pet prairie dogs exposed to an ill Gambian giant rat.[6] These molecular epidemiology-based techniques were also useful in the detection of a novel coronavirus as the causative agent of severe acute respiratory syndrome (SARS) during a worldwide outbreak originating from a single health care worker in China.[7,8]

Strain typing techniques are now used for other clinical applications as well. To determine if isolates of the same genus and species cultured from a patient weeks or months apart represent reinfection with a new strain or recrudescence of a previous infection, they might be typed by molecular methods. In one report, an immunocompromised child had episodes of bacteremia 4 months apart with the same uncommon gram-negative bacterium, *Flavobacterium meningosepticum*. Molecular analysis by pulsed-field gel electrophoresis (PFGE) showed the isolates to be indistinguishable. The two episodes of sepsis likely resulted from an indwelling central catheter that harbored small numbers of organisms.[9] In another example, 1 year after having been adequately treated for an *M. tuberculosis* infection, a patient with human immunodeficiency virus (HIV) was again found to have active disease. Was the therapy inadequate or had the patient been reinfected? Molecular studies showed the second strain recovered to be the same as the first, except for a mutation rendering it resistant to rifampin. The strain was presumed to have become resistant in vivo during rifabutin prophylaxis to prevent infection with *Mycobacterium avium*. Hence, molecular analysis proved reactivation of disease with a new antibiotic resistance in the patient's original strain.[10]

Additionally, molecular techniques may be used to determine if multiple blood cultures drawn over 1 or more days yielding coagulase-negative staphylococci or other skin flora represent a true bacteremia or culture contamination. Multiple strains isolated from a true bacteremia generally have the same molecular type, whereas skin contamination will likely produce heterogeneous strains.[11,12]

Finally, as important pathogens such as *S. aureus* and *S. pneumoniae* evolve, acquiring new antimicrobial resistance genes, or as new microbial pathogens emerge, molecular typing techniques can be used to investigate these strains within the health care environment and community at large.

Definitions and Background

Throughout this chapter, vocabulary known to the microbiologist and molecular biologist will be used. To create a framework for the reader, some basic concepts with respect to strain relatedness will be defined. Strain typing methods that preceded molecular techniques will be discussed. An overview of microbial nucleic acids and ways in which the genetic content of a microbe can vary will be given. The laboratory techniques used to detect genetic change will also be explained in this section before specific molecular typing methods are presented.

Relevant Concepts and Conventional Strain Typing Methods

An *isolate* refers to the bacterium or other microbe recovered from a primary microbiology culture. Typically, an isolate is characterized only by its source and its genus and species. The word *strain* is applied after some further testing is performed. Isolates may be grouped as a single strain based upon characteristics they have in common. They can be considered unique strains if the typing technique distinguishes them from other strain types tested. *Clones* are isolates that have been derived from the same parent strain. Strains are considered clones if they are indistinguishable from one another. Although progeny strains are produced from indistinguishable isolates, normally occurring genetic mutations will cause them to diverge gradually. Therefore, after multiple generations, daughter strains may no longer be identical, but will likely be clonally related.

Relationships among strains are to some extent relative. They may depend on which test is used for characterization. Different techniques provide information about different aspects of the organism. Also, isolates may be related to varying degrees depending on the amount of mutation within a species and the number of generations between the isolates.[13]

Before the advances in molecular biology of the past 20–30 years, the techniques used to characterize microorganisms were based on their phenotypic characteristics. The phenotype of an organism is derived from the expression of the genetic material. Biotyping, antimicrobial susceptibility patterns, serotyping, phage typing, bacteriocin typing, and protein-based methods are all examples of phenotypic tests. Each of these measures varies within a species and each has observable properties. Although more discriminatory molecular methods have replaced these for accurate strain typing, the information provided by phenotypic results should not be minimized.

As part of the speciation of bacteria and yeasts, organisms are tested for the expression of various metabolic functions such as biochemical reactions and growth under selected environmental conditions. The results produced in these tests provide characteristic patterns for identification, and they are referred to as the "biotype." Sometimes isolates of a particular species will be observed with an unusual biochemical marker distinguishing them from other strains of that species. However, biotyping is usually not a sensitive indicator of strain differences.

As bacteria are speciated, the clinical laboratory performs susceptibility testing of that microbe to a panel of antibiotics appropriate for therapy. The susceptibility results are reported as susceptible, intermediate, or resistant to each antibiotic. The susceptibility of the organism to the panel of antibiotics is termed the "antibiogram." Two isolates found to have the same atypical antibiogram may be an early indicator that clonal dissemination is occurring. For highly resistant nosocomial species, such as vancomycin-resistant enterococci (VRE) or methicillin-resistant *S. aureus* (MRSA), antibiograms are of limited use because few changes will be seen in the susceptibilty profile between isolates. Isolates with vastly different antibiograms are most likely unrelated. Sometimes two antibiograms may differ by only one or a few antibiotic susceptibilities. Strains producing such patterns may be clonally related. Bacteria can become antibiotic resistant depending on the selective pressure of antibiotics in the environment or the presence of other resistant species that can transfer resistance genes. Conversely, organisms can also lose antibiotic resistance genes carried on extra-chromosomal DNA called plasmids. Overall, antibiograms provide highly standardized, prospective data and are an excellent place to start in making strain comparisons.

Some bacteria can be differentiated by serotype. Antigenic determinants (e.g., cell surface carbohydrates, membrane proteins, and lipopolysaccharides) are variable and can be detected with specific antibodies. Serotyping continues to be a useful method for species such as *Haemophilus influenzae*, *S. pneumoniae*, *Neisseria meningitidis*, *Salmonella* and *Shigella* species, *Escherichia coli*, and some viruses. Not only can serotyping differentiate strains, but certain serotypes are markers of virulence. For example, *H. influenzae* type B causes severe invasive disease and *E. coli* O157:H7 can cause hemolytic uremic syndrome. Influenza viruses can be typed to determine which hemagglutinin (H) and neuraminidase (N) serotypes are circulating, for inclusion in yearly vaccine development. Serotyping, however, is limited as an epidemiologic typing method, because the discriminatory power is less than other, molecular methods. Additionally, serotyping can be expensive and is useful for only a limited number of organisms for which antisera have been developed.[14]

Bacteriophage typing had long been the standard typing method for *S. aureus*. A bacteriophage is a viral particle that is capable of infecting bacterial cells and causing cell lysis. The isolates to be typed can be tested for susceptibility to a panel of different bacteriophages to produce a pattern known as the "phage type." This method, however, is technically demanding and requires stock strains of bacteriophages, which are generally available only in reference laboratories. Bacteriocin testing is similar to phage typing. A bacteriocin is a toxin to which a bacterium may be susceptible. Strains to be typed are tested with a set of bacteriocins to achieve a bacteriocin profile. As with phage typing, this method is expensive and technically difficult.[14]

The presence, size, and function of proteins can be used to distinguish strains of bacteria. Proteins can be isolated from whole cell preparations or from cell wall fractions. Sodium dodecyl sulfate–polyacrylamide gel electrophoresis (SDS–PAGE) is then used to separate the protein extracts based on molecular mass. Protein bands can be visualized with radioactive labels, by stain, or by the Western immunoblotting technique. For the latter method, the proteins in the gel are transferred to a nitrocellulose membrane. Antibody is added, which will bind to specific proteins of interest on the membrane. The first antibody is detected with a second conjugated antibody that gives a signal with an enzyme–substrate system.[15] A drawback of this method is the numerous bands that are often detected, making interpretation difficult. Electrophoretic protein typing is rarely used for outbreak investigations today.

A second protein-based method is multilocus enzyme electrophoresis (MLEE). Extracts containing metabolic enzymes from the bacteria are separated by electrophoresis in starch gels. The location for each enzyme in the gel is detected with a colorimetric substrate specific to that enzyme. Because the electrophoretic mobility of the enzymes depends on their exact amino acid content, it is strain specific. Evaluated as a profile, the electrophoretic mobilities or isoenzyme patterns are referred to as an "electrophoretic type." Moderately discriminatory, this technique is not in widespread use because it is technically demanding.[15]

As with all living forms, microbes are composed of nucleic acid, protein, lipid, and carbohydrate. Methods exist for identifying intraspecies differences for each of these four categories, some of which have been discussed above. However, in the last two decades, methods based upon the presence, size, and sequence of nucleic acids have come to predominate in the field of molecular epidemiology. These methods are referred to as "genotypic" because they are based on the genetic content of the microbe.

The Basics of Microbial Nucleic Acids and Mutational Change

The primary location of the genetic content of a microorganism is its chromosome. Bacteria are classified as prokaryotes, and they generally contain a single, circular chromosome comprised of double-stranded DNA (dsDNA). Fungi are eukaryotes and carry multiple linear chromosomes. An understanding of the components of DNA is essential to the basic theory of molecular epidemiology. All dsDNA has two complementary strands, which pair by hydrogen bonding. A sugar–phosphate backbone and the nucleotide bases adenine (A), guanine (G), thymidine (T), and cytosine (C) comprise each strand. Adenine pairs with thymidine and guanine with cytosine. It is the order or sequence of these base pairings that determines the genetic content. Molecular biologists measure chromosomes, specific genes, or other DNA fragments by their length in base pairs (bp). In fact, many genome-sequencing projects have been completed, allowing for the determination of the number of base pairs in the chromosome, and complete DNA sequence for these species. On average, bacterial chromosomes range in size from 800 kilobases (kb) to 10,000 kb. In addition to the chromosome, there may be extra-chromosomal segments of DNA known as episomes or plasmids. Such DNA elements usually range in size from 1 to 200 kb. The organism's total genetic content (i.e., chromosomal and episomal DNA together) is referred to as the genome. Molecular epidemiologists determine strain relatedness by detecting changes in the genome. Several ways exist in which variations in the genetic content of a bacterium can occur (Exhibit 9-1).

> **Mutations in chromosomal DNA**
> - DNA point mutations
> - DNA insertions
> - DNA deletions
> - DNA rearrangements
>
> **Mobile genetic elements**
> - Insertion sequences
> - Transposons
> - Conjugative plasmids
> - Lysogenic phages
>
> **Excessory genetic material**
> - Multicopy plasmids
> - Single copy plasmids
> - Accessory chromosomes

Exhibit 9-1 Types of alterations in DNA that can be detected by molecular epidemiology.

Mutational Changes

Mutations are mistakes in copying the DNA of a parent bacterial strain during the replication process. The basal mutation rate for most bacterial species is about one error in 10^8 bp per generation. Hence, in an organism that has a genome size of 10^7 bp, a base pair replication error will be made once every 10 generations. Two general types of mutations are seen: (1) the substitution of one base for another is a point mutation; and (2) rearrangements of fragments of DNA including insertions or deletions from the chromosome. Substitutions are further divided into two classes: synonymous and nonsynonymous single nucleotide polymorphisms (sSNPs and nsSNPs, respectively). sSNPs do not alter the amino acid sequence of a protein; however, nsSNPs lead to an amino acid replacement.[16] Most mutations are inconsequential or silent (i.e., they do not lead to physiologic or functional changes in the mutated progeny cell). In organisms that replicate quickly and are present in large environmental reservoirs, significant genetic drift is observed. If the basal rate of genetic replication errors is assumed to be constant, then the more genetic differences between two isolates of the same species, the more time has passed since the two originated from a common ancestor. Hence, it is possible to identify numerous changes of subspecies of most bacterial organisms, and to estimate the distance in evolutionary time between isolates.

Mobile Genetic Elements

Most bacterial species contain mobile genetic elements that create variability in the genome. These pieces of DNA are referred to as "jumping genes" because they are capable of moving themselves around the chromosome. A common type of mobile genetic element is the transposon. Duplicative transposons are capable of copying themselves and inserting a second copy at another site within the bacterial chromosome. Mobile genetic elements, such as transposons, lead to more easily detectable changes in the bacterial chromosome than point mutations resulting from the basal rate of mutation. Later in this chapter we will review how transposable elements may be used as part of a strain typing system.

Plasmids

Finally, accessory genetic elements can be used to identify differences between species. In addition to the chromosome, many species contain small, circular pieces of self-replicating DNA known as plasmids, which are present in single or multiple copies in the cytoplasm of the bacterial cell. Often these plasmids are nonessential and may come and go over time within a particular bacterial subpopulation. Some plasmids, however, carry elements that code for functional genes (e.g., metabolic enzymes, virulence factors, or antibiotic resistance). Antibiotic use can create selective pressure to maintain a plasmid. Likewise, absence of antibiotic can lead to loss of plasmids. Plasmids carried by a species (and their type and size) may be useful in identifying subspecies of the same strain.

Molecular Biology Tools Available to the Molecular Epidemiologist

Some understanding of molecular biology laboratory techniques will be useful before the discussion of specific typing methods is presented. The next section is a brief overview of selected "tools." The reader is referred to *Molecular Cloning: A Laboratory Manual*[17] or *Molecular Microbiology: Diagnostic Principles and Practice*[18] for more detail on specific procedures.

Restriction Endonucleases

Restriction endonucleases or restriction enzymes are "workhorses" for strain identification techniques. These are enzymes that scan dsDNA searching for specific sequences. When a specific recognition sequence innate to the restriction enzyme is found, the enzyme cleaves the dsDNA. Table 9-1 shows several restriction enzymes and the sequences at which they cut.

In addition to having different recognition site sequence specificities, restriction endonucleases also have different restriction site length specificities. This information is illustrated in Table 9-1, which shows restriction enzyme *Hae*III and *Sau*3AI. Both of these are four base pair recognition endonucleases, which are sometimes called four-base cutters. Table 9-1 also shows six-base cutters, *Eco*RI and *Hind*III, as well as two 8-base cutters, *Pac*I and *Not*I.

As also shown in Table 9-1, four-base cutters will cleave DNA much more frequently than do six- or eight-base cutters. In DNA that is evenly distributed in its AT and GC content (50:50) a four-base cutter will be expected to cleave every 256 bp on average, whereas a six-base cutter every 4096 and an eight-base cutter every 65,530 bp. Hence, four-base cutters or "frequent-cutters" cleave chromosomal DNA into many small pieces distributed around 250 bp, whereas six-base cutters cleave DNA into a moderate number of intermediate-size fragments of approximately 4000 bp, and finally

TABLE 9-1 Some Common Restriction Endonucleases and Their Recognition Site Specificities

Restriction Enzyme	Recognition Sequence	Base Pairs Recognized (N)	Approximate Frequency of Cutting (bp)
*Hae*III	5′—GG↓CC—3′ 3′—CC↑GG—5′	4	256
*Sau*3AI	5′—↓GATC—3′ 3′—CTAG↑—5′	4	256
*Eco*RI	5′—G↓AATTC—3′ 3′—CTTAA↑G—5′	6	4,096
*Hind*III	5′—A↓AGCTT—3′ 3′—TTCGA↑A—5′	6	4,096
*Pac*I	5′—TTAAT↓TAA—3′ 3′—AAT↑TAATT—5′	8	65,530
*Not*I	5′—GC↓GGCCGC—3′ 3′—CGCCGG↑CG—5′	8	65,530

Note: Arrows indicate the place in the DNA sequence where cutting occurs.

eight-base cutters or "infrequent-cutters" create very large fragments of approximately 65,000 bp in size.

In addition, the frequency of cutting is not only dependent upon the number of bases in the recognition site but is also dependent on the percent GC and percent AT of the organism. If a bacterial species is GC rich, a restriction endonuclease whose recognition site is biased toward AT will be an infrequent cutter and a restriction endonuclease whose recognition site has a heavy GC content will be much more common than expected. A good example of this occurs in *M. tuberculosis*, which is 67% GC and 33% AT in its DNA content. The eight-base cutter *PacI*, which recognizes the AT-rich sequence TTAATTAA is expected to cut DNA, containing equal amounts of AT and GC base pairs about every 65,537 bp. However, because of the heavy GC content of *M. tuberculosis* DNA, *PacI* fails to cut even once within its 4.7 million bp.

If a mutation has occurred at a restriction endonuclease site, the alteration of bases will prevent the enzyme from cutting. This is illustrated in Table 9-2, where a change from an AT base pair to a CG base pair in an *Eco*RI restriction site destroys the recognition sequence and prevents *Eco*RI cleavage. Likewise, insertion or deletion of DNA may lead to the creation or elimination of a restriction site. The use of restriction enzymes is fundamental to many molecular typing tests. Isolates that are clones will have the same DNA base sequence and, therefore, share the same spacing of restriction sites.

When the chromosome of a microbe is cut with a restriction enzyme, many DNA fragments of a variety of lengths are produced according to the spacing of the restriction enzyme recognition sites for that restriction endonuclease. Base mutations (insertions, deletions, or point mutations) that alter restriction enzyme recognition sites will change the number and size of some of the restriction fragments. Also, nucleotides inserted or deleted between restriction sites will alter the length of restriction fragments.

Changes in the genome sequence (which may be detected by altered patterns of restriction enzyme cleavage) are called "polymorphisms." *Restriction fragment length polymorphism (RFLP)* refers to variations in the lengths of restriction fragments; different RFLP patterns indicate genetic differences between strains and suggest that the strains are not clonal. Figure 9-1 is a schematic diagram of the bacterial chromosome illustrating this principle. Organisms 1 and 2 are clones and, therefore, have an identical restriction site distribution as depicted by the lines cutting the circular chromosome. Organ-

TABLE 9-2   Sequence Recognized by Restriction Enzyme *Eco*RI

5′—G↓AATTC—3′ 3′—CTTAA↑G-5′	Recognition sequence for *Eco*RI. **Arrows** indicate site of enzyme cleavage.
5′—GCATTC—3′ 3′—CGTAAG—5′	A point mutation occurs. AT base pair changed to CG. Restriction site specificity is lost.
5′—G**AAGC**AATTC—3′ 3′—C**TTCG**TTAAG—5′	A DNA insertion occurs. Addition of four base pairs. Restriction site specificity is lost.

Note: Point mutations or DNA insertions or deletions cause loss of restriction specificity as shown.

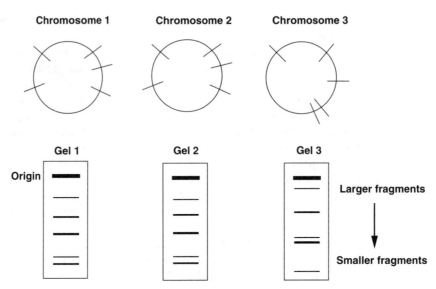

FIGURE 9-1   Restriction fragment length polymorphism of three bacterial chromosomes. Lines on circles indicate sites for cutting with a restriction enzyme. Organisms 1 and 2 share restriction endonuclease sites and, therefore, have identical banding patterns on gel electrophoresis as depicted. Bacterium 3 has different restriction sites. The fingerprint for organism 3 is different from the other two.

ism 3 is unrelated and has a different restriction site pattern. The differences between organisms may be visualized by separating the fragments resulting from restriction enzyme digestion by gel electrophoresis. Nucleic acid probes and Southern hybridization can also be used to identify specific restriction fragment differences. Only restriction fragments with specificity for the probe are detected (highlighted bands on Figure 9-1). Southern hybridization using a DNA probe to a region known to be highly variable is an efficient, sensitive way of detecting RFLPs.

Gel Electrophoresis

A technique known as gel electrophoresis is used to separate DNA molecules. Agarose gels are formed with wells into which small amounts of solutions containing DNA are placed. Agarose is a polysaccharide derived from seaweed, which forms a large matrix through which DNA fragments must migrate. DNA is negatively charged and, when a positive electrode is placed at the distal end of the gel and a negative electrode at the proximal end, the DNA migrates in a lane toward the positive charge (Figure 9-2). Usually, this migration occurs on the basis of size; small fragments run more rapidly than large fragments. After the separation under an electric charge, the gel is removed from the electrophoresis apparatus and stained using a variety of intercalating fluorescent chemicals such as ethidium bromide, which enables visualization of the DNA bands. Cameras attached to computer systems capture gel images and store or print these files. A molecular weight marker or size standard is always run on the same gel to determine DNA band size.

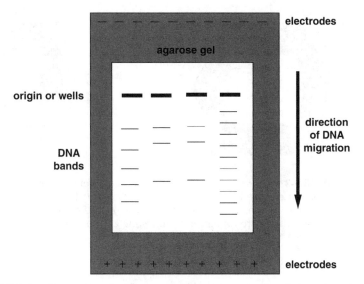

FIGURE 9-2 Conventional agarose gel electrophoresis. Fourth lane from left indicates molecular weight marker.
Source: Copyright © 2000, Susan M. Harrington.

Standard agarose gel electrophoresis enables the separation of fragments of DNA ranging from 50 bp to about 15,000 bp. Beyond 15,000 bp, the DNA molecules are too large to fit easily through the agrose gel matrix and the fragments fail to migrate proportionally to their size. Thus, segments greater than 15,000 bp tend to accumulate at the origin of the agarose gel.

A modification of standard agarose gel electorphoresis is pulsed-field gel electrophoresis (PFGE). PFGE is an adaptation that enables large fragments of DNA ranging from 10,000 bp to 5 million bp to be separated on the basis of size. The technique uses standard agarose gels; however, the electric field in which the DNA migrates is not applied in only one direction as in conventional electrophoresis. PFGE utilizes alternating electric fields, in which the current is applied for varying lengths of time in each direction, depending on the size of fragments to be separated. Several electrode configurations have been used by investigators, the most popular system is the contour-clamped homogeneous electric field (CHEF). The CHEF apparatus consists of a hexagonal array of electrodes producing two electric fields at 120° angles to one another (Figure 9-3). The length of time that the current is applied in each direction is referred to as the "switch time" or "pulse time." Larger DNA molecules require longer pulse times and smaller fragments are separated adequately with shorter pulse times. PFGE can be used to separate the fragments created by restriction endonuclease digestion of bacterial or fungal genomic DNA. Such digestion generally yields approximately 10 to 20 bands that have a range of fragment sizes. The array of small, medium, and large size fragments is separated by "ramping" the pulse time. With ramping, the pulse time is increased incrementally from just a few seconds up to several minutes over the course of the run.[19] Most users of PFGE purchase CHEF equipment, which can perform these intricate electrical switches with

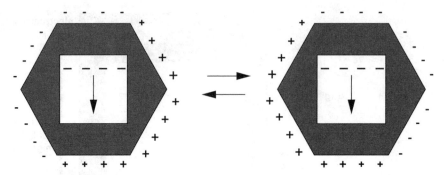

FIGURE 9-3 Schematic diagram of pulsed-field gel electrophoresis (PFGE) by the contour-clamped homogeneous electric fields (CHEF) technique. Alternation of current is shown. The figure on the left indicates current from northwest to southeast. The figure on the right shows the current from northeast to southwest. *Source:* Copyright © 2000, Susan M. Harrington.

little programming by the operator. However, such CHEF equipment can be expensive.

Handling pieces of DNA that are large requires great care because such DNA fragments are fragile. For PFGE, DNA is extracted from cells that have been immobilized in agarose so that the DNA is not broken by agitation, vibration, or excessive pipetting.

Hybridization and Nucleic Acid Probes

Hybridization refers to the pairing or annealing of nucleic acid, both RNA and DNA, to complementary nucleic acid strands. Because of the rules of base pairing (A pairs with T and C pairs with G), single strands of nucleic acid will anneal or hybridize to complementary strands that have the correct sequence of matching base pairs in order to form a complete set of Watson–Crick pairs. Nucleic acid probe technology is based on the principle of hybridization. Sequences derived from specific genes or other DNA sequences can be used as probes to find places in the genome where their complementary sequences occur. The probe anneals to the genomic target sequences creating new, hybrid dsDNA.

In the process of Southern hybridization, target DNA, which has been digested with a restriction enzyme, is separated by size with agarose gel electrophoresis. The DNA bands are transferred by capillary action or "blotted" onto a nylon or nitrocellulose membrane and immobilized so that they will not come off even in liquid solutions (Figure 9-4A). The target DNA, now on the membrane, is chemically treated to permit access to probe DNA. Probe DNA is then added and hybridization is allowed to occur at the appropriate temperature. The probe DNA seeks out sequences that are complementary to it, and anneals to the target DNA bands immobilized on the membrane. Probe DNA is typically labeled with a radioisotope, or a fluorescent or chemiluminescent substrate. Following hybridization, the membrane is used to expose X-ray film (for radioisotope labeled DNA) or treated with appropriate reagents (for fluorescent or chemiluminescent labeled DNA) to develop the indicator on the probe. This permits visualization of the target bands among all the bands on the membrane (Figure 9-4).

Polymerase Chain Reaction

Polymerase chain reaction (PCR) is a tool used to amplify short sequences from among a diverse DNA pool such as a bacterial chromosome. The DNA length limits of PCR are sequences approximately 10,000 bp long; beyond this, amplification methods fail and other techniques are necessary to obtain large quantities of longer pieces of DNA. In a standard PCR reaction, two specific oligonucleotide primers are mixed with template DNA. Oligonucleotides are very short segments of DNA, typically 15 to 30 bp in length. The template is the DNA that contains the sequences to be amplified. Template DNA is generated by lysing bacteria, fungi, or viral particles to release their respective genome. The oligonucleotides are chosen based on the target

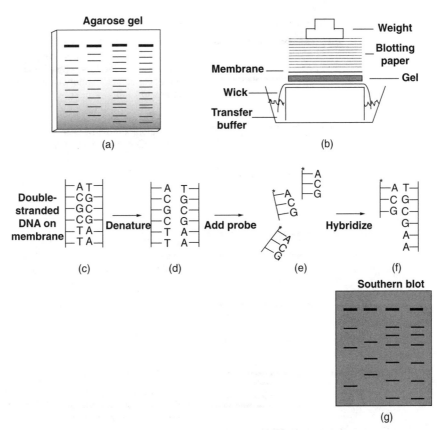

FIGURE 9-4   (a) Agarose gel electrophoresis. (b) Southern transfer of DNA from agarose gel to nylon membrane, steps involved in hybridization of probe DNA to target DNA on nylon membrane. Double-stranded DNA (c) is separated to the single-stranded form (d). Labeled probe (*) is added (e). Probe hybridizes to complementary DNA to form labeled dsDNA (f). Only bands from the agarose gel (a) with DNA sequence complementary to probe will hybridize. The hybridized Southern blot (g) shows target bands detected by labeled probe.
Source: Copyright © 2000, Susan M. Harrington.

sequence to be amplified within the template DNA. One oligonucleotide primer is complementary to the top strand at one end of the target sequence and the second oligonucleotide is complementary to the bottom strand at the opposite end of the target sequence (Figure 9-5).

Polymerases are enzymes that facilitate DNA replication. Because PCR requires high and low temperatures, thermostable polymerases (e.g., the DNA polymerase enzyme from *Thermus aquaticus* [Taq]) are used to amplify the target sequence. A typical PCR reaction mix contains template DNA, oligonucleotide primers, polymerase, magnesium, deoxyribonucleotide triphosphate bases, and a suitable buffer. Approximately 30 cycles are usually conducted in which first the template DNA is dissociated by heating to 94°C. Annealing occurs by cooling to 55°C; at this stage, the oligonucleotides have an

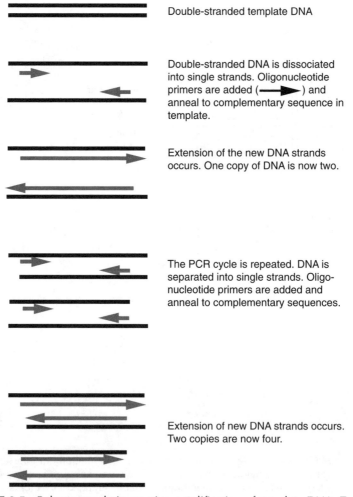

FIGURE 9-5 Polymerase chain reaction amplification of template DNA. Two cycles of PCR are shown. Double-stranded DNA is separated into single strands. Primers anneal. New DNA strands are created through extension. Typical PCR reactions are 30 to 40 cycles long, creating millions of copies of double-stranded DNA.

advantage because of their high concentration and they bind to the target more quickly than the original complementary strand. Finally, an extension phase occurs at 72° C where the polymerase adds the correct nucleotides to the short primer oligonucleotide strand to create a new complementary strand. The result after 30 cycles of dissociation, annealing, and extension is a large amplification of the target sequence, namely, the sequence between the two oligonucleotide primers called the PCR product from the diverse and low concentration template DNA (Figure 9-5). The amplified PCR product DNA, referred to as the "amplicon," can then be analyzed by gel electrophoresis, restriction endonuclease analysis, or Southern hybridization.

A common application of PCR is the detection of microbial DNA in clinical specimens. PCR is particularly useful when the microbe of interest either grows slowly or cannot be cultivated by conventional techniques. PCR has the power to turn one copy of dsDNA into more than a billion copies. This power brings with it an important drawback: DNA from other samples or DNA from previous PCR reactions can contaminate the test, causing false-positive results. In recent years, a number of advancements in PCR methodologies have helped investigators minimize contamination. Most important among these is the physical separation of the steps involved. Processing, PCR reaction setup, and analysis of postamplification products are performed in different rooms. Protocols also call for the addition of chemicals, photochemicals, and enzymes, which inactivate contaminating nucleic acids. Finally, laboratory technicians take particular care with technique, including working in biologic safety hoods, wearing gloves and gowns, cleaning surfaces, and using specialized equipment. With appreciation of the intricacies of the method, PCR is a robust and indispensable tool.

Microarrays

An oligonucleotide microarray (i.e., DNA chip) is an efficient method for detecting DNA sequences of interest. For this technique greater than 10,000 different oligonucleotides can be attached to a $1 \, cm^2$ solid surface. Each DNA's location on the surface acts as an identifier. Unknown sequences that are complementary to known oligonucleotides on the DNA-chip hybridize, allowing for their subsequent identification. Some examples of different formats for single nucleotide polymorphism (SNPs) typing with microarrays include hybridization arrays and arrays with enzymatic processing. For hybridization arrays, alleles of known SNPs located at specific regions of a "chip" are allowed to hybridize with query SNPs present in fluorescently labeled PCR products. Hybridization results in positive signals that are detected by computer leading to identification of unknown SNPs. During arrayed primer extension, PCR products containing unknown SNPs are hybridized to the arrayed oligonucleotides. Bound oligonucleotides act as primers for a DNA polymerase extension reaction that incorporates fluorescently labeled dideoxynucleotides. The addition of enzymatic discrimination increases the specificity of the latter method.[20]

As typing methods are the focus of this chapter, the next section will examine how these techniques use frequent and infrequent cutting enzymes, PFGE, hybridization, PCR, and microarrays to detect strain differences based on DNA sequence and/or restriction site specificities.

Specific Techniques of Molecular Epidemiology

In this section the methodologies of the most commonly used nucleic acid molecular methods are described. Strengths and weaknesses of each method and some examples are included. With the exception of DNA sequencing, all of these methods rely on visualization of DNA bands, whether they are from plasmids, restriction digests, hybridization, or PCR products. These banding patterns are the "DNA fingerprints" used to compare one isolate to another.[21]

Evaluation of Typing Systems

It is important to keep in mind that typing systems measure different biologic properties and perform with varying degrees of success depending on the organism and technical requirements. No one system is best for all species, although several newer methods can be applied to almost all bacterial species, especially those causing the majority of hospital-associated outbreaks. As with other clinical laboratory methods, strain typing techniques must be carefully evaluated before they are used to answer epidemiologic questions. The specific question that needs to be answered may lead to the selection of one method over another.

To be widely useful, a typing system must give an interpretable result for every isolate of a given species. This is referred to as "typeability." Plasmid analysis, one of the earliest typing methods, detects the extra-chromosomal DNA of bacteria. However, not all strains within a species will contain plasmids, rendering them nontypeable by this method.

Additionally, reproducibility is a critical factor. An assay cannot be considered reliable if the same results are not obtained when an isolate is tested multiple times in the system. Some molecular methods are highly technique-dependent in this sense. For example, the reaction conditions, reagents, and template DNA used in the arbitrary primed PCR reaction must be carefully standardized or a different result could be obtained with each run. Standardization is another important component. Interpretation of results is much more reliable when methods are performed in the same way from batch to batch.[14]

Discriminatory power is the ability of the typing technique to distinguish unrelated isolates from epidemiologically related strains. It is critical to include epidemiologically unrelated strains in the evaluation of new typing systems as controls. Many methods are able to link closely clustered isolates; however, the more difficult aspect is to exclude unassociated strains. Often some isolates are found with a molecular link for which no epidemiologic link exists. The key is to minimize this phenomenon with the most powerful typing tool available.[14] It must also be understood that to some degree the ability to discriminate related from unrelated isolates is species dependent. For example, the number of different clones of MRSA is much more limited than for methicillin-susceptible strains. This is a result of the way the methicillin resistance gene was acquired by some strains of the species.[22] The limited number of clones could cause one to falsely link strains that are truly unrelated. For MRSA it is important to compare isolates over a short time frame and to combine laboratory results with careful epidemiologic analysis.

The ease of interpretation or readability of DNA fingerprints varies. Some methods, such as chromosomal restriction endonuclease analysis, produce many bands that are difficult to distinguish because they are so close together. Faint or very bold bands can be equally difficult to discern. Interpretability can vary between methods or even between applications of a single method. For example, in Southern hybridization methods one probe may yield a much more readable RFLP than another.

Issues of cost-effectiveness, ease of use, ease of interpretation, and turn-around time must also be considered. As molecular methods have become more discriminatory, they have required more expensive and sophisticated machinery, including PCR thermocyclers, PFGE equipment, DNA sequencers, and computer software for archiving data and comparing run-to-run results. The time to results for these powerful techniques may be from 1 or 2 days for PCR to approximately 4 days for PFGE. The technical expertise needed to perform molecular techniques also varies from simple DNA extraction to lengthy hybridization procedures. Finally, interpretation of banding patterns and results is method-dependent as well.

The choice of a typing method is dependent on all of these parameters; it will vary with the needs and capabilities of individual laboratories. As each method is presented, it will be evaluated based on these criteria.

Plasmid Analysis

As described, some bacterial strains harbor extra-chromosomal DNA called plasmids. Plasmids are frequently found in the Enterobacteriaceae and in gram-positive organisms responsible for many hospital-associated infections such as staphylococci and enterococci. Analysis of plasmid DNA is one of the oldest of the nucleic acid-based methods for strain typing and has been used in the evaluation of many outbreaks.[23] Plasmids are easily extracted from bacterial cells in a process that takes only several hours. The plasmid preparation can then be evaluated by agarose gel electrophoresis to analyze the number and size of the plasmid(s) from each strain. Because plasmids are frequently present in bacterial cells and easily extracted for analysis with inexpensive electrophoresis equipment found in many laboratories, this method can easily be applied in many investigations.

Practically, some difficulties may be encountered when plasmid gel electrophoresis is performed. Plasmid DNA can range in size from just a few kilobases to almost 200 kb. The larger DNAs separate poorly, tending to accumulate at the top of the gel. Moreover, different plasmids of the same size could have different sequences, a characteristic unappreciated if size alone is evaluated. During extraction, the supercoiled, covalently closed, circular nature of plasmids is often disturbed, yielding relaxed, nicked, circular and linear forms. A single plasmid could appear as three bands by gel analysis, because these forms migrate differently in the gel. Hence, plasmid gels can have poor reproducibility and can be difficult to interpret. These problems can be overcome by cutting the plasmid DNA with a restriction enzyme. Often referred to as plasmid restriction enzyme analysis (REA), this method creates smaller, linear fragments that migrate faithfully according to size, and they are more easily interpreted. Restriction enzyme cutting is dependent on DNA sequence; therefore, REA can distinguish if single, large plasmids are the same in both DNA content and size. The number of REA bands will increase proportionately with the number of plasmids. However, as band number increases, interpretation becomes more difficult.

When applying this method, the variable nature of plasmids must be appreciated. Depending on the environment and the antibiotic resistance genes or virulence factors encoded by the plasmids that a bacterium harbors, plasmids can be gained or lost because of selective pressures. Hence, depending on what antibiotic therapy is in use, strains involved in an outbreak can evolve through changes in plasmid content even as the outbreak is being evaluated.[24] Movement of plasmids (or the transposable elements that they carry) between strains of the same species and even between species has been observed.[25,26] Thus, a plasmid epidemic could be encountered.[27] Plasmid results must be evaluated carefully in comparison to the susceptibility profiles of the organisms isolated at the time of an outbreak.

Two other factors should be considered when using plasmid analysis. First, not all strains will give a result because some do not carry plasmids. Second, since plasmid analysis focuses on only a small part of the genome, two bacteria strains can have the same plasmid content, but unique chromosomes. With all of this in mind, it is probably best to apply this typing technique to studies that are relatively limited in time span and to combine plasmid analysis with other methods.

Restriction Endonuclease Analysis of Chromosomal DNA

Analysis of chromosomal DNA is an alternative to plasmid typing methods. The chromosome is the more stable genetic element, not subject to gain and loss as is the plasmid. Chromosomal restriction endonuclease analysis (REA) is performed by extracting genomic DNA and cutting it with a restriction enzyme. Hundreds of fragments approximately 0.5 to 50 kb in length are produced, which are separated by gel electrophoresis. To produce these relatively small fragments "frequent cutting" restriction enzymes such as *Bam*HI, *Hind*III, and *Eco*RI are used. As with plasmid analysis, this method does not require specialized equipment. DNA can be extracted and restriction digested in just a few hours with minimal technical expertise. Gels are usually run overnight to achieve the best possible separation of bands. The major advantage to chromosomal REA is that with the correct selection of restriction enzyme all bacterial species are typeable. However, the large number of bands produced makes interpretation difficult. Multiple fragments can migrate together and very large bands can group together at the top of the gel.[15] Some investigators preferentially analyze the high molecular weight (top) portion of the gel, which is usually most interpretable.[28] The extraction procedures used do not separate plasmid from chromosomal DNA. Two isolates with the same chromosome, but distinct plasmids, could have slightly different patterns. Chromosomal REA has largely been replaced by newer methods.

RFLP Analysis Using REA with Southern Hybridization

The interpretability of chromosomal REA has been improved with the addition of nucleic acid probes targeted to specific multicopy genes, insertion sequences, or mobile genetic elements such as transposons. First, DNA cut with a frequent cutting restriction enzyme is separated in agarose as described above. The DNA fragments are transferred from agarose to a membrane by the Southern blotting technique. The DNA fragments immobilized on the membrane can then be hybridized with a nucleic acid probe. Only a small portion (ideally 10 to 20) of the thousands of restriction fragments will have specificity for the probe and will be detected. This is the technique referred to as restriction fragment length polymorphism. RFLP detects the number of copies of sequence homologous to the probe and reflects the size of the restriction fragments containing those sequences. The number of bands will be proportional to the number of copies of the target as long as the target does not contain a restriction site. When a single restriction site is present within the target sequence, the probe will hybridize along both sides of the restriction site and two bands will be produced for each copy of target. Several probes are most commonly used for RFLP typing; however, theoretically, any repetitive sequence with species specificity can work. For example, the *mec* gene, which encodes methicillin resistance, and Tn554, a transposon, have both been used as probes of chromosomal digests for *S. aureus*.[22,29] Other types of probes have included insertion sequences, toxin-producing genes, and even random chromosomal sequences.[18] However, most of these probes are specific to only a single species and sometimes only to strains within a species carrying the gene of interest.

Ribotyping is a popular approach, almost universally applicable to all bacterial species. Ribosomal RNA (rRNA) or DNA homologous to the ribosomal operon is used as the probe. The ribosomal operon, which encodes the rRNA transcripts essential to make a ribosome, is highly conserved within bacterial species and is usually present in multiple copies in the chromosome. Organisms such as *E. coli*, *Klebsiella*, and *Staphylococcus* species have from 5 to 7 copies of this element, producing easily interpreted ribotype patterns with 10 to 15 bands.[30] In a study comparing 12 typing methods for *S. aureus*, ribotyping was highly sensitive, identifying all outbreak-associated strains. However, as demonstrated in this study, unrelated isolates are sometimes grouped with an outbreak strain.[29]

Although ribotyping uses a commercially available standardized probe, the choice of restriction enzyme is not standardized. In fact, the most discriminatory enzyme varies between species. An increase in discrimination can be obtained by combining the results with two or more enzymes.[29] Although ribotyping results are easily interpreted and very reproducible, other more discriminatory methods are now available for many organisms.[31,32]

Ribotyping is not of value for strain delineation of *M. tuberculosis* because only one copy of the ribosomal operon is present. Several repetitive elements have been studied as probes for RFLP.[33,34] Currently, the method of choice proposed by an international expert panel uses IS6110, an insertion sequence present in 1 to 26 copies in *M. tuberculosis* complex organisms, to probe *Pvu*II digested genomic DNA.[35] This method has been applied in many studies, including transmission in large cities and HIV-infected populations, epidemiology between nations, laboratory contamination, and outbreaks.[36-40] Figure 9-6 is an example of an IS6110-probed Southern blot of *M. tuberculosis*. Matched pairs are found in lanes 6 and 7, as well as in 8 and 9. Lanes 1 and 10 contain DNA from a well-characterized *M. tuberculosis* strain that is used as a standard molecular weight marker. Inclusion of a bacterium as a

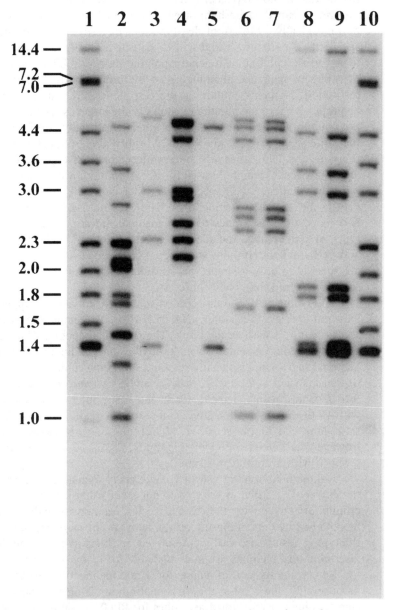

FIGURE 9-6　Restriction fragment length polymorphism of *Mycobacterium Tuberculosis* with IS6110 probe. Lanes 2 to 9 contain clinical isolates. Lanes 1 to 10 are the molecular weight marker Mt 14323. Molecular weights are shown in kilobase pairs.

marker instead of purchasing one commercially is highly desirable. Not only does using DNA from a live organism serve as a determiner of molecular size, it is also a useful extraction control. To be confident of the extraction process in the laboratory, every time this strain's DNA is extracted and cut with the indicated restriction enzyme, the same number and size of bands must be obtained.

Rarely, *M. tuberculosis* or related organisms will lack IS6110. Most of these strains have come from cases in Southeast Asia. Additionally, up to 25% of isolates have fewer than six IS6110 bands.[41] Isolates with low band numbers are shown in lanes 3 and 5 of Figure 9-6. It follows that the fewer the bands, the less reliable is the discrimination. For IS6110 typing or for other methods, isolates with few bands should be repeated with a second probe or by another procedure.

Ribotyping and other RFLP techniques generally produce interpretable banding patterns that are highly reproducible. An advantage of these tests is that they do not require a lot of expensive equipment. However, they may take up to a week to perform and require considerable technical expertise. An automated ribotyping instrument, The Riboprinter (DuPont-Qualicon), is now available. Up to 32 organisms may be typed in a single day. However, the cost of the instrument and associated reagents is prohibitive for many laboratories.

Pulsed-Field Gel Electrophoresis

First described in 1984 by Schwartz and Cantor, PFGE is one of the most widely used and discriminatory typing techniques.[19] Developed to separate large DNA molecules, PFGE is ideal for electrophoresis of the fragments created by digestion of a genomic DNA extract with infrequent cutting restriction enzymes. Optimally, 10 to 20 bands are produced. A major strength of PFGE is that probes and Southern blotting are usually not needed. The low number of bands can be visualized by staining and gel documentation with a computer imaging system.

With the appropriate restriction enzyme, PFGE can be used to type most bacteria and a number of fungal species. Rarely, DNA from isolates will be degraded and an uninterpretable pattern will result.[28] As with all strain typing methods, no one restriction enzyme is considered standard. Choice of restriction enzyme depends on the percent GC content of the organism, as previously described. Some enzymes inherently work better than others do. Lists of organisms and restriction enzymes used for PFGE have been published.[13,18]

Fungi have multiple individual chromosomes that vary in size. These may be extracted for separation as whole chromosomes or cut with restriction enzymes. Both the number and size of chromosomes can also vary within a particular fungal species. Separation of such intact chromosomes generates a type of fingerprint referred to as an electrophoretic karyotype. Interpreting karyotypes can be difficult if the chromosomes migrate closely to one another. Some investigators digest these DNAs with restriction enzymes, yielding smaller, more distinguishable bands.[42,43]

PFGE is the method most frequently used for outbreak investigations involving common hospital-associated pathogens. It has been shown to be highly discriminatory in outbreaks caused by many organisms such as *Staphylococcus, Candida, E. coli, Enterococcus,* and *Enterobacter.*[44-48] Figure 9-7 shows some examples of VRE from a hospital ICU outbreak. A total of 13 VRE isolates were obtained from patient cultures over a 5-week period. Seven of these were characterized as belonging to the outbreak cluster. Lanes 2 to 4 in Figure 9-7 are indistinguishable outbreak isolates. The VRE isolate in lane 5 was considered a clonally related strain within the outbreak because it has only two bands different from the main outbreak strain. Lane 6 contains an environmental strain isolated from the surface of a bedside infusion pump. Because it shares many bands with the outbreak strain, this strain is also possibly related to the outbreak cluster. The strains in lanes 7 and 8 are from patients unrelated to the outbreak. It was believed that these two patients were colonized before admission. The isolate in lane 9 was recovered 4 months after the outbreak; its banding pattern suggests that it is a progeny isolate that has diverged from the outbreak strain. The end lanes contain *Not*I-digested *E. faecalis* (ATCC 47077) as a molecular weight marker.[13]

Because PFGE fingerprints are highly reproducible, interpretation is fairly straightforward. However, two major disadvantages of PFGE are the

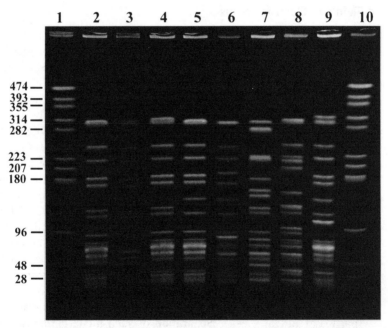

FIGURE 9-7   Pulsed-field gel electrophoresis of vancomycin-resistant *Enterococcus faecium.* Lanes 2 to 5, 7, and 8 are patient isolates recovered during an outbreak in an ICU. Lane 6 contains an isolate cultured from the surface of an IV machine. Lane 9 is a strain isolated 4 months later. The molecular weight maker, *Not*I-digested *E. faecalis* ATCC 47077, is in lanes 1 and 10. Molecular weights are in kilobase pairs.

difficulty of comparing results obtained from different laboratories[49] and the lack of a convenient method of measuring genetic relationships among strains with unrelated PFGE patterns.[50] In addition, interpretation can become time-consuming when several isolates, which differ by only a few bands, are compared as illustrated in Figure 9-7. When many isolates are compared, it is often necessary to run those with similar fingerprint patterns side by side on the same gel. Some investigators are using computer database and analysis sofware to compare large numbers of strains run on multiple gels. It should be kept in mind, however, that no software can substitute for visual comparison of isolates run in adjacent lanes.

In addition to the expense of the PFGE apparatus, the total time required to perform the test is a disadvantage of this method. DNA extraction procedures take about 2 to 3 days, although more rapid methods have been developed.[51,52] The electrophoresis time is also lengthy; 24 hours is a typical running time, and a fair amount of technical expertise is necessary. To prevent mechanical breakage of chromosomal DNA, all extraction steps must be carefully performed with preparations embedded in agarose.

PCR-Based Methods

All of the methods presented to this point need a fairly large amount of DNA for gel electrophoresis. PCR-based strain typing techniques require only a small amount of DNA from the clinical isolate. In addition, DNA from organisms that cannot be grown by conventional culture methods can be amplified and used to delineate strain differences. Compared with RFLP and PFGE, PCR fingerprinting is rapid with results available within a day.

Three basic variations of PCR fingerprinting have been described. The first, PCR-RFLP utilizes PCR to amplify known variable regions of the genome. A restriction endonuclease is then used to digest these PCR products, yielding several smaller DNA fragments. For example, in a method called Vir typing, the gene for the antiphagocytic M protein in *Streptococcus pyogenes* is amplified and digested with HaeIII, producing characteristic RFLP patterns.[53] The DNA fragments are visualized by conventional gel electrophoresis. No hybridization or PFGE equipment is needed. Species-specific virulence genes such as the M protein gene of *S. pyogenes*, the coagulase gene of *S. aureus*,[54] or genes coding for rRNA have been useful for this method. Multilocus restriction fragment typing is a recently described method in which housekeeping genes are PCR amplified and digested with restriction enzymes.[50] This method will be described further in a later section. Only well-characterized regions specific to a given species will be discriminatory by PCR-RFLP. Hence, the discriminatory power of PCR-RFLP varies, depending on the organism and the gene being amplified. This method does, however, generate easily interpreted, reproducible fingerprints.[14]

The second method, repetitive element PCR (rep-PCR), uses PCR to amplify regions between known sequences.[55] Oligonucleotide primers homologous to the ends of sequences that are present in multiple copies prime PCR reactions to amplify the sequences between repeats. Repetitive sequences may be spaced somewhat randomly throughout the chromosome. It follows that the DNA fragment lengths between the repetitive elements are also variable. Amplification of the sequences between the repeats, therefore, produces a range of fragment lengths (or a DNA fingerprint) that is size fractionated by agarose gel electrophoresis. The repetitive extrapalindromic sequences of *E. coli* (rep), the enterobacterial repetitive intergenic consensus (ERIC) elements of Enterobacteriaceae, the BOX elements of gram-positive bacteria and regions between rRNA genes are some of the repetitive elements used for this technique.[18,56] Applicable to many bacterial species, rep-PCR is a discriminatory method. Discriminatory power can be enhanced with multiple primer sets.[57] In addition, more recently the DiversiLab System (Bacterial Barcodes [Spectral Genomics Inc., Houston, TX]), a commercial variant of rep-PCR has been described. This technique utilizes rep-PCR; however, after the amplification step the PCR products are size fractionated on a micro-fluidics detection platform ("chip"). The newer technology allows for highly accurate, automated, reproducible data that can be archived allowing for outbreak comparison.

Arbitrary primed PCR (AP-PCR) or random amplified polymorphic DNA (RAPD) is the third PCR fingerprinting technique. A single, short oligonucle-otide primer (8 to 10 bp) is selected and is not intended to be specific for defined target sequences. The number of recognition sites for this primer in the template DNA is generally not known. PCR is performed at a low anneal-ing temperature to facilitate binding of oligonucleotide to the template in the regions that may lack perfect sequence homology. When primers anneal sufficiently close to each other (within ~1 kb), in the correct orientation and on opposite DNA strands, amplification of the region between the arbitrary primers takes place. These primers will anneal at multiple locations through-out the template. As with rep-PCR, products of various sizes will result. The PCR products can be separated by gel electrophoresis yielding a fingerprint pattern.[58] An advantage of this method is that no sequence information about the organism is required. Many bacterial species, fungi, and some parasites have been typed successfully with AP-PCR.[57] An example of a RAPD or AP-PCR fingerprint pattern is given in Figure 9-8.

Whereas typeability is excellent for this method, batch-to-batch repro-ducibility is sometimes poor. Alteration in concentration of primers, template DNA, *Taq*, or magnesium will influence results. Different lots of *Taq* or primer, or use of a different thermocycler, can affect fingerprints, as can contamina-tion with a product from a previous run. Frequently, nonspecific bands will be produced when any of these variables are changed. To show if nonspecific bands are present, inclusion of a control tube that lacks template DNA is recommended. This sample should not have any visualized bands. Although a strength of AP-PCR is its ability to type strains with a small amount of nucleic acid that may not be very pure, results are much more reproducible if DNA is used at a standardized quantity and of fairly high quality.[56] Unfor-tunately, quantification and DNA purification increase the technical difficulty and time required to perform this test.

In general, AP-PCR is a more rapid method and is less technically demanding than RFLP or PFGE because fewer steps are involved. However, AP-PCR can be more difficult to interpret than either RFLP or PFGE. The bands seen on AP-PCR gels generally vary in intensity, depending on reaction conditions, the ability of the arbitrary primers to anneal to template, and the efficiency of the elongation step. AP-PCR is probably best used with relatively small numbers of isolates compared within the same run on the same day.[14,26] A number of studies have demonstrated AP-PCR to have discriminatory power similar to PFGE and better than some other methods. Multiple primer sets have been used to increase discriminatory power.[59]

Various primers, whether for arbitrary or intergenic amplification, and different restriction enzymes have been used for PCR strain typing methods. Interlaboratory comparisons are problematic because there is run-to-run variability.[56] Standardized PCR reactions, electrophoretic conditions, and data analysis such as those of the DiversiLab System (Bacterial Barcodes [Spectral Genomics Inc., Houston, TX]) can significantly improve the variability encountered with these methods.

DNA Sequencing

DNA sequencing is a strain typing method that is rapidly becoming very useful for epidemiologic analyses. Well-characterized genes or DNA sequences that are relatively variable are PCR amplified. Following amplification, the nucleotide sequences (i.e., the order of the A, T, C, G bases) are determined by gel electrophoresis or with an automated computer-based sequencing instrument. The nucleotide sequences can then be aligned, usually in a computerized database to find base differences between isolates. DNA sequence typing has been described for some bacteria and for viruses.[14] Two recently described techniques, sSNP Genotyping and multilocus sequence typing, make use of sequencing with novel methodologies and will be described in the following sections.

sSNPs Genotyping

Whole-genome DNA sequencing has opened the door for designing new methods for the typing of bacteria. Proteins capable of being produced from such DNA can be identified with computer programs (e.g., Gene Locator and Interpolated Markov Modeler [GLIMMER]). Analysis of the DNA sequence of different strains of bacteria and their predicted proteins allows for the discovery of numerous polymorphisms, of which synonymous single nucleotide polymorphisms (sSNPs) show distinct promise as a typing method. Once identified, sSNPs are verified by repeating DNA sequencing or use of mass spectrometry. Verified sSNPs for a particular organism can then be assayed for by microarray (e.g., GeneChip [Affymetrix Inc., Santa Clara, CA]), mass spectrometry (e.g., Masscode [Qiagen Inc., Valencia, CA]), gel electrophoresis (e.g., RFLP), and other methodologies.[16,20,60,61] Data generated from comparisons of sSNPs from different strains of a particular genus are then utilized for epidemiologic and phylogenetic studies.

sSNPs genotyping is efficient, amenable to automation, applicable to large bacterial populations, and is predicted to have a significant impact particularly in the epidemiology and evolution of *M. tuberculosis*. This method, however, is limited by its cost, need for prior DNA sequence knowledge, and effort required for establishing an assay. Likely the future widespread use of sSNPs as a genotyping method will depend on cheaper, higher throughput technologies.[20,60,61]

Multilocus Sequence Typing

Multilocus sequence typing (MLST) is a promising technique that has been used for the typing of a number of bacterial genera. For *S. aureus*, genomic DNA is characterized based on the similarities and differences within PCR-derived short sequences (segments approximately 450 bp) of seven conserved housekeeping genes (*arcC, aroE, glp, gmk, pta, tpi, yqiL*). Amplicons obtained are sequenced by computer-based analysis and variation within the internal segments is used for assigning different alleles. Strains are then defined as sequence types (STs) by the specific alleles present for the queried genes. As there are an average of 42 alleles present at each locus (providing the ability to define greater than 200 billion STs), isolates are unlikely to be identical by chance, and when identical, strains can be considered to represent the same clone.[49,62]

As with other typing methods MLST has its pros and cons. MLST is highly discriminatory and identifies changes that accumulate slowly. It overcomes the difficulty of comparing results between laboratories without exchanging reference strains and allows for inter-laboratory comparison through the Internet at MLST Web sites (http://mlst.zoo.ox.ac.uk or http://www.mlst.net). These Web sites have the added advantage of banking linked epidemiological associations by STs[49,62,63] and contain allelic data from at least 25 countries, representing over 1000 *S. aureus* isolates.[64] MLST is suited for local and worldwide long-term epidemiology.[65] The cost and technically demanding nature of necessary experiments are part of its limitations. Also, MLST is intolerant of errors in DNA sequencing, which can result in mistyping. In addition, epidemiologists need to be aware that this technique is dependent on a combination of results from different experiments on seven genes, allowing for several steps for human and nonhuman error, which can impact data included in the MLST Web site.[65]

Multilocus Restriction Fragment Typing

Diep et al.[66] have described a method for *S. aureus* typing called multilocus restriction fragment typing (MLRFT), based on the theory behind MLST.[50] In this method sequence variations in the same housekeeping genes used for MLST are detected by restriction fragment analysis (as opposed to sequencing). PCR is performed on the MLST defined housekeeping genes, but the amplicons obtained are directly cut (without a purification step), by up to two restriction endonucleases, then analyzed by banding pattern after gel electrophoresis. Restriction alleles are assigned by banding patterns expected from primary MLST banked sequences. It is predicted that MLRFT has the ability to detect 95% of the diversity available by MLST.

Compared to MLST, MLRFT is less expensive, more time efficient, and requires less specialized equipment. It may, therefore, be more suitable for use in the routine clinical setting and the developing world. In addition, because MLRFT is based on the same sequences used for MLST, its results are capable of being linked to the MLST Internet database. MLRFT has high discriminatory power and is believed to be portable between laboratories, because it is based on primary sequence data, with specific restriction endonuclease sites. In contrast to PFGE, MLRFT tends to detect slow changes in the genome and MLRFT is unable to make fine strain distinctions, therefore its use in local outbreaks has been questioned.[50] Despite these potential limitations MLRFT has been used in combination with PFGE and MLST in local molecular epidemiological investigations.[66,67]

Interpretation of Results

As molecular typing methods have been described, the interpretability or readability of the fingerprint has also been discussed. This is not the same as the interpretation of results. With the exception of DNA sequencing, all of these methods produce a DNA fingerprint, or banding pattern, for each isolate. As the fingerprints are compared, the similarity or differences between them must be evaluated. All of the bands from an isolate are compared with those in the other lanes on the gel.

The simplest comparison is that of two isolates having the same DNA fingerprint. These are more accurately described as "indistinguishable" rather than identical. Each of the molecular typing methods evaluates only a portion of the genome (i.e., restriction endonuclease sites, a specific gene, or amplified sequence). It is impossible to say that two microorganisms are exact clones based on these types of tests. Clearly, mutations in the genome will occur that will not be detected by these methods. At the opposite end of the spectrum, it is fairly easy to decide that two isolates having vastly different fingerprints are not clonally related. The difficult interpretations are those in which isolates vary by just a few bands. Such strains may be related to each other, but how closely?

The relative relatedness of organisms can be expressed in terms of the number of genetic events or changes to the chromosome that occur from one generation to the next. For example, two organisms that demonstrate changes in the chromosome produced by one genetic event may be categorized as "probably related." Strains that differ by two genetic events are characterized as "possibly related." Isolates differing by three or more genetic events are most likely "unrelated." It seems reasonable to categorize strains based on these definitions of relative relatedness.[13] However, it is much more difficult to decide the number of fingerprint band differences that place strains into these categories. Tenover et al. present a detailed discussion of molecular typing methods and the way in which mutations affect banding patterns.[26] Additionally, the way in which changes in fingerprint patterns are evaluated varies widely between laboratories.

Some interpretive criteria used by investigators in molecular epidemiology can be found in the literature. The guidelines for PFGE have probably been those most widely applied. For example, it is possible for one genetic change to cause up to a three-band difference between two isolates. Hence, isolates with one- to three-band differences are probably related. Two genetic events would alter the PFGE pattern by anywhere from four to six bands. Strains with four- to six-band differences are possibly related. Unrelated strains differ by more than six bands. Most investigators evaluating strain typing data in an outbreak will designate the most common type by a letter or number, as in strain A. Isolates that differ from A by one to three bands are subtypes of A. Isolates with more than three band differences are given new letter designations. In practice, as numerous fingerprints are compared, categorizing strains that "may be related" becomes complex. For example, two isolates may each be subtypes of strain A and vary from one another by more than four bands. These subtype strains would represent new type strains B and C if evaluated apart from the type A strain. This emphasizes the importance of evaluating strain types over a limited time period relative to an outbreak. Differences between epidemiologically unrelated strains will occur randomly. Two such strains could, therefore, have only minor molecular differences and be grouped as subtypes if no epidemiologic information is considered. Hence, interpretive guidelines can give misleading information if applied in a larger context without epidemiologic data.[13]

These interpretive criteria are valid for PFGE because the whole chromosome is assessed. For other typing systems interpretation is less easily defined. Many genetic events can occur that will not be detected. For example, substitution mutations of DNA that do not alter restriction sites or target areas for probes will not be detected by RFLP methods.[26] Although no standard approach to RFLP interpretation has been proposed, some investigators have designated isolates with one-band differences subtypes of one another. Isolates with two or more band differences represent new strain types.[29]

For rep-PCR and AP-PCR, no standard approach is found for analyzing minor differences in band patterns such as changes in intensity or a one-band size shift. Frequently, a second set of PCR primers is used to see if similar results are consistently obtained. Any mutational event may be responsible for the alterations seen in PCR fingerprints if that mutation occurs at a primer binding site. Additionally, insertions or deletions of DNA between primer binding sites will alter the banding pattern. However, not all mutations will be detected by this method. In a manner similar to interpretation of RFLP, isolates having a one-band difference by PCR fingerprinting may be considered subtypes of each other. PCR patterns having two or more bands different are generally categorized as different strains.[26,68]

Using plasmid analysis, strains with three or more plasmids that are the same by gel electrophoresis are considered indistinguishable. Confidence in the discriminatory ability of this method declines if fewer than three plasmids are present. Although strains containing only one identical plasmid have been helpful in elucidating outbreaks, better discrimination can also be achieved with plasmid REA.[26]

Computer-Assisted Analysis

Sometimes the molecular epidemiologist needs to compare isolates in large populations or over a lengthy period of time. This circumstance requires between-gel comparisons, which cannot be done without strict standardization of the method (i.e., the same DNA extraction procedure, electrophoresis conditions, molecular weight standards). Computer system assistance, therefore, becomes helpful. Such systems allow gels, photographs, or autoradiographic images to be scanned and stored as digitized images. A molecular size standard with a well-characterized pattern is included in the two end lanes and often in the middle of every gel. The bands in the other lanes are then "normalized" to the standard to account for variability between gels. Depending on the computer program used either band sizes or band positions relative to the standard are stored for subsequent comparisons. Analysis software finds bands automatically, but allows the user the flexibility to add, delete or move bands after visual inspection. Within-gel and between-gel band matching can then be accomplished as desired. The user can also set deviation or percent tolerance for matching around each band, which further minimizes within-gel and between-gel differences and enhances strain matching. The microprocessors use various numerical indices (e.g., Dice coefficients) to assign percent similarities to selected isolates. Finally, graphical representation of strain relatedness can be accomplished in the form of dendrograms based upon several grouping methods (e.g., Underweighted Pair Group Method with Arithmetic Mean [UPGMA], neighbor joining). A dendrogram links isolates according to percent similarity in a manner similar to a phylogenetic tree. Currently, three popular computer fingerprinting systems are available: Dendron (Solltech Inc., Oakdale, IA), Whole Band Analysis (BioImage, Ann Arbor, MI), and GelCompar or Molecular Analyst Fingerprinting Plus (Biorad Laboratories, Hercules, CA). Each of these systems uses unique software, but each performs the basic functions outlined.[69]

When done in a rigorously standardized fashion, fingerprinting software allows the user to accomplish many comparisons that would otherwise be very time consuming. Computerized analysis does have limitations, however. Although these systems can correct for differences that arise between gels, they do so imperfectly. They are unable to correct for great variability. The degree of matching is determined by the percent deviation around the bands selected by the operator. Overmatching or undermatching can occur, depending on this setting. Because the systems use mathematical methods to match strains, isolate 1 may match perfectly to isolate 2 and isolate 3, but isolates 2 and 3 may not match each other with 100% similarity. However, all three of these may be grouped together in a mathematical cluster. Such cluster analysis must be carefully interpreted. It is best to allow the computer program to find strains that are closely related and then run these strains on the same gel in adjacent lanes. Visual inspection of banding patterns is often better to determine relatedness than computer software. Finally, software-derived dendrograms must also be interpreted with caution. The tree structure is highly dependent on the grouping method chosen and can lead to false conclusions. Some grouping methods give different tree structures, depending on the order in which strains are added to the tree. Distance between strains on the tree may be relative, not absolute. It is probably best to use dendrograms only as graphical representations of large groupings of strains. The distance between individual isolates or small clusters should not be interpreted as representative of genetic distance.

In summary, computer software is very helpful in archiving fingerprint data from a large number of strains. Although computer systems can be good at finding similar or matching indistinguishable isolates in the database, closer comparison should be performed by testing related isolates on the same gel.

Conclusion

Before strain typing is initiated, epidemiologic investigations should always start with simple questions based on current case findings and microbiology. Controls known to be epidemiologically unrelated to cases should be included to ensure adequate discrimination and the most appropriate strain typing method for that species applied. The method chosen will also depend on the epidemiologic question to be answered and practical issues such as cost, ease of use, equipment availability, and time to results. By definition, various typing methods measure different biological properties, and they sometimes group isolates differently, which is to be expected. For this reason, a combination of molecular tests is sometimes utilized. This can be in the form of two different primers for RAPDs, two different restriction enzymes for PFGE, two RFLP probes, or two different methods altogether.

Currently, PFGE-, MLST-, and PCR-based tests have the highest discriminatory power for strain delineation of most common hospital-associated pathogens and many fungal species. They have largely replaced plasmid fingerprinting, chromosomal REA, and even ribotyping. Exceptions exist, however, such as for *M. tuberculosis*, where IS6110 RFLP is still a recommended method. Unfortunately, high equipment costs and the need for technical expertise render the most discriminatory methods unsuitable for small laboratories. However, a number of larger hospitals and academic centers are offering fingerprinting services on a per isolate basis.

Molecular strain typing has truly advanced the field of infectious disease epidemiology. As part of a classic epidemiologic investigation, molecular epidemiology has been used to determine the source of an outbreak and distinguish cases from noncases. Potential sources of infection (e.g., fomites or the environment) can be surveyed during an outbreak. Pathogens recovered can then be analyzed with these methods to determine any links to patient infections. Molecular methods are now considered standard to ongoing infectious disease outbreak investigations. Additionally, strain typing has been used to answer clinical questions such as if therapy should be altered because of relapse of an infection or if a new strain or resistance gene was acquired. Whether multiple isolates of the same species are indistinguishable or represent various contaminants has also been a recent application of these methods.

The future of DNA fingerprinting is exciting. Many genome-sequencing projects are completed and others are under way. As detailed DNA sequence information is published, the structure and function of many more genetic elements may be determined. This information will likely be useful for the rapid assessment of strain differences, which should have even more impact on intervention and outcomes.

References

1. Pfaller MA. Molecular approaches to diagnosing and managing infectious diseases: practicality and costs. *Emerg Infect Dis.* 2001;7: 312–318.

2. Byington CL, Spencer LY, Johnson TA, et al. An epidemiological investigation of a sustained high rate of pediatric parapneumonic empyema: risk factors and microbiological associations. *Clin Infect Dis.* 2002;34:434–440.

3. La Scola B, Fournier P, Musso D, et al. Pseudo-outbreak of listeriosis elucidated by pulsed-field gel electrophoresis. *Eur J Clin Microbiol Infect Dis.* 1997;10:756–760.

4. Michele T, Cronin W, Graham N, et al. Transmission of *Mycobacterium tuberculosis* by a fiberoptic bronchoscope. *JAMA.* 1997;278:1093–1095.

5. Spika J, Waterman S, Soo Hoo G, et al. Chloramphenicol-resistant *Salmonella newport* traced through hamburger to dairy farms. *New Engl J Med.* 1987;316:565–570.

6. Reed KD, Melski JW, Graham MB, et al. The detection of monkeypox in humans in the Western Hemisphere. *N Engl J Med.* 2004;350:342–350.

7. Ksiazek TG, Erdman D, Goldsmith CS, et al. A novel coronavirus associated with severe acute respiratory syndrome. *N Engl J Med.* 2003;348:1953–1966.

8. Drosten C, Gunther S, Preiser W, et al. Identification of a novel coronavirus in patients with severe acute respiratory syndrome. *N Engl J Med.* 2003;348:1967–1976.

9. Sader H, Jones R, Pfaller M. Relapse of catheter-related *Flavobacterium meningosepticum* bacteremia demonstrated by DNA macrorestriction analysis. *Clin Infect Dis.* 1995;21:997–1000.

10. Bishai W, Graham N, Harrington S, et al. Rifampin-resistant tuberculosis in a patient receiving rifabutin prophylaxis. *N Engl J Med.* 1996;334:1573–1576.

11. Zaidi A, Harrell L, Rost J, et al. Assessment of similarity among coagulase-negative staphylococci from sequential blood cultures of neonates and children by pulsed-field gelelectrophoresis. *J Infect Dis.* 1996;174:1010–1014.

12. Hartstein A, Valvano M, Morthland V, et al. Antimicrobic susceptibility and plasmidprofile analysis as identity tests for multiple blood isolates of coagulase-negative staphylococci. *J Clin Microbiol.* 1987;25: 589–593.

13. Tenover F, Arbeit R, Goering R, et al. Interpreting chromosomal DNA restriction patterns produced by pulsed-field gel electrophoresis: criteria for bacterial strain typing. *J Clin Microbiol.* 1995;33:2233–2239.

14. Arbeit R. Laboratory procedures for the epidemiologic analysis of microorganisms. In: Murray P, Jo Baron E, Pfaller M, et al, eds. *Manual of Clinical Microbiology.* 6th ed. Washington, DC: ASM Press; 1995:190–208.

15. Maslow J, Mulligan M, Arbeit R. Molecular epidemiology: application of contemporary techniques to the typing of microorganisms. *Clin Infect Dis.* 1993;17:153–164.

16. Gutacker MM, Smoot JC, Lux Migliaccio CA, et al. Genome-wide analysis of synonymous single nucleotide polymorphisms in *Mycobacterium tuberculosis* complex organisms: resolution of genetic relationships among closely related microbial strains. *Genetics.* 2002;162:1533–1543.

17. Sambrook J, Russel D, eds. *Molecular Cloning: A Laboratory Manual.* 3rd edition. Cold Spring Harbor, NY: Cold Spring Harbor Laboratory Press; 2001.

18. Persing D, Tenover F, Versalovic J, eds. *Molecular Microbiology: Diagnostic Principles and Practice.* Washington, DC: ASM Press; 2003.

19. Schwartz D, Cantor C. Separation of yeast chromosome-sized DNAs by pulsed field gradient gel electrophoresis. *Cell.* 1984;37:67–75.

20. Gut IG. Automation in genotyping of single nucleotide polymorphisms. *Hum Mutat.* 2001;17:475–492.

21. Pfaller M, Herwaldt L. The clinical microbiology laboratory and infection control: emerging pathogens, antimicrobial resistance, and new technology. *Clin Infect Dis.* 1997;25:858–870.

22. Kreiswirth B, Kornblum J, Arbeit R, et al. Evidence for a clonal origin of methicillin resistance in *Staphylococcus aureus. Science.* 1993;259:227–230.

23. Mayer L. Use of plasmid profiles in epidemiologic surveillance of disease outbreaks and in tracing the transmission of anitibiotic resistance. *Clin Microbiol Rev.* 1988;1:228–243.

24. Locksley R, Cohen M, Quinn T, et al. Multiple antibiotic-resistant *Staphylococcus aureus*: introduction, transmission, and evolution of nosocomial infection. *Ann Intern Med.* 1982;97:317–324.

25. Rubens C, Farrar W, McGee Z, et al. Evolution of a plasmid mediating resistance to multiple antimicrobial agents during a prolonged epidemic of nosocomial infections. *J Infect Dis.* 1981;143:170–181.

26. Tenover F, Arbeit R, Goering R. How to select and interpret molecular strain typing methods for epidemiological studies of bacterial infections: a review for healthcare epidemiologists. *Infect Control Hosp Epidemiol.* 1997;18:426–439.

27. Tompkins L, Plorde J, Falkow S. Molecular analysis of R-factors from multiresistant nosocomial isolates. *J Infect Dis.* 1980;141:625–636.

28. Kristjansson M, Samore M, Gerding D, et al. Comparison of restriction endonuclease analysis, ribotyping, and pulsed-field gel electrophoresis for molecular differentiation of *Clostridium difficile* strains. *J Clin Microbiol.* 1994;32:1963–1969.

29. Tenover F, Arbeit R, Archer R, et al. Comparison of traditional and molecular methods of typing isolates of *Staphylococcus aureus. J Clin Microbiol.* 1994;32:407–415.

30. Hinojosa-Ahumada M, Swaminathan B, Hunter S, et al. Restriction fragment length polymorphisms in rRNA operons for subtyping *Shigella sonnei. J Clin Microbiol.* 1991;29:2380–2384.

31. Gordillo M, Singh K, Murray B. Comparison of ribotyping and pulsed-field gelelectrophoresis for subspecies differentiation of strains of *Enterococcus faecalis. J Clin Microbiol.* 1993;31:1570–1574.

32. Martin I, Tyler S, Tyler K, et al. Evaluation of ribotyping as epidemiologic tool for typing *Escherichia coli* serogroup 0157 isolates. *J Clin Microbiol.* 1996;34:720–723.

33. van Soolingen D, Hermans P, de Haas P, et al. Occurrence and stability of insertion sequences in *Mycobacterium tuberculosis* complex strains: evaluation of an insertion sequence-dependent DNA polymorphism

as a tool in the epidemiology of tuberculosis. *J Clin Microbiol.* 1991;29:2578–2586.

34. van Soolingen D, DeHaas W, Petra E, et al. Comparison of various repetitive DNA elements as genetic markers for strain differentiation and epidemiology of *Mycobacterium tuberculosis*. *J Clin Microbiol.* 1993;31:1987–1995.

35. van Embden J, Cave M, Crawford J, et al. Strain identification of *Mycobacterium tuberculosis* by DNA fingerprinting: recommendations for a standardized methodology. *J Clin Microbiol.* 1993;31:406–409.

36. Small P, Hopewell P, Singh S, et al. The epidemiology of tuberculosis in San Francisco. *New Engl J Med.* 1994;330:1703–1709.

37. Alland D, Kalkut G, Moss A, et al. Transmission of tuberculosis in New York City. *New Engl J Med.* 1994;330:1710–1716.

38. Yang Z, Mtoni I, Chonde M, et al. DNA fingerprinting and phenotyping of *Mycobacterium tuberculosis* isolate from human immunodefiency virus (HIV)-seropositive and HIV-seronegative patients in Tanzania. *J Clin Microbiol.* 1995;33:1064–1069.

39. Yang Z, de Haas P, van Soolingen D, et al. Restriction fragment length polymorphism of *Mycobacterium tuberculosis* strains isolated from Greenland during 1992: evidence of tuberculosis transmission between Greenland and Denmark. *J Clin Microbiol.* 1994;32:3018–3025.

40. Small P, McClenny N, Singh S, et al. Molecular strain typing of *Mycobacterium tuberculosis* to confirm cross-contamination in the mycobacteriology laboratory and modification of procedures to minimize occurrence of false-positive cultures. *J Clin Microbiol.* 1993;31:1677–1682.

41. Burman W, Reves R, Hawkes A, et al. DNA fingerprinting with two probes decreases clustering of *Mycobacterium tuberculosis*. *Am J Respir Crit Care Med.* 1997;155:1140–1146.

42. King D, Rhine-Chalberg J, Pfaller M, et al. Comparison of four DNA-based methods for strain delineation of *Candida lusitaniae*. *J Clin Microbiol.* 1995;33:1467–1470.

43. Merz W. *Candida albicans* strain delineation. *Clin Microbiol Rev.* 1990;3:321–334.

44. Roman R, Smith J, Walker M, et al. Rapid geographic spread of a methicillin-resistant *Staphylococcus aureus* strain. *Clin Infect Dis.* 1997;25:698–705.

45. Diekema D, Messer S, Hollis R, et al. An outbreak of *Candida parapsilosis* prosthetic valve endocarditis. *Diagn Microbiol Infect Dis.* 1997;29:147–153.

46. Keene W, Sazie E, Kok J, et al. An outbreak of *Escherichia coli* 0157:H7 infections traced to jerky made from deer meat. *JAMA.* 1997;277: 1229–1231.

47. Shi Z, Liu P, Lau Y, et al. Epidemiological typing of isolates from an outbreak of infection with multidrug-resistant *Enterobacter cloacae* by repetitive extragenic palindromic unit b1-primed PCR and pulsed-field gel electrophoresis. *J Clin Microbiol.* 1996;34:2784–2790.

48. McDougal LK, Steward CD, Killgore GE, et al. Pulsed-field gel electrophoresis typing of oxacillin-resistant *Staphylococcus aureus* isolates from the United States: establishing a national database. *J Clin Microbiol.* 2003;41:5113–5120.

49. Enright MC, Day NPJ, Daves CE, et al. Multilocus sequence typing for characterization of methicillin-resistant and methicillin-susceptible clones of *Staphylococcus aureus*. *J Clin Microbiol.* 2000;38:1008–1015.

50. Diep BA, Perdreau-Remington F, Sensabaugh GF. Clonal characterization of *Staphylococcus aureus* by multilocus restriction fragment typing, a rapid screening approach for molecular epidemiology. *J Clin Microbiol.* 2003;41:4559–4564.

51. Matushek M, Bonten M, Hayden M. Rapid preparation of bacterial DNA for pulsed-field gel electrophoresis. *J Clin Microbiol.* 1996;34: 2598–2600.

52. Leonard RB, Carroll KC. Rapid lysis of gram-positive cocci for pulsed-field gel electrophoresis using achromopeptidase. *Diagn Mol Pathol.* 1997;6:288–291.

53. Hartas J, Hibble M, Sriprakash K. Simplification of a locus-specific DNA typing method (vir typing) for *Streptococcus pyogenes. J Clin Microbiol.* 1998;36:1428–1429.

54. Goh S, Byrne S, Zhang J, et al. Molecular typing of *Staphylococcus aureus* on the basis of coagulase gene polymorphisms. *J Clin Microbiol.* 1992;30:1642–1645.

55. Versalovic J, Koeuth T, Lupski JR. Distribution of repetitive DNA sequences in eubacteria and application to fingerprinting of bacterial genomes. *Nucleic Acids Res.* 1991;19:6823–6831.

56. Tyler K, Wang G, Tyler S, et al. Factors affecting reliability and reproducibility of amplification-based DNA fingerprinting of representative bacterial pathogens. *J Clin Microbiol.* 1997;35:339–346.

57. van Belkum A. DNA fingerprinting of medically important microorganisms by use of PCR. *Clin Microbiol Rev.* 1994;7:174–184.

58. Welsh J, McClelland M. Fingerprinting genomes using PCR with arbitrary primers. *Nucleic Acids Res.* 1990;18:7213–7218.

59. van Belkum A, Kluytmans J, van Leeuwen W, et al. Multicenter evaluation of arbitrarily primed PCR for typing of *Staphylococcus aureus* strains. *J Clin Microbiol.* 1995;33:1537–1547.

60. Fleishmann RD, Alland D, Eisen JA, et al. Whole-genome comparison of *Mycobacterium tuberculosis* clinical and laboratory strains. *J Bacteriol.* 2002;184:5479–5490.

61. Alland D, Whittmam TS, Murray MB, et al. Modeling bacterial evolution with comparative-genome-based marker systems: application to *Mycobacterium tuberculosis* evolution and pathogenesis. *J Bacteriol.* 2003;185:3392–3399.

62. Enright MC, Robinson DA, Randle G, et al. The evolutionary history of methicillin-resistant *Staphylococcus aureus* (MRSA). *Proc Natl Acad Sci USA.* 2002;99:7687–7692.

63. Monk AB, Curtis S, Paul J, et al. Genetic analysis of *Staphylococcus aureus* from intravenous drug user lesions. *J Med Microbiol.* 2004;53:223–227.

64. Enright MC. The evolution of a resistant pathogen—the case of MRSA. *Curr Opin Pharmacol.* 2003;3:474–479.

65. Peacock SJ, de Silva GDI, Justice A, et al. Comparison of multilocus sequence typing and pulsed-field gel electrophoresis as tools for typing *Staphylococcus aureus* isolates in a microepidemiological setting. *J Clin Microbiol.* 2002;40:3764–3770.

66. Diep BA, Sensabaugh GF, Somboona NS, et al. Widespread skin and soft-tissue infections due to two methicillin-resistant *Staphylococcus aureus* strains harboring the genes for Panton-Valentine leucocidin. *J Clin Microbiol.* 2004;42:2080–2084.

67. Carleton HA, An Diep B, Charlebois ED, et al. Community-adapted methicillin-resistant *Staphylococcus aureus* (MRSA): population

dynamics of an expanding community reservoir of MRSA. *J Infect Dis.* 2004;190:1730–1738.

68. Woods C Jr, Versalovic J, Koeuth T, et al. Analysis of relationships among isolates of *Citrobacter diversus* by using DNA fingerprinting generated by repetitive sequence-based primers in the polymerase chain reaction. *J Clin Microbiol.* 1992;30:2921–2929.

69. Gerner-Smidt P, Graves L, Hunter S, et al. Computerized analysis of restriction fragment length polymorphism patterns: comparative evaluation of two commercial software packages. *J Clin Microbiol.* 1998;36:1318–1323.

CHAPTER TEN

THE IMMUNE SYSTEM AND HOST DEFENSE AGAINST INFECTIONS

Joseph B. Margolick, Richard B. Markham, and Alan L. Scott

Introduction

The human immune system is a diverse array of cells that permeate the human body (Box 10-1) and protect it against the pathogenic effects of infectious organisms that may enter and threaten the body. The goal of this chapter is to describe (at a level appropriate for a nonimmunologist) how this protection is provided. Astonishing insights into immunity have accrued in the last few decades, more than can be encompassed by a chapter that assumes little prior knowledge of immunology or cell biology. Therefore, although we provide here a basic outline, we also provide supplemental details in text boxes, and we refer to other sources for those who may want to learn more detail. The last 30 years have been an exciting and challenging time for both immunology and infectious disease epidemiology. In this chapter, you will have the best of both worlds!

Research on immune functions uses many experimental methods, both in vivo and in vitro. In many cases, cells perform the same functions in tissue culture, where they are relatively easy to measure, that they do in the body. Because these functions are generally similar across the immune systems of humans and of other animals, inferences from animal models of disease often have direct applicability to human host defense and immune function. Finally, the advent of modern molecular microbiology and recombinant DNA methods have made it possible to isolate and characterize many of the molecules produced by immune cells to regulate and/or mediate the functions of the immune system. These same innovations have also allowed us to gain insight into the functions of these molecules in animal models by inserting or deleting ("knocking out") the genes that code for these molecules.

Studies have revealed a complex and dynamic interaction between cells of the immune system and pathogens. Two distinct but interrelated systems—one

Box 10-1   Cells of the immune system

Cells of the immune system include lymphocytes, mononuclear phagocytes, macrophages, and dendritic cells. These cells are derived from bone marrow precursors.

In the peripheral blood, about one fourth of the white blood cells are lymphocytes and about one twentieth are monocytes, the circulating form of mononuclear phagocytes. Less than 1% are dendritic cells. At any given time, only about 2% of lymphocytes are in the peripheral blood.

general and one highly specific—have evolved for the recognition of pathogens and foreign molecules. Both systems involve a complex of cell surface receptors and soluble molecules that work in concert to identify a pathogen through unique aspects of its molecular makeup, and tag it for elimination. One system is designed to work within minutes after a pathogen establishes residency in the vertebrate host. This response utilizes receptors that are constitutively expressed on mononuclear and polymorphonuclear phagocytic cells and on "killer" cells and that recognize pathogen-associated molecular patterns (PAMPS). These receptors provide a general signal that certain types of microorganisms are present, and they initiate cellular mechanisms that can clear the foreign pathogen from the body. This ready-to-use capacity to rapidly recognize pathogens is referred to as the innate immune response. (The term *innate* refers to the fact that these responses do not require time to develop but rather are ready to go at any time.)

Most encounters with microorganisms and toxins are unapparent because the innate immune response is able to eliminate the threat of infection. However, in those situations where cells and molecules of the innate immune response fail to control and eliminate a pathogenic organism, the role of the innate response shifts to one of initiating, modulating, and mediating the second, highly specific arm of the vertebrate defense system—the *adaptive* immune response. (The term *adaptive* refers to the fact that these responses take time to develop in the infected host.) The cells that regulate and carry out most of the major effector functions of the adaptive immune response are lymphocytes called T cells and B cells. These lymphocytes provide the inducibility and specificity that are hallmarks of the adaptive immune response through antigen-specific surface receptors. In addition, after clearing the pathogen, the cells of the adaptive immune response develop a long-lived "memory" of the exposure that can be quickly mobilized upon reexposure to the same antigens. In the following review, we will expand on the description and roles of the cells and molecules that play key roles in the functions of the innate and adaptive immune responses.

Pathogens that reside within cells pose a special challenge to the immune system, because they are not directly accessible to detection by the immune system. However, cells containing pathogens are themselves altered at the cell surface, and these alterations can be recognized by both the innate and the adaptive immune systems. As mentioned above, the innate immune system can recognize molecular patterns present on the pathogen itself. It can also recognize patterns on the infected cell, which may be generically altered as a result of being infected. (For example, infection of a cell may cause a normal surface molecule to be expressed at abnormally high or low levels.) Thus, innate immunity does not depend primarily on the identity of the infecting pathogen. (Innate immunity is also triggered by other processes that affect integrity of cells, such as heat injury, radiation, or toxic exposures.) The main cell types involved in innate immunity are macrophages, dendritic cells, and natural killer (NK) cells (see Boxes 10-2 and 10-3).

Box 10-2 Macrophages and dendritic cells

Mononuclear phagocytes circulate in the peripheral blood as monocytes and migrate into tissues where they become macrophages.[1] Their functions are to ingest and eliminate infectious agents,[2] process and present antigens, and help regulate the functions of other immune cells, both innate and adaptive.

Dendritic cells have a characteristic shape with many long cytoplasmic processes (dendrites). They home through the peripheral blood to tissues, where they persist in an immature form. When stimulated to mature, by infection or injury, they are avid inducers of innate immunity. The mature cells also migrate to lymphoid organs carrying antigens bound to their cell surface and function as potent antigen-presenting cells. Uniquely, these cells can induce a primary immune response. They also affect the cytokine secretion pattern of the antigen-activated T cells.

Box 10-3 Types and names of lymphocytes

There are three types of lymphocytes in the peripheral blood—T cells, B cells, and natural killer (NK) cells. These cells are morphologically indistinguishable by conventional techniques, although NK cells are often a bit larger and have more granules in their cytoplasm than T or B cells. T and B cells are lymphocytes that are named after the organs that are necessary for their maturation.

T cells mature in the thymus, a gland located underneath the breastbone or sternum, in mammals and rodents. B cells received their name from the bursa of Fabricius, an organ found in birds that is essential for B-cell maturation. Humans do not have this organ, and B cells appear to mature in the bone marrow. NK cells are described in Box 10-6.

Lymphocyte biology is a relatively new field. Only in 1960 was it discovered (by Peter Nowell) that resting lymphocytes could be triggered to become activated and only in 1964 (by John Gowans) that lymphocytes recirculated in the body from blood to lymph and back to blood, even though recirculation of red cells had been demonstrated in 1628 by William Harvey.

The immune system is traditionally considered to have three defining characteristics. The first is that it can discriminate between self and nonself, meaning what is normally present in the host and what is not. The second is that it remembers what it has encountered (memory). Memory allows the immune system to react more quickly and effectively to a stimulus it has encountered previously. The third characteristic is that it responds only to the pathogen that is at hand (specificity). In this chapter, we will also explain how the immune system attains these characteristics.

Recognition of Pathogens

The first step in the immune response to a pathogen is the recognition of the pathogen. It has long been known that the immune system can distinguish self from nonself or foreign antigens. How this was accomplished was a fascinating mystery for many years, but the essential mechanisms have now been clarified in work that resulted in at least six Nobel prizes.

What does the immune system actually recognize, or react to? Substances that can trigger an immune response are called *antigens*. More specifically, the receptors on cells of the immune response recognize small subregions on each antigen, termed *epitopes* or *antigenic determinants*. A single antigen molecule can have many epitopes that can be recognized by different receptors. Epitopes can be made up of amino acids, sugars, lipids, or nucleotides. In adaptive immunity, lymphocyte receptors recognize highly unique epitopes on pathogen-derived antigens. In contrast, the receptors used in the innate immune response recognize pathogen-derived antigens that are not species specific, but are representative of a class of microorganism, such as virus, bacteria, fungi, or parasite. In adaptive immunity, cells of the immune system recognize specific antigens that are not normally present in the body, such as those that belong to particular bacteria, viruses, parasites, or other organisms. In innate immunity, antigens are not pathogen specific, but are still recognized by receptors. In recent years, much work has been directed at defining the precise chemical nature of antigens and what characteristics a substance must have in order to elicit an effective immune response. This work has been motivated by very practical concerns, such as developing needed vaccines and understanding immune responses to dangerous organisms.

Antigen Recognition in Adaptive Immunity (T and B Cells)

The cells that are responsible for specific recognition of foreign antigens (i.e., adaptive immunity) are B and T lymphocytes (see Box 10-3). These cells have surface proteins that bind to (recognize) antigens with high specificity and affinity: each protein can recognize one antigen and that one only. These surface recognition proteins are called *antigen receptors*, and it is the precise binding characteristics of these receptors (they bind strongly to only one epitope out of all possible epitopes) that is responsible for the amazing specificity of the immune system. For T cells the epitope is usually a small peptide; for B cells it is frequently more than a small peptide that is recognized. (Indeed, for many years the specificity of antibodies produced by immunizing experimental animals has been exploited to identify substances in experiments and in clinical medicine.) When the antigen receptor binds its antigen, the B or T cells become activated, and the immune response is triggered (as will be described in more detail below).

Both B and T cell receptors can recognize any antigen that can be encountered. This includes synthetic antigens that don't exist in nature. How such a vast array of receptors could exist puzzled immunologists for many years, because there isn't enough DNA in the entire body to code for one gene for each possible antibody! The answer to this problem was worked out for B cells and subsequently shown to apply for T cells as well: it involves the combining of conserved areas of the receptor, which require only small numbers of genes, with several highly variable gene segments, thus generating a huge number of possible permutations of the final receptor molecule (see Box 10-4).

Box 10-4   Generation of receptor diversity

The receptors for both T and B cells have a number of functional domains or regions. A large proportion of both these receptors have common functions such as anchoring the receptor to the cell membrane, binding to a number of accessory proteins both at the cell surface (to stabilize cell–cell interactions) and in the cytoplasm (where they act as a binding point for the proteins that participate in the transduction of signals to the nucleus that results in cell activation and differentiation). Both T-cell and B-cell receptors have a domain that is designed to specifically bind to a small portion of an antigen (i.e., an epitope). Some aspects of these receptors are illustrated in Figures 10-1 through10-3. This antigen-binding site is unique for each different B-cell receptor (i.e., antibody) or T-cell receptor and is the source of antigen specificity for a B cell or a T cell, respectively.

The vast number of unique specificities used by the receptors of the adaptive immune response is generated by a random combinatorial mechanism that is independent of antigen. T-cell and B-cell receptors are composed of multiple protein chains. (See Figures 10-1 through 10-3.) Each chain is encoded by a number of gene segments that are spliced together at the DNA level to form genes for specific receptors. There are a large number of germ line gene segments that encode the domains that form the sites for antigen recognition. These segments are assembled in a random fashion that, along with random insertions and deletions of nucleotides at splicing junctions, determines the final amino acid sequence of this variable region of the receptor protein, which in turn determines the specificity of each receptor chain. Following molecular events that assemble the variable region of the receptor to the constant regions, the multiple protein chains are joined by the cell to make the mature receptor. It is the interactions of the variable regions of these multichain molecules that determines the fine specificity of each receptor. Current estimates of the number of different T-cell and B-cell receptors that are generated by the random use of multiple germ line variable genes, imprecise joining of gene segments, and random use of different chains generates approach 10^{18}! This vast array of receptor molecules accounts for the astounding ability of the immune system to recognize any possible antigen.

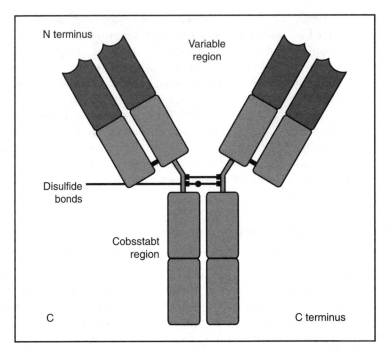

FIGURE 10-1 Diagrammatic representation of an antibody (immunoglobulin) molecule, showing the variable and constant regions, and the four protein chains (2 light [short] and 2 heavy [long] chains) that are linked together by disulfide bonds.
Source: Janeway CA et al. Immunobiology: the Immune System in Health and Disease, 6th ed. (Garland, New York, 2005).

B- and T-cell antigen receptors work in different ways. The B-cell receptor recognizes antigens in their native form, meaning as they exist in nature. This means that the antigen does not need to be manipulated in any way, and the B cell can recognize an antigen by itself without the help of any other cells. (This is true whether the B-cell receptor, which is an antibody molecule, is attached to the membrane of the B cell or has been secreted and is free of the B cell entirely.)

The T-cell antigen receptor differs from the B-cell antigen receptor in two ways. First, it cannot recognize native antigen. Rather, it recognizes only antigens that have been broken down into short, epitope-sized peptide fragments. This process is referred to as *antigen processing* and can be carried out by many types of cells. Thus, T-cell antigen recognition requires *antigen-processing cells*. Second, the T-cell receptor recognizes not just the processed peptide, but also a protein on the antigen processing cell that carries the peptide. The host cell proteins that do this are called *major histocompatibility (MHC) proteins*. On the surface of the antigen-processing cell, the processed peptide can be seen by the T cell, a process that is called *antigen presentation*. In other words, the T-cell antigen receptor, even though it is specific for one peptide, is also specific for one MHC protein, and T cells therefore recognize antigen only in the context of the correct MHC protein.

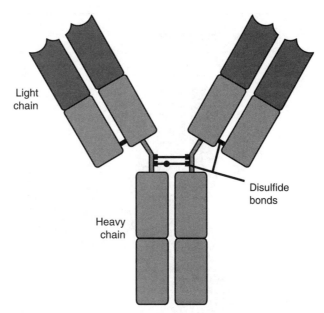

FIGURE 10-2   Diagrammatic representation of an antibody molecule showing the two heavy and two light chains.
Source: Janeway CA et al. Immunobiology: the Immune System in Health and Disease, 6th ed. (Garland, New York, 2005).

For this reason, antigen recognition by T cells is said to be MHC restricted, and antigen-presenting cells and T cells must be *histocompatible* for T-cell activation to occur. Because of MHC restriction, one person's T cells will not recognize any antigens unless that person's own antigen-presenting cells (or antigen-presenting cells from another person who happens to have some of the same particular MHC proteins) are doing the presenting. In summary, then, T-cell responses require the processing and presentation of antigen by an antigen-presenting cell to a histocompatible T cell.

MHC proteins are highly variable from person to person and in fact are among the most variable proteins known (see Box 10-5). It is this variability from person to person that allows the immune system to distinguish self from nonself, meaning one's own cells and antigens from someone else's. There are two broad classes of MHC molecules: class I, which are expressed on all nucleated cells in the body, and class II, which are primarily expressed by cells of the immune system (monocyte/macrophages, dendritic cells, B cells, and activated T cells). In the human, MHC proteins are also called human leukocyte antigens (HLA).

It may seem arcane to speak of all these different molecules, but they are fundamental to viral immune processes. MHC class I proteins are the primary antigens responsible for graft rejection and also must be expressed by a target cell in order for this cell to be killed by an antigen-specific CD8 T cell.[3] MHC class II must be the same on the antigen-presenting cell and the CD4 T cells in order for the latter to be triggered.[4] In fact, all of the cells listed above as expressing class II MHC are important antigen-presenting cells, even B

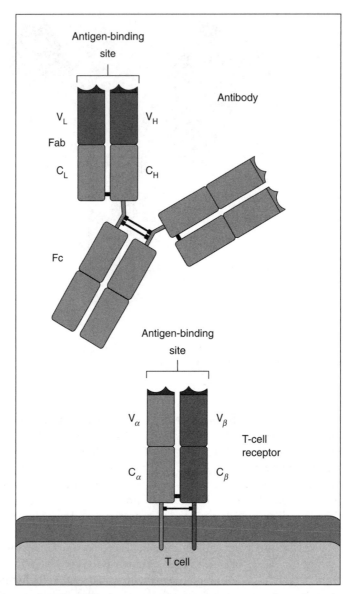

FIGURE 10-3 Diagrammatic representation of the structural similarity between the B-cell receptor (antibody molecule) and the T-cell receptor. Both have large constant regions and smaller variable regions, with the antibody-binding sites in the variable regions. Both are composed of disulfide-linked protein chains, called heavy and light for the B-cell receptor and chains for the T-cell receptor, which also have variable and constant regions.
Source: Janeway CA et al. Immunobiology: the Immune System in Health and Disease, 6th ed. (Garland, New York, 2005).

cells. Of note, activated B cells can use their antigen-specific surface receptor to facilitate antigen uptake as the first step in antigen processing. For this reason, B cells can process antigens that are present in very low concentrations and are important cells for presentation of antigen to T cells during mature immune responses.[5] However, B cells specific for a given antigen are

Box 10-5   Diversity of MHC proteins

In humans, more than 2100 distinct MHC allele sequences have been described. Human class I MHC proteins include HLA-A, -B, and -C proteins, which have 319, 609, and 161 known variants, respectively. Class II MHC proteins include HLA-DR, -DQ, and -DP; these have 406, 72, and 120 variants, respectively. The number of distinct protein molecules that can be generated is not precisely known, but is certainly very large.

MHC proteins contain indentations or clefts that can accommodate small peptides (about 9–15 amino acids long). The characteristics of the amino acids in the MHC cleft determine the characteristics of the peptides that can be bound in the cleft and thus will be presented to T cells.Each person inherits one set of class I (A, B, C) and one of class II (HLA-DR, -DR, and -DP) from each parent; all six class I and all six class II are expressed in a *codominant* fashion, meaning all forms of a given gene are expressed equally. The mix of MHC molecules inherited and expressed is called an immunological *hapoltype*.

much are less numerous than other antigen-presenting cells, which is why the nonspecific-antigen presenting cells are essential.

Because MHC proteins vary so widely among individuals, the MHC proteins from different individuals will interact differently with the foreign proteins or peptides encountered by those individuals. Most of the antigens associated with pathogens are complex molecules that can be degraded by antigen-processing cells into many different peptides. Among individuals with different MHC proteins, therefore, different peptides may bind most efficiently to a given individual's repertoire of MHC proteins. For example: if a protein contains epitopes A, B, and C, only epitope A may be presented by antigen-presenting cells in an individual of one MHC type and only epitope B in an individual of another MHC type. Some individuals may be of an MHC type that will not bind any of these epitopes, and such individuals will not recognize any of these peptides. This means that immunizing T cells for a human population is much more complicated than immunizing B cells, because B cells recognize native antigen, which is the same for everybody. Given the enormous diversity of MHC proteins in the human population, vaccines that will induce general T-cell immunity represent an extremely formidable challenge. It is not a coincidence that almost all successful vaccines generated to date have depended largely on B-cell responses (i.e., antibodies) rather than T-cell responses.

Antigen Recognition in Innate Immunity

A third type of lymphocyte, termed natural killer (NK) cells, plays a key role in triggering innate immunity (see Box 10-6).

The mechanism by which NK cells are triggered to kill has only recently been elucidated. Although they do not have antigen receptors, NK cells have surface receptors that inhibit their killing function. These inhibitory receptors, termed killer inhibitory receptors (KIRs), recognize abnormal levels of MHC class I molecules on all other nucleated cells in the body. This means that if the target cell expresses MHC class I to a normal degree, the NK cell is not triggered and the target cell is not killed. On the other hand, down-regulation of MHC class I molecule expression (which is common in some virally infected cells and some tumor cells) removes the inhibition of the NK cell, and the target cell is killed.

This mechanism appears to be an important component of host defense against certain viral infections.[6,7] Many viruses interfere with expression of MHC molecules by the host cell (possibly as a means of evading cytotoxic CD8+ T cells, which require MHC class I molecules to be expressed on the target cell, as discussed above). Thus, NK cells help prevent the virus from getting away with this trick. This mechanism elegantly explains the function of NK cells. (Then, in a surprise, stimulatory NK receptors were discovered. Although the precise mechanisms and importance of these receptors are not well understood, it appears that the function of NK cells is regulated by the balance of signals coming from the KIR and activating receptors. It has been hypothesized that stimulatory receptors on NK cells may be important in situations in which MHC proteins are overexpressed, which is uncommon in infectious diseases but may occur in neoplastic or preneoplastic conditions.)

Macrophages and dendritic cells have been described in Box 10-2. How do they recognize antigens? In contrast to the specific recognition of particular antigens by T cells, as described above, macrophages and dendritic cells recognize molecules common to multiple pathogens or structures derived from such antigens. For this reason, antigen receptors on these cells are referred to as pattern recognition receptors[10] (see Box 10-7).

After Antigen Binding: Immune Activation

Lymphocytes in the blood are generally in a *resting* state. That means the cell is structurally and functionally quiescent or inactive. B and T lymphocytes

Box 10-6   History of natural killer (NK) cells

NK cells were discovered as the cells responsible for the background killing that was detectable when peripheral blood cells were tested for cytotoxicity against various target cells. It was found that there was usually some level of cytotoxicity in such assays that did not depend on the presence of antigen in the assay, did not require priming of the cells, and was not mediated by the cytotoxic lymphocytes that were known at the time (i.e., the cytotoxic T cells discussed above). The cytotoxic cells turned out to be large granular lymphocytes, and these were named natural killer or NK cells because they did not need to be induced (primed) by in vitro treatments of the cells.

Box 10-7 Examples of pattern recognition in innate immunity

Examples of molecules that are recognized by their pattern are certain carbohydrates and lipopolysaccharides, including endotoxins. Another example is nonmethylated GpC motifs in bacterial DNA; these motifs are not present in mammalian DNA. These patterns are recognized by a family of receptors called toll-like receptors, so named because they resemble a type of receptor found in fruit flies called a toll receptor.[8,9]

have the morphology one would expect of such cells (see Box 10-8). But when the lymphocyte encounters the antigen it is programmed to recognize (through its antigen receptor), the cell becomes transformed into an activated cell. Activated cells can make important immune regulatory and effector molecules and can also proliferate, or multiply, by mitosis. So, the resting state in which most lymphocytes that we see in the peripheral blood exist is just a temporary phase, at least potentially. NK cells also circulate in a resting state, though with slightly more cytoplasm and preexisting effector molecules than B or T cells.

The fact that immune cells generally exist in the resting state, along with the specificity of T- and B-cell receptors, allows the immune system to aim its weapons only where they are needed. As discussed further below, the immune system includes powerful responses that can cause great damage to the host if it is not carefully controlled. This means that activation must be limited to those cells needed to neutralize a particular threat, and also that activation should be turned off as soon as possible after the threat has been removed or neutralized.

Activation of Adaptive Immunity

Both T- and B-cell receptors are anchored in the cell membrane and are associated with adjacent molecules that cross through the cell membrane into the cytoplasm of the cell. When the antigen receptor binds its antigen, the associated molecules are altered in such a way that intracellular enzymes are activated that cause the lymphocyte to begin to carry out its preprogrammed functions.

Box 10-8 Morphology of lymphocytes

Resting cells are characterized by condensed nuclear chromatin (i.e., nuclear DNA coiled and inaccessible to genetic machinery of the cell) and a minimal amount of cytoplasm (where cellular products such as antibodies and cytokines are made). In contrast, in activated cells the nuclear DNA is dispersed and available for transcription into RNA, and the cytoplasm is more abundant and contains more organelles.

The ability of an *extracellular* antigen to cause activation of *intracellular* processes requires the carrying of a signal across the cell membrane, a process called *signal transduction*. This requires the antigen receptor to be present on the surface of the cell. Signal transduction is not as simple as just binding of the antigen to the receptor; factors such as the affinity of the antigen for the receptor are important, and in most cases an additional signal besides the antigen receptor-induced signal is required for the cell to become fully activated. The second signal is not antigen specific but can be mediated by binding of molecules on the antigen-presenting cell to other molecules on the surface of the lymphocyte.[11] The sequence of biochemical events in lymphocyte signal transduction has been extensively researched, and reviews can be found in textbooks of immunology, such as those listed at the end of this chapter.

The B and T cells that have been activated undergo cell division and begin to proliferate, giving rise to a clonal expansion of just the cells that are responding to the immune stimulus. This process is called *clonal selection* and is one of the most important mechanisms by which careful control is maintained over immune reactions.

Activation of Innate Immunity

Activation of phagocytic cells through their pattern recognition receptors and of NK cells through their activation and inhibitory receptors occurs via a cascade of receptor-linked biochemical events similar to that which activates T cells through the T-cell receptor.

Dealing with the Pathogen: Immune Effector Mechanisms

Once a foreign antigen enters the body, innate immunity is the first line of defense and the humoral and cellular arms of the adaptive immune response the second. There is an important time element to these responses. Several days are required for the full development of protective immunity in a naive host, because a very low number of antigen-specific T cells must be activated, clonally expanded, and converted from naive cells into activated effector cells and, eventually, into memory cells. One of the functions of the innate response is to fill the lag period between infection and the development of a mature adaptive immune response with a defense mechanism that can blunt the capacity of the pathogen to expand.

Broadly speaking, the effector functions of adaptive immunity include antibody production, the activation and arming of immune cells capable of direct or indirect killing of microorganisms, killing of appropriate organisms and cells (such as cells infected with a virus), generation of delayed type hypersensitivity responses, and regulation (induction and suppression) of these functions. Each of these aspects of adaptive immunity is carried out by specific subsets of cells, under the regulation of specific cytokines.

In innate immunity, NK cells and macrophages become activated, and in adaptive immunity T and B cells become activated through their receptors. All of these processes are regulated or effected by a complex tapestry of interconnecting cellular activations. These are finely regulated by hormone-like proteins (termed *cytokines*; see below and Box 10-9) that are produced

Box 10-9   Cytokines

Cytokines are small proteins that function like hormones, except that as a general rule they do not circulate in the blood in meaningful quantities, but rather act over a distance of a few cell diameters. In other words, they act on cells adjacent, or in close proximity, to the secreting cell (this is called *paracrine* regulation, as distinguished from *endocrine* regulation, which implies circulation in the blood and action on distant cells). An example of paracrine function would be secretion by activated helper T cells of cytokines that help nearby B cells differentiate into antibody-secreting cells, or cytokines that activate macrophages or killer T cells to become much more potent at killing microorganisms. In some cases, cytokines act on the secreting cell itself, which is called *autocrine* regulation. An example of autocrine regulation is the secretion by activated helper T cells of cytokines that allow the activated T cells to proliferate and expand clonally.

The first cytokine was described in 1970, and this was followed by the description of many immune functions (and other functions) that were mediated by possible cytokines. A major stumbling block to these early studies was the fact that, as mentioned above, cytokines are generally not present in the blood and in fact are extremely potent molecules whose physiological concentrations are tiny. This made biochemical purification and isolation of these molecules difficult technically and greatly hampered the working out of cytokine networks. It was only with the advent of molecular biology, genetic cloning, and recombinant DNA methods that cytokines could be studied efficiently, because now genes for cytokines can be isolated and large quantities of pure proteins (i.e., uncontaminated by small amounts of other cytokines) can be generated. This allowed the identities, modes of action, and functional properties of unique cytokines to be defined.

by the activated cells and act on the same or other cells. Another way in which the actions of cytokines are controlled is through the regulation of expression of *cytokine receptors* (i.e., the proteins to which cytokines bind on target cells). These receptors are responsible for transduction of regulatory signals across cell membranes.

In other words, immune effector mechanisms, such as immune activation, are stringently regulated by tight control of (1) the amount and type of cytokines that are produced, (2) the level of expression of cytokine receptors on cells of the immune response, (3) the different types of cells concerned, whose numbers can expand or contract by up to several orders of magnitude in a just few days, and (4) immunoglobulin proteins (termed *antibodies*) that can recognize and bind to the offending antigens. Cytokines are antigen independent; that is, their structure and function do not depend on the antigen that elicits their production. There are now more than 100 known cytokines, and the number is still growing. Some of the most important cytokines are described below.

Many cytokines have been given the name interleukin, because they facilitate interactions between white blood cells (*leuko* meaning *white*). For example, interleukin-2 (IL-2) is a cytokine that promotes proliferation and growth of activated T cells, as well as other functions such as activation of natural killer cells to become more cytotoxic. Other related terms include *lymphokine* to describe cytokines made by lymphocytes, and *monokine* to refer to those made by mononuclear phagocytes. (The interleukin nomenclature is much simpler than naming proteins for their function. This is untenable because cytokines have many functions. For example, a cytokine that stimulates growth of B cells and one that stimulates metabolic activity of hepatocytes both turned out to be IL-6.)

Adaptive Immune Effector Mechanisms

Almost all T cells belong to one of two major subsets. The first is helper T cells, which induce or permit functions of other immune cells. These cells express a protein called CD4 (see Box 10-10) on their cell surface, and thus are called CD4 lymphocytes. CD4 lymphocytes produce cytokines that increase the ability of macrophages to kill ingested organisms[12] and facilitate B cells to differentiate into antibody-producing cells,[13] activate other helper T cells to expand clonally as mentioned above, and potentiate the cytotoxic functioning of killer T cells and NK cells. The other major subset of T cells is cytotoxic T cells, which generally inhibit other cells or kill them, and express a surface protein called CD8.[14] Adaptive immune mechanisms differ for extracellular versus intracellular pathogens.

Extracellular Immune Effector Mechanisms

Protection against free-living extracellular organisms is provided mainly by antibodies and phagocytic cells. As mentioned above, the production of antibodies is mediated by B cells. When B cells become activated, they begin rearranging the genes that code for antibodies, and the cells begin to differentiate into cells that are actually tiny antibody factories. These cells are called plasma cells. They are produced in the secondary lymphoid tissues (lymph nodes, spleen, Peyer's patches, etc.) and eventually migrate to the bone marrow to secrete antibodies.

Antibodies produced by plasma cells are secreted proteins, though they are structurally similar to, and have the same antigen specificity as, the antibody molecules that are present in the membrane of the progenitor B cell. The function of antibodies is to bind to whole antigens in their native

Box 10-10   CD nomenclature

The letters *CD* stand for *cluster designation* and are used to denote proteins defined by being recognized by sets or clusters of monoclonal antibodies. CD numbers have been assigned through CD339 based on data presented at several international workshops. CD4 was the fourth protein to be assigned a CD number.

forms as mentioned above. Antibodies are thus well designed to provide host defense against extracellular antigens, such as bacteria that can grow outside cells. In many cases, these bacteria can grow quite rapidly, and it is important for host defense to be able to mount a vigorous immune response as quickly as possible. The main host defense against bacterial infection is ingestion of bacteria by white blood cells known as neutrophils. This process of ingestion (termed *phagocytosis*) is made hugely more efficient if the bacteria have been coated with antibodies, because neutrophils have receptors on their cell surfaces that recognize a conserved structural part of the antibody molecule that is part of the constant portion of the antibody molecule. The phenomenon of coating of bacteria by antibodies to facilitate phagocytosis is called *opsonization*. Other host proteins also facilitate phagocytosis and lysis of extracellular pathogens. For example, complement is the name given to a series of proteins that can bind to the surface of microorganisms and to each other. The result is a cascade of reactions that generates membrane-bound proteins on the microorganism that can be recognized by phagocytic cells through complement receptors. (However, in general complement proteins are not as efficient as antibodies in facilitating phagocytosis.) Antibodies can also directly interfere with replication of pathogens, binding of obligate intracellular pathogens to their target cells, and binding of toxins to their target molecules.

Antibodies come in five different classes—immunoglobulins M, D, G, A, and E—which have different chemical structures, localization in the body, and functions (Figure 10-4). As might be expected from this, these antibodies serve different roles in host defense against infections, and this is described below in the section on B-cell immune deficiency.

Intracellular Immune Effector Mechanisms

As discussed above, MHC class I proteins, which are produced inside the cell and then move to the cell surface, carry with them peptides that are being produced inside the cell. If the cell has been infected by a virus and viral proteins are being produced, peptides derived from these viral proteins will be carried to the cell surface in this way. There, the MHC I viral peptide complex can be recognized ("seen," in immunological parlance) by virus-specific CD8+ T cells that come in contact with the infected cell. These in turn are activated by the interaction between the MHC class I viral peptide complex and the specific T-cell receptors, and the T cells kill the infected cell (see Box 10-11).

Because antigen processing and presentation occur faster than viral production after the virus enters a cell, the infected cell can be recognized and killed even before new virus is produced or expressed on the cell surface. This is key to controlling the viral infection. This pathway also explains why MHC class I is expressed on all (nucleated) cells in the body: this allows the immune system to see the internal state of all cells, creating a form of immune surveillance.

In contrast to this intracellular pathway of antigen processing, class II MHC molecules become loaded with peptides from antigens ingested from outside the cell, and this is referred to as the *extracellular pathway*. This

Functional Activity	IgM	IgD	IgG1	IgG2	IgG3	IgG4	IgA	IgE
Neutralization	+	−	++	++	++	++	++	−
Opsonization	+	−	+++	*	++	+	+	−
Sensitization for killing by NK cells	−	−	++	−	++	−	−	−
Sensitization of mast cells	−	−	+	−	+	−	−	+++
Activates complement system	+++	−	++	+	+++	−	+	−

Distribution	IgM	IgD	IgG1	IgG2	IgG3	IgG4	IgA	IgE
Transport across epithelium	+	−	−	−	−	−	+++ (dimer)	−
Transport across placenta	−	−	+++	+	++	+/−	−	−
Diffusion into extravascular sites	+/−	−	+++	+++	+++	+++	++ (monomer)	+
Mean serum level (mg ml^{-1})	1.5	0.04	9	3	1	0.5	2.1	3×10^{-5}

FIGURE 10-4 Schematic representation of the functions and distributions of different types of antibodies (immunoglobulins).
Source: Janeway CA et al. Immunobiology: the Immune System in Health and Disease, 6th ed. (Garland, New York, 2005).

Box 10-11   T-cell killing mechanisms

Two mechanisms by which T cells kill cells are known. In the first, a T-cell product, perforin, binds to the target cell membrane and causes pores to form in it. A second T-cell product, granzyme, facilitates this process and also induces programmed cell death in the target cell. (Programmed cell death is a mechanism by which cells can self-destruct.) In the second mechanism, T-cell molecules termed *Fas ligand* bind to Fas proteins on the target cell, again inducing programmed cell death. Which mechanism kills the target cell is influenced by many factors, including the nature of the infection in the cell.[15]

explains why class II is expressed primarily by antigen-presenting cells, as mentioned above.

Killing of microorganisms occurs by several mechanisms. Cytotoxic T cells kill target cells expressing microbial antigens through the mechanisms outlined in Box 10-11. Macrophages kill microorganisms they have ingested, but do so poorly if not activated by cytokines, of which the most important is interferon gamma (IFN-γ). In addition, a T-cell product called granulolysin can inhibit growth of both intracellular and extracellular microorganisms.[16] (This is an example of how the immune system tends to defy generalizations: it is not always true that antibodies protect against extracellular infections and cellular immunity against intracellular infections.)

During the course of a viral infection, CD8+ T cells may be activated in very large numbers. Because of their activated morphology, they look very different from the usual circulating lymphocyte, which, as has been mentioned, is a resting cell. For example, in acute infection with Epstein-Barr virus, there are so many of these "atypical lymphocytes" in the blood that this disease has been called infectious mononucleosis. (Other viruses can cause this disease, too, and for the same reason—the florid activation of viral-specific T cells, primarily CD8+.)

Innate Immune Cell Effector Mechanisms

NK cells become much more effective killers when exposed to certain cytokines and can be stimulated to differentiate into lymphokine-activated killer cells after exposure to IL-2.[17-19] The cytotoxic mechanism of NK cells is similar to that by which cytotoxic T cells kill, meaning perforin/granzyme-mediated and Fas/Fas Ligand–mediated induction of programmed cell death (apoptosis) of the target cells.[20] NK cells also play an immunoregulatory role through the production of cytokines, especially interferon-g, which exerts an important effect against viruses and other intracellular pathogens by activating macrophages.

Other effector mechanisms also contribute to innate immunity. Neutrophils and macrophages can ingest microorganisms, especially those that have been coated with antibody. (Because antibody is produced by the adaptive immune system, this is an example of cooperation of innate and adaptive immunity.) Antibody molecules can also bind to antibody receptors on the surface of killer cells (such as NK cells); this binding is by the constant end of the antibody molecule, so that the antigen receptor is free and can bind to antigen. This enables the antibody-effector cell unit to recognize and kill a target cell, a process known as *antibody-dependent cellular cytotoxicity (ADCC)*. Finally, a series of serum proteins called *complement proteins* can bind to microorganisms and other target cells, either killing the cells outright (by forming large pores in their outer membranes) or rendering them susceptible to phagocytosis, as mentioned above.

Cytokines of the Innate and Adaptive Immune Systems

Up to this point we have described innate and adaptive immunity separately. This is convenient conceptually, but there is substantial overlap in these systems, and this is certainly true for the cytokines involved in these aspects of immunity. Therefore, in this section we describe the most important cytokines in each system, but also point out how these cytokines overlap in function between innate and adaptive immunity.

Cytokines have several important characteristics. They are produced in tiny amounts and are meant to be short lived. For example, they are synthesized only for short periods of time, due to transient gene expression and instability of RNA intermediates. Cytokines have many different activities, and many cytokines may have the same activity (i.e., the cytokine network is redundant). Cytokines typically bind to their receptors with very high affinity, although in some cases there are intermediate- or low-affinity receptors that are activated only when very high concentrations of cytokine are present. (It is these latter receptors that are responsible for most of the toxicity that occurs when cytokines are administered pharmocologically.) Cytokine receptors also share the ability to bind more than one cytokine in some cases and also share component structures in many cases. Among the many actions of cytokines on target cells are activation; stimulation of proliferation; production of other proteins including other cytokines, cytokine receptors, or antibodies; selection of the type of antibody to be produced; differentiation; and death. These processes may be either stimulated or inhibited depending on the combination and concentration of cytokines produced.

Cytokines of the Innate Response

Cells of the innate immune system produce cytokines in response to pattern recognition stimuli as described above. These cells include macrophages, NK cells, epithelial cells, endothelial cells (cells that form the blood vessel wall), dendritic cells, platelets, mast cells, and fibroblasts. Some of these cytokines, and some of their actions, are mentioned here.

Tumor Necrosis Factor (TNF)

TNF is produced primarily by macrophages in response to lipopolysaccharides of gram-negative bacteria. It is also produced by T cells and NK cells. TNT receptors are expressed on most cell types, and binding of TNF to these receptors can lead to either cell activation or cell death (death occurs by activating cellular enzymes that cause the cell to self-destruct and undergo programmed cell death, like a spy who has been caught). TNF recruits monocytes and neutrophils to sites of infection where it also activates them to kill pathogens and to secrete other molecules that attract anti-inflammatory cells. TNF is one of the most important mediators of septic shock, a life-threatening condition characterized by hypotension and intravascular coagulation. TNF also activates lipoprotein lipase in adipocytes, and for this reason chronic production of TNF can result in wasting. Indeed, a cachexia-inducing protein (termed cachexin) that was described as a unique factor turned out, when its gene was cloned and its amino acid sequence determined, to be identical to TNF. Drugs that inhibit TNF have been reported to reduce tissue damage in inflammatory diseases such as rheumatoid arthritis but can increase susceptibility to tuberculosis.[21]

Interleukin-1 (IL-1)

The actions of IL-1 have considerable overlap with TNF. Both are produced by macrophages in response to microbial products and activate innate immune responses. Both also induce fever and cause cachexia. Unlike TNF, IL-1 is produced by epithelial cells and endothelial cells and does not induce programmed cell death in cells exposed to it. IL-1 helps to activate T cells. IL-1 release is stimulated by TNF. IL-1 exists in two agonistic forms, α and β, and a third form that is antagonistic to the first two at the level of the IL-1 receptor, to which all three forms bind. The receptor is present on T cells, fibroblasts, and epithelial and endothelial cells.

Interleukin-6 (IL-6)

This cytokine is also produced by macrophages, but also by fibroblasts and endothelial cells. Production is enhanced by IL-1 and TNF. Receptors for IL-6 are present on activated B cells and hepatocytes, and IL-6 serves as a growth and differentiation factor for B cells and a potent stimulator of production of acute phase reactants by the liver.

Interleukin-12 (IL-12)

This cytokine is produced by macrophages and dendritic cells stimulated by lipopolysaccharide, viral infections, and intracellular pathogens. Production is also stimulated by interferon α from NK cells and T cells. IL-12 is a major stimulator of the cell-mediated adaptive immune response and so is critical for the control of intracellular pathogens. This effect appears to be mediated through stimulation of production of interferon gamma by NK cells and T cells, which in turn activates the cytotoxic function of macrophages. IL-12 is considered one of the main cytokines that directs the adaptive cellular immune response as opposed to the humoral response. (IL-18 appears to enhance these functions of IL-12.) The IL-12 receptor is present on NK and T cells exposed to interferon-γ and dendritic cells exposed to IL-15. Deficiency of this receptor has been associated with exacerbation of mycobacteria infections.[22]

Interleukin-15 (IL-15)

This cytokine is produced by immune (macrophages, dendritic cells) as well as nonimmune cells (osteoblasts, fibroblasts) in response to lipopolysaccharide and intracellular antigens. Its major action is to stimulate proliferation of NK cells during the first stages of an infection (a function performed by IL-2 in later stages of the infection). IL-15 receptors are expressed by T cells, NK cells, and antigen-presenting cells; the latter are activated by IL-15. Mice that have had the IL-15 gene deleted have reduced numbers of NK cells and impaired memory responses of CD8+ T cells.[23]

Chemokines

Chemokines are small proteins secreted by a variety of cells, not just immune cells, to attract or recruit immune cells to the site of an infection or inflammatory response. Lymphocytes and other immune cells respond to chemokines, as you might expect by now, through the expression of chemokine receptors on their cell surface. (Chemokine receptors have become famous as the second receptors that human immunodeficiency virus uses to enter cells.) Chemokines can be secreted in the extravascular tissues. They then diffuse into the bloodstream, where they activate endothelial cells so that intravascular cells such as lymphocytes, monocytes, and neutrophils can receive a signal telling them to exit the blood at that location.

Interleukin-10 (IL-10)

We have taken the dramatic step of listing this cytokine out of numerical order because, unlike the preceding cytokines, it was first described as an inhibitor, rather than a stimulator, of immune reactions. Specifically, it inhibits the functions of activated antigen-presenting cells, such as the production of IL-12 and IFN-γ and the expression of class II MHC molecules and costimulatory molecules. Thus, it has a major effect on antigen presentation and T-cell activation.[24] Interestingly, no fewer than seven viruses, including Epstein-Barr virus and cytomegalovirus, produce proteins that mimic the effects of IL-10 by binding to IL-10 receptors.[25] Presumably the inhibition thereby induced helps favor viral replication. In mice that lack IL-10, immune regulation is abnormal, and a condition resembling inflammatory bowel disease develops.[26,27]

Cytokines of the Adaptive Response

These cytokines are released primarily by T cells. They help T cells proliferate and differentiate into effector cells and thus are critical for cell-mediated immunity.

Interleukin-2 (IL-2)

IL-2 is produced primarily by antigen-activated CD4+ T cells, with a peak in secretion at about 8–12 hours after activation. Antigen-induced activation also results in the expression of high-affinity IL-2 receptors, so that antigen-activated T cells can preferentially respond to IL-2 production by proliferating. Thus, IL-2 is an autocrine T-cell growth factor (and can be used to expand the numbers of T cells for several weeks in vitro). Lower affinity IL-2 receptors are expressed by naive T cells, NK cells, and B cells.

Interleukin-4 (IL-4)

This cytokine, like IL-2, is produced by antigen-activated CD4+ T cells, but it is also produced by mast cells, eosinophils and basophils. IL-4 mediates expansion of CD4+ cells with a type 2 cytokine secretion pattern (see below for a description of type 1 and type 2 cytokine patterns). To this end, it also inhibits type 1 responses such as interferon-γ production. IL-4 stimulates B cells to produce IgE and one subclass (4) of IgG.

Interleukin-5 (IL-5)

This T-cell-derived cytokine stimulates the growth and differentiation of eosinophils, and it also promotes production of IgA by B cells.

Interferon Gamma (IFN-γ)

This cytokine is produced by T cells and NK cells. Th1 helper T cells produce it in response to antigen and NK cells after exposure to pathogens. Both responses are amplified by IL-12, which for T cells can come from the antigen-presenting cell. The functions of IFN-γ favor inflammation:

- activation of cells that kill pathogens (macrophages, NK cells, neutrophils),
- activation of antigen presentation including up-regulation of expression of MHC molecules (both class I and class II),
- stimulation of production of IL-12, which in turn amplifies Th1 responses,
- stimulation of recruitment of immune cells by endothelial cells (along with TNF-α),
- stimulation of production of IgG1 and inhibition of IgG4 and IgE, and
- inhibition of Th2 responses.

Deficiency of IFN-γ, or its receptor, increases susceptibility to intracellular pathogens, pathogens that are killed by macrophages, or pathogens that are controlled by being walled off in granulomas.[28,29]

Type 1 and Type 2 Cytokine Patterns

The cytokine response to pathogen challenge is complex and variable depending on a number of factors including the genetics and immunological history of the host. However, within this variable response patterns can be observed, and these patterns have been used to help us structure our understanding of the dynamics of the immune response. These two main cytokine secretion patterns have been designated type 1 and type 2 or, for helper T cells, Th1 and Th2. Although T cells make a significant contribution to the regulation and production of these cytokines, many cells participate in the response. In type 1 responses, cells produce predominantly IL-2, IL-12, and IFN-γ and are associated with cell-mediated immunity. Type 2 responses are dominated by the production of IL-4, IL-5, IL-6, and IL-10, and the general outcome is to promote humoral rather than cellular immunity. Type 1 and type 2 responses are counterregulatory, meaning type 1 cytokines inhibit type 2 cytokines and vice versa. For example, IFN-γ inhibits the production of IL-4, and IL-4 and IL-10 inhibit the production of IL-12 and IFN-γ. This ability to counterregulate has important physiological consequences. A healthy immune response has a proper balance between type 1 and type 2 responses. Highly polarized type 1 and type 2 responses are typically associated with pathology. For example, autoimmunity is generally driven by polarized type 1 responses, and allergy is a manifestation of a highly skewed type 2 response against environmental antigens. In certain infections, which pattern predominates can affect the outcome of that infection. The determinants of which pattern will predominate are not well defined, but early production of IL-12 by macrophages and dendritic cells favors the Th1 pattern, while early production of IL-4 favors Th2.

Tolerance and the Regulation of the Immune Response

One of the most remarkable qualities of the immune system is that it recognizes and responds to a seemingly infinite array of foreign and pathogen-associated molecules, but it does not respond to self-molecules. This immunological unresponsiveness to self is referred to as *tolerance* or *self-tolerance*. Tolerance is maintained by several mechanisms. First, lymphocytes with receptors for self-antigens are eliminated in the thymus or bone marrow before they fully mature (this is referred to as *central tolerance*). Second, self-reacting lymphocytes are rendered functionally nonresponsive (*anergy*) or induced to self-destruct (by *apoptosis*, a form of *programmed cell death*) when their receptors engage self-antigens without proper costimulation (this is referred to as *peripheral tolerance*). Imbalances in the regulation of tolerance can lead to autoimmune disorders.

Another important aspect of immune regulation is the down-regulation of the scope and duration of inflammatory responses. Again, multiple mechanisms come into play. Although immune-mediated elimination of antigen is important in limiting inflammatory responses, it has recently become clear that there are also active mechanisms of limiting these responses. In particular, a subclass of T cells referred to as *T-regulatory cells (Treg)* also suppresses self-reactivity, thus playing a key balancing role between reactivity and tolerance. Perturbation of Treg function can lead to prolonged exuberant immune responses, tissue damage, and immune-mediated pathology.

Selective Immune Deficiencies: Windows into the Normal Functioning of the Immune System

As in other areas of medicine and biology in general, much of what we know about the function of specific types of cells and specific proteins is derived from clinical syndromes in which these cells or proteins are absent or not functional (or experimental conditions designed to mimic these syndromes).

B-Cell Immune Deficiency

Syndromes exist in which B cells fail to develop, and the patient is unable to produce antibodies. The primary symptom of this type of immune deficiency is recurrent bacterial infections with common bacteria such as *Staphylococcus* or *Streptococcus*. Pneumonia and sinusitis are especially common. The reason why a lack of antibodies predisposes to this type of infection is that opsonization of these bacteria by antibodies is so important in allowing host phagocytic cells to ingest and kill the bacteria. Without antibodies, the phagocytic cells are outpaced by the rapidly growing bacteria and cannot do their job of clearing the infection. Conversely, if the missing antibodies are replaced by periodic injections of pooled antibodies, the clinical consequences of the underlying antibody deficiency can be prevented.

T-Cell Immune Deficiency

Based on early animal experiments in which the thymus was removed, and on the clinical manifestations in human syndromes when the thymus fails to develop, the picture of selective T-cell deficiency has long been known to consist of recurrent infections with parasites, viruses, and intracellular bacteria. A similar picture has been recognized in transplant recipients whose cellular immunity is pharmacologically suppressed to prevent rejection of the graft (although this can also be complicated by recurrent extracellular bacterial infections if neutrophils are depleted by the therapy). These clinical manifestations of cellular immune deficiency were sufficiently established that when the first cases of AIDS in the United States occurred in the late 1970s and early 1980s, it was immediately recognized that there was a new cause of cellular immune deficiency.[30-32] Notably, only a few cases of *Pneumocystis carinii* pneumonia and other opportunistic illnesses were required for this recognition, because these illnesses were (and are) exceedingly rare in people with no known reason to be immunocompromised. In fact the manifestations of AIDS are a perfect illustration of the consequences of cellular immune deficiency. No further description will be given here, because there is a very thorough description of AIDS elsewhere in this book.

NK Cell Immune Deficiency

For a long time after NK cells were discovered, it was controversial whether they had any clinical importance. As so often happens, this question was answered by a clinical case.[33] The patient was a girl presented at age 13 with a life-threatening infection with varicella virus. The patient had a history of recurrent ear infections and low white blood cell counts. At age 17 she had disseminated cytomegalovirus infection, and at 19 an infection with herpes simplex virus with fever and generalized rash. Between infections, antibody levels, T-cell subset ratios, and T-cell responses in vitro (including the response to varicella-zoster virus) were normal, and live vaccines had caused no clinical problems for her. The patient was shown to have a complete absence of NK cells, with no detectable NK cell function in vitro. This case implicated NK cells in host defense against herpes viruses. It is still the only case of NK cell deficiency that has been reported, and the only clear demonstration of in vivo functioning of NK cells. Other functions of NK cells in host defense are believed to occur, however, and are under active investigation. NK cell function is reduced in HIV infection, and NK cells can directly lyse some intracellular pathogens such as *Toxoplasma gondii* and *Trypanosoma cruzi*.[34-36] NK cells also have antitumor activity in vitro.

Other Immune-Mediated Diseases Related to Infectious Organisms

Why do most lymphocytes circulate in a resting state? As discussed above, immune reactivity is a double-edged sword. The same mechanisms that kill microorganisms or infected cells can severely damage normal cells and body constituents. A good example of this is toxic shock syndrome.

This syndrome is characterized by circulatory collapse, hypotension, shock, and in some cases death. Bacterial proteins can cause this by a variety of mechanisms. The common denominator of these mechanisms is the activation of very high numbers of T cells, resulting in excessive production of cytokines that in turn lead to vasodilation and shock (see Box 10-12).

Another example of the risks of having an activated immune system is autoimmune disease. Autoimmunity in the thyroid gland and the pancreas, for example, can cause hypothyroidism and diabetes (due to lack of insulin), respectively. Infections have been postulated to cause some autoimmune diseases (see Box 10-13). Inflammation due to infections has also been postulated to contribute to the etiology of, if not cause, other diseases not traditionally considered infectious, such as atherosclerosis and certain cancers.[37-39]

Box 10-12   Consequences of diffuse activation of cellular immunity

In some infections, the reason why the bacterial proteins are able to activate so many T cells is that instead of binding only to antigen receptors specific for these proteins (present only on a tiny proportion of T cells, maybe 0.01% or less), they bind to a relatively nonpolymorphic region of the T-cell antigen receptor (present on many T cells—as much as 5–10%). For this reason, proteins that can bind to the T-cell receptor in this way are called *superantigens*. Superantigens can activate a wide variety of T-cell receptors, far more than could be activated through the antigen-specific part of the receptor, which as mentioned above is highly polymorphic. This results in an enormous immune activation with release of huge amounts of cytokines, which in turn cause the symptoms of the syndrome.

Box 10-13   Etiology of autoimmune disease

What triggers autoimmune disease is not known, but it has been intensively investigated since description of the first autoimmune disease (thyroiditis leading to destruction of the thyroid gland and thus to hypothyroidism) in 1956. It is now clear, however, that immune reactions normally involve self-recognition (through the requirement for MHC recognition in antigen presentation), so the problem is likely one of regulation rather than purely a failure to distinguish between self and nonself. There is clear evidence that some genetic factors are associated with a higher incidence of autoimmune disease (e.g., certain MHC alleles, female sex) and environmental factors also play a role.

Some autoimmune diseases have been postulated to result from infectious organisms whose antigens are very similar to normal host antigens. Thus, the immune system is "tricked" by an infection into reacting against normal host antigens. This mechanism of initiation of autoimmune disease is called *molecular mimicry*.

Conclusion

This chapter should be seen as an introduction to the immune system and its role in host defense against infections. By necessity we have had to omit many, if not most, of the details of how immune reactions are regulated, and most, if not all, of the principles and generalizations described have exceptions, sometimes important ones. But interested readers can pursue their interests, which we hope have been stimulated (in a non-MHC-restricted way, of course!).

Recommended Textbooks of Immunology

Paul WE. *Fundamental Immunology.* Baltimore, Md: Lippincott Williams and Wilkins; 2003. Especially Chapter 1, "The Immune System—An Introduction." A very detailed text.

Janeway CA, Travers P, Walport M, Schlomchik M. *Immunobiology: The Immune System in Health and Disease.* 6th ed. New York, NY: Garland; 2005. A good introductory text.

Roitt IM, Delves PJ. *Essential Immunology.* 10th ed. London: Blackwell; 2001.

References

1. Gordon S. Macrophages and the immune response. In: Paul WE, ed. *Fundamental Immunology.* Lippincott-Raven; Baltimore, MD: 1999.
2. Ismail N, Olano JP, Feng HM, Walker DH. Current status of immune mechanisms of killing of intracellular microorganisms. *FEMS Microbiol Lett.* 2002;207:111–120.
3. Rouse BT, Norley S, Martin S. Antiviral cytotoxic T lymphocyte induction and vaccination. *Rev Infect Dis.* 1988;10:16–33.
4. Katz DH, Hamaoka T, Benacerraf B. Cell interactions between histoincompatible T and B lymphocytes. II. Failure of physiologic cooperative interactions between T and B lymphocytes from allogeneic donor strains in humoral response to hapten-protein conjugates. *J Exp Med.* 1973;137;1405–1418.
5. Lanzavecchia A. Antigen-specific interaction between T and B cells. *Nature.* 1985;314:537–539.
6. Lorenzo ME, Ploegh HL, Tirabassi RS. Viral immune evasion strategies and the underlying cell biology. *Semin Immunol.* 2001;13:1–9.
7. Ploegh HL. Viral strategies of immune evasion. *Science.* 1998;280:248–253.
8. Hornung V, Rothenfusser S, Britsch S, et al. Quantitative expression of toll-like receptor 1-10 mRNA in cellular subsets of human peripheral blood mononuclear cells and sensitivity to CpG oligodeoxynucleotides. *J Immunol.* 2002;168:4531–4537.
9. Takeuchi O, Sato S, Horiuchi T, et al. Cutting edge: role of toll-like receptor 1 in mediating immune response to microbial lipoproteins. *J Immunol.* 2002;169:10–14.
10. Uthaisangsook S, Day NK, Bahna SL, Good RA, Haraguchi S. Innate immunity and its role against infections. *Ann Allergy Asthma Immunol.* 2002;88:253–264.
11. Carreno BM, Collins M. The B7 family of ligands and its receptors: new pathways for costimulation and inhibition of immune responses. *Annu Rev Immunol.* 2002;20:29–53.
12. Silva RA, Florido M, Appelberg R. Interleukin-12 primes CD4+ T cells for interferon-gamma production and protective immunity during *Mycobacterium avium* infection. *Immunol.* 2001;103:368–374.
13. Cantor H, Shen FW, Boyse EA. Separation of helper T cells from suppressor T cells expressing different Ly components. II. Activation by antigen: after immunization, antigen-specific suppressor and helper activities are mediated by distinct T-cell subclasses. *J Exp Med.* 1976;143:1339–1340.

14. Littman DR, Thomas Y, Maddon PJ, Chess L, Axel R. The isolation and sequence of the gene encoding T8: a molecule defining functional classes of T lymphocytes. *Cell.* 1985;40:237–246.
15. Mullbacher A, Hla RT, Museteanu C, Simon MM. Perforin is essential for control of ectromelia virus but not related poxviruses in mice. *J Virol.* 1999;73:1665–1667.
16. Stenger S, Hanson DA, Teitelbaum R, et al. An antimicrobial activity of cytolytic T cells mediated by granulysin. *Science.* 1998;282:121–125.
17. Carson WE, Giri JG, Lindemann MJ, et al. Interleukin (IL) 15 is a novel cytokine that activates human natural killer cells via components of the IL-2 receptor. *J Exp Med.* 1994;180:1395–1403.
18. Zhang T, Kawakami K, Qureshi MH, Okamura H, Kurimoto M, Saito A. Interleukin-12 (IL-12) and IL-18 synergistically induce the fungicidal activity of murine peritoneal exudate cells against *Cryptococcus neoformans* through production of gamma interferon by natural killer cells. *Infect Immun.* 1997;65:3594–3599.
19. Rayner AA, Grimm EA, Lotze MT, Chu EW, Rosenberg SA. Lymphokine-activated killer (LAK) cells. Analysis of factors relevant to the immunotherapy of human cancer. *Cancer.* 1985;55:1327–1333.
20. Smyth MJ, Thia KY, Cretney E, et al. Perforin is a major contributor to NK cell control of tumor metastasis. *J Immunol.* 1999;162:6658–6662.
21. Keane J, Gershon S, Wise RP, et al. Tuberculosis associated with infliximab, a tumor necrosis factor alpha-neutralizing agent. *N Engl J Med.* 2001;345:1098–1104.
22. Altare F, Durandy A, Lammas D, et al. Impairment of mycobacterial immunity in human interleukin-12 receptor deficiency. *Science.* 1998;280:1432–1435.
23. Kennedy MK, Glaccum M, Brown SN, et al. Reversible defects in natural killer and memory CD8 T cell lineages in interleukin 15-deficient mice. *J Exp Med.* 2000;191:771–780.
24. Moore KW, de Waal MR, Coffman RL, O'Garra A. Interleukin-10 and the interleukin-10 receptor. *Annu Rev Immunol.* 2001;19:683–765.
25. Fickenscher H, Hor S, Kupers H, Knappe A, Wittmann S, Sticht H. The interleukin-10 family of cytokines. *Trends Immunol.* 2002;23:89–96.
26. Chmiel JF, Konstan MW, Saadane A, Krenicky JE, Lester KH, Berger M. Prolonged inflammatory response to acute *Pseudomonas* challenge in interleukin-10 knockout mice. *Am J Respir Crit Care Med.* 2002;165:1176–1181.
27. Takahashi I, Matsuda J, Gapin L, et al. Colitis-related public T cells are selected in the colonic lamina propria of IL-10-deficient mice. *Clin Immunol.* 2002;102:237–248.
28. van Schaik SM, Obot N, Enhorning G, et al. Role of interferon gamma in the pathogenesis of primary respiratory syncytial virus infection in BALB/c mice. *J Med Virol.* 2000;62:257–266.
29. Dorman SE, Picard C, Lammas D, et al. Clinical features of dominant and recessive interferon gamma receptor 1 deficiencies. *Lancet.* 2004;364:2113–2121.
30. Masur H, Michelis MA, Greene JB, et al. An outbreak of community-acquired *P. carinii* pneumonia: initial manifestation of cellular immune dysfunction. *N Engl J Med.* 1981;305:1431–1438.
31. Gottlieb MS, Schroff R, Schander HM, et al. *Pneumocystis carinii* pneumonia and mucosal candidiasis in previously healthy homosexual men: evidence for a new acquired cellular immunodeficiency. *N Engl J Med.* 1981;305:1425–1431.

32. Siegal FP, Lopez E, Hammer GS, et al. Severe acquired immunodeficiency in male homosexuals manifested by chronic perianal ulcerative herpes simplex lesions. *N Engl J Med.* 1981;305:1439–1444.

33. Biron CA, Byron KS, Sullivan JL. Severe herpesvirus infections in an adolescent without natural killer cells. *N Engl J Med.* 1989;320: 1731–1735.

34. Hauser WE Jr, Tsai V. Acute toxoplasma infection of mice induces spleen NK cells that are cytotoxic for *T. gondii* in vitro. *J Immunol.* 1986;136:313–319.

35. Cantor H, Boyse EA. Functional subclasses of T-lymphocytes bearing different Ly antigens. I. The generation of functionally distinct T-cell subclasses is a differentiative process independent of antigen. *J Exp Med.* 1975;141:1376–1389.

36. Martinez-Marino B, Shiboski S, Hecht FM, Kahn JO, Levy JA. Interleukin-2 therapy restores CD8 cell non-cytotoxic anti-HIV responses in primary infection subjects receiving HAART. *AIDS.* 2004;18:1991–1999.

37. Arcari CM, Gaydos CA, Nieto FJ, Krauss M, Nelson KE. Association between *Chlamydia pneumoniae* and acute myocardial infarction in young men in the United States military: the importance of timing of exposure measurement. *Clin Infect Dis.* 2005;40:1123–1130.

38. Danesh J, Whincup P, Walker M, et al. *Chlamydia pneumoniae* IgG titres and coronary heart disease: prospective study and meta-analysis. *BMJ.* 2000;321:208–213.

39. Houghton J, Wang TC. *Helicobacter pylori* and gastric cancer: a new paradigm for inflammation-associated epithelial cancers. *Gastroenterology.* 2005;128:1567–1578.

VACCINES: PAST, PRESENT, AND FUTURE

Anita M. Loughlin and Steffanie A. Strathdee

Introduction

A vaccine is any biologically derived substance that elicits a protective immune response when administered to a susceptible host. The first documented account of vaccination is attributed to a Buddhist nun who described how smallpox scabs were dried, ground, and blown into the nostrils of susceptible persons in approximately AD 1000 to protect them from disseminated disease.[1] The first trial to evaluate the effects of vaccination occurred in 1796, when Edward Jenner proved that persons inoculated with cowpox were resistant to challenge with *Variola* virus, the etiologic agent of smallpox.

Worldwide improvements in sanitation and vaccination led to impressive declines in the incidence and mortality of many infectious diseases throughout the 1900s. Perhaps the greatest public health achievement of the modern era is the global eradication of smallpox in 1977 and the near elimination of polio. Despite these achievements, a significant proportion of the estimated 11.5 million deaths attributed to infectious and parasitic diseases in 1998 could have been prevented by existing vaccines (Figure 11-1). Barriers to achieving protective immunity in populations at highest risk leave us far short of reaping the full potential of vaccines. In the world, one million children die from measles each year, 50% of whom live in Africa, despite the existence of highly effective vaccine. For tuberculosis, the less than fully efficacious vaccines coupled with poor distribution and the emergence of HIV have resulted in an uncontrolled epidemic throughout the world even though a vaccine has been available since 1927.

In this chapter, we describe various types of traditional and experimental vaccines, the role of vaccines in the eradication of specific infectious diseases (e.g., smallpox, polio), and recent technological advances in vaccine development. We also summarize fundamental concepts relating to vaccine efficacy and effectiveness and barriers to achieving adequate vaccine coverage.

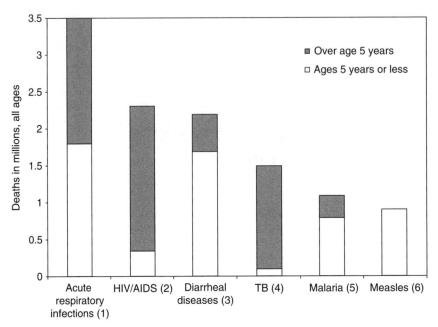

FIGURE 11-1 Leading causes of death worldwide from infectious diseases in 1998.
Notes:
1. Acute respiratory infections include influenzae and bacterial causes of pneumonia (such as *Haemophilus influenzae* b and *Streptococcus pneumoniae*) for which vaccine are available.
2. HIV-positive people who died with TB have been included among AIDS deaths, no licensed vaccine is available.
3. Among diarrheal diseases vaccines are currently available for cholera and typhoid; shigella and rotavirus vaccines are being developed.
4. BCG vaccine first licensed in 1927 given to prevent *Mycobacterium tuberculosis* infection.
5. Malaria vaccines are in development.
6. Licensed measles vaccines have been available since 1964 and are efficient at preventing disease.
Source: © World Health Organization 1999 Online [http://www.who.int/infectious-disease-report/pages/graph5.html]

Active Versus Passive Immunization

Protection from many infectious diseases can be conferred by either passive or active immunization. Passive immunity refers to protection conferred to a susceptible host through the transfer of animal or human antibody (immunoglobulin), usually by injection. Passive antibody transfer from mother to child in utero or through breast-feeding plays an important role in preventing disease in newborns. Although maternal antibodies do not necessarily provide full protection from infection, immunization of pregnant women against tetanus has led to dramatic reductions in the incidence of neonatal tetanus.[2] A disadvantage of passive immunity is that it is typically short lived. Protection conferred by immunoglobulin lasts only a few weeks; maternal antibodies can protect newborns for up to six months.

Active immunity refers to protection produced by the host's own immune system and relies on the ability of the host to generate an immune response following exposure to specific antigen(s). In the field of immunology antigens are described as being *self* if they are from the host or person, and *nonself* if they are from someone or something else. Immunogenic antigens are foreign bodies—commonly proteins or polysaccharides—that are recognized by the immune system as nonself and which then elicit a response. The goal of immunization is to elicit a protective immune response that confers protective immunity against natural infection with a wild-type (i.e., pathogenic) microorganism without causing serious clinical illness. For many pathogens the immunologic response of people who have had natural infection and survived without chronic morbidity can guide in the development of a vaccine. Features of an ideal vaccine are tabulated in Exhibit 11-1.

Factors that affect the host immune response include the type and dose of antigen, the route of administration (e.g., intramuscular, subcutaneous, or oral), the presence or absence of maternal antibody, host factors (e.g., age, immunosuppression, genetics), and specific characteristics of the vaccine (Exhibit 11-1). Timing of immunization is also an important consideration. For most vaccines, immunization must take place before natural infection occurs, allowing for several weeks to generate an adequate immune response. During some outbreaks (e.g., hepatitis A, measles) passive immunization offers effective short-term protection, especially when there is insufficient time for susceptibles to mount an adequate immune response following active immunization. The extent of the host's immune response has an important bearing on vaccine efficacy, which is discussed in detail later in this chapter.

Types of Vaccines

Traditionally, vaccines have been considered to fall into two main groups. The antigenic agent used in active immunization can be: (1) a live organism that has been attenuated (i.e., weakened); or (2) an inactivated form that is either whole or fractionated (e.g., protein or polysaccharide component).

Exhibit 11-1   Characteristics of an Ideal Vaccine

1. Produces a good humoral, cell-mediated, and local immune response, similar to natural infection, in a single dose.
2. Elicits protections against clinical disease and reinfection.
3. Provides protection for several years, preferably a lifetime.
4. Results in minimal immediate adverse effects or mild disease with no delayed effects that predispose to other diseases.
5. Induced immunity confers protections to multiple strains of organisms.
6. Can be administered simply in a form that is practically, culturally, and ethically acceptable to the target population.
7. Vaccine preparations do not require special handling (e.g., a cold chain).
8. Does not interfere significantly with the immune response to other vaccines given simultaneously.
9. Costs and benefits associated with receiving the vaccine clearly outweigh the costs and risks associated with natural infection.

Recombinant vaccines are developed through genetic manipulation, and these can be either live or inactivated. Below, we describe characteristics of the various types of vaccines, as well as a newer experimental approach involving vaccination with naked DNA. A diagram of how vaccines are made and examples of specific types are found in Exhibit 11-2.

Whereas vaccines are imagined to prevent infection, many vaccines prevent or minimize the consequences of infection. Toxoid vaccine prevents tissue damage from bacterial toxins (e.g., tetanus or diphtheria toxin) but does not actually act against the bacteria themselves. Inactivated poliovirus vaccine does not prevent wild type poliovirus from multiplying in the intestinal tract, but immune barriers induced by this vaccine prevent the virus from causing central nervous system disease.

Exhibit 11-2   Vaccine Manufacturing

Parent Organism	Process	Vaccine Types	Examples
	Serial passage attenuate organism →	**Live, attenuated vaccine**	Measles, mumps, rubella, oral polio, yellow fever
	Kill organism by heat, chemical, or radiation →	**Inactivated "killed" vaccines**	Hepatitis A, *H. influenzae* inactivated polio, cholera, rabies
	Grow organism → Purify toxin → Formalin "detoxify" →	**Toxoids**	Tetanus, diphtheria
	Inactivate → Disrupt → Purify antigens →	**Subunit vaccines**	Pertussis
	Inactivate disrupt → Purify antigens → Antigen-protein link →	**Conjugate vaccines**	*H. influenzae* b, pneumococcal
	Attenuate → Remove essential genes →	**Recombinant vaccines**	Hepatitis B (recombinant subunit vaccine)
	Identify essential antigens → Extract genes coding for antigens → Insert gene in vector →	**Vector vaccines**	Clinical trials HIV vaccines with canarypox vector and vaccinia vector
	Identify essential antigens → Extract genes coding for antigens → Naked DNA →	**DNA vaccines**	Clinical trials malaria, herpes, HIV

The public health burden of specific cancers may be also considerably reduced through the introduction of preventive or therapeutic vaccines. The inclusion of hepatitis B (HBV) vaccine in several national immunization programs will prevent primary disease but is also hoped to reduce the incidence of liver cancer. However, overcoming the barriers to achieving adequate coverage will be necessary. Preventive vaccines are near licensure for human papillomavirus (HPV) infection, which is highly prevalent among young men in the United States (25%) and accounts for approximately 95% of all cervical cancers. In the future, it is hoped that antitumor vaccines can be used to boost host immune responses to promote tumor destruction.[3]

Live Attenuated Vaccines

Bacteria and viruses are referred to as being *attenuated* if they have been rendered nonpathogenic. Bacteria can be attenuated through laboratory culture, and viruses through serial passaging in tissue culture or animal hosts. Both bacteria and viruses can be attenuated through genetic manipulation. The potential role of attenuated organisms in vaccination was identified soon after Jenner's landmark smallpox vaccination study in 1796. In the 1870s, Louis Pasteur recognized that inoculating a weakened form of chicken cholera protected chickens against challenge with the wild type virus. Pasteur then developed an attenuated anthrax bacilli vaccine that was first administered to livestock in 1881, and an attenuated live rabies vaccine that was used to immunize two human volunteers in 1885.[4] In 1909, the Bacille Calmette-Guerin (BCG) tuberculosis vaccine was the first live attenuated bacterial vaccine developed for humans.

Live attenuated organisms must replicate, or multiply, in the host to induce an adequate immune response. Live vaccines typically generate a stronger immune response than inactivated vaccines, and immunity is considered lifelong due to immunologic memory. Live vaccines have the advantage of inducing both humoral and cell-mediated immunity. In simple terms, humoral immunity refers to antibody, specifically immunoglobulin (Ig), production. Antigen recognition by lymphocytes (T cells and B cells) leads to clonal expansion of specific antibodies that are directed against a particular antigen and the generation of memory cells. The primary humoral immune response to a new antigen involves short-term production of IgM antibodies, which is replaced by longer-lasting, higher-affinity IgG antibodies. If the host is reexposed to the same antigen, a rapid expansion of memory cells results in a secondary immune response involving IgG but not IgM antibodies. Cell-mediated immunity includes both nonspecific first-line responses against invading organisms, such as phagocytes, natural killer cells, complement and antigen-specific activation of cytotoxic T lymphocytes (T cells that express CD8+ on their cell surface). These responses may be induced by live attenuated viral vaccines and potentially from naked DNA vaccines. Figure 11-2 depicts humoral and cellular immune response pathways. For a detailed account of the humoral and cell-mediated response to infectious agents, the reader is referred to Chapter 10 and the following text.[5–8]

Another potential advantage of live vaccines is the possibility of horizontal transmission, which refers to the transmission of vaccine virus to other susceptible individuals. Horizontal transmission of vaccine virus has

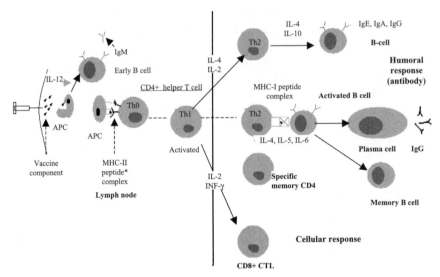

FIGURE 11-2   Antigen-specific immune response.
* Peptide is the processed vaccine component expressed on MCH II
APC = Antigen-presenting cell (a dendritic cell or macrophage) processes vaccine
component to present it as peptides to lymphocytes.
IL = The cytokine interleukin.
INF = The cytokine interferon.
CD4+ = T lymphocyte helper T cell. Function is to activate other lymphocytes (T
cells, B cells).
CD8+-CTL = Cytotoxic T lymphocyte. Function is targeted cell killing all cells
manufacturing vaccine (e.g., virus infected cells).

been described for live oral polio vaccine (OPV).[9] Indirect vaccination has
the significant benefit of enhancing vaccine coverage by exposing unvaccinated persons to the vaccine strain. However, the vaccine strain of polio
can revert to the virulent strain in the gut of vaccinated patients. This has
resulted, rarely, in vaccine-associated paralytic polio (VAPP) among the nonimmune contacts of OPV recipients.[10] For this reason, horizontal transmission
of vaccine strains requires careful monitoring and surveillance, should it be
known to occur. In countries where polio is no longer endemic, inactivated
polio vaccine is recommended. In the United States OPV has not been used
since 1999.[10]

Although attenuated vaccine strains may be controlled by immune com-
petent persons, they may be poorly controlled by those with compromised
immune systems (e.g., the elderly, infants, those on immune suppressive
drugs, or persons with HIV/AIDS). In these populations, severe adverse events
can occur. All unintended consequences of vaccination must be carefully
assessed by clinical trials before approval and through surveillance mechanisms postlicensure.

Antibodies induced by live attenuated vaccines can sometimes be rendered inactive by circulating antibodies that cross-react with the attenuated
organism. Interference can be caused by antibody produced during concurrent natural infections, immune globulin administered during recent passive
immunization, or maternal antibodies. Measles vaccine is particularly sensitive to circulating maternal antibodies, which has complicated measles immu-

nization schedules in preschool children.[11] In rare cases, antibodies induced by one vaccine can inhibit the immune response to another, a situation that bears consideration when several vaccines are administered simultaneously. Previous concerns that administering yellow fever and cholera vaccines simultaneously could reduce the long-term immune response to both have not been borne out[12]; however, the Centers for Disease Control and Prevention (CDC) still recommends that these vaccines be administered at least three weeks apart. In addition, some antimalarial drugs (e.g., chloroquine) do interfere with live cholera vaccine.[12]

Immunization programs that incorporate live vaccines also need to take appropriate measures to protect the vaccine from environmental conditions (e.g., heat, light). The system of vaccine storage and transport from manufacturer to client is called the *cold chain*. Although stabilizing agents (e.g., magnesium chloride) can be used to safeguard the viability of live vaccines, failure to maintain the cold chain can compromise vaccine efficacy. When appropriate, simultaneous administration of several live virus vaccines (e.g., measles, mumps, rubella [MMR]) reduces cost and minimizes cumbersome handling, shipping, and storage requirements.[13]

Inactivated Vaccines

Inactivated vaccines are either whole viruses or bacteria that are "killed" using heat or chemicals (e.g., formalin), as well as extracted or purified components of the organism. As early as 1888, it was discovered that the diphtheria bacillus (*Corynebacterium diphtheriae*) produced a powerful toxin that caused the disease pathology.[14] In the early 1900s, chemical inactivation of bacterial toxins led to the first toxoids for diphtheria and tetanus that could be used for vaccination. Another type of inactivated vaccine is based on polysaccharides that are typically derived from bacterial cell walls (e.g., pneumococcus, meningococcus, *Haemophilus influenza* type b [Hib]). These vaccines primarily induce short-lived nonspecific IgM and no immunologic memory. Polysaccharide-based vaccines are not consistently immunogenic for the elderly, immunocompromised persons, or infants, and are not recommended for children under two years of age. In some cases, polysaccharides can be chemically linked, or conjugated, to a protein carrier that can boost the immune response. This approach has been successfully used to maximize the immune response to Hib, which was the first conjugate licensed for use in humans. A newer conjugate 7-serotype vaccine (PCV7) prevents many invasive *Streptococcus pneumoniae* infections, which replaced Hib as the most common bacterial cause of meningitis, bacteremia, and pneumonias.[15]

By definition, inactivated vaccines are not alive, and, therefore they cannot replicate in the host or revert to virulence. They are not rendered ineffective by circulating antibody and require less stringent handling procedures. Inactivated vaccines are associated with fewer adverse effects, which are usually localized to the injection site. Although these properties are favorable, the immune response associated with inactivated vaccines is typically restricted to humoral immunity. Several doses are usually required to boost the specific antibody level, or *titre*. Immunity produced by inactive vaccines also wanes with time, therefore necessitating booster doses.

In cases where the antigenic component of the organism has not easily been isolated, whole inactivated viruses and bacteria have formed the basis of vaccine preparations. These vaccines are more likely to induce adverse effects, in which case they are referred to as being *reactogenic*. This was a common problem with whole cell pertussis vaccine, which led to the development of an acellular form that is associated with fewer side effects.

Recombinant Vaccines

In the last two decades, much attention has focused on genetic manipulation of organisms to generate either live attenuated or inactivated vaccines. Several different approaches have been used. Hepatitis B vaccine was the first recombinant DNA vaccine, and was licensed in 1986. There was substantial interest in developing a new hepatitis B vaccine as an earlier vaccine; while it was highly efficacious, it was derived from human blood products, and it was known that some donors later developed the, at that time, newly recognized AIDS syndrome. The recombinant vaccine harnessed the ability of *Saccharomyces cerevisiae,* yeast cells, to make proteins. The hepatitis B surface antigen (HBsAg) genes were inserted into the yeast cell genome in a process known as *transvected*. Once the genes were inserted, the yeast cells could be clonally expanded so that large quantities of HBsAg could be produced. This technique allows for high production of antigen without the use of human-derived materials and evolved rapidly to generate many new vaccines. For example, *Escherichia coli* has been used to express lipoprotein from *Borrelia burgdorferi*, the arbovirus responsible for Lyme disease.[16] The first human vaccine for Lyme disease was licensed in 1998.

Another approach to developing a recombinant vaccine involves deletion or modification of genes that are known to confer pathogenicity. This method has been used to construct an oral typhoid vaccine and numerous others. Recently, genetic manipulation of rhesus monkey and human rotavirus genomes enabled the development of vaccines for rotavirus, the major etiologic agent responsible for diarrheal deaths in children. Development of rotavirus vaccines took advantage of the fact that human and animal (i.e., bovine, rhesus) strains of the virus readily underwent reassortment. The resultant multivalent vaccine increases the potential to provide protection against serotypes.[17]

A third approach to recombinant vaccine development involves insertion of a gene from one organism to another, usually a live virus. The modified virus subsequently acts as a carrier, or vector, that expresses the foreign gene. Using this innovative approach, canarypox virus has been used to express HIV glycoproteins. This modified canarypox virus is currently being evaluated in clinical trials as a candidate HIV vaccine.[18] Vaccinia virus and adenovirus have been used to express rabies G protein.[19,20] This vaccine vector has been used to immunize wildlife against rabies in a novel program in the southwestern United States.[19] Because the vaccine could be administered orally, the vaccine was put into meat sticks that were distributed in an aggressive campaign that used airplane drops as well as ground distribution to surround known cases of rabies. Coupled with an immunization campaign for domestic animals and an education campaign about the purpose and safety of the immunization meat sticks, the campaign was successful in slowing the spread of rabies in Texas.[19]

DNA Vaccines

DNA vaccines differ from traditional vaccines in that the naked DNA coding for a specific component of a disease-causing organism is injected directly into the body. The delivery system is either a saline solution injected through a hypodermic needle, or DNA-coated gold beads propelled into the body using "gene guns." Although no DNA vaccine is currently licensed, DNA vaccination represents a considerable technological advance that may revolutionize immunization. Developed extensively throughout the 1990s, this approach offers the possibility of safer and cheaper vaccines, even for diseases where there has been only limited success with traditional vaccines. DNA vaccines are currently under development for malaria, rotavirus, and HIV, among others.

There are several potential advantages associated with DNA vaccines. First, the actual production of the immunizing protein takes place in the cells of the vaccinated host. This theoretically eliminates the risk of the vaccine causing the infection it is intended to prevent, which is a concern with traditional live attenuated vaccines. Second, like live vaccines, DNA vaccines have the ability to elicit a wide range of humoral and cell-mediated immune responses that are potentially long term. Third, DNA vaccines are very stable and can be stored under a vast array of conditions, which eliminates the need for a cold chain. For this reason, they may be particularly suitable in developing countries. Finally, DNA vaccines may lend themselves to generic production methods that will simplify and standardize vaccine production.

An important shortcoming of DNA vaccines is that they are limited to developing immune responses against protein components. Therefore, they cannot substitute for traditional polysaccharide-based vaccines (e.g., pneumococcal vaccine). There are also novel safety concerns posed by these vaccines. DNA from the vaccine incorporates into host chromosomes and could be oncogenic if the incorporation turned on oncogenes or turned off tumor suppressor genes. Therefore, the safety and efficacy of DNA vaccines need to be carefully evaluated to ensure that the potential risks of these new vaccines can be understood.

Novel Vaccines

Novel approaches in vaccine development include the identification of new targets, new adjuvants, and new vaccine delivery methods, as well as the development of new vaccine types and combination vaccines. Both disease severity and disease burden remain important criteria for selecting an organism for vaccine development. Notable infections influencing vaccine development include HIV, tuberculosis, and malaria; a virus, bacterium, and parasite, respectively. *The Jordan Report* lists many infectious agents for which vaccines are in the pipeline.[21] Viral vaccines include those focused on the hepatitis C virus, herpes (HSV-1 and HSV-2), and human papillomavirus (HPV). In addition to HSV and HPV vaccines, other vaccines are in development to prevent sexually transmitted infections including gonorrhea, syphilis, and chlamydia. Vaccines to prevent *Escherichia coli, Salmonella typhi, Shigella* species, and rotavirus infections are among the many vaccines being developed to prevent diarrheal diseases that account for 4.0% of all deaths and 5.7% of all disease burden worldwide.[22]

Enhancing the specific and protective immune response to a vaccine remains a significant challenge. Adjuvants, such as aluminum salt (alum) have been used since the 1920s to increase immunogenicity. The mechanism of action of these older adjuvants was to inhibit clearance of an antigen from the site of injection allowing better recognition of the antigen by antigen-presenting cells (APC). Newer adjuvants that improve the delivery of antigens to APCs in the lymphoid tissue have been developed. For example, particulate adjuvants, such as liposomes and microspheres, protect antigens from being destroyed in the stomach and present antigens to macrophages in the gut to enhance mucosal immunity. Other adjuvants are being developed to direct the immune response toward either a cellular-mediated (Th1) or an antibody (Th2) immune response. These adjuvants include immunomodulatory cytokines, such as interleukin and interferon gamma, and chemokines.[23-25] Vaccines that target intracellular infections, such as HIV and *Mycobacterium tuberculosis* or parasites such as *Plasmodium* sp. (malaria) need to produce a strong Th1 response. Strong antibody (Th2) responses are the best defense for extracellular bacterial infections (e.g., *Haemophilus influenzae* type b) or toxin-mediated diseases (*Bordetella pertussis*).[23-25] The incorporation of an adjuvant in a vaccine's formulation may increase the risk of an adverse reaction; therefore, separate animal studies and safety studies are needed to evaluate the adjuvant effects. For more in-depth discussion of adjuvants, the reader is referred to the article by Vogel and Alving in the 2002 *Jordan Report*.[24]

The way vaccines are administered is also changing. Combination vaccines have been developed to reduce the number of overall injections. The measles, mumps, and rubella vaccine (MMR) and the diphtheria-tetanus-acellular pertussis vaccine (DTaP) are combination vaccines currently being administered. New vaccines in clinical trials include the addition of varicella vaccine to the MMR vaccine and the combination of *Haemophilus influenza* type b and hepatitis B vaccine (Hib-HepB). The newly licensed live attenuated influenzae vaccine administered intranasally aims to produce both local (mucosal) and systemic immune responses. Likewise, orally administered vaccines (e.g., polio and cholera vaccines) are advantageous in that they produce mucosal immunity.

In the foreseeable future, edible vaccines may be used to administer vaccines more widely, safely, and cheaply. Transgenic plants such as potatoes, tomatoes, and bananas are being developed such that the plant gene will encode for the targeted vaccine antigens.[22,23] Among the edible vaccines in development are vaccines that target measles, *E. coli*, and hepatitis B. It is hoped that such plants can be developed for the delivery of multivalent vaccines for protection against a broad range of diseases. Last, transcutaneous immunization systems, including skin patches and gene guns, aim to deliver vaccine antigen and adjuvant across the epidermis to Langerhans cells, a specific class of dendritic APC.[23,25]

The development of DNA and other gene-based vaccines holds promise that new mechanisms to deliver antigen-encoding genomes to the host will result in novel vaccine types: vector vaccines, such as simple plasmids or more complex modified viral vaccines (e.g., vaccinia or adenovirus) or bacterial vectors.[25] Newer HPV vaccines include a piece of the HPV genome enclosed in a nonenveloped capsid creating a virus-like-particle (VLP).[26] VLP vaccines are not infectious but are capable of eliciting a strong immune response. Two HPV vaccines against different combinations of HPV subtypes are near licensure.

Immunization Schedules

The goal of an effective immunization program is to vaccinate a high proportion of susceptible persons early in life (i.e., before they are potentially exposed to the infectious agent). In the United States, infants and children are immunized against hepatitis B, diphtheria, tetanus, pertussis, Hib, polio, measles, mumps, rubella, and varicella virus (Exhibit 11-3). Alternative immunization schedules are available from other sources for children who have missed primary immunization series or who were inadequately immunized.[27,28]

Immunization schedules differ from country to country, depending on the burden of disease in the population, the availability of an efficacious and effective vaccine, economic factors, and the level of priority that is placed on vaccine preventable diseases. Prevention of hepatitis B infection has become a worldwide priority; therefore, an HBV vaccine has been added to the World Health Organization (WHO) Expanded Program on Immunization recommendations. The routine vaccinations recommended by the WHO are diphtheria, tetanus, and pertussis vaccine (DTP); oral polio vaccine (OPV); and measles, mumps, rubella vaccine (MMR). In addition, the WHO recommends vaccination against tuberculosis (i.e., BCG) and yellow fever in countries where these diseases are endemic.

Target Populations

Vaccine programs must identify individuals before exposure to natural infection and must boost vaccination before immunity wanes to nonprotective levels. A failure to maintain vaccine levels has resulted in outbreaks of disease among school-aged children. Assessment of adolescents at routine health care visits is warranted to ensure completion of primary vaccine series for newer vaccines (e.g., varicella, hepatitis B vaccine) and to provide boosters for MMR and tetanus toxoid.[28] In 2005, two new vaccines will be licensed and recommended for adolescents including a conjugate meningococcal vaccine and a diphtheria-tetanus-acellular pertussis vaccine.[28] Vaccines to prevent sexually transmitted infections, including herpes simplex virus type 2 (HSV-2), human papillomavirus (HPV), and the human immunodeficiency virus (HIV), will likely be offered to adolescents in the future to assure vaccination prior to exposure to these viruses.

Adult vaccination is an important part of preventive medical care. Routine adult vaccines include pneumococcal vaccine, influenza, and tetanus toxoid. In higher risk individuals, MMR, hepatitis B, hepatitis A, and varicella vaccines are recommended. The US Public Health Service and the CDC also provide immunization recommendations for international travelers, depending on endemic disease in the destination country (e.g., MMR, hepatitis A and B, yellow fever, meningococcal, typhoid, polio, rabies, plague, and Japanese

Exhibit 11-3   Recommended Childhood and Adolescent Immunization Schedule, United States: July–December 2004

Age → / Vaccine	Birth	1 mos	2 mos	4 mos	6 mos	12 mos	15 mos	18 mos	24 mos	4-6 yrs	11-12 yrs	13-18 yrs
Hepatitis B	HepB #1	HepB #2			HepB #3						HepB Series*	
Diphtheria, tetanus, pertussis			DTaP	DTaP	DTaP		DTaP			DTaP	Td	Td
Haemophilus influenzae type b			Hib	Hib	Hib	Hib						
Inactivated poliovirus			IPV	IPV	IPV					IPV		
Measles, mumps, rubella						MMR #1				MMR #2	MMR*	
Varicella						VAR				VAR*		
Pneumococcal			PCV	PCV	PCV	PCV			PCV		PPV	
Influenza					Influenza (yearly)					Influenza (yearly)		
Hepatitis A									HepA series			

* Immunization status of older children and adolescents should be reviewed and necessary vaccines administered as needed.

---- Vaccines below this line are for selected high-risk populations.

Hep B vaccine is given to infants of positive mothers in the first 12 hours of life, second dose is given at age 1–2 months.

   If mother is negative first doses is gives in the first 2 months of life.

PPV = Pneumococcal polysaccharide vaccines are recommended in addition to conjugate PCV vaccine in certain high-risk groups.

encephalitis).[29] Hib, pneumococcal, and meningococcal vaccinations are recommended for immunosuppressed persons who are at high risk of invasive bacterial infections. However, vaccine-induced immune responses may not be optimal in immune-suppressed people and some may remain susceptible.

Conditions That Contraindicate Vaccination

Immunization schedules are modified when an individual has a contraindication to a particular vaccine (Exhibit 11-4). Mild illnesses (e.g., low-grade fever, upper respiratory infection, otitis media, and mild diarrhea) or breastfeeding are not contraindications for immunization. Previous or suspected anaphylactic reaction to a vaccine component is the strictest contraindication to immunization. When a concurrent moderate or severe illness may be exacerbated by a vaccine-induced immune response, immunization can be delayed. Contraindications are specific to live attenuated vaccines, which pose a threat to immunosuppressed individuals or to a fetus. Because measles can be a severe illness in an HIV-infected person, MMR immunization is recommended for HIV-infected individuals before they become severely immunocompromised. Among blood product recipients, circulating antibody present in transfused blood components can interfere with the replication of live vaccine virus. Therefore, it is recommended that MMR and varicella vaccinations be postponed for a period following blood or blood product transfusions.

Vaccine Development

Vaccine innovation includes identification and characterization of antigens that induce neutralizing antibody or humoral response, identification of genetic clones that produce these antigens, vaccine biochemical formulation, numerous animal studies, and extensive manufacturing innovation to mass-produce vaccine. Vaccine science, innovation, and manufacturing are critical components in the development of safe and efficacious vaccines for all national immunization programs.

Licensure of any new vaccine requires that efficacy be demonstrated from preclinical studies. The vaccine manufacturer begins this process upon filing an Investigational New Drug (IND) application with the US Food and Drug Administration (FDA). All information concerning vaccine formulation, vaccine manufacturing, stability and sterility testing, and results of animal

Exhibit 11-4   Contradictions for Vaccination

---

1. Severe allergy to any vaccine component
2. Severe illness
3. Immunosuppression (live vaccines only)
4. HIV infection (live virus vaccines except measles)
5. Pregnancy (especially live vaccines)
6. Encephalopathy
7. Recent receipt of blood products (MMR and varicella)

testing is submitted to the FDA. The FDA approves the implementation of human studies only if the new vaccine demonstrates preliminary potency, safety, and effectiveness in animal studies. The following section outlines the hierarchical process of preclinical and clinical research. At each point, the decision to progress to the next phase is based upon promising results from the previous set of studies.

Preclinical Studies

Animal testing is used to develop assays that assess the humoral and cellular immune response to candidate vaccines. Through a series of studies, appropriate animal models are used to determine the dose-response relationship, to identify the optimal routes of administration, and the dosing schedule necessary to achieve the maximum beneficial dose (i.e., the dose that maximizes the protective immune response and minimizes serious adverse events). Animal studies represent the first step in evaluating vaccine safety. A list of vaccine-induced toxicities is established, which may include severe systemic effects and organ systems damage, as well as the unlikely potential of a vaccine to be carcinogenic or teratogenic. Provided that potential benefit is deemed to outweigh potential harms, the products proceed to human studies.

Phase I: Dose Finding and Safety

Following FDA review and approval by an institutional review board (IRB), early vaccine studies in humans are conducted to evaluate vaccine dose and safety and to assess whether the vaccine is biologically active. Specific toxicities (e.g., local and systemic reactions and hematological abnormalities) are evaluated in both phase I and phase II safety and immunogenicity studies. Rules for stopping an immunization series are established from the onset and are adapted as more data are collected.

Most preventive vaccine clinical trials begin with trials in healthy, adult volunteers. Childhood vaccines are first tested in healthy adults and older children, prior to testing in infants. For some vaccines (i.e., HIV vaccines), initial clinical trials may be conducted in previously infected persons and subsequently among uninfected healthy adults. Adult studies typically begin with a single fixed dose of vaccine in a small number of volunteers (e.g., 5 to 10 subjects). Postinoculation serologic assays measure the level and duration of the immune response. Adverse events are carefully enumerated and graded for severity, duration, and the relationship to vaccination. Small sequential studies may be conducted whereby the vaccine dose is increased until a beneficial dose is established. Additional phase I or phase I/II safety and immunogenicity studies are performed in children and infants to fine-tune the dose, define the vaccine schedule, and continue monitoring immune response and vaccine safety in these age groups.

Phase II: Safety and Immunogenicity Trials

In phase II studies, safety, benefit, and evidence of efficacy are the primary end points. Safety and immunogenicity end points are predefined based on preclinical and phase I studies. The vaccine is tested in healthy persons representing the population for which the vaccine is indicated. Sample size needs to be sufficiently large to measure benefit (i.e., evidence of efficacy) without compromising the ability to estimate rates of adverse events. Studies of 50 to 100 persons can measure adverse events at a rate of 10 in 100 doses and estimate the beneficial effect that occurs in 10% or more of the population. As in phase I studies, postinoculation serologic assays are performed to measure the level and duration of the immune response. Participants are closely evaluated for severity and duration of adverse events. Expected adverse events and severity grades are listed in toxicity tables used to standardize safety evaluations. Correlates of protection provide evidence of vaccine clinical efficacy. These are immunologic markers of immune response to the vaccine, such as seroconversion (i.e., development of neutralizing antibodies), rise in antibody titer (i.e., booster response), and development of cell-mediated immune response (e.g., cytotoxic T lymphocytes).

Phase III: Comparative Efficacy Trials

Comparative efficacy trials determine the impact of vaccination on prevention of infection and begin to assess the feasibility of administering vaccinations in at-risk populations. Vaccines that are shown to be safe and immunogenic in phase I and II trials advance to phase III randomized comparative trials to assess true vaccine efficacy. Phase III trials involve large numbers of susceptible persons in more generalizable settings. The definitive study design for determining vaccine efficacy is the randomized, double-blinded, placebo-controlled trial. Often, multiple clinic sites are required to recruit a large enough sample to demonstrate vaccine efficacy with adequate study power. Sample size requirements depend upon the incidence of infection in an unvaccinated population (or a similar vaccinated population if a standard vaccine is already available), as well as the reduction in incidence one expects to observe in the vaccinated population. In phase III trials, vaccine efficacy is calculated as the observed reduction in incidence (I) in the vaccinated (vac) versus the unvaccinated (unv) population, expressed as a percentage.

Randomization strives to achieve comparability between vaccinated and unvaccinated groups with respect to demographic characteristics and risk factors for natural infection. Theoretically, randomization of a sufficient number of persons will ensure that characteristics that could affect the safety and efficacy of a vaccine will be evenly distributed between the arms of the study. However, many factors that could affect immunization response are known. For example, risk factors for most childhood infections include other immunizations, attendance in day care or school, exposure to infected individuals, and general health status. In vaccine trials of HIV, HBV, and hepatitis C virus, risk factors that require consideration include the number of unprotected sexual acts and/or sharing of potentially contaminated injection equipment. For infections such as malaria that are transmitted by a vector (e.g., *Aedes* sp.), it is important to take into account the level of endemicity of *Plasmodium* sp. and participants' use of mosquito nets and insect repellents. Appropriate adjustment for these potential confounders is crucial, because differential exposure to the infectious agent across the vaccinated and unvaccinated (control) groups can bias estimates of vaccine efficacy. Adjustment can be made in the design or analysis phase. By design, a trial may strive to have equal distribution of key factors in each arm by blocking participants prior to randomization. For example, a trial may separate participants by age groups and then randomize participants within each age group. This would ensure that the arms of the trial had a similar age distribution. Adjustments may also be made in the analysis to account for known characteristics that, despite randomization, may not have been evenly distributed between the study arms.

Vaccine Efficacy and Vaccine Effectiveness

Measures of vaccine efficacy (VE) are calculated from prelicensure, randomized, double-blind, clinical trials. Results from postlicensure observational studies associate disease outcomes with vaccine failure in fully vaccinated and inadequately vaccinated individuals, and in populations with low vaccine coverage. Whereas vaccine trials measure efficacy, the overall estimate of protective effect calculated from an observational epidemiologic study is more accurately defined as vaccine effectiveness (VE*).[30,31] Overall vaccine effectiveness is the result of both the vaccine's direct effect, which refers to its ability to protect individuals from infection, and its indirect effect, which is its ability to reduce the spread of the infection in a population.[31,32] For a discussion of the ways in which vaccines can indirectly decrease the duration of disease, alter susceptibility, or reduce the infective period of an organism in a given population, refer to Halloran et al.[32-34]

In any given population, spread of disease is a function of the rate of contact (C), the probability of exposure to an infectious agent (E), and the probability that exposure leads to infection (P) (see Figure 11-3). Determination of VE* generally assumes that infected, immune, and susceptible persons are randomly mixed in the population and that the population is sufficiently dense so that contact (C) will be equal.[32-34] The probability of exposure is related to both the prevalence of disease and the number of immune persons in the population. *Herd immunity*, which refers to the level of immunity in a population, depends upon the extent of immunity acquired from previous epidemics, as well as other factors, such as vaccine coverage. The probability that contact with an infected person will result in infection is a function of an individual's susceptibility and the virulence of the organism. Individual susceptibility can be lower in those with protective immunity from either previous infection or vaccination.

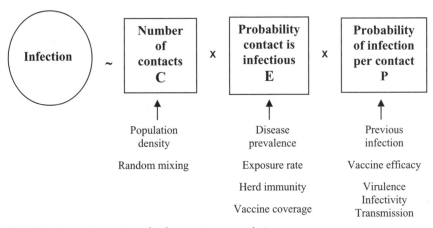

FIGURE 11-3 Dynamics of infection in a population.

In a randomized clinical trial, vaccine efficacy (VE) is the percent reduction in the incidence of disease in the vaccinated (I vac) compared to the incidence of disease in the unvaccinated (I unv).

$$VE = \frac{I_{unv} - I_{vac}}{I_{unv}} \times 100$$

The following equation is derived from dividing by the incidence in the unvaccinated:

$$VE = 1 - \frac{I_{vac}}{I_{unv}} = 1 - RR$$

As demonstrated by these equations, the ratio of incidence in the vaccinated to unvaccinated groups is a measure of relative risk (RR). The equation VE = 1 − RR, is useful in epidemiological studies where vaccine effectiveness (VE*) can be assessed. Vaccine effectiveness (VE*) approximates vaccine efficacy (VE) when exposure (E) to the infectious agent is not dependent upon vaccination status and does not differ across comparison groups, and when the vaccinated and unvaccinated persons arise from the same population, such that the rate of contact (C) is equivalent.

$$VE^* = 1 - \frac{C_{vac} \times E_{vac} \times P_{vac}}{C_{unv} \times E_{unv} \times P_{unv}} = 1 - \frac{P_{vac}}{P_{unv}} = 1 - RR$$

If the comparison groups are similar, then vaccine effectiveness, VE* = 1 − P_{vac} / P_{unv}, is a function of the ratio of individual immunity in the vaccinated and unvaccinated groups, and can be estimated by VE* = 1 − RR.[32-34] Table 11-1 summarizes equations for calculating vaccine effectiveness.

Epidemiologic Studies

After licensure, vaccines are distributed among heterogeneous populations at risk of disease, who will vary in age, infirmity, access to health care, and risk of exposure. At this point, observational studies play an important role in assessing vaccine effectiveness. In contrast to randomized clinical trials evaluating vaccine efficacy, case-control and cohort studies evaluate the combination of vaccine efficacy and the success of a given immunization program. A significant decline in the overall incidence of disease is one indicator that the vaccine itself and the immunization campaign have contributed to the prevention of disease. However, vaccine effectiveness can be suboptimal because of a variety of factors. For example, the potency of an inactivated vaccine can be reduced if a specific lot of vaccine was less antigenic, whereas the potency of a live attenuated vaccine can be compromised if the cold chain was not maintained. Vaccine effectiveness can also be low due to incomplete vaccine coverage.

Seldom, if ever, do vaccine efficacy and/or coverage attain 100%. Therefore, outbreaks among vaccinated populations can and do occur. Observational studies are often used to determine whether vaccine failures contribute

TABLE 11-1   Vaccine Efficacy Equations

Prospective Studies	**Cohort**	$VE^* = 1 - RR$
	Outbreak investigation (Attack rates or cumulative incidence)	$VE^* = 1 - AR_{vac}/AR_{unv}$
	Household spread (Secondary attack rate)	$VE^* = 1 - SAR_{vac}/SAR_{unv}$
	Longitudinal follow-up with time to event data	
	Life-table (Hazard ratio)	$VE^* = 1 - H_{vac}/H_{unv}$
	Person-time (Cumulative incidence)	$VE^* = 1 - CI_{vac}/CI_{unv}$
Retrospective Studies	**Case-control studies**	$VE^* = 1 - OR$
	Unmatched	$VE^* = 1 - (a/c)/(b/d)$ ratio of the odds of vaccination in cases and controls.
	Matched	$VE^* = 1 - b/c$ ratio of discordant pairs
	Logistic regression model or proportional hazard model	$VE^* = 1 - e^{\beta vac}$

Source: Halloran ME, Struchiner CJ, and Longini IM, Study designs for evaluating different efficacy and effectiveness aspects of vaccines, *Am J Epidemiol* 1997; 146(10): 789–803, by permission of the Oxford University Press.

to epidemics in the general population or within subgroups, and lend themselves to the study of risk factors for vaccine failure. Vaccine effectiveness can be measured within a population experiencing an outbreak, special populations at risk of infection (e.g., the elderly, children in day care, people in refugee camps), or as part of community-wide surveillance of vaccine-preventable diseases.

Vaccine effectiveness can be determined by comparing risk of disease among vaccinated and nonvaccinated groups. In general, an ideal study includes groups of comparable susceptibility before vaccination, equal exposure to disease before and after vaccination, and equal risk of being diagnosed with disease during the study period.[31] As in randomized trials of vaccine efficacy, it is important to ensure that these groups are comparable with respect to exposure, risk of infection, access to the vaccine, and opportunity for diagnosis. Potential bias may occur if any of the following occur:

1. There is unequal exposure to disease that causes individuals to self-select for vaccination.
2. Vaccination status systematically differs between healthy and diseased persons.
3. Infection or disease is differentially diagnosed in the vaccinated versus the unvaccinated.[31-34]

Essential components to any epidemiologic study include definition of a case, standardized case finding, ascertainment of vaccine status, and level of exposure.

An a priori case definition of infection or disease should be sensitive and specific. A case definition that poorly represents the disease in question may lead to imprecise estimates of vaccine effectiveness.[34,35] For invasive infections (e.g., bacteremia and meningitis), the organism is isolated and cultured; such laboratory confirmation yields a sensitive and specific case definition. Although it is not essential for every observational study, laboratory confirmation of cases generally increases the point estimate of vaccine effectiveness.[31,32]

In any study, it is crucial to assure that case finding occurs with the same degree of rigor in both the vaccinated and unvaccinated groups. Vaccination may prevent clinical disease but not infection or it may reduce the severity of disease, resulting in a differential disease diagnosis in the vaccinated versus unvaccinated groups. Therefore, to avoid bias, a case definition must detect a spectrum of mild, moderate, and severe disease. The point estimate of vaccine effectiveness will be biased by the extent to which groups differ in assessment, medical care and diagnosis, validity of self- or parental report of disease, and quality of medical records. Even among those who receive medical care for a vaccine-related event or breakthrough illness, the diligence of medical providers to report diseases is proportional to their perception of the severity of the condition. Thus, studies that rely on passive reporting systems may have bias in the assessment of cases of disease among the vaccinated and unvaccinated.

Equal effort must be made to confirm vaccination status in diseased and nondiseased persons. Reliance upon the self-reporting of vaccination status or inaccurate vaccination records (e.g., school records) may result in misclassification. When possible, self-reported vaccine histories should be confirmed through provider records, which are also important in confirming vaccination dates, vaccine type, manufacturer and lot number, and expiration dates.

The definition of *vaccination* must also be clear. When multiple doses of vaccine are required to develop full protection, the appropriate comparison is between persons who receive no vaccine and those who receive a complete course. If it is assumed that one or two doses induce some immunity, inclusion of these persons in the unvaccinated group would enrich that group with nonsusceptibles, thereby lowering the attack rates in the unvaccinated group relative to attack rates in the vaccinated. This, in turn, lowers the estimate of vaccine effectiveness. Alternatively, if the vaccinated group includes persons receiving less than the full series, the vaccinated group would be enriched with susceptibles, resulting in increased attack rates. This would result in decreased estimates of vaccine effectiveness.[31,32] Vaccine effectiveness for one, two, and three doses compared to no vaccination can be calculated from prospective cohort and case-control studies.

Observational studies evaluating vaccine effectiveness are vulnerable to selection factors that can cause rates derived from diseased and nondiseased or vaccinated and unvaccinated groups to differ systematically. Factors such as age, sex, race, socioeconomic status, place of work or residence, attendance in school, day care, and residence in jail or nursing homes may independently be related to both risk of disease and to vaccination status. Therefore, these studies must diligently control for confounding factors in the design (e.g., through stratification or matching), or preferably by ensuring sufficient sample size so that appropriate adjustments in the analysis may be made.

In highly endemic areas and/or where there are adequate resources, surveillance is conducted among cohorts of vaccinated and unvaccinated persons. Upon establishing vaccination status at baseline, the cumulative incidence of infection in vaccinated persons (CI vac) is compared to the cumulative incidence of infection in unvaccinated persons (CI unv), estimating the relative risk.[33] Other types of epidemiologic study designs that are used to evaluate vaccine effectiveness are described in detail below. In-depth discussion on these field methods is found in Halloran et al.[32-34]

Seroprevalence Cross-Sectional Studies

Evidence of vaccine efficacy and effectiveness are often correlated with a protective level of antibody in serum. In a cross-sectional study, a single serum sample is drawn and antibody levels are correlated with past records of vaccination and disease. The comparison of the proportion of subjects who have been vaccinated with protective antibody with the proportion of subjects not vaccinated with protective antibody is a prevalence ratio (PR). In this case, the calculation of vaccine effectiveness is $VE^* = 1 - PR$. One advantage of seroprevalence studies is the ability to quickly assess vaccine-induced immunity, measured according to the length of time since vaccination. These results should be interpreted with caution, because antibody responses wane over time, and the absence of antibody does not necessarily indicate susceptibility.

Prospective Studies

Populations at high risk of infection can be defined during an outbreak investigation, a household contact study, or in a highly endemic area. Using methods such as personal interviews and medical records review, vaccination status can be confirmed and a cohort of vaccinated and unvaccinated persons followed for the purpose of identifying new cases of disease. Prospective studies yield valid estimates of RR when the disease is common and exposure (i.e., vaccination status) is rare. In situations where the attack rate (AR) is expected to be high and the population is a mix of vaccinated and unvaccinated persons, a prospective study is useful for evaluating vaccine effectiveness.

In outbreak studies, vaccination status is established at baseline, and the RR is used to compare the AR in the vaccinated (AR vac) and the unvaccinated (AR unv). Households of primary cases represent highly exposed populations that warrant close observation. As high-risk households are identified, vaccination status is confirmed for each member, and any secondary cases are identified. To estimate vaccine effectiveness, the RR is calculated as the ratio of vaccinated secondary cases (SAR vac) to unvaccinated secondary cases (SAR unv) from all households. Time-to-event analyses (i.e., survival analysis) are also useful for estimating RR. Using Cox proportional hazards models, the hazard ratio is an estimate of the instantaneous relative risk, which is the ratio of the probability of disease in the vaccinated group at some time point (H vac) relative to the probability of disease in the unvaccinated (H unv) at the same time point.[32–34]

In prospective studies, factors that erroneously increase the attack rate in the vaccinated, relative to the unvaccinated, will cause vaccine effectiveness to be underestimated, whereas any erroneous increase in the attack rate in the unvaccinated, relative to the vaccinated, will lead to an overestimate of vaccine effectiveness.

Case-Control Studies

Case-control studies can be an appropriate study design for assessing vaccine effectiveness when the disease is rare. One advantage is that data pertaining to multiple risk factors of vaccine failure can be collected and evaluated. Cases are often identified through a surveillance system, such as direct laboratory reporting or national surveillance databases. To avoid bias, controls should be selected from the same population as cases and should not significantly differ with respect to their probability of vaccination or exposure to infection. As in other case-control studies, a matched or unmatched design may be used. The odds ratio (OR) is used to estimate RR or, in this case, VE*. The OR is calculated as the ratio of the odds of vaccination in the cases relative to the odds of vaccination in the controls, or the ratio of discordant pairs for unmatched and matched designs, respectively. Vaccine effectiveness is calculated as $VE^* = 1 - OR$. When logistic models are used to calculate the OR for disease in the vaccinated, the equation $VE^* = 1 - e^\beta vac$ is the measure of vaccine effectiveness, where $e^\beta vac$ is the expotentiated log OR of disease in the vaccinated population. In case-control studies, VE* is underestimated when vaccination rates are erroneously overreported in the cases, relative to the controls, and overestimated when controls are more likely to be misclassified as being vaccinated, relative to cases.[34,35]

Monitoring Adverse Events and Vaccine Safety

In most cases, the risk of disease trumps the risk of vaccination. Some vaccines have been developed to avoid potential risks of vaccination. For example, recombinant hepatitis B vaccine replaced the theoretical risk of infection from the human serum-derived vaccine. Oral polio vaccine, which carried a rare risk of paralysis, has been replaced by inactivated polio vaccine in countries at low risk of natural infection. Most recently, acellular pertussis vaccines have replaced more reactinogenic whole cell pertussis vaccines. As vaccine-preventable diseases become more rare, the perceived risk of severe adverse events from vaccine can appear to outweigh the risk of natural infection among an uninformed public.

Comparative studies continue to collect information on adverse events. Additional postlicensure monitoring is achieved through the use of surveillance systems to track vaccine-related adverse events, which is a mandate of the National Childhood Injury Act of 1986. By 1998, a nationwide vaccine adverse event reporting system (VAERS) was established by the US Department of Health and Human Services.[36,37] VAERS is a passive reporting system designed to collect case-series data to detect rare events, to identify trends in commonly reported adverse events, and to detect early warning signals and generate hypotheses about possible new adverse events.[38] The strength of VAERS is its demonstrated feasibility as a cost-effective public health system for identifying potential harmful effects of mass vaccination. Health care providers and vaccine manufacturers are required to report all adverse events associated with the administration of a US licensed vaccine. VAERS is especially important with newly licensed vaccines and in the assessment of new indications for vaccinations.

Like many passive reporting systems, VAERS case-series data are biased due to underreporting and/or overreporting of suspected vaccine reactions.[36-38] Rates of adverse events cannot be calculated because the system does not collect denominator data (i.e., number of persons vaccinated or number of doses given).[38] However, VAERS data can be used to identify clusters of rare adverse events, such as associations between oral polio vaccine and poliomyelitis, and DTP with sudden infant death syndrome (SIDS). More recently, after the licensure of rotavirus vaccine, the VAERS system detected a cluster of intussusception cases following vaccine (see Figure 11-4).[39,40] Following identification of adverse event clusters or signals, clinical, epidemiologic, and laboratory investigations are required to assess causality. Studies that substantiate severe adverse effects may lead to the withdrawal of vaccine, the development of safer vaccines, or compensation for persons who experienced adverse event. The investigations of intussusception following rotavirus vaccine led the CDC to recommend suspension of its use on July 16, 1999,[40] which was followed by voluntary withdrawal of the vaccine from the market.[38] However, it is important to note that neither of these preliminary findings were confirmed. In further analysis, DTP has been cleared of an association with SIDS, and while there was an increased risk of intussusception following rotavirus vaccination, overall rates of intussusception were dramatically reduced among vaccinated infants.

The Vaccine Safety Datalink (VSD) Project is another effort to improve postlicensure monitoring of vaccine-related adverse events. Beginning in 1991, the CDC, in partnership with health maintenance organizations (HMOs), established large cohorts of vaccinated children.[41] Subsequently, the VSD has expanded to monitor vaccine-related adverse events in adolescents and adults. VSD data are generated during routine health care visits and contain adverse event as well as denominator data (number vaccinated and doses administered) on large, stable populations. As such, the system is less subject to underreporting or other biases common to passive surveillance systems. The VSD thus provides a rapid and economical means of conducting postlicensure comparative studies of vaccine safety.[41]

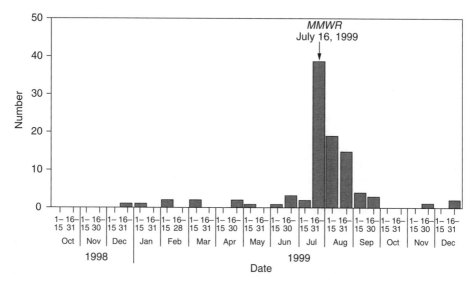

*n = 98.

FIGURE 11-4   Number* of confirmed cases of intussusception after implementation of rhesus-human rotavirus reassortant-tetravalent vaccine, by date reported to the Vaccine Adverse Event Reporting System—United States, October 1, 1998–December 31, 1999. *Source:* Suspension of rotavirus vaccine after reports of intussusception—United States, 1999; MMWR. 2004 Sep 3;53(34):786–9.

In a review of research tools to evaluate the causal association between vaccines and adverse events, Dr. Robert Chen, a CDC researcher, lists four criteria to establish causality. First, laboratory confirmation (e.g., isolating vaccine virus strain from the pathogenic lesion) is required. Second, unique clinical syndromes specific to a vaccine (e.g., acute flaccid paralysis following OPV vaccine) must be identified. Third, there is a need to demonstrate that the adverse event recurs on rechallenge with the vaccine. Fourth, it should be demonstrated that the adverse event occurs more often in the vaccinated than in the unvaccinated group.[42] Adverse events that meet the first three criteria are rare. Clinical trials are often not powered for safety studies to identify events that are rare; for example, intussusception occurs once per 10,000 doses of rotavirus vaccine, and acute encephalopathy occurs once in 100,000 doses of whole-cell pertussis vaccine. Despite the limitations of epidemiologic studies to quantify extremely rare events, they serve to define an upper limit of risk of adverse events.[42] Consistency in observational studies must be coupled with evidence of a biological mechanism by which a vaccine may cause the adverse event. Both of these criteria define the plausibility criteria set forth by the Institute of Medicine's (IOM) Immunization Safety Review Committee, which was convened to evaluate the plausibility and significance of many alleged vaccine adverse events.[42]

The association between autism and vaccines, specifically MMR vaccine, was one of the many vaccine-adverse events scrutinized by the IOM committee. Two observations supported the hypothesis linking autism with MMR.

First, an increased number of autism cases were being reported in the same time period when an increasing number of children were being vaccinated against measles (ecological association). Second, the signs of autism (e.g., loss of language skills) in the second year of life occurred close to the time when MMR was given. The latter factor indicated a temporal association between vaccine and disease, but it remained possible that the events are coincident and unrelated.[43]

The IOM investigated two potential causes of autism, the measles vaccine virus and the mercury-containing preservative, thimerosal.[44,45] In a 1998 study by Wakefield et al., researchers found measles virus RNA in the intestines of 8 of 12 children with neurological disorders, specifically autism. These findings presented a potential biologic link between measles vaccine and autism, but not specific evidence of a biologic mechanism.[46] The IOM considered this link along with the body of epidemiological data including nine controlled-observational studies, three ecological studies, and two studies based on the passive surveillance of systems, which consistently demonstrated no evidence of an association between MMR vaccine and autism. The committee concluded that the evidence favored rejection of a causal association between MMR vaccine and autism.[44]

The situation with thimerosal was less clear. It has been well known that high doses of mercury exposure cause neurological damage. Studies of low-dose mercury exposure, ingested in seafood, on neurologic development have been inconclusive. The committee reported that no published or unpublished study that they reviewed linked thimerosal to autism. Despite this finding, the committee was concerned that children received many vaccines containing thimerosal and a cumulative effect was possible. The committee concluded that there was insufficient evidence to accept or reject the causal association between thimerosal and autism.[44]

For many rare and potential vaccine-related adverse events, the actual biological mechanisms are not yet known. Surveillance and epidemiologic studies may suggest a mechanism, but further research is needed to establish the biologic bases for any event. In the United States, the CDC has funded seven Clinic Immunization Safety Assessment (CISA) centers. A stated goal of these centers is to develop standard assessments of individuals with vaccine-adverse events to advance the scientific understanding of the pathophysiology and risk factors associated with these reactions. This network will further augment the VAERS and VSD systems in the evaluation of vaccine safety.[42,47]

Direct Impact of Vaccination

"The impact of vaccination on the health of the people worldwide is difficult to exaggerate. With the exception of safe water, no modality, not even antibiotics, has had such a major effect upon reducing mortality and subsequent population growth."[48] The direct impact from widespread use of vaccines can be easily understood when one examines the incidence rates of specific diseases over time. Below, we highlight disease trends in poliomyelitis, measles, and invasive *Haemophilus influenzae* type b to illustrate the impact of effective vaccines and vaccine programs.

Polio

The increased incidence of paralytic poliomyelitis coincided with improvement in hygiene and societal development in the 1930s and 1940s (Figure 11-5). Prior to the development of sanitation systems, children acquired protective immunity when exposed to polio virus in infancy. Polio infection in infants is restricted to the gastrointestinal tract because the human receptors necessary for polio virus infection of neurons are not expressed until later in childhood. Between 1940 and 1952, the incidence of paralytic polio in the United States rose from less than 12 cases per 100,000 persons to about 37 cases per 100,000 persons. Although the total number of cases declined before the first vaccine was introduced in 1955, the proportion of paralytic cases increased from a rate of 66% to 88% of all cases.[49]

In 1955, the Salk inactivated polio vaccine (IPV) was the first vaccine licensed. After licensure, the United States began a mass immunization campaign, and the incidence of poliomyelitis cases fell dramatically as more and more children were immunized. A 90% reduction in the number of poliomyelitis cases was attained with the Salk IPV alone. As a result, the death rate declined from 1.9 per 100,000 cases between 1915 and 1924 to 0.1 per 100,000 cases in 1961. The Salk IPV did not induce sufficient mucosal immunity to protect against reinfection, and outbreaks continued to occur, including a high number of cases in persons that were fully vaccinated.[49,50]

The Sabin oral live attenuated vaccine (OPV) was licensed for human use in 1961–1962, after which the incidence of poliomyelitis continued to decline further; in 1964, only 59 polio cases were reported in the United States. In 1960, a total of 2525 paralytic cases were reported, compared to 61 in 1965.[49,50] Thus, the Sabin OPV quickly became the vaccine of choice in the United States and in most other parts of the world. In the United States, the last indigenously acquired poliovirus infection occurred in 1979,[51] and the last imported case occurred in 1993.[52]

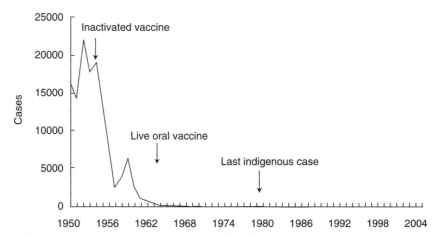

FIGURE 11-5 Poliomyelitis cases reported in the United States, 1950–2004. *Source:* Poliomyelitis. In: Atkinson W, and Wolfe C, eds. Epidemiology and Prevention of Vaccine Preventable Diseases. 7th ed. GA: Public Health Foundation; 2002; p. 75.

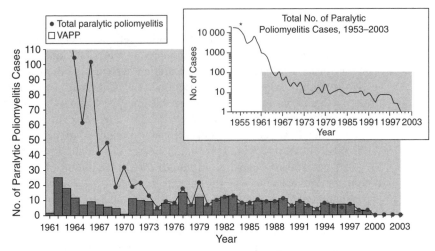

FIGURE 11-6 Reported cases of paralytic poliomyelitis, United States 1953–2003.
Source: Alexander, L. N. et al. JAMA 2004;292:1696–1701.

Vaccine-associated paralytic poliomyelitis (VAPP) was recognized as early as 1962. Since the early 1970s, VAPP accounted for almost all of the paralytic polio cases identified in the United States (see Figure 11-6). Alexander et al. reviewed the United States paralytic polio cases between 1990 and 2003 and estimated VAPP incidence to be 0.34 cases per 1 million OPV vaccine distributed to immunocompetent children, and demonstrated that the risk of VAPP increased with increasing number of OPV doses received.[52] Persons with primary immunodeficiency who were indirectly vaccinated with vaccine poliovirus were at highest risk for VAPP. The authors estimated VAPP incidence with this population to be 3077 cases per 1 million immunocompromised population.[52] In 1999, the United States vaccine recommendation changed from an all OPV immunization schedule to a 2-dose IPV followed by OPV schedule. This resulted in a 54% decline in VAPP. In 2000, an all-IPV schedule was implemented. The last case of VAPP in the United States occurred in 1999.[52]

Measles

Measles was an extremely important cause of childhood morbidity and mortality up to five years prior to vaccine licensure (1958–1962). At that time the average annual number of reported measles cases in the United States was 503,282 with approximately 500 deaths per year.[53] Epidemic cycles of measles occurred every 2–3 years, and the actual annual number of cases of measles was estimated to be about 3 to 4 million. More than 50% of the population had experienced measles by age 6, and more than 90% had measles by age 15, with the highest incidence between ages 5 to 9 years.[54] The first live attenuated measles vaccine (Edmonston B strain) was licensed for use in 1963; the currently available vaccine, the Enderson-Edmonston strain, was licensed in 1968. Following initial licensure, the incidence of measles decreased by more than 98%, and the 2–3 year epidemic cycles no longer occurred (Figure 11-7).[54]

Regional elimination of measles began in 1989, when the World Health Assembly resolved to reduce measles morbidity and mortality by 90% and 95%, respectively, by 1995. The goal to eliminate indigenous measles in the United States was set in 1978. In September 1999, the CDC reported a record low number of measles cases in the United States; only 100 measles cases were confirmed in 1998, most of which were imported or associated with an imported case.[53,55] In 2002, measles was recognized as nonendemic in the United States with only 44 imported cases.[56]

In the United States, between 1985 and 1988, 42% of measles cases occurred in children who were vaccinated on or after their first birthday, and 68% of cases were in school-aged children who had been appropriately vaccinated. However, of the latter group, only 16% had been appropriately vaccinated. The measles outbreaks in 1985 and 1986 led to a recommendation in 1989 of universal reimmunization of children against measles, either at school entry or at entry into middle school or junior high school.[57]

A resurgence of measles occurred between 1989 and 1991. There were 18,193 cases in 1989, 27,786 in 1990, and 9643 in 1991. During this resurgence, the age distribution changed, and children 5 years and younger accounted for 45–48% of the new cases. The principal cause of the measles epidemic of 1989 to 1991 was failure to vaccinate children at the recommended age.[58,59] Pockets of low-immunization coverage were observed in

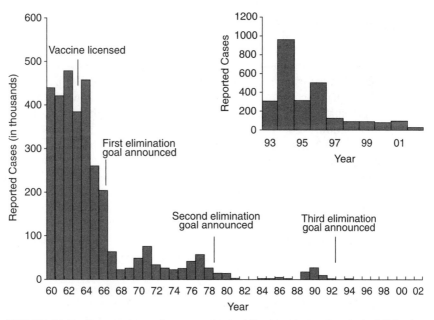

FIGURE 11-7   Reported measles cases, United States, 1960–2002 (unpublished data from the Centers for Disease Control and Prevention).
Source: Meissner, H. C. et al. Pediatrics 2004;114:1065–1069.

inner-city communities, and the highest measles incidence occurred among Hispanic and African-American children. Surveys conducted in areas experiencing preschool measles outbreaks indicated that as few as 50% of children had been vaccinated for measles by their second birthday, particularly among African-American and Hispanic children. Intensive efforts to vaccinate preschool-age children were successful and coverage among 2-year-old children increased from 70% in 1990 to 91% in 1996. Since 1993, fewer than 1000 cases have been reported annually.[54]

Outbreaks of measles still occur, primarily among communities with religious and philosophic exemptions to vaccination. Smaller outbreaks were reported in unvaccinated preschool populations, vaccinated school populations (vaccine failures), college students, and adult communities. To enhance immunity levels, the CDC targets young adults born after January 1957 by encouraging MMR booster vaccination at colleges or other postsecondary educational institutions.

In contrast, some developing countries have not yet achieved high rates of measles immunization coverage, and measles accounts for nearly 50% of the 1.6 million vaccine-preventable deaths annually in children.[60] The 1990 World Summit for Children adopted a goal of vaccinating 90% of children worldwide against measles by the year 2000.[53] By 2002, immunization rates had increased worldwide, yet barriers remain to preventing high immunization rates in some countries. For example, war and complex emergencies such as the devastating tsunami that hit Asia in late 2004 have been associated with outbreaks of measles, tetanus, and water-borne diseases that are also vaccine preventable (e.g., cholera). Work is needed to address barriers, including the public's perception of unsafe vaccines, building political and financial commitments, and development of effective partnerships.[43]

Haemophilus Influenzae Type B

Prior to the advent of an effective vaccine, it was estimated that 1 in every 200 children would develop an invasive *Haemophilus influenzae* type b (Hib) infection before the age of 5 years.[61] Subsequently, 60% of infected children developed bacterial meningitis, and 10% of these children died while many more suffered permanent impairments, ranging from hearing loss to mental retardation.

By 1993, invasive Hib disease had decreased by 95%, and the disease has been practically eliminated in the United States (see Figure 11-8). This decline began with the introduction of bacterium capsular polysaccharide Hib vaccine in 1985. However, the vaccine was recommended for children over 2 years as it was poorly immunogenic in those less than 18 months. Yet young infants are at greatest risk of disease.[61] To overcome poor immunogenicity of polysaccharide-only vaccine, particularly in young infants, Hib polysaccharide-protein conjugates were developed. The first Hib conjugate vaccine was licensed in 1987 for children age 18 months and older. In 1988, similar vaccines were licensed for children as young as 2 months of age, based on clinical trials showing over 90% efficacy of these vaccine in fully immunized infants.[62] By 1997, 93% of all 2-year-old children in the United States completed the Hib vaccine series. From 1989 to 1997, the race-adjusted incidence of Hib invasive disease among children younger than 5 years of

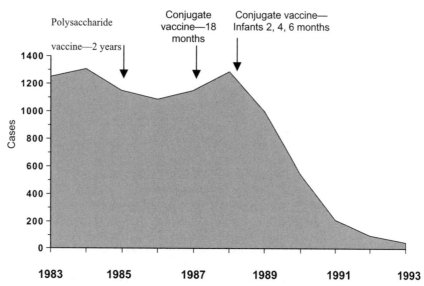

FIGURE 11-8 *Haemophilus influenzae* type b cases per year, United States 1983–1993.
Source: NIH. *The Jordan Report 1998: Accelerated Development of Vaccines.* Division of Microbiology and Infectious Diseases, National Institute of Allergy and Infectious Diseases.

age decreased by 99%, from 34 cases to 0.4 cases per 100,000 children.[63] Progress toward complete elimination continues in the United States and in Europe. Hib vaccines against strains circulating in the developing world have recently been tested in clinical trials.

The Role of Vaccines in Eradication of Specific Diseases

Eradication of a given communicable disease implies total control over morbidity, disability, mortality, and subclinical disease, beyond control of the etiologic agent(s) itself. As suggested by Evans, eradication is achieved when there is no risk of infection or disease in the absence of vaccination or any other control measures.[64] The need to immunize susceptibles before natural infection occurs is a formidable obstacle in the case of many childhood diseases. Factors that favor the eradication of a communicable disease are provided in Exhibit 11-5.

An immunization program need not achieve 100% coverage to provide protection against disease in a community. Herd immunity implies that some level of immunity in a community can provide protection to susceptible (unimmunized) persons. This collective immunologic protection represents an indirect effect of a vaccine beyond the level of the individual to that of the population. As long as susceptible persons do not contact infected persons, transmission can be interrupted. However, the concept of herd immunity assumes that susceptible persons mix randomly within the population, which

Exhibit 11–5   Factors Associated with Potential for Eradication of a
Communicable Disease

Factors Associated with the Disease
  Ease of diagnosis and treatment
  Low prevalence of subclinical disease
  High disease burden and economic impact
  Immunity is long term or lifelong
  Disease cannot be reactivated
  Disease has predictable seasonality
Factors Associated with the Etiologic Agent
  Lack of an animal reservoir or vector
  Only one causative agent or serotype
  Short incubation period
Factors Associated with the Host or Target Population
  Correlates or protection can be demonstrated
  Host cannot be reinfected with the agent
  Host cannot shed the organism once infection is resolved
  Public acceptance of the vaccine and other control measures is
high
Factors Associated with the Vaccine
  Can confer long-lasting protection in a few injections
  Minimal handling and storage requirements (e.g., cold chain)
  Simple administration
  Can be administered simultaneously with other vaccines or adapted
to schedules and timing of the national childhood immunization
programs
  Few short- or long-term adverse effects
  Low cost to produce and purchase vaccine

Source: Adapted from Evans, AS. Am J Epidemiol 1985;122(2):199–207, by
permission of the Oxford University Press.

is often not the case. Groups of unimmunized persons who share common characteristics (e.g., age, religion, culture) often cluster together in relatively restricted geographic settings. The degree of herd immunity required to prevent an epidemic varies according to the specific disease, the extent to which an infected individual is capable of transmitting the infection, the duration of the infectious period, the size of the population, and mixing patterns within and between other populations.

The global eradication of smallpox provides the gold standard against which other eradication programs are judged. Systematic application of smallpox vaccine began in Mexico and in Guatemala around 1805, and elsewhere in North America and Europe.[65] Initially, smallpox vaccine was offered to all age groups, but only those at risk (e.g., health care workers, travelers) were specifically targeted. As a result, incomplete coverage caused outbreaks to continue throughout the world.

The first attempt at global immunization of smallpox was in 1956, but this effort was not successful in containing the disease. In 1967, there were still 10–15 million cases of smallpox per year causing at least 2 million deaths and 100,000 cases of blindness.[65] In 1967, the global smallpox eradication program was enhanced to utilize enhanced surveillance and containment. Smallpox cases were always symptomatic, and always symptomatic before they were infectious. The vaccine prevents the development of symptomatic, or infectious disease, even after exposure to an infectious case. This approach emphasized extensive case-finding and tracking of the origin of the outbreak, coupled with immunization of remaining susceptibles.[65] In addition, a standardized, lyophilized ("freeze-dried") vaccine had become available, and rapid, effective administration of vaccine was made possible through the development of the bifurcated needle. These factors, combined with leadership, political will, and adequate resource allocation, ended the smallpox pandemic. The last known case was observed in Somalia in 1977. Vaccination in the United States waned in the mid-1960s and was no longer recommended for the general population in 1965. US military recruits were vaccinated for smallpox until 1982 although actual vaccination coverage was low. In 1980, the WHO officially declared that smallpox had indeed been eradicated, representing the most significant public health achievement of the 1900s. The threat of biologic weapons containing smallpox virus, after September 11, 2001, led the United States government to once again recommend smallpox vaccine for all medical care providers, emergency first responders, and members of the US military.

Toward Global Eradication of Polio

Although incidence and prevalence of polio-induced paralysis decreased after the introduction of the Salk (IPV) and Sabin (OPV) vaccines in the 1950s, polio continued to take its toll in developing countries. In 1988, the World Health Assembly set a target to eradicate polio from the world by the year 2000, a goal which unfortunately was not met. From the outset, eradication of polio appeared more difficult compared to smallpox. Three serotypes of polio virus exist with no considerable cross-immunity. Polio infection is associated with a higher prevalence of subclinical infections, a longer incubation period, and multiple routes of exposure. Moreover, several doses of OPV or IPV are usually needed to induce immunity. Despite these obstacles, progress toward eradication of polio over the last 10 years has been impressive. The virus was eradicated from the Western Hemisphere in 1991. In 1998, the WHO estimated that global routine immunization coverage with three doses of OPV was 82%. Globally, numbers of cases have decreased by 80% since 1988. By 2003, the number of countries with endemic polio decreased from 125 to 7, suggesting that eradication of polio may soon be a reality.[66,67]

A setback to the Global Polio Eradication Initiative was announced in June 2004, when the WHO announced that western and central Africa were at risk of a large polio outbreak. The vulnerable countries included those that border Nigeria, a country where the polio immunization programs were suspended in 2003 due to public fear of the vaccine's safety. At the beginning of 2003, only two sub-Saharan African countries had endemic polio.

In 2004, paralytic polio cases had been identified in 10 previously polio-free countries across the continent. The WHO began massive immunization campaigns across the continent in October and November of 2004, during the peak season for polio.[66] The campaign was successful in all but the poorest and most densely populated developing countries, where health delivery systems are inadequate, and where armed conflicts have interrupted routine vaccination campaigns. The major remaining reservoirs of polio are South Asia, and West and Central Africa.[67]

Appropriate evaluation of an immunization program is essential for establishing whether control has been attained and whether a pool of susceptibles exists that could represent the potential for new outbreaks. Evaluation should include surveys to assess vaccine coverage, coupled with clinical and/or serological confirmation of immunity. Sentinel surveillance should be maintained to identify the persistence of wild type, indigenous, or imported virus, as well as live vaccine virus.[68] The use of highly specific serology tests can be used when available, but simpler measures that are highly sensitive markers of polio such as acute flaccid paralysis and lameness are important surveillance tools. Only with systematic application of these methods will it be possible to determine whether polio or any other agent has been successfully eradicated.

Potential for Eradication of Other Communicable Diseases

The ability to control or attempt eradication of a communicable disease varies by country, according to demographic, environmental, hygienic, and economic factors. Apart from criteria that need to be taken into account when considering a specific communicable disease for eradication, such programs require political will, financial resources, and unwavering commitment to meet defined goals. In 1974, the WHO created an Expanded Programme on Immunization (EPI), which initially aimed to eliminate six diseases: tuberculosis, diphtheria, neonatal tetanus, whooping cough, poliomyelitis, and measles (Table 11-2). Prior to this initiative, less than 5% of children in developing countries were being immunized against these preventable childhood diseases. In more recent years, new vaccines have been added to EPI (e.g., TB, HBV, yellow fever), although the number of countries participating in the various programs varies considerably. Since the establishment of EPI, major progress has been made toward the elimination of other communicable diseases in various parts of the world. For example, routine administration of tetanus toxoid has virtually eliminated neonatal tetanus.

In a response to poor vaccine coverage in preschool children, the United States launched the Childhood Immunization Initiative in 1993. Its five strategies include the following

1. Improve the quality and quantity of immunization services.
2. Reduce vaccine costs.
3. Increase community participation, education, and partnerships.
4. Improve systems for monitoring diseases and vaccinations.
5. Improve vaccines and vaccine use.

Following establishment of this program, measles, diphtheria, mumps, pertussis, tetanus, Hib, and congenital rubella have been virtually eliminated from

TABLE 11-2   Year of Introduction of Selected First-Generation Vaccines for Use in Humans, and Year of First National and Expanded Immunization Programme (EPI)

Vaccine*	Year First Introduced	Year of First National Immunization Program	Year Beginning EPI
Smallpox	1798	1804	1956
Plague	1897	—	—
Diphtheria	1923	mid-1940s[†]	1974
Pertussis	1926	mid-1940s[†]	1974
Tuberculosis (BCG)	1921	1949	1974
Tetanus	1927	mid-1940s[†]	1974
Yellow fever	1935	1989	1989 (endemic countries)
Oral polio vaccine	1962	1974	1974
Measles	1964	1974	1985
Mumps	1967	1977	—
Rubella	1969	1970	—
Hepatitis B	1981	1990	1995
Haemophilus influenza type b	1985	1985	pending
Varicella-zoster	1984	1989	—

Note: In 1974, EPI was established with six targeted diseases: diphtheria, pertussis, tetanus, measles, polio, and tuberculosis (BCG). Rubella and mumps vaccines were never adapted into the EPI as single antigen vaccines.
*Not necessarily the vaccine currently in use.
[†]Approximate time period of wide use in the United States.

the United States. However, there are known subpopulations of unimmunized persons that represent the potential for new outbreaks.

Despite the successes described above, characteristics of some infectious agents make it unlikely they will be eradicated. In general, measles meets the criteria for eradication. By 2003 only 105 cases of measles were reported in the Western Hemisphere, raising hopes that measles may soon be eradicated in the Americas.[69] However, global eradication has proven to be difficult as there is only a narrow window in time to vaccinate after loss of protective maternal antibodies and exposure to natural infection. Control of influenza is hampered by the multiplicity of antigenic types, high contagiousness of the disease, and the persistence of multiple reservoirs (i.e., swine, fowl) for the origin of new recombinant viruses. Yellow fever does not have the diversity of influenza, and an effective vaccine is in use. Yellow fever remains endemic due to the sylvan cycle, where mosquitoes transmit the virus to primates and commonly humans, making eradication unlikely.

Barriers to Vaccine Implementation and Coverage

Seemingly insurmountable barriers are encountered in the attempt to deliver proven vaccines to those who need them the most. Because most vaccines are developed and manufactured in developed countries, steps must be taken to ensure that live vaccine can be transported and stored in a developing country in a viable form, maintaining the cold chain where appropriate. Staff must be trained in vaccine administration, safe injection techniques, and program management. To increase vaccine acceptability, public education campaigns are required, using materials that are sensitive to local language and culture.

Even in developed countries, proven vaccines do not necessarily reach those individuals who are at highest risk of infection. Although hepatitis B vaccine has been added to childhood immunization schedules in many developed countries, immunization levels are low and risk of infection is high among injection drug users and homosexual/bisexual men, particularly those old enough to have missed the vaccine in childhood (Exhibit 11-6).

Pockets of low coverage in most, if not all, countries are capable of perpetuating disease transmission. Even when adequate coverage has been achieved, births, immigration, waning immunity, and requirements for multiple doses mean that diligence is required to maintain herd immunity. Threats to achieving and maintaining coverage include wars, civil unrest, natural disasters, and other complex emergencies that can destroy the health infrastructure supporting immunization programs. The possibility of changes in the natural history of some diseases (e.g., new route of infection, new reservoir or host, reactivation of latent disease) underscores the need for continued sentinel surveillance in national and global immunization programs. The high cost of many proven vaccines also prevents many countries from adding them to their national immunization programs. Apart from biologic

Exhibit 11-6   Barriers to Achieving High Coverage with Recombinant Hepatitis B Vaccine in the United States

1. One quarter of HBV-infected persons deny known risk factors for HBV infection.
2. Access to high-risk populations (e.g., homosexual/bisexual men, injection drug users, illegal aliens from endemic countries) is difficult because populations are "hidden"; high-risk behaviors are highly stigmatized.
3. Low awareness of HBV infection and consequences of disease (i.e., hepatitis, liver cancer).
4. Low acceptability of vaccine schedule.
5. Lack of third-party reimbursement to cover vaccine costs.
6. Rapid acquisition of HBV infection among high-risk populations.
7. Age-specific decline in immunogenicity of vaccine.
8. Waning of induced immunity over time (i.e., protection estimated to last 13 years).

considerations, some vaccines that have been proven both efficacious and effective have not been licensed, due to high cost, low public health priority, or lack of endorsement from pharmaceutical companies. If global eradication of major vaccine-preventable diseases is to be upheld as a realistic goal, developed countries, nongovernmental organizations, and pharmaceutical companies must fulfill their obligation to support immunization programs in resource-poor countries.

References

1. Hume EH. *Vaccines*. Baltimore, Md: W.B. Saunders Company; 1940.
2. Rappouli R. New and improved vaccines against diphtheria and tetanus. In: Levine MM, Woodrow GC, Kaper JB, Cobon GS, eds. *New Generation Vaccines*. 2nd ed. New York, NY: Marcel Dekker, Inc; 1997: 417–436.
3. Hellstrom KE, Helstrom I, Chen L. Antitumor vaccines. In: Levine MM, Woodrow GC, Kaper JB, Cobon GS, eds. *New Generation Vaccines*. 2nd ed. New York, NY: Marcel Dekker, Inc; 1997:1095–1116.
4. Pasteur L. *Vaccines*. Paris: W.B. Saunders Company; 1885.
5. Abbas A, Lichtman A, Pober J. *Cellular and Molecular Immunology*. 3rd ed. Philadelphia, Pa: W.B. Saunders Company; 1997.
6. Janeway C, Travers P. *Immunobiology*. 3rd ed. New York, NY: Garland Publishers; 1997.
7. Huston DP. The biology of the immune system. *JAMA*. 1997;22: 1804–1814.
8. McDonnell WM, Askari FK. Immunization. *JAMA*. 1998;22:2000–2007.
9. Levine MM, Tacket CO, Galen JE, et al. Progress in the development of new attenuated strains of *Salmonella typhi* as live oral vaccines against typhoid fever. In: Levine MM, Woodrow GC, Kaper JB, Cobon GS, eds. *New Generation Vaccines*. 2nd ed. New York, NY: Marcel Dekker, Inc; 1997:437–446.
10. Alexander LN, Seward JF, Santibanez TA, et al. Vaccine policy changes and the epidemiology of poliomyelitis in the United States. *JAMA*. 2004;292:1692–1701.
11. Black F. Measles in acute viral infections. In: Evans AS, ed. *Viral Infections of Humans: Epidemiology and Control*. 2nd ed. New York, NY: Plenum Medical Co; 1989:521–522.
12. Kollaritsch H, Que JU, Kunz C, Wiedermann G, Herzog C, Cryz SJ. Safety and immunogenicity of live oral cholera and typhoid vaccines administered alone or in combination with antimalarial drugs, oral polio vaccine, or yellow fever vaccine. *J Infect Dis*. 1997;175:871–875.
13. Guess HA. Combination vaccines: issues in evaluations of effectiveness and safety. *Epidemiol Rev*. 1999;2:89–95.
14. Roux E, Yersin A. Contribution a l'etude de la diptherie. *Ann Inst Pasteur*. 1888;2:629–661.
15. Black S, Shinefield H, Fireman B, et al. Efficacy, safety and immunogenicity of hepavalent pneumococcal conjugate vaccine in children. *Pediatr Infect Dis J*. 2000;19:187–195.
16. Steere AC, Sikand VK, Meurice F, et al. Vaccination against Lyme disease with recombinant *Borrelia burgdorferi outer-surface lipoprotein A with adjuvant*. *N Engl J Med*. 1998;339:209–215.

17. Kapikian AZ, Hoshino Y, Chanock RM, Perez-Schael I. Efficacy of a quadrivalent rhesus rotavirus-based human rotavirus vaccine aimed at preventing severe rotavirus diarrhoea in infants and young children. *J Infect Dis*. 1996;174:S65–S72.

18. Clements-Mann ML, Weinhold K, Matthews TJ, et al. Immune responses to human immunodeficiency virus (HIV) type 1 induced by canarypox expressing HIV-1MN gp120, HIV-1SF2 recombinant gp120, or both vaccines in seronegative adults. *J Infect Dis*. 1998;177:1230–1246.

19. Brochier B, Kieny MP, Costy F, et al. Large-scale eradication of rabies using recombinant vaccinia-rabies vaccine. *Nature*. 1991;354: 520–522.

20. Prevec L, Campbell JB, Christie BS, Belbeck L, Graham FL. A recombinant human adenovirus vaccine against rabies. *J Infect Dis*. 1990;161:27–30.

21. National Institutes of Health (NIAID). *The Jordan Report* 20th Anniversary: Accelerated Development of Vaccines 2002, Appendix C: Status of Vaccine Research and Development. Available at: http://www .niaid.nih.gov/dmid/vaccines/jordan20/. Accessed January 13, 2005.

22. Pruss A, Kay D, Fewtrell L, Bartram J. Estimating the burden of diseases from water, sanitation, and hygiene at the global level. *Environ Health Perspect*. 2002;110:537–542.

23. Ada G. Vaccine and vaccination. *N Engl J Med*. 2001;345:1042–1053.

24. Vogel FR, Alving CR. Progress in immunologic adjuvant development: 1982–2002. *The Jordan Report* 20th Anniversary: Accelerated Development of Vaccines 2002, Appendix C: Status of Vaccine Research and Development. Available at: http://www.niaid.nih.gov/dmid/ vaccines/jordan20/. Accessed January 13, 2005.

25. Liu MA, Ulmer JB, O'Hagan D. Vaccine technologies. *The Jordan Report* 20th Anniversary: Accelerated Development of Vaccines 2002, Appendix C: Status of Vaccine Research and Development. Available at: http://www.niaid.nih.gov/dmid/vaccines/jordan20/. Accessed on January 13, 2005.

26. Pinto LA, Edwards J, Castle PE, et al. Cellular immune responses to human papillomavirus (HPV)-16 L1 in healthy volunteers immunized with recombinant HPV-16 L1 virus-like particles. *J Infect Dis*. 2003;188:327–338.

27. Recommended Childhood and Adolescent Immunization Schedule–United States, July–December 2004. *MMWR*. 2004;53:Q1–Q3.

28. Recommended childhood and adolescent immunization schedule: United States, 2005. *Pediatrics*. 2005;115:182.

29. National Center of Infectious Disease. Traveler's health. Available at: http://www.cdc.gov/travel. Accessed January 4, 2005.

30. Comstock GW. Vaccine evaluation by case-control or prospective studies. *Am J Epidemiology*. 1990;131:205–207.

31. Ornestein WA, Bernier RH, Hinman AR. Assessing vaccine efficacy in the field: further observations. *Epidemiol Rev*. 1988;10:212–241.

32. Halloran ME, Haber M, Longini IM, Struchiner CJ. Direct and indirect effects in vaccine efficacy and effectiveness. *Am J Epidemiology*. 1991;133:323–331.

33. Halloran ME, Struchiner CJ, Longini IM. Study designs for evaluating different efficacy and effectiveness aspects of vaccines. *Am J Epidemiology*. 1999;146:789–803.

34. Halloran ME, Longini IM, Struchiner CJ. Design and interpretation of vaccine field studies. *Epidemiol Rev*. 1999;21:73–88.

35. Rodrigues LC, Smith PG. Use of the case control approach in vaccine evaluation: efficacy and adverse effects. *Epidemiol Rev.* 1999;21:56–72.

36. Chen RT, Rastogi SC, Mullen JR, et al. The Vaccine Adverse Event Reporting System (VAERS). *Vaccine.* 1994;5:542–549.

37. Braun MM, Ellenberg SS. Descriptive epidemiology of adverse events after immunization: reports of the Vaccine Adverse Event Reporting System (VAERS) 1991–1994. *J Pediatr.* 1997;131:529–535.

38. Varricchio F, Iskander J, Destefano F, et al. Understanding vaccine safety information from the Vaccine Adverse Event Reporting System. *Pediatr Infect Dis J.* 2004;23:287–294.

39. Haber P, Chen RT, Zanardi LR, Mootrey GT, English R, Braun MM. An analysis of rotavirus vaccine reports to Vaccine Adverse Event Reporting System: more than intussusception alone? *Pediatrics.* 2004;114:e353–e359.

40. Suspension of rotavirus vaccine after reports of intussusception–United States, 1999. *MMWR.* 2004;53:786–789.

41. Chen RT, Glasser JW, Rhodes PH, et al. Vaccine Safety Datalink Project: a new tool for improving vaccine safety monitoring in the United States. *Pediatrics.* 1997;99:765–773.

42. Chen RT. Evaluation of vaccine safety after the events of 11 September 2001: role of cohort and case control studies. *Vaccine.* 2004;22:2047–2053.

43. Meissner HC, Strebel PM, Orenstein WA. Measles vaccines and the potential for worldwide eradication of measles. *Pediatrics.* 2004;144:1065–1069.

44. Institute of Medicine. Immunization safety review. Available at: http://www.iom.edu/project.asp?id=4705. Accessed January 9, 2005.

45. McCormack MC. The autism "epidemic"; impressions from the perspective of immunization safety review. *Ambulatory Pediatrics.* 2003;3:119–120.

46. Wakefield AJ, Murch SH, Anthony A, et al. Illeal-lymphoid-nodular hyperplasia, non-specific colitis, and pervasive developmental disorders. *Lancet.* 1998;351:631–637.

47. Plotkin SL, Plotkin SA. A short history of vaccination. In: Plotkin SA, Mortimor EA, eds. *Vaccines.* 3rd ed. Philadelphia, Pa: W.B. Saunders Company; 1999.

48. Pless R, Casey C, Chen R. CISA: improving the evaluation, management and understanding of adverse events possibly related to immunizations. National Immunization Program, Centers for Disease Control and Prevention. Available at: http://www.cdc.gov/nip/vacsafe/cisa/intro-cisa.html. Accessed January 3, 2005.

49. Ogra PL. Poliomyelitis as a paradigm for investment in the success of vaccination programs. *Pediatr Infect Dis J.* 1999;18:10–15.

50. Atkinson W, ed. Poliomyelitis. In: *Epidemiology and Prevention of Vaccine Preventable Diseases.* Atlanta, Ga: Centers for Disease Control and Prevention; 1997:81–99.

51. Centers for Disease Control. Poliomyelitis–United States: 1975–1984. *MMWR.* 1986;35:180–182.

52. Alexander LN, Seward JF, Santibanez TA, et al. Vaccine policy changes and epidemiology of poliomyelitis in the United States. *JAMA.* 2004;292:1696–1701.

53. Atkinson W, et al. Measles. In: *Epidemiology and Prevention of Vaccine Preventable Diseases.* Atlanta, Ga: Centers for Disease Control and Prevention, Department of Health and Human Services; 1997:117–137.

54. The National Vaccine Advisory Committee. The measles epidemic: the problems, barriers, and recommendations. *JAMA.* 1991;266:1547–1552.
55. Centers for Disease Control and Prevention. Epidemiology of measles—United States, 1998. *MMWR.* 1999;48:749–753.
56. Centers for Disease Control and Prevention. Measles—United States 2000. *MMWR.* 2002;51:120–123.
57. Centers for Disease Control and Prevention. Impact of vaccine universally recommended for children 1999. Available at: http://www.cdc.gov/od/oc/media/fact/impvacc.htm. Accessed November 12, 1999.
58. George P. Childhood immunizations. *N Engl J Med.* 1992;327:1794–1800.
59. Centers for Disease Control and Prevention. Progress toward global measles control and regional elimination, 1990–1997. *MMWR.* 1998;47:1049–1054.
60. Strebel P, Cochi S, Grawbowski M, et al. The unfinished measles immunization agenda. *J Infect Dis.* 2003;187:S1–S7.
61. Cochi SL, Broome CV. Vaccine prevention of *Haemophilus influenzae* type b disease, past, present, and future. *Pediatr Infect Dis.* 1985;5:12–19.
62. Santosham M, Wolff M, Reid R, et al. The efficacy in Navajo infants of conjugate vaccine consisting of *Haemophilus influenzae* type b polysaccharide and *Neisseria meningitides* outer membrane protein complex. *N Engl J Med.* 1991;324:1767–1772.
63. McCollough M. Update on emerging infections from the Centers for Disease Control and Prevention. *Ann Emerg Med.* 1999;334:109–111.
64. Evans AS. The eradication of communicable diseases: myth or reality? *Am J Epidemiology.* 1985;122:1999–2007.
65. Fenner F, Henderson DA, Arita I, Jesek Z, Ladnyi ID. *Vaccines.* Philadelphia, Pa: W.B. Saunders Company; 1994.
66. World Health Organization. Polio experts warn of largest epidemic in recent years, as polio hits Darfur. Available at: http://www.who.int/mediacentre/news/releases/204/pr45/en. Accessed January 4, 2005.
67. World Health Organization. The *World Health Report—Shaping the Future*: Chapter 4, Polio Eradication—the final challenge. Available at: http://www.who.int/whr/2003/chapter4/en/. Accessed January 4, 2005.
68. Evans A. Criteria for control of infectious diseases with poliomyelitis as an example. *Prog Med Virol.* 1984;29:141–165.
69. Pan American Health Organization. Progress towards measles elimination, Western Hemisphere, 2002–2003. *Wkly Epidemiol Rec.* 2004;79:149–151.

NUTRITION AND INFECTION

Alice M. Tang, Ellen Smit, and Richard D. Semba

Introduction

This chapter provides a practical introduction to the relationship between nutrition and infectious diseases. Over the past few decades, our knowledge of the interactions between nutrition, infection, and immune function has steadily expanded. It has been established that adequate nutritional status is necessary for the normal functioning of various components of the immune system.[1-3] Malnutrition may affect the course of infectious diseases through a variety of mechanisms, including compromising host immune function, diminishing response to therapies, and promoting comorbidities.[4]

The relationship between nutrition, infection, and immune function is generally cyclical in nature[5] (Figure 12-1). Even in a well-nourished host, the course of an infection will adversely affect nutritional status. If an infection is left untreated or becomes chronic, nutritional deficiencies will develop that further compromise the immune system, leading to more severe disease and increased susceptibility to other infections. If the host is already malnourished, acquiring an infection leads to further nutritional deficiencies, and the host can rapidly progress into a downward spiral leading to increased morbidity and mortality.

The nutritional consequences of infection, no matter what microorganism is causing the infection, tend to be predictable. Any infection, whether symptomatic or asymptomatic, is accompanied by losses of some nutrients from the body and redistribution of other nutrients. The magnitude of these changes is dependent on the severity and duration of the infection. Metabolic and nutritional responses that are specific to certain organisms occur when the infection becomes localized within a single organ system. For example, diarrheal infections cause sizeable losses of fluid and electrolytes, while paralytic forms of infection result in wasting of bone and muscle. If the infection can be cured or eliminated naturally by the host immune system, lost body

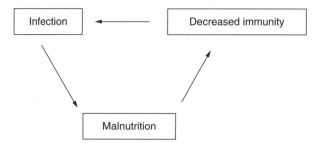

FIGURE 12-1 The cyclic relationship between infection, malnutrition, and immune function.

nutrients can then be replenished over a period of weeks to months. However, if the infectious process is not eliminated and becomes chronic, body composition can become markedly altered, and a new equilibrium of body nutrient balances is reached at a cachectic, or extremely wasted, level.

Effects of Infection on Nutritional Status

Acute infections cause metabolic rates and oxygen consumption to increase. Both anabolic and catabolic processes are involved. The cells in the liver and lymphoid tissues rapidly increase their rates of synthesis of proteins needed for host defense mechanisms, and the proliferation of phagocytic and lymphoid cells is speeded up. To support these anabolic requirements and to maintain high metabolic rates in the presence of anorexia and a diminished food intake, catabolic processes are accelerated also. The stores of available protein in muscle fibers and other tissues provide the additional supply of amino acid substrate. These are used for glucose production and the synthesis of new proteins required for host defense. To fuel the increased metabolic activity required to fight off the infection, the body appears to increase its utilization of glucose, but not lipids. As a result of the catabolic processes, the body loses weight and muscle mass, as nutrient stores are consumed in excess of intake. If the infection becomes chronic, available nitrogen stores are used up, fat depots are consumed, and a wasted, cachectic state develops. During the acute phase of fever, the body also retains water and salt.

Effects of Malnutrition on Host Defense Mechanisms

Malnutrition is best understood as a syndrome associated with variable losses of protein, carbohydrate, and fat stores, along with changes in micronutrients such as vitamins and minerals. It is often complicated by infection-induced anorexia and catabolism. A common finding in malnourished patients is the depletion of lymphocytes, particularly in T-cell regions of the thymus, spleen, and lymph nodes. Studies suggest that there is a relative reduction in circulating mature T lymphocytes (both helper T and suppressor T cells) so that plasma is enriched with immature and functionally defective cells.[5] As a result, there is a reduction in the efficacy of all host defenses that depend on T-cell function. Serum antibody levels are usually normal or elevated in the presence of malnutrition. This may be due in part to the numerous infections and high antigenic loads faced by malnourished individuals in impoverished areas, and at the same time, a defect in suppressor T-cell function, which normally inhibits antibody production. One exception is that secretory IgA levels are often depressed in Protein Energy Malnutrition (PEM) causing more frequent mucosal infections of the gut and urinary tract. As a result, malnourished patients usually exhibit increased frequency and/or severity of certain bacterial, viral, fungal, and parasitic infections.

Malnutrition and Specific Infectious Diseases

Malnutrition is a major determinant of morbidity and mortality for many major infectious diseases, particularly among young children in developing countries who often suffer from multiple serial infections.

Diarrheal Disease

Diarrheal disease causes an estimated 19% of all child deaths worldwide.[6] Malnutrition and associated immunodeficiency are important risk factors for diarrheal disease among infants and young children in developing countries.[7] Children who are malnourished (low weight-for-age, low mid-upper arm circumference) have an increased prevalence of diarrhea and a higher mortality rate.[8] Micronutrient deficiencies that have been described during diarrheal disease include that of vitamins A, D, B_{12}, folate, copper, iron, magnesium, selenium, and zinc.[8,9] Several clinical trials show that supplementation with vitamin A[9-11] or zinc can reduce the morbidity and mortality of diarrheal disease in children.[12-15]

Lower Respiratory Infections

Worldwide, lower respiratory infections account for 19% of all child deaths.[6] Vitamin A deficiency causes pathologic alterations in the mucosal epithelium of the respiratory tract, including keratinization and loss of ciliated cells, mucus, and goblet cells. Epidemiologic studies demonstrate that vitamin A deficiency is associated with lower respiratory infections[9]; however, vitamin A supplementation appears to have little effect upon reducing lower respiratory infections in children and respiratory syncytial virus infection.[16,17,18] Vitamin D and calcium deficiency may be important risk factors for lower respiratory infections in children.[19]

Measles

Measles causes an estimated 2 million deaths per year, and despite measles immunization, periodic and serious outbreaks occur due to lapses in immunization programs, vaccine failure, and problems related to optimal timing of immunization.[20] Case-fatality rates during acute, complicated measles infection are often 10–30%, depending on age and nutritional status of the children. Low serum vitamin A levels are associated with higher mortality in acute, complicated measles infection.[21] Randomized, placebo-controlled clinical trials show that vitamin A supplementation can reduce the mortality of measles by 50% or more, and high-dose vitamin A supplementation is now recommended as standard therapy for measles both in developing countries and in the United States.[9] Vitamin A supplementation for measles is one of the most important examples of the use of micronutrients as disease-targeted therapy.

Tuberculosis

About 1.8 billion individuals, or about one third of the world's population, are infected with *Mycobacterium tuberculosis*, and most of these individuals have latent infection. Malnutrition is a major risk factor for the progression of tuberculosis[22]; however, tuberculosis control programs tend to focus upon chemoprophylaxis and chemotherapy alone, rather than upon improvement of host nutritional status. Cod-liver oil, a rich source of vitamins A and D, was used as treatment for tuberculosis for over 100 years prior to the development of antibiotics.[23] The role of nutrition and tuberculosis remains a major area of neglect, despite the promise that micronutrients have shown as therapy for other types of infections and the long record of the use of vitamins A and D for treatment of pulmonary and miliary tuberculosis in both Europe and the United States.

Malaria

Malaria affects about 400 million individuals each year, resulting in 1 to 2 million deaths worldwide,[24] and malaria is reemerging worldwide.[25] Vector control and antimalarial drugs have been the traditional strategy against malaria, and little attention, until recently, has been paid to improving host nutritional status. Low levels of vitamin A, zinc, iron, and folate have been shown to be responsible for a substantial proportion of malaria morbidity and mortality.[26,27] Two separate randomized, placebo-controlled clinical trials conducted in Papua New Guinea demonstrated that vitamin A supplementation or zinc supplementation can reduce malarial morbidity in preschool children by 30–50%.[28,29]

Human Immunodeficiency Virus Infection

Malnutrition may impact the course of HIV infection through a variety of mechanisms, including compromising host immune function, diminishing response to therapies, and promoting comorbidities.[4] Wasting and malnutrition have been routinely observed in AIDS patients since the beginning of the AIDS epidemic.[30,31] HIV wasting syndrome has been associated with increased opportunistic infections (OIs), lower CD4 counts, and hyperactivation of the immune system.[32-35] Weight loss of as little as 5% is predictive of death.[36,37] Prior to the advent of highly active antiretroviral therapy, HAART, specific micronutrient abnormalities were more common in HIV-positive than HIV-negative individuals.[38-40] Low serum levels of many of these nutrients (particularly, vitamins A, B_6, B_{12}, and zinc) were associated with more rapid disease progression,[41] increased mortality,[42] impaired neurologic function,[43] diminished lymphocyte response to mitogens,[39] and increased maternal-fetal transmission.[44] In observational studies of dietary intake, increased intakes of specific nutrients have been associated with decreased progression to AIDS.[45,46] Two recent randomized controlled trials have examined the effects of vitamin supplementation on HIV disease progression and mortality. In Thailand, multivitamin supplementation (twice daily) significantly reduced death rates after 48 weeks among a subgroup of participants with CD4 cell counts less than 100 cells/μl.[47] In Tanzania, HIV-positive pregnant women randomized to a megadose multivitamin supplement (B_1, B_2, B_6, B_{12}, niacin, C, and E), but not megadose beta-carotene plus vitamin A, were 30% less likely to progress to late-stage disease or death than those randomized to a placebo.[48] These results have direct implications for delaying HIV progression among populations that currently have little or no access to antiretroviral agents.

Micronutrients and Immunity to Infectious Diseases

The role of micronutrients in the immunity to different infections is a rapidly growing and promising area of investigation. Micronutrients can influence immunity to infectious diseases through their roles in the immune function (Table 12-1).[3] Micronutrient deficiencies, such as those of vitamin A and zinc, can have a major impact upon T- and B-cell function, the generation of antibody responses, and function of other immune effector cells. Micronutrients such as vitamin E, vitamin C, zinc, and selenium can play a role as strong antioxidants and influence the clinical course of infections. Oxidative stress, which occurs during infections, refers to the condition when the balance between pro-oxidants and antioxidants is upset, and there is overproduction of free radicals and resulting pathology.[49] Activated macrophages and neutrophils have important roles in the killing of microorganisms through the generation of free radicals. Host bystander cells can also be damaged by free radicals, which can cause oxidation of nucleic acids, chromosomal breaks, peroxidation of lipids in cell membranes, and damage to collagen, proteins, and enzymes.

Investigators who want to study the relationship between micronutrients and infectious diseases must often focus on one or two micronutrients for practical reasons. There is considerable cost and complexity in providing a comprehensive study of micronutrient status during infection, although a comprehensive approach would be ideal as micronutrient deficiencies often occur simultaneously. A brief overview of the relationship of specific micronutrients in immunity to infection follows.

Vitamin A

Vitamin A, or all-*trans* retinol, is an essential micronutrient for immunity, growth, cellular differentiation, maintenance of mucosal surfaces, reproduction, and vision.[9] There are two main dietary forms of vitamin A: preformed vitamin A, found in foods such as butter, egg yolks, and cod-liver oil; and provitamin A carotenoids, found in foods such as spinach, carrots, mangoes, and papayas. About 90% of the vitamin A in the body is stored in the liver, and the adult liver can contain enough vitamin A to last over one year.

TABLE 12-1   Selected Micronutrients and Their Functions

Vitamin A, carotenoids	Vitamin A refers to three types of compounds that exhibit biologic activity: the alcohol (retinol), the aldehyde (retinal or retinaldehyde), and the acid (retinoic acid). Plants contain a group of compounds called *carotenoids* that are converted to retinol in the body. Beta-carotene is the most biologically active carotenoid. Has essential roles in vision and various systemic functions, including normal cell differentiation and cell recognition, growth and development, bone development, immune functions, and reproduction.
Vitamin B_6	Coenzyme in numerous enzyme reactions particularly amino acid transport and metabolism. Direct effect on immune system through its role in protein and nucleic acid synthesis. Deficiency leads to a reduction in nucleic acid synthesis that restricts proliferation of lymphocytes.
Vitamin B_{12}	Coenzyme involved in transmethylation from methylfolate to homocysteine. Released unmethylated folate becomes available for nucleic acid synthesis.
Vitamin E	Most important lipid-soluble antioxidant in cell membranes. Protects unsaturated phospholipids of the membrane from oxidative degradation from ROS by donating a hydrogen (called free-radical scavenging). Is important component of the cellular antioxidant defense system, which involves other enzymes (e.g., superoxide dismutases, glutathione peroxidases, glutathione reductase, catalase), many of which depend upon adequate levels of other antioxidants. Therefore the antioxidant function of vitamin E can be affected by the levels of other nutrients (zinc, selenium, copper, vitamin C).
Selenium	Active form functions as selenoenzyme. Major function as part of glutathione peroxidase that reduces cellular peroxides to H_2O and alcohol and Prevents oxidative damage to proteins, lipid, lipoproteins, and DNA.
Zinc	Zinc binds to protein, forming zinc fingers that are involved in DNA transcription factors, hormone receptors, and enzymes. Zinc deficiency has been shown to impair a variety of immune functions: ↓ lymphocyte counts, loss of helper T-cell function, ↓ killer T lymphocyte activities, delayed dermal hypersensitivity responses, depressed humoral and cell-mediated immunity. Excess levels of zinc intake can have toxic effects on the immune system and may promote viral replication.

Source: Tang AM, Lanzillotti J, Hendricks K, Gerrior J, Ghosh M, Woods M, Wanke C. Micronutrients: current issues for HIV care providers. *AIDS.* 2005;19:847–861 (Table 1).

Vitamin A acts as a regulator of over 300 genes through its active metabolites, all-*trans* and 9-*cis* retinoic acid, and specific nuclear receptors that are in the steroid and thyroid hormone receptor superfamily.[50]

Vitamin A exerts a wide-ranging effect upon different compartments of the immune system, including the growth, maturation, and function of T and B lymphocytes, the expression of certain cytokines, and the maintenance of mucosal surfaces of the respiratory, gastrointestinal, and genitourinary tracts.[51,52] A hallmark of vitamin A deficiency is an impaired ability to mount an antibody response to protein antigens.[52] Traditionally, it has been considered that the main clinical manifestations of vitamin A deficiency are night blindness and xerophthalmia (changes in the conjunctiva and cornea of the eye),[9] although it is becoming apparent that increased incidence and severity of infections are part of the spectrum of vitamin A deficiency. Infants, preschool children, pregnant women, and lactating women are at the highest risk of developing vitamin A deficiency.[9] Abnormal urinary losses of vitamin A can occur during infections and can accelerate the depletion of the body's vitamin A stores.[53] Because vitamin A is a fat-soluble vitamin, steatorrhea can interfere with intestinal absorption of vitamin A.

Methods for the assessment of vitamin A status include serum or plasma vitamin A levels by high-performance liquid chromatography (HPLC), the relative dose response and modified relative dose response tests (which indirectly measure liver reserves of vitamin A), measurement of breast milk vitamin A, dark adaptometry, pupillary responses, and conjunctival impression cytology.[54]

Vitamin D

Vitamin D includes steroids with the biological activity of vitamin D_3. Vitamin D is produced in the skin upon exposure to sunlight and is also available in dietary sources such as egg yolks and fish liver oils. Vitamin D regulates calcium and phosphorus metabolism and bone mineralization, and the clinical syndrome of vitamin D deficiency is rickets in children and osteomalacia in adults.[55] Vitamin D acts to regulate genes via specific nuclear receptors. Vitamin D receptors may interact with nuclear retinoic acid receptors, providing some basis for interaction between vitamins A and D.[50] Vitamin D plays a role in monocyte function, and this has been most extensively studied in tuberculosis.[56] An epidemiologic study in Ethiopia suggested a link between pneumonia and vitamin D deficiency.[19] Methods for the assessment of vitamin D status include measurements of serum vitamin D levels (25-hydroxyvitamin D) by HPLC.[57]

Vitamin E

Vitamin E refers to tocopherol and tocotrienol compounds, of which α-tocopherol is the most active and abundant isomer. Rich dietary sources of vitamin E include seeds, nuts, margarine, and vegetable oils. Vitamin E is a strong antioxidant that protects against cellular damage by inhibiting peroxidation of polyunsaturated fatty acids in cell membranes. A clear-cut deficiency syndrome of vitamin E has not been described in humans.[58] Vitamin E may protect immune effector cells against free-radical reactions.[59-61] Methods for assessment of vitamin E status include measurements of serum vitamin E levels by HPLC.[57]

B Complex Vitamins

The B complex vitamins include thiamin, riboflavin, niacin, vitamin B_6, vitamin B_{12}, and folate. These vitamins participate in the metabolism of carbohydrates, fats, and proteins, and in hematopoiesis and synthesis of DNA. There is some evidence that vitamins B_6, B_{12}, and folate may play a role in immune function[62,63]; the possible role of these micronutrients in the pathogenesis of infectious disease needs further clarification.

Vitamin C

Vitamin C, or ascorbic acid, is involved in a variety of biological reactions, including conversion of dopamine to norepinephrine, carnitine synthesis, iron absorption, and folate metabolism. Citrus fruits, peppers, green vegetables, potatoes, and berries contain high amounts of vitamin C. Deficiency of vitamin C results in scurvy, a syndrome characterized by skin lesions, hemorrhages, joint effusions, and weakness. The therapeutic efficacy of vitamin C as treatment for symptoms of the common cold remains controversial.[64] The evidence that vitamin C is involved in immune function is limited.[65] Most current investigations of vitamin C in infectious diseases are concerned with the role of vitamin C as a potent antioxidant.

Iron

Iron plays an important role in oxygen transport, as an electron carrier in cytochromes, and in certain iron metalloenzymes.[66] Iron deficiency is associated with anemia,[67] impaired psychomotor development,[68,69] lower work capacity,[70] prematurity,[71] and higher maternal mortality.[72,73] An estimated 2 billion people suffer from iron deficiency anemia worldwide.[74] Pregnant women, women of childbearing age, infants, and children are at higher risk of developing iron deficiency anemia. A high-cereal diet (which can interfere with iron absorption), chronic diarrhea, malabsorption, and blood loss from pregnancy, menstruation, and intestinal parasites can contribute to iron deficiency.[75] Although iron deficiency may adversely affect neutrophil and lymphocyte function, the relationship between iron deficiency and infection is unclear.[76] Some early studies suggested that iron supplementation could increase susceptibility to malaria; however, recent studies show that iron deficiency should be corrected in children with malaria.[77] Oral iron therapy does not appear to exacerbate infections in most areas of the world,[76] and reducing iron deficiency still remains a formidable challenge worldwide.

Selenium

Selenium, an essential trace element, is contained in the enzyme glutathione peroxidase and protects cells against oxidative damage.[78] Selenium is found in seafood, some meats, and, depending on the selenium content of the soil, grain products. Keshan's disease, a cardiomyopathy, and Kashin-Beck disease, an osteoarticular disorder, occur in areas where the soil is low in selenium. Selenium appears to influence the function of T lymphocytes.[79] Recent studies with a murine model for coxsackie B-induced myocarditis suggests that selenium deficiency can increase virulence of the coxsackie B virus.[80] The biological importance of selenium is being established; whether selenium status is important during infections in humans needs further clarification.

Iodine

Iodine deficiency can result in goiter and a wide spectrum of mental, psychomotor, and growth abnormalities.[81] Iodine functions as a component of thyroxine (T_4), and 3,5,3'-triiodothyronine (T_3), two hormones that are required for normal growth, development, and metabolism. Nuclear thyroid hormone receptors can bind with retinoic acid receptors, suggesting that there may be interaction between vitamin A and thyroid status.[50] Rich sources of iodine include seafood and iodized salt. An estimated 1.6 billion people worldwide may consume inadequate amounts of iodine.[82] Increased rates of stillbirths, abortions, and infant mortality have been noted in areas with endemic iodine deficiency. Studies suggest that iodine supplementation or iodination of irrigation water can reduce infant mortality.[83-85] The role of iodine deficiency in immune function is not well established and further studies of the relationship between iodine deficiency and infections are needed.[83]

Zinc

Zinc is an important trace element that is needed for the function of over 300 metalloenzymes, including those involved in metabolism of proteins, fats, and carbohydrates; for regulation of RNA synthesis through zinc fingers; for synaptic transmission; and for the function of protein kinase C.[86] Rich dietary sources of zinc include shellfish, beef, chicken, fish, nuts, and beans. Zinc deficiency is characterized by growth retardation, reproductive abnormalities, increased infections, and skin and neurological disorders. Zinc deficiency usually arises because of inadequate dietary intake of zinc. Pregnant and lactating women, infants, and preschool children are at the highest risk of zinc deficiency.

Zinc plays an important role in the growth, development, and function of neutrophils, macrophages, natural killer cells, and T and B lymphocytes.[87] A large series of randomized, placebo-controlled clinical trials suggests that zinc supplementation can reduce the morbidity of diarrheal disease, respiratory disease, and malaria.[12-15,20] These studies suggest that the importance of zinc status in resistance to infections is only just being realized. The measurement of zinc status remains somewhat problematic, and plasma or serum zinc levels can be measured using atomic absorption spectroscopy and specialized trace element handling techniques.[57]

Assessment of Nutritional Status

The previous sections briefly illustrated the interrelationships between nutritional status, infection, and immune function. Due to the cyclical nature of the relationships, epidemiological studies can examine nutritional status as either a risk factor (exposure or determinant) of infectious diseases or as an outcome of infections. The tools used to assess nutritional disorders are at the core of a study's success in obtaining quality data, minimizing misclassification, and accurately estimating disease associations. The remainder of this chapter will review the most common methods used in assessing nutritional status in epidemiologic studies.

Dietary Intake Assessment

Dietary intake assessments are based on information supplied by the study participants themselves, or by a surrogate. Most assessments focus on what foods were consumed, how much of it was consumed, how the foods were prepared, and how often they were consumed during a specific reference period. Some methods will try and collect all of this information, while others focus on a few of these aspects. During the study design phase, it is best to try and select the method that will be the best in getting the information needed for the specific research goals and for the specific study population. Sometimes a tool is selected because it is what others are using (good for comparisons across studies) or it is the only one available. Although there is disagreement in the field about which tool is better, it is generally agreed that there is no perfect tool. The most commonly used methods for assessing dietary intake are reviewed below.

Food Records

A food record is a method of intake assessment where a subject is asked to write down all foods and beverages he or she consumes for a period of days (usually 3 to 7 days). Subjects are generally instructed on how to give an estimate of the amount or serving size of each food item consumed, and this can either be weighed or described. The food record is used as a quantitative way to describe the intake during the recording days. Often this method is used as the gold standard in validation or calibration studies. It is thought that portion sizes are more accurately recorded because they are written down at the time of consumption rather than relying on recall. Participants may, however, alter what they eat while reporting their intake. In addition, keeping a food record requires participants to be literate and compliant in recording everything they eat. Other disadvantages of this method are that the records need to be legible, returned to the study investigator, and that data entry of the food records can be time consuming. Some studies have shown that food records tend to underestimate dietary intake.[88,89]

In deciding to use food records as a dietary assessment tool in a study of nutrition and infectious diseases, the following questions need consideration: How many days of record keeping will be sufficient to give an estimate of the usual intake of the study population? Will the study participants be compliant in keeping the records? Can the participants write legibly? Will participants not lose the food record? How will participants return the food records to the study investigators? Will study investigators (ideally, trained nutritionists) be able to review the records with each participant for completeness and clarity? Other methods of record keeping, such as using tape recorders or dictaphones, may be an option in some studies, but the increased cost of this may be prohibitive. Thus, while food records may be a good method for the general population, it may not be a feasible option for specialized populations.

24-Hour Recall

A 24-hour recall is a method of intake assessment where the subject is asked to recall everything consumed during the previous day or 24 hours. It is usually administered by a trained interviewer and may be done in person or by telephone. An advantage of the 24-hour recall is that the recall period is only one day, so most subjects are able to accurately recall their intake. Also, if the 24-hour recall is unannounced or unsuspected, there is not the influence in food selection that can be observed with food records. Data entry can be completed after the interview if it has been recorded in pen and paper format, or it can be entered during the interview using a computer. The 24-hour recall can be completed on one occasion, or multiple 24-hour recalls can be completed on several days for each participant. While the 24-hour recall is simpler and requires less burden on the participants, a single 24-hour recall does not provide good information on individual intake. Therefore, dietary information collected from 24-hour recalls should not be used to classify participants into deficient and nondeficient diets due to day-to-day variation within each person's diet. It can, however, be used to obtain reasonable estimates of average intakes of groups.[90,91]

For studies that require participants to be ranked individually according to nutrient intake, the single 24-hour recall is not the ideal method. Multiple 24-hour recalls may be considered, but this requires participants to return to the study site for additional visits. This also eliminates the "unexpectedness" of the assessment, and participants may then alter their food intake accordingly. Conducting 24-hour recalls over the phone may be feasible if study participants are accessible by telephone. It is important that the 24-hour recall includes a full 24 hours. Many people consume foods during the middle of the night, and important nutrient data would be missed if one assumes that all food intake occurs between morning and evening hours. It is also important to customize serving sizes to the study population. In some populations, serving sizes may be described by the price or brand of the product, rather than the actual amount. It is important to customize any dietary intake assessment tool to the target population; therefore, prior knowledge of eating and food buying habits in that community is essential.

Food Frequency Questionnaire

A food frequency questionnaire (FFQ) aims to get an estimate of usual intake by recalling intake from a list of a specific number of foods for a defined reference period, usually one year. It generally asks subjects how often they ate certain foods, thinking back over the reference period. Some FFQs also include serving sizes, often as a specified portion or as a small, medium, or large portion size. Based on all the foods in the food list, their frequency of intake, and serving size, nutrient intake values are calculated. FFQs can be self- or interviewer-administered. The processing time of FFQ versus food records or 24-hour recalls is generally shorter. Due to its ease of use, the method is now commonly used in epidemiologic studies. However, FFQs depend on recollection of food intake during the reference period, and participants must have fairly regular eating habits. It also depends heavily on the food list used. Some FFQs have been shown to provide reasonable estimates of group intakes, and some have been shown to be able to rank individual intake. Several investigators have described in detail issues to be considered when selecting, developing, and/or validating an FFQ.[92-98]

FFQs do not work well among study populations that have irregular eating habits, such as populations with extended periods of hospitalization, incarcerations, and/or homelessness. Irregular intakes, large variations in places of intake (e.g., relative's house, friend's house, soup kitchens, restaurants), and seasonal variations in intake all make it difficult for participants to recall and average their food intake over a 12-month or even a 6-month recall period. Some FFQs allow study investigators to adapt the food list to their specific population. For example, based on pilot studies, an investigator may decide to eliminate some foods from the food list that the population does not generally consume and/or add foods commonly consumed. Foods on the food list may also be grouped or ungrouped, depending on the frequency of consumption of each of the items. When altering the food list on an FFQ, the food and nutrient database must be updated according to the new food list. An FFQ should not be used indiscriminately with all populations.

Diet History

The original diet history (Burke's method) includes general eating and health questions, a 24-hour recall, and a food record.[99] The diet history method is used to reflect any assessment of past diet, with a reference period ranging from one month to one year. Obtaining a diet history entails a lengthy interview and is expensive to process. It can provide good information about usual intake and correlates well with biochemical measures, but it does have a tendency to overestimate intake.[100]

Translating Foods into Nutrients

The information obtained using any of the dietary intake assessments discussed above are translated into nutrients through the use of databases that contain nutrient information for a range of foods. Foods consumed are first translated into food codes that link the consumed foods to a nutrient database. A nutrient database contains the food codes and nutrient values for each code. After the food code and the amount of food consumed have been entered, nutrient intakes can be computed.

There are a variety of government and commercial nutrient databases available, and results may vary depending on which database is used. Not only can databases differ between methods, for example, the 24-hour recall and the FFQ, but different databases may also be used for the same method, such as a 24-hour recall completed by different investigators. As with the assessment tools, no database is perfect. During the food coding process, because there are often many similar food items in the database, there may be incorrect selection or incorrect coding of the food items. Databases also do not include all nutrients and nonnutrients. In addition, databases need to be updated according to product availability in the food supply. For example, recent changes in trans-fatty acids contents of some foods and the introduction of low-carbohydrate foods need to be captured in the dietary assessment methods and then become part of the databases.

Other Intake Assessment Issues

Cognitive processes affect dietary intake assessments.[101] Although the impact of cognitive processes has been studied in the general US population to some degree, little is known about the implications for specialized or international populations. For example, research indicates that asking questions and probes in neutral ways in the general US population improves the quality of recalling dietary intake.[102] However, the effects of this on the quality of dietary intake assessment in other populations remain to be investigated.

Often, investigators are interested in the use of vitamin and mineral supplementation in addition to dietary intake. Assessing supplement use can be done for a 24-hour recall period, for the same reference period as the FFQ, or recorded as part of the food record. There is no standard method for collecting this information, and although several dietary intake assessment tools have questions on vitamin-mineral supplementation, it is important to adapt these to the population of interest. Ideally, it is best to include detailed questions on type, brand name, frequency, and amount of each supplement used. Furthermore, multivitamins should be distinguished from single vitamin supplements. However, people are often unable to recall brand names, other than the generic multivitamin, and may have difficulty answering questions on separate vitamins. For example, a participant who takes only a multivitamin and answers *yes* to taking a multivitamin may also answer *yes* to taking a vitamin C supplement as vitamin C is included as part of the multivitamin. Participants may also have difficulty recalling the amount or dose of individual vitamins. When designing a questionnaire on vitamin and mineral supplements, questions should be carefully pilot tested among the study population before incorporating them into the final questionnaire.

The analysis of dietary data can be complex, especially when trying to decide whether to adjust for energy intake and/or other dietary variables. This topic continues to be of great epidemiologic debate, and there is not always a clear answer.[103–105] Many dietary variables are collinear, and one needs to take great care when using adjustment methods. For more detailed information, several good resources are available.[98,106]

Although the limitations of intake assessment may seem discouraging, it would be more discouraging to let the limitations stop us from doing important dietary intake research. We do need to be aware of the limitations of the tools we use and pretest our tools in the study population. Moreover, it is important for us to strive to improve current dietary intake assessment tools.

Body Composition

Measuring body composition can be as difficult as measuring dietary intake. Each method measures a different body compartment and each has its advantages and disadvantages. The most common methods used in research settings are height, weight, and body mass index (BMI) (weight in kilograms divided by height in meters squared), which is a height and weight index used as a measure of obesity. For example, the National Heart, Lung, and Blood Institute Obesity Education Initiative uses the following classification of overweight and obesity by BMI: <18.5 underweight; 18.5–24.9 normal weight; 25.0–29.9 overweight; 30.0–39.9 obese; and ≥40 extreme obesity.[107] Ideally, weight should be measured rather than self-reported, although self-reported weights can be reasonably used in some populations.[108-110] Interpreting weight as well as BMI can be problematic when there is edema or ascites, or, for example, in an obese patient who is protein-energy malnourished, yet still is overweight. The waist circumference is used as a measure of abdominal fat content. For men, a waist of greater than 102 centimeters and for women a waist of greater than 88 centimeters is associated with an increased risk for obesity-associated factors.[107] This measurement requires locating the waist consistently for all subjects, which tends to be more difficult in obese individuals.

Densitometry measures the density of the body, which is then used to calculate percent body fat. One method to determine body density is underwater weighing, which is a measure of body volume and is often used as the gold standard. The major limitation of this method is that it is cumbersome and expensive. Another method of densitometry is the whole body plethysmograph (BODPOD), where body volume is measured in a sealed chamber rather than underwater. This method appears to be as accurate as underwater weighing, but the equipment is complex and costly.[111]

Skinfold measurements are used as a measure of subcutaneous fat (Figure 12-2). The measurements are obtained at a number of different body sites using special calipers. It requires trained, certified personnel who are regularly retrained, as the measure is only as good as the measurer (Figure 12-3).[112] Measurements from three to seven sites on the body (usually a combination of triceps, subscapular, suprailiac, thigh, abdomen, chest, and midaxillary) are then combined using validated equations to obtain a measure of subcutaneous fat. When performed correctly, these measurements can correlate highly with underwater weighing.[113]

Bioelectrical impedance analysis (BIA) is a method used to estimate body cell mass, fat, and fat free mass. The method is based upon the principle that lean tissues, composed primarily of electrolyte-containing water, are highly conductive and represent a low-impedance pathway. Fat and bone, on the other hand, are nonconductive and have high impedance to current flow.[114] In practice, to obtain the BIA measurement, an imperceptible current (800 μA at a signal frequency of 50 KHz) is passed between the foot and hand of the subject and two components of impedance are measured: resistance and reactance. These values are entered into any of several prediction equations to obtain estimates of total body water, fat, fat free mass, and body cell mass. The validity of BIA, particularly the equations used to calculate body fat, has been debated and continues to be investigated.[115,116] For optimal accuracy of measurements, subjects should not have taken any alcohol within 12 hours or exercised vigorously within 8 hours of testing. The measurements should be taken on subjects 4 hours after eating and at least 1 hour after the last drink of water and within 30 minutes of voiding. Subjects are clothed with the exception of shoes and socks and lie supine with limbs not touching

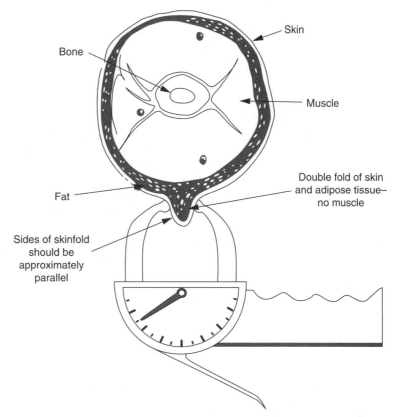

FIGURE 12-2   Skinfold measurement as measurement of subcutaneous fat.
Source: Lee RD and Nieman DC. Nutritional Assessment. Copyright McGraw-Hill Publishers.

their bodies. The subject should not be diaphoretic or soaked in urine as the analyzer measures this fluid as fat free mass. Gel electrodes are placed on the wrist, metacarpal region, ankle, and metatarsal region on the right side of the body. BIA is a quick, inexpensive, and portable method for assessing body composition, and appears to be reproducible.[117] However, results may be altered when hydration is abnormal (e.g., dehydration or edema).

Dual energy X-ray absorptiometry (DEXA) has become more popular in recent years for the measurement of body composition. DEXA scanners generate X-rays at two energy levels in order to differentiate body weight into the components of fat, muscle, and bone mineral content. The results from DEXA scans have been shown to correlate well with underwater weighing.[118,119] The advantages of the DEXA method are that it is based on a three-compartment model rather than a two-compartment model as in most other methods. It can also distinguish regional as well as whole body parameters of body composition. However, the disadvantages are that the equipment is expensive and often requires trained radiology personnel to operate. Computed tomography (CT) scanning is another method for determining body composition. CT scans provide measures of body fat distributions and are used to obtain ratios of intra-abdominal to extra-abdominal fat. In addition

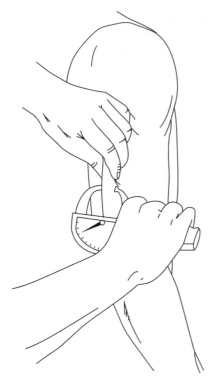

Grasp a double fold of skin and subcutaneous adipose tissue with the thumb and index finger of the left hand.

Place the caliper tips on the site where the sides of the skinfold are approximately parallel and 1 cm distal to where the skinfold is grasped.

Position the caliper dial so that it can be read easily. Obtain the measurement about 4 sec after placing the caliper tips on the skinfold.

FIGURE 12-3   Measurement of triceps skinfold using a caliper.
Source: Lee RD and Nieman DC. Nutritional Assessment. Brown & Benchmark Publishers, Madison, WI 1993. page 37.

to being costly, the radiation dose from a CT scan is higher than that from DEXA.[120] Other methods for determining body composition include magnetic resonance imaging (MRI), total body electrical conductivity (TOBEC), and near infrared interactance (NIR). The equipment needed for these methods is also complex and costly.

When deciding what method to use to assess body composition in studies of nutrition in infectious diseases, consider using a combination of methods, as this can strengthen the results. For example, to assess changes and redistribution of body fat in HIV infection, a DEXA could be used to assess total body fat and a CT scan to assess the intra-abdominal to extra-abdominal fat ratio. For studies other than those with relatively small numbers of participants, some methods (e.g., underwater weighing) are clearly not feasible. Some methods, such as DEXA and CT scan, may not be available within close vicinity to the study clinic. Some studies may require methods that are quick and readily available, such as skinfolds and BIA, in order to maximize the number of participants willing to participate.

In children, malnutrition has been defined as mildly underweight, or weight-for-age less than two standard deviations below the National Center for Health Statistics (NCHS) reference population mean.[121] Z-scores for weight-for-age, height-for-age, and weight-for-height are also used to classify malnutrition in children, and there are a wide variety of classification systems and cut-off points for malnutrition.[57] Mid-upper arm circumference can be used in screening for malnutrition when weight and height are difficult to obtain and the exact age of the child is unknown.[57]

Biochemical Measurements

Biochemical measurements may be of a nutrient or its metabolite. A test may be used for examining metabolic pathways, such as a particular dose is orally administered and the appearance of metabolites in urine is measured.[122] Ideally, a measurement that reflects nutrient status (the amount available to the body) should be used so that deficiency, excess, or adequacy can be defined. Some measurements can detect deficiencies before signs and symptoms appear, while others can reflect recent intake. For some nutrients, levels in the blood may also be used as an assessment of dietary intake.[123] Measures are most commonly done on samples of blood (whole blood, white cells, serum, or plasma) and urine, but for some nutrients, samples have included saliva, hair, nails, or tissue biopsies.

Many factors affect a measurement, and little is known about the exact influence of nonnutritional factors such as lifestyle, recreational drug use, medications, and the influence of disease. Quality control of any laboratory procedure needs to be stringent so that measures can be reliable and valid. Many times there are multiple methods or assays available for the same nutrients, and it is important to keep in mind when comparing study results what methods were used.

The same debate about the number of days necessary to determine average dietary intake may be argued for biochemical measures of nutrients as well, as intra-individual variation of a measure may require repeated measures. In addition, what may be an abnormal level for a healthy person may not be an abnormal level for a person with disease. For example, changes in biochemical measures can occur with infection or inflammation, which may not reflect real changes in general tissue nutrient status or dietary intake. It is also important to know how quickly changes in dietary intake affect changes in biochemical measurements (i.e., does the measurement respond within days or hours after changes in intake). Other factors, such as lifestyle or genetics, may also affect serum levels. The ability to control factors that affect the measurements need to be evaluated. For example, if a fasting specimen is needed, can the study participants reasonably be expected to come in fasting? If fecal or urinary analyses are required, can cooperation from study participants be expected? Biochemical measurements are useful when combined with other indicators of nutritional status. Again, more research is needed to discover better biochemical markers of nutritional status.

Conclusion

Nutrition is a major determinant of the morbidity and mortality caused by infectious diseases. Several micronutrients play essential roles in the growth, development, and function of the immune system and influence oxidative stress. Epidemiological studies of infectious diseases should include characterization of nutritional status. At a minimum, basic anthropometric indices such as weight and height should be a basic part of any epidemiological investigation of infectious diseases. Nutritional assessment can be expanded into more sophisticated measures of specific micronutrients, dietary intake, and body composition. Major indicators of health such as child mortality, birth weight, and maternal mortality are influenced by host nutritional status. Micronutrients have been shown to influence the clinical course of diarrheal and lower respiratory disease, measles, malaria, and HIV. However, supplementation with micronutrients may have varying effects depending on whether levels are for correcting deficiencies or at pharmacological doses. The potential role of micronutrients in the clinical course of tuberculosis, a major reemerging disease, remains neglected.

Although a variety of nutrition assessment tools are available, limited information is available on the appropriateness of their use in specialized populations. The decision on what tool(s) to use should be based on the study population and the specific research goals. Each tool should, to the extent possible, be customized to the target population. Few studies currently focus on improving nutrition assessment methodology. Further research is needed toward improving the tools used to assess nutritional status by developing innovative new tools or improving existing tools.

References

1. Hughes DA, Darlington LG, Bendich A, eds. *Diet and Human Immune Function.* Totowa, NJ: Humana Press; 2004.
2. Calder PC, Field CJ, Gill HS, eds. *Nutrition and Immune Function.* New York, NY: CABI Publishing; 2002.
3. Beisel WR. Single nutrients and immunity. *Am J Clin Nutr.* 1982;35(suppl):417–468.
4. Guenter P, Muurahainen N, Simons G, et al. Relationships among nutritional status, disease progression, and survival in HIV infection. *J Acquir Immune Defic Syndr.* 1993;6:1130–1138.
5. Keusch GT. The history of nutrition: malnutrition, infection and immunity. *J Nutr.* 2003;133:336S–340S.
6. UNICEF. *The State of the World's Children 1998.* Oxford and New York: Oxford University Press; 1998.
7. Caulfield LE, de Onis M, Blossner M, Black RE. Undernutrition as an underlying cause of child deaths with diarrhea, pneumonia, malaria, and measles. *Am J Clin Nutr.* 2004;80:193–198.
8. Schroeder DG, Brown KH. Nutritional status as a predictor of child survival: summarizing the association and quantifying its global impact. *Bull World Health Organ.* 1994;72:569–579.
9. McLaren DS, Frigg M. *Sight and Life Manual on Vitamin A Deficiency Disorders (VADD).* 2nd ed. Basel, Switzerland: Task Force Sight and Life; 2001.
10. Beaton GH, Martorell R, L'Abbe KA, et al. *Effectiveness of Vitamin A Supplementation in the Control of Young Child Morbidity and Mortality in Developing Countries.* New York, NY: United Nations; 1993.
11. Bhandari N, Bahl R, Sazawal S, Bhan MK. Breast-feeding status alters the effect of vitamin A treatment during acute diarrhea in children. *J Nutr.* 1997;127:59–63.

12. Sazawal S, Black RE, Bhan MK, et al. Zinc supplementation reduces the incidence of persistent diarrhea and dysentery among low socioeconomic children in India. *J Nutr.* 1996;126: 443–450.
13. Ninh NX, Thissen JP, Collette L, Gerard G, Khoi HH, Ketelslegers JM. Zinc supplementation increases growth and circulating insulin-like growth factor I (IGF-I) in growth-retarded Vietnamese children. *Am J Clin Nutr.* 1996;63:514–519.
14. Rosado JL, Lopez P, Munoz E, Martinez H, Allen LH. Zinc supplementation reduced morbidity, but neither zinc nor iron supplementation affected growth or body composition of Mexican preschoolers. *Am J Clin Nutr.* 1997;65:13–19.
15. Sazawal S, Black RE, Bhan MK, Jalla S, Sinha A, Bhandari N. Efficacy of zinc supplementation in reducing the incidence and prevalence of acute diarrhea—a community-based, double-blind, controlled trial. *Am J Clin Nutr.* 1997;66:413–418.
16. Potential interventions for the prevention of childhood pneumonia in developing countries: a meta-analysis of data from field trials to assess the impact of vitamin A supplementation on pneumonia morbidity and mortality. The Vitamin A and Pneumonia Working Group. *Bull World Health Organ.* 1995;73:609–619.
17. Dowell SF, Papic Z, Bresee JS, et al. Treatment of respiratory syncytial virus infection with vitamin A: a randomized, placebo-controlled trial in Santiago, Chile. *Pediatr Infect Dis J.* 1996;15:782–786.
18. Bresee JS, Fischer M, Dowell SF, et al. Vitamin A therapy for children with respiratory syncytial virus infection: a multicenter trial in the United States. *Pediatr Infect Dis J.* 1996;15:777–782.
19. Muhe L, Lulseged S, Mason KE, Simoes EA. Case-control study of the role of nutritional rickets in the risk of developing pneumonia in Ethiopian children. *Lancet.* 1997;349:1801–1804.
20. Walker CF, Black RE. Zinc and the risk for infectious disease. *Annu Rev Nutr.* 2004;24:255–275.
21. Markowitz LE, Nzilambi N, Driskell WJ, et al. Vitamin A levels and mortality among hospitalized measles patients, Kinshasa, Zaire. *J Trop Pediatr.* 1989;35:109–112.
22. Whalen C, Semba RD. Tuberculosis. In: Semba RD, Bloem NW, eds. *Nutrition and Health in Developing Countries.* Totowa, NJ: Humana Press; 2001:209–235.
23. Williams CJB, Williams CT. *Pulmonary Consumption, Its Etiology, Pathology, and Treatment.* London: Longmans, Green, and Company; 1989.
24. Murphy GS, Oldfield EC III. *Falciparum malaria. Infect Dis Clin North Am.* 1996;10:747–775.
25. Krogstad DJ. Malaria as a reemerging disease. *Epidemiol Rev.* 1996;18:77–89.
26. Caulfield LE, Richard SA, Black RE. Undernutrition as an underlying cause of malaria morbidity and mortality in children less than five years old. *Am J Trop Med Hyg.* 2004;71:55–63.
27. Friis H, Mwaniki D, Omondi B, et al. Serum retinol concentrations and *Schistosoma mansoni*, intestinal helminths, and malarial parasitemia: a cross-sectional study in Kenyan preschool and primary school children. *Am J Clin Nutr.* 1997;66:665–671.
28. Shankar AH, Genton B, Semba RD, et al. Effect of vitamin A supplementation on morbidity due to *Plasmodium falciparum* in

young children in Papua New Guinea: a randomised trial. *Lancet.* 1999;354:203–209.

29. Shankar AH, Genton B, Baisor M, et al. The influence of zinc supplementation on morbidity due to *Plasmodium falciparum*: a randomized trial in preschool children in Papua New Guinea. *Am J Trop Med Hyg.* 2000;62:663–669.

30. Kotler DP, Goetz H, Lange M, Klein EB, Holt PR. Enteropathy associated with the acquired immunodeficiency syndrome. *Ann Intern Med.* 1984;101:421–428.

31. Kotler DP, Wang J, Pierson RN Jr. Body composition studies in patients with the acquired immunodeficiency syndrome. *Am J Clin Nutr.* 1985;42:1255–1265.

32. Graham NMH, Munoz A, Bacellar H, Kingsley LA, Visscher BR, Phair JP. Clinical factors associated with weight loss related to infection with human immunodeficiency virus type 1 in the multicenter AIDS cohort study. *Am J Epidemiol.* 1993;137:1–8.

33. Graham NMH, Rubb S, Hoover DR, McCall LD, Palenicek JG, Saah AJ. Beta2-microglobulin and other early predictors of human immunodeficiency virus type 1–related wasting. *Ann Epidemiol.* 1994;4:32–39.

34. Zangerle R, Reibnegger G, Wachter H, Fuchs D. Weight loss in HIV-1 infection is associated with immune activation. *AIDS.* 1993;7:175–181.

35. Grunfeld C, Feingold KR. Metabolic disturbances and wasting in acquired immunodeficiency syndrome. *N Engl J Med.* 1992;327:329–337.

36. Wheeler DA, Gibert CL, Launer CA, et al, The Terry Beirn Community Programs for Clinical Research on AIDS. Weight loss as a predictor of survival and disease progression in HIV infection. *J Acquir Immune Defic Syndr.* 1998;18:80–85.

37. Tang AM, Forrester J, Spiegelman D, Knox TA, Tchetgen E, Gorbach SL. Weight loss and survival in HIV-positive patients in the era of highly active antiretroviral therapy. *J Acquir Immune Defic Syndr.* 2002;31:230–236.

38. Beach RS, Mantero-Atienza E, Shor-Posner G, et al. Specific nutrient abnormalities in asymptomatic HIV-1 infection. *AIDS.* 1992;6:701–708.

39. Baum MK, Mantero-Atienza E, Shor-Posner G, et al. Association of vitamin B6 status with parameters of immune function in early HIV-1 infection. *J Acquir Immune Defic Syndr.* 1991;4:1122–1132.

40. Bogden JD, Baker H, Frank O, et al. Micronutrient status and human immunodeficiency virus (HIV) infection. In: Bendich A, Chandra RK, eds. *Micronutrients and Immune Functions.* Vol. 587. New York, NY: New York Academy of Sciences; 1990:189–195.

41. Graham NMH, Sorenson D, Odaka N, et al. Relationship of serum copper and zinc levels to HIV-1 seropositivity and progression to AIDS. *J Acquir Immune Defic Syndr.* 1991;4:976–980.

42. Semba RD, Graham NMH, Caiaffa WT, Margolick JB, Clement L, Vlahov D. Increased mortality associated with vitamin A deficiency during HIV-1 infection. *Arch Intern Med.* 1993;153:2149–2154.

43. Mantero-Atienza E, Baum MK, Morgan R, et al. Vitamin B12 in early human immunodeficiency virus-1 infection. *Arch Intern Med* 1991;151:1019–1020.

44. Semba RD, Miotti PG, Chiphangwi JD, et al. Maternal vitamin A deficiency and mother-to-child transmission of HIV-1. *Lancet.* 1994;343:1593–1597.

45. Tang AM, Graham NMH, Kirby AJ, McCall LD, Willett WC, Saah AJ. Dietary micronutrient intake and risk of progression to AIDS in HIV-1 infected homosexual men. *Am J Epidemiol.* 1993;138:937–951.

46. Abrams B, Duncan D, Hertz-Picciotto I. A prospective study of dietary intake and acquired immune deficiency syndrome in HIV seropositive homosexual men. *J Acquir Immune Defic Syndr.* 1993;6:949–958.

47. Jiamton S, Pepin J, Suttent R, et al. A randomized trial of the impact of multiple micronutrient supplementation on mortality among HIV-infected individuals living in Bangkok. *AIDS.* 2003;17:2461–2469.

48. Fawzi WW, Msamanga GI, Spiegelman D, et al. A randomized trial of multivitamin supplements and HIV disease progression and mortality. *N Engl J Med.* 2004;351:23–32.

49. Baruchel S, Wainberg MA. The role of oxidative stress in disease progression in individuals infected by the human immunodeficiency virus. *J Leukoc Biol.* 1992;52:111–114.

50. Chambon P. A decade of molecular biology of retinoic acid receptors. *FASEB J.* 1996;10:940–954.

51. Semba RD. Vitamin A, immunity, and infection. *Clin Infect Dis.* 1994;19:489–499.

52. Semba RD. The role of vitamin A and related retinoids in immune function. *Nutr Rev.* 1998;56:S38–S48.

53. Alvarez JO, Salazar-Lindo E, Kohatsu J, Miranda P, Stephensen CB. Urinary excretion of retinol in children with acute diarrhea. *Am J Clin Nutr.* 1995;61:1273–1276.

54. International Vitamin A Consultative Group. A brief guide to current methods of assessing vitamin A status. Washington, DC: The Nutrition Foundation; 1993.

55. Fraser DR. Vitamin D. *Lancet.* 1995;345:104–107.

56. Crowle AJ, Ross EJ. Comparative abilities of various metabolites of vitamin D to protect cultured human macrophages against tubercle bacilli. *J Leukoc Biol.* 1990;47:545–550.

57. Gibson RS. *Principles of Nutritional Assessment.* 2nd ed. New York, NY: Oxford University Press; 2005.

58. Meydani M. Vitamin E. *Lancet.* 1995;345:170–175.

59. Meydani SN, Barklund MP, Liu S, et al. Vitamin E supplementation enhances cell-mediated immunity in healthy elderly subjects. *Am J Clin Nutr.* 1990;52:557–563.

60. Meydani M, Meydani SN, Leka L, Gong J, Blumberg JB. Effect of long-term vitamin E supplementation on lipid peroxidation and immune responses of young and old subjects. *FASEB J.* 1993;7:A415.

61. Meydani SN. Vitamin E enhancement of T cell-mediated function in healthy elderly: mechanisms of action. *Nutr Rev.* 1995;53:S52–S58.

62. Rall LC, Meydani SN. Vitamin B6 and immune competence. *Nutr Rev.* 1993;51:217–225.

63. Dhur A, Galan P, Hercberg S. Folate status and the immune system. *Prog Food Nutr Sci.* 1991;15:43–60.

64. Hemila H. Vitamin C supplementation and common cold symptoms: problems with inaccurate reviews. *Nutrition.* 1996;12:804–809.

65. Weber P, Bendich A, Schalch W. Vitamin C and human health—a review of recent data relevant to human requirements. *Int J Vitam Nutr Res.* 1996;66:19–30.

66. Beard JL, Dawson H, Pinero DJ. Iron metabolism: a comprehensive review. *Nutr Rev.* 1996;54:295–317.

67. Viteri FE. Iron supplementation for the control of iron deficiency in populations at risk. *Nutr Rev.* 1997;55:195–209.

68. Lozoff B, Brittenham GM, Wolf AW, et al. Iron deficiency anemia and iron therapy effects on infant developmental test performance. *Pediatrics.* 1987;79:981–995.

69. Walter T, De Andraca I, Chadud P, Perales CG. Iron deficiency anemia: adverse effects on infant psychomotor development. *Pediatrics.* 1989;84:7–17.

70. Basta SS, Soekirman, Karyadi D, Scrimshaw NS. Iron deficiency anemia and the productivity of adult males in Indonesia. *Am J Clin Nutr.* 1979;32:916–925.

71. Scholl TO, Hediger ML, Fischer RL, Shearer JW. Anemia vs iron deficiency: increased risk of preterm delivery in a prospective study. *Am J Clin Nutr.* 1992;55:985–988.

72. Alauddin M. Maternal mortality in rural Bangladesh: the Tangail District. *Stud Fam Plann.* 1986;17:13–21.

73. Harrison KA. Tropical obstetrics and gynaecology. 2. Maternal mortality. *Trans R Soc Trop Med Hyg.* 1989;83:449–453.

74. Viteri FE. Iron supplementation for the control of iron deficiency in populations at risk. *Nutr Rev.* 1997;55:195–209.

75. Stoltzfus RJ, Dreyfuss ML, Chwaya HM, Albonico M. Hookworm control as a strategy to prevent iron deficiency. *Nutr Rev.* 1997;55:223–232.

76. Walter T, Olivares M, Pizarro F, Munoz C. Iron, anemia, and infection. *Nutr Rev.* 1997;55:111–124.

77. Menendez C, Kahigwa E, Hirt R, et al. Randomised placebo-controlled trial of iron supplementation and malaria chemoprophylaxis for prevention of severe anaemia and malaria in Tanzanian infants. *Lancet.* 1997;350:844–850.

78. Foster LH, Sumar S. Selenium in health and disease: a review. *Crit Rev Food Sci Nutr.* 1997;37:211–228.

79. Roy M, Kiremidjian-Schumacher L, Wishe HI, Cohen MW, Stotzky G. Supplementation with selenium restores age-related decline in immune cell function. *Proc Soc Exp Biol Med.* 1995;209:369–375.

80. Levander OA, Beck MA. Interacting nutritional and infectious etiologies of Keshan disease. Insights from coxsackie virus B-induced myocarditis in mice deficient in selenium or vitamin E. *Biol Trace Elem Res.* 1997;56:5–21.

81. Delange F. The disorders induced by iodine deficiency. *Thyroid.* 1994;4:107–128.

82. Hetzel BS, Pandav CS. *S.O.S. for a Billion: The Conquest of Iodine Deficiency Disorders.* New York, NY: Oxford University Press; 1994.

83. Cobra C, Muhilal K, Rusmil K, et al. Infant survival is improved by oral iodine supplementation. *J Nutr.* 1997;127:574–578.

84. Ren Q, Gu D, Cao X, et al. Effect of environmental supplementation of iodine on infant mortality and growth in children in Xinjiang, China. *Zhonghua Liu Xing Bing Xue Za Zhi.* 2002;23:198–202.

85. DeLong GR, Leslie PW, Wang SH, et al. Effect on infant mortality of iodination of irrigation water in a severely iodine-deficient area of China. *Lancet.* 1997;350:771–773.

86. Walsh CT, Sandstead HH, Prasad AS, Newberne PM, Fraker PJ. Zinc: health effects and research priorities for the 1990s. *Environ Health Perspect.* 1994;102(suppl 2):5–46.

87. Shankar AH, Prasad AS. Zinc and immune function: the biological basis of altered resistance to infection. *Am J Clin Nutr.* 1998;68: 447S–463S.

88. Livingstone MB, Prentice AM, Strain JJ, et al. Accuracy of weighed dietary records in studies of diet and health. *BMJ.* 1990;300:708–712.

89. Mertz W, Tsui JC, Judd JT, et al. What are people really eating? The relation between energy intake derived from estimated diet records and intake determined to maintain body weight. *Am J Clin Nutr.* 1991;54:291–295.

90. Karvetti RL, Knuts LR. Validity of the 24-hour dietary recall. *J Am Diet Assoc.* 1985;85:1437–1442.

91. Gersovitz M, Madden JP, Smiciklas-Wright H. Validity of the 24-hr. dietary recall and seven-day record for group comparisons. *J Am Diet Assoc.* 1978;73:48–55.

92. Briefel RR, Flegal KM, Winn DM, Loria CM, Johnson CL, Sempos CT. Assessing the nation's diet: limitations of the food frequency questionnaire. *J Am Diet Assoc.* 1992;92:959–962.

93. Sempos CT. Invited commentary: some limitations of semiquantitative food frequency questionnaires. *Am J Epidemiol.* 1992;135:1127–1132.

94. Rimm EB, Giovannucci EL, Stampfer MJ, Colditz GA, Litin LB, Willett WC. Authors' response to 'Invited commentary: some limitations of semiquantitative food frequency questionnaires.' *Am J Epidemiol.* 1992;135:1133–1136.

95. Kushi LH. Gaps in epidemiologic research methods: design considerations for studies that use food-frequency questionnaires. *Am J Clin Nutr.* 1994;59:180S–184S.

96. Thompson FE, Byers T. Dietary assessment resource manual. *J Nutr.* 1994;124:2245S–2317S.

97. Cade J, Thompson R, Burley V, Warm D. Development, validation and utilisation of food-frequency questionnaires—a review. *Public Health Nutr.* 2002;5:567–587.

98. Willett WC. *Nutritional Epidemiology.* New York, NY: Oxford University Press; 1998.

99. Burke BS. The dietary history as a tool in research. *J Am Diet Assoc.* 1947;23:1041–1046.

100. Jain M, Howe GR, Johnson KC, Miller AB. Evaluation of a diet history questionnaire for epidemiologic studies. *Am J Epidemiol.* 1980;111:212–219.

101. Dwyer JT, Coleman KA. Insights into dietary recall from a longitudinal study: accuracy over four decades. *Am J Clin Nutr.* 1997;65:1153S–1158S.

102. Friedenreich CM. Improving long-term recall in epidemiologic studies. *Epidemiology.* 1994;5:1–4.

103. Willett WC, Howe GR, Kushi LH. Adjustment for total energy intake in epidemiologic studies. *Am J Clin Nutr.* 1997;65:1220S–1228S.

104. Freedman LS, Kipnis V, Brown CC, Schatzkin A, Wacholder S, Hartman AM. Comments on "Adjustment for total energy intake in epidemiologic studies." *Am J Clin Nutr.* 1997;65(suppl):1229S–1231S.

105. Spiegelman D, McDermott A, Rosner B. Regression calibration method for correcting measurement-error bias in nutritional epidemiology. *Am J Clin Nutr.* 1997;65:1179S–1186S.

106. Margetts BM, Nelson M, eds. *Design Concepts in Nutritional Epidemiology.* Oxford, UK: Oxford University Press; 1991.

107. US Dept of Health and Human Services, National Heart, Lung, and Blood Institute. Clinical guidelines on the identification, evaluation, and treatment of overweight and obesity in adults: the evidence report. Washington, DC: Public Health Service; 1998.

108. Kuczmarski MF, Kuczmarski RJ, Najjar M. Effects of age on validity of self-reported height, weight, and body mass index: findings from the Third National Health and Nutrition Examination Survey, 1988–1994. *J Am Diet Assoc.* 2001;101:28–34.

109. Villanueva EV. The validity of self-reported weight in US adults: a population based cross-sectional study. *BMC Public Health.* 2001;1:11.

110. Spencer EA, Appleby PN, Davey GK, Key TJ. Validity of self-reported height and weight in 4808 EPIC-Oxford participants. *Public Health Nutr.* 2002;5:561–565.

111. Gundlach BL, Visscher GJ. The plethysmometric measurement of total body volume. *Hum Biol.* 1986;58:783–799.

112. Ruiz L, Colley JR, Hamilton PJ. Measurement of triceps skinfold thickness. An investigation of sources of variation. *Br J Prev Soc Med.* 1971;25:165–167.

113. Jackson AS, Pollock ML. Practical assessment of body composition. *Physician Sports Med.* 1985;13:76–90.

114. Ellis KJ. Human body composition: in vivo methods. *Physiol Rev.* 2000;80:649–680.

115. Chumlea WC, Guo SS. Bioelectrical impedance and body composition: present status and future directions. *Nutr Rev.* 1994;52:123–131.

116. Houtkooper LB, Lohman TG, Going SB, Howell WH. Why bioelectrical impedance analysis should be used for estimating adiposity. *Am J Clin Nutr.* 1996;64:436S–448S.

117. Baumgartner RN. Electrical impedance and total body electrical conductivity. In: Roche AF, Heymsfield SB, Lohman TG, eds. *Human Body Composition.* Champaign, Ill: Human Kinetics Books; 1996: 79–108.

118. Roubenoff R, Kehayias JJ, Dawson-Hughes B, Heymsfield SB. Use of dual-energy x-ray absorptiometry in body-composition studies: not yet a "gold standard." *Am J Clin Nutr.* 1993;58:589–591.

119. Svendsen OL, Haarbo J, Hassager C, Christiansen C. Accuracy of measurements of body composition by dual-energy x-ray absorptiometry in vivo. *Am J Clin Nutr.* 1993;57:605–608.

120. Lohman TG. Advances in body composition assessment: current issues. In: Roche E, Heyensfield SB, Lohman TG, eds. *Exercise Science.* Monograph 3. Champaign, Ill: Human Kinetics Publishers; 1992.

121. Mason JB, Musgrove P, Watson F, Habicht JP. Undernutrition. In: Murray CJL, Lopez AD, eds. *Quantifying Global Burden Health Risks: The Burden of Disease Attributable to Selected Risk Factors.* Cambridge, Mass: Harvard University Press; 1996.

122. Lee RD, Nieman DC. *Nutrition Assessment.* St Louis, Mo: Mosby-Year Book Inc; 1996.

123. Hunter D. Biochemical indicators of dietary intake. In: Willett WC, ed. *Nutritional Epidemiology.* New York, NY: Oxford University Press;1998:174–243.

EMERGING AND NEW INFECTIOUS DISEASES

Kenrad E. Nelson

However secure and well-regulated civilized life may become, bacteria, protozoa, viruses, infected fleas, lice, ticks, mosquitoes, and bedbugs will always lurk in the shadows ready to pounce when neglect, poverty, famine, or war lets down the defenses. And even in normal times they prey on the weak, the very young, and the very old, living along with us, in mysterious obscurity waiting their opportunities. About the only genuine sporting proposition that remains unimpaired by the relentless domestication of a once free-living human species is the war against these ferocious little creatures, which lurk in the dark corners and stalk us in the bodies of rats, mice, and all kinds of domestic animals; which fly and crawl with the insects, and waylay us in our food and drink and even in our love.

−Hans Zinsser, *Rats, Lice and History*, 1934

Introduction

Despite the optimistic forecasts often made in the 1960s and 1970s about the eventual control or even elimination of most of the major infectious diseases of developed Western countries, the outlook has changed in the 1980s and 1990s. Most dramatic has been the appearance of the acquired immune deficiency syndrome (AIDS) pandemic, which most likely arose from human contact with a modified or recombinant primate retrovirus from an infected chimpanzee in central Africa. Infections with this new human virus spread around the world within a decade.[1] The targeting of critical cells of the immune system by the human immunodeficiency virus (HIV), such as the CD4 T lymphocytes, macrophages, and Langerhans cells, has led to the emergence of a large number of important secondary pathogens, or opportunistic infections, that cannot be controlled by the damaged immune system of infected individuals. The HIV-1 pandemic has allowed the dramatic explosion of infections with several pathogens that had been rare or were under good control prior to the AIDS epidemic.

Some Important HIV/AIDS-Related Infections

Tuberculosis

Worldwide, the most important opportunistic infection associated with the HIV/AIDS epidemic is tuberculosis.[2] In a matter of a few years after the report of the first cases of AIDS in the United States, the downward trend in new cases of tuberculosis that had been uninterrupted since the licensure of INH in 1952 was reversed. Between 1989 and 1995, 75,000 cases in excess of the number that had been estimated to occur in the absence of the AIDS epidemic were reported in the United States. However, the global impact of the HIV pandemic has been even more striking. Tuberculosis is the most important opportunistic infection associated with HIV and is second only to AIDS as a cause of infectious disease mortality worldwide.[2]

The increase in tuberculosis cases has commonly involved young adults who are HIV infected. Many of these cases of tuberculosis represent reactivation disease, but some are progressive primary infections. Patients who are HIV-positive more often develop disseminated tuberculosis. It has been estimated that persons who are immunosuppressed because of HIV have a 20–30% risk of developing active tuberculosis in the first year after they are infected with *M. tuberculosis* and a 40–50% lifetime risk, in contrast with an estimated 5% risk in the year after infection and an overall lifetime risk of 10% among HIV-negative persons who are not seriously immunosuppressed.[3] This is evidence that an HIV infection converts many otherwise asymptomatic infections with the tubercle bacillus into clinically active and often contagious tuberculosis.

Cryptococcosis and Other Systemic Fungal Infections

One of the early hallmarks of the HIV/AIDS epidemic in Africa was a dramatic increase in the incidence of cryptococcal meningitis.[4] Because tuberculosis had been a common infection in African and Asian populations prior to the AIDS epidemic, an increase in cryptococcosis was more noticeable to clinicians and public health officials. As with many other AIDS-associated opportunistic infections, it was possible to treat cryptococcal meningitis in AIDS patients with amphotericin-B (ambisome), even though the acute mortality remained at a rate of about 20%.[5] However, in contrast to cryptococcal meningitis in patients who were immunosuppressed from diseases other than AIDS or who were not obviously immunosuppressed, patients with AIDS were highly likely to relapse in the months following effective therapy.[6] It soon became apparent that chronic suppressive therapy with antifungal drugs would be necessary in AIDS patients to prevent the frequent relapses. Several other systemic fungal infections, including histoplasmosis, coccidioidomycosis, and disseminated *Penicillium marneffei* infections in Southeast Asia, were found to be common in patients with AIDS.[7] Curiously, the rates of blastomycosis and paracoccidioidomycosis, a fungal infection endemic in Colombia, seem not to be increased in patients with AIDS.[8]

Kaposi's Sarcoma

One of the early hallmarks of the AIDS epidemic was a dramatic increase in the number of patients with Kaposi's sarcoma (KS). The epidemic of AIDS in homosexual men was first recognized as an outbreak of KS with/or without *Pneumocystis carinii* pneumonia (PCP) in homosexual men in Los Angeles, San Francisco, and New York.[9] The intensive investigation of these KS and PCP cases led first to the discovery that these men were immunosuppressed and later that HIV was the viral infection causing the underlying immunosuppression in AIDS patients.[10,11] Subsequently, studies of the epidemiology of KS provided data suggesting that the disease might be due to a sexually transmitted infection other than (or in addition to) HIV. This hypothesis arose from studies of the distribution of KS, which was seen primarily in populations whose HIV infection was acquired sexually, rather than those with drug use, transfusion, or perinatal transmission as risk factors. Also, women in the United States who developed AIDS because of heterosexual contact with a male partner had significantly higher rates of KS than did women who were injection drug users.[12] Recently, studies of Chang, Moore, and colleagues have identified the sequences of a new human herpes virus (HHV-8) in the tissues of patients with KS.[13,14] Further studies of HHV-8 have shown it to be associated with KS, even among patients who are not HIV infected.[14] Data indicating that infection with HHV-8 usually precedes the occurrence of KS by months to years have been obtained by several investigators.[15,16] It is now accepted by most experts that the association between HHV-8 and KS is causal, although immunosuppression and various hormonal factors appear to modify whether or not KS will result from an HHV-8 infection and when it will occur after an infection with HHV-8.

Pneumocystis carinii Pneumonia

The other opportunistic infection that was originally identified as the hallmark of AIDS before the identification of HIV was PCP occurring in a person without a malignancy or congenital immunodeficiency syndrome. Prior to the use of active antiretroviral therapy and specific prophylaxis for PCP, the disease occurred in nearly 75% of AIDS patients.[17] The fact that AIDS patients often had both PCP and KS led to the original hypothesis that AIDS was due to generalized immunosuppression, especially involving cell-mediated immune function. Although PCP has been reported from all risk groups of AIDS patients, it has been reported rarely among patients in Africa.[18] The reasons for this are unclear. However, some investigators have carefully studied African AIDS patients with bronchoscopy and autopsy, and have found the organism to be uncommon among these patients.[19]

Mycobacterium avium and Other Nontuberculous Mycobacteria

Mycobacterium avium infections are especially common in patients with severe immunosuppression from AIDS. Typically, *M. avium* complex (MAC) infections occur in patients with CD4 cell counts below 50/mL. Recently, clinical trials have shown that prophylaxis with clarithromycin or rifabutin is effective in preventing MAC infections in AIDS patients with severe immunosuppression. In addition to preventing clinical symptoms from MAC infections, the use of these drugs appears to prolong the survival of AIDS patients when prophylaxis is successful.[20] Infection with several other non-tuberculous mycobacterial species, especially *M. kansasii*, also has been reported in AIDS patients.

Cytomegalovirus, Herpes Simplex Virus Type 2, and Varicella-Zoster Virus

Persistent and recurrent infections with many herpes viruses are quite common in AIDS patients. Typically, cytomegalovirus (CMV) infections occur and present as CMV retinitis in patients with CD4 cell counts below 50 cells/mL. If immunosuppression cannot be reversed with effective antiretroviral therapy, prophylactic therapy is necessary to prevent relapse and further retinal damage from occurring after successful treatment. Recent studies indicate that the risk of primary or recurrent CMV retinitis has been greatly reduced by treatment with combination antiretroviral drugs that include protease inhibitors. Studies also indicate that continuation of CMV prophylaxis may not always be necessary to prevent relapses in patients with good immune recovery. Infections with CMV can also manifest as gastrointestinal or central nervous system infections. Herpes simplex virus type 2 (HSV-2) infections are commonly seen in patients with HIV infection and often occur in patients prior to severe immunosuppression. Genital ulcerations from HSV-2 infections in AIDS patients can be difficult to treat effectively and are very prone to recurrence. Similarly, dermatomal or disseminated herpes zoster VZV infections often occur in patients with HIV infection who have only moderately decreased CD4 counts in the range of 200 to 400 cells/mL.

Other Infections

Patients with AIDS are at risk of developing a number of different opportunistic infections in addition to those described above. Infections with pneumococci are especially common. Increases in the rates of invasive pneumococcal infections (pneumonia, sepsis, and meningitis) have been proposed as a sentinel marker for the spread of HIV in a population.[21] It is characteristic of HIV infections and AIDS that clinically significant infections with an endemic pathogen increase in frequency if they are normally controlled by cellular immune mechanisms in persons exposed to the organisms. For example, in several countries in southern Europe, visceral leishmaniasis is a common manifestation of AIDS.[22] AIDS often presents as disseminated histoplasmosis among patients in the histoplasmosis belt in the midwestern United States.[8] In Southeast Asia, especially in northern Thailand and southern China, disseminated *P. marneffei* infections (a fungal organism) are common clinical presentations in patients with AIDS.[7] Toxoplasmosis, cryptosporidiosis, and microsporidiosis are quite common parasitic infections in patients with AIDS.

AIDS-Associated Malignancies

In addition to a large number of opportunistic infections, AIDS patients also are at high risk of developing several malignancies. Kaposi's sarcoma is one of the most frequent AIDS-associated conditions and has been reviewed above. In addition, AIDS patients are at increased risk of non-Hodgkin's lymphoma (NHL), Hodgkin's disease, squamous cell carcinoma of the anus or penis, and cervical cancer.[23] Studies of the natural history of oncogenic human papillomavirus (HPV) in AIDS patients are under way. Chronic carriage of oncogenic HPV strains, especially HPV types 16, 18, and 31, appear to be more common in AIDS patients.[24] Typically, NHL occurs in severely immunosuppressed AIDS patients and is disseminated, commonly involving the central nervous system at the time of diagnosis.[25]

Other Conditions

Some patients with AIDS present with chronic diarrhea and severe weight loss, with or without chronic diarrhea, termed *slim disease* in Africa.[26] Such patients may or may not be infected with specific intestinal pathogens that cause chronic diarrheal disease. A number of other opportunistic pathogens, in addition to those discussed above, are relatively common in patients with HIV/AIDS.

Factors in the Emergence of Infectious Diseases

Although there has been a marked decline in the morbidity and mortality from infectious diseases during the 1900s related to the development and use of effective vaccines and antibiotics and a more hygienic environment, new infectious diseases have emerged, and old ones, such as tuberculosis, have reemerged. Some of the important factors favoring the emergence and growing importance of infectious diseases, in addition to the HIV/AIDS pandemic, will be reviewed here briefly (Exhibit 13-1).

Population Growth

Perhaps the most important factor globally in the emergence of infectious diseases has been the growth of the human population that started in the latter half of the 1800s. The human population had been stable for several centuries, then increased gradually with the urbanization and concentration of the labor force required for industrialization.

However, in the last several decades of the 1900s there has been an accelerated increase in the population of the planet. Along with this increase in population, there has been a dramatic growth in large urban populations. Some large urban centers have inadequate sanitary infrastructure, such as sewage disposal, water supply, and food distribution and storage. Nearly all large cities in both the developed and developing world have substantial populations living in crowded slums. The resultant crowding and marginal sanitary conditions have been associated with increases in infectious diseases. Most experts predict that the population increase will continue, as will the growth of megacities, in the current century. Some experts predict that the global population will grow from the current 6.5 billion to 12 to 15 billion—2.5 times the current population—by the middle of the century.

Exhibit 13-1   Emerging Infectious Diseases and Changes in Environment, Host, or Organism That Have Promoted Their Emergence

SARS	Human contact with exotic animals (civet cats), international travel
Monkey Pox	Human contact with exotic animals, animal contact
Anthrax	Bioterrorism

Arenaviruses
   Junin virus (Argentine
      hemorrhagic fever [HF])
   Machupo virus (Bolivian HF)
   Guanarito virus
      (Venezuelan HF)
	Changes in agriculture allowing closer contact with infected rodents

Hantavirus Sin Nombre virus (HPS)	Climatic changes allowing mice expansion
Rift Valley fever	Dams, irrigation, climate change
Filoviridae species Ebola-Marburg virus	Increased contact between infected primates and man; nosocomial spread, importation of animals
Dengue	Increased global travel, urbanization, increase in mosquito reservoir
Influenza	Integrated pig–duck agriculture, increase in global travel
HIV/(AIDS) HTLV	Changes in sexual behavior, urbanization, increase in illicit drug use, global shipment of blood products
Raccoon rabies	Shipment of infected raccoons
Cyclospora cayetanensis	International shipment of raspberries
Cholera	El Niño climate change, international travel, shipment of foods
Borrelia burgdorferi (Lyme disease)	Increased deer population, increased human contact with ticks in nature
Malaria	Growth and movement of human populations, declining use and effectiveness of insecticides, crowding
Escherichia coli O157:H7 (enterohemorrhagic *E. coli*)	Growth-centralized agriculture promoting cross-contamination, global distribution of foods
Pfisteria pisticida	Changes in agricultural practices leading to pollution of rivers and estuaries, overgrowth of dinoflagellates
Quinolone-resistant *Campylobacter*	Overuse and misuse of antibiotics in agriculture and in clinical settings
Multidrug-resistant *Mycobacterium tuberculosis*	Misuse of antibiotics, crowding in prisons, slums, hospitals, etc., allowing transmission
Cryptosporidium parvum	Contamination of municipal water supplies, increases in immunocompromised populations

Population growth to these levels could severely test our ability to control the emergence and spread of infectious diseases. More optimistic projections predict a global population of about 10 billion. Wherever the current population growth settles, the public health problems will be more severe than they are today. Limiting population growth is a critical public health issue that underlies our ability to control infectious diseases and other health and social problems.

Speed and Ease of Travel

Dramatic changes in the ability and ease of travel occurred in the 1900s. In the last several decades, with modern airplane travel, it has been possible to get from a tropical rain forest in Africa or South America to a suburban or rural area in the United States during the incubation period of a disease such as Lassa fever, dengue, malaria, West Nile virus (WNV), encephalitis, and most other infectious diseases.[27] This has facilitated the introduction and spread of diseases from one area to another. In fact, autochthonous transmission of malaria has occurred occasionally in the temperate zone of the United States, secondary to the introduction of malaria by a visitor from an endemic area and subsequent focal transmission by local anopheline mosquitoes.[28]

In addition to the movement of people, the food supply of the United States and most developed countries has become very international. The repeated introduction of *Cyclospora* on raspberries imported into the United States or Canada from Guatemala,[29,30] the importation of *Escherichia coli* O157:H7 into Japan on radish sprouts from the United States,[31] and the importation to the United States of chickens contaminated with quinolone-resistant *Campylobacter* from Mexico are recent examples of the global transport of infectious pathogens.[32,33]

Dam Building

The construction of large dams to provide hydroelectric power to growing populations and irrigation for rural crops has had adverse consequences in the emergence of infectious diseases. The number of large dams that were constructed in the United States, Asia, Africa, and elsewhere in the 1900s has increased in parallel with the population growth (Figure 13-1).

The construction of dams often has displaced rural and semirural populations and has provided a propitious environment for the growth of mosquitoes and other vector species. The construction of the Aswan high dam in upper Egypt was accompanied by a large expansion of the snail population and hundreds of thousands of *Schistosoma haematobium* infections in the populations that were exposed to the water supply.

Expansion of Human Populations into Previously Uninhabited Forested and Suburban Areas

The redistribution of the human population into areas that were previously uninhabited has had a major impact on the emergence of infectious diseases in both developed and developing countries.

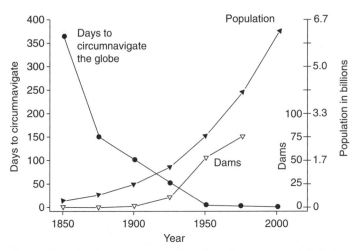

FIGURE 13-1   Over the last 150 years, there have been many global changes that have enhanced the probability of the emergence of new infectious diseases of humans and animals. This chart depicts three examples of such trends: The increase in the human population; the increased construction of large dams (over 75 meters high) built in the United States, 1890–1975; and the decrease in time needed to circle the globe.
Source: Reprinted with permission from F.A. Murphy and N. Nathanson, *Seminars in Virology,* Vol. 5, p. 88, © 1994, Academic Press, Inc.

The emergence of Lyme disease, human granulocytic ehrlichiosis (HGE), human monocytic ehrlichiosis (HME), babesiosis, and Rocky Mountain spotted fever (RMSF) in various areas of the United States is directly linked to the growth of suburbia and recreation in tick-infested areas. In tropical Africa, the emergence of Ebola virus, Lassa fever, monkey pox, and HIV-1 and HIV-2 infections are related to the expansion of the human population into wilderness areas and increased close exposures of humans to nonhuman primate populations.

Relocation of Animals

In addition to international travel and shipment of food, some infectious diseases have emerged because of shipment and relocation of animals. An epidemic of raccoon rabies was recognized in the northeastern United States, which was initiated by the intentional transportation of raccoons from the South, especially Georgia, Alabama, Florida, and the Carolinas, to Virginia and West Virginia for hunting by sportsmen.[34] Unfortunately, the raccoons were obtained from a population of animals in which an epizootic of rabies was occurring. Subsequently, raccoon rabies has spread widely to many states in the northeastern United States; currently, most human postexposure rabies vaccine prophylaxis in this area is given because of exposures to rabid or possibly rabid raccoons. For reasons that are unclear, there has only been one documented transmission of rabies to humans from rabid raccoons, despite over 1000 instances of human exposures annually in New York State and similar extensive use of vaccine after raccoon exposure in other Atlantic coastal states.

The epidemic of Ebola virus infections in rhesus macaques (*Macaca fascicularis*), monkeys imported from the Philippines to the United States Army primate facility in Reston, Virginia, is another example of transportation of a new infectious disease with infected animals.[35] An outbreak of Marburg virus infection in laboratory workers occurred in Germany from exposure to infected monkeys imported from Africa.[36]

Global Climate Change

A major environmental factor that potentially could lead to the emergence of infectious diseases is global climate change. The changes in climate that have occurred during the past 100 years or so and are predicted to continue in the future are often termed *global warming*. Although this term is accurate, it doesn't completely capture the total complexity of global climate change. Some areas of the Earth are becoming warmer; others are not. Nevertheless, there has been an overall measured increase in average surface temperatures of the Earth during the last century. Three research programs have analyzed available data from over 7000 stations that have recorded surface temperature around the globe. These data have been compiled and plotted by three different research groups: the National Oceanic and Atmospheric Administration (NOAA), the National Aeronautic and Space Administration (NASA), and the Climate Research Unit (CRU) of the University of East Anglia, Norwich, in the United Kingdom. Overall, these data have measured a warming of about 1°F (0.4°C) since the late 1800s (Figure 13-2). Although global warming during the past century seems to have been well documented, not all areas of the Earth's surface have been equally affected, and the causes of the warming and predictions for the future have been debated. However, most climatologic researchers believe that human activities that have increased greenhouse gases, such as carbon dioxide, methane, and nitrous oxide, have played a major role in the climate change of the Earth during recent decades. Data collected by Oak Ridge National Laboratory showed dramatic increases in carbon dioxide emissions during the 1900s from the use of fossil fuels (Figure 13-3).

Although it is difficult to predict with certainty how global climate change will affect the emergence of new infectious diseases, several recent epidemics have occurred in which climate change is believed to have been an important factor. One example is the infectious diseases consequent to the recent El Niño event that warmed the surface of the South Pacific Ocean in 1993. This severe El Niño is believed to have led to an algal boom in the surface waters along the Pacific coast of South America. The subsequent zooplankton expansion was believed to have spread the ocean reservoir of *Vibrio cholera* along coastal South America.[37] The consequence was a new emergence of cholera, which had not been epidemic in South America during the previous century.

In the Four Corners area of New Mexico, Colorado, Arizona, and Utah, the increased rainfall associated with El Niño climate conditions is believed to have led to an expansion of the deer mouse population because of the availability of a markedly increased food supply of pinon nuts. The mice that were chronically infected with Sin Nombre hantavirus infected the human population when they invaded their homes. The outbreak of hantavirus

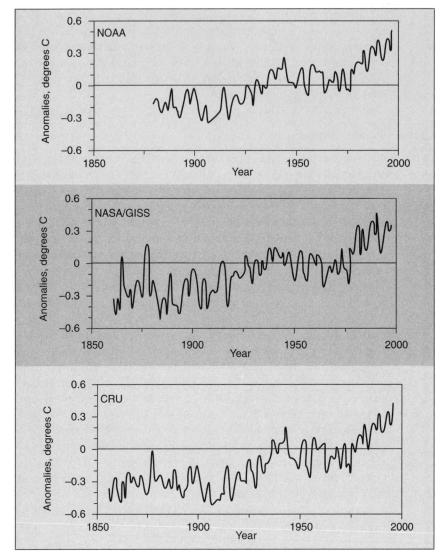

Sources: NOAA, NASA/GISS, AND CRU.

FIGURE 13-2 Global temperature anomalies.
Source: Reprinted from NOAA Web site.

pulmonary syndrome is believed to have been the first outbreak of infections with this virus in a human population. Serologic surveys of populations in New Mexico who might have been exposed previously did not yield evidence of previous unrecognized epidemics. The unique environmental conditions that occurred at this time allowed this virus to emerge as a significant human pathogen (Table 13-1).

An epidemic of Rift Valley fever (RVF) occurred in Tanzania and countries in east Africa between December 1997 and April 1998 that is believed to have been caused by an unusually large rainfall and subsequent expansion of the mosquito vector population. At least 478 deaths occurred, and

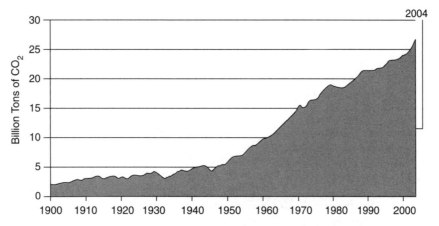

Sources & Notes: WRI estimates based on IEA, 2004; EIA 2004; Marland et al., 2005; and BP, 2005.
Emissions include fossil fuel combustion, cement manufacture, and gas flaring.

FIGURE 13-3 Global emissions of CO_2 from fossil fuels, 1900–2004.
Source: Baumert, Kevin A. Herzog, Timothy and Pershing, Jonathan. 2005. Navigating the Numbers: Greenhouse Gases and International Climate Change Agreements. Washington, DC: World Resources Institute. Emissions include fossil fuel combustion, cement manufacture, and gas flaring.
Source & Notes: WRI estimates based on IEA, 2004; EIA 2004; Marland et al., 2005; and BP, 2005.

TABLE 13-1 Ecologic Features of Different Virus Complexes Within the Genus *Hantavirus*

Virus Complex	Wildlife Host (rodent subfamily)	Geographic Distribution	Human Disease (severity)
Hantaan	*Apodemus agrarius,* striped field mouse (Murinae)	Eastern Asia, Eastern Europe	Hemorrhagic fever (severe)
Seoul	*Rattus* species, wild/ laboratory rat (Murinae)	Eastern Asia, seaports worldwide	Hemorrhagic fever (moderate/mild)
Puumala	*Clethrionomys glareolus,* bank vole (Arvicolinae)	Europe, European Russia	Nephropathia epidemica (mild)
Prospect Hill	*Microtus pennsylvanicus,* meadow vole (Arvicolinae)	United States	Unknown
Sin Nombre	*Peromyscus maniculatus,* deer mouse (Sigmodontinae)	Western United States	Hantavirus pulmonary syndrome (HPS) (severe)

Notes: Hemorrhagic fever is also known as hemorrhagic fever with renal syndrome (HFRS). In the United States, two other hantaviruses have been associated with a few cases of HPS (Black Creek Canyon virus, carried by *S. hispidus*, and Bayou virus, carried by *O. palustris*), and other new hantaviruses will probably be defined (Nichol et al., 1996).
Source: Fields, Knipe and Hally, Virology, p. 1485, © 1996, Lippincott-Raven Publishers.

approximately 89,000 persons were estimated to have been infected in this epidemic.[38] Analysis of previous RVF virus epidemics in east Africa has determined that they have nearly always been associated with unusually high rainfall, leading to the expansion of an infected mosquito population.[39]

Many climatologists and epidemiologists are concerned that global warming associated with an increase in environmental pollution from greenhouse gases could lead to an expanded range of anopheline mosquitoes with epidemics of malaria in previously uninfected populations. Also, the expansion of the range of *Aedes aegypti* and *Aedes albopictus* could occur with modest increases in mean temperatures. This could lead to epidemics of dengue, yellow fever, and viral encephalitis (such as eastern encephalitis [EE]). Another effect of global warming is the extrinsic incubation period of dengue virus in the mosquito vector is shortened by elevated temperatures, which increases the size of dengue epidemics.[40]

Significant global climate change could have major effects on the epidemiology of infectious diseases. One concern of climatologists is that global climate change might lead to both droughts in some areas and major increased rainfall with flooding in other areas. Warming of the Earth's surface could affect the hydrologic cycle, with increases in both drought and severe rainstorms and floods. Both droughts and floods could promote the emergence and spread of infectious diseases from contaminated water, expansion of vector populations, and food shortages. Whether global warming will continue at an accelerated rate, as some have predicted, and whether this will lead to an expansion of infectious diseases is not certain. However, the evolving scenario has sufficient biologic plausibility to be taken seriously.

War and Societal Disruption

Nearly every major war has been accompanied by significant epidemics of infectious disease that involve both the military combatants and the civilian populations. Often, the epidemics of infectious disease overshadow military factors in the outcome of the conflict.[41]

There are many examples of this interaction. However, the "swine influenza" pandemic of 1918–1919 that occurred during World War I in Europe may be the most graphic example. This epidemic was unlike any influenza epidemic seen before or since, in that it targeted healthy young adults, often with a fatal outcome. It was estimated to have killed over 20 million persons worldwide and at least 43,000 US military personnel. Over 80% of the American war casualties were due to influenza.[41]

Germany's General Erich Von Rudendroff blamed the defeat of the German army directly on the influenza epidemic. He noted that more than 2000 men in each of his army divisions were ill with the flu in June 1918.[41] It has been estimated that 20% of the world's population and one of every four persons in the United States were infected during this epidemic. It is now believed that the virus was transmitted to humans from a bird source in Kansas and was transported to the European War theater by infected US troops.[42]

During World War II, a major common source outbreak of hepatitis B infection was caused by the immunization of troops with a contaminated yellow fever vaccine. The source of the contamination was human serum that had been added to the vaccine as a stabilizer. It had been prepared from an

HBV carrier, unfortunately. Also, malaria, diarrheal disease, and other infections were common in the troops during World War II. After the war, malaria was introduced into the United States.

During the Korean conflict, Korean hemorrhagic fever caused by Hantaan virus became a significant health problem among US Army troops. Many US soldiers serving near the demilitarized zone developed fever, hemorrhagic phenomenon, and renal failure. The cause of the disease was not discovered for another decade. In the Gulf War of 1993, visceral leishmaniasis due to *Leishmania tropica* occurred in US troops. During World War II, large epidemics of dengue were experienced by military troops and civilian populations in the South Pacific.

Civilian refugees who are displaced when fleeing political crisis in their homeland often are even more vulnerable than are military populations. Malnutrition, accompanied by outbreaks of cholera, shigellosis, and malaria, is frequent among refugees in tropical areas in Africa and Asia. The United Nations High Commission on Refugees estimates that there are currently over 16 million refugees and 5.4 million internally displaced persons throughout the world.[43] Many of these refugees are highly vulnerable to epidemics of infectious diseases.

Growth of Day Care for Infants and Children Outside the Home

In the last 30 years, more and more women with dependent infants and children have been employed full time outside the home. This includes single parents and families in which both parents work. Currently, over two thirds of women with children under 18 years of age are in the workforce.[44] This has necessitated a dramatic growth in the use of day-care facilities to care for preschool children. Clustering of children in day-care centers has facilitated the transmission of a number of infectious agents from one child to another, day-care staff, and, eventually, to others living in the households of children attending day care. Because many day-care centers have substantial populations of children in diapers, the transmission of pathogenic organisms by the fecal–oral route is facilitated. Infections from organisms such as rotavirus, *Giardia lamblia, Campylobacter jejuni, Shigella* species, and hepatitis A virus (HAV) have been transmitted in the day-care setting. In fact, a substantial change in the epidemiology of hepatitis A virus infections was reported in the late 1970s in Maricopa County (Phoenix), Arizona. A significant increase in patients with jaundice due to HAV infection was related to HAV transmission in day-care settings between children, which was subsequently spread to household contacts.[45] Outbreaks of HAV infections in day-care centers average 12 cases in size and last 3 months in duration.[46] Typically, young children are asymptomatic or have mild infections; adults in the household or the day-care center have more severe clinical illnesses. Outbreaks are more often associated with larger centers that accept children in diapers.

Infections spread by the respiratory route and by direct contact are also common among children attending day-care centers. It has been estimated that about 10 respiratory infections per year occur among children at the peak age for respiratory infections, i.e., the second 6 months of life.[47] Most respiratory infections are viral, but day care facilitates the transmission of some bacterial infections, as well.[47]

Recently, increased attention has been directed toward reducing the transmission of infections in day care by improved hand washing and disinfection of fomites, such as toys. Also, the development and licensure of new vaccines, including HAV, varicella, *Haemophilus influenzae* B, acellular pertussis, and *Streptococcus pneumoniae,* have allowed improved strategies for the prevention of some day-care infections. However, public health strategies of excluding infants and children with active infections have been difficult to implement successfully, due to economic pressures on parents to work.

Increase in Nursing Home Population

The increase in the elderly population in nursing homes has been another factor promoting the transmission of infectious agents. Not uncommonly, residents of nursing homes may be given antibiotics or be admitted to a hospital where they become infected or colonized with a nosocomial pathogen, such as staphylococci, enterococci, or gram-negative organisms that are resistant to multiple antibiotics. The population in nursing homes may be an important reservoir in the community for these nosocomial pathogens. Clearly, this population is at increased risk of infectious diseases due to declining immunity, limited mobility, and crowding in extended-care facilities.

Antibiotic Use and Abuse

An important selective force in the emergence of pathogenic microorganisms is the widespread use of antibiotics in both the human and animal populations. Antibiotics are used for the therapy and prophylaxis of infections in humans and animals and for growth promotion in domestic animals. A recent study of *C. jejuni* infections in Minnesota between 1992 and 1998 linked many human infections with quinolone-resistant organisms to the use of these effective antibiotics as a growth factor in chickens by the poultry industry.[32] This widespread practice, which began in the United States in 1995 and earlier in Mexico, led to the emergence of these difficult-to-treat infections in humans in only a few years.[33] This illustrates the need for ecologic and public health–based decision making in agricultural industries to avoid promoting the emergence of new antibiotic-resistant human pathogens. Some studies suggest that restriction of the use of antibiotics in clinical settings might sometimes favor the reemergence of an antibiotic-sensitive flora.[48] However, such strategies often are not entirely successful. This important topic is covered more completely in Chapter 14.

Bioterrorism

In the past few years, especially since the attack on the World Trade Center in New York on September 11, 2001, and the subsequent epidemic of anthrax transmitted through the postal system, bioterrorism has become a major public health concern in the United States. Surveillance systems have been designed to recognize the next episode as early as possible. Early medical responders, such as nurses, physicians, and other medical personnel working in emergency rooms throughout the United States, have been offered smallpox vaccine. Theoretically, they would likely be the first to see a case or cases and need protection. Intensive research has been funded by the National Institutes of Health to develop more effective vaccines or anti-infective agents to prevent or treat anthrax, smallpox, plague, tularemia, botulism, and other potential bioterrorism agents.

There have been a few documented intentional attacks on populations using biologic agents in the past. During the Revolutionary War in America, Indians were repeatedly given blankets intentionally contaminated with smallpox scabs containing variola virus in the hopes of causing disease in the recipients.[49] Although less well documented, it is likely that some form of biologic warfare was practiced by ancient civilizations. One such episode was the trebucheting (catapulting) of corpses of persons who had died of plague over the walls of the city of Caffa in the Crimea. A memoir by an Italian, Gabriel de Mussi, who was alive at the time, traces this event to the introduction of the Black Death.[50] Recently, a large community outbreak of salmonellosis in Oregon was found to be due to the intentional contamination of salad bars in multiple restaurants by followers of Bhagwan Shree Rajneesh, with the purpose of influencing the local election, whose results could have affected the group.[51] Interestingly, intentional precipitation of an epidemic was not suspected or proven until nearly a year after its occurrence in this episode.

Prior to the occurrence of the epidemic of anthrax transmitted via the postal service, it was commonly feared by most experts that when an attack came it would be with *Bacillus anthracis* (anthrax) spores. The most commonly stated scenario was a bioterrorist dropping a vial of anthrax spores in a crowded area with a recirculating air supply, such as a subway in a large city. In fact, what really happened was perhaps even more devastating in a way, because the attacks continued and were geographically diffuse. Anthrax spores were sent through the mail to persons throughout the United States, including several United States senators, newscasters, and others. This resulted in five deaths and 22 cases of anthrax, but also several large postal facilities and public buildings were contaminated with *B. anthracis* spores and had to be decontaminated at considerable expense. Occupants of the buildings experienced a great deal of anxiety as to whether decontamination had been complete when the buildings were reopened.

Large numbers of persons were given prophylactic Ciprofloxacin based on a possible exposure. An analysis of the outbreak concluded that the antibiotic prophylaxis probably was effective in preventing 40 additional cases of anthrax.[52] The episode accomplished its goal of instilling deep concerns, even panic, as to where and when the next letter containing anthrax would appear and who was the enemy. Although the attacks soon stopped, the culprit(s) have still not been identified or apprehended. This episode has instilled fear as to when the next biologic attack would occur, with which organism, and where.

To plan for and detect the next biologic attack early or to limit the morbidity and mortality as much as possible, federal and local public health officials and other scientists have developed plans for research, detection, and response to outbreaks. Substantial federal funds have been provided for the effort to prevent, detect, and respond to another bioterrorist attack.

Prioritizing Bioterrorism Candidates

The possibility of a biologic attack on the United States population had been considered and feared a few years before the World Trade Center attack on September 11, 2001. The fear that a bioterrorism attack might actually occur increased considerably after learning that Iraq had prepared large stockpiles of biologic weapons, especially anthrax, and that bioweapons were used in the war with Iran and to quell a Kurdish uprising. Of even greater concern were the reports of a defector from the Soviet Union, who reported that the Soviet military had developed a major industry to test and produce biologic weapons, including smallpox, plague, anthrax, and other agents, during the 1960s through 1980s.[53] The massive size and scope of the Russian program could allow significant dispersal of bioweapons that were ready to be used to other states or dissident groups, as well.

In 1999, the Congress designated the Centers for Disease Control and Prevention (CDC) as the lead agency for overall public health planning to combat bioterrorism. The CDC has worked with many other governmental and nongovernmental agencies to develop plans to deal with bioterrorism.

In June 1999, the CDC convened a group of experts to develop a list of possible agents that might be used in a terrorist attack.[54] Organisms were placed in three categories based on the following criteria: (1) public health import based on morbidity and mortality, (2) ability to deliver the agent plus secondary person-to-person transmission, (3) public perceptions and fear, and (4) special needs to deal with an attack, such as vaccine, drugs to treat illness, and surveillance needs. Opinions and data collected by the military, the biologic weapons convention list of WHO, and other sources were consulted to develop a list of possible agents to consider and rank into three categories: category A for agents of greatest potential, category B for agents that posed a significant threat but with less serious outcomes, and category C for other possible agents.

The final classification placed 6 organisms in category A and another 10 organisms or groups of organisms into category B (Table 13-2). The criteria used to classify the organisms according to their utility as a bioweapon are shown in Table 13-3. These criteria include potential to cause disease and/or death, potential to produce and disseminate the agent widely, person-to-person transmissibility, public perceptions, and requirement for public health preparedness for prevention.

The Anthrax Epidemic of 2001

On October 4, 2001, the first bioterrorism-related anthrax case in the United States was identified in Florida.[55] The patient was a 63-year-old man who worked in a national newspaper printing office. He became ill with a febrile illness that progressed to vomiting, confusion, and incoherent speech within 2 days. Large numbers of *Bacillus anthracis* organisms were seen on the GRAM stain of his spinal fluid. Among 1076 nasal cultures obtained from his coworkers, two persons, a coworker and a mail handler, were found to be positive. Environmental samples were positive for anthrax spores at his workplace and at six county postal facilities. All of the 1076 workers at this news publishing company were offered prophylactic treatment with Ciprofloxacin, and no other clinical illnesses occurred among them.

TABLE 13-2   Bioterrorism Agents and Diseases

- **Category A (See definition in Table 13-3)**
- **Anthrax** (*Bacillus anthracis*)
- **Botulism** (*Clostridium botulinum* toxin)
- **Plague** (*Yersinia pestis*)
- **Smallpox** (variola major)
- **Tularemia** (*Francisella tularensis*)
- **Viral hemorrhagic fevers** (filoviruses [e.g., Ebola, Marburg] and arenaviruses [e.g., Lassa, Machupo])
- **Category B (See definition in Table 13-3)**
- **Brucellosis** (*Brucella* species)
- Epsilon toxin of *Clostridium perfringens*
- **Food safety threats** (e.g., *Salmonella* species, *Escherichia coli* O157:H7, *Shigella*)
- Glanders (*Burkholderia mallei*)
- Melioidosis (*Burkholderia pseudomallei*)
- Psittacosis (*Chlamydia psittaci*)
- **Q fever** (*Coxiella burnetii*)
- **Ricin toxin** from *Ricinus communis* (castor beans)
- Staphylococcal enterotoxin B
- Typhus fever (*Rickettsia prowazekii*)
- Viral encephalitis (alphaviruses [e.g., Venezuelan equine encephalitis, eastern equine encephalitis, western equine encephalitis])
- Water safety threats (e.g., *Vibrio cholerae*, *Cryptosporidium parvum*)
- **Category C (See definition in Table 13-3)**
- Emerging infectious diseases such as Nipah virus and hantavirus

Source: http://www.bt.cdc.gov/agent/agentlist-category.asp

After the recognition of the case in Florida and the convincing evidence that the infections occurred because an envelope containing anthrax spores was mailed to the newspaper office, the CDC began a nationwide investigation to find additional cases. After a comprehensive investigation involving thousands of public health and criminal justice personnel a total of 22 cases of anthrax with five deaths were identified among persons living in seven states in the eastern United States.[56]

The cases occurred in two clusters from envelopes mailed from Trenton, New Jersey (Figure 13-4). The first envelopes were postmarked September 18, 2001, and the second batch was postmarked on October 9, 2001. Each envelope contained a letter referring to the September 11 World Trade Center attacks, such as "09-11-01. You can not stop us, we have this anthrax. You die now. Are you afraid?"

The envelopes went through various US postal facilities and mail-sorting machines before they were delivered. Letters had been mailed to America Media, Inc., in Florida, to Tom Brokaw at Columbia Broadcasting System in New York, to the American Broadcasting Company in New York, the

TABLE 13-3   Category Definitions

Category A Diseases/Agents

The US public health system and primary health care providers must be prepared to address various biologic agents, including pathogens that are rarely seen in the United States. High-priority agents include organisms that pose a risk to national security because they can do the following:

- Be easily disseminated or transmitted from person to person
- Result in high mortality rates and have the potential for major public health impact
- Cause public panic and social disruption
- Require special action for public health preparedness

Category B Diseases/Agents

Second highest priority agents include those that do the following:

- Are moderately easy to disseminate
- Result in moderate morbidity rates and low mortality rates
- Require specific enhancements of CDC's diagnostic capacity and enhanced disease surveillance

Category C Diseases/Agents

Third highest priority agents include emerging pathogens that could be engineered for mass dissemination in the future because of the following:

- Availability
- Ease of production and dissemination
- Potential for high morbidity and mortality rates and major health impact

Source: http://www.bt.cdc.gov/agent/agentlist-category.asp

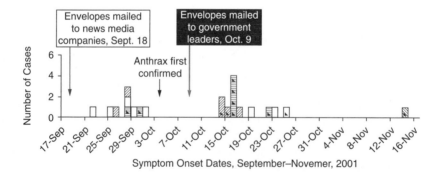

FIGURE 13-4   Epidemic curve for 22 cases of bioterrorism-related anthrax, United States, 2001.
Source: Jernigan DB et al. Investigation of bioterrorism-related anthrax, United States, 2001: epidemiologic findings. *Emerg Infect Dis.* 2002 Oct;8(10):1019–28.

National Broadcasting Company in New York, offices of the *New York Post*, and Senators Tom Dashle and Patrick Leahy at the Senate office building in Washington, DC.

Twelve anthrax patients (55%) were mail handlers, including 9 US Postal Service employees, one government mail processing staffmember, and 2 media company mailroom workers. Eight of these workers developed inhalational anthrax and 4 developed cutaneous anthrax (Table 13-4).

Among the 11 persons who developed inhalational anthrax 5 died (45%); there were no deaths among the 11 persons with cutaneous anthrax. One case of inhalational anthrax occurred in a 94-year-old female who lived in Oxford, Connecticut; the onset of her disease was on November 14, 2001, a couple of weeks after the last cluster of cases (Figure 13-4).[57] No anthrax spores were identified at her home, but *B. anthracis* spores were identified at the US Postal Service center in Wallingford, Connecticut. This postal facility received mail from the contaminated postal facility in Hamilton, New Jersey. This case has been explained as being caused by cross-contamination in the mail distribution system.

The median number of days from the postmark date in the first cluster was 10 days (range 4–13 days). The illness onset of all of the cases in the first cluster occurred prior to the recognition of *B. anthracis* in the cerebrospinal fluid of the Florida case. The second case cluster began approximately 5 days after the envelopes had been mailed. Starting on October 15 nasal swab specimens were obtained from 625 persons potentially exposed to the letters at the Hart Senate office building in Washington, DC, and 28 were found to be positive for anthrax.[56] Environmental sampling from the Hart Senate office building and the Brentwood postal facility found both buildings to be heavily contaminated with *B. anthracis* spores. Also at least 25 other government postal or mail-receiving facilities affiliated with Brentwood had environmental samples positive for anthrax spores. Some of these facilities did not receive the implicated envelopes but processed other mail from Brentwood. Eventually both the Brentwood postal facility and the Hart Senate office building were closed and underwent decontamination using chlorine gas. Mail handled by critical US Postal Service facilities was irradiated in an attempt to disinfect it in several key postal facilities in the Washington, DC, area. Overall, an estimated 32,000 persons instituted postexposure antibiotic prophylaxis, and 10,300 persons were recommended to complete a 60-day course of antibiotics following exposure or possible exposure to contaminated aerosols.

B. anthracis isolates were obtained from four powder-containing envelopes, 17 clinical specimens from cases, and 106 environmental samples. All had identical antibiotic sensitivities and were identical genetically by multiple-locus variable-number tandem repeat analysis (MLVA).[58,59]

Issues Raised and Lessons Learned from This Outbreak

- *B. anthracis* is a very effective biologic terrorism agent.
- The US mail is an effective system to distribute a biologic weapon like anthrax anonymously. These cases occurred from sending only five contaminated letters through the mail.

TABLE 13-4   Demographic, Clinical, and Exposure Characteristics of 22 Cases of Bioterrorism-Related Anthrax, United States, 2001

Case No.	Onset Date, 2001	Date of Anthrax Diagnosis by Lab Testing	State[a]	Age (yrs)	Sex	Race	Occupation	Case Status	Anthrax Presentation	Outcome	Diagnostic Tests
1	9/22	10/19	NY	31	F	W	*NY Post* employee	Suspect	Cutaneous	Alive	Serum IgG reactive
2	9/25	10/12	NY	38	F	W	NBC anchor assistant	Confirmed	Cutaneous	Alive	Skin biopsy IHC+/ serum IgG reactive
3	9/26	10/18	NJ	39	M	W	USPS machine mechanic	Suspect	Cutaneous	Alive	Serum IgG reactive
4	9/28	10/15	FL	73	M	W, H	AMI mailroom worker	Confirmed	Inhalational	Alive	Pleural biopsy IHC+/ serum IgG reactive
5	9/28	10/18	NJ	45	F	W	USPS mail carrier	Confirmed	Cutaneous	Alive	Skin biopsy IHC+ and PCR+/ serum IgG reactive
6	9/28	10/12	NY	23	F	W	NBC TV news intern	Suspect	Cutaneous	Alive	Serum IgG reactive

continued

TABLE 13-4   continued

Case No.	Onset Date, 2001	Date of Anthrax Diagnosis by Lab Testing	State[a]	Age (yrs)	Sex	Race	Occupation	Case Status	Anthrax Presentation	Outcome	Diagnostic Tests
7	9/29	10/15	NY	0.6	M	W	Child of ABC employee	Confirmed	Cutaneous	Alive	Skin biopsy IHC+ / blood PCR+
8	9/30	10/4	FL	63	M	W	AMI photo editor	Confirmed	Inhalational	Dead	Cerebrospinal fluid culture +
9	10/1	10/18	NY	27	F	W	CBS anchor assistant	Confirmed	Cutaneous	Alive	Skin biopsy IHC+ / serum IgG reactive
10	10/14	10/19	PA	35	M	W	USPS mail processor	Confirmed	Cutaneous	Alive	Blood culture +/serum IgG reactive
11	10/14	10/28	NJ	56	F	B	USPS mail processor	Confirmed	Inhalational	Alive	Blood PCR+ / pleural fluid cytology IHC+ / serum IgG reactive
12	10/15	10/29	NJ	43	F	A	USPS mail processor	Confirmed	Inhalational	Alive	Pleural fluid IHC+ / bronchial biopsy IHC+/ serum IgG reactive

continued

TABLE 13-4 continued

Case No.	Onset Date, 2001	Date of Anthrax Diagnosis by Lab Testing	State[a]	Age (yrs)	Sex	Race	Occupation	Case Status	Anthrax Presentation	Outcome	Diagnostic Tests
13	10/16	10/21	VA	56	M	B	USPS mail worker	Confirmed	Inhalational	Alive	Blood culture +
14	10/16	10/23	MD	55	M	B	USPS mail worker	Confirmed	Inhalational	Dead	Blood culture +
15	10/16	10/26	MD	47	M	B	USPS mail worker	Confirmed	Inhalational	Dead	Blood culture +
16	10/16	10/22	MD	56	M	B	USPS mail worker	Confirmed	Inhalational	Alive	Blood culture +
17	10/17	10/29	NJ	51	F	W	Bookkeeper	Confirmed	Cutaneous	Alive	Skin biopsy IHC+ and PCR+ / serum IgG reactive
18	10/19	10/22	NY	34	M	W, H	NY Post mail handler	Suspect	Cutaneous	Alive	Skin biopsy IHC+
19	10/22	10/25	VA	59	M	W	Government mail processor	Confirmed	Inhalational	Alive	Blood culture +
20	10/23	10/28	NY	38	M	W	NY Post employee	Confirmed	Cutaneous	Alive	Skin biopsy culture +
21	10/25	10/30	NY	61	F	A	Hospital supply worker	Confirmed	Inhalational	Dead	Pleural fluid and blood culture +
22	11/14	11/21	CT	94	F	W	Retired at home	Confirmed	Inhalational	Dead	Blood culture +

Source: Jernigan DB et al. Investigation of bioterrorism-related anthrax, United States, 2001: epidemiologic findings. Emerg Infect Dis. 2002 Oct;8(10):1019–28.
Race: W = white, B = black, H = Hispanic, A = Asiar

- Anthrax spores can penetrate sealed unopened letters, making it difficult to gauge who has had a significant exposure.
- Postexposure antibiotic prophylaxis is likely to have been effective, but it probably needs to be continued for 60 days because of delayed germination of anthrax spores after they are inhaled in some cases.[52,60] None of 28 Capitol Hill employees who were given antibiotics because of positive nasal swabs after exposure to an opened envelope containing *B. anthracis* spores developed clinical disease or antibodies to anthrax protective antigen. Reaerosolization of anthrax spores in buildings can occur, so effective disinfection of buildings is mandatory before they are reoccupied. More knowledge about how to disinfect buildings is needed.
- Cross-contamination of the mail from unopened letters containing anthrax spores is possible. The risk is low, but cross-contamination can occur.
- The efficacy of the existing licensed vaccine in the prevention of inhalation anthrax is unknown, although it is probably somewhat effective. However, a more effective vaccine is needed that can elicit a protective immune response quickly and with fewer doses; immunization with the current licensed vaccine requires six doses.
- Despite extensive criminal investigation, the perpetrator has not been found. Current use of bioterrorism is more likely to be done or directed by dissident small groups or carried out by unbalanced individuals, rather than by an army or state during warfare, as in the past. This likely will make it more difficult to prevent and to find the perpetrator after it has occurred.

Other Emerging Infectious Diseases

In addition to the infectious diseases that have emerged as opportunistic pathogens in patients with HIV-related immunosuppression and AIDS, other infections have emerged in recent years because of factors favoring the increased exposure or susceptibility of human populations to infectious agents, which have been reviewed above. Several examples of recent experiences with specific emerging infectious diseases and some of the factors promoting their emergence will be reviewed.

Severe Acute Respiratory Syndrome (SARS)

The best example of the emergence of a new infectious disease among humans since the emergence of AIDS in the early 1980s is the SARS epidemic of 2003.[61,62] In contrast to other infections like Dengue or tuberculosis, which have reemerged in the past couple of decades, or West Nile virus or monkey pox, which have spread to a new area, the first cases of SARS among humans occurred in 2003.

Evolution of the Epidemic

In November 2002, an outbreak of an unusually severe atypical pneumonia occurred in Foshan, Guangdong Province, China. In January 2003, the outbreak spread to Guangzhou, the capital city of the province. In February 2003, Chinese authorities reported to WHO that the outbreak included 305 cases with five deaths. Initially, WHO was concerned that the epidemic might be caused by the H5N1 strain of influenza, which had caused human respiratory infections with a high mortality rate in Hong Kong a few years earlier among persons having contact with poultry at live markets.

On February 21, 2003, a 65-year-old physician checked into "Hotel M" in Hong Kong. He had been ill for 6 days and had traveled to Hong Kong from Guangdong province. The following day his health deteriorated, and he was admitted to a hospital in Hong Kong. While in the hotel, he transmitted his infection to 13 other guests and visitors in the hotel (Figure 13-5). The hotel guests had no direct contact with the index patient.[63] On February 26, a former guest at Hotel M became ill and was admitted to a hospital in Hanoi; he was the source of an outbreak that included seven health care workers. A

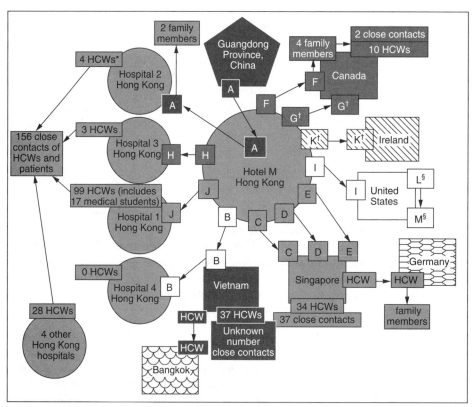

* Health care workers.
† All guests except G and K stayed on the 9th floor of the hotel. Guest G stayed on the 14th floor, and Guest K stayed on the 11th floor.
§ Guests L and M (spouses) were not at Hotel M during the same time as index Guest A but were at the hotel during the same times as Guests G, H, and I, who were ill during this period.

FIGURE 13-5 Chain of transmission among guests at Hotel M—Hong Kong, 2003.
Source: Update: Outbreak of Severe Acute Respiratory Syndrome—Worldwide, 2003. MMWR Weekly. March 28, 2003 / 52(12);241–248.

physician working with WHO in Vietnam, Dr. Carlo Urbani, acquired SARS in Vietnam and died a few days later in a Bangkok hospital.[64] Subsequently, cases were reported from Singapore and Toronto among former guests at the hotel during the index patient's stay.[65,66] Eventually the SARS epidemic spread to many other countries throughout the world when travelers from the epidemic countries in Asia returned home.[67-69]

When patients with SARS were hospitalized for treatment, there were some instances of extensive spread of the disease to medical personnel, other patients, and visitors.[65,69-71] One patient who was infected when he was a hotel guest at Hotel M was admitted to the Prince of Wales hospital in Hong Kong on March 4 after being ill since February 24.[71,72] During his hospitalization, he transmitted SARS to 47 health care workers on the ward to which he was admitted. SARS developed in all but one of the 16 nurses and all 6 physicians on the ward. In addition, other health workers, medical students, and patients became ill. There were an estimated 112 secondary cases and 26 tertiary cases in this outbreak. These cases included 20 doctors, 34 nurses, 15 allied health workers, and 16 medical students, as well as 53 patients or visitors to the same ward as the patient.

A more detailed study of the exposures leading to SARS was done among 66 medical students who visited the ward during the patients' hospitalization.[71] These exposures occurred prior to the diagnosis of SARS in the index patient and his isolation. Among the students who remembered entering the patient's cubicle, 10 developed SARS; 4 of 18 students who couldn't remember whether or not they entered the cubicle became ill, and only 1 of 20 students who didn't enter the cubicle developed SARS. None of the remaining 268 medical students who didn't enter the patient's ward developed SARS.

Students were assigned to examine patients on the ward on March 6 and 7. Among 19 students who spent about 40 minutes examining patients on the ward, all 3 students who examined patients in beds adjacent to the index patient developed SARS. Four of 8 students who examined patients in the same cubicle (but who were not in adjacent beds to the index patient) and none of 8 students who examined patients in other cubicles became ill with SARS (Fishers exact test, $P = .003$). These data suggest that, despite the very large number of secondary cases related to this hospitalized index case, fairly close contact may have been required in order for transmission to occur. This episode also illustrates the potential for very widespread transmission of SARS-CoV when the disease is not recognized and the patient not effectively isolated in a busy modern hospital.

The World Health Organization responded quickly to this pandemic and organized a network of international laboratories and a surveillance system to evaluate and control the disease. In late March and early April 2003, laboratories in Germany, Hong Kong, Canada, and the CDC identified the agent as the SARS coronavirus, a newly discovered human pathogen that was unrelated to other known human coronaviruses (Figure 13-6).[73-76] Intensive epidemiologic studies subsequently isolated the SARS coronavirus (SARS-CoV) from civet cats in Guangdong Province; about 13% of workers in "wet markets" in China that sell live civet cats and other exotic species of animals were found to be seropositive for SARS-CoV.[77] Among animal traders, the highest prevalence of antibody (72.7%) was found in those who traded primarily in masked palm civets.[77] Another study reported the isolation of SARS-CoV from four Himalayan civets and a raccoon dog and neutralizing antibodies from 40% of wild animal traders in the market.[78]

Although patients with clinical symptoms of SARS seroconverted to SARS-CoV, healthy contacts and controls from the areas of epidemic spread remained seronegative. Subclinical infections were rarely documented. After the implementation of public health control measures to isolate cases and quarantine contacts of SARS patients, the last case of SARS in this epidemic was reported in Taiwan on July 5, 2003. WHO declared the end of the SARS pandemic when no further cases occurred among the contacts of this case after more than two incubation periods (i.e., 20 days) had passed. However, during the SARS pandemic over 8450 persons became ill and 850 died in 26 countries on five continents. This was a devastating pandemic.

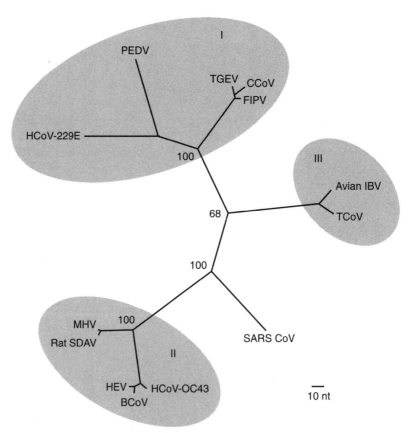

FIGURE 13-6 Estimated maximum-parsimony tree based on the sequence alignment of 405 nucleotides of the coronavirus polymerase gene open reading frame 1b (nucleotide numbers 15173 to 15578 based on bovine coronavirus complete genome accession number NC_003045) comparing SARS coronavirus with other human and animal coronaviruses.
Source: Ksiazek et al. A Novel Coronavirus Associated with Severe Acute Respiratory Syndrome. NEJM. Volume 348:1953–1966. Copyright 2003 by the Massachusetts Medical Society.

Hong Kong Epidemic

The epidemic in Hong Kong involved 1755 cases, of which 302 (17.2%) patients died, between February 15 and May 31, 2003 (Figure 13-7).[79] Hong Kong was also the critical link between the earlier outbreak in Guangdong Province and the subsequent global spread of the disease. The cases in Hong Kong were especially well studied, and SARS-CoV was identified either by reverse transcriptase polymerase chain reaction (RT-PCR) of serum, respiratory secretions, or stool samples or by antibody testing from 83.6% of the reported cases. The Hong Kong cases were carefully studied in detail in order to document the clinical and epidemiologic characteristics of the disease.[79,80] This investigation found that:

- The mean incubation period was 6.4 days; 95% of patients became symptomatic within 12.5 days of infection.
- Most cases clustered in hospitals, clinics, nursing homes, and residential buildings; 23.1% of cases occurred in health care workers, most of whom were nurses. A large outbreak of over 300 cases occurred in one large housing complex: the Amoy Gardens (see detailed description below).
- There was a relative deficit of children and adolescents but an excess of elderly persons (older than 75 years of age) among the cases (Figure 13-8). In the SARS outbreak in Beijing, only 23 (0.9%) of 2521 cases occurred in children under 10 years old.[81]
- The first generation RT-PCR assay was positive in only 54% of cases[82]; however, a second-generation nested RT-PCR assay was positive in 88% of respiratory specimens obtained during the first 3 days of illness.[83]

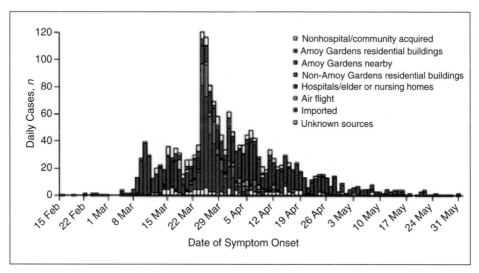

FIGURE 13-7   Severe acute respiratory syndrome epidemic curve in Hong Kong, 2003, by infection cluster.
Source: Leung GM. Epidemiology of Severe Acute Respiratory Syndrome in the 2003 Hong Kong Epidemic: An Analysis of All 1755 Patients. Ann Intern Med. Volume 141 Issue 9 | Pages 662–673.

- The peak rate of RT-PCR positivity occurred 9–11 days after the first symptoms (Figure 13-8), and gastrointestinal specimens gave higher yields of viral RNA than respiratory specimens. The delay in the peak viral load and the common absence of pneumonia or early definitive respiratory symptoms could have increased the risk of transmission in the hospital because of a false negative screening test and misdiagnosis.

- No transmission was documented to have occurred from infected patients prior to the onset of symptoms.

Amoy Gardens Epidemic

One of the most dramatic outbreaks of SARS occurred among residents of the Amoy Gardens housing complex in Hong Kong. A patient recovering from SARS visited the Amoy Gardens housing complex unit 7 on a middle floor in building E on March 14 and again on March 19. The patient, who had chronic renal disease, stayed with his brother. He had diarrhea and used the toilet on both days. This housing complex includes 7 buildings with 36 floors each and 8 apartments on each floor (Figure 13-9). Subsequently, an epidemic of SARS occurred among the residents of the Amoy Gardens, which eventually included 330 persons living in the complex and 128 persons who lived in other nearby buildings.[84] Overall the Amoy Gardens outbreak accounted for 26.1% of the 1755 SARS cases in Hong Kong (Figure 13-9).

The cases of SARS that occurred in the Amoy Gardens appeared to be a large common source outbreak initially with some subsequent person-to-person spread (Figure 13-10). The outbreak peaked on March 24 and most new cases occurred between March 24 and 26; the last case occurred in

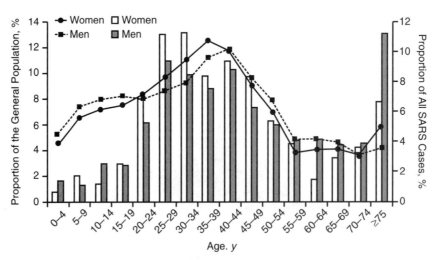

FIGURE 13-8   Age and sex distributions of patients with severe acute respiratory syndrom (SARS) compared with the Hong Kong general population. The solid and dotted lines refer to the proportion of the general population, and the bars refer to the proportion of all SARS cases.
Source: Leung GM. The Epidemiology of Severe Acute Respiratory Syndrome in the 2003 Hong Kong Epidemic: An Analysis of All 1755 Patients. Ann Inter Med. Volume 141 Issue 9 | Pages 662–673.

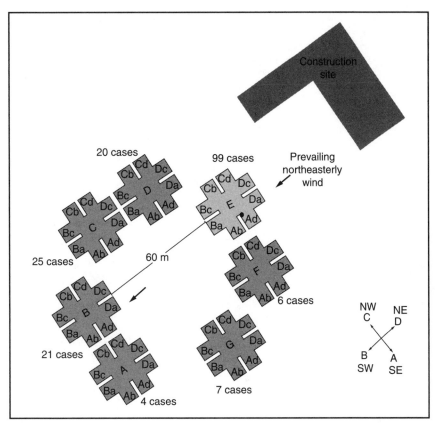

FIGURE 13-9 Distribution of cases of SARS infection in buildings A to G in the Amoy Gardens housing estate. The prevailing wind (arrows) during the period of possible exposure was northeasterly, or roughly perpendicular to the exterior walls of apartment units Dc and Da in building E. The distance between buildings E and B is 60 m. The direction from which the wind blew shifted from nearly north to east and even southeast. The dot in building E indicates the unit that the index patient visited. The directional indicator for the units at the lower righthand corner indicates the direction each unit faced. In the directional code (Ab, Ad, Ba, Bc, Cb, Cd, Da, Dc) used to designate an apartment unit, uppercase letters denote front-facing windows and lowercase letters side-facing windows.
Source: Yu, IT. Evidence of Airborne Transmission of the Severe Acute Respiratory Syndrome Virus. N Engl J Med. 2004 Apr 22;350(17):1731–9. Copyright 2004 by the Massachusetts Medical Society.

mid-April. More than half of the initial 187 cases occurred in building E (99 cases), but cases also occurred among the residents of each of the 7 buildings in the complex (Figure 13-9). However, the greatest proportion of cases occurred among persons living on the upper floors and in those living in other buildings in apartments facing building E. The wind direction was northeasterly during the time of the outbreak, which would have blown an infectious aerosol from building E toward the other buildings in the complex. The bathrooms in the complex were aligned vertically with an exhaust fan and a soil stack outside the bathrooms. Traps in the floor drains, which should have been filled with water, had often dried out allowing air from

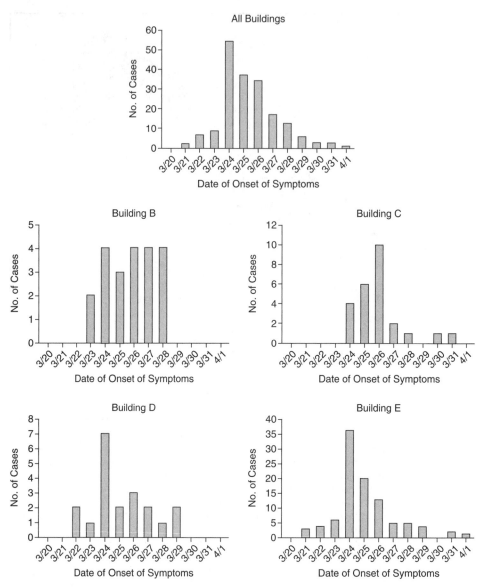

FIGURE 13-10 Epidemic curves for all buildings and for buildings B, C, D, and E. *Source:* Yu, IT. Evidence of Airborne Transmission of the Severe Acute Respiratory Syndrome Virus. N Engl J Med. 2004 Apr 22;350(17):1731–9. Copyright 2004 by the Massachusetts Medical Society.

the soil stack readily to enter and leave the bathrooms. An infectious aerosol containing the virus could have been generated when the toilet was flushed. This aerosol could have exited the apartment out the soil stack and entered other apartments above the index case through the vent. The infectious aerosol could have exited building E and traveled to other buildings in the complex that were downwind, resulting in infections in the residents of other buildings of the complex. Analysis and confirmation of this possible scenario was done using computational fluid-dynamics modeling and other modeling methods.[84] This outbreak, and a few other clusters of cases, emphasize the potential for extensive spread of SARS infection by airborne spread under some circumstances, even though most transmission probably occurred by close contact with an infectious case from droplet transmission.

The Singapore SARS Outbreak

The epidemic of SARS in Singapore followed closely that in Hong Kong. On March 6, 2003, the Singapore Ministry of Health (MOH) was notified that three persons who had traveled to Hong Kong in February had been admitted to local hospitals for treatment of pneumonia. They had been guests at Hotel M in Hong Kong on February 20 and 21, coinciding with the stay of the index case, previously described. On March 14, the MOH was notified about six persons, including two health care workers, who were admitted to a local hospital after having had close contract with the first case in the traveler index case.

In the ensuing Singapore outbreak there were five SARS patients who were identified as "superspreaders," meaning that they had transmitted the infection to 10 or more persons (Figures 13-11 and 13-12). Most of these cases resulted in continued transmission of the virus to one or more secondary cases and an expanded chain of cases. The secondary cases did not also become superspreaders. Generally, the infected contacts spread the virus to only one or two persons (Figure 13-11). This suggests that severe illness in these superspreaders (with excretion of large amounts of virus, coupled with delayed recognition of the infection) rather than an increase in infectivity of the virus probably was responsible for these large clusters. In contrast to these large clusters, 81% of SARS cases did not result in transmission to any of their contacts (Figure 13-13).

Spread of SARS due to delayed diagnosis of infection was characteristic of the last three superspreaders in the Singapore outbreak. Case 3 was a 53-year-old with diabetes and ischemic heart disease who was admitted to a hospital in March with a diagnosis of polymicrobial sepsis with diarrhea. He was not isolated on March 20, and he died on March 29. He was directly linked to probable SARS in 23 persons (18 health care workers and 5 family members and visitors). Case number 4 had chronic kidney disease, diabetes, and gastrointestinal bleeding and developed *E. coli* bacteremia. Case number 5 had ischemic heart disease with congestive heart failure. These other medical conditions caused a delay in the diagnosis of SARS and led to the spread of SARS to a total of 62 persons (Figure 13-12).

The occasional superspreaders played a major role in the propagation of the SARS outbreak and were involved in each of the cities that had large outbreaks. It was found that 71.1% and 74.8% of SARS cases were attributable to superspreaders in Hong Kong and Singapore, respectively.[85] Superspreaders of SARS also played a major role in transmission of SARS-CoV in the Beijing outbreak.[70]

The Toronto Outbreak

The largest outbreak of SARS in North America occurred in Toronto, Canada; between February 23, 2003, and June 8, 2003, a total of 225 patients were

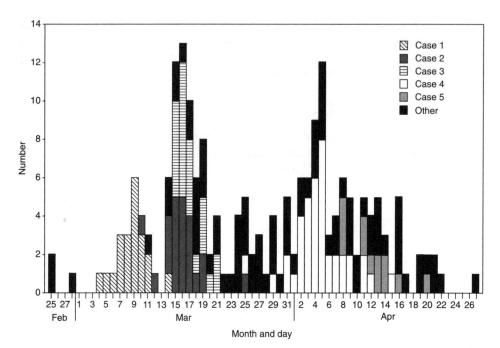

FIGURE 13-11 Number of probable cases of severe acute respiratory syndrome, by date of fever onset and reported source of infection—Singapore, February 25–April 30, 2003. *Source:* Severe Acute Respiratory Syndrome—Singapore, 2003. MMWR Weekly. 52(18);405–411.

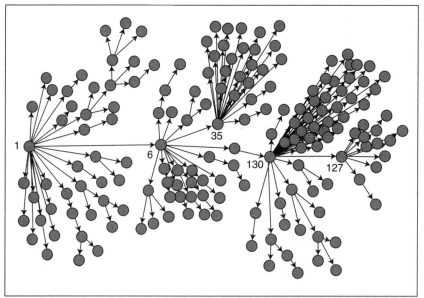

* Patient 1 represents Case 1; Patient 6, Case 2; Patient 35, Case 3; Patient 130, Case 4; and Patient 127, Case 5. Excludes 22 cases with either no or poorly defined direct contacts or who were cases translocated to Singapore and the seven contacts of one of these cases.
Reference: Bogatti SP. Netdraw 1.0 Network Visualization Software. Harvard, Massachusetts: Analytic Technologies, 2002.

FIGURE 13-12 Probable cases of severe acute respiratory syndrome, by reported source of infection—Singapore, February 25–April 30, 2003. *Source:* Severe Acute Respiratory Syndrome—Singapore, 2003. MMWR Weekly. 52(18);405–411.

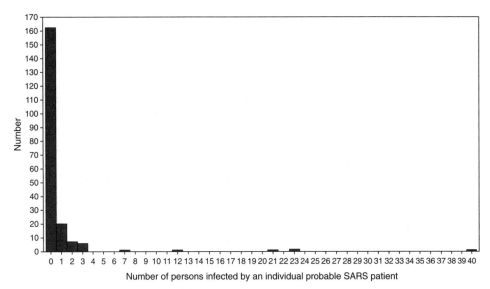

FIGURE 13-13 Number of reported secondary cases from probable cases of severe acute respiratory syndrome, Singapore, February 25–April 30, 2003.
Source: Severe Acute Respiratory Syndrome—Singapore, 2003. MMWR Weekly. 52(18);405–411.

diagnosed as having SARS (Figure 13-15). However, the Toronto Public Health Department investigated 2132 potential cases of SARS and identified 23,103 contacts of SARS patients who required quarantine.[86,87] The epidemic in Toronto was linked to a woman who returned from Hong Kong on February 23 and had stayed in the same hotel (Hotel M) as the index case in the Hong Kong outbreak. She became severely ill and died at home on March 5, 2003. Her son developed severe respiratory illness and was admitted to a hospital on March 7 and died on March 13. Four other family members became febrile and developed abnormal chest radiographs. All were admitted to three different hospitals on March 13. On March 12, the World Health Organization alerted the global community to a severe respiratory outbreak in Hanoi, Vietnam, and Hong Kong that was spreading to other countries.

Subsequently all except three travel-related cases were linked by chains of transmission from the index case. Most of the spread occurred either in hospitals or in household contacts of SARS cases. Only 20 cases were acquired in the community outside of a hospital or household contact with a case. However, transmission of the virus occurred in 11 (58%) of the acute care hospitals in Toronto.[87]

One unique feature of the Toronto epidemic was that it was bimodal, with a cluster of 128 probable or suspect cases occurring between February 23, 2003, and April 20, 2003, and then the number of cases declined dramatically.[87] This was followed by another cluster of cases occurring between April 27, 2003, and June 8, 2003, which peaked on about May 25, 2003 (Figure 13-14).

On April 23, 2003, the World Health Organization issued an advisory against travel to Toronto and Beijing. The advisory for Toronto was lifted on

April 30, but it had a profound economic impact on the business community and tourism industry.[87] Rigorous infection control procedures were imposed in all ICUs in Toronto area hospitals, and infectious SARS cases were isolated and their contacts quarantined for 10 days, the outer limit of the incubation period. In response to these public health measures the number of cases declined after April 10, 2003. In early May 2003, the Department of Public Health declared that the epidemic was over.

However, soon thereafter the numbers of cases increased again. After the decreased number of cases was recognized in early and mid-April in one hospital rigorous infection control procedures established to control the outbreak were relaxed on the general wards of the hospital, although they were kept in place in the ICU and Emergency Department. Staff were no longer required to wear masks or respirators, except in high-risk areas and when caring for known SARS patients.

On May 20, five patients in a rehabilitation hospital in Toronto were reported with febrile respiratory illness. Two patients had been hospitalized on an orthopedic ward at hospital A; one was found to be positive for SARS CO-V nucleic acid. Subsequently, eight additional patients with previously unrecognized SARS from the general wards of hospital A were recognized. The index case was a 96-year-old man who was admitted to the hospital on March 22 with a fractured pelvis. On April 2, he was transferred to the orthopedic ward with a fever and an infiltrate on a chest radiograph. However, he had had no known contact with a SARS patient, and his condition appeared to respond initially to antibiotic treatment. He also had *Clostridium difficile*-associated diarrhea. However, subsequently 78 new cases of SARS occurred among hospital staff, other patients, and visitors. On May 23, the hospital was closed to all new admissions other than patients with SARS, an increased level of infection control was reinstituted, and health care workers were placed on a 10-day work quarantine. These procedures

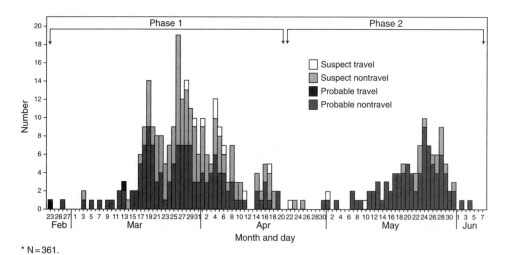

* N = 361.

FIGURE 13-14 Number of reported cases of severe acute respiratory syndrome, by classification and date of illness onset—Ontario, February 23–July 7, 2003.
Source: Update: Severe Acute Respiratory Syndrome—Toronto, Canada, 2003. 52(23);547–550.

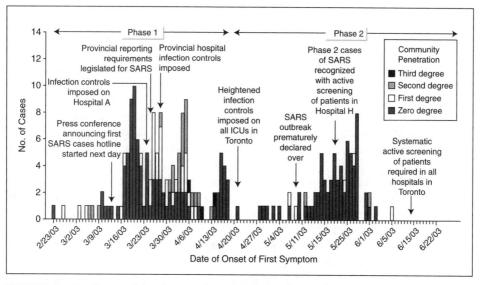

FIGURE 13-15   Onset of SARS in residents of Toronto in relation to the implementation of control measures. The onset of the last case of SARS in Toronto that was not travel-related was on June 8, 2003. The World Health Organization designated Toronto as a region not affected by SARS 20 days after a case with an onset on June 12, 2003, outside of Toronto. Community penetration quantifies the extent of transmission beyond the hospital or travel-related setting, and the levels are as follows: zero degree (cases that were related to travel or patients who were exposed in the hospital), first degree (cases among household contacts of persons with zero-degree cases; cases among contacts of persons with first-degree cases in the same household were also considered first-degree cases), second degree (cases among contacts of persons with zero-degree or first-degree cases outside households of persons with zero-degree cases [e.g., work and school contacts]), and third degree (cases among contacts of persons with second-degree cases). ICU denotes intensive care unit.
Source: Svoboda T. Public Health Measures to Control the Spread of the Severe Acute Respiratory Syndrome during the Outbreak in Toronto. NEJM. 350:2352–2361. Copyright 2004 by the Massachusetts Medical Society.

eventually were successful in controlling the second wave of the SARS outbreak in Toronto.[87]

Public Health Interventions

The pandemic of SARS eventually was controlled largely through several public health interventions to interrupt transmission in countries experiencing epidemics. Fundamental public health interventions included (1) isolation of cases of SARS when they were ill and infectious, (2) use of personal protective equipment (PPE) including N-95 fitted masks, gloves, and gowns by health care personnel caring for SARS patients, and (3) quarantine of exposed healthy contacts until it was clear that they weren't infected (for one incubation period after their last exposure). The procedures for detection of cases, their isolation, and quarantine of contacts varied among the different countries experiencing SARS epidemics. However, evaluation of the successes and failures elucidated several important epidemiologic features of SARS.

Beijing

The epidemic in Beijing between March and July of 2003 was the most severe of any city; 2591 probable cases of SARS were reported for an attack rate of 19/100,000 population.[81] In contrast to the epidemics in Singapore and Toronto that spread from a single infected case, multiple introductions of SARS occurred in Beijing.[81] To control the epidemic, the health department instituted enhanced surveillance to detect cases; isolation of SARS patients; use of personal protective equipment including double surgical masks, N95 masks, gloves, and gowns for health care workers; quarantine of contacts of SARS patients; and prohibition of public events (Figure 13-16).[88] To effectively isolate infectious SARS patients the government rapidly built a special isolation hospital. Overall, about 30,000 Beijing residents were quarantined in their homes or another quarantine site for 14 days after possible exposure to a SARS patient.[88,89]

Exposure was defined as a 30-minute exposure to a SARS or possible SARS case as follows:

1. Health care workers who did not use PPE while treating a SARS patient
2. Others who provided care for a SARS patient
3. Persons who shared the same living quarters with a SARS patient
4. Persons who visited a SARS patient
5. Persons who worked in the same office or worksite with a SARS patient
6. Classmates or teachers of a SARS patient
7. Persons who used the same public conveyance as a SARS patient

An evaluation of the efficacy of these quarantine procedures among 5186 persons quarantined in the Haidian district of Beijing March 1–May 23 found that only persons who had direct contact with a SARS patient developed SARS.[89] No cases occurred among persons who were quarantined because of contact with a contact of a SARS patient or in those whose contact with a

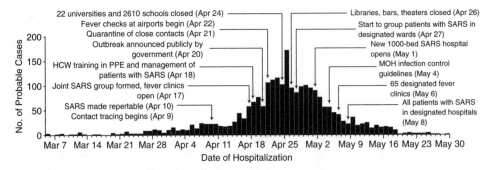

FIGURE 13-16 Epidemic curve for Beijing SARS outbreak and timeline of major control measures from March 5 to May 29, 2003.
Source: Pang X, et al. Evaluation of control measures implemented in the severe acute respiratory syndrome outbreak in Beijing, 2003. JAMA. 2003 Dec 24;290(24):3215–21.

SARS patient was only during the incubation period. Overall, the attack rate in those who had cared for a SARS patient without precautions was 31.1%, 8.9% in those visiting a SARS patient, and 4.6% in those living with a SARS patient (Table 13-5).

Taiwan

As of July 9, 2003, a total of 671 probable cases of SARS had been reported from Taiwan. The government instituted quarantine regulations for 10–14 days on March 18 for those who had been in close contact with a SARS patient. The definition of *close contact* included similar criteria to that used in Beijing, but in addition persons traveling on an airplane and sitting within three rows of a SARS patient were added to those requiring level A quarantine.[90] After the number of SARS patients increased in mid-April, persons were quarantined if they arrived from a country having a SARS epidemic (level B quarantine). Overall 131,132 persons were quarantined; of 50,319 persons held in level A quarantine 78 cases of suspect SARS and 34 with probable SARS occurred (0.22% total). Among 80,813 persons in level B quarantine, 10 suspect SARS and 11 probable SARS occurred (0.03% total). Taiwan was the last country to be declared SARS free by WHO, on July 5, 2003 (Table 13-6).[90]

Airline Travel

Transmission of SARS from an infected person to others during travel on an airline has been documented.[91] In a study of three flights that included a passenger with SARS, in only one was there evidence of transmission of the virus.[92] After this flight, carrying a symptomatic person and 119 other persons, SARS developed in 22 other persons.

Illness in passengers was related to the physical proximity to the index patient, with illness reported in 8 of the 23 persons who were seated in the rows in front of the index patient, as compared with 10 of the 88 persons seated elsewhere. However, several passengers who developed SARS were seated at considerable distance from the index case. This distribution suggests that transmission of SARS on the plane was by small particle aerosol (Figure 13-17). In contrast, another flight carrying four symptomatic persons resulted in transmission to at most one other person. Another flight that carried a person incubating SARS resulted in no transmissions.

Other Public Health Interventions

In addition to isolation of cases, personal protective equipment for health care workers caring for SARS patients, and quarantine of exposed persons, several other procedures were instituted by some countries:

- Screening of persons leaving or arriving from SARS endemic countries for fever or other SARS-related symptoms, often using infrared "fever sensors" at airports
- Use of surgical masks in public
- Cancellation of all public events where crowds might gather

TABLE 13-5 Attack Rates for Probable Severe Acute Respiratory Syndrome (SARS)* among Persons Quarantined for Direct Contact with a Probable SARS Patient, by Nature of Contact—Haidian District, Beijing, March–May 2003†

Nature of Contact	Contact During Symptomatic Period (n = 383)				Contact Only During Incubation Period (n = 167)			
	Contacts		Attack Rate		Contacts		Attack Rate	
	%	(95% CI§)	%	(95% CI)	%	(95% CI)	%	(95% CI)
Cared for SARS patient¶	15.9	(12.5–20.1)	31.1	(20.2–44.4)	2.4	(0.8–6.4)**	0	NC††
Visited SARS patient§§	11.7	(8.8–15.5)	8.9	(2.9–22.1)	4.2	(1.8–8.8)	0	NC
Lived in same residence¶¶	50.9	(45.8–56.0)	4.6	(2.3–8.9)	31.1	(24.3–38.8)	0	(0–8.6)
Lived in same building***	26.9	(22.5–31.7)	0	(0–4.5)	13.7	(9.1–20.2)	0	NC
Worked with SARS patients†††	2.0	(0.8–3.9)	0	NC	38.9	(31.6–46.8)	0	(0–7.0)
Other manner of contact	6.0	(3.9–9.0)	0	NC	13.2	(8.6–19.5)	0	NC
Total	100.0	(98.8–100.0)	6.3	(4.1–9.3)	100.0	(97.2–100.0)	0	(0–2.8)

*Defined by using the case definition of the Chinese Ministry of Health (CMoH), which is similar to the World Health Organization case definition (1). The CMoH case definition differs principally by including pneumonia patients whose contacts acquired SARS and by requiring radiographic evidence of atypical pneumonia.

† N = 550. Excludes 80 persons with direct contact who did not answer specified question.

§Confidence interval.

¶ Both at home and in the hospital.

**Cared for patients who had other medical conditions during these patients' incubation period.

†† Not calculated because proportion exposed was too small.

§§ Includes some persons who lived in the same residence or building.

¶¶ Includes some persons who lived in the same residence as a SARS patient.

***Includes some persons who visited or cared for a SARS patient and excludes persons who lived in the same residence as a SARS patient.

†††Excludes persons who visited, cared for, lived with, or lived in the same building as a SARS patient.

Source: MMWR Weekly. 52(43);1037–1040.

TABLE 13-6 Number of Persons Quarantined, Number of Persons with Suspect or Probable Severe Acute Respiratory Syndrome (SARS),* and Percentage of Persons Quarantined with Suspect or Probable SARS, by Level and Reason for Quarantine—Taiwan, March–July 2003

Level/Reason for Quarantine	No. Persons Quarantined	No. Patients with Suspect SARS	No. Patients with Probable SARS	% Persons Quarantined with Suspect or Probable SARS
Level A quarantine				
Health care workers	1,751	6	0	(0.34)
Family members	6,663	14	8	(0.33)
Coworkers and friends	4,351	5	1	(0.14)
Classmates and teachers	14,919	7	2	(0.06)
Passengers on an airplane who sat in the same row as, or adjacent three rows from, a SARS patient	1,380	5	0	(0.36)
Other†	18,273	32	23	(0.30)
Discharged suspect and probable SARS patients§	1,796	9	0	(0.50)
Missing information	1,186	0	0	(0)
Total	50,319	78¶	34**	(0.22)
Level B quarantine				
Travel from SARS-affected areas	80,813	10††	11§§	(0.03)
Total	131,132	88	45	(0.09)

*Persons with suspect SARS were defined as those who had a temperature of ≥100.4°F (≥38°C) and cough or shortness of breath and, within the 10 days before onset of symptoms, had one or more of the following contact exposures: (1) close contact with a person with probable or suspect SARS, (2) history of travel to an area with recent local transmission of SARS, or (3) residence in an area with recent local transmission of SARS. Persons with probable SARS were defined as those having suspect SARS plus one or more of the following: (1) chest radiograph consistent with findings of pneumonia, (2) acute respiratory distress syndrome (ARDS), (3) an unexplained respiratory illness resulting in death, with an autopsy consistent with ARDS and without another identifiable cause, or (4) laboratory confirmation, including one or more of the following: two oropharyngeal swab specimens positive by polymerase chain reaction (PCR) for SARS-associated coronavirus (SARS-CoV), serologic specimen positive by enzyme-linked immunosorbent assay for SARS antibody, serologic specimen positive by indirect immunofluorescence antibody for SARS antibody, or any specimen positive by viral culture for SARS-CoV.

†Includes passengers and drivers of internal public transportation who traveled for ≥1 hour in the same bus or train cabin with a SARS patient, persons who had contact with a person under quarantine who received care in a medical facility in which a cluster of SARS occurred, and homeless persons.

§Discharged suspect and probable SARS patients were required to remain isolated for 10 days after their last symptom. If they were discharged to home, they were monitored by quarantine personnel.

¶Oropharyngeal swab specimens were obtained for 60 patients; 5 (8%) specimens were PCR positive.

**Oropharyngeal swab specimens were obtained for 32 patients; 15 (47%) specimens were PCR positive.

††Oropharyngeal swab specimens were obtained for 8 patients; no specimen was PCR positive.

§§Oropharyngeal swab specimens were obtained for 8 patients; 1 (13%) specimen was PCR positive.

Source: MMWR Weekly. 52(29);680–683.

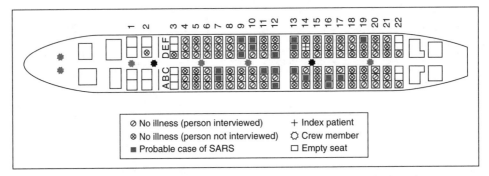

FIGURE 13-17   Schematic diagram of the Boeing 737-300 aircraft on flight 2 from Hong Kong to Beijing. Two flight attendants and two Chinese officials also reportedly had illness that met the WHO criteria for a probable case of SARS. The flight attendants are shown here as members of the crew. The seat locations of the two Chinese officials are unknown, and they are not included in the diagram.
Source: Olsen SJ et al. Transmission of the severe acute respiratory syndrome on aircraft. NEJM. 2003 Dec 18;349(25):2416–22. Copyright 2003 by the Massachusetts Medical Society.

- Notification of visitors at airports to alert health authorities if they developed a fever soon after arrival
- Quarantine of all visitors arriving from countries having an active SARS epidemic was implemented in Taiwan
- Cancellation of classes and work-related events involving crowds
- Twice daily fever monitoring of quarantined persons
- Fever monitoring of the general public

It is difficult to evaluate the effectiveness of these additional measures. Although they increased the public awareness of the epidemic, they probably were not very effective as prevention measures.[93]

The epidemic was controlled after July 5, 2003. Since that time there have only been three cases of SARS related to exposures in a laboratory.

Conclusions

Several epidemiologic features of SARS enhanced the effectiveness of public health control of the epidemic, namely:

- In contrast to many other respiratory viral infections, SARS is not contagious during the incubation period.
- Maximal infectiousness occurs about 7 days after the onset of symptoms when viral load is highest and when diagnosed patients should be isolated.
- SARS is unusual in young children.
- SARS coronavirus can be excreted in stool as well as respiratory secretions, but chronic excretion is uncommon.
- The Ro, or proportion of secondary cases of SARS transmitted by a single infected case, has been estimated to be 2.7, excluding superspreaders, by one group[93] and 2.2–3.6 by another group.[94]
- On the other hand, SARS can be quite contagious and the occasional superspreaders can effectively propagate an epidemic. Modern air

travel was very effective in spreading the infection on a global scale. Aside from the occurrence of 8450 cases and 850 deaths, the SARS epidemic of 2003 caused major disruptions and panic in many modern societies, especially in Asia.

Lyme Disease

Lyme disease was first recognized by Steere and colleagues in 1975, following the identification of a group of children living in Old Lyme, Connecticut, who were diagnosed with juvenile rheumatoid arthritis.[95] The geographic clustering of cases, the seasonal distribution with onset of illness in the summer, and a history of a prior distinctive skin lesion, erythema chronica migrans (ECM), eventually led to the hypothesis that Lyme disease was due to an infectious agent that was transmitted by ticks.[96] Subsequently, the causative spirochete organism was identified in the salivary glands of the tick *Ixodes scapularis* by Willy Burgdorfer in studies of ticks on Shelter Island, New York. When the patients with classic Lyme disease showed evidence of specific immuno-fluorescent antibodies to this new organism, the conclusion was reached that Lyme disease was caused by infection with this new organism, which was subsequently named *Borrelia burgdorferi*.[97]

In the 20 years since the recognition of Lyme disease, the number of reported cases has increased progressively, and the geographic areas of endemicity of the disease have expanded to include the coastal northeastern and mid-Atlantic states, several states in the Midwest (especially Minnesota, Wisconsin, and Michigan), and coastal California.[98,99] Although the clinical suspicion that a patient may have Lyme disease has increased among physicians because of the potential for chronic sequelae, there has clearly been an increase in the incidence of the disease.[100] Factors promoting the emergence of Lyme disease include the encroachment of human populations into areas infected with tick vectors and the growth of the deer populations, allowing for an increased survival and density of *Ixodes scapularis* ticks.[101] The epidemiology of Lyme disease is reviewed in more detail in Chapter 25.

Other Tick-Borne Infections

Other tick-borne infections that are endemic in the United States have been described in recent years, and these diseases may have increased in frequency as well. However, the data on temporal trends of their incidence are less clear because the only reportable tick-borne infections in the United States are Lyme disease and RMSF. The number of reported patients with RMSF increased from about 200 to 400 cases in the 1950s and 1960s to over 1000 cases in the late 1970s and 1980s.[61] Increased opportunities for human exposure to the vectors, primarily the Rocky Mountain wood tick (*Dermocenter andersonii*) in the western United States and the American dog tick (*Dermocenter variabilis*) in the eastern United States, occurred because of the expansion of suburban housing into wooded, tick-infested areas and the increased opportunities for exposure associated with recreational activities.

Two forms of human ehrlichiosis, HME due to infection with *Ehrlichia chaffeeinsis* and HGE due to infection with *Ehrlichia ewingii*, have also been recognized with increased frequency in the past few years.[103-106] These diseases are also transmitted by ticks: HME by the dog tick and HGE by the deer tick.

Another tick-borne disease, babesiosis, an infection of red blood cells with *Babesia microti*, can be transmitted to humans by tick bites in the endemic areas in the coastal northeastern United States.[107] It is not unusual for a patient to be seen who has both Lyme disease and ehrlichiosis after exposure to tick habitats in an endemic area. It seems likely that these other tick-borne diseases have increased in frequency, similar to increases documented with Lyme disease. However, the documentation of this increased incidence has been difficult, because these diseases have not been routinely reported to health authorities.

Cholera

Cholera has reemerged as an epidemic disease in the 1990s. In 1991, cholera occurred in Latin America after an absence of over 100 years.[81] Within 2 years, cholera spread from Peru to Mexico. In 1992, a new epidemic strain, *Vibrio cholerae* 0139, appeared for the first time in India and Bangladesh.[108] There is lack of cross-immunity between classic or El Tor *V. cholerae* 01 strains and the newly recognized *V. cholerae* 0139 strain. Therefore, major outbreaks of cholera, estimated at more than 200,000 cases, occurred in India, Bangladesh, and several other countries in Southeast Asia. Travel-associated, imported cases were reported in the United States, Europe, and Japan.[109]

In addition, a massive outbreak of El Tor cholera occurred among Rwandan refugees in Goma, Zaire, during the war in Rwanda, resulting in 20,000 cases and 12,000 deaths in July 1994.[110] This outbreak, once again, demonstrated the potential for cholera to cause severe mortality in a situation of extreme civil disruption. In contrast, the cholera mortality was under 1% in Latin American countries, where good diagnostic and medical services and oral dehydration therapy were readily available. These cholera epidemics demonstrate the potential for modern societies to disseminate a potent epidemic pathogen globally. Also, *Shigella* dysentery spread in epidemic fashion in the refugee camps in Zaire.

One theory of how cholera was introduced into Latin America reported that a ship from the Orient released contaminated bilge water into a Peruvian harbor, which contaminated local shell fish and established an epidemic focus.[111] However, more recently, Colwell has reported studies indicating that the effects of global warming associated with recent El Niño conditions may have been critical in the resurgence of cholera.[37] These intriguing studies indicate that warmer seawater temperatures could expand the environmental reservoir of the organism. Warming of seawater temperatures promotes a phytoplankton expansion, followed by a zooplankton bloom. These zooplankton copepods can carry *V. cholerae* on their surfaces and in their guts in high concentration, up to 10^4 organisms per copepod. The warming of seawater temperatures and spread of the environmental reservoir of *V. cholerae* by copepods could explain the rapid widespread dissemination of cholera along coastal areas of Latin America soon after its reintroduction.[37] Because of the rapid spread of cholera recently among coastal populations of South America, copepods may have played a major role in the emergence of cholera in this area.

Escherichia coli O157:H7

E. coli O157:H7 is a recently emerged pathogen that was first incriminated as causing infections in humans in 1982.[112] This organism is now recognized as a major cause of large-scale epidemics and sporadic cases of gastrointestinal illness in North America, Europe, and Japan.[78-80] Infections with this organism are estimated to cause about 79,000 illnesses and 61 deaths each year in the United States.[113] In contrast, infections with the organism have not been recognized to be a significant problem in most developing countries. Infections with *E. coli* O157:H7 produce a clinically distinct illness with bloody diarrhea and, in some patients, hemolysis and acute renal failure, called the *hemolytic-uremia syndrome.* This organism evolved from the ordinary intestinal flora of cattle. It emerged as a human pathogen after acquiring genetic material that would allow increased intestinal adherence, a large plasmid coding for a hemolysin, and a gene coding for severe cytotoxicity, the Shiga toxin. Also, the organism acquired the ability to withstand an acid environment.[114] This trait allowed the organism to survive the normally protective action of stomach acid and to survive in the environment in the presence of acid rain. In addition to the increased resistance to acid, the infectious dose is very small, only 50 to 100 organisms are required to infect an individual.

These genetic changes in the organism, acid stability, and the ability to produce the potent Shiga toxin allowed this organism to emerge as a new "superbug." The organism is usually not pathogenic to cattle, which carry the organism in their intestinal tract without having symptoms. It has been isolated from 1% to 10% of healthy cattle and from sheep in the United States and throughout the world.[114] The organism can be transmitted by food, raw milk, water, and by direct person-to-person spread. Large outbreaks have occurred in the United States from improperly cooked hamburgers. These outbreaks occurred because beef was commonly contaminated with these organisms, acquired during the slaughtering process, and thorough cooking was required to disinfect the food from an organism that is highly pathogenic with small numbers of organisms. Rare or incompletely cooked hamburgers could contain an infectious inoculum of *E. coli* O157:H7 in the center of the sandwich. The modern food processing and distribution networks, collectively known as *corporate agribusiness*, promote the cross-contamination of cattle in the slaughtering process and disseminate meat widely. Now the only defense is thorough cooking of the meat. The cultural preference for rare beef, translated into poorly cooked hamburger, increases the risk of exposure. The organism has also been transmitted by other foods, including vegetables such as alfalfa sprouts that have been contaminated with cow manure used as fertilizer or with fruit juices, such as apple cider. Often, apples used to produce cider may be harvested from the fruit that has fallen from the tree. Contamination with a small inoculum of organisms on the surface of the apples from cow manure on the ground can survive the acid environments of apple juice and the stomach. This has led to several outbreaks and recommendations are that apple juice be pasteurized to avoid this risk.[115]

After a large outbreak related to hamburgers from a commercial fast-food chain, the industry established standard cooking procedures and microbiologic monitoring of beef. Consequently, no cases related to the fast-food industry have been reported since about 1995.[116]

Waterborne Parasitic and Viral Infections and *Cryptosporidium* Species

The resurgence of cholera has primarily involved populations in developing countries in Asia, Latin American, and Africa. However, it has been appreciated recently that waterborne infections from newly recognized parasitic agents are a significant and increasing problem in the United States. The risk of waterborne infections was appreciated when a massive outbreak of diarrhea occurred in the spring of 1993 in Milwaukee.[117] This outbreak involved an estimated 403,000 people who received water from one of two municipal water treatment plants in the city where the water had been treated with chlorination and filtration. Between March 23 and April 9, the water treated at the city's southern treatment plant had shown marked increases in turbidity. In early April, the Wisconsin Department of Health received reports of large numbers of persons who were experiencing diarrhea that resulted in widespread absenteeism among hospital employees, students, and school teachers. At this time, little information was available about the organism involved in the outbreak. However, two laboratories identified *Cryptosporidium* oocysts in stool samples from a number of adults with typical illnesses. A survey of laboratories in the area showed no reported increased isolation of *Salmonella*, *Shigella*, *Campylobacter*, *E. coli* 0157:H7, or other common bacterial causes of diarrhea. The epidemiologists investigating this outbreak were able subsequently to isolate *Cryptosporidium parvum* from ice that had been frozen during the period of the contamination of the water supply. A subsequent analysis of the data from the Milwaukee water system and clinical occurrences of diarrhea in the population suggests that endemic contamination of the water supply with *C. parvum* oocysts may have occurred prior to the large outbreak in April 1993.[118] This large outbreak was followed by prospective surveillance of several municipal water supplies in the United States to evaluate the risks of waterborne cryptosporidiosis. These studies have shown that contamination of domestic water supplies with *C. parvum* oocysts is not uncommon.[119-121] Several large municipal water supplies in the United States do not filter the water to remove *C. parvum* oocysts.[122] Although chlorination of municipal water supplies is routinely practiced by most municipal water systems in the United States, *C. parvum* oocysts are resistant to chlorination. The potential for waterborne disease is increased by the fact that the infectious dose necessary to cause human disease is quite low, probably in the range of 10 to 100 oocysts per liter of water.[119] Furthermore, clinical laboratories do not routinely screen stool samples from diarrhea patients for *C. parvum* unless the clinician requests this evaluation. The detection of *C. parvum* in stools requires staining the stool with an acid-fast stain and examining the sample microscopically for *C. parvum* oocysts. Consequently, in the Milwaukee epidemic, which involved an estimated 403,000 persons, only about 12 cases were confirmed in the laboratory.[117] This has led epidemiologists to question whether waterborne outbreaks of cryptosporidiosis might be much more common than appreciated.[117]

Another issue raised by this outbreak is the risk to the subset of the population who are immunosuppressed, such as persons with AIDS, those on chemotherapy, and those with malignancies. Cryptosporidia is known to be a significant pathogen in AIDS patients. The infection is not effectively treatable in this population.[93] Contamination of a municipal water supply, even at a fairly low level, could cause significant morbidity and even mortality at the population level. Other parasitic pathogens that are resistant to chlorine and could cause disease in humans with exposure to a few organisms include *Microsporidia* species, *Cyclospora*, and *Giardia lamblia*.[121] Studies are beginning to estimate the risk of waterborne infections from these pathogens in the United States and to evaluate various strategies to prevent these infections.

Cyclosporiasis

Another parasitic organism that has emerged recently as an important human pathogen in the United States is *Cyclospora cayetanensis*. Before 1996, most documented cases of cyclosporiasis in North America occurred in travelers returning from overseas, and only three small US outbreaks had been reported.[122] However, in 1998, several health departments reported cases of cyclosporiasis to the Centers for Disease Control and Prevention (CDC). Ultimately, 978 laboratory-confirmed cases occurring in the spring and summer of 1996 were reported to the CDC and the Canadian Health Department. A total of 1465 cases was eventually reported. Extensive investigation of multiple outbreaks in the United States and Canada eventually implicated raspberries imported from Guatemala as the source of these outbreaks.[29] Raspberries were first cultivated in Guatemala as a commercial crop in 1987. They were first exported in 1988, and exports markedly increased in the mid-1990s. Another outbreak of cyclosporiasis related to Guatemalan raspberries occurred in 1997 (Figure 13-18).[30] Although the exact mode of contamination of the raspberries is unclear, it is likely that rinsing of the implicated raspberries with contaminated water prior to their export had occurred. These outbreaks emphasize the potential infection problems associated with importation of a food product that is eaten uncooked and is not easily monitored or disinfected before it is consumed. With the expansion of international commerce and importation of foods from many countries, this type of problem is certain to become even more frequent in the future.

Hantaviruses

A new viral infection first came to the attention of Western medicine during the Korean War in 1951, when US troops stationed in Korea developed a new disease that was subsequently named *Korean hemorrhagic fever*. The disease was manifested by a febrile course with influenza-like symptoms. In about a third of the cases, hemorrhagic symptoms and hypertension, followed by severe renal failure, occurred. Over 3000 troops were infected, and the mortality rate was about 5%.[123] The etiologic agent was not identified until 1976, after Lee et al. working in Seoul, Korea, identified the etiologic agent as a virus when it was isolated in Vero cell cultures.[124] The virus was named Hantaan virus after the Hantaan River, which transects the epidemic area at the demilitarized zone separating North and South Korea. The virus was isolated from the lungs of the striped field mouse, *Apodermus agrarius*. This common animal is now recognized as the major rodent host of the Hantaan virus in rural Korea. These rodents commonly acquire the infection early in life and continuously excrete the virus in their urine for the rest of their

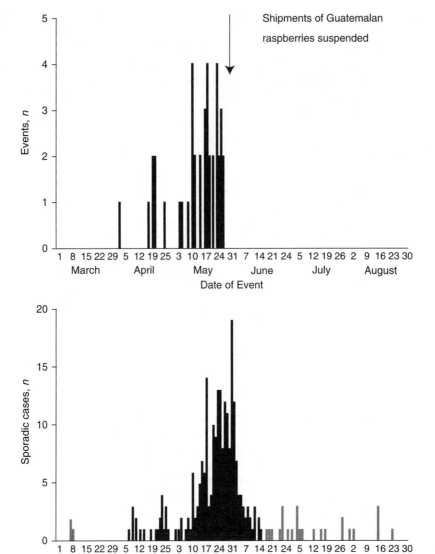

FIGURE 13-18 Dates of 41 events associated with clusters of cases of cyclosporiasis (*n* = 762 cases) in the United States and Canada in April and May 1997. For multiday events, the date of the first day of the event is shown. The last shipment of Guatemalan raspberries in the spring of 1997 was on May 28. Bottom. Dates of symptom onset for laboratory-confirmed sporadic cases of cyclosporiasis in the United States and Canada in 1997. The gray bars represent 31 case-patients who became ill during the period from March through August but not during the outbreak period of April through 15 June. The black bars represent 250 case-patients whose cases were classified as having occurred during the outbreak period. The median date of symptom onset for the 250 case-patients was May 26 (range, April 6 to June 15). Only 22 persons (8.8%) became ill in April, and most (225 [90.0%]) became ill by June 4. The date selected as the last date of the outbreak period was June 15 because Guatemalan raspberries exported in late May could still have been available for consumption in early June and because infected persons would have become symptomatic an average of 1 week after exposure. Not all of the sporadic cases of cyclosporiasis were necessarily due to consumption of raspberries.
Source: Herwaldt BL, et al. The return of Cyclospora in 1997: another outbreak of cyclosporiasis in North America associated with imported raspberries. Cyclospora Working Group. Ann Intern Med. 1999 Feb 2;130(3):210–20.

lives. Persons who may be exposed to infected urine, such as a soldier in a foxhole, are at risk of infection. There was no evidence of person-to-person spread of infection or of water- or food-borne transmission of Hantaan virus in Korea.

Subsequently, another rodent-associated virus with some similarities to Hantaan virus was isolated from urban rats (*Rattus norwegicus* and *Rattus rattus*). Isolated cases of hemorrhagic fever were identified in urban residents and in laboratory workers who were exposed to these rats; the virus was named *Seoul virus*. It has now spread worldwide with infected rodents as passengers on commercial ships. This virus has been identified in Baltimore and has been shown in a preliminary case-control study to have an association with hypertension and chronic renal disease[125]; however, these data are awaiting further confirmation.

Another related virus, Puumala virus, was isolated from patients in Sweden and voles in Finland. This virus caused a syndrome, termed Nephropathica epidemica, which is an acute febrile disease with renal involvement.[126] Subsequently, the World Health Organization grouped the syndromes caused by these three related viruses together under the rubric *hemorrhagic fever with renal syndrome* (HFRS).

In May 1993, an apparently new disease was recognized among previously healthy young Native Americans and Caucasians in New Mexico. This new disease consisted of an abrupt onset of fever, myalgia, headache, and cough, followed by the rapid development of acute pulmonary edema and acute respiratory distress syndrome. The overall mortality in this outbreak was about 5%.[127] Eventually, 100 cases occurred among persons living in New Mexico, Arizona, and Colorado (Figure 13-19). Most patients were previously healthy young adults; the median age was 32 years, 33% were Native Americans, and 66% were Caucasians.[128] Pathologically, the disease was characterized by interstitial pneumonitis with a mononuclear cell infiltrate and focal hyaline membranes. Testing of acute and convalescent sera from these patients demonstrated seroreactivity to various hantaviruses, with the strongest reaction to Puumala virus. This finding was unexpected because, at that time, hantaviruses had not been seen in the United States, and the clinical syndrome associated with infection with other hantaviruses had included renal disease, rather than pulmonary failure. Following the serologic evidence, reverse transcriptase PCR studies of hantaviruses revealed a DNA sequence similar but 30% different from Prospect Hill virus (another hantavirus).[129] The virus was eventually grown in cell culture, using Vero E-6 cells and named Sin Nombre virus.[131]

The rodent reservoir was eventually identified as the deer mouse, *Peromyscus maniculatus*, which had expanded 10-fold because of extraordinary climatic conditions with large amounts of precipitation in the preceding winter and spring that provided an abundant supply of pinon nuts used as food by the mice.[130] Satellite photos of vegetation accurately identified hot spots where cases occurred and where high concentrations of deer mice were located. Apparently, this "new" infectious disease arose because of a dramatic expansion of the deer mouse population, often chronically infected with Sin Nombre virus, and invasion into the homes in the area, allowing human contact with infected aerosolized urine. Interestingly, there was no evidence of person-to-person transmission of the agent among household or hospital

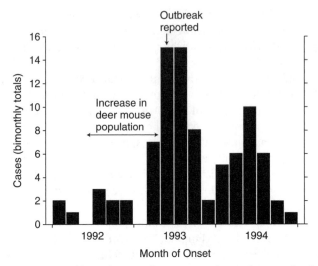

FIGURE 13-19 Cases of hantavirus pulmonary syndrome by month of onset, United States, 1992–1994, omitting 16 cases with onsets prior to 1992.
Source: N. Nathanson and S. Nichol, Korean and Hemorrhagic Fever and Hanta Virus Pulmonary Syndrome: Two Examples of Emerging Pathoviral Diseases, in *Emerging Infections*, p. 370, R.M. Krause, ed., © 1998, with permission from Elsevier.

contacts. Population-based serologic surveys found very few asymptomatic cases. Nearly all infected cases were ill and had classic hantavirus pulmonary syndrome.

Ebola and Marburg Viruses

Ebola and Marburg viruses are recently emerging viruses in the Filoviridae family that have elicited serious concern because of their high infectivity and mortality rates in human populations (Table 13-7). The first recognition of filoviruses was in 1967, when an epidemic of 31 cases and 7 deaths from viral hemorrhagic fever occurred in Marburg, Germany, among persons having contact with vervet or African green monkeys or their tissues that had been imported from Uganda.[132,133] The virus, named *Marburg virus*, was cultivated from the blood of sick humans who had become ill after exposure to the monkeys. The very unusual morphology of the Marburg virus and the potential for human-to-human transmission of this severe infection underscored the fact that this was a serious threat to human health.

In 1976, two outbreaks of infection with Ebola virus occurred in Zaire and the Sudan; together, there were more than 550 cases and 430 deaths.[134–136] In the next 20 years, an additional 18 outbreaks of Ebola virus infections in humans have been recognized.[137] Although most of these human epidemics have been initiated by contact with monkeys or other nonhuman primates, it is felt to be unlikely that monkeys are the primary reservoir for Ebola virus, because they also have experienced high mortality from infection.[137] The disease is characterized by an abrupt onset with fever, diarrhea, dysphagia, severe weakness and hemorrhagic phenomena, and, in most outbreaks, high mortality.[138] In Africa, where most of these epidemics have occurred, human-

TABLE 13-7   Filovirus Hemorrhagic Fever Outbreaks in Humans

Virus	Contact	Location
Marburg	Imported African green monkeys (23% mortality)	Marburg, Germany 1967
Ebola, Zaire strain (EBO-2)	Unknown origin, close contact, and needles, 318 cases (88% mortality)	Zaire 1976
Ebola, Sudan strain (EBO-5)	Unknown origin, nosocomial transmission, 284 cases (53% mortality)	Sudan 1976, 1979
Ebola, Reston strain (EBO-R)	Infected monkeys imported from Philippines, 4 asymptomatic human cases	Reston, Virginia, USA 1989
Ebola, Zaire strain	Contacts with chimpanzees, monkeys, other primates, and nosocomial spread; multiple outbreaks	Gabon, Zaire, Cote d'Ivore 1994–1999; Largest in Kikwit, Zaire, 317 cases (78% mortality)

to-human transmission has been common. In the large outbreak in 1995 in Kikwit, Zaire (now the Congo), health care workers and relatives of cases acquired the disease and often succumbed.[139] Among the first 283 cases, 90 (32%) occurred in health care workers, and 28 (16%) of 173 members in the first 27 households developed disease. However, the institution of routine barrier precautions (including gowns and gloves) and the discontinuation of the ritual of bathing and cleaning of the corpse after death limited contact with infectious secretions and appeared to control further transmission.

The concept that good barrier practices in nursing are adequate to control nosocomial transmission of Ebola is supported by the experience in Gabon in 1996, where 32 patients were cared for without any infections in house staff or nurses caring for the patients. A survey of family members of 27 patients who developed Ebola infection in Kikwit found a secondary attack rate of 16%; however, only those household members who had direct contact with body fluids of ill patients developed infection.[140–142]

Another outbreak of Ebola virus infection occurred in a monkey colony in Reston, Virginia. In this outbreak, the infected cynomolgus monkeys (*M. fascicularis*) had been imported from the Philippines, an area not known to be endemic for Ebola or other filoviruses. The monkeys were coinfected with another virus, Simian hemorrhagic fever (SMF) virus. In this outbreak, in contrast with previous outbreaks of Ebola virus, there was some evidence of aerosol transmission among the monkeys.[35,141–143] Also, four laboratory workers who had used barrier precautions in handling the monkeys developed serologic evidence of infection but remained asymptomatic.[35,143] These outbreaks underscore the potential importance of differences between strains of Ebola virus in their infectivity and pathogenicity; four subtypes of Ebola virus have been identified to date.[137,144]

One apparent feature of persons who survive Ebola virus infections is that they appear not to develop high titers of neutralizing antibodies.[110] Therefore, an immune serum has not been developed for the therapy of persons with acute infections. A chronic carrier state of Ebola virus has not been identified in any animal species.[145] The natural interepidemic reservoir of Ebola virus has not been defined. The genetic structures of Ebola isolates from the various outbreaks have considerable diversity, suggesting that they are not directly linked with one another, for example, through continued human-to-human transmission.[145]

Fever cases and outbreaks of Marburg hemorrhagic fever (MHF) infections other than those from Ebola virus have been reported since the original isolation of the Marburg virus in 1967. A large outbreak began in 1998 in northeastern Democratic Republic of Congo (DRC) that eventually involved over 150 cases and a high mortality rate.[146] A cross-sectional serologic survey was done in a village population in the DRC after the outbreak was controlled. Overall, 15 (2%) of 912 participants were seropositive for Marburg virus antibodies, and 13 (87%) of the seropositives had worked in a local gold mine.[147] However, no other risk factors for Marburg seropositivity were identified in this study.

In 2005, another large outbreak of MHF occurred in Uige, Angola. In this outbreak, 374 cases were reported to the WHO, of which 329 (88%) were fatal.[148] This epidemic has generated great fear in the involved communities. Because of the high mortality rates in the patients seeking treatment, ill persons often come to the hospital late and after other members of the household have been exposed and infected.

Arenaviruses

The arenaviruses are a group of negative-stranded, RNA viruses that are important causes of epidemic infections in tropical areas of Africa and South America. The prototype arenavirus, lymphocytic choriomeningitis virus (LCM), was discovered in 1933 and causes benign aseptic meningitis in humans in temperate areas of North America, as well as the tropics (Table 13-8). Junin virus was recovered from patients with Argentine hemorrhagic fever (AHF) in 1958, and Machupo virus, the cause of Bolivia hemorrhagic fever (BHF), was discovered in 1960.[149,150] Another disease, Venezuela hemorrhagic fever (VHF), was initially described in 1964.[151] Recently, VHF has been recognized as a distinct human disease caused by an arenavirus carried by rodents.[150,151] The extent of the public health problem from infections with the Guanarito virus is not clear.

In 1969, Lassa fever virus was isolated from a missionary nurse stationed in rural northeastern Nigeria. Following her admission to the hospital, two additional cases developed in nurses who were caring for her, and two of the three original cases died.[152] In one outbreak, 13 of 17 health care workers contracted the disease and died.[152] Subsequently, outbreaks occurred in Nigeria, Liberia, and Sierra Leone, with mortality of 20% to 60% of those infected.[152] Infections have occurred among persons working with this virus in a laboratory in the United States.[152] There was great concern after Lassa fever was first described that this virus might be the "Andromeda strain" that would spread rapidly to all human contacts, with high mortality. However, subsequent investigation suggests that spread is preventable with ordinary respiratory precautions. Various rodent species are the reservoir for the arenaviruses. These include *Mus musclus* (the house mouse) for LCM, *Mastomys* species for Lassa fever, and *Calomys* species for AHF, BHF, and VHF.

TABLE 13-8 Ecologic Features of Arenaviruses Pathogenic for Humans

Virus	Natural Host	Geographic Distribution	Disease
Lymphocytic choriomeningitis virus	*Mus musculus* (house mouse)	Europe, America	Aseptic meningitis
Junin virus	*Calomys musculinus*	Argentina	Argentine hemorrhagic fever
Machupo virus	*Calomys callosus*	Bolivia	Bolivia hemorrhagic fever
Guanarito virus	*Sigmodon alstoni*	Venezuela	Venezuela hemorrhagic fever
Lassa virus	*Mastomys natalensis*	West Africa	Lassa hemorrhagic fever

These diseases have emerged because of man-made changes in the environment that favor higher density of virus-infected rodents that have close contact with humans. Junin virus emerged as an important human pathogen in Argentina when the pampas grassland that had been a grazing area for cattle was converted into cultivated farm land for the production of maize. This led to a major expansion of the population of a mouse, *Calomys musculinus*, that fed on the grain. Because these mice were frequently chronically infected with Junin virus, which they shed in their urine, the harvesting of the maize allowed humans to come into contact with the virus.

In Bolivia, an epidemic of BHF occurred in 1960 and was caused by a related virus, Machupo virus, when an area in eastern Bolivia was converted from cattle raising to subsistence agriculture. This ecologic change provided a suitable environment for the expansion of the population of a small mouse, *Calomys callosus*. This mouse invaded the homes and gardens of the local inhabitants and spread the virus that caused BHF. However, unlike AHF, this epidemic is now under control, due in part to the greater pathogenicity of the virus for the carrier mouse and the more limited contact of the population with the reservoir host.[149]

Monkey Pox

During May and June of 2003, the first cluster of human cases of monkey pox in the United States was reported.[153] Monkey pox in humans was first identified in 1970 in the Democratic Republic of the Congo.[154] The virus is an Orthopox virus that is related to the smallpox (variola) virus and a number of other human and animal viruses.

Clinically, the disease resembles smallpox but is milder. After an incubation period of about 12 days, patients develop fever, headache, muscle aches and backaches, and the lymph nodes swell. Lymphadenopathy is apparently more marked in monkey pox than in smallpox. Then 1 to 3 days later a rash appears on the face, chest, and trunk. The rash evolves through stages of papule, vesicle, pustule, and scabs. Like smallpox, but different from chickenpox, all of the rash lesions are in the same stage. When the rash heals it often leaves scars.

The illnesses occurred among persons who had contact with various animals, especially prairie dogs (*Cynomys* sp.). The first diagnosed case had been seen at the Marshfield Clinic in Marshfield, Wisconsin, where the diagnosis was made based on identifying a virus morphologically consistent with a pox virus from a skin lesion biopsy. Subsequently, the clinic identified a similar virus in lymph node tissue from the patient's pet prairie dog and isolated the virus on culture of these tissues.[155] The virus was confirmed to be monkey pox at the CDC.

All of the cases were associated with prairie dogs that had been purchased from an animal distributor in Illinois. These prairie dogs appear to have been infected with monkey pox virus through contact with Gambian rats and deer mice that originated and were purchased on April 21 by the distributor in Illinois (Figure 13-20). Approximately 200 prairie dogs had been at the Illinois facility during April and May. Some overlapped with the purchase of animals that had been imported from Africa. A total of 93 prairie dogs were traced from the Illinois facility to six states. Also an unknown number had died or were sold or exchanged at "animal swap" events to be used as pets; no records were available from these events.

A trace back investigation was done to identify the source of introduction of monkey pox into the United States. This investigation identified a Texas animal distributor who had imported a shipment of approximately 800 small mammals from Ghana on April 9 that contained 762 African rodents. Several animals from this shipment were tested for monkey pox virus infection by CDC and found to be positive. Included among the infected animals was one Gambian rat, three deer mice, and one rope squirrel.[156] A total of 178 (28%) African rodents could not be traced from the Texas facility because records were not available. However, no cases of monkey pox were detected as a result of contact with these African rodents. All of the 71 suspect, confirmed, or possible human cases of monkey pox infection had contact with an infected prairie dog (Figure 13-20). There were no cases of human-to-human transmission of monkey pox that could not be explained by direct contact with an infected prairie dog. The 71 cases were reported from six states: Wisconsin (39 cases), Indiana (16 cases), Illinois (12 cases), Missouri (2 cases), Kansas (1 case), and Ohio (1 case).[156] The epidemic terminated in early July 2003.

Public health strategies that were implemented to control this outbreak by the Food and Drug Administration, CDC, and state regulatory authorities included a joint order banning importation and movement of the implicated animal species; states enacted measures to further prohibit intrastate shipment and trade, establish premises quarantine, and begin animal euthanasia. Additionally, smallpox vaccine was given to 30 persons who had been exposed to infected animals to prevent infection. One of these 30 persons developed a rash confirmed to be monkey pox within 2 weeks of immunization.[156]

Monkey pox has reemerged in Africa in the past two decades since smallpox has been eliminated and routine vaccinia immunization has been stopped. Studies of monkey pox in humans in Africa have detected sporadic outbreaks in the 1970s and 1980s with only occasional human-to-human spread of infection, usually not beyond two generations.[157,158] In fact, monkey pox is much less infectious by person-to-person contact than smallpox; the

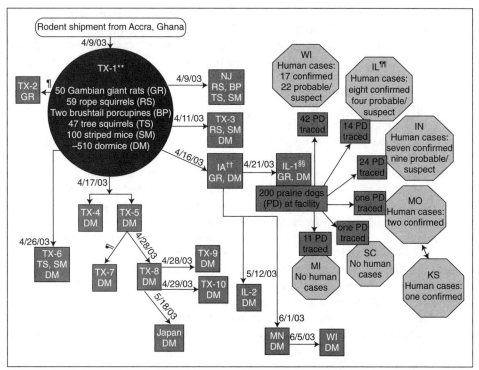

* Illinois (IL), Indiana (IN), Iowa (IA), Kansas (KS), Michigan (MI), Minnesota (MN), Missouri (MO), New Jersey (NJ), South Carolina (SC), Texas (TX), and Wisconsin (WI). Japan is included among sites having received shipment of rodents implicated in this outbreak.

† As of July 8, 2003.

§ Does not include one probable human case from Ohio; investigation is ongoing.

¶ Date of shipment unknown.

** Identified as distributor C in *MMWR* 2003; 52:561–564.

†† Identified as distributor D in *MMWR* 2003; 52:561–564.

§§ Identified as distributor B in *MMWR* 2003; 52:561–564.

¶¶ Includes two persons who were employees at IL-1.

FIGURE 13-20 Movement of imported African rodents to animal distributors and distribution of prairie dogs from an animal distributor associated with human cases of monkeypox—11 states, 2003.
Source: Update: Multistate Outbreak of Monkeypox—Illinois, Indiana, Kansas, Missouri, Ohio, and Wisconsin, 2003. MMWR. 52(27);642–646.

longest transmission chain of human-to-human transmission reported has been four transmission cycles.[159] Although severe, even fatal, disease can occur, it is much less common than in smallpox infection; mortality in Africa has ranged from 1% to 15%.

Smallpox vaccine is effective in preventing monkey pox, and breakthrough cases are milder and have fewer vesicles or pustules than unvaccinated individuals. However, since routine smallpox vaccination was discontinued in most African countries between 1981 and 1985, after the elimination of smallpox, most of the younger members of the population in an endemic area have not been vaccinated. Surveillance of monkey pox in several African countries has been done by WHO, since the disease was recognized. The first human case occurred in a child in the Democratic Republic of the Congo in

1970. Between 1970 and 1980 a total of 59 cases of monkey pox in humans were detected in Cameroon, Cote d'Ivoire, Liberia, Nigeria, Sierra Leone, and the Democratic Republic of the Congo.[158] Of the 47 cases in the Congo, all occurred in areas bordering the two tropical rain forests and 8 (17%) of the infections were fatal. Serologic surveys in unvaccinated children done after 1980 in the endemic areas suggested that about 12–15% had antibodies to monkey pox, but most of the antibody-positive persons did not have a history of a compatible illness.[160]

Based partly on these data, expert committees of WHO recommended against re-institution of smallpox vaccine to control monkey pox. In 1996–1997, Medicens sans Frontiers reported an outbreak of monkey pox in the Congo to WHO.[161] Studies of the populations suggested that as many as 511 cases may have occurred. The reemergence of monkey pox in the Congo was facilitated by an ongoing war; the hostilities forced many persons to seek refuge in the forest. However, most incidences of the disease were fairly mild, and the secondary attack rate was estimated to be 18%; it was 3% among those with a history of vaccination and 26% in those without a history of vaccination.[162] The possibility of reinstitution of smallpox vaccine to control monkey pox in the endemic area was reconsidered by WHO. However, it was decided not to use the vaccine in the general population in part because the prevalence of HIV infection was 7–10% or higher, and a fatal reaction to smallpox vaccine had been reported in a soldier in the United States.[163]

Issues Raised by Monkey Pox

The monkey pox epidemic has emphasized, in a dramatic way, the potential for animal-to-human transmission of an unusual pathogen made possible by the unimpeded ability to transport animals from remote areas into the United States. The risk of introducing and spreading exotic diseases into a new environment by importation of infected animals has likely increased in the last few decades. A similar scenario, which has not yet been recognized, could have been responsible for the introduction of West Nile virus into the United States in 1999. How are future importations of new diseases to be prevented? It may not be easy to prevent a similar problem from recurring in the future because of global trade and commerce.

What should be done to prevent an increased incidence of monkey pox among African populations where the disease is endemic? Clearly, ongoing surveillance will be important in order to guide any future public health activities. Perhaps diluted smallpox vaccine might be useful to control outbreaks of monkey pox among isolated populations, but decisions should be made based on continued surveillance data. Do subjects need to be screened for HIV before giving smallpox vaccine? If so, what about their household contacts?

The rapid diagnosis of monkey pox and coordinated public health response by CDC and FDA was effective in preventing the establishment of monkey pox as an epizootic disease in the United States. Many animals are susceptible to monkey pox, including squirrels, which are believed to be an important natural reservoir in Africa.[164]

Zoonotic Paramyxovirus Infections

Several epidemics of human paramyxovirus infection have occurred in recent years. These epidemics have occurred in Australia and Asia from reservoirs in domestic animals.

Hendra Virus Epidemic in Australia

In September 1994, an outbreak of respiratory disease affected 18 horses, their trainer, and a stable hand in Queensland, Australia. Fourteen horses and one human died. A novel virus was isolated from the horses and humans, and originally was named *equine morbili-virus*.[165] One of the persons who had aseptic meningitis during the original outbreak recovered but became ill with encephalitis and died 13 months later.[166] During this illness, he developed seizures with distinctive changes on magnetic resonance imaging and histologic changes in the cerebral cortex. PCR of spinal fluid, brain, and serum yielded sequences identical to those obtained during the original outbreak. Subsequently, a second, unrelated outbreak was identified in Queensland, in which two horses died and one human became infected.[167] Laboratory studies have suggested that fruit bats (*Pteropus* species) in Australia and Papua New Guinea may be infected and serve as the natural reservoir for this newly recognized virus, which has been renamed *Hendra virus*.[168]

Nipah Virus

Between February and April 1999, a severe outbreak of viral encephalitis occurred in the Bakit Pelandok area of peninsular Malaysia that affected more than 200 individuals and a large number of pigs.[169] The outbreak was initially thought to be due to Japanese encephalitis virus (JE) because it involved people in close contact with pigs, a known reservoir of JE virus. However, several features of this outbreak differed from the usual clinical and epidemiologic characteristics of JE. Namely, the outbreak involved only men who were in direct contact with pigs. The illness had a very high attack rate in this population. Many of the pigs also were sick, and most of the human cases had been immunized against JE. Among the 91 patients admitted to the University of Malaya Medical Center in Kuala Lumpur, there were 28 deaths.[169] A virus was isolated from the cerebrospinal fluid (CSF) of several patients that stained positively with antibodies against Hendra virus by indirect immunofluorescence. IgM capture ELISA showed that several patients had IgM antibodies in CSF against Hendra virus antigens. There was no clinical evidence of pulmonary involvement; however, inclusion bodies of probable viral origin were present in neurons. Electron microscopy revealed viruslike structures resembling paramyxoviruses, and nucleotide sequencing indicated that the virus was related but not identical to Hendra virus.[170] All cases had been working on pig farms and had direct contact with ill pigs. Subsequently, 11 cases were reported from Singapore among workers on pig farms. These outbreaks were controlled by culling all of the pigs from farms with infected animals.

In 2001 and 2003, outbreaks of Nipah virus encephalitis were reported from Bangladesh.[171] In these outbreaks no contact with pigs was reported.

However, fruit bats were positive for Nipah virus antibodies, and there was evidence of household clustering, suggesting human-to-human transmission.

Legionnaires' Disease

An outbreak of a new infectious disease was recognized in July 1976 that affected 182 persons in Philadelphia.[172] Most had attended the American Legion Convention in Philadelphia that was held July 21–24 and had stayed at one hotel. However, 39 persons had not actually stayed at the hotel but had exposure to the air emanating from the hotel. No evidence of human-to-human transmission was found during this outbreak. Laboratory investigation eventually isolated gram-negative bacteria by inoculating hamsters with infectious material. The organism would not grow in standard media, such as blood agar, thioglycollate broth, or tryptocase soy agar. This organism was named *Legionella pneumophila*.[173] Attack rates of illness were higher in persons staying at the hotel who had underlying illnesses or were cigarette smokers. Attack rates were 4.0% among those attending the convention, and mortality was 15.9% among those who were ill.

Another outbreak of an airborne infection had occurred 8 years previously in a county health department in Pontiac, Michigan, that affected 95 of 100 persons employed in the health department and numerous visitors, including the epidemiologists from CDC who were sent to investigate the outbreak.[174] This illness, which was called Pontiac fever, was characterized by self-limited symptoms of fever, chills, headache, and myalgia, lasting 2 to 5 days. In contrast to the Legionnaires' disease outbreak, none of those involved in the Pontiac fever outbreak developed pneumonia.

Subsequent to the identification of *Legionella pneumophila*, methods have been developed to diagnose infections with this bacteria and related agents. The organism can be grown on charcoal yeast extract agar, and serologic methods are also available for diagnosis. A number of outbreaks have been identified that usually involved exposure to aerosols generated by cooling towers, mist machines, shower heads, and other aerosols.[175–178] Over 30 different species of *Legionella* have been identified, and 19 have been found to infect humans. The organisms have been found to replicate in freshwater amoeba and protozoa.[179–181] They grow at temperatures of 40° to 50°C and survive in chlorinated water. However, they can be eliminated by hyperchlorination or heating water to higher temperatures.[134–136] Recent studies have shown that *Legionella* strains are a common cause of endemic pneumonia, both in the community and in health care settings.

Influenza Viruses

Perhaps the most important emerging virus infection of humans is influenza. This highly contagious acute respiratory illness has caused epidemics in humans since ancient times. One influenza epidemic was recorded by Hippocrates in 412 BC, and numerous epidemics were described in the Middle Ages.[182] Epidemics of influenza that occurred between AD 1500 and

1800 were reviewed by Noble.[183] He noted the following features of these epidemics:

- Epidemics were sudden in onset and occurred frequently but at irregular intervals.
- Epidemics varied in severity but usually caused mortality, primarily in older persons.
- Some epidemics spread worldwide from their origins in Russia or China.

Influenza is the principal infectious disease that has been severe enough to cause major increases in mortality in the total population of the United States and Europe in the 1900s, prior to the advent of the epidemic of HIV/AIDS in the early 1980s. The most severe epidemic of the 1900s was the "Spanish Influenza" pandemic of 1918–1919. An estimated 20 to 40 million persons died in this pandemic. This epidemic is believed to have been caused by a new H1/N1 swine influenza virus, to which none of the human population was immune.

A limited epidemic in humans of a totally new strain of influenza, due to an H5N1 influenza virus, occurred in Hong Kong in the winter of 1997. Infections with this virus were fatal in a high proportion (about 30%) of the humans that were infected and caused disseminated viremia in infected persons.[184] The virus was epidemic in chickens in Hong Kong at the time. However, there was no evidence of person-to-person transmission of this new human virus; all human cases had direct contact with chickens and probably acquired their infection as a zoonotic infection. Public health authorities slaughtered a large number of infected chickens to prevent further chicken-to-human transmission of this H5N1 virus and control this epidemic. Recently, outbreaks of H5N1 influenza have been widespread among aquatic and domestic birds with occasional spread to humans, and rare human-to-human transmission.[185] Since the human population lacks immunity to these viruses, there is great concern that these viruses may cause the next influenza pandemic.

Staphylococcal Toxic Shock Syndrome

Infections with *Staphylococcus aureus*, a gram-positive organism, are quite common. The organism is a well-known cause of food poisoning, abscesses, pneumonia, endocarditis, and the scalded skin syndrome in humans, and causes mastitis and other infections in cattle and sheep. However, in 1978, Todd et al. reported an outbreak of a new staphylococcal disease, a severe systemic illness in young children, called *toxic shock syndrome* (TSS).[186] The illness was characterized by high fever, hypotension or shock, a generalized erythematous rash that progresses to desquamation, and multiorgan system dysfunction. Toxin-producing strains of *S. aureus* were recovered from various sites in these children with TSS.

Two years later, TSS cases suddenly appeared, first in Wisconsin and Minnesota, then nationwide, among young adult women during their menstrual period.[187,188] The disease was serious and caused substantial mortality; however, recovery was complete among survivors. Recurrences were common during a subsequent menses unless the offending *S. aureus* vaginal infection was effectively treated with antibiotics. Eventually, 941 cases were reported from every state in the United States; however, 247 (26%) of the cases occurred in women in Minnesota and Wisconsin.[188]

The pathogenesis of TSS involved the use of "superabsorbent" tampons made of a blend of synthetic materials, including polyacrylate fibers, carboxymethyl cellulose, high-absorbency rayon-cellulose, and polyester foam. Previously, tampons had been made of rayon or a blend of rayon and cotton. These superabsorbent tampons were much more absorbent than the traditional tampons marketed previously and could be left in place for longer periods. However, they tended to cause abrasions of the vaginal mucosa, and the blood-soaked tampons were a very good culture medium for the proliferation of *S. aureus*, which produced a chromosomally encoded toxin, designated *toxic shock syndrome toxin-1* (TSST-1). Studies have shown that over 90% of *S. aureus* strains recovered from vaginal cultures of women with TSS synthesized TSST-1, whereas the toxin is found much less frequently in other *S. aureus* isolates.[189,190] The TSST-1 is a member of the class of structurally related molecules called *superantigens*. TSST-1 and other superantigens bind to the major histocompatibility complex (MHC) class II molecules of antigen-presenting cells. This results in the stimulation of production of a number of cytokines, including several interleukins–tumor necrosis factors (TNFs) alpha, beta, and interferon gamma–leading to multiple systemic symptoms.

Importantly, the public health response in removing these highly absorbent tampons from the market as soon as they were implicated in TSS effectively controlled this devastating epidemic.[191] However, occasional sporadic cases that were not related to tampon use continued to be reported (Figure 13-21).

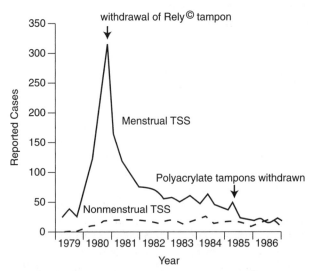

FIGURE 13-21   Number of reported cases of toxic shock syndrome in the United States, by year (1979–1986), based on passive surveillance.
Source: C.V. Broome, Epidemiology of Toxic Shock Syndrome in the United States: Overview, *Review of Infectious Disease*, Vol. 11, Suppl. 1, p. S17, © 1989, University of Chicago Press.

Streptococcal Infections

Infections from group A streptococci in the 1800s often were quite severe, even fatal. However, the mortality from scarlet fever, a common manifestation of toxigenic group A streptococcal infections, declined dramatically in the United States, beginning in the early 1900s. During World War II, acute rheumatic fever, a chronic complication of group A streptococcal infections, was quite common, especially among troops stationed in crowded military barracks.[192] During this time, extensive epidemiologic studies were done to define the risk factors associated with clinical or subclinical infection with group A streptococci and subsequent acute rheumatic fever.[192]

Antibiotic treatment regimens were evaluated in carefully controlled clinical trials to develop regimens that eradicated pathogenic group A streptococci from the pharynx and prevented rheumatic fever.[193,194] This was followed by a dramatic decrease in the incidence of severe streptococcal infections, acute rheumatic fever (ARF), and poststreptococcal glomerulonephritis between the 1960s and early 1980s. Although group A streptococci were still commonly cultured from the throat in persons with and without pharyngitis, severe inflammation was uncommon, and the risk of subsequent rheumatic fever seemed to be very low. Most experts believe that the attenuated severity of acute streptococcal infections and decrease in the incidence of acute rheumatic fever during this period was not due to the widespread use of therapeutic antibiotics. Instead, the change in virulence was believed to be due to poorly understood changes in the epidemiology, the infectivity, or the virulence factors of streptococci causing human infections.

Suddenly, in 1985, a substantial increase in the number of cases of ARF occurred in Salt Lake City and surrounding areas; 136 cases of ARF were reported from persons living in this area in 1985 and 1986.[195] Most of the patients had typical full-blown rheumatic fever, and most were middle- or upper-class suburban or urban residents. Poor, lower-class populations from the inner cities were overrepresented in rheumatic fever patients earlier in the century.

Subsequently, Stevens and colleagues described 20 patients from the Rocky Mountain region (Utah, Idaho, Montana, and Nevada) with an unusually severe form of systemic group A streptococcal infection.[196] These patients had extensive local tissue destruction and signs and symptoms of severe systemic toxicity. Nineteen of these patients had shock, 80% had renal impairment, many had an acute respiratory distress syndrome, and six died. In some patients, necrotizing fasciitis (soft tissue and muscle necrosis) was a prominent feature. The group A streptococci that were isolated from these patients produced an exotoxin that was similar to the TSS toxin (TSST-1) produced by *S. aureus* strains isolated from patients with the staphylococcal TSS. Subsequently, a dramatic increase in the number of patients with streptococcal TSS and necrotizing fasciitis occurred throughout the United States, Canada, several European countries, Australia, and New Zealand.[197] The organisms associated with necrotizing fasciitis were termed *flesh-eating bacteria* by the lay press.

Investigation of this resurgence of severe streptococcal disease in the past 15 years has found that most strains contain M-protein types 1 or 3 (over 80 M-protein types of streptococci have been identified). Group A streptococci are often classified on the basis of their M-protein, which is a known virulence factor. Perhaps more important, most of the organisms associated with the TSS or necrotizing fasciitis produce streptococcal exotoxin types A, B, or C. So, for unknown reasons, there appeared to be an emergence of new types of streptococci that commonly infected human populations with increased pathogenicity and virulence during the last decade of the 1900s. The factors leading to the emergence of these more virulent streptococci are poorly understood, as was the decreased pathogenicity of group A streptococci in the previous few decades. Possibly, host factors, such as low levels of herd immunity to these more virulent strains or genetic changes in the organisms, may have played a significant role in the emergence of these serious infections.

Transmissible Spongiform Encephalopathies

In the last 30 years, a radically new class of infectious agents, the spongiform encephalopathies, has been recognized as the cause of several diseases of man and animals (Exhibit 13-2). The infectious agents causing these diseases appear to differ from viruses, in that they do not contain nucleic acids but only proteins; they have been labeled *prions*, or *proteinaceous infectious particles* by Stanley Prusiner.[198,199] The spongiform encephalopathies are unique among the infectious diseases in that they exhibit none of the traditional hallmarks of an infectious disease. The brain tissue of animals with these infections show spongiform changes in the cytoplasm of nerve cells without an inflammatory infiltrate; the patient or animal does not have a fever, high white cell count, or a rise in acute phase reactants or cytokines; nor is there a measurable immune response to the infectious agent.[200] Therefore, these

Exhibit 13-2 Transmissible Spongiform Encephalopathies of Animals and Humans (Prion Diseases)

A. Animal Diseases
- Scrapie (sheep and goats)
- Transmissible mink encephalopathy
- Wasting disease of deer and elk
- Bovine spongiform encephalopathy*
- Transmissible spongiform encephalopathy of captive wild ruminants*
- Feline spongiform encephalopathy*

B. Human Diseases
- Kuru
- Sporadic Creutzfeldt-Jakob disease
- Familial Creutzfeldt-Jakob disease
- Gerstmann-Straussler-Scheinker disease
- Fatal familial insomnia
- New variant Creutzfeldt-Jakob disease*

*These diseases all appear to have a common source.
Source: R. T. Johnson and C. J. Gibbs, Greutzfeldt-Jakob Disease and Selected Transmissable Spongiform Encephalopathies, *New England Journal of Medicine*, Vol. 339, pp. 1994-2004, Copyright © 1998, Massachusetts Medical Society. All rights reserved.

diseases originally were felt to be degenerative, rather than infectious, and due to genetic factors, rather than infectious agents.

Scrapie

The disease of sheep called *scrapie* has been known for at least 200 years. It is widespread among sheep in Europe, Asia, and the Americas, and is also seen among goats cohabiting with affected sheep. The Scottish term *scrapie* comes from the characteristic feature of the disease, which is marked by areas of the skin denuded of fleece, due to the animals rubbing their irritated skin against fixed objects. The disease is insidious in onset but is characterized eventually by a progressive, eventually fatal, ataxia that leads to death of the affected animals in a matter of months. The affected sheep are afebrile and have normal CSF and no overt signs of infection. Pathologic lesions are limited to the central nervous system and show the characteristic noninflammatory spongiform lesions with nerve loss, cytoplasmic vacuolization of degenerating nerves, and a striking astrocytosis. The disease initially was felt to be an autosomal dominant genetic disease until two French investigators transmitted the disease to uninfected animals and found the agent to be a filterable agent.[201] Subsequently, it was demonstrated that the disease also could be transmitted to mice.[202]

The scrapie agent is unusual in that it contains no nucleic acids and is resistant to chemicals that normally inactivate nucleic acids, such as formaldehyde, ethanol, UV radiation, alkylating agents (such as B-propriolactone), proteases, and nucleases. However, the organism can be inactivated by autoclaving at 121°C under pressure or by exposure to extremes of pH, detergents, or phenol. The infectious agent has been felt to be an infectious protein, or prion, which is a proteinase-resistant isoform of a normal cellular protein that is characterized by abnormal folding.[198,199]

Kuru

In the 1950s, a disease was recognized among primitive Fore people living in a remote area of highland New Guinea. The disease was called *Kuru*, meaning *shivering* or *trembling* in the Fore language. The disease was characterized by an insidious onset of truncal ataxia. The ataxia progressed and became incapacitating. Eventually, ataxia occurred with every effort of voluntary movement, and death occurred uniformly 3 to 24 months after the onset of symptoms. The pathology showed spongiform changes in the brain similar to that caused by scrapie. Because of the transmission of scrapie to laboratory animals, William Hadlow, a veterinarian who had worked with the scrapie agent, suggested that Kuru might also be due to a transmissible agent.[203] Subsequently, brain tissue from Kuru patients was inoculated into chimpanzees and transmitted the disease.[204] Epidemiologic studies indicated the likelihood that Kuru was due to ritual cannibalism of the victims after their death, usually by the Fore adult women and children (Table 13-9).[204,205] 5 Consequently, the disease was more common in adult women, but male and female children were affected equally, because the women, fed infectious material to their children, regardless of their sex. With the suppression of cannibalism by Australian missionaries and settlers, the disease has virtually disappeared.[206]

Creutzfeldt-Jakob Disease

Creutzfeldt-Jakob disease (CJD) presents as a dementia, characterized by rapidly progressive mental deterioration, myoclonic jerking, and other neurologic signs. Classic CJD commonly begins between 55 and 70 years of age, but rare cases have occurred in younger adults, even in adolescents. The disease often begins with fatigue, insomnia, and other nonspecific signs or sometimes with focal signs, such as ataxia, visual loss, or aphasia. These symptoms are followed by progressive and relentless dementia, myoclonus, and other neurologic signs. The mean duration of survival is only 5 to 6 months, and over 80% of patients die within 12 months. As in the other spongiform encephalopathies, there is no fever or other signs of infection, the spinal fluid is normal, and the brain has characteristic spongiform changes.

About 10% of patients with CJD have a family history consistent with an autosomal dominant inheritance. In most but not all of these affected families, persons with CJD have a point mutation in the gene coding for the prion protein. The majority of CJD cases (90%) have no other affected family members. CJD occurs at a rate of about 1 per million persons per year without evident clustering, aside from the 10% of familial cases, in virtually all populations.

The disease has been inadvertently transmitted by the transplantation of dural and corneal grafts from infected donors. Over 80 cases have been recognized to be due to such exposures in the last 16 years.[207] It has also

TABLE 13-9 Transmission of Prion Diseases from Human to Human

Mode of Transmission	Example (no. of cases reported)	Incubation Period (years)
1. Intracranial transplantation or inoculation	a. Dural grafts (>80 cases)	1.3–17
	b. Inadequately sterilized instruments (several cases)	0.6–2.2 1.3–1.8
2. Extracranial transplantation	Corneal grafts (2 cases)	1.3–1.5
3. Extracranial inoculation of neural tissue	a. Human growth hormone and gonadotropin (>100 cases)	4–19*
	b. Arterial embolization with lyophilized dura mater (2 cases)	3.5–7.5
4. Extracranial inoculation or oral exposure	a. Possible exposure to bovine spongiform encephalopathy prion (40 cases)	5–10*
	b. Transmission of Kuru by ritual cannibalism (several thousand cases)	4.40 or more

*Numbers represent minimum incubation periods since hormone was given over periods of years (time from midpoint of treatment to onset = 12 years).
Source: R.T. Johnson and C.J. Gibbs, Creutzfeldt-Jakob Disease and Selected Transmissible Spongiform Encephalopathies, New England Journal of Medicine, Vol. 339, pp. 1994–2004, Copyright © 1998, Massachusetts Medical Society. All rights reserved.

been transmitted by the intracerebral use of a sterotactic electrode to control an epileptogenic focus. This electrode had been used previously in a CJD patient and subsequently was disinfected only by soaking in alcohol; the CJD prion, like the prion causing scrapie, is resistant to disinfection by virucidal compounds. The largest number of iatrogenic cases, however, has been transmitted by the use of human growth hormone (HGH) prepared from a large pool of human pituitary tissue. The first three cases of CJD due to growth hormone were reported in 1985. Subsequently, 16 cases have occurred in the United States, 25 cases in the United Kingdom, 53 cases in France, and scattered cases elsewhere.[208] Fortunately, HGH is now prepared synthetically, rather than by extraction from pools of human pituitary glands, so no further patients should acquire CJD by this route. However, additional clinical cases may still appear from previous exposure, due to the long incubation period of CJD; the incubation period has ranged up to 40 years in Kuru.

Bovine Spongiform Encephalopathy and Variant Creutzfeldt-Jakob Disease (vCJD)

In April 1985, a dairy farmer in the south of England observed a previously healthy cow that became apprehensive, ataxic, and developed aggressive behavior. Progressive ataxia developed, and, eventually, the cow died. When tissues were sent to the central veterinary laboratory in the United Kingdom, the brain exhibited the typical features of bovine spongiform encephalopathy (BSE), a disease of cattle known to be caused by infection with a prion. Over the next few years, the number of cases of BSE in cattle in the United Kingdom grew rapidly. Sixteen cases were found in 1986, and more than 7000 cases were found in 1989. The epidemic peaked in 1992, when 36,000 cases of BSE were reported throughout Great Britain, Scotland, and Ireland (Figure 13-22).[10]

Eventually, over 220,000 cases of BSE were reported from more than 34,000 herds in the United Kingdom.[209] The cattle herds with cases of BSE were scattered throughout the United Kingdom, and there was no evidence of horizontal transmission of the disease between cattle in the same herd. The epidemiologic pattern of disease was that of a common source, food-borne outbreak. It was eventually concluded that the most likely source was from contaminated meat and bone meal that had been used for cattle feed. Meat and bone meal (MBM) had been prepared in the United Kingdom from the rendered carcasses of sheep and other livestock, including cattle. Sheep had long been known to have an endemic level of infection with a prion disease, scrapie, in the United Kingdom. But not until the 1980s had BSE appeared in cattle. On investigation, it was concluded that prion from scrapie-infected sheep and cattle with BSE were identical.[210-211] The epidemic followed changes in the rendering process that had occurred in the late 1970s. At that time, changes were introduced into the rendering process for the preparation of bone meal from animal remains (offal), due in part to an oil crisis in the Middle East. The use of continuous heating of offal, as opposed to batch heating, was substituted to save fuel. Also, the sale of tallow became no longer profitable because of public concern about the health effects of animal fat consumption. The collapse of the tallow market resulted in most of the rendered fat remaining with the offal. Previously, it had been separated from the offal to be sold. The added fat content probably acted to prevent

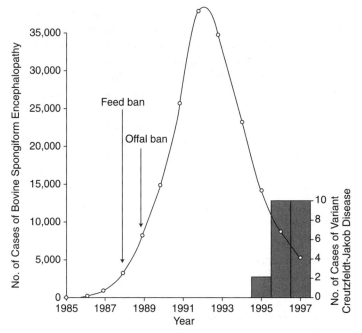

FIGURE 13-22 Cases of bovine spongiform encephalopathy (linear graph) and new-variant Creutzfeldt–Jakob disease (bar Graph) in the United Kingdom. The decline in the incidence of bovine spongiform encephalopathy began five years after the imposition of the ban on feeding ruminant-derived protein to ruminants. Cases of new-variant Creutzfeldt–Jakob disease have been reported since February 1994. It has been postulated that these patients were exposed to contaminated meat products before the ban on cattle offal in human food was imposed in 1989. In the absence of knowledge of the duration of the incubation period in humans, this cluster of cases provides little information on the possible future incidence of the disease. Dates represent the years when cases were reported rather than years of onset or death.
Source: Johnson RT et al. Creutzfeldt-Jakob disease and related transmissible spongiform encephalopathies. N Engl J Med. 1998 Dec 31;339(27):1994–2004. Copyright 1998 by the Massachusetts Medical Society.

the disinfection of prion proteins in the animal carcasses. Further amplification of the epidemic was probably related to the use of animal carcasses, including neural tissues from animals, such as cattle, and sheep that succumbed to BSE or scrapie, for the preparation of animal feed. So the dose of BSE/scrapie prions in cattle feed probably had increased dramatically in the late 1970s. Bovine spongiform encephalopathy and other prion diseases have been transmitted experimentally to a number of species by the oral route; oral transmission has been accomplished with various species of rodents and nonhuman primates.[212] These experimental data supported the hypothesis that BSE could be a food-borne outbreak in the cattle. The theory that the BSE agent in cattle had originated from sheep scrapie was strengthened considerably when molecular genetic studies of the BSE prion protein found it to be identical to the scrapie protein.[211]

Concern about the growing epidemic of BSE grew until the UK government instituted a ban against the use of carcasses from animals at risk to spongiform diseases for the preparation of animal feed. In 1988, a ban on feeding animal-derived feed (such as meat and bone meal from rendered sheep, goats, or cattle) to ruminants was instituted in the United Kingdom (Figure 13-22). This intervention was most likely the critical public health strategy to control the BSE epidemic. Nevertheless, as the epidemic evolved, disturbing evidence appeared suggesting cross-species infection from the BSE prion may have occurred. Domestic cats, as well as captive and exotic ruminants, died of BSE after eating animal feed containing possibly infected cattle tissues.[213] However, the public health actions that were taken, especially the animal feed ban in 1988, had a dramatic effect on controlling the epidemic after a lag period of about 5 years, which is the median incubation period of the disease in cattle. The epidemic peaked in 1992 and has declined progressively since then (Figure 13-22).

The occurrence of BSE in species other than cattle heightened concerns as to whether humans might also be susceptible.[213,214] Although there was no evidence that humans were susceptible to scrapie, which had been endemic in sheep in the United Kingdom for two centuries, passage of prions through another animal may have altered the host range. There is good evidence in other prion diseases that passage of a prion through one species may alter the host susceptibility in a third species. Experimentally, mouse-adapted strains of scrapie passed through hamsters altered their transmissibility to other rodents,[215] human strains of Kuru or CJD could not be transmitted to ferrets until passed through primates or cats,[216] and a bovine strain of BSE could not be transmitted to hamsters until it was passed through mice.[217] Although the reasons for the species barrier in prion diseases is not known, the theory is that the likelihood of successful interspecies transmission is influenced by the degree of homology between the pathologic prion protein and the host endogenous prion protein. The pathogenesis of prion disease is believed to be related to an abnormal folding of a prion protein that accumulates in neural tissues.

In 1989, specified bovine offals (including brain, spinal cord, and organ meats) were banned from human food in the United Kingdom. However, because of concern about the potential transmission of BSE to humans, national surveillance of CJD was instituted in the United Kingdom in 1990. During the interval between 1990 and 1994, no unusual cases or clusters of CJD in humans were encountered.[215] However, beginning in 1994, patients with CJD with an unusual clinical presentation, course, laboratory findings, and brain histopathology appeared. Furthermore, these cases of atypical CJD were much younger than the classic cases. Because of their unusual demographic, clinical, and pathologic features, they were called *variant Creutzfeldt-Jakob disease* (vCJD).[218,219] The clinical and pathologic differences between classic and variant CJD made it possible to classify patients (Table 13-10). The cases could then be classified definitively by molecular analysis of their prion to determine whether it was a BSE or classic prion protein. Between 1995 and 2004, 148 deaths from vCJD occurred in the United Kingdom, seven deaths occurred in France, and one death each occurred in Ireland, Italy, Canada, Japan, and the United States (Table 13-11). Importantly, the numbers of cases of classic CJD and hereditary CJD in the United Kingdom remained about the same during this interval (Table 13-12).

TABLE 13-10 Comparison of New-Variant and Sporadic Creutzfeldt-Jakob Disease

Characteristic	Variant*	Sporadic
Mean age at onset (yr)	29	60
Mean duration of disease (mo)	14	5
Most consistent and prominent early signs	Psychiatric abnormalities, sensory symptoms	Dementia, myoclonus
Cerebellar signs (% of patients)	100	40
Electroencephalographic periodic complexes (% of patients)	0	94
Pathological changes	Diffuse amyloid plaques	Sparse plaques in 10%

Source: Johnson RT et al., Creutzfeldt-Jakob disease and related transmissible spongiform encephalopathies. N Engl J Med. 1998 Dec 31;339(27):1994–2004. Copyright 1998 by the Massachusetts Medical Society.

TABLE 13-11   vCJD Cases Worldwide

• France	15
• Italy	1
• Netherlands	1
• Portugal	1
• Spain	1
• Republic of Ireland	2
○ Republic of Ireland	2
○ USA	1
○ Canada	1
○ Japan	1
○ Saudi Arabia (source uncertain)	1
• Probably acquired in UK ○ Probably non-UK.	

Source: R. Knight. CJD Surveillance Unit, Edinburgh.

Variant Creutzfeldt-Jakob Disease

The patients with vCJD are strikingly different from those with classic CJD. They are quite young with a mean age of 29 years versus 60 years for sporadic, classic CJD patients. They present with prominent psychiatric and behavioral manifestations, and have persistent painful paresthesia; the skin sensations may be similar to the sensory abnormalities leading to the scrapie lesions in sheep. Cerebellar ataxia uniformly develops, and the clinical course is prolonged, with an average survival of 14 months, compared with only 5 months in classic sporadic CJD.[199,219] The electroencephalogram fails to show the typical periodic complexes of classic CJD, although some EEG abnormalities may occur. The histopathology of the brain lesions in vCJD differs from

TABLE 13-12 Deaths from Definite and Probable CJD, 1990–2004

	Referrals of Suspect CJD		Deaths of Definite and Probable CJD					
Year	Referrals	Year	Sporadic	Iatrogenic	Familial	GSS	vCJD	Total Deaths
1990	[53]	1990	28	5	0	0	—	33
1991	75	1991	32	1	3	0	—	36
1992	96	1992	45	2	5	1	—	53
1993	78	1993	37	4	3	2	—	46
1994	118	1994	53	1	4	3	—	61
1995	87	1995	35	4	2	3	3	47
1996	134	1996	40	4	2	4	10	60
1997	161	1997	60	6	4	1	10	81
1998	154	1998	63	3	3	2	18	89
1999	170	1999	62	6	2	0	15	85
2000	178	2000	50	1	2	1	28	82
2001	179	2001	58	4	3	2	20	87
2002	163	2002	72	0	4	1	17	94
2003	162	2003	76	5	4	2	18	105
2004	112	2004	46	1	2	1	9	59
Total Referrals	**1920**	**Total Deaths**	**757**	**47**	**43**	**23**	**148**	**1018**

Source: CJD Surveillance Unit, Edinburgh.

that in classic CJD in containing diffuse amyloid plaques called *florid plaques* (or daisy plaques) (Table 13-10). When brain tissue from patients with vCJD is inoculated into mice by the intracerebral route, the incubation period of vCJD and BSE are identical and differ from classic CJD.[220]

All of the patients with vCJD had a history of eating meat prior to their illnesses. One patient reported becoming a vegetarian within 1 year of onset of symptoms of vCJD, but he had eaten beef previously. None reported eating cattle brains but, prior to the ban on the inclusion of cattle brain tissues (or specific bovine offals—SBOs) in human food in 1989, these tissues were commonly included in sausages, meat pies, and other human foods. As a result of the epidemiologic, clinical, histopathologic, and animal inoculation data cited above, it is now clear that variant Creutzfeldt-Jakob disease represents human infection with the prions of BSE, due to oral ingestion of the agent in food.[220] If this theory is correct, it raises several difficult public health issues. How many cases of vCJD will eventually occur in the United Kingdom after the limit of the incubation period has been reached? How many people are now incubating the disease in the United Kingdom, where over 200,000 cases of BSE in cattle have been reported?

Predicting the number of cases of vCJD that might eventually occur in the United Kingdom has been extremely problematic. Different scientists have used different sets of data at various times during the epidemic and different assumptions about the biology, transmissibility, and incubation period of BSE to predict the eventual numbers of cases of vCJD that might occur.[221-224] These estimates have ranged from high estimates of 6.1–13.7 million cases, a prediction made in the late 1990s, to about 300–400 cases in the most recent and probably most realistic prediction in 2003. The difficulties for epidemiologists in agreeing on a similar prediction are several. First, the number of cattle infected with BSE was large; 200,000 cases were diagnosed and reported but also several million asymptomatic cattle over 30 months of age were consumed prior to the report of the first human cases of vCJD. What the risk to humans is of consuming meat from an infected cow is unknown. However, the risk likely varies greatly by whether neurologic tissue or organ meats are consumed or not, since the BSE prion is not present in muscle but is localized to neural tissue and lymphoid-containing organs. However, several popular cuts of meat, such as T-bone steak, often contain intercostal nerves and if the animal has been killed by first stunning the cow with an air gun, this could drive brain and CNS tissue into blood vessels and muscle; also mechanically recovered meat often contains neural tissue.[225] When meat is mechanically recovered, instruments are used to scrape the meat from the bone after the carcass has been cut into steaks, and this often results in the inclusion of nerve tissue.

The second problem is that the incubation period can be quite long in prion diseases. It is assumed that vCJD probably has an incubation period of 10–15 years, with some cases occurring after much longer periods, perhaps up to 40 years, as has been observed with Kuru.

Third, it appears that only a proportion of the human population is fully susceptible to vCJD. Susceptibility is related to the amino acid composition of the prion protein gene in humans; all of the human cases studied to date have been homozygous for methionine at the prion protein codon (codon 129). Only about 40% of the British population is homozygous for methionine (Met/Met) at prion codon 129; 50% are heterozygous methionine/valine, and 11% are homozygous for valine at the prion protein codon 129 (Table 13-13). Among cases of sporadic CJD in the United Kingdom that occurred between 1990 and 2001, 69% were Met/Met, 15% were Met/Val, and 17% were Val/Val. Also in the 51 cases of iatrogenic CJD in France, who were infected by contaminated human growth hormone, 32 (61%) were Met/Met, 6 (12%) were Met/Val, and 13 (25%) were Val/Val at codon 129; the non-Met/Met cases were smaller in number and had a 5-year longer incubation period.[226] Therefore, it is possible that persons who are not homozygous for Met/Met at codon 129 will have reduced susceptibility to vCJD but a longer incubation period. Nevertheless, the number of cases of vCJD have declined since peaking in 2000 when 28 cases were diagnosed, while sporadic, iatrogenic, and familial CJD have remained stable (Table 13-12). These data suggest that the eventual number of cases will be in the hundreds, rather than the thousands or millions as was predicted earlier. The declining number of BSE cases in the United Kingdom and the extensive public health procedures to eliminate human exposure to BSE-infected cattle has probably limited any human exposure in persons in the United Kingdom to the period 1980–1996 (Figure 13-23).

However, since the BSE epidemic among cattle in the United Kingdom was recognized, other countries have reported BSE in their cattle.[227] From 1986 through 2001, more than 98% of BSE cases worldwide were reported from the United Kingdom where the disease was first described. During this period, four other European countries reported at least one indigenous case. By 1998, the number of countries with cattle BSE increased to 8 and then to 18 by 2001. From 2001 to 2003, three countries outside Europe, Canada, Japan, and Israel, reported cases of BSE. In 2004, a case of BSE was reported in a cow in the United States that had been imported from Canada. By the year 2003, more than 55% of BSE cases worldwide were reported outside the United Kingdom.[227] This apparent diffusion of BSE cases reflected a marked decline of BSE among cattle in the United Kingdom, as well as improved surveillance for the disease and larger number of cases in many other countries. It is also possible that contaminated cattle feed, such as meat and bone meal (MBM), had been imported from the United Kingdom by several other countries after the laws were enacted prohibiting the use of MBM in the United Kingdom. Also, cattle from the United Kingdom may have been imported by other countries. The US FDA denies that either MBM or cattle from the United Kingdom were ever imported into the United States, however.

TABLE 13-13 Percentage of Codon 129 Genotypes in CJD and in the Normal Population

	Met/Met	Met/Val	Val/Val
Normal population	39%	50%	11%
Sporadic CJD	68%	15%	18%
hGH-related CJD	48%	20%	32%
vCJD	100%	—	—

Source: Will, RG. Acquired prion disease: iatrogenic CJD, variant CJD, kuru. British Medical Bulletin. 2003,66:255–65, by permission of the Oxford University Press.

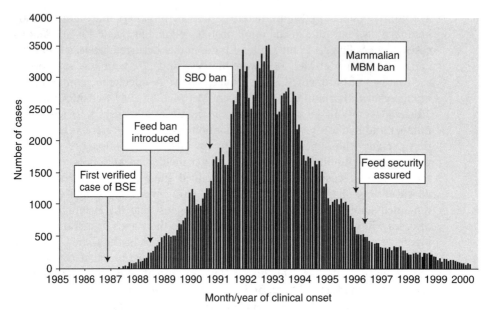

FIGURE 13-23 Time course of epidemic bovine spongiform encephalopathy in the United Kingdom, 1986–2000, with dates of major precautionary interventions. The mammalian ban on meat and bone meal in March 1996 extended a 1994 ban for farmed food animal species to include *all* mammalian species. SBO = specified bovine offals (brain, spinal cord, thymus, tonsil, spleen, and intestines from cattle >6 months of age); MBM = meat and bone meal (protein residue produced by rendering).
Source: Brown P. Bovine spongiform encephalopathy and variant Creutzfeldt-Jakob disease: background, evolution, and current concerns. Emerg Infect Dis. 2001 Jan–Feb;7(1):6–16.

An interesting study to estimate the number of UK residents who may be incubating vCJD but are now asymptomatic is being done by Hilton and colleagues.[228–230] They are collecting samples of appendices and tonsils from the general population of the United Kingdom and testing the tissues for the presence of the abnormal scrapie prion protein PRP[sc]. They have detected PRP[sc] in 3 of 12,674 appendix samples to date.[229] This gives an estimate of 237 possibly infected persons/million in the United Kingdom, with a 95% confidence interval of 49–692/million (Table 13-14).

Studies of tissues from diagnosed vCJD cases taken 3 years and 4 years prior to the onset of clinical vCJD were positive for PRP[sc] using their methods, but a sample 11 years prior to clinical vCJD from another patient was negative.[228] Clearly, more data of this type are needed to estimate the number of persons who might have subclinical BSE infections, given the wide confidence interval of currently available data. Nevertheless, these data suggest that the vCJD epidemic may well continue for at least another decade or so.

Possible Transfusion-Transmitted vCJD

Soon after the recognition of vCJD, concerns were expressed that the infection might be more likely than classic CJD to be spread by blood or blood

TABLE 13-14   PrP^{sc} in Appendix and Tonsils: Association with vCJD

Postmortem vCJD	19/20
Preclinical vCJD*	2/3
1st Surgical Survey	1/8318
2nd Surgical Survey	3/12,674

Estimated UK prevalence of abnormal PrP in lymphoid tissues.
1st survey: ~120/million (95% CI 0.5–900/million).
2nd survey: ~237/million (95% CI 49–692/million).
*1 yr, 2 yr, 10 yr (neg) before onset of symptoms; 3 yr, 4 yr, 11 yr (neg) before death.

product transfusion. Patients with vCJD routinely have evidence of prions in lymphatic tissues of the gastrointestinal tract, such as the appendix and tonsils. In contrast, in patients with classic CJD infectious prions are concentrated in the central nervous system. No evidence has been obtained to suggest that classic CJD was spread by transfusion,[231,232] despite the fact that one study found it possible to transfer CJD to mice by intracerebral injection of buffy coat cells from an infected animal.[233] A few investigators have also detected the CJD agent in the buffy coat cells of experimentally infected guinea pigs or mice. However, the prion is usually not present in human blood in patients with classic CJD. In addition, no cases of classic CJD have been reported from multiply transfused patients with clotting disorders or hemoglobinopathies. If an infectious CJD agent was present in the blood of patients prior to symptoms, patients with hemophilia and related disorders would have been transfused with infected blood during the era when factor 8 pools contained blood from up to 10,000 donors. Furthermore, recipients of blood transfusions from over 200 persons who donated blood shortly prior to the onset of clinical classic CJD have remained free of the disease, some for many years.[232] Despite this reassuring data from persons transfused with blood from patients with classic CJD, substantial concern was expressed about the possible risks of the transfusion transmission of vCJD due to the different distribution of PRP^{sc}, involving peripheral lymphatic tissues, in infected patients who are incubating the disease.

The United Kingdom transfusion service made efforts soon after the epidemic of vCJD was recognized to obtain all of their blood products from sources outside the United Kingdom to reduce this risk. In 1999, the US FDA recommended that potential blood donors who had lived in the United Kingdom 6 months or more between 1980 and 1996 be excluded as donors, while the potential risk of the transfusion transmission of vCJD was being evaluated.[210] The choice of 6 months residency in the United Kingdom to exclude donors was made in order to limit the exposure of transfusion recipients to potentially infected donors while maintaining an adequate donor pool. A survey of donors from several large Red Cross blood banks found that the 6-month deferral would exclude about 80% of donors who had lived or visited the United Kingdom, while reducing the total donor pool by only 2–3%.[210] Subsequently, BSE was reported among cattle from many other countries in Europe, however at rates far lower than in the United Kingdom

(Table 13-15). The apparent spread of BSE to other European countries led the FDA to subsequently recommend the exclusion of blood donors who had visited or lived in the United Kingdom for 3 months and also persons who had lived or visited other European countries for a total of 5 years between 1980 and 1996. The decision to exclude blood donors based on the theoretical risk of transmission of the vCJD agent was quite difficult and controversial when it was made, since it was based solely on the distribution of the prion in peripheral tissues, presumably including circulating blood cells and the theoretical risk that transfusion transmission might be possible. No transfusion-transmitted cases had occurred from vCJD, and there was fairly convincing data that the risk of transfusion transmission of classic CJD was very low or absent when the decision was being considered. However, there was a substantial concern that a large proportion of the UK population could be incubating vCJD and be infectious. The stakes of a delayed decision that was later found to be incorrect were felt to be quite high in light of the prognosis of vCJD infection after clinical symptoms appeared.

TABLE 13-15   Reported Cases of Bovine Spongiform Encephalopathy in the United Kingdom and Other Countries, as of December 2000

Country	Native Cases	Imported Cases	Total Cases
United Kingdom	180,376[a]	—	180,376
Republic of Ireland	487	12	499
Portugal	446	6	452
Switzerland[b]	363	—	363
France[b]	150	1	151
Belgium	18	—	18
Netherlands	6	—	6
Liechtenstein	2	—	2
Denmark	1	1	2
Luxembourg	1	—	1
Germany	3	6	9
Oman	—	2	2
Italy	—	2	2
Spain[c]	—	2	2
Canada	—	1	1
Falklands (UK)	—	1	1
Azores (Portugal)[d]	—	1	1

[a] Includes 1287 cases in offshore British islands.
[b] Includes cases detected by active surveillance with immunologic methods.
[c] Origin and dates of imported cases are under investigation.
[d] Case imported from Germany.
Source: Brown P. Bovine spongiform encephalopathy and variant Creutzfeldt-Jakob disease: background, evolution, and current concerns. Emerg Infect Dis. 2001 Jan–Feb;7(1):6–16.

To evaluate the risk of transfusion-transmitted vCJD, the data from the CJD surveillance unit and the UK blood donor services were linked in 1997. This study identified 48 recipients of blood from a total of 15 donors who later developed vCJD.[234] In one of these cases, transfusion transmission of vCJD probably occurred. The recipient was a 62-year-old who had been transfused with red cells from a 24-year-old donor in 1996. The donor developed vCJD in 2000, 3 years and 4 months after the donation. The recipient developed symptoms of vCJD in late 2002, 6.5 years after the blood transfusion.

Subsequently another probable transfusion-transmitted infection occurred in the United Kingdom.[235] This patient had received a unit of nonleukodepleted red blood cells from a donor who developed vCJD 18 months after his donation. Five years after the transfusion the recipient died from a ruptured aortic aneurysm. At postmortem the protease-resistant scrapie protein was detected in his spleen and cervical lymph node, but not in the brain of this patient. So the patient was infected but had not yet developed vCJD. He was found to be heterozygous at prion protein codon 129; the codon contained both methionine and valine. This raises the possibility that heterozygotes are susceptible to infection but may have longer incubation periods prior to clinical vCJD.

Remaining Questions

There are several important outstanding questions abut this continuing epidemic. First, how many vCJD cases will eventually occur in the United Kingdom? Will cases occur among persons who are heterozygous, or have Val/Val amino acids at codon 129? Will additional cases occur in countries outside the United Kingdom? Will additional transfusion-transmitted cases of vCJD be detected? Will human cases of vCJD occur in populations outside the United Kingdom where cattle BSE has been identified? Is there a risk of nosocomial transmission by contaminated instruments used for surgery in patients who are incubating vCJD but are not yet clinically ill? How long will this tragic epidemic persist?[236]

Chronic Wasting Disease of Mule Deer and Elk

Several prion diseases affect animals but have not been found to be transmissible to humans to date. One such disease of concern is chronic wasting disease (CWD). This disease affects only deer (*Odocoileus* species) and Rocky Mountain elk (*Cervus elaphus nelsoni*).[237] CWD was first identified as a fatal wasting syndrome of captive mule deer in the 1960s in research facilities in Colorado and was recognized to be a transmissible spongiform encephalopathy in 1978.[238] The disease was first recognized in wild, free-ranging elk in Colorado in 1981.[239] Subsequently, it was found among deer and elk in a contiguous area in northeastern Colorado and southeastern Wyoming (Figure 13-24). Based on surveillance of hunter-harvested animals from 1996–1999, it has been estimated that 5% of mule deer, 2% of white-tailed deer, and <1.0% of elk may be infected.[240] The diagnosis of preclinical or clinical CWD can be made based upon immunohistochemical studies.[241,242]

The disease can be transmitted horizontally from one animal to another, in contrast to BSE. Also the environment can be contaminated with prions

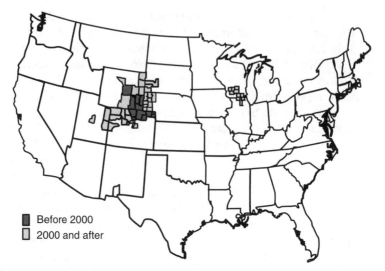

Before 2000
2000 and after

FIGURE 13-24 Chronic wasting disease among free-ranging deer and elk by county, United States.
Source: Belay, ED et al. Chronic wasting disease and potential transmission to humans. Emerg Infect Dis. 2004 Jun;10(6):977–84.

from an animal that has died. This can cause recurring epidemics among captive animals that are housed in an area where CSW-positive animals have previously died.

In the past few years the disease has spread beyond its previous locale to include areas in Utah, southern Wisconsin, and New Mexico.[243] It isn't clear how the disease spread, but it could have been by migration or transport of animals for hunting. Out of concern about CWD spread among wild deer and elk in Wisconsin and the fear that CWD could eventually be spread to humans, the Wisconsin Department of Natural Resources launched a culling program by providing special hunting permits to eliminate the disease in the area where it was detected.[243] Thus far no humans have been found to have been infected with the CWD prion. However, public health officials remain concerned because of the example of BSE, the long incubation period of prion disease, the difficulty of diagnosing prion diseases prior to symptoms, and the frequent human consumption of venison among persons living in the endemic area for CWD. A few cases of encephalopathy in young persons exposed to venison have been reported, but on careful study they were found to be classic CJD with onset at a young age and not infection with the CWD prion.[244] However, it is not certain at this point that CWD could not be spread to humans if larger numbers of persons consumed CWD-infected animals. Continued surveillance is essential.

Responses to the Threat of Emerging Infections

Institute of Medicine

As with any public health problem, an effective plan to deal with the reality of new and emerging infections depends on the official recognition of the problem. The recognition that emerging infections constituted a substantial threat to the health of the American public and the population of the world was fostered by a meeting and report of the problem by a committee on emerging microbial threats to health. This committee was chaired by Nobel Laureate Dr. Joshua Lederberg, professor at Rockefeller University, and Dr. Robert E. Shope, professor of epidemiology and director of the Arbovirus Research Unit at Yale University School of Medicine. The committee of the Institute of Medicine (IOM) met in February 1991 and convened an expert multidisciplinary committee to conduct an 18-month study of emerging microbial threats to health. The charge to the committee was "to identify significant emerging infectious disease, determine what might be done to deal with them, and recommend how similar future threats might be confronted to lessen their impact on public health."[245]

After reviewing evidence on the emergence of infectious disease presented by numerous experts, the committee made a series of recommendations, including the following:

1. The need for strengthened surveillance of infectious disease through CDC, National Institutes of Health (NIH), and the US Department of Agriculture (USDA)
2. Expansion of the National Nosocomial Infection Surveillance (NNIS) system managed by the CDC
3. Development by the US Public Health Service of a computerized database on infectious disease surveillance and vaccine and drug availability
4. Increase of creative and coordinated international infectious disease surveillance through the CDC, Department of Defense, NIH, and USDA
5. Increased research on agent, host, vector, and environmental factors leading to the emergence of infectious disease and expansion of the Epidemic Intelligence Service (EIS) and Field Epidemiology Training Program of the CDC
6. Congressional funding of a program installed in the National Health Service Corps for training in public health and related disciplines
7. Development of a means for generating stockpiles of selected important vaccines
8. Development of procedures to ensure availability and usefulness of critical antibiotics to maintain human health
9. Development and implementation by the Environmental Protection Agency of procedures for the licensing of critical pesticides for use in infectious disease emergencies and giving of priority for funding to develop new pesticides
10. Focus of attention on developing more effective ways to use education to enhance behavior change in groups at high risk of particular infectious diseases

Other National and International Agencies

Subsequent to the recommendation of the Institute of Medicine committee, several national and international health agencies have developed plans for dealing with the threat of new and emerging infections. The CDC plan focuses on more effective surveillance, improvements in the public health infrastructure, and applied research in public health prevention activities.[246] The NIH focuses on research and training. The Department of Defense plan focuses on surveillance and detection of new and emerging infectious disease, especially in international settings, and the development of better vaccines. The World Health Organization plans to improve international surveillance and communication to detect and monitor emerging infectious diseases.

Newly Discovered Pathogens

Traditionally, infectious agents have been linked to specific diseases by the isolation of an organism on artificial media, a tissue culture, recovery of the organism after inoculation of infectious material into an animal, or visualization of the organism in tissues or excretions of an infected patient. However, in the last decade or so, molecular biologists have developed methods to identify the genetic material (DNA or RNA) of infectious organisms and even sequence the genome of pathogenic organisms without ever isolating the entire intact organism in vitro. One of the first examples of the genetic characterization of an organism using molecular methods solely was the amplification of the nucleic acid of the hepatitis C virus (HCV) and the identification of this important cause of human hepatitis in 1989.[247] Recently, additional successes have been reported in the use of molecular methods to identify the causative agents of infectious diseases. Also, epidemiologic methods have been applied to link new agents to well-studied chronic diseases. Both of these approaches have revolutionized thinking about infectious diseases and have identified "new" infectious diseases. Several examples will be reviewed briefly.

Whipples Disease

In 1907, George Whipple described a disease characterized by chronic diarrhea, with malabsorption, weight loss, polyarticular arthritis, and lymphadenopathy.[248] The intestines and lymph nodes of patients with the disease had abnormal fat deposits, and the disease was often called *intestinal lipodystrophy*. However, Whipple also noted bacilli in the walls of the intestines, but repeated attempts to isolate and characterize the organisms by in vitro culture failed. Although steroids produced some temporary benefit, long-term antibiotic use sometimes was curative. With the advent of modern methods of molecular biology, it was possible to amplify the bacterial 16SrRNA gene and identify the causative organism as an actinomycete, which has been named *Tropheryma whippelii*.[249]

Cat Scratch Fever, Bacillary Angiomatosis, and Trench Fever

The clinical disease cat scratch fever has been known to clinicians for some time. It is characterized by fever and unilateral necrotizing lymphadenopathy involving the epitrochlear and axillary nodes that appear after a cat scratch. Recently, another syndrome, bacillary angiomatosis (BA), has been recognized in AIDS patients. This disease is characterized by nodular vascular proliferative lesions in the skin, bone, or other organs. Infection of the liver results in the formation of angiomatous lesions known as *bacillary peliosis hepatis*. Using both molecular techniques and cultures, an organism, *Bartonella henselii*, has been isolated from patients with cat scratch fever and with BA. Apparently, the organism causing the two diseases is similar, and host factors determine the clinical appearance of the resultant disease after infection. The organisms are sensitive to macrolide antibiotics, but the response is somewhat dependent on the immune competence of the infected patient. The reservoir for BA is the domestic cat, and the organisms are spread to humans by the cat flea.[250]

A related organism, *Bartonella quintana*, is the cause of trench fever, a disease that was common among soldiers serving in World War I; the disease was transmitted from one person to another by the body louse.[251] Although the disease has become very rare, cases have been described recently among homeless men.[252,253]

Helicobacter pylori: Peptic Ulcer and Gastric Cancer

Spiral bacteria have been found in the human stomach since 1906.[254] At one time, they were believed to lead to chronic inflammation and gastritis, but this theory was abandoned in favor of chronic stress, leading to acid and pepsin hypersecretion, as an explanation for the pathogenesis of chronic peptic ulcer disease. However, Warren and Marshall in Australia revived interest in the hypothesis that peptic ulcer disease might be caused by an infection when they cured a patient with chronic peptic ulcer disease by treatment with tetracycline.[255] Subsequently, they isolated the putative causative organism, which was originally called *Campylobacter pyloridis* but was later renamed *Helicobacter pylori*. The organism was linked to peptic ulcer disease and chronic gastritis, and they demonstrated that these diseases could be treated successfully with antibiotics.[256] Because some antacid regimens contain bismuth, a compound now known to be active against *H. pylori*, some of the reported successes with antacid therapy could have occurred because of the effect of bismuth on the organism. In response to skepticism about the importance of *H. pylori* as the etiologic agent of gastritis, Marshall had himself gastroscoped to prove that his stomach was normal, then ingested *H. pylori* after neutralizing his stomach acid with histamine blockers. After about 7 days, he developed epigastric discomfort and vomiting. Repeat gastroscopy showed that the organism had colonized the stomach and led to acute inflammation.[257] The organism and the pathology could be cleared with antibiotic therapy. This experiment was repeated subsequently by another investigator, but the antibiotics failed to clear the *H. pylori*, and the gastritis persisted.[258] These self-experiments were followed with hundreds of studies of the association of *H. pylori* and gastric pathology. The studies have clearly and consistently shown a strong association between infections with *H. pylori* and dyspepsia, peptic ulcer disease involving both gastric and duodenal ulcers, hypertrophic gastritis, gastric cancer, and gastric lymphoma. As a result of these data, a consensus conference sponsored by the NIH in 1994 concluded that *H. pylori* infection was a major cause of peptic ulcer disease and recommended that antibiotic therapy become the mainstay of treatment.[259]

Infections with *H. pylori* are not systemic but involve only the superficial areas of the gastric mucosa. The organism secretes large amounts of urease, an enzyme that hydrolyzes urea to CO_2 and ammonia.[260] It has been hypothesized that the large amounts of ammonia produced by the urease may protect the organism from the deleterious effects of stomach acid.[261] The organism prefers to live in a neutral environment, such as is found beneath the gastric mucosa, but it can survive in an acid environment with a pH of 1.5. Infections with *H. pylori* can be detected by culture, histologic examination, or with the urease test of gastric aspirates, or it can be documented serologically by an ELISA antibody test or by using the carbon-labeled urea breath test.[262] In the breath test, the subject ingests C^{13}- or C^{14}-labeled urea, and the breakdown of the urea into C^{13} or C^{14} CO_2 by the urease-producing organisms is detected in the exhaled air.

Studies of the epidemiology of gastric cancer are also consistent with an etiologic role for *H. pylori* in this disease. Such studies have shown higher rates of *H. pylori* infection in populations living in areas with higher rates of gastric cancer. Furthermore, the prevalence of *H. pylori* is higher at early ages, especially in childhood, in countries with high gastric cancer rates. In addition, gastric cancer patients have higher rates of *H. pylori* infection than do controls.[263,264] *H. pylori* infection precedes cancer by many years.[264] The association between *H. pylori* and gastric cancer is restricted to tumors distal to the gastric cardia. Although other factors, such as smoking, may also affect the risk of gastric cancer, *H. pylori* is now believed to be of critical importance.

Gastric lymphoma is a rare disease because the stomach is not a lymphoid organ; the incidence is estimated to be about seven cases per million population per year.[265] The pathogenesis of gastric lymphoma and the association with *H. pylori* are believed to be related to the chronic inflammatory response to the infection.[266]

The theory that gastric cancer could be etiologically related to *H. pylori* infections helps to explain the epidemiology of this tumor over the last several decades in the United States.[264] Mortality from gastric cancer has shown dramatic reductions in incidence during the last several decades (Figure 13-25). This could be explained by the changes in hygiene that occurred during the 1900s that have afforded less opportunity for high rates of infections with *H. pylori* during childhood and gastric cancer several decades later. In contrast, in areas of the world with greater opportunities for fecal–oral transmission of *H. pylori*, the rates of gastric cancer remain high.

Chlamydia pneumoniae, CMV, *Helicobacter pylori* and Other Organisms, and Atherosclerosis

A recent hypothesis that is more controversial and uncertain than the *H. pylori*–peptic ulcer/gastric cancer association is that infections with one of several organisms may initiate or be a cofactor in coronary atherosclerosis.[267] In reality, the idea that heart attacks might be caused by a specific infection is an old idea that was popular at the end of the 1800s and early in the 1900s.[268,269] However, infections have not been considered to be relevant cofactors or even evaluated systematically in the many epidemiologic studies of coronary heart disease (CHD) that have been done during the last

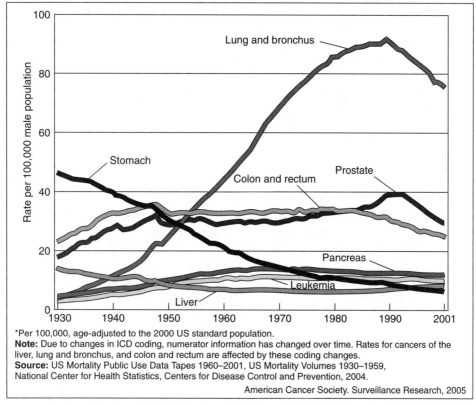

FIGURE 13-25 Age-adjusted cancer death rates, males by site, US, 1930–2001.
Source: Cancer Facts and Figures, 2005. American Cancer Society.

four decades. The Framingham study of the NIH concluded that there were three primary factors in the pathogenesis of CHD, namely, elevated serum cholesterol and triglycerides, elevated blood pressure, and tobacco smoking. Some studies have found that other factors also could be important, such as stress, sedentary lifestyle, obesity, and dietary biochemical factors other than cholesterol, such as homocystine. Many epidemiologic studies of CHD have identified the same risk factors. Therefore, public health programs for the prevention of CHD have emphasized reduction in animal fat in the diet and reduction of serum cholesterol by diet or with the use of cholesterol-lowering drugs, blood pressure control, and prevention/cessation of cigarette smoking. The implementation of these public health programs has been accompanied by significant reduction in mortality from CHD. Nevertheless, CHD remains the number one cause of death in the United States.

Only recently has the role of infections in the etiology of CHD been suggested and studied. Most studies have focused on one of three organisms: *H. pylori*, CMV, or *C. pneumoniae*.

H. pylori *Infection*

An association between *H. pylori* infections and CHD was first reported in 1994.[270] Since that time, a few additional studies have been reported. Most, including all of the prospective studies, have shown a modestly (and non-significant) elevated risk of CHD in patients with *H. pylori* infection. Many of the studies have not adequately adjusted for confounders, such as low socioeconomic status.[271] *H. pylori* leads only to a localized infection in the gastric mucosa. How, then, could it cause heart disease? It has been postulated that the pathogenetic mechanism is an autoimmune reaction between the heat shock protein 60 of *H. pylori* and a similar antigen in the endothelium of cardiac vessels.[272] Although this is an intriguing hypothesis, clearly, more data are needed on this possible association.

Cytomegalovirus

One group of investigators has reported an association between coronary stenosis, or restenosis after balloon angioplasty, and CMV antibody prevalence.[272] Another study found a significant association between carotid artery intimal narrowing and CMV antibodies.[273] Also, the CMV genome has been identified in coronary atheroma or in smooth muscle cells of coronary arteries by PCR by some investigators.[274] It is believed by some investigators that a human herpes virus might be involved in atherogenesis, because a related herpes virus causes Marek's disease, an atherosclerotic disease in chickens.

Chlamydia Pneumoniae

Chlamydia pneumoniae was first described as a distinct organism and originally named the *TWAR agent* by Grayston et al. in 1986.[275] It is now believed to be an important cause of community-acquired pneumonia in adults; it was associated with about 15% of pneumonia cases in a health maintenance organization in Seattle.[276]

Several studies have been done, and most reported a rate of *C. pneumoniae* antibodies that are twofold or more higher in patients with CHD than in matched controls.[277] The organism is an intracellular pathogen that is capable of replication in human smooth muscle cells, endothelial cells, and macrophages.[278] It has been found in about half of the atherosclerotic lesions in the 13 pathologic studies in which it has been looked for, and it is almost never present in normal arterial walls.[271,279] However, it has also been found in other tissues and, thus, could be merely an innocent bystander that infects already damaged tissue, in some cases.

Nevertheless, because a few studies have demonstrated the organism inside the cells at the base of an atheroma, it could be the nidus that initiated atheroma formation.[279] More evidence is needed before the role of *C. pneumoniae* in the genesis of coronary heart disease can be assessed, as the evidence on the role of *C. pneumoniae* in early CHD is conflicting.[280] Two large randomized controlled trials of antibiotic therapy of persons with established coronary heart disease found no evidence that the antibiotics were effective in preventing recurrent disease.[281,282] It is currently believed that *C. pneumoniae* infection may have a role as an etiologic cofactor early in the pathogenesis of coronary atherosclerosis but be less important in established disease.[283,284] However, because of the importance of CHD as a cause of morbidity and mortality, the modest elevation in risk associated with the traditional risk factors, and the intriguing preliminary data, further studies of the role of C. *pneumoniae* as an initiator or cofactor in the pathogenesis of CHD are important.

Hodgkin's Disease and Epstein-Barr Virus

Epstein-Barr virus (EBV) is known to be associated with nasopharyngeal carcinoma, a tumor that is especially common among populations living in south China. The virus has also been associated with Burkitt's lymphoma, a malignant B-cell lymphoma that is highly prevalent in children living in tropical Africa. The DNA of EBV is present in multiple copies in each cell of most African Burkitt's lymphomas.

Recently, studies have been done of EBV infection in patients with Hodgkin's disease, a common tumor of unknown etiology.[285] Earlier studies had demonstrated that persons with a history of infectious mononucleosis, a common clinical manifestation of primary EBV infection in older children and young adults, had an increased risk of developing Hodgkin's disease later in life.[286] Also, patients with Hodgkin's disease commonly have elevated antibody titers to EBV viral antigens. However, these antibodies might simply be due to reactivation of latent EBV after persons develop Hodgkin's disease. However, the recent report of increased antibody titers to EBV capsular antigen, nuclear antigen, and early antigen 4 or more years prior to the appearance of Hodgkin's disease, in comparison with matched controls, suggests that EBV infections may often precede the onset of the disease, which is one criterion for a causal association.[285] More data are needed on the association of EBV and Hodgkin's disease. The age distribution of Hodgkin's disease, with bimodal peaks in incidence, led to the suggestion by MacMahon that the disease might have two etiologies and that Hodgkin's disease occurring among young adults could be a sequelae of an infection, whereas disease with an older age of onset might have a different etiology.[286]

Other Chronic Diseases

An infectious etiology of a number of chronic diseases has been sought for many years. Several diseases of unknown etiology are believed likely to have an infectious etiology. Among the diseases considered most likely to be caused by infection are systemic lupus erythematosis, Kawasaki disease, multiple myeloma, multiple sclerosis, idiopathic aplastic anemia, juvenile diabetes mellitus, rheumatoid arthritis, and chronic myelogenous leukemia. Many other chronic diseases could have an infectious etiology. An enigmatic disease that spread across the globe in the 1920s was von Economo encephalitis.[160] It was followed by a form of Parkinsonism after an incubation period of 6 months to several years in about a third of the survivors. It is likely that von Economo disease was caused by an infectious agent; some have postulated that the swine influenza virus of 1918 was responsible, because nearly all cases of this type of encephalitis had previously had influenza during the 1918 epidemic. However, von Economo disease has disappeared.[205] Most current cases of Parkinson's disease are idiopathic, although occasionally the disease may follow acute viral encephalitis due to WE, SLE, or JE viruses or encephalitis due to coxsackie B viruses.

Criteria for Causality

The classic criteria for establishing a causal relationship between an infectious agent and a disease was developed by Robert Koch in the 1880s, at a time when microbiology was a new science. When new organisms were being isolated from sick patients and animals, it was necessary to develop a set of standardized criteria to determine whether a given organism was causative, rather than an incidental isolate or even a contaminant. The criteria that were developed became known as the *Henle-Koch postulates*, shown in the following list:

1. A causative organism had to be consistently isolated from patients or animals with the disease.
2. It was not present in patients with other diseases or as a harmless parasite.
3. The disease could be induced in another animal or person if the organism was inoculated in pure culture after it was isolated and grown in the laboratory.
4. The organism could then be found or isolated from the experimentally infected subject.

However, new technologies are now available that often make the Henle-Koch postulates less important criteria of causality. Modern molecular biology has required that the roles of causation be modified.[287] For example, molecular techniques such as consensus PCR allow the identification of conserved genetic sequences in the tissues of infected persons that are shared by closely related organisms. It may then be possible to demonstrate antibodies to proteins from organisms that have not been isolated. It may be possible to use such techniques to build a case for a causative relationship by establishing that the antibodies or the DNA or RNA are consistently present in persons with the disease and precede the clinical illness.[287] Another new PCR-based technique is called *representational difference analysis* (RDA). In this technique, healthy and diseased tissues are analyzed by a variant of PCR that subtracts sequences common to both specimens to find the genome of the infectious agent. The technique of RDA was utilized by Chang and colleagues to discover the human herpes virus type 8 that has been shown to cause KS.[13] HCV was discovered by scientists at CDC, NIH, and the Genetech Corporation, who created a cDNA library from the sera of HCV-infected chimpanzees and demonstrated that persons with non-A, non-B hepatitis had specific antibodies to the expressed proteins.[288] Subsequent PCR studies of blood from infected humans were done to characterize the sequence of the HCV genome. These new organisms were established as the cause of a human disease without isolating the agent in vitro and, in the example of HHV-8, without the availability of an animal model. It was impossible to fulfill Koch's postulates to establish these organisms as the cause of a human disease.

Nevertheless, the evidence for causality is strong for each of these pathogen–disease associations. Perhaps a modification of the general criteria of causation originally developed by Bradford Hill and initially applied to assess the evidence of the etiologic association between tobacco and smoking and lung cancer should be considered in evaluating the evidence of a causal association between an organism and a disease.[289] The Bradford Hill criteria that might be used to establish the causal relationship between an organism and an infectious disease are as follows:

- Temporal association: Infections with the organism precedes the development of the disease.
- Biologic plausibility: It is biologically plausible and consistent with existing knowledge that the organism could cause the disease.
- Consistency: Evidence of infection with the organism is consistently found in patients with the disease by various investigators, using a variety of different techniques.
- Strength of the association: The relative risks of the disease are high in persons who are infected with the agent, in comparison with persons in whom no evidence of infection can be found.
- Dose-response relationship: Often, the relative risk of the disease or the length of the incubation period after infection and disease onset is related to the infectious dose.
- Removing, preventing, or decreasing the exposure is followed by a reduction in the risk of disease.

Although all of these criteria have some relevance to the determination of whether an organism is directly causative of an infectious disease, an appropriate temporal relationship, consistency of the association found by several laboratories, the specificity of the relationship, and the prevention of the disease by eliminating exposure to the putative causal organism are the most compelling. These criteria have been applied successfully to establish several new infectious diseases described in the last 20 years, including HIV/AIDS, HCV/hepatitis, and *H. pylori*/peptic ulcer.

The last two decades of the 1900s provided dramatically new challenges and understanding of the complex multiplicity of factors, leading to the emergence and spread of new infectious diseases. Almost certainly, this century will bring even greater challenges to the understanding and control of infectious diseases as the population grows and our relationship with the environment becomes even more complex and better understood than it is at present.

References

1. Gao F, Bailes E, Robertson DL, et al. Origin of HIV-1 in the chimpanzee, *Pantroglodytes troglodytes*. *Nature*. 1999 Jun;196(3): 336–341.
2. Sepkowitz KA, Raffalli J, Riley C, Kiehu TE, Armstrong D. Tuberculosis in the AIDS era. *Clin Micro Rev*. 1995;8:180–199.
3. Selwyn PA, Hartell D, Lewis VA, et al. A prospective study of the risk of tuberculosis among intravenous drug users with human immunodeficiency virus infection. *N Engl J Med*. 1989;320: 545–550.
4. Mitchell TG, Perfect JR. Cryptococcosis in the era of AIDS–100 years after the discovery of *Cryptococcus neoformans*. *Clin Micro Rev*. 1995;8:515–548.
5. Dismukes WE. Cryptococcal meningitis in patients with AIDS. *J Infect Dis*. 1988;157:624–628.

6. Bozette SA, Carsen RA, Chiu J, et al. A placebo controlled trial of maintenance therapy with fluconazole after treatment of cryptococcal meningitis in the acquired immunodeficiency syndrome. *N Engl J Med*. 1991;324:580–584.

7. Supparatpinyo K, Khamwan C, Baosoong V, Uthammachi C, Nelson KE, Sirisanthana T. Disseminated *Penicillium marneffei* infection: an emerging HIV-associated opportunistic infection in Southeast Asia. *Lancet*. 1994;344:110–113.

8. Wheat J. Endemic mycoses in AIDS: a clinical review. *Clin Micro Rev*. 1995;8:146–159.

9. Centers for Disease Control. *Pneumocystis* pneumonia, Los Angeles and Kaposi's sarcoma and *Pneumocystis* pneumonia. *MMWR*. 1981;30: 250–252,305–308.

10. Barre-Sinoussi F, Chermann JC, Rey F, et al. Isolation of a T-lymphocyte retrovirus from patient at risk for acquired immunodeficiency syndrome (AIDS). *Science*. 1983;220:868–871.

11. Gallo RC, Salahudin SZ, Popovic M, et al. Frequent detection and isolation of cytopathic retroviruses (HTLVIII) from patients with AIDS and at risk for AIDS. *Science*. 1984;224:500–503.

12. Beral V, Peterman TA, Berkelman RL, et al. Kaposi's sarcoma among persons with AIDS: a sexually transmitted infection. *Lancet*. 1990;1:123.

13. Chang Y, Cesarman E, Pessin MS, et al. Identification of herpes virus-like DNA sequences in AIDS-associated Kaposi's sarcoma. *Science*. 1994;266:1864–1865.

14. Moore PS, Chang Y. Detection of herpes virus-like DNA sequences in Kaposi's sarcoma in patients with and those without AIDS. *N Engl J Med*. 1995;332:1181–1185.

15. Melbye M, Cook PM, Hjalgram H, et al. Risk factors for Kaposi's sarcoma-associated herpes virus (KSHV/HHV-8) seropositivity in a cohort of homosexual men, 1981–1996. *Int J Cancer*. 1998;77: 543–548.

16. Grulich AE, Olsen SS, Luo K. Kaposi's sarcoma-associated herpes virus: a sexually transmissible infection. *J AIDS Hum Retro*. 1999;30: 387–393.

17. Phair J, Muñoz A, Detels R, et al. The risk of *Pneumocystis carinii* pneumonia among men infected with human immunodeficiency virus type 1: multicenter AIDS Cohort Study Group. *N Engl J Med*. 1990;322:161–165.

18. Allen S, Batongwanayo J, Kerlikowski K, et al. Two-year incidence of tuberculosis in cohorts of HIV-infected and uninfected urban Rwandan women. *Am Rev Respir Dis*. 1992;146:1439–1444.

19. Sande M, Volberding PA. *Pneumocystis carinii* pneumonia—current concepts. In: Saude MA, Volberding PA, eds. *The Medical Management of AIDS*. 3rd ed. Philadelphia, Pa: WB Saunders Company; 1992:261–282.

20. Pierce M, Crampton S, Henry D, et al. The effect of MAC and its prevention on survival in patients with advanced HIV infection (Abstract/CB-18). *35th Interscience Conference on Antimicrobial Agents and Chemotherapy*. San Francisco, Calif; 1995.

21. Schuchat A, Broome CV, Hightower A, Costa SJ, Parkin W. Use of surveillance for invasive pneumococcal disease to estimate the size of the immunosupressed HIV-infected population. *JAMA*. 1991;265:3275–3279.

22. Montalban C, Calleja JC, Erice A, et al. Visceral leishmaniasis in patients infected with human immunodeficiency virus. *J Infect.* 1990;21:261–270.

23. Kaplan CD, Northfelt DW. Malignancies associated with AIDS. In: Sande MA, Volberding PA, eds. *The Medical Management of AIDS.* 6th ed. Philadelphia, Pa: WB Saunders Company; 1999:467–496.

24. Sillman FH, Sedlis A. Anogenital papilloma virus infection and neoplasia in immunodeficient women. *Obstet Gynecol Clin North Am.* 1987;14:537–558.

25. Levine AM, Sullivan-Halley J, Pike MC, et al. Human immunodeficiency virus-related lymphoma: prognostic factors predictive of survival. *Cancer.* 1995;683:2466–2472.

26. Serwadda D, Mugerwa RD, Sewankambo NK, et al. Slim disease: a new disease in Uganda and its association with HTLV-III infection. *Lancet.* 1985;2:849–852.

27. Murphy FA, Nathanson N. The emergence of new virus diseases: an overview. *Semin Virol.* 1994;5:87–102.

28. Zucker JR. Changing pattern of autochthonous malaria transmission in the United States. *Emerg Infect Dis.* 1996;2:37–43.

29. Herwaldt B, Ackers MC, and the Cyclospora Working Group. An outbreak in 1996 of cyclosporiasis associated with imported raspberries. *N Engl J Med.* 1997;336:1548.

30. Herwaldt B, Beach MJ, and the Cyclospora Working Group. The return of *Cyclospora* in 1997: another outbreak of cyclosporiasis in N. America associated with imported raspberries. *Ann Int Med.* 1999;130:210–220.

31. Izumiya H, Terjama J, Wada A, et al. Molecular typing of enterohemorrhagic *E. coli* O157:H7 isolates in Japan using pulse-field gel electrophoresis. *J Clin Microbiol.* 1997;35:1675–1680.

32. Smith KE, Besser JM, Hedberg CW, et al. Quinolone-resistant *Campylobacter jejuni* infections in Minnesota, 1992–1998. *N Engl J Med.* 1999;340:1525–1532.

33. Wegener HC. The consequences for food safety of the use of fluoroquinolones in food animals. *N Engl J Med.* 1999;340:1581–1582.

34. Rupprecht CE, Smith JJ. Raccoon rabies: the reemergence of an epizootic in a densely populated area. *Semin Virol.* 1994;5:155–164.

35. Jahrling PB, Geisbert TW, Dalgard DW, et al. Preliminary report: isolation of Ebola virus from monkeys imported to the USA. *Lancet.* 1990;335:502–505.

36. Kissling RE, Robinson RQ, Murphy FA, Whitfield SG. Agent of disease contracted from green monkeys. *Science.* 1968;160:888–890.

37. Colwell RR. Global climate and infectious disease: the cholera paradigm. *Science.* 1996;274:2025–2031.

38. Centers for Disease Control. Rift Valley fever–East Africa, 1997–1998. *MMWR.* 1998;74:261–264.

39. Linthicum KJ, Anyamba A, Tucker CJ, Kelley PW, Myers MF, Peters CJ. Climate and satellite indicators to forecast Rift Valley fever epidemics in Kenya. *Science.* 1999;285:397–400.

40. Watts DM, Burke DS, Harrison BA, et al. Effect of temperature on the vector efficiency of *Aedes aegypti* for dengue 2 virus. *Am J Trop Med Hyg.* 1987;36:143–152.

41. Crosby AW. *Epidemic and Peace, 1918.* Westport, Conn: Greenwood Press; 1976.

42. Taobenberger JK, Reid AH, Krafft AE, et al. Initial genetic characterizations of the 1918 "Spanish" influenza virus. *Science.* 1997;275:1793.

43. United Nations High Commission for Refugees. *The State of the World's Refugees: In Search of Solutions.* New York, NY: Oxford University Press; 1995.

44. Aronson SS, Osterholm MT. Infectious diseases in child day care: management and prevention, summary of the symposium and recommendation. *Rev Infect Dis.* 1986;8:672–679.

45. Hadler SC, Webster HM, Erben JJ, Swanson JE, Maynard JE. Hepatitis A in day-care centers: a community-wide assessment. *N Engl J Med.* 1980;302:1222–1227.

46. Hadler SC, McFarland L. Hepatitis in day care centers: epidemiology and prevention. *Rev Infect Dis.* 1986;8:548–557.

47. Denny FW, Collier AM, Henderson FW. Acute respiratory infections in day care. *Rev Infect Dis.* 1986;8:523–532.

48. Langlois BE, Dawson KA, Cromwell GI, Stahly TS. Antibiotic resistance in pigs following a 13 year ban. *J Anim Sci.* 1986;62:18–32.

49. Fenner F. *The History of Smallpox and Its Spread Around the World.* Geneva, Switz: World Health Organization; 1988.

50. Wheelis M. Biological warfare at the 1346 siege of Caffa. *Emerg Infect Dis.* 2002;8:971–975.

51. Torok TJ, Tauxe RV, Wise RP, et al. A large community outbreak of salmonellosis caused by intentional contamination of restaurant salad bars. *JAMA.* 1997;278:389–395.

52. Brookmeyer R, Blades N. Prevention of inhalational anthrax in the U.S. outbreak. *Science.* 2002;295:1861.

53. Alibek K. *Biohazard.* New York, NY: Random House; 1999.

54. Rotz LD, Khan AS, Lillibridge SR, Ostroff SM, Hughes JM. Public health assessment of potential biological terrorism agents. *Emerg Infect Dis.* 2002;8:225–230.

55. Traeger MS, Wiersma ST, Rosenstein NE, et al. First case of bioterrorism-related inhalational anthrax in the United States, Palm Beach County, Florida, 2001. *Emerg Infect Dis.* 2002;8:1029–1034.

56. Jernigan DB, Raghunathan PL, Bell BP, et al. Investigation of bioterrorism-related anthrax, United States, 2001: epidemiologic findings. *Emerg Infect Dis.* 2002;8:1019–1028.

57. Griffith KS, Mead P, Armstrong GL, et al. Bioterrorism-related inhalational anthrax in an elderly woman, Connecticut, 2001. *Emerg Infect Dis.* 2003;9:681–688.

58. Hoffmaster AR, Fitzgerald CC, Ribot E, Mayer LW, Popovic T. Molecular subtyping of *Bacillus anthracis* and the 2001 bioterrorism-associated anthrax outbreak, United States. *Emerg Infect Dis.* 2002;8:1111–1116.

59. Keim P, Price LB, Klevytska AM, et al. Multiple-locus variable-number tandem repeat analysis reveals genetic relationships within *Bacillus anthracis. J Bacteriol.* 2000;182:2928–2936.

60. Hsu VP, Lukacs SL, Handzel T, et al. Opening a *Bacillus anthracis*-containing envelope, Capitol Hill, Washington, D.C.: the public health response. *Emerg Infect Dis.* 2002;8:1039–1043.

61. Poutanen SM, Low DE. Severe acute respiratory syndrome: an update. *Curr Opin Infect Dis.* 2004;17:287–294.

62. Peiris JS, Guan Y, Yuen KY. Severe acute respiratory syndrome. *Nat Med.* 2004;10:S88–S97.

63. Update: outbreak of severe acute respiratory syndrome—worldwide, 2003. *MMWR*. 2003;52:241–246,248.
64. Reilley B, van Herp M, Sermand D, Dentico N. SARS and Carlo Urbani. *N Engl J Med*. 2003;348:1951–1952.
65. Severe acute respiratory syndrome—Singapore, 2003. *MMWR*. 2003;52:405–411.
66. Update: severe acute respiratory syndrome—Toronto, Canada, 2003. *MMWR*. 2003;52:547–550.
67. Varia M, Wilson S, Sarwal S, et al. Investigation of a nosocomial outbreak of severe acute respiratory syndrome (SARS) in Toronto, Canada. *CMAJ*. 2003;169:285–292.
68. Severe acute respiratory syndrome—Taiwan, 2003. *MMWR*. 2003;52:461–466.
69. Cluster of severe acute respiratory syndrome cases among protected health-care workers—Toronto, Canada, April 2003. *MMWR*. 2003;52:433–436.
70. Shen Z, Ning F, Zhou W, et al. Superspreading SARS events, Beijing, 2003. *Emerg Infect Dis*. 2004;10:256–260.
71. Wong TW, Lee CK, Tam W, et al. Cluster of SARS among medical students exposed to single patient, Hong Kong. *Emerg Infect Dis*. 2004;10:269–276.
72. Leung GM, Hedley AJ, Ho LM, et al. The epidemiology of severe acute respiratory syndrome in the 2003 Hong Kong epidemic: an analysis of all 1755 patients. *Ann Intern Med*. 2004;141:662–673.
73. Peiris JS, Lai ST, Poon LL, et al. Coronavirus as a possible cause of severe acute respiratory syndrome. *Lancet*. 2003;361:1319–1325.
74. Rota PA, Oberste MS, Monroe SS, et al. Characterization of a novel coronavirus associated with severe acute respiratory syndrome. *Science*. 2003;300:1394–1399.
75. Marra MA, Jones SJ, Astell CR, et al. The genome sequence of the SARS-associated coronavirus. *Science*. 2003;300:1399–1404.
76. Drosten C, Gunther S, Preiser W, et al. Identification of a novel coronavirus in patients with severe acute respiratory syndrome. *N Engl J Med*. 2003;348:1967–1976.
77. Prevalence of IgG antibody to SARS-associated coronavirus in animal traders—Guangdong Province, China, 2003. *MMWR*. 2003;52:986–987.
78. Guan Y, Zheng BJ, He YQ, et al. Isolation and characterization of viruses related to the SARS coronavirus from animals in southern China. *Science*. 2003;302:276–278.
79. Lee N, Hui D, Wu A, et al. A major outbreak of severe acute respiratory syndrome in Hong Kong. *N Engl J Med*. 2003;348:1986–1994.
80. Donnelly CA, Fisher MC, Fraser C, et al. Epidemiological and genetic analysis of severe acute respiratory syndrome. *Lancet Infect Dis*. 2004;4:672–683.
81. Liang W, Zhu Z, Guo J, et al. Severe acute respiratory syndrome, Beijing, 2003. *Emerg Infect Dis*. 2004;10:25–31.
82. Tang P, Louie M, Richardson SE, et al. Interpretation of diagnostic laboratory tests for severe acute respiratory syndrome: the Toronto experience. *CMAJ*. 2004;170:47–54.
83. Poon LL, Chan KH, Wong OK, et al. Early diagnosis of SARS coronavirus infection by real time RT-PCR. *J Clin Virol*. 2003;28:233–238.

84. Yu IT, Li Y, Wong TW, et al. Evidence of airborne transmission of the severe acute respiratory syndrome virus. *N Engl J Med.* 2004;350:1731–1739.

85. Li Y, Yu IT, Xu P, et al. Predicting superspreading events during the 2003 severe acute respiratory syndrome epidemics in Hong Kong and Singapore. *Am J Epidemiol.* 2004;160:719–728.

86. Booth CM, Matukas LM, Tomlinson GA, et al. Clinical features and short-term outcomes of 144 patients with SARS in the greater Toronto area. *JAMA.* 2003;289:2801–2809.

87. Svoboda T, Henry B, Shulman L, et al. Public health measures to control the spread of the severe acute respiratory syndrome during the outbreak in Toronto. *N Engl J Med.* 2004;350:2352–2361.

88. Efficiency of quarantine during an epidemic of severe acute respiratory syndrome—Beijing, China, 2003. *MMWR.* 2003;52:1037–1040.

89. Pang X, Zhu Z, Xu F, et al. Evaluation of control measures implemented in the severe acute respiratory syndrome outbreak in Beijing, 2003. *JAMA.* 2003;290:3215–3221.

90. Use of quarantine to prevent transmission of severe acute respiratory syndrome—Taiwan, 2003. *MMWR.* 2003;52:680–683.

91. Olsen SJ, Chang HL, Cheung TY, et al. Transmission of the severe acute respiratory syndrome on aircraft. *N Engl J Med.* 2003;349:2416–2422.

92. Bell DM. Public health interventions and SARS spread, 2003. *Emerg Infect Dis.* 2004;10:1900–1906.

93. Riley S, Fraser C, Donnelly CA, et al. Transmission dynamics of the etiological agent of SARS in Hong Kong: impact of public health interventions. *Science.* 2003;300:1961–1966.

94. Lipsitch M, Cohen T, Cooper B, et al. Transmission dynamics and control of severe acute respiratory syndrome. *Science.* 2003;300:1966–1970.

95. Steere AC, Malawista SE, Saydman DR, et al. Lyme arthritis: an epidemic of oligoarticular arthritis in children and adults in three Connecticut communities. *Arthritis Rheum.* 1977;20:7–17.

96. Steere AC, Malawista SE, Hardin JA, Ruddy S, Askenase W, Andiman WA. Erythema chromium migrans and lyme arthritis: the enlarging clinical spectrum. *Ann Intern Med.* 1977;86:685–698.

97. Burgdorfer W, Barbour AG, Hayes SF, Benach JC, Grunwaldt G, Davis JP. Lyme disease, a tick-borne spirochetosis. *Science.* 1982;216:1317–1319.

98. Steere AC. Lyme disease. A growing threat to urban populations. *Proc Natl Acad Sci USA.* 1994;91:2378–2383.

99. Centers for Disease Control. Lyme disease United States, 1995. *MMWR.* 1996;45:481–484.

100. Steere AC. Lyme disease. *N Engl J Med.* 1989;321:586–596.

101. Woodward TE, Dumler JS. Rocky Mountain spotted fever. In: Evans AS, Brachman PS, eds. *Bacterial Infections of Humans.* 3rd ed. New York, NY: Plenum Press; 1998:597–612.

102. Maeda K, Markowitz N, Harley RC, Ristic M, Cox D, McDade JE. Human infection with *Ehrlichia canis*, a leukocytic rickettsia. *N Engl J Med.* 1987;310:853–856.

103. Anderson BS, Dawson JE, Jones DC, Wilson K. *Ehrlichia chaffeensis*, a new species associated with human ehrlichiosis. *J Clin Microbiol.* 1991;29:2838–2842.

104. Dumler JS, Bakken JS. Ehrlichial diseases of humans: emerging tick-borne infections. *Clin Infect Dis.* 1995;20:1102–1110.
105. Bakken JS, Dumler JS, Chen SM, Eckman MR, Van Etta LL, Walker DH. Human granulocytic ehrlichiosis in the upper Midwest United States: a new species emerging? *JAMA.* 1994;272:212–218.
106. Ruebush TR, Juranek DD, Chisholm ES, et al. Human babesiosis on Nantucket Island: evidence for self-limited and subclinical infections. *N Engl J Med.* 1977;297:825.
107. Sack DA, Sack RB, Nair GB, Siddique AK. Cholera. *Lancet.* 2004;362:223–233.
108. Cholera Working Group, International Center for Diarrheal Disease Research, Bangladesh. Large epidemic of cholera-disease in Bangladesh caused by *Vibrio cholerae* O139. *Lancet.* 1993;342:387–390.
109. Siddigue AK, Salam A, Islam MS, et al. Why treatment centers failed to prevent cholera deaths among Rwanda refugees in Goma, Zaire. *Lancet.* 1995;345:359–361.
110. Anderson C. Cholera epidemic traced to risk miscalculation. *Nature.* 1991;354:255.
111. Riley LW, Remis RS, Helgerson SD, et al. Hemorrhagic colitis associated with a rare *Escherichia coli* serotype. *N Engl J Med.* 1983;308:681–685.
112. Armstrong GL, Hollingsworth J, Morris JG Jr. Emerging food-borne pathogens: *Escherichia coli* O157:H7 as a model of entry of a new pathogen into the food supply of the developed world. *Epidemiol Rev.* 1996;18:29–51.
113. Griffin PM, Tauxe RV. The epidemiology of infections caused by *Escherichia coli* O157:H7, other enterohemorrhagic *E. coli* and the associated hemolytic uremic syndrome. *Epidemiol Rev.* 1991;13:60–98.
114. Feng P. *Escherichia coli* O157:H7: novel vehicles of infection and emergence of phenotypic variants. *Emerg Infect Dis.* 1995;1:47–52.
115. Mead PS, Slutsker L, Dietz V, et al. Food-related illness and death in the United States. *Emerg Infect Dis.* 1005;5:607–625.
116. Whittam TS, McGraw EA, Reid SD. Pathogenic *Escherichia coli* O157:H7: a model for emerging infectious diseases. In: Krause RM, ed. *Emerging Infections.* New York, NY: Academic Press; 1998.
117. Steele BT, Murphy N, Rance CP. An outbreak of homolytic uremic syndrome associated with ingestion of fresh apple juice. *J Pediatr.* 1982;101:963–965.
118. Rangel JM, Sparling PH, Crowe C, Griffin PM, Swerdlow DC. Epidemiology of *Escherichia coli* O157:H7 outbreaks, United States 1982-2002. *Emerg Infect Dis.* 2005;11:603–609.
119. Mackenzie WR, Hoxie NJ, Proctor ME, et al. A massive outbreak in Milwaukee of *Cryptosporidium* infection transmitted through the public water supply. *N Engl J Med.* 1994;331:161–167.
120. Morris RD, Naumora EN, Griffiths JK. Did Milwaukee experience water-borne cryptosporidiosis before the large outbreak in 1993? *Epidemiology.* 1998;9:264–270.
121. Current WL, Garcia LS. Cryptosporidiosis (review). *Clin Microbiol Rev.* 1991;4:325–358.
122. Griffiths JK. Human cryptosporidiosis. Epidemiology, transmission, clinical disease, treatment and diagnosis. *Adv Parasitol.* 1998;40:37–85.

123. Morris RD, Levin R. Estimating the incidence of waterborne infectious diseases related to drinking water in the United States. In: Reichard EG, Zappeni G, eds. *Assessing and Managing Health Risks from Drinking Water Contamination: Approaches and Applications.* Great Britain: International Association of Hydrological Sciences Press; 1995.

124. Huang P, Weber JJ, Sosin DM, et al. The first reported outbreak of diarrheal illness associated with *Cyclospora* in the United States. *Ann Intern Med.* 1995;123:409–414.

125. Earle D. Symposium on epidemic hemorrhagic fever. *Am J Med.* 1954;16:619–709.

126. Lee H, Lee PW, Johnson KJ. Isolation of the etiologic agent of Korean hemorrhagic fever. *J Infect Dis.* 1978;137:298–308.

127. Glass GE, Watson AJ, Leduc J, Kelen GD, Quinn TC, Childs J. Infection with a rat-borne hantavirus in U.S. residents is consistently associated with hypertensive renal disease. *J Infect Dis.* 1993;167:614–620.

128. Niklasson B, Leuc J. Epidemiology of nephropathica epidemica in Sweden. *J Infect Dis.* 1987;155:269–276.

129. Hughes JM, Peters LJ, Cohen MC, et al. Hantavirus pulmonary syndrome: an emerging infectious disease. *Science.* 1993;262:850–851.

130. Khan AS, Khabbaz RF, Armstrong CR, et al. Hantavirus pulmonary syndrome: the first 100 cases. *J Infect Dis.* 1996;173:1297–1303.

131. Nichol ST, Spiropoulou CF, Morzuno SP, et al. Genetic identification of a hantavirus associated with an outbreak of acute respiratory illness. *Science.* 1993;262:914–917.

132. Stone R. The mouse-pinon nut connection. *Science.* 1993;262:833.

133. Pini N. Hantavirus pulmonary syndrome in Latin America. *Curr Opin Infect Dis.* 2004;17:429–431.

134. Smith CEG, Simpson DIH, Bowen ETW. Fatal human disease from vervet monkeys. *Lancet.* 1967;2:1119–1121.

135. Kissling RE, Robinson RQ, Murphy FA, Whitfield SG. Agent of disease contracted from green monkeys. *Science.* 1968;160:888–890.

136. Bowen ETN, Lloyd G, Harris WJ, Platt GS, Baskerville A, Vella EE. Viral hemorrhagic fever in southern Sudan and northern Zaire. *Lancet.* 1977;1:571–573.

137. World Health Organization. Ebola haemorrhagic fever in Sudan 1976. Report of World Health Organization International Study Team. *Bull WHO.* 1978;56:247–270.

138. World Health Organization. Ebola haemorrhagic fever in Zaire, 1976. Report of an international commission. *Bull WHO.* 1978;56:271–293.

139. Murphy FA, Peters CJ. Ebola virus: where does it come from and where is it going? In: Krause RM, ed. *Emerging Infections.* New York, NY: Academic Press; 1998:375–410.

140. Bwaka MA, Bonnet MJ, Calain P, et al. Ebola hemorrhagic fever in Kikwit, Democratic Republic of Congo: clinical observations in 103 patients. *J Infect Dis.* 1999;179(suppl 1):S1–S7.

141. Roels TH, Bloom AS, Buffington J, et al. Ebola hemorrhagic fever, Kikwit, Democratic Republic of the Congo, 1995: risk factors for patients without a reported exposure. *J Infect Dis.* 1999;179(suppl 1):S92–S97.

142. Dowell SE, Mukunu R, Ksiazek TG, Khan AS, Rollin PE, Peters CJ. Transmission of Ebola hemorrhagic fever: a study of risk factors in family members, Kikwit, Democratic Republic of the Congo, 1995. *J Infect Dis.* 1999;(suppl 1):S87–S91.

143. Preston R. *The Hot Zone*. New York, NY: Random House; 1994.
144. Le Guenno B, Formenty P, Wyers M, Govnon P, Walker F, Boesch C. Isolation and partial characterization of a new strain of Ebola virus. *Lancet*. 1996;345:1271–1274.
145. Jezek Z, Szczeniowski MY, Mayembe-Tamfom JJ, McCormick JB, Heymann D. Ebola between outbreaks: intensified Ebola hemorrhagic fever surveillance in the Democratic Republic of the Congo, 1981–1985. *J Infect Dis*. 1999;(suppl 1):S60–S64.
146. World Health Organization. Marburg fever, Democratic Republic of the Congo. *Wkly Epidemiol Rec*. 1999;74:145.
147. Bausch DG, Borchert M, Grein T, et al. Risk factors for Marburg hemorrhagic fever, Democratic Republic of the Congo. *Emerg Infect Dis*. 2003;9:1531–1537.
148. Marburg hemorrhagic fever in Angola update 26. *World health Organization*, August 2005. Available at: http: www.who.org.
149. Johnson KM, Halstead SB, Cohen SN. Hemorrhagic fevers of Southeast Asia and South America: a comparative appraisal. *Prog Med Virol*. 1967;9:105–158.
150. World Health Organization. International symposium on arena viral infections of public health importance. *Bull WHO*. 1975;52:318–766.
151. Salas R, Manziona N, Tesh RB, et al. Venezuelan hemorrhagic fever. *Lancet*. 1991;338:1033–1036.
152. Buckley SM, Casals J. Lassa fever, a new disease of man from West Africa III: isolation and characterization of the virus. *Am J Trop Hyg Med*. 1970;19:680–691.
153. Multistate outbreak of monkeypox—Illinois, Indiana, and Wisconsin, 2003. *MMWR*. 2003;52:537–540.
154. Ladnyj ID, Ziegler P, Kima E. A human infection caused by monkeypox virus in Basankusu Territory, Democratic Republic of the Congo. *Bull WHO*. 1972;46:593–597.
155. Reed KD, Melski JW, Graham MB, et al. The detection of monkeypox in humans in the Western Hemisphere. *N Engl J Med*. 2004;350:342–350.
156. Update: multistate outbreak of monkeypox—Illinois, Indiana, Kansas, Missouri, Ohio, and Wisconsin, 2003. *MMWR*. 2003;52:642–646.
157. Breman JG, Kalisa R, Steniowski MV, Zanotto E, Gromyko AI, Arita I. Human monkeypox, 1970–79. *Bull WHO*. 1980;58:165–182.
158. Breman JG, Nakano JH, Coffi E, Godfrey H, Gautun JC. Human poxvirus disease after smallpox eradication. *Am J Trop Med Hyg*. 1977;26:273–281.
159. Jezek Z, Arita I, Mutombo M, Dunn C, Nakano JH, Szczeniowski M. Four generations of probable person-to-person transmission of human monkeypox. *Am J Epidemiol*. 1986;123:1004–1012.
160. Jezek Z, Grab B, Szczeniowski MV, Paluku KM, Mutombo M. Human monkeypox: secondary attack rates. *Bull WHO*. 1988;66:465–470.
161. Hutin YJ, Williams RJ, Malfait P, et al. Outbreak of human monkeypox, Democratic Republic of Congo, 1996 to 1997. *Emerg Infect Dis*. 2001;7:434–438.
162. Heymann DL, Szczeniowski M, Esteves K. Re-emergence of monkeypox in Africa: a review of the past six years. *Br Med Bull*. 1998;54: 693–702.
163. Redfield RR, Wright DC, James WD, Jones TS, Brown C, Burke DS. Disseminated vaccinia in a military recruit with human immunodeficiency virus (HIV) disease. *N Engl J Med*. 1987;316: 673–676.

164. Khodakevich L, Szczeniowski M, Manbu MD, et al. The role of squirrels in sustaining monkeypox virus transmission. *Trop Geogr Med.* 1987;39:115–122.

165. Selrey LA, Wells RM, McCormick JG, et al. Infection of humans and horses by a newly described morbilli-virus virus. *Med J Aust.* 1995;162:642–645.

166. O'Sullivan JD, Allworth AM, Paterson DL, et al. Fatal encephalitis due to novel paramyxovirus transmitted from horses. *Lancet.* 1997;349: 93–95.

167. Rogers RJ, Douglas IC, Baldock FC, et al. Investigation of a second focus of equine morbillivirus infection in a coastal Queensland. *Aust Vet J.* 1996;24:243–245.

168. Williamson MM, Hooper PT, Selleck PW, et al. Transmission studies of Hendravirus (equine morbillivirus) in fruit bats, horses and cats. *Aust Vet J.* 1996;76:813–818.

169. Chua KB, Gohk J, Wong KT, et al. Fatal encephalitis due to Nipah virus among pig farmers in Malaysia. *Lancet.* 1999;354:1257–1259.

170. Centers for Disease Control. Outbreak of Hendra-like virus—Malaysia and Singapore, 1998–1999. *MMWR.* 1999;48:265–269.

171. Hsu VP, Hossain MJ, Parashar UD, et al. Nipah virus encephalitis reemergence, Bangladesh. *Emerg Infect Dis.* 2004;10:1082–1087.

172. Fraser DW, Tsai TR, Orenston W, et al. Legionnaires' disease: description of an epidemic of pneumonia. *N Engl J Med.* 1977;297:1189–1197.

173. McDade JE, Shepard CC, Fraser DW, Tsai TR, Redus MA, Dowdle WR. Legionnaires' disease: isolation of a bacterium and demonstration of its role in other respiratory disease. *N Engl J Med.* 1977;297:1197–1203.

174. Glick TH, Gregg MB, Berman B, Mallison G, Rhodes WW Jr, Kassanoff I. Pontiac fever: an epidemic of unknown etiology in a health department: 1. Clinical and epidemiologic aspects. *Am J Epidemiol.* 1978;107:149–160.

175. Dondero TJ Jr, Rendtorff RC, Mallison GF, et al. An outbreak of Legionnaires' disease associated with a contaminated air-conditioning cooling tower. *N Engl J Med.* 1980;302:365–370.

176. Myerowitz RL, Pasculla AW, Dowling JW, et al. Opportunistic lung infection due to Pittsburgh pneumonia agent. *N Engl J Med.* 1979;301:958–958.

177. Beatty HN, Miller AA, Broome CV, Goings S, Phillips CA. Legionnaires' disease in Vermont, May to October 1977. *JAMA.* 1978;240:127–137.

178. Breiman RF, Fields BS, Sanden GN, Volmer CJ, Meier A, Spika JS. Association of shower use with Legionnaires' disease, possible role of amoebae. *JAMA.* 1990;263:2924–2926.

179. Muder RR, Yu VC, Woo AH. Mode of transmission of *Legionella pneumophila*: a critical review. *Arch Intern Med.* 1986;146:1607–1612.

180. Aibeiro CD, Burge S, Palmer S, et al. *Legionella pneumophila* in a hospital water system following a nosocomial outbreak: prevalence, monoclonal antibody subgrouping and effect of control measures. *Epidemiol Infect.* 1987;98:253–259.

181. Plouffe JF, Webster CR, Hackman B. Relationship between colonization of hospital buildings with *Legionella pneumophila* and hot water temperatures. *Appl Environ Microbiol.* 1983;46:769–790.

182. Webster RG. Influenza: an emerging viral pathogen. In: Krause RM, ed. *Emerging Infections.* New York, NY: Academic Press; 1998:275–300.

183. Noble GR. Epidemiological and clinical aspects of influenza. In: Beare AS, ed. *Basic and Applied Influenza Research*. Boca Raton, Fla: RCC Press; 1982:18–50.

184. Centers for Disease Control. Isolation of avian influenza A (H5N1) viruses from humans—Hong Kong, May–December, 1997. *MMWR*. 1997;46:1204–1207.

185. Ungchusak K, Auewarakul P, Dowell SF, et al. Probable person-to-person transmission of avian influenza A (H5N1). *N Engl J Med*. 2005;352:333–340.

186. Todd J, Fishart M, Kapral F, Welch T. Toxic shock syndrome associated with phase-group 1 staphylococci. *Lancet*. 1978;2:1116–1118.

187. Davis JP, Chesney PJ, Wand PJ, et al. Toxic-shock syndrome: epidemiologic features, recurrence, risk factors and prevention. *N Engl J Med*. 1980;303:1429–1435.

188. Osterholm MT, Forfang JC. Toxic-shock syndrome in Minnesota: results of an active-passive surveillance system. *J Infect Dis*. 1982;145:458–464.

189. Broome CV. Epidemiology of TSS in the United States: overview. *Rev Infect Dis*. 1989;2(suppl S1):S14–S21.

190. Musser JM, Schlievert PM, Chow AW, et al. A single clone of *Staphylococcus aureus* causes the majority of cases of toxic shock syndrome. *Proc Natl Acad Sci USA*. 1990;87:225–299.

191. Centers for Disease Control. Reduced incidence of menstrual toxic-shock syndrome—United States, 1980–1990. *MMWR*. 1990;39:421–423.

192. Rammelkamp CH, Denny FW, Wannamaker LW. Studies on the epidemiology of rheumatic fever in the armed services. In: Thomas C, ed. *Rheumatic Fever*. Minneapolis, Minn: University of Minnesota Press; 1952:72–89.

193. Stollerman GH, Rusoff H, Hirshfield I. Prophylaxis against group A streptococci in rheumatic fever. The use of single monthly injections of benzathine penicillin G. *N Engl J Med*. 1955;252:787–791.

194. Wood HF, Stollerman GH, Feinstein AR, et al. A controlled study of three methods of prophylaxis against streptococcal infection in a population of rheumatic children. *N Engl J Med*. 1957;257:394–399.

195. Reasy CG, Wiedmeier SE, Osmond GS, et al. Resurgence of acute rheumatic fever in the inter-mountain area of the United States. *N Engl J Med*. 1987;316:421–427.

196. Stevens DL, Tanner MH, Winship J, et al. Severe group A streptococcal infections associated with a toxic shock-like syndrome and scarlet fever toxin A. *N Engl J Med*. 1989;321:1–7.

197. Musser JM, Krause RM. The revival of group A streptococcal diseases, with a commentary on staphylococcal toxic shock syndrome. In: Krause RM, ed. *Emerging Infections*. New York, NY: Academic Press; 1998:185–281.

198. Prusiner SB. Novel proteinaceous infectious particles cause scrapie. *Science*. 1982;216:136–144.

199. Prusiner SB. Prions and neurodegenerative diseases. *N Engl J Med*. 1987;317:1571–1581.

200. Johnson RT, Gibbs CJ. Creutzfeldt-Jakob disease and related transmissible spongiform encephalopathies. *N Engl J Med*. 1998;339:1994–2004.

201. Cuille J, Chelle PL. La maladic die "tremblante du mouton" est-elle inoculable. *CR Acad Sci (Paris)*. 1936;203:1552–1554.

202. Chandler RC. Encephalopathy in mice produced by inoculation with scrapie brain material. *Lancet.* 1961;1:378–379.
203. Hadlow WJ. Scrapie and kuru. *Lancet.* 1959;2:289–290.
204. Gajdusck DC, Gibbs CJ, Alpers M. Experimental transmission of a kuru-like syndrome to chimpanzees. *Nature.* 1966;209:794–796.
205. Glasse R. Cannibalism in the kuru region of New Guinea. *Trans NY Acad Sci.* 1967;29:748–754.
206. Johnson RT. *Viral Infections of the Nervous System.* 2nd ed. Philadelphia, Pa: Lippincott-Raven Press; 1998:356.
207. Brown P. Environmental causes of human spongiform encephalopathy. In: Baker HF, Ridley RM, eds. *Prion Diseases.* Totowa, NJ: Humana Press; 1996:139–154.
208. Brown P, Gajdusek DC, Gibbs C, Asher DM. Potential epidemic of Creutzfeldt-Jakob disease from human growth hormone therapy. *N Engl J Med.* 1985;313:728–731.
209. Nathanson N, Wilesmith J, Griot C. Bovine spongiform encephalopathy (BSE): causes and consequences of a common source epidemic. *Am J Epidemiol.* 1997;145:959–969.
210. Collinge J, Sidle KC, Meads J, Ironside J, Hill AF. Molecular analysis of prion strain variation and the aetiology of 'new variant' CJD. *Nature.* 1996;383:685–690.
211. Bruce ME, Will RG, Ironside JW, et al. Transmissions to mice indicate that 'new variant' CJD is caused by the BSE agent. *Nature.* 1997;389:498–501.
212. Gibbs CJ Jr, Amyx HL, Bacote A, Masters CL, Gajdusek DC. Oral transmission of kuru, Creutzfeldt-Jakob disease, and scrapie to nonhuman primates. *J Infect Dis.* 1980;142:205–208.
213. Wyatt JM, Pearson GR, Smerdon T, Gruffyold-Jones TJ, Wells GAH. Spongiform encephalopathy in a cat. *Vet Rec.* 1990;126:513.
214. Kirkwood JK, Wells GA, Wilesmith JW, Cunningham AA, Jackson SI. Spongiform encephalopathy in an arabian oryx (*Oryx leucoryx*) and a greater kudu (*Tragelaphus strepsiceros*). *Vet Rec.* 1990;127:418–420.
215. Kimberlin RH, Walker CA, Fraser H. The genomic identity of different strains of mouse scrapie is expressed in hamsters and preserved on reisolation in mice. *J Gen Virol.* 1989;70(Pt 8):2017–2025.
216. Gibbs CJJ, Gajdusek DC, Amyx H. Strain variation in viruses of Creutzfeldt-Jakob Disease and Kuru. In: Hadlow WJ, ed. *Slow Transmissible Diseases of the Nervous System.* New York, NY: Academic Press; 1979:87–110.
217. Foster JD, Hope J, McConnell I, Bruce M, Fraser H. Transmission of bovine spongiform encephalopathy to sheep, goats, and mice. *Ann N Y Acad Sci.* 1994;724:300–303.
218. Cousens SN, Zeidler M, Esmonde TF, et al. Sporadic Creutzfeldt-Jakob disease in the United Kingdom: analysis of epidemiological surveillance data for 1970-96. *BMJ.* 1997;315:389–395.
219. Will RG, Ironside JW, Zeidler M, et al. A new variant of Creutzfeldt-Jakob disease in the UK. *Lancet.* 1996;347:921–925.
220. Scott MR, Will R, Ironside J, et al. Compelling transgenetic evidence for transmission of bovine spongiform encephalopathy prions to humans. *Proc Natl Acad Sci U S A.* 1999;96:15137–15142.
221. Cousens SN, Vynnycky E, Zeidler M, Will RG, Smith PG. Predicting the CJD epidemic in humans. *Nature.* 1997;385:197–198.
222. Ghani AC, Ferguson NM, Donnelly CA, Hagenaars TJ, Anderson RM. Epidemiological determinants of the pattern and magnitude of the vCJD epidemic in Great Britain. *Proc Biol Sci.* 1998;265:2443–2452.

223. Donnelly CA, Fisher MC, Fraser C, et al. Epidemiological and genetic analysis of severe acute respiratory syndrome. *Lancet Infect Dis.* 2004;4:672–683.
224. Ghani AC, Ferguson NM, Donnelly CA, Anderson RM. Predicted vCJD mortality in Great Britain. *Nature.* 2000;406:583–584.
225. Bruce ME, McConnell I, Will RG, Ironside JW. Creutzfeld-Jakob disease infectivity in extraneural tissues. *Lancet.* 2001;358:208–209.
226. Deslys JP, Jaegly A, d'Aignaux JH, Mouthon F, de Villemeur TB, Dormont D. Genotype at codon 129 and susceptibility to Creutzfeldt-Jakob disease. *Lancet.* 1998;351:1251.
227. Will RG. Acquired prion disease: iatrogenic CJD, variant CJD, kuru. *Br Med Bull.* 2003;66:255–265.
228. Hilton DA, Ghani AC, Conyers L, et al. Accumulation of prion protein in tonsil and appendix: review of tissue samples. *BMJ.* 2002;325:633–634.
229. Hilton DA, Ghani AC, Conyers L, et al. Prevalence of lymphoreticular prion protein accumulation in UK tissue samples. *J Pathol.* 2004;203:733–739.
230. Hilton DA, Fathers E, Edwards P, Ironside JW, Zajicek J. Prion immunoreactivity in appendix before clinical onset of variant Creutzfeldt-Jakob disease. *Lancet.* 1998;352:703–704.
231. Wilson K, Code C, Ricketts MN. Risk of acquiring Creutzfeldt-Jakob disease from blood transfusions: systematic review of case-control studies. *BMJ.* 2000;321:17–19.
232. Esmonde TF, Will RG, Slattery JM, et al. Creutzfeldt-Jakob disease and blood transfusion. *Lancet.* 1993;341:205–207.
233. Manuelidis EE, Kim JH, Mericangas JR, Manuelidis L. Transmission to animals of Creutzfeldt-Jakob disease from human blood. *Lancet.* 1985;2:896–897.
234. Llewelyn CA, Hewitt PE, Knight RS, et al. Possible transmission of variant Creutzfeldt-Jakob disease by blood transfusion. *Lancet.* 2004;363:417–421.
235. Peden AH, Head MW, Ritchie DL, Bell JE, Ironside JW. Preclinical vCJD after blood transfusion in a PRNP codon 129 heterozygous patient. *Lancet.* 2004;364:527–529.
236. Head MW, Ironside JW. Mad cows and monkey business: the end of vCJD? *Lancet.* 2005;365:730–731.
237. Williams ES, Miller MW. Chronic wasting disease of deer and elk: a review with recommendations for management. *J Wildl Manage.* 2002;66:551–563.
238. Williams ES, Young S. Chronic wasting disease of captive mule deer: a spongiform encephalopathy. *J Wildl Dis.* 1980;16:89–98.
239. Spraker TR, Miller MW, Williams ES, et al. Spongiform encephalopathy in free-ranging mule deer (*Odocoileus hemionus*), white-tailed deer (*Odocoileus virginianus*) and Rocky Mountain elk (*Cervus elaphus nelsoni*) in northcentral Colorado. *J Wildl Dis.* 1997;33:1–6.
240. Miller MW, Williams ES, McCarty CW, et al. Epizootiology of chronic wasting disease in free-ranging cervids in Colorado and Wyoming. *J Wildl Dis.* 2000;36:676–690.
241. O'Rourke KI, Baszler TV, Besser TE, et al. Preclinical diagnosis of scrapie by immunohistochemistry of third eyelid lymphoid tissue. *J Clin Microbiol.* 2000;38:3254–3259.
242. Wild MA, Spraker TR, Sigurdson CJ, O'Rourke KI, Miller MW. Preclinical diagnosis of chronic wasting disease in captive mule deer

(*Odocoileus hemionus*) and white-tailed deer (*Odocoileus virginianus*) using tonsillar biopsy. *J Gen Virol.* 2002;83:2629–2634.

243. Belay ED, Maddox RA, Williams ES, Miller MW, Gambetti P, Schonberger LB. Chronic wasting disease and potential transmission to humans. *Emerg Infect Dis.* 2004;10:977–984.

244. Belay ED, Gambetti P, Schonberger LB, et al. Creutzfeldt-Jakob disease in unusually young patients who consumed venison. *Arch Neurol.* 2001;58:1673–1678.

245. Institute of Medicine. *Emerging Infectious: Microbial Threats to Health in the United States.* Washington, DC: National Academies Press; 1992.

246. Centers for Disease Control. Preventing emerging infectious diseases: a strategy for the 21st century. *MMWR.* MMWR Recomm Rep. 1998 Sep 11;47(R8-15):1–14.

247. Choo QL, Kuo G, Weiner AJ, et al. Isolation of a cDNA clone derived from a blood-borne non-A non-B hepatitis genome. *Science.* 1989;244:359–362.

248. Whipple GH. A hitherto undescribed disease characterized anatomically by deposits of fat and fatty acids in the intestinal and mesenteric lymphatic tissues. *Johns Hopkins Hosp Bull.* 1907;18:382–391.

249. Relman DA, Schmidt TM, MacDermott RP, Falkow S. Identification of the uncultured bacillus of Whipples disease. *N Engl J Med.* 1992;327:293–301.

250. Koehler JE, Glaser CA, Tappero JW. *Rochalimaea henselae* infection: a new zoonosis with the domestic cat as reservoir. *JAMA.* 1994;271:531–535.

251. Strong RP, ed. *Trench Fever: Report of Commission, Medical Research Committee American Red Cross.* Oxford, England: Oxford University Press; 1918:40–60.

252. Drancourt M, Mainard JC, Brouqui P, et al. *Bartonella (Rochalimaea) quintana* endocarditis in three homeless men. *N Engl J Med.* 1995;332:419–423.

253. Spach DH, Kanter AS, Dougherty MJ, et al. *Bartonella (Rochalimaea) quintana* bacteremia in inner-city patients with chronic alcoholism. *N Engl J Med.* 1995;332:424–428.

254. Kreinitz W. Uber das Auftreten von Spirochaeten verschiedener form in Mageninhatl bei carcinoma ventricul. *Dtsch Med Wochenschr.* 1906;38:872.

255. Marshall BJ. History of the discovery of *C. pylori.* In: Campylobacter pylori *in Gastritis and Peptic Ulcer Disease.* New York, NY: Igaku-Shoin; 1989.

256. Marshall BJ, Armstrong JA, McGeche DB, Glany RJ. Attempt to fulfill Koch's postulates for pyloric *Campylobacter. Med J Aust.* 1985;142:436–439.

257. Morris A, Nicholson G. Ingestion of *Campylobacter pyloridis* causes gastritis and raises fasting gastric pH. *Gastroenterology.* 1987;82:192–194.

258. NIH Consensus Development Panel on *Helicobacter pylori* in peptic Ulcer Disease. *JAMA.* 1994;272:65–69.

259. Torbett GR, Hoj PB, Horne R, Mee BJ. Purification and characterization of the urease enzymes of *Helicobacter* species from humans and animals. *Infect Immunol.* 1992;60:5259–5266.

260. Marshall BJ, Barrett LJ, Prakash C, McCallum RW, Guerrant RL. Urea protects *Helicobacter (Campylobacter)* from the bactericidal effect of acid. *Gastroenterology.* 1990;99:697–702.

261. Brown KE, Perra DA. Diagnosis of *Helicobacter pylori* infection. *Gastroenterol Clin North Am.* 9193;22:106–118.

262. Taylor DN, Blaser MJ. The epidemiology of *Helicobacter pylori* infection. *Epidemiol Rev.* 1991;13:42–59.

263. Howson C, Hiyama T, Wynder E. The decline in gastric cancer: epidemiology of an unplanned triumph. *Epidemiol Rev.* 1986;8: 1–27.

264. Parsonnet J, Friedman GD, Vandersteen DP, et al. *Helicobacter pylori* infection and the risk of gastric cancer. *N Engl J Med.* 1991;325:1127–1131.

265. Severson RK, Davis S. Increasing incidence of primary gastric lymphoma. *Cancer.* 1990;66:1283–1287.

266. Parsonnet J, Hansen S, Rodriguez L, et al. *Helicobacter pylori* infection and gastric lymphoma. *N Engl J Med.* 1994;330:1267–1271.

267. Ross R. Atherosclerosis: an inflammatory disease. *N Engl J Med.* 1999;340:115–126.

268. Frothingham C. The relation between acute infectious diseases and arterial lesions. *Arch Intern Med.* 1911; 8:153–162.

269. Nieto JF. Infections and atherosclerosis: new clues from an old hypothesis? *Am J Epidemiol.* 1998;148:937–940.

270. Murry LJ, Bamford KB, O'Reilly DPJ, McCrum EE, Evans AE. *Helicobacter pylori* infection: relation with cardiovascular risk factors, ischemic heart disease, and social class. *Br Heart J.* 1995;74: 497–501.

271. Danesh J, Collins R, Peto R. Chronic infections and coronary heart disease: is there a link? *Lancet.* 1997;350:430–436.

272. Carlson J, Miketic S, Mueller KH, et al. Previous cytomegalovirus or *Chlamydia pneumonia* infection and risk of restenosis after transluminal coronary angioplasty. *Lancet.* 1998;350;1225.

273. Nieto FJ, Adam E, Sorlie P, et al. A cohort study of cytomegalovirus infection as a risk factor for carotid intimal-media thickening, a measure of subclinical atherosclerosis. *Circulation.* 1996;94:922–927.

274. Melnick JL, Hu CH, Burck J, Adam C, DeBakey ME. Cytomegalovirus DNA in arterial walls of patient with atherosclerosis. *J Med Virol.* 1994;42:396–404.

275. Grayston JT, Kuo CC, Wang SP, Altman J. A new *Chlamydia psittaci*, strain TWAR, isolated in acute respiratory infection. *N Engl J Med.* 1986;315:161–168.

276. Grayston JT, Campbell LA, Kuo CC, et al. A new respiratory pathogen: *Chlamydia pneumonia*, strain TWAR. *J Infect Dis.* 1990;161:618–625.

277. Arcari C, Gaydos C, Nieto JF, Krauss M, Nelson KE. Association between *Chlamydia pneumonia* and acute myocardial infarction in young men in the United States military: importance of timing of exposure measurement. *Clin Infect Dis.* 2005;40:1123–1130.

278. Gupta S, Leatham EW, Carrington D, Mendall MA, Kaski JC, Camm AJ. Elevated *Chlamydia pneumoniae* antibodies, cardiovascular events, and azithromycin in male surviving of myocardial infarction. *Circulation.* 1997;96:404–407.

279. Gaydos CA, Summergill JT, Sabney NN, Ramirez JA, Quinn TC. Replication of *Chlamydia pneumoniae* in vitro in human macrophages, endothelial cells, and aortic artery smooth muscle cells. *Infect Immunity.* 1996;64:1614–1620.

280. Hansson GK. Inflammation, atherosclerosis, and coronary artery disease. *N Engl J Med.* 2005;352:1685–1695.

281. Grayston Jt, Kronmal RA, Jackson LA, et al. Azithromycin for the secondary prevention of coronary events. *N Engl J Med.* 2005;352:1637–1645.

282. Cannon CP, Braunwald E, McCabe CH, Grayston JT, Muhlestein JB, Giugliano RP. Antibiotic treatment of *Chlamydia pneumoniae* after acute coronary syndrome. *N Engl J Med.* 2005;352:1646–1654.

283. Acari C, Gaydos C, Nieto FJ, Krauss M, Nelson KE. Association between Chlamydia pneumoniae and Acute Myocardial Infarction in Young Men in the United States Military; The Importance of Timing of Exposure Measurement *ClinInfect Dis* 2005;40:1123–1130.

284. Grayston JT. Chalamydia pneumoniae and Atherosclerosis, *ClinInfect Dis* 2005;40:1131–1132.

285. Mueller N, Evans A, Harris NC, et al. Hodgkin's disease and the EBV: altered antibody pattern before the diagnosis. *N Engl J Med.* 1989;320:696–701.

286. MacMahon B. Epidemiologic evidence on the nature of Hodgkin's disease. *Cancer.* 1957;10:1045–1054.

287. Fredericks DN, Relman DA. Sequence-based identification of microbial pathogens: a reconsideration of Koch's postulates. *Clin Micro Rev.* 1996;9:18–33.

288. Kuo G, Choo Q-L, Alter HJ, et al. An assay for circulating antibodies to a major etiologic virus of non-A, non-B hepatitis. *Science.* 1989;244:362–364.

289. US Public Health Service. *Smoking and Health: Report of the Advisory Committee to the Surgeon General of the Public Health Service.* Publication no. 1103. Washington, DC: US Public Health Service; 1964:19–21.

CHAPTER FOURTEEN

NOSOCOMIAL INFECTIONS

Rashid A. Chotani, Mary-Claire Roghmann, and Trish M. Perl

Introduction

The problems associated with nosocomial infections–hospital-acquired or health care–associated infections–have undoubtedly existed since sick people were gathered in health care environments. Interest in the fate of patients at health care facilities has existed for centuries. In only recent decades has the rather new discipline of hospital (health care) epidemiology, which studies infectious and noninfectious adverse events, developed into an accepted medical science.

As modern medicine develops new cutting-edge diagnostic and therapeutic technologies for prolonging life and as the population ages or has compromised defenses, nosocomial infections will become one of the primary medical and public health problems that we will face. Currently in the United States, approximately 2.5 million nosocomial infections occur annually, resulting in about 250,000 deaths.[1] These numbers may significantly underestimate the problem's magnitude as more patients are discharged early, and infections are being diagnosed and cared for in nontraditional medical settings. The Centers for Disease Control and Prevention (CDC) estimates that nosocomial infections contribute to 0.7% to 10.1% of deaths and cause 0.1% to 4.4% of all deaths occurring in hospitals.[2] In fact, following some medical procedures, such as cardiac surgery, nosocomial infections are the most significant contributors to prolonged hospital stay and increased hospital mortality.[3]

Nosocomial infections also cause considerable morbidity and cost. In 1992, a nosocomial infection added an average of four extra hospital days and $2100 to the patient's costs (Table 14-1).[1] In total, these infections added approximately $4.5 billion to the cost of the health care system.[4] Thus, hospitals or health care institutions witness a financial loss when a patient develops an infection associated with health care.

TABLE 14-1 Nosocomial Infection Morbidity and Cost per Patient, 1992

Type of Infection	Excess Hospitalization Days	Extra Cost	Attributable Mortality
UTI	1	$680	Very Low
SSI	7	$3,152	Low
Pneumonia	6	$5,683	10%
BSI	7	$3,517	9%

Source: S. K. Fridkin et al., The Role of Understaffing in Central Venous Catheter-Associated Bloodstream Infections, Infection Control and Hospital Epidemiology, Vol. 17, pp. 150–158, Copyright © 1996, Slack, Inc.

Nosocomial infections occur for four essential reasons:

1. Host factors: Patients may have a compromised immune system due to underlying disease(s), which increases their risk of developing infections from both high- and low-virulence organisms.
2. Environment: The hospital environment promotes the spread of microbial pathogens. The proximity to other patients, contamination of common equipment, exposure to water contaminated with microorganisms, presence of construction and renovation, and the often-unwashed hands of health care workers contribute to create the ideal conditions for transmission of infectious organisms.
3. Technology: Technologic advances in health care provide sophisticated methods of monitoring and caring for patients. These advances provide new portals of entry, alter normal host flora, and may increase antibiotic resistance, thus increasing the risk of nosocomial infections.
4. Human factors: With tremendous cutbacks in the health care industry, the number and skill level of caregivers have decreased. Support staff now provide previously specialized nursing functions. Health care workers are busier than ever, allowing them little time to observe simple infection control practices, such as hand washing. These changes may contribute substantially to nosocomial transmission of organisms and development of infections.

In the United States, the type and number of infections are estimated by several surveillance systems; one of them is the National Nosocomial Infections Surveillance (NNIS) system, which was established in 1970.[5] Currently, 231 self-selected hospitals participate voluntarily and collect data using the following four standardized protocols for surveillance:

1. All patients (hospital-wide)
2. Adult and pediatric intensive care unit (PICU) patients
3. High-risk nursery (HRN) patients
4. Surgical procedures[6,7]

In the United States, based on NNIS data (January 1990 to March 1996), urinary tract infections (UTIs) accounted for 34.5% of nosocomial infections; surgical site infections (SSIs) for 17.4%; bloodstream infections (BSIs) for 14.2%; lower respiratory tract infections (LRIs) for 13.2%; and others for 20.8%.[5] This represents a change from the past when SSIs represented 25%

and BSIs 10% of nosocomial infections. These changes most likely reflect institutional-based surveillance strategies that do not capture changes in health care delivery patterns.

Approximately 90% of the nosocomial infections are caused by bacteria, with viral, fungal, protozoal, and other classes of microorganisms associated with the remaining infections.[8] Based on NNIS data, the most common pathogens isolated from any nosocomial infections are *Staphylococcus aureus* (13%), *Escherichia coli* (12%), coagulase-negative staphylococci (CNS, 11%), enterococcus (10%), and *Pseudomonas aeruginosa* (9%).[5] Like community-acquired infections, the most commonly isolated organism depends on the site of infection. *E. coli* most commonly causes UTI (24%), *S. aureus* most commonly causes SSI (20%), CNS most commonly causes BSI (31%), and *S. aureus* and *P. aeruginosa* cause 19% and 17% of nosocomial LRI.

Keeping these facts in mind, infection control programs should be organized to reduce nosocomial infections as well as the spread of resistant organisms and their associated morbidity and mortality. The ultimate goal of these programs is to improve patient care, reduce hospital stays, and reduce health care–related costs. It is estimated that one third of nosocomial infections can be prevented by well-organized infection control programs; however, less than one tenth (6% to 9%) are actually prevented.[9,10] The following components of these programs are crucial in reducing nosocomial infections:

- A trained infection control physician (hospital epidemiologist)
- At least one infection control nurse per 250 beds
- A computerized surveillance system
- A system of reporting infection rates of hospitalized patients to practicing physicians and surgeons[9,10]

History

The earliest advice regarding hospital hygiene was probably written in the fourth century BC, in the *Charaka-Samhita*, a Sanskrit textbook of medicine, based on Indian Vedic medicine. The following extract demonstrates the early principles of hospital infection control:

> In the first place a mansion must be constructed under the supervision of an engineer well conversant with the science of building mansions and houses. It shall be spacious and roomy. . . . One portion at least should be open to the current wind. It should not be exposed to smoke, or dust, or injurious sound or touch or taste or form or scent. . . . After this should be secured a body of attendants of good behavior, distinguished for purity and cleanliness of habits.[11,12]

In medieval and Renaissance Europe, hospitals were overcrowded. Pioneers such as Theodoric of Bologna and Casper Stromayr tried to reform hospital practice by bathing their patients or shaving the site of operation, yet met with little success.[13,14] Toward the end of the 1700s, Madam Necker proposed "nursing the sick in a single bed."[15] Prior to this time, up to eight patients were nursed in a bed amid appalling squalor.

Simpson, a Scottish surgeon, demonstrated that mortality following amputation was proportional to the size of the hospital and the degree of overcrowding.[16,17] In the mid-1800s, Florence Nightingale published a dramatic report after her Crimean War experiences at the military hospitals. Her report demonstrated that far more soldiers died of hospital-acquired infections than died from the primary effects of battle injuries.[18] Florence Nightingale,[19] with the help of John Farr, demonstrated a direct relationship between sanitary conditions at a hospital and postoperative complications. She proposed that ward sisters maintain records of hospital patients who developed infections and introduced broad hospital hygiene, thus pioneering the concept of nosocomial infection surveillance.

During the same era, Dr. Ignatz Semmelweis, the head of obstetrical service at the Royal Lying-In Hospital of Vienna, investigated the high maternal mortality rate. He probably undertook the first hospital-based epidemiologic study.[20] He recognized that puerperal fever was higher in the ward staffed by physicians. The physicians participated in autopsies of women with puerperal sepsis and would then return to the wards to care for women in labor. He linked the increased rates to a lack of hand washing. Once hand washing was instituted as a control measure, the ward-specific excess rate of puerperal sepsis and mortality declined.[20] (See Chapter 1.)

Louis Pasteur demonstrated that air is contaminated with living germs and that growth of germs leads to spoilage.[21-23] Hence, Lister reasoned that microbes were responsible for wound suppuration and introduced antisepsis to surgery.[24] He proposed controlling suppuration by preventing contaminated air from coming in contact with a wound. Similarly, in 1895, George Emerson Brewer,[25] an American surgeon, recognized the problem of infections after surgery and undertook an intensive surveillance project to estimate the frequency of SSIs. He reported that SSI rates among patients with clean surgery were not 5% or less, but actually 39%. These findings initiated a review of surgical techniques and environmental risk factors. In 1915, Brewer reported in a follow-up a steady decline of SSIs to 1.2% among patients undergoing clean surgical procedures.[26]

In 1937, with the introduction of penicillin to treat serious staphylococcal and streptococcal infections, misconceptions developed that antibiotics could control and eventually eliminate all infectious diseases. Some physicians worried less about infections because nontoxic drugs could prevent serious complications and cure infections. In the 1940s, the concept of postsurgical antibiotic prophylaxis was introduced, and the widespread use of penicillin occurred. Shortly after this widespread use of penicillin began, strains of resistant staphylococci emerged. In the late 1950s, the first epidemics of nosocomial penicillinase-producing *Staphylococcus* were reported in Europe and North America. In these outbreaks, patients, primarily neonates admitted to hospital nurseries without infections, subsequently developed staphylococcal sepsis.[27]

In the 1970s, gram-negative organisms emerged as the most frequent cause of nosocomial infections. In the 1980s, new gram-positive organisms, specifically, CNS, methicillin-resistant *Staphylococcus aureus* (MRSA), and fungi, primarily *Candida* species,[28] emerged as important nosocomial pathogens. Since then, organisms, both bacteria and fungi, that cause nosocomial infections have become increasingly resistant to antimicrobial agents.

For example, the prevalence of MRSA among nosocomial *S. aureus* isolates has increased from 2.4% in 1975 to 29% in 1991.[5] Infections caused by

MRSA are similar to those caused by methicillin-sensitive *S. aureus* (MSSA), in that they are life threatening. However, the only therapeutic option is vancomycin, which is the only effective antibiotic against these resistant organisms. The frequent empiric use of vancomycin has contributed to the development of vancomycin resistance among other organisms, especially enterococci. In recent years, strains of *S. aureus* with intermediate susceptibility to vancomycin or other glycopeptide antibiotics have been documented. Should glycopeptide-intermediate susceptibility (GISA) emerge as a major pathogen, we would essentially reenter the preantibiotic era with respect to their control.

In 1959, the first infection control practitioner (ICP) was appointed in England to control hospital-acquired *Staphylococcus* infections.[29] It was not until 1963 that a full-time practitioner was hired to control hospital infections in the United States.[30] In 1964, Boston City Hospital conducted some of the first modern prevalence studies and reported that 15% of inpatients had nosocomial infections.[10,31] By 1968, the CDC was training ICPs in surveillance, prevention, and control of nosocomial infections, and in 1969, the Joint Commission for Accreditation of Healthcare Organizations mandated that all hospitals support an infection control nurse.

The NNIS system, created in 1970, is composed of nonrandomly selected hospitals. One of the first studies, the Study on Efficacy of Nosocomial Infection Control (SENIC) was to determine whether infection surveillance and control programs reduce the rate of nosocomial infections.[32] Data from this sentinel study estimated that 2.1 million nosocomial infections occurred per year, approximately four times the number of admissions for acute myocardial infarctions. The SENIC project demonstrated that 32% of all nosocomial infections (urinary tract, surgical site, lower respiratory tract, and bloodstream) could be prevented by well-organized surveillance and control efforts.[33] In fact, those hospitals without an established infection control and surveillance program had nosocomial infection rates 30% higher than hospitals with established programs. This study concluded that the following four factors were essential in decreasing nosocomial infections:

1. Surveillance
2. Adequate numbers of trained ICPs
3. Reports that "feed back" infection rates to health care providers
4. An effective and trained infection control physician (hospital epidemiologist)

Methods for Surveillance of Nosocomial Infections

Definition

Nosocomial infections develop in patients exposed to hospitals or to medical and surgical procedures that occur in a health care environment. An infection is considered nosocomial if it develops in a patient who has been hospitalized for 48 to 72 hours and was not incubating the infection at the time of admission. Nosocomial infections may also develop after surgical procedures. Nosocomial infections may be present on admission if they were acquired during a previous admission or outpatient medical/surgical procedure. Patients can

also develop nosocomial infections in long-term care facilities and be subsequently transferred to an acute care facility. Increasingly, an infection
acquired in the hospital may manifest after discharge because of shorter
hospital stays and more frequent outpatient surgical procedures.

Infections are defined using a set of standard criteria that have been
developed over the years. The CDC has assumed a primary role in developing
definitions.[34] These definitions have been tested and validated in many acute
care settings. Separate definitions have been developed for long-term care
facilities. Uniform definitions are critical to following trends within hospitals
and to comparing infection rates between hospitals or data systems. Although
the definitions are often based on positive culture results, these definitions
may also use clinical criteria to distinguish between organisms that have
colonized a body site versus those that are causing infections.

Measures of Occurrence

Nosocomial infections are evaluated by calculating rates, not the number of
nosocomial infections. For instance, the presence of six nosocomial infections
at a large institution (bed size >500) has different implications than the same
number at a small institution (bed size <25).

Crude Infection Rate

The most common measure of occurrence, the crude infection rate, is the
ratio of infections per 100 admissions or discharges:

$$\text{Crude infection rate} = \frac{\text{Number of infections}}{100 \text{ admissions or discharges}}$$

The crude infection rate can also be site specific. For example:

$$\text{Crude BSI} = \frac{\text{Number of BSI}}{100 \text{ admissions or discharge}}$$

Adjusted Infection Rate

To derive a rate that represents changes in the nosocomial infection rate from
one period to another, the crude infection rate is often adjusted by patient-
days or number of procedures. This corrects for a patient being admitted in
one month and discharged in another. An example of an adjusted infection rate is the ratio of infections per 1000 patient-days or 100 surgical
procedures.

$$\text{Adjusted infection rate} = \text{Number of infections}/1000 \text{ patient-days}$$

or

$$= \text{Number of infections}/100 \text{ surgical procedures}$$

The crude infection rate does not adjust for risk factors for nosocomial infections that vary among patients. The risk-adjusted infection rate adjusts the rate by the major risk factor for the infections by the number of days that a medical device (central venous catheter, urinary catheter, ventilator) is used. A recent study demonstrated that data collected for institutional nosocomial infection rates should be adjusted for risk factors in order to correct for severity of illness.[35]

Risk-adjusted infection rate = Number of infections in question/Number of days that a device is in place

Device-Associated Infection Rates

A device-associated infection rate is a specific example of a risk-adjusted infection rate. This method also allows the calculation of the device-associated, device-day rate, which is usually expressed per 1000 device-days:

$$\frac{\text{Number of device-associated infections for specific site}}{\text{Number of device-days}} \times 1000$$

Before calculating the risk-adjusted infection rate, certain steps should be followed:

1. Decide on the time period for the analysis (week, month, quarter, half, or year).
2. Select the patient population (ICU, HRN).
3. Choose the site of infection that is to be calculated (numerator).

The infection selected should be site specific and should occur in the selected population; the infection onset days should occur during the time period selected. Once the device-days are determined, infections such as urinary catheter-associated UTIs would be calculated using the following formulation:

$$\frac{\text{Number of urinary catheter-associated UTIs}}{\text{Number of urinary catheter-days}} \times 1000$$

How to Calculate the Number of Days That a Device Is in Place

In January 1998, 20 patients on the first day of the month had urinary catheters; 19 on day 2; 15 on day 3; 25 on day 4; 20 on day 5; 15 on day 6; and 15 on day 7. The number of patients with urinary catheters from days 1 to 7 is added (20 + 19 + 15 + 25 + 20 + 15 + 15), yielding 129 urinary catheter-days for the first week (Table 14-2). The total catheter-days for the entire month is the sum of the daily counts.

Device-Day Utilization

To determine the percentage of patient-days to device-days, the device utilization ratio can be calculated. The device utilization day is specifically useful for measuring infection risk among patients in ICUs or HRNs.

TABLE 14-2   Device Utilization Days

Number of Day	Number of Device-Days	Patient-Days
1	20	20
2	19	20
3	15	18
4	25	25
5	20	24
6	15	20
7	15	18
TOTAL	129	145

Device utilization = Number of device-days/Number of patient-days

To calculate the number of patient-days, let us use an example: In January 1998, 20 patients were in the unit on the first day; 20 on day 2; 18 on day 3; 25 on day 4; 24 on day 5; 20 on day 6; and 18 on day 7. To calculate the patient-days, add the number of patients in the unit from day 1 to day 7. The total number of patient-days for the week is 145 (Table 14-2). Thus, the patient-days are the total number of days that patients are in a unit during a selected time period. We had calculated above the total urinary catheter-days to be 129. Thus:

$$\text{Device utilization } = \frac{129}{145} = 0.8897, \text{ or } 89\%$$

Eighty-nine percent of patient-days were also urinary catheter-days for the first week of the month. Calculating the device-associated, device-day rate and utilization ratio helps ICPs to evaluate how their hospital compares with the mean rates, such as those reported by the NNIS system. Some caveats apply. If the denominator is small (<50 device-days or patient-days), this ratio will not be a good estimate of the "true" device utilization. Therefore, a longer time period should be chosen. Also, not all hospitals are similar to the hospitals included in the comparison group (i.e., NNIS hospitals). If huge variations in hospital infection rates are noted, reasons for these variations should be explored.

Risk Stratification for Surgical Procedures

To understand better the epidemiology of nosocomial transmission, stratification of measures of occurrence by patient or surgery characteristics can be used. In 1964, a National Research Council study stratified the risk of developing an SSI and devised the traditional wound classification.[36] Based on the probability of wound contamination at the time of surgery, this classification segregates all surgical procedures into four categories: clean, clean-contaminated, contaminated, and dirty. Experts believed that clean procedures (e.g., a coronary artery bypass graft) should be associated with a low risk of SSI, whereas dirty procedures (e.g., a ruptured appendicitis) are considered infected and should have a higher risk of becoming clinically infected. However, high rates from clean SSI were encountered in some institutions, where surgeons operated on sicker and older patients or where surgeons performed more complex procedures. The traditional wound classification fails to account for host-intrinsic susceptibility and the differences in the complexity of a surgical procedure.

To account for these two components, the SENIC risk index was developed and predicted the risk of SSI twice as well as the traditional wound classification had (Table 14-3).[37] These higher-risk patients represented 50% of the surgical population and included 90% of the SSI. However, the SENIC risk index measured the host susceptibility to infection, with discharge diagnoses obtainable only upon discharge of the patient, thus precluding prospective surveillance from the date of surgery.[38] Furthermore, all surgical procedures were considered equivalent, and the index did not account for the complexity of some procedures or their duration (Figure 14-1).[38]

In 1991, the CDC modified the SENIC risk index and renamed it the *NNIS risk index*. Three components were included in the NNIS risk index (Table 14-4). According to the NNIS risk index, the risk of infection varies from a low of 1.5%, if a patient has a score of 0, to a high of 13%, if a patient has a score of 3. Nonetheless, recent data have revealed that even these more detailed indices fail to predict the risk of SSI after certain procedures.[39] For example, these indices may not reflect an increase in the infection risk associated with prolonged hospital stay or increased exposure to procedures. Other limitations include the decrease in admissions due to more outpatient procedures and early hospital discharges, which may alter the true rate, due to a change in the denominator (the number of procedures may decrease if outpatient procedures are not included in routine surveillance) or a change

TABLE 14-3 SENIC Risk Index

Risk Factors	Regression Coefficients	Score
Intra-abdominal procedure	1.12	
Surgical procedure lasting longer than 2 hours	1.04	
Surgical procedure classified as either contaminated or dirty by the traditional wound classification	1.04	Score up to 4 (one point for each risk factor)
Patient with three or more discharge diagnoses	0.86	

Source: L. Haley et al., Identifying Patients at High Risk of Surgical Wound Infections: A Simple Ultivariate Index of Patient Susceptibility and Wound Contamination, American Journal of Epidemiology, Vol. 121, pp. 206–215, 1985, by permission of the Oxford University Press.

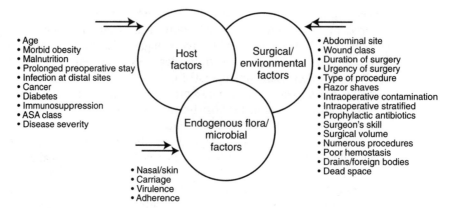

FIGURE 14-1   Risk factors for surgical site infections. ASA, American Society of Anesthesia.
Source: T.M. Perl and M.C. Roy, Post-Operative Wound Infections: Risk Factors and Role of *Staphylococcus Aureus* Nasal Carriage, *Journal of Chemotherapy*, 7: Suppl. 3:29–35, © 1995.

TABLE 14-4   NNIS Risk Index

Risk Factors	Total Score	Risk of Infection
ASA preoperative score of 3, 4, or 5	0	1.5%
Surgical procedure lasting longer than T hours*	1	2.9%
Surgical procedure classified as either contaminated or dirty by the traditional wound classification	2	6.8%
	3	13.0%
Score up to 3 (1 point for each risk factor).		

Notes: ASA, American Society of Anesthesia.
*T hours depends on the procedure being performed.
Source: C. Salemi, D. Anderson, and D. Flores, American Society of Anesthesiology Scoring Discrepancies Affecting the National Nosocomial Infection Surveillance System: Surgical-Site-Infection Risk Index Rates, Infection Control and Hospital Epidemiology, Vol. 18, pp. 246–247, © 1997, Slack, Inc.

in the numerator (the number of infections may decrease because infections after discharge are more difficult to detect).

Incidence and Prevalence

To measure the nosocomial infection frequency at an institution, meaning the incidence and prevalence, surveillance surveys are performed. Incidence surveys determine the rate of new infections during a given time, whereas prevalence surveys determine the proportion of patients with infections at a given point in time. To calculate the incidence rate (I), the number of nosocomial infections (during a given month) is divided by the number of patients discharged or admitted (during the same month), or by the number of patient-days[29,40]:

$$I = \frac{\text{Number of new nosocomial}}{\text{Number of patients discharged or admitted}}$$
$$\text{(during the same month), or patient-days}$$

In addition, incidence rates can be site or organism specific, using the number of infections at a given site in the numerator, with the denominator described above.

Prevalence surveys are designed to measure all current nosocomial infections. A prevalence survey requires planning and usually produces higher rates than do incidence surveys. This is because nosocomial infections generally are associated with longer hospitalization, so infected patients will be overrepresented in a cross-sectional survey. However, prevalence surveys are useful in large populations of high-risk patients. During a prevalence survey, infection control personnel examine all patients' medical records and interview clinical staff to identify nosocomial infections. The prevalence rate (P) is calculated by dividing the number of active (current) nosocomial infections present on a given day in hospitalized patients by the number of patients hospitalized on the same day:

$$P = \frac{\text{Number of active nosocomial}}{\text{Number of patients present}}$$
$$\text{(on the same day)}$$

The prevalence rate traditionally overestimates infection rates, compared with incidence rates, but provides a picture at a single point in time.[41]

Methods to Evaluate Risk Factors for Nosocomial Infections and the Impact of Interventions

Both observational and interventional epidemiologic studies can be used to study nosocomial infections. Observational studies, such as case-control studies and cohort studies, are used to identify risk factors in outbreak investigations or epidemiologic studies and to assess outcomes. Intervention studies, such as clinical trials, are used to evaluate whether a given intervention is effective. Surveillance and outbreak investigations are routinely performed in most infection control programs. Randomized clinical trials are usually performed in infection control programs with active research programs.

Surveillance is a key component of infection control programs and is "a dynamic process for gathering, managing, analyzing, and reporting data on events which occur in specific populations."[42] The building blocks of surveillance are the following:

1. Collecting relevant data systematically for a specified purpose and during a defined period of time
2. Managing and organizing the data
3. Analyzing and interpreting the data
4. Communicating the results to those empowered to make beneficial changes

A more complete discussion of surveillance is available in chapter 4. Also, several excellent reviews have been published recently.[1,42] Surveillance is also a method used to measure the rate of nosocomial events. The purpose of measuring the event is to determine what the baseline rate of an event is in order to compare the rate after an intervention has been instituted. Hence, surveillance may be a component of an intervention study.

The method by which cases or nosocomial infections are detected may be based on the following factors:

- Total chart review
- Selective medical record review (e.g., chart summaries—either hand-written, such as the nursing Kardex, or stored in hospital databases)
- Reports of clinical symptoms from providers
- Review of microbiology reports
- Extraction of data from pharmacy records, such as antibiotic use
- Computer-based models that identify high-risk patients

Sensitivity and specificity vary for detecting nosocomial infections when compared with the gold standard—total chart review. However, total chart review has not been shown to improve the sensitivity of detecting nosocomial infections, compared with selective review of charts, based on review of microbiology reports and the nursing Kardex (74–94% versus 75–94%) and is very time intensive.[43] Case-finding methods must be applied systematically so that results are comparable over time. Most infection control practitioners choose the surveillance strategies depending on the type of hospital, the patient population served, and the "local" epidemiology.

Outbreak investigations are the epidemiologic studies most closely identified with infection control programs, even though epidemic-related infections constitute fewer than 5% of overall nosocomial infections.[44] Outbreak investigations begin with identifying an unusual occurrence or an excessive rate of infections. Cases are defined and described in place, person, and time. Organisms should be speciated and compared for similarity, using antibiotic susceptibility and molecular technologies. If the cause of the outbreak is not overtly apparent or if a study is required to confirm the cause, a case-control study is usually performed to determine risk factors.

Information on the risk factors for and the outcomes of nosocomial infection is often obtained through different types of studies. For example, knowledge of the risk factors for SSIs was obtained through a series of cohort studies in which surgical patients were followed postoperatively for SSI.[37] Information on any possible risk factors for SSI was collected on all patients in the cohort, then relative risks were calculated. The costs of nosocomial infections have been measured, using matched case-control methods and cohort studies. For example, patients with nosocomial UTI were matched to controls with similar diagnoses and severity of illness, then costs and lengths of stay were compared.[45,46]

Randomized controlled trials are the best study method to prove causation; they have been used to show that sterilization and disinfection, closed urinary drainage systems, intravascular catheter care, dressing techniques, and care of respiratory therapy equipment are effective.[47] However, clinical trials have been equally important in showing what does not work. For example, a randomized clinical trial of antibiotic prophylaxis for patients with chronic urinary catheters demonstrated no difference in the rate of UTIs and febrile episodes, compared with the control group.[48]

Risk Factors

Hospitalized patients, in general, are at high risk for infection, due to their underlying illness (immunosuppression, diabetes); hospitalization circumstances (trauma, burns); environmental, microbiologic, and virulence factors; procedure-related interventions, such as surgery or medical care (urinary catheter, vascular catheter, ventilators); and the process of care (patient/nurse ratios, inappropriate antibiotic use). Because patient characteristics are beyond our control, reduction in nosocomial infections is best achieved by altering health care worker behaviors, procedure-related techniques and conditions, or other processes of care.

Host Factors

Host factors that contribute to hospitalized patients developing infections are extremes of age, severity of underlying illnesses, immune dysfunction (T- or B-cell mediated), poor nutrition, genetic factors, and loss of the body's normal protective functions (skin integrity, microbial imbalance). Extremes of age have been found to be a major significant risk factor for nosocomial infections.[35,49-52] The NNIS study indicated that 54% of the infections in adults appeared in patients aged 65 years or older.[5] Interestingly, only 23% to 24% of discharges occurred in those over 60 years of age; however, 37% to 64% of all nosocomial infections appear in this age group.[53,54]

Several studies have shown that nosocomial infections are related to underlying illness. Underlying disease, such as cancer, that causes immunosuppression can make the host highly prone to nosocomial infections. In a 2-year study[55] conducted in an oncology ICU, the overall infection rate was 50 per 100 patients, or 91.7 per 1000 patient-days. Patients with granulocytopenea or acquired immune deficiency syndrome (AIDS) are immunosuppressed, exposed to many antibiotics, and hospitalized frequently for prolonged periods of time. These patients may be at a higher risk of developing nosocomial infections due to bacterial colonization and catheter placement.[56-59] Other underlying diseases put some patients at high risk for nosocomial infections. Examples are pulmonary, cutaneous, and hematologic diseases that alter host defenses by changing or modifying normal flora, breaching normal anatomic barriers, suppressing inflammatory responses, and modifying the reticuloendothelial system.[60-62]

Many different methods are currently being used to measure severity of illness; however, none is adequately validated, making nosocomial infection rates in critically ill persons difficult to use as indicators of quality of care.[63] Although one would suspect that altering the host underlying illness is important, this is rarely feasible and has not been studied. Until better measures of host factors and underlying illness can be developed, this important factor in nosocomial infections will be poorly understood.

Environment

Air, water, and the inanimate surfaces surrounding the patient are referred to as the *environment*. Contamination of the floor, walls, bed frames, chairs, water, and air of the patient's environment may lead to nosocomial infection.

Air

Malfunctioning or inadequate ventilation systems in health care facilities may not adequately filter air. *Aspergillus* species, one of the most invasive fungi, under appropriate environmental conditions can produce and disseminate several thousand spores per cubic meter of air.[64,65] These can remain suspended for long periods. Eventually, the spores settle and can contaminate surfaces. These spores remain viable for months and can become airborne when dust-generating activities are performed, such as construction or demolition. If walls or surfaces become wet and are not replaced, molds can flourish and become sources of infection.

Water

Since the etiologic agent of Legionnaires' disease was first identified in 1977,[66] numerous outbreaks of nosocomial Legionnaires' disease have been identified.[67] *Legionella* can colonize the water systems of large buildings and hospitals.[68] Hospital hot water distribution systems and water cooling towers for air conditioners have been implicated as sources of legionellosis outbreaks in patients.[69,70] Other pathogens, such as *Pseudomonas* species, *Acinetobacter* species, *Acromobacter* species, *Aeromonas hydrophila*, *Flavimonas*, certain nontuberculosis mycobacteria, and *Flavobacterium meningosepticum* have been associated with water contamination leading to infection.

Inanimate Objects

More recently, spread of resistant organisms has been linked to a contaminated environment or a fomite.[71] Both vancomycin-resistant enterococcus and MRSA have been cultured in the environment.[72-74] Also, contaminated fomites have been found to be a source of nosocomially transmitted viral respiratory infections.[75]

Microbiologic Factors

The microbiologic factors that contribute to nosocomial transmission include virulence factors, their ability to survive in the hospital environment, and antimicrobial resistance. *S. aureus* and *Pseudomonas aeruginosa* are highly virulent nosocomial pathogens; however, pathogens of low virulence can cause nosocomial infections in immunocompromised patients. Bacteria that can survive in the hospital environment can be transmitted to patients on ventilators or to those with urinary and vascular catheters. Coagulase-negative staphylococci adhere to prosthetic devices and vascular catheters; this has become a major cause of nosocomial BSIs in patients with foreign bodies, such as prosthetic joints, valves, or permanent central venous catheters. Moreover, these pathogens live in water and soil, where they are exposed to antimicrobial substances and may develop an inherent resistance to common antibiotics. Microorganisms such as *Pseudomonas*, *Acinetobacter*, *Serratia*, and *Enterobacter* species can survive in hospital environments and can be relatively resistant to disinfectants.[76-79]

Extrinsic Factors

The extrinsic factors that contribute to nosocomial infections include medical treatment and interventions, including placement of invasive devices and operative procedures. Therapy of the patient through use of chemotherapy may cause immunosuppression and mucosal disruption and allow organisms a port of entry into the host. Equipment, such as dialysis machines or ventilators, may have complicated reservoirs, filters, or mechanisms to prevent backflow; these can malfunction and lead to organisms entering the body. Once organisms enter the body, infection may ensue. Nasogastric and endotracheal tubes have been shown to increase the risk of acquiring nosocomial pneumonia.[80] Although all of the above-mentioned extrinsic elements contribute to nosocomial infections, the most frequently implicated extrinsic factors are surgical operations and invasive devices.

In addition, the use of antibiotics can lead to imbalance in the normal symbiotic relationship of organisms in the gastrointestinal (GI) tract. As the normal state of human endogenous flora is altered, there is selective pressure in favor of antibiotic-resistant organisms. In fact, patients who received norfloxacin or fluconazole for GI tract decontamination during episodes of neutropenia developed resistant organisms as a result of selective pressure.[81,82] Organisms such as vancomycin-resistant enterococcus can proliferate when broad-spectrum antibiotics have killed the normal gastrointestinal tract gram-negative and anaerobic flora.[83]

Etiology and Transmission

Endogenous vs. Exogenous Organisms

There are four potential sources that can transmit microorganisms and lead to infections. Three of these are exogenous sources—fixed structures of the hospital, devices or instruments used at the hospital, and health care personnel—and one is endogenous—the (source) patients. Exogenous infections are a direct result of pathogenic or nonpathogenic organisms directly acquired from the environment. Exogenous infections can be transmitted via the airborne route, through fomites or direct contact with carriers, by ingesting contaminated foods, or by parenteral inoculation. Endogenous source infections are divided into primary or secondary infections. Organisms that are a part of a patient's normal flora cause primary endogenous infections. Organisms that become part of the patient's flora during the hospital stay cause secondary endogenous infections.

Transmission of Microorganisms

Nosocomial transmission of organisms can be described by five routes: contact, droplet, airborne, common vehicle, and vector-borne.

Contact

The first and the most frequent route of nosocomial infections occurs by direct or indirect contact. Direct contact between body surfaces results in the transfer of microorganisms between a susceptible host and a colonized or infected individual. Direct-contact transmission usually requires personal contact. This type of transmission can occur between patient and health care provider or between two patients, with one serving as the source of the infectious microorganisms and the other as a susceptible host. Health care workers (HCWs) are significant reservoirs of microorganisms. They can carry potentially infectious organisms on their hands, which can colonize their hands or nails. For example, increases in SSIs due to nasal carriage of *S. aureus* have been traced to HCWs who carry the organism.[84] Furthermore, outbreaks of *S. aureus*, *Candida albicans*, and *Rhodococcus* have also occurred from colonized or infected HCWs.

Indirect-contact transmission involves contact of a susceptible host with a contaminated, usually inanimate object or with fomites (porous fungi capable of storing and transmitting infections). Fomites can be medical devices (e.g., resuscitation bags, endotracheal tubes, suction devices, ventilators, endoscopes), instruments (e.g., rectal thermometers, blood pressure cuffs, stethoscopes), dressings (especially in burn units), and toys (especially stuffed animals).[85] For example, Hughes and colleagues in 1986 demonstrated that stuffed teddy bears used in a hand washing promotional campaign were heavily contaminated and colonized by organisms causing nosocomial infections.[86]

Droplet

Infections can also be transmitted by respiratory droplets. Coughing, sneezing, and talking can produce droplets containing microorganisms. Droplets are propelled a short distance through the air and can deposit on the nasal mucosa, conjunctiva, or mouth of the host. Likewise, respiratory secretions may contain organisms that can be transmitted to HCWs or other patients while performing such tasks as suctioning or bronchoscopy. Respiratory syncitial virus and influenza are transmitted by droplets.

Airborne

Organisms are also transmitted via air (airborne), by the spread of either the evaporated airborne droplets (5 μm or smaller in size) that contain microorganisms or the dust particles with the infectious agent. These small particles can remain suspended in the air for a long period of time and can be propelled to greater distances than droplets. Tuberculosis and viruses such as rubella and varicella are transmitted in this fashion.

Common Vehicle

Organisms can be transmitted extrinsically through common vehicles, such as food, water, medications, intravenous fluids, contaminated blood products, and medical equipment or devices.

Vector-Borne

Vector-borne transmission of microorganisms within hospitals or health care settings is unusual in the United States. Vectors such as mosquitoes, flies, ticks, and others can transmit microorganisms. This mode of transmission still remains a significant problem in some developing and underdeveloped countries.

Types of Infection

Urinary Tract Infection

Definition/Impact

Nosocomial UTIs are the most common nosocomial infection in both acute and long-term health care facilities. UTIs are generally defined as bacteriuria (a single positive urine culture in patients with a urinary catheter or two positive cultures in patients without) and can be further stratified by the presence or absence of symptoms (fever, increased frequency of urination, dysuria, or suprapubic tenderness). The natural history of UTIs in patients in acute care hospitals has been well documented.[87] The majority of bacteriuric ($>10^6$ organisms/mL of urine) patients (67%) are asymptomatic; 28% have fever or symptoms attributed to a UTI, and 5% have cultured blood growing the same organism.

Risk Factors

UTIs are predominantly a device-associated infection. Approximately 5–10% of UTIs are associated with genitourinary manipulations, such as urologic surgery. Over 80% of UTIs are associated with indwelling urinary (Foley) catheters. The risk of UTI increases with the length of time that a urinary catheter remains in place. These catheters increase the risk for developing a UTI because they avert the normal defenses of the urologic system in multiple ways. First, bacteria can be directly inoculated into the bladder during insertion of the catheter. Second, both the inside and outside walls of the catheter serve as conduits from the external environment to the bladder. Third, a biofilm that forms within the internal lumen of a catheter protects bacteria from antibiotics. Fourth, the catheters damage the glycosaminoglycan layer of the bladder and blunt the white blood cell immune response to infection. Finally, residual urine from the bladder that does not completely drain serves as a reservoir for bacterial growth.

Microbiology

Aerobic gram-negative rods, such as *Escherichia coli*, are the most common cause of urinary tract infection. They are usually acquired from the endogenous colonic flora of the patient. However, bacteria that are acquired after exposure to the health care environment and become part of the colonic flora, such as multiple antibiotic-resistant enterococci, can also cause UTI. The most common organisms causing urinary tract infections are shown in Table 14-5.[1,5]

Interventions

Preventing UTI in acute and long-term care patients involves preventing bacteriuria. This can be done by doing the following:

1. Avoid using indwelling urinary catheters and alternatives, including condom catheters, suprapubic catheters, and intermittent catheterization.
2. Maintain a closed drainage system for the urinary catheter.
3. Minimize the duration of the catheterization.

Interestingly, neither treating meatal colonization nor suppressing bacteriuria through bladder irrigation with polymyxin-neomycin or through the addition of hydrogen peroxide into the collection bag has been shown to decrease the risk of urinary infection.[89-91] In fact, antibiotic treatment of bacteriuria did not alter the rate of febrile episodes in a randomized control trial but increased the numbers of antibiotic-resistant bacteria isolated from urine cultures.[48] Therefore, the treatment of asymptomatic bacteriuria is not recommended.

In summary, UTIs are the most common nosocomial infection in both acute care and long-term care facilities. The overwhelming majority of UTIs is

TABLE 14-5   Most Common Organisms Causing UTIs

Setting	Microorganism(s) in Descending Order
Hospital	*Escherichia coli*
	Enterococci
	Pseudomonas aeruginosa
	Candida species
Intensive care unit	*Candida* species
	E. coli, enterococci
	P. aeruginosa
Long-term care facility	*E. coli*
	P. aeruginosa
	Proteus mirabilis
	Providencia stuartii

Source: W.T. Hughes et al, The Nosocomial Colonization of Teddy Bears, Infection Control, Vol. 7, pp. 495–500, © 1986.

associated with use of a urinary catheter. Prevention should be aimed at minimizing urinary catheter use and decreasing the duration of catheterization.

Lower Respiratory Infection or Pneumonia

Impact

Approximately 300,000 cases of LRI (of the bronchi and lungs) occur each year in the United States.[92] One percent of all patients admitted to an acute care institution developed pneumonia or bronchitis.[93,94] Nosocomial pneumonia occurs in 6 per 1000 discharges and is the second most common nosocomial infection.[1,95,96] Of all the nosocomial infections in the United States, 18% involve the lower respiratory tract.[1,95,97,98] Up to 28.7% of patients in ICUs develop pneumonia.[99] The crude mortality rate of nosocomial pneumonia is between 20% and 50%, and the attributable mortality rate is between 30% and 33%,[94,100–107] making it one of the most fatal nosocomial infections (Table 14-1).

Microbiology

The most common pathogens isolated from the lower respiratory tract are *S. aureus* (19%), *P. aeruginosa* (17%), and *Enterobacter* species (11%).[1,5] Trends of common pathogens isolated from 1980 to 1996 are shown in Table 14-6. Nosocomial pneumonia among immunocompromised hosts can be caused by inhalation of aerosols or droplets contaminated with *Legionella* species, *Aspergillus* species, respiratory syncytial virus (RSV), or influenza virus.[108–110] RSV and influenza A have emerged as important pathogens in recent years,[111,112] and outbreaks of nosocomial pneumonia have been documented from both of these agents.[111,113]

Risk Factors

Risk factors for developing nosocomial pneumonia include severe underlying illness, extremes of age, chronic lung disease, immunosuppression, depressed sensorium, use of histamine type 2 blockers, large volume aspiration, mechanically assisted ventilation, frequent changes of ventilator circuits

TABLE 14-6   Hospital-Acquired Pneumonia: Microbiology, Nosocomial Infection Surveillance (NNIS) System

Pathogen	1980–1995	1986–1990	1990–1996
Pseudomonas aeruginosa	17%	17%	17%
Staphylococcus aureus	13%	16%	19%
Enterobacter spp.	6%	11%	11%
Klebsiella spp.	12%	17%	8%

Source: Data from National Nosocomial Infections Surveillance (NNIS) Report, data summary from October 1986–April 1996. American Journal of Infection Control, Vol. 24, p. 380, © 1996, Mosby, Inc.

(24 hours versus 48 hours), cardiopulmonary disease surgery (particularly high abdominal or thoracic incisions), presence of an intracranial pressure monitor, and fall or winter season.[94,114-121] Patients at highest risk of infection are mechanically ventilated, although they do not represent the majority of nosocomial pneumonias. Intubation increases the risk of developing nosocomial pneumonia at least fourfold and increases mortality by 55%.[121,122] Once the first lines of host defenses are breached by intubation and placement of an endotracheal tube, patients tend to aspirate nonpathogenic bacteria that colonize the oropharynx or upper GI tract.[123]

Definition

Defining pneumonia has been a challenge because the findings are frequently nonspecific, and laboratory and radiographic findings may lag behind other physical findings or mimic other diseases. Furthermore, colonization of the trachea with normal pathogenic organisms frequently occurs in hospitalized patients, many of whom are febrile for other reasons. Patients who develop a nosocomial pneumonia while in an acute care hospital may develop a cough, purulent sputum with potential pathogenic bacteria in significant numbers, radiograph abnormalities, temperature of above 38°C, and physical findings consistent with pneumonia. Any of the aforementioned criteria, including radiograph and clinical findings, are sufficient to diagnose an LRI. In neonates, radiograph findings with evidence of pneumonia alone are sufficient for the diagnosis of LRI.

Interventions

To prevent nosocomial pneumonia, the CDC recommends interventions to decrease aspiration by the patient (raising the head of bed) and prevent colonization or cross-contamination by hands of heath care workers, appropriate disinfection, appropriate sterilization of devices (especially respiratory therapy), timely vaccination, and education of patient and hospital staff.[124] The role of oral decontamination and empiric antibiotics remains controversial.

Surgical Site Infection

Impact

Each year, over 23,000,000 people undergo surgery in the United States.[125] In the United States, SSI is the third most frequent nosocomial infection, responsible for 29% of all nosocomial infections and 14% of all nosocomial adverse events.[126] SSIs cause significant morbidity and account for 55% of all the extra hospital days attributed to nosocomial infections.[127] Recent studies have demonstrated that the average SSI prolongs the hospital stay by 7.4 days.[128] These infections are estimated to cost $3152 per infection and contribute to 42% of total extra charges attributed to nosocomial infections (Table 14-1).[129] Furthermore, SSI causes almost 2% of all deaths in the United States.[130] These numbers highlight the tremendous burden of these infections and the importance of controlling them. Because of the frequency, morbidity, mortality, and economic burden of these infections, Haley and colleagues[33] recommended that SSI should be given the highest priority for surveillance, and at least 50% of the infection control time should be directed to this activity.

Microbiology

Only 33% to 67% of infected wounds are cultured.[131] Among those, 15% to 20% of SSI are caused by *S. aureus*; enterococcus and CNS species account for 15% each.[130] The remainder of SSIs are caused by gram-negative organisms and yeast. The infecting organisms vary according to the site of the surgical incision.

Risk Factors

Risk factors (Figure 14-1) that increase a patient's risk of developing an SSI can be categorized as those associated with the host, those related to the surgical procedure or to the environment, and those related to the organism.[132] The patient's risk may increase if he or she has more than one risk factor. Some mathematical models have been developed, but because they have not been validated, their widespread use in clinical medicine has not occurred.

Host Risk Factors

Patient characteristics, including the underlying medical condition(s) and the severity of the underlying disease, can increase the risk of developing an SSI. Very few controlled studies have examined the relative importance of these risk factors. Those risk factors that definitely increase the risk of developing an SSI include morbid obesity, old age, diabetes mellitus, severe underlying illness, a prolonged preoperative hospital stay, or a preoperative infection.[132,133] Several studies show that patients who are malnourished, have low albumin, have cancer, or are receiving immunosuppressive therapy are at increased risk.[134] Unfortunately, it is frequently difficult to ameliorate these risks. Occasionally, the patient's surgery is not urgent, and the health problems, such as diabetes, can be controlled or the patient surgery can be delayed until the patient's health improves. Nonetheless, studies demonstrating that reversal of these conditions reduces SSI rates have not been done.

Operative and Perioperative Risk Factors

Certain practices and procedures that occur in the operating room or during the perioperative period can increase the risk of SSI. In some cases, health care workers can alter their practices and possibly the patient's outcome. Those surgical and environmental factors that may alter the patient's risk of developing an SSI include a wound classified as contaminated or dirty, a surgical procedure involving the abdomen, a long surgical procedure, hair removal by razor (especially the night before surgery, so that preoperative colonization occurs), multiple surgical procedures, poor hemostasis during the procedure with blood loss and the need for transfusions, presence of drains, dead space, a less-skilled or inexperienced surgeon, a low intraoperative body temperature, internal fixation of fractures, and spine fusion.[135]

Although the definition of an SSI has been debated for years, for the purposes of surveillance, a reasonable definition is used to analyze rates and to examine for trends over time. Ideally, the definition chosen should remain unchanged in order to compare data throughout the years and to see that interventions implemented reduce these rates. In 1992, a consensus group that included the Centers for Disease Control (CDC), the Society for Hospital Epidemiology of America (SHEA), and the Surgical Infection Society (SIS) modified how SSI was defined and changed the name to surgical site infection.[136] SSIs are divided into incisional and organ-space SSIs. Incisional SSIs are further classified as involving only the skin and subcutaneous tissue (superficial incisional SSIs) or involving deep soft tissues of the incision (deep incisional SSIs). Superficial infections require that at least one of the following occur within 30 days of the operation:

- Pus appears from incision
- Organisms are isolated aseptically from cultured fluid or tissue
- At least one of the following: pain or tenderness, localized swelling, redness, or heat when the surgeon deliberately opens the surgical wound
- The surgeon or attending physicians diagnose the infection

SSI secondary to prosthetic devices can occur up to 1 year after the operation.

Interventions

The single most important intervention is the appropriate use and timing of perioperative antibiotic prophylaxis.[137] Pathogens that infect surgical sites during surgical procedures can be acquired from the patient, the hospital environment, or health care personnel. The patient's endogenous flora is responsible for most infections. In surgical procedures involving the GI, respiratory, genital, and urinary tracts, antibiotic prophylaxis has proven efficacious in reducing SSI. For most clean wound procedures, antibiotic prophylaxis is still controversial, although experts suggest giving patients prophylactic antibiotics when a foreign body implant is inserted or if an infection occurring in a clean procedure would be associated with severe or life-threatening consequences (e.g., valve replacement). Finally, if the perioperative antibiotic is administered after the incision, the risk of an SSI increases sixfold above the risk when it is administered 2 hours or less before the incision.[137]

Most exogenous wound contamination occurs during the operation through contact or airborne transmission of organisms; hence, events occurring after the operation (e.g., ward dressings and isolation techniques) are less likely to contribute to SSI.

Perhaps the single most important intervention to reduce nosocomial SSI is reporting surgeon-specific SSI rates. Programs that perform surveillance of wound infection rates may reduce SSI rates as much as 35% by reporting the rates associated with specific surgical teams.[136] To save resources, some programs have adopted methods that group the entire surgical population into patients who are at high or low risk of developing SSI.

One of the major challenges in infection control is deciding when to include postdischarge surveillance for detecting SSI. Recent studies show that patients are developing SSI after their discharge from the hospital (Table 14-7).[38,131,138-141] Thus, surveying each patient for a defined period after his or her surgery should be incorporated into surveillance strategies. Telephone surveys and questionnaires sent to patients and/or physicians have been used. It is still unclear which method provides the most accurate data.[136] These studies show that SSI after either clean or clean-contaminated procedures is most likely to occur after hospital discharge, thus supporting the need for continuing surveillance after discharge.

Bloodstream Infections

Impact

Nosocomial BSIs cause about 14.2% of all nosocomial infections,[5] leading to 62,500 deaths per year and accounting for $3.5 billion in cost related to excess hospital stay.[142,143] Between 1977 and 1981, Bryant and colleagues reviewed bacteremias in over 300,000 patients discharged from four major acute care hospitals[144]; 51% of the bacteremias were acquired nosocomially and carried a 50% higher risk of mortality, compared with the community-acquired BSI. The crude mortality is between 25% and 50%, and the direct or attributable mortality averages about 27% to 35% in critically ill patients.[143,145] Nosocomial BSIs are more common in ICUs, occurring two to seven times more often than on the ward.[34,145,146] Furthermore, the risk of developing nosocomial BSI increases in patients admitted to a surgical ICU (SICU), compared with those admitted to other ICUs.[34,107,145] Pittet and colleagues estimated the cost attributable to a nosocomial BSI in a SICU patient to be $40,000.[145]

TABLE 14-7 Percentage of SSI Detected After Discharge

Author (Year) Reference	Patient Population	% SSI Detected After Discharge
Sands (1996)[138]	Nonobstetrical	84
Roy (1994)[139]	CABG*[88]	52
Simchen (1992)[419]	Herniography	51
Hulton (1992)[420]	Caesarian section	59
Weigelt (1992)[421]	General surgery	35
Law (1990)[422]	Elective procedures	59
Manian (1990)[131]	All procedures	20
Olson (1990)[423]	All procedures	30
Krukowski (1988)[424]	Appendectomy	50
Reimer (1987)[425]	All procedures	71
Brown (1987)[426]	Major procedures	46

*CABG, coronary artery bypass graft.

The rates of nosocomial BSI vary by the following:

- The type of population admitted to the hospital
- The size of the hospital
- The type of hospital (teaching vs. nonteaching)
- The length of hospital stay
- The location within the hospital

NNIS data[147] from 1980 to 1989 demonstrated that BSI rates were the highest for large teaching facilities and lowest for small nonteaching facilities. During the 9-year study period, significant increases ($P < .0001$) in nosocomial BSI were observed, regardless of hospital size. Although the rates were reported to be the highest in large teaching facilities, the overall increase in primary nosocomial BSI was the highest in small nonteaching hospitals (279%), followed by large nonteaching (196%), small teaching (124%), and large teaching hospitals (70%). The increase in overall nosocomial BSI could be due to a variety of factors, including host and laboratory factors and changes in health care delivery patterns. Studies have demonstrated that elderly patients are at higher risk for nosocomial BSI.[52,53,148,149] Populations are living longer, and there is an increase in older patients being admitted to hospitals who have severe underlying conditions, poor nutritional status, limited mobility, and poor host defenses, making them susceptible for developing nosocomial BSI. Another factor accounting for the higher rates could be increased recognition of BSI through improved culture techniques in laboratories and increased frequency of blood cultures.

Definitions

Nosocomial BSI can be divided into primary and secondary types of infections. Primary BSI is caused by an unrecognized focus of infection. Bloodstream infections that are secondary to intravenous (IV) or arterial lines are considered primary bacteremias.[150] It is estimated that 50,000 to 100,000 catheter-related BSIs occur in the United States each year.[151] Two thirds of BSIs are primary in origin, and 19% of them are caused by an IV or arterial line.[152] Staphylococci cause 74% of the IV or arterial line–related BSI. About 90% of intravenous catheter–related BSIs are associated with central lines.[151] Secondary sources cause 38% of nosocomial BSI. Secondary BSIs develop following a documented infection with the same organism at another anatomic site.[150] Sources for secondary BSI include LRIs, UTIs, SSIs, and infections of GI origin.[152] Nosocomial BSIs can be further subdivided as the following:

- Transient, or that which follow manipulation of a nonsterile mucosal surface (perhaps associated with acute infection)
- Intermittent, or that which clear, then recur (e.g., undrained abdominal abscess)
- Continuous, such as those due to endocarditis or suppurative thrombophlebitis

Microbiology

Coagulase-negative *Staphylococcus* is the most common pathogen causing BSI (NNIS, January 1990–March 1996) and is isolated 31% of the time. *S. aureus* caused 16% of infections, enterococcus 9%, *Candida* species 8%,

Klebsiella pneumoniae 5%, *Enterobacter* species 4%, and others 27%.[99] The most common nosocomial fungal cause of BSIs is *Candida* species, with an estimated overall crude mortality rate of 40% to 60%.[153] *Candida* has become the fourth most common isolate recovered from blood cultures in recent years.[153] Also, a noticeable shift toward non-*albicans Candida* species has been observed.[154-156] The attributable mortality of nosocomial BSI associated with IV catheters is between 12% and 28%.[157,158] The mortality attributable to nosocomial BSI due to particular organisms has been studied using matched case-control studies. A 38% attributable mortality is reported for *Candida* species, 31% for enterococcus, and 14% for CNS.[157,159,160] All cultured blood-growing organisms should be evaluated carefully, even in the absence of clinical signs or symptoms. *Candida* species, gram-negative rods, and *S. aureus* in the blood should always be considered true pathogens. Coagulase-negative staphylococci, *Corynebacterium* species, and enterococci may represent skin contaminants. Helpful clues include cultured blood that grows organisms within 48 hours, at least 2 bottles growing the organisms, and isolation of the identical organism from another sterile body fluid.

Risk Factors

Risk factors for BSI vary with underlying disease and include age greater than 65 years or less than 1 year, preexisting comorbid illness (or illness severity),[161] immunosuppression, a diagnosis of cancer, malnutrition, having multiple trauma, burns, being admitted to an ICU, long hospital stay, a surgical operation, a complicated surgery,[161] receiving antimicrobial therapy, a decreased nurse/patient ratio, and male gender.[162] One study in adults at a cancer center using a multivariate analysis model showed that having a central venous catheter, poor performance status, weight loss, hematologic disease, and receiving previous antimicrobial therapy were risk factors that independently influenced outcome.[163] Central lines have been found to be a risk factor in many settings. Among neonates in HRNs, umbilical or central IV catheters are major risk factors for BSI.[164] *Candida* species infections, for example, are more common in children with a central venous catheter placed in the femoral vein, a tunneled central venous catheter, and prolonged hyperalimentation.[165] In all patients, predisposing factors for candidemia are similar and include acute leukemia, leukopenia, burns, GI disease, prematurity, treatment with multiple antibiotics, having a Hickman catheter, hemodialysis, and isolation of *Candida* species from anatomic sites other than the blood. A reduction in the nurse/patient ratio has been shown to be an independent risk factor for central line–associated BSIs.[166]

Interventions

Control measures for minimizing nosocomial BSI include meticulous care of intravenous catheters. Meier and colleagues demonstrated that primary BSI decreased by 35% (from 1.1 to 0.7 infections per 1000 patient-days) after the introduction of a dedicated IV therapy team.[167] Another study showed that the introduction of an IV therapy team decreased IV-related bacteremias from 4.6 to 1.5 per 1000 patient discharges.[166] The best approach is to use principles of basic asepsis, such as appropriate hand washing, proper disinfection of site of entry using maximum sterile barriers while inserting lines, the use of topical antimicrobials at the insertion site, timely checking and changing of dressing, and the use of subcutaneous tunnel insertion for central venous catheters. Technique has also been shown to be important in preventing catheter-related infections. Currently, central catheters are left in place unless the patient develops systemic signs and symptoms of an infection or the site becomes erythematous, tender, or purulent. Changes over guide wires of non-infected lines are permitted. However, all central catheters should be placed using maximal barrier precautions (gown, gloves, and mask).[161] In contrast, peripheral catheters are changed every 72 hours and are placed under sterile conditions, but maximal barriers are not used. The CDC recommendations for the prevention of vascular catheter–related infections contain pertinent information that could help reduce such infections.[161] Finally, the procedures that ensure sterile preparation of infusates and resources that provide patient-specific equipment are also important in preventing BSIs.

In summary, nosocomial BSIs are associated with high morbidity and mortality, as well as cost. Infection control staff must perform active surveillance of patients with central venous catheters and report the rates of these infections to health care providers. Surveillance helps to identify potential infection clusters, which promotes timely intervention as well as aiding in determination of endemic rates of nosocomial BSI. Finally, and most important, clinicians must be aware of the clinical, epidemiologic, and microbiologic features of device-related BSI. These strategies might help to reduce nosocomial BSIs.

Other Sites

Gastroenteritis and GI Infections

Nosocomial GI tract infections (unexplained diarrhea with or without an etiologic agent lasting 2 or more days in a hospitalized patient) are a major source of morbidity and mortality, especially in children and in patients in the developing world.[150,168] Hospitalized patients with diarrhea can become dehydrated, which may lead to a prolonged hospital stay. In the United States, nosocomial gastroenteritis infections occur in 10.5 per 10,000 patients discharged in the NNIS study (1985–1994 data). The infection rate varies by service and subspecialty service (Tables 14-8 and 14-9). In the underdeveloped world, the rate of this infection is substantially higher.

Definitions

As with other nosocomial infections, one must determine the incubation period of the suspected agent. Diarrhea should be defined using appropriate information about stool frequency and consistency. Other common causes of diarrhea must be ruled out, such as antacids, laxatives, cytotoxic drugs, and enteral hyperalimentation fluids.

Microbiology

Nosocomial diarrhea can be infectious or related to antibiotics. The etiologic agent can be identified in 97% of the patients who are appropriately

TABLE 14-8 Nosocomial Gastroenteritis Infection Rate by Service, Nosocomial Infection Surveillance (NNIS) System Hospitals 1985–1994

Service	Number of Infections	Rate per 10,000
Medicine	3610	15.0
Surgery	2201	12.0
Pediatric	392	10.7
Gynecology	138	5.1
Newborn	185	2.8
Obstetrics	78	1.0

Source: S.T. Cookson, J.M. Hughes, and W.R. Jarvis, Nosocomial Gastroenteritis Infections, In Prevention and Control of Nosocomial Infections, 3rd edition, R.P. Wenzel, ed., © 1997, Lippincott, Williams & Wilkins.

TABLE 14-9 Nosocomial Gastroenteritis Infection Rate by Subspecialty Service, Nosocomial Infection Surveillance (NNIS) System Hospitals 1985–1994

Subspecialty Service	Number of Infections	Rate per 10,000
Burn/trauma	53	23.5
General surgery	1365	20.2
High-risk nursery	120	19.2
Oncology	365	19.1
Cardiac surgery	189	17.1
Medicine	3245	14.9
Orthopedic surgery	325	7.9
Genitourinary surgery	111	6.4
Neurosurgery	95	6.1

Source: S.T. Cookson, J.M. Hughes, and W.R. Jarvis, Nosocomial Gastroenteritis Infections, In Prevention and Control of Nosocomial Infections, 3rd edition, R.P. Wenzel, ed., © 1997, Lippincott, Williams & Wilkins.

investigated; 93% of nosocomial gastroenteritis is caused by bacterial agents, of which *Clostridium difficile* and rotavirus cause most infections. However, in pediatric hospitals or hospitals with immunocompromised patients, the role of viral agents is underestimated unless the institution has access to laboratory methods to diagnose viral agents.[169-172] Bacterial agents such as *Salmonella* can cause severe nosocomial outbreaks and are more common outside of North America and Europe.[173,174]

Risk Factors

Risk factors for nosocomial GI tract infections include extremes of age, achlorhydria, gastrectomy and antacid use (reduction in gastric acidity helps pathogens reach the small bowel), reduced intestinal motility, alterations in the normal intestinal flora (antimicrobial therapy), and placement of a naso-gastric feeding tube. The major route of transmission is fecal-oral, typically involving either spread of pathogens from person to person (direct or indirect) or in a common vehicle. Contamination of the environment has been demonstrated to be a risk factor for nosocomial transmission of agents such as *C. difficile.* In outbreaks, common vehicle transmission has been documented, but contact spread remains the most important route for endemic disease.

Interventions

The fecal-oral route is the most important mode of transfer of enteric infections. Thus, the most important control measure is hand washing. Hand washing with soap alone can reduce enteric contaminants to a level that might not be harmful to healthy individuals. Hand washing with antiseptic soap can be used when caring for debilitated or immunocompromised patients or newborn infants, because these patients are susceptible to low doses of inoculum. Surveillance of food-handling facilities must be carried out routinely by ICPs. Surveillance must include observation of food preparation, disinfection of kitchen devices, and education of food handlers. Food handlers with active diarrhea must be removed from food handling until diarrhea resolves and stool cultures are negative. Pathogens such as enterotoxigenic *E. coli* are transmitted by food and water; thus, proper food-handling techniques and chlorination of water supplies can prevent disease. *Shigella* are primarily transmitted by person-to-person contact. All persons who are culture-positive for *Shigella* should be treated with antibiotics. Salmonellosis outbreaks have been associated with contaminated colonoscopes and biopsy forceps.[175,176]

Eye Infections

Impact

Infections of the eye account for 0.5% of all nosocomial infections (0.24 per 10,000 discharges) and primarily occur in specialized hospitals.[177] Still, because they involve a sensory organ and can cause long-term debilitating effects, they are important. These infections are most frequent on pediatric units and occur at a rate of 1.8% per 10,000 discharges.

Microbiology

The most common pathogens include *S. aureus* (24%), coagulase-negative staphylococci (23%), *P. aeruginosa* (13%), *Streptococcus* species (8%), and *E. coli* (7%).

Definitions

Ocular infections are categorized as surgical or nonsurgical. Surgical nosocomial eye infections are further classified into five categories: preseptal or orbital cellulitis, dacryocystitis, episcleritis, keratitis, and endophthalmitis. Endophthalmitis is the most devastating infectious complication of ocular surgery.[178] Non-surgical-related nosocomial eye infections are further divided into five categories: blepharitis, conjunctivitis, keratitis, retinochoroiditis, and endophthalmitis. Conjunctivitis is the most commonly encountered nonsurgical nosocomial eye infection and most frequently occurs in the newborn.[179,180] The pathogens most commonly identified as causing nosocomial conjunctivitis include *Chlamydia trachomatis, Staphylococcus* species, and *Neisseria gonorrhoeae.* Outbreaks of nosocomial conjunctivitis usually have a viral etiology and are usually concurrent with community epidemics.[181] The most common causative agent is adenovirus type 8.[182]

Interventions

A formal set of infection control policies and procedures has been shown to reduce the number of nosocomial ocular outbreaks.[183] Thus, implementation of routine infection control guidelines and appropriate disinfection of instruments can be effective control measures.

Central Nervous System Infections

Nosocomial infections involving the central nervous system are very serious, if not life threatening. These infections can arise from superficial wounds, foreign bodies (ventricular shunts), and the deep structures of the brain parenchyma. The overall incidence is 0.56 per 10,000 hospital discharges. However, the rates are higher on pediatric services (3.3 per 10,000 discharges), high risk nurseries (2.1 per 10,000 discharges), and neurosurgical services (1.7 per 10,000 discharges). NNIS data (1975–1982) demonstrated a 15% mortality rate in patients with nosocomial central nervous system infections. Mortality related to nosocomial meningitis not associated with prosthetic devices ranges between 20% and 67% [184-189] The most common pathogens causing central nervous system injection include coagulase-negative staphylococci (31%), gram-negative bacilli (27%), and streptococci (18%), and *S. aureus* (11%).[1]

Definitions

Nosocomial central nervous system infections can be divided into surgical or device-related and non-surgical-related infections. The surgical or device-related infections are SSIs and can be further categorized into three groups: organ space infections, such as meningitis/ventriculitis; superficial infections involving the skin; or deep infections involving the brain.[136] Meningitis/ventriculitis is associated with ventriculostomies; superficial and deep SSIs with subarachnoid bolts, brain abscess, subdural empyemas, and epidural abscess; and meningoencephalitis with corneal/dural implants. Nosocomial meningitis can be associated with parameningeal infections and brain abscesses that occur after head trauma, neuroinvasive procedures, sepsis, high-risk neonates, and immunosuppression.

Risk Factors

Risk factors for nosocomial central nervous system infections are age, gender, poor physical status, underlying disease, poor nutritional status, presence of other remote infections, long preoperative stay, emergency surgical procedure, hair removal by shaving, surgeon, type of operation and skill of the surgeon, site of surgery, whether gloves were punctured, postoperative cerebrospinal fluid leak, paranasal entry, placement of a foreign body, and use of postoperative drains.[189-192]

Interventions

Control measures include strict antiseptic preparation of skin and the use of clippers rather than shaving, meticulous surgical technique, minimization of the duration of surgery, limiting of preoperative stay, and proper use of drains. Prophylactic use of antibiotics such as cefazolin is indicated for some neurosurgical procedures and in institutions with infection rates greater than or equal to 10%.[193] Finally, adherence to infection control practices should decrease the rates of these infections.

Emerging and Reemerging Pathogens

Emerging and reemerging pathogens encompass both community-acquired and hospital-acquired microorganisms and include bacteria, fungi, and viruses. New organisms are becoming important causes of nosocomial infections, old organisms have reemerged as nosocomial agents, and nonbacterial organisms are assuming an increasingly important role. Increased resistance or changes in resistance patterns frequently appear first in health care settings. Resistance develops under the selective pressure of antibiotics, by transfer of plasmids or chromosomal DNA, or by genetic mutation. Resistance can occur as a result of a single genetic change or can require a series of changes. Gram-positive bacteria, such as *S. aureus, Enterococcus faecium, Staphylococcus epidermidis*, and *Streptococcus pneumoniae*, have become resistant to commonly used antimicrobial agents such as oxacillin, penicillin, and vancomycin. Resistance tends to occur to multiple antibiotics. In fact, once an organism is resistant to one antibiotic in a class, it usually is resistant to all antibiotics in that class. Gram-negative bacteria, such as *Enterobacter cloacae, Klebsiella pneumoniae, P. aeruginosa*, and *E. coli*, have also become resistant to antimicrobial agents such as imipenem and ceftazidime. Fungi such as *C. albicans* are becoming resistant to some antifungal agents. The epidemiology of MRSA, vancomycin-resistant *E. faecium* (VRE), and *S. pneumoniae* are discussed, then general measures to prevent the emergence of resistant bacteria are reviewed.

Methicillin-Resistant *S. aureus*

Staphylococcus aureus is a gram-positive bacteria that colonizes the anterior nares and is a common cause of skin and soft tissue infections, BSIs, and nosocomial pneumonia. MRSA is similar to methicillin-sensitive *S. aureus* (MSSA) in its transmission and ability to cause infection, but it is resistant to oxacillin, nafcillin, commonly used cephalosporins, and erythromycin. The prevalence of MRSA continues to increase. Among *S. aureus* isolates causing nosocomial infections, MRSA increased from 2.4% in 1975 to 29% in 1991 in NNIS hospitals.[5] MRSA is more common in large hospitals with more than 500 beds, where 38% of *S. aureus* isolates are resistant to methicillin.[1] Risk factors for acquiring MRSA include prolonged hospitalization, exposure to antibiotics, and the presence of other patients with MRSA colonization or infection in the hospital.

MRSA are of interest to ICPs because they increase the overall nosocomial infection rate.[194] Infections with MRSA do not replace MSSA infections. Second, MRSA causes life-threatening infections; mortality from MRSA infections may be greater than that from MSSA infections. Third, vancomycin, a glycopeptide antibiotic, is the only drug useful to treat MRSA infections. The continued use of vancomycin may promote the growth of vancomycin-resistant organisms, such as vancomycin-resistant enterococci (VRE) and *S. aureus* with intermediate susceptibility to vancomycin or other glycopeptide antibiotics (VISA/GISA). The high prevalence of MRSA in a facility increases the use of vancomycin. Finally, a large burden of infectious MRSA represents a failure of infection control practices.

Vancomycin-Resistant Enterococcus

Vancomycin-resistant enterococci are another emerging pathogen that cause an increasing proportion of nosocomial enterococcal infections, of which two species are primary human pathogens, *E. faecalis* and *E. faecium* (most VRE are *E. faecium*). NNIS reports a 20-fold increase in VRE nosocomial infections from 1989 to 1993.[195] The overall percentage of nosocomial enterococcal isolates resistant to vancomycin increased from 0.3% to 7.3% and from 0.4% to 13.6% among ICU patients. Most nosocomial isolates resistant to vancomycin have been reported in patients in the Northeast and the Mid-Atlantic regions of the United States. Furthermore, recent data from the SCOPE hospital consortium report that 17% of nosocomial enterococcal bloodstream isolates were vancomycin resistant.[196] Although this study found the highest prevalence in the northeast United States, it also found that 16% of enterococcal isolates from the southwest United States, 5% from the northwest United States, and 4% from the southeast United States were resistant to vancomycin. Among bone marrow transplant patients, the attributable mortality of VRE bacteremia is estimated to be 38%.[197]

Enterococci are normal inhabitants of the GI tract and cause nosocomial urinary tract, bloodstream, wound, and intra-abdominal infections. Although less virulent than *S. aureus*, enterococci are intrinsically resistant to multiple antibiotics. Treatment of infected patients using a penicillin and an aminoglycoside are required to kill the organism and to improve clinical outcomes.

Numerous outbreaks of VRE infection or colonization have been reported,[198-202] most commonly in patients on oncology services. Patients with serious underlying illness who have received multiple antibiotics, including vancomycin, cephalosporins, and antianaerobic drugs and who are colonized with VRE are at risk for developing a clinically significant VRE infection. Other risk factors for infection include underlying disease (AIDS, *C. difficile* diarrhea, mucositis, malignancies, immonosuppression, neutropenia), having received a bone marrow transplant, extended duration of vancomycin and antibiotic therapy, surgery, having a central line, characteristics of the patient's hospitalization (duration, ICU, transplant service, oncology, nursery), and contamination of the environment (proximity to VRE-colonized patient, equipment, electronic thermometer, ear oximeter).[200-205]

One of the primary reasons that VRE is worrisome is the potential to transfer vancomycin or glycopeptide resistance genes to other bacteria. If glycopeptide resistance spreads to MRSA, the resulting organism, glycopeptide-resistant *S. aureus*, would be a virulent organism, resistant to all available antibiotics. Transfer of glycopeptide resistance genes to *S. aureus* has occurred in the laboratory, although this phenomenon has not been documented in the clinical setting. However, *S. aureus* is already developing increased resistance to vancomycin. Six patients with infection caused by *S. aureus* isolates showing intermediate susceptibility to vancomycin have been reported.[206-211] The first case was reported in Japan in 1997, when a young boy's SSI did not respond to 29 days of vancomycin treatment.[207,208] Subsequently, three other cases were reported in the United States and one in France. The sixth case was reported in February of 1999 in Hong Kong. In all cases, patients had been on long-term vancomycin or teichoplanin for MRSA infections.[206] More recent data, however, suggest these organisms evolved from MRSA.

Streptococcal Pneumonia

Streptococcus pneumoniae is a gram-positive bacteria that colonizes the naso- and oropharynx and causes respiratory infections, otitis media, sinusitis, BSI, pneumonia, and meningitis. Traditionally, pneumococci have been exquisitely susceptible to penicillin and other beta-lactams. However, penicillin-resistant pneumococcal isolates have been detected and are becoming increasingly prevalent.[212] Adults who had received a beta-lactam antibiotic during a previous hospitalization have been shown to be at increased risk for colonization or infection with penicillin-resistant *S. pneumoniae*.[213] Also, attendance in a day-care center and frequent antibiotic use are risk factors for penicillin-resistant *S. pneumoniae* colonization or infection.[214]

SARS

The SARS coronavirus is the most recent example of the dramatic emergence of a new pathogen that can be transmitted extensively as a nosocomial infection. In February, 2003 a 65 year old physician from Guangdong, province in China visited Hong Kong during his illness with an acute respiratory infection due to the SARS coronavirus. He stayed at a hotel in Hong Kong briefly during which time he infected 13 other hotel guests, who then travelled to 6 other countries and spread their infection after they arrived and were hospitalized. The SARS pandemic eventually spread to 26 countries and infected 8450 persons of whom 850 died before the epidemic was controlled in July, 2003. The majority of infections (>80%) with the SARS coronavirus were nosocomial. This epidemic illustrates the risk of the transmission of serious respiratory infection by droplet or aerosol in the hospital environment. Of even greater concern at present is the potential for the emergence of a new virulent influenza virus, which could be spread extensively in hospitals. A detailed discussion of the SARS epidemic can be found in the chapter on Emerging Infections (Chapter 13).

Control Measures

Several themes recur throughout this discussion of emerging and resistant pathogens: the control of antibiotic use and the prevention of nosocomial transmission. Controlling antibiotic use is difficult. Antibiotics are prescribed in the inpatient and outpatient settings by individual physicians, and physician behavior has been notoriously difficult to change. Clinicians tend to focus their interest on prescribing antibiotics that have maximal efficacy and safety in treating or preventing an infection in an individual patient and often are less cognizant of ecologic or epidemiologic factors of importance to infection control. There is evidence that changing antibiotic prescribing patterns can influence antibiotic resistance of specific pathogens. Reducing the use of ceftazidime has led to a reduction in ceftazidime-resistant *K. pneumoniae* infections during an outbreak, and reducing the use of cephalosporins and vancomycin have reduced VRE infections.[205,215]

In an era of health care reform, controlling nosocomial transmission of antibiotic-resistant pathogens has new challenges. Several recent outbreak investigations have identified a reduction in nursing staff as a risk factor associated with an increase in nosocomial infections and resistant organisms.[216,217] Infection control activities, such as hand washing and isolation, take time but are critical to reducing the transmission of these emerging pathogens.

In order to control the spread of respiratory pathogens in the hospital, it is important that hospital epidemiologists are aware of epidemics in the community and institute appropriate and effective screening patients and hospital visitors isolation together with precautions. After the SARS epidemic was recognized isolation of infectious cases effectively controlled further spread when they were rigorously enforced. However, control of nosocomial respiratory transmission is much more difficult when patients are highly infectious early in their illness or prior to becoming symptomatic.

Control and Prevention Measures

Control and prevention of nosocomial infections can occur at many levels. The SENIC study demonstrated the utility of well-developed infection control programs that include ICPs. Antibiotic control programs are of increasing importance and should now be included in infection prevention programs. Surveillance and notifying clinicians of infection rates in their patients have been shown to enhance the effectiveness of infection control. Finally, the development of policies and procedures to ensure infection prevention at all levels is necessary. Examples of such practices include hand washing among HCWs, immunization of HCWs, isolation of patients with communicable disease, infectious hospital vistors from patient contact, antibiotic control, cleaning of the environment, and installation and maintenance of water, heating, and air-conditioning systems.

Presence of an Integrated Program

The key to controlling nosocomial infections is the presence of an integrated program that includes the following:

- Department of epidemiology and infection control
- Microbiology laboratory
- Occupational health services
- Pharmacy
- Computers/information systems

Department of Epidemiology and Infection Control

The role of this department is to measure the rates of nosocomial infections, understand their epidemiology, and devise and evaluate effective strategies for their control and prevention. The components of this program are surveillance, outbreak investigation, education, health care system employee health, antibiotic utilization, product evaluation, cost-benefit analysis, and policy and procedure guidelines. The organizational structure should include a trained hospital epidemiologist; nurse epidemiologist(s) or ICP; computer(s); microbiology and administrative support; an infectious disease fellow; and an infection control committee. The infection control committee should be chaired by the hospital epidemiologist and should have representatives from the medical and surgical staff, hospital administration, employee health, pharmacy, microbiology, housekeeping, central supply, and engineering, as well as the ICPs.

Microbiology Laboratory

Active involvement of the microbiology laboratory is crucial for a successful infection control program. Culture reports from the microbiology laboratory are one of the most important pieces of data included in surveillance. The infection control department and the microbiology laboratory must have a close working relationship. This interaction not only provides the ICPs with timely microbiologic information but also helps the laboratory to determine the clinical significance of isolates and to differentiate patients who are colonized from those with clinical infection. The microbiology laboratory can support the infection control department in the following ways:

- Ensure high-quality performance in the laboratory.
- Designate a person to be a consultant to the infection control department.
- Report relevant results in a timely, organized, and accessible way.
- Provide basic microbiologic training to infection control staff.
- Monitor isolates of unusual pathogens, clusters of pathogens that might indicate an outbreak, and the emergence of multidrug-resistant pathogens.
- Characterize antimicrobial susceptibility.
- Perform special procedures and molecular fingerprinting studies.
- Store isolates of epidemiologic importance.
- Conduct environmental microbiologic studies.
- Monitor commercial products, devices, or equipment that might become contaminated during manufacturing or transportation, when indicated.

Employee Health Services

Exposure events are defined when patients or hospital employees are exposed to infectious microorganisms or ectoparasites. When an individual is exposed, the goal of the infection control department is to prevent further transmission. In the event of an exposure, all patients, visitors, and staff who might have been exposed must be identified, and appropriate measures should be initiated immediately. In most institutions, an employee health department evaluates whether an employee has been exposed to or remains susceptible to a contagious disease, examines them, enforces work restrictions, and allows personnel to return to work. Infection control staff must collaborate with employee health services and develop protocols for triage, evaluation, prophylaxis, and follow-up after exposures to communicable diseases. Roles and responsibilities of both departments should be identified and clear lines of communication established.

Pharmacy Service

Pharmacy is also an essential partner in infection control. This service identifies the quality, efficacy, safety, and cost-effectiveness of drugs.[218] Antimicrobials account for 15% to 30% of the overall pharmacy budget,[219] of which 25% is used in the hospital. The use and availability of antimicrobial drugs may alter the susceptibility patterns of nosocomial pathogens. Studies have demonstrated that 23% to 37.8% of hospitalized patients receive antibiotics,[220-223] of which 40–50% of the antibiotics are used inappropriately.[219-221] One of the easiest and the most cost-effective ways to determine the gross antibiotics utilization is based on pharmacy data. High-risk drugs, units, and patients whose antibiotic utilization rates are above those expected or that correlate with resistant organisms can be identified. Antibiotic use is the number of units, or defined daily doses, per 1000 population in a primary health setting or per patient-days in hospital settings. This allows comparisons for trends in antibiotic use to be evaluated and to be evaluated and stratified by unit or service.

Computers

With limited resources, resulting in limited time to perform surveillance activity, computers can help ICPs manage their time more effectively. Administrative databases that contain patient demographics, clinical and pharmacy data, and microbiology and radiology reports are an important adjunct to surveillance. These data can be merged into a surveillance data system that can be stored and manipulated to facilitate surveillance. Such systems help to identify problems such as outbreaks, antibiotic susceptibility trends, nosocomial pneumonias, SSIs, UTIs, BSIs, and the emergence of important pathogens, such as MRSA and VRE. These infection control management systems need to be custom developed with infection control and hospital informatics and the hospital information system department.

Hand Washing

Hand washing is the single most important preventive strategy and remains the cornerstone of infection control.[224-228] The normal microbial flora of the skin helps to prevent colonization of hospital-acquired microorganisms. Skin flora is composed of resident and transient microorganisms. Resident microorganisms are most frequently found on the superficial skin layers, where they can survive, multiply, and be cultured. The density of normal resident microorganism populations on hands ranges between 10^2 and 10^3 colony-forming units (cfu)/cm^2.[229] They usually consist of staphylococcal species (*S. epidermidis, S. hominis,* and *S. capitis*) and micrococci. Moreover, organisms such as *S. aureus, Klebsiella-Enterobacter* group, and *Acinetobacter* species have been reported to colonize the hands of HCWs.[230-235] Larson has shown that 21% of HCWs persistently carry microorganisms from the *Acinetobacter* and *Klebsiella-Enterobacter* groups.[234] About 10–20% of the resident microorganisms inhabit deep epidermal layers.[236,237]

In general, resident microorganisms tend not to be highly virulent but can cause infections in patients who are immunocompromised or who have implanted foreign devices. Transient microorganisms are acquired through accidental contamination and are characterized by their inability to multiply and persist. The hands of HCWs may acquire transient microorganisms from colonized or infected patients.

Many outbreaks have been reported in the ICU due to breakdowns in infection control practices.[238-242] Routine hand washing before and after contact with a patient; before and after performing invasive procedures; before and after touching wounds; and after contact with inanimate sources, such as urine-measuring devices that are potentially contaminated with microorganisms, could prevent many nosocomial infections. This simple practice substantially reduces the risk of microbial transmission from one patient to another by HCWs, as well as transmission from a contaminated site to a clean site of a patient. A brief, vigorous rubbing together of all surfaces of lathered hands, followed by rinsing under a stream of water, is adequate hand washing. Various products are available for hand washing, ranging from plain soap to detergents to antimicrobial-containing products. Microorganisms can either be removed mechanically, by washing hands with soap or detergents and rinsing; or chemically, by washing hands with antimicrobial products that can inhibit the growth or kill the microorganisms. In high-risk health care settings (such as an ICU), effective hand washing with antimicrobial agents (containing chlorhexidine), compared with washing with soap and water, was shown to reduce nosocomial infections.[243] Transient microorganisms, in contrast to resident flora, are easily removed by mechanical means. Antimicrobial soaps should be used in nurseries, neonatal units, ICUs, and when dealing with patients with immunodeficiencies or who are at risk of developing infections with resistant organisms. The hand washing facilities should be conveniently accessible—ideally, one sink per patient, located either in or immediately outside the room, with either elbow, knee, foot, or automatic temperature-adjustable taps and easy-to-use, appropriate cleansing products and dispensers. In places where sinks are not available, antimicrobial disinfectants such as foam or rinses that do not require water should be used.

Unfortunately, hand washing is not performed as frequently as recommended. Factors that predict hand washing compliance are profession, hospital ward, time of day, patient/nurse ratio, and type of care provider.[244] Donowitz examined breaks in hand washing technique among health care providers in a PICU and demonstrated that physicians did not wash their

TABLE 14-10   Hand Washing Compliance by Hospital Profession

Physicians	10–59%
Nurses	25–66%
Respiratory therapists	76%
Radiology technicians	44%
Nurses' aides	13%
Others	10–73%

Source: Data from R.K. Albert and F. Condie, Hand-Washing Patterns in Medical Intensive-Care Units, *The New England Journal of Medicine*, Vol. 304, pp. 1465–1466, © 1981, Massachusetts Medical Society and W.R. Jarvis, Handwashing—the Semmelweis Lesson Forgotten? *The Lancet*, Vol. 344, pp. 1311–1312, © 1994, with permission from Elsevier.

hands 79% of the time that hand washing was indicated.[245] In this prospective study, failure to wash hands following direct patient or support equipment contact was seen 70% of the time.[245] A study examining the frequency of hand washing in an emergency department demonstrated that nurses had the highest hand washing frequency (58.2%), which was significantly more frequent than residents (18.6%) and faculty (17.2%).[246] Compliance with hand washing rarely exceeds 40% of the times it is indicated under study conditions and is particularly poor among physicians.[247,248-251] The hand washing compliance of different hospital professions is shown in Table 14-10. Factors leading to poor hand washing compliance include lack of education, poor hygienic habits, perceived lack of importance, lack of time, dry skin, skin irritation or dermatitis, absence of suitable cleansing agent, and inadequate hand washing facilities.[246,248,252-254]

Even in today's highly technical hospital environment, adequate hand washing is still the most crucial strategy to decrease nosocomial infections. This lack of adherence and inadequate hand washing place patients at risk for acquiring nosocomial infections. Hand washing is a mundane, tedious, and repetitive task that will remain suboptimal without strict implementation of infection control practices and monitoring. The fact remains that, unless HCWs are trained to wash their hands thoroughly and without exception, the use of antimicrobial soaps and alcohol-based hand rinses, location of the sinks, and mechanism of scrubbing have little effect. Hospitals should make monitoring compliance and feedback of hand washing compliance a high priority. New and efficient techniques to improve hand washing should be evaluated because they are desperately needed.

Isolation

To transmit disease-causing organisms, a source of organisms, a susceptible host, and a mode of transmission are necessary. In a hospital setting, a source of organisms can be patients, HCWs, or visitors.

The CDC and Hospital Infection Control Practices Advisory Committee (HICPAC) have recently proposed two levels of isolation guidelines for hospitalized patients: standard and transmission-based precautions. This new system replaces the previous disease-specific systems and has integrated universal precautions and body-substance isolation.

Standard precautions are a combination of universal precautions—designed to reduce the risk of transmission of blood-borne pathogens from patients to HCWs—and body-substance isolation—designed to reduce transmissions of body fluid microorganisms between patients and HCWs. Standard precautions state that blood; all patients' body fluids (except sweat), secretions, and excretions; mucous membranes; and nonintact skin be treated as potentially infectious. The components of standard precautions include the following:

- Hand washing
- Wearing gloves
- Wearing mask, eye protection, face shield, and gowns when appropriate
- Cleaning patient-care equipment
- Enforcing environmental control
- Cleaning linen
- Enforcing occupational health and blood-borne pathogen protocols
- Cohorting patients

Transmission-based precautions are used for infected or colonized patients (confirmed or suspected) with transmittable microorganisms. These precautions should be used in conjunction with standard precautions and are divided into airborne, droplet, and contact precautions (Table 14-11).

Empiric isolation is crucial and based on clinical presentation and symptoms at the time of admission, before a definitive diagnosis is made. Depending on different clinical scenarios, empirical isolation, using airborne precautions (e.g., cough, fever, maculopapular, vesicular rash, tuberculosis), droplet precautions (e.g., meningitis, pertussis, influenza), and contact precautions (e.g., acute infectious diarrhea, history of previous colonization with multidrug-resistant microorganism, such as MRSA or VRE) should be implemented, pending definite diagnosis. Hospitals should have a system in place to ensure that proper empirical precautions are implemented.

Epidemic Investigation and Control

In general, nosocomial infections are endemic in nature, although approximately 5% of them occur in epidemics.[255] Wendt and Herwaldt reviewed 555 published reports of outbreaks in health care institutions.[256] Their review demonstrated that most of the outbreaks were due to bacteria (71%); however, viruses caused 12%, fungi 5%, and parasites 3%. Among bacteria, nearly half of the outbreaks were caused by gram-negative organisms. Gram-positive bacteria were associated with 36% of the outbreaks.

An increase in the incidence of nosocomial infections over the expected rates in a specified area within a time period defines an epidemic. Epidemic nosocomial infections are due either to an increase in person-to-person transmission or to a common source and are usually clustered temporally or geographically. To identify outbreaks, reliable and sensitive surveillance is crucial. Once the existence of an outbreak is established, the infection control personnel need to take certain steps, detailed in Table 14-12.

TABLE 14-11   Hospital Epidemiology: New Isolation Guidelines

Transmission of Organisms

Common Mechanisms	How?	Examples
Direct and Indirect Contact	contaminated hands, contaminated equipment	MRSA
Droplet	large droplets (>5–10 µm) generated by talking	Influenza
Airborne	small droplet nuclei (1–10 µm) waft on air currents	Tuberculosis

Standard Precautions—used on all patients

Universal Precautions	Body Substance Isolation
• gloves for contact with blood or any body fluid contaminated with blood	• same as universal precautions but for any moist body substance, i.e., urine, saliva, nonintact skin
• gowns and goggles for splashes	

Transmission-Based Precautions—used for patients known or suspected to have epidemiologically important diseases

VA/CDC Name:	Examples:
Airborne (AFB)	Tuberculosis
• private room	Disseminated Zoster
• negative pressure room	Zoster in IC Host
• 6–12 air exchanges/hr	Varicella
• respiratory protection	Measles
1. TB-PAPR	
2. Varicella or measles—nonimmune staff should not enter	
Droplet Precautions	Influenza
• private room or cohort	RSV, Adenovirus
• regular masks	Mumps, Rubella
• do not need negative pressure	Pneumonia due to *S. aureus*, DRSP during first 48 hours of treatment Invasive Meningococcus or *H. flu*
Contact Precautions (acute and nonacute)	MRSA-resistant gram-negative rods
• private room or cohort or low-risk roommate	Shigella, hepA if diarrhea
• gloves for entry into room or per Standard Precautions	*C. difficile* if diarrhea Wounds that cannot be covered
• gowns for any contact with patient or immediate environment or per Standard Precautions	Scabies

Source: Courtesy of University of Maryland, Department of Hospital Epidemiology.

TABLE 14-12 Steps for Outbreak Investigation

a. Determine the nature, location, and severity of the problem.

b. Identify cases.

c. Document notes regarding the outbreak in an orderly fashion.

d. Conduct a literature search.

e. Create a preliminary questionnaire.

f. Review medical records to establish a case definition.

g. Save isolates from cases, as well as suspected cases and/or source.

h. Summarize data into an easy-to-read line listing.

i. Form a hypothesis (source, mode of transmission, cause).

j. Test the hypothesis by either a case-control or cohort study.

k. Create an epidemic curve.

l. Demonstrate biologic plausibility.

m. Inform the appropriate agencies.

n. Institute emergency control measures:
   i. Eliminate the source, which could be environment, patient, or an HCW.
   ii. Protect exposed individuals by administering chemoprophylaxis or immunization.

o. Evaluate the control measures.

p. Document and report the outbreak.

Immunization

An estimated 8.8 million people work in the health care industry.[257] Health care workers are at risk for exposure to a diverse group of occupational infectious diseases, including vaccine-preventable diseases. Diseases such as diphtheria, hepatitis A and B, influenza, measles, mumps, pertussis, rubella, and varicella result in unnecessary and preventable morbidity and mortality. Nonimmune HCWs can acquire these infections from patients or can introduce vaccine-preventable diseases into the health care environment, causing outbreaks.[258-262] A recent study demonstrated that physicians can contract measles, hepatitis B, pertussis, varicella, and influenza following patient exposure.[263] The importance of HCW vaccination and screening for vaccine-preventable diseases is briefly discussed.

Diphtheria

Although an extremely rare disease in the United States, a few cases of nosocomial transmission have been reported in the literature.[264-266] Diphtheria is reemerging in some areas of the world where immunization rates are low. In recent years, epidemics have occurred in the new independent states of the former Soviet Union, and other areas of the world.[267-270]

Diphtheria is caused by *Corynebacterium diphtheriae* and is transmitted from infected patients by respiratory droplets or contact with skin lesions. The incubation period for diphtheria is 1 to 4 days. If diphtheria remains untreated, infected individuals are usually contagious for less than 2 weeks. Rarely, patients may shed the bacteria for 6 months or more.

Immunization with tetanus and diphtheria toxid (Td) is recommended every 10 years for adults who have received a complete immunization series. Foreign-born individuals from endemic areas without documentation of immunization should receive a primary 3-dose series. Prophylaxis of unimmunized workers after contact with a patient with diphtheria with benzathine penicillin (1.2 million units intramuscular) single dose, or erythromycin (1 g/day orally) for 7 days is recommended.[271] Two weeks after the initiation of antimicrobial therapy, nasopharyngeal cultures for *C. diphtheriae* should be obtained, and, if cultures are positive, patients should receive 10 days of erythromycin. Exposed and previously immunized HCWs who have not received Td in the past 5 years should be vaccinated.[271] Exposed susceptible HCWs should be excluded from duties until completion of therapy and a negative nasopharyngeal culture.

Hepatitis A Virus

Hepatitis A virus (HAV) is a rare cause of nosocomial infection, transmitted primarily through the fecal-oral route and, rarely, by transfusion of blood products.[272-276] Infectivity is highest 2 weeks prior to the onset of clinical symptoms or jaundice. Ninety percent of infants remain asymptomatic after HAV infection, although most adults develop jaundice (see Chapter 22).

Nosocomial outbreaks of HAV are rare but have been reported following exposure to infected neonates or children, adult patients with diarrhea or fecal incontinence, or an infected HCW. Transmission has been associated with breaks in standard hygienic practices.[241,277-280] Employees who are (1) exposed to stools of infected patients, (2) consume food prepared by infected employees, and (3) have close contact to a patient with HAV are at risk of acquiring infection. Risk factors identified for HCWs who acquired the disease were failure to comply with basic infection control practices, such as hand washing, wearing gloves, and eating, drinking, or smoking in the patient care area.[241,277,279,280]

The FDA licensed hepatitis A vaccines in 1995. Two inactivated hepatitis A vaccines are available in the markets; both have efficacy greater than 94%.[281-284] Both are well tolerated and have no serious side effects. The vaccine is not routinely recommended for HCWs in the United States. Nevertheless, vaccines should be given for HCWs in high-risk areas, such as neonatal and PICUs, food service, or personnel working with HAV-infected primates or in an HAV research laboratory. In case of direct exposure to the stools of a serologically confirmed case of HAV, postexposure prophylaxis with immunoglobulin (0.02 mL/kg intramuscular) is 80–90% efficacious if given within 2 weeks of exposure. HCWs with suspected HAV infection should not work until jaundice or clinical symptoms subside.

Hepatitis B Virus

Hepatitis B virus (HBV) carries a serious nosocomial transmission risk for HCWs who come in contact with blood or body fluids.[285-291] HCWs represent 2% of all reported cases of HBV infection in the United States.[292] It is estimated that approximately 1000 HCWs became infected with HBV in 1994, which was a 90% decline from 1985.[293]

Prior to vaccine availability, it was estimated that 10–25% of HCWs had evidence of prior HBV infection.[294] This decline has been attributed to vaccine use and adherence to infection control practices. The virus is transmitted parenterally, sexually, and perinatally. The most important mode of occupational transmission is percutaneous exposure to infected blood or serum-derived body fluids. The infectious state is determined by the presence of hepatitis B surface antigen (HBsAg) and hepatitis Be antigen (HBeAg) in the blood. Anyone with a positive HBsAg is considered potentially infectious and is deemed to be highly infectious if HBeAg is positive. HBeAg is a marker for active viral replication, and the risk for transmission from parenteral exposure from a HBeAg-positive patient is greater than 40%.[294] The incubation period is 45 to 180 days (average 60 to 90 days).

There is clear evidence suggesting that patient-to-HCW and HCW-to-patient transmission have occurred, and many nosocomial outbreaks have been documented.[295-303] The risk of transmission depends on the infected person's HBeAg status and level of viremia. An HCW with percutaneous, mucous membrane, or nonintact skin exposure to blood or body fluid of any patient should be considered to have been exposed to HBV until proven otherwise. A positive HBsAg in the source patient confirms exposure.

The Occupational Safety and Health Administration mandates that hepatitis B vaccine be made available to all HCWs at their employers' expense, and universal vaccination of HCWs should be the cardinal goal of occupational health services. Prevaccination serology is not necessary prior to being vaccinated, although postvaccination screening for antibody to the surface antigen (anti-HBs) is recommended. Exposed, unvaccinated HCWs should receive intramuscular hepatitis B immunoglobulin (HBIG) (0.06 mL/kg) within 24 to 48 hours with the first dose of hepatitis B vaccine (1 mL intramuscular) at a different site,[304] followed by additional doses at 1 and 6 months. Exposed, vaccinated HCWs should have their anti-HBs level measured; an antibody level of 10 mLU/mL or more indicates no need for prophylaxis. Workers whose levels have fallen below this level with a previously documented protective level should receive HBIG and a booster vaccine dose.[285,304] If an antibody response has been demonstrated after the HBV vaccine series, HBIG is not needed; these exposed HCWs can be given a booster dose of HBV vaccine alone.

Influenza

Influenza is a major nosocomial pathogen, and transmission has been well documented from patients to HCW, HCW to patients, and HCW to HCW.[305-312] It has been associated with increased morbidity and mortality among patients in long-term as well as acute care facilities. The transmission predominantly occurs through person-to-person contact via large, virus-laden droplets during close contact with infected individuals and by small-particle aerosols or droplet nuclei.[313-316] The incubation period is 1 to 2 days, and viral shedding begins approximately 1 day prior to onset of symptoms and continues up to 10 days.

Nosocomial outbreaks of influenza often occur during community epidemics and can occur in a hospital or health care setting. Numerous outbreaks have been reported in the literature, demonstrating the infectivity of influenza.[317-327] Persons at greatest risk of serious disease are: (1) people older than 65 years, (2) residents of nursing homes and chronic care facilities, (3) persons with chronic pulmonary or cardiac conditions, and (4) persons with diabetes mellitus.[328]

Influenza vaccine is recommended for HCWs each year. HCW vaccination has been shown to decrease mortality among elderly patients in long-term care facilities.[329] In the United States, influenza activity peaks between late December and early March. Thus, the ideal time to vaccinate with influenza vaccine is between October and mid-November. Vaccinating HCWs can be highly cost-effective, can reduce the risk to HCWs, and can prevent transmission from HCWs to high-risk patients.[330] During an outbreak, prophylaxis with antiviral agents (amantadine, rimantadine) for 2 weeks in conjunction with vaccine is recommended.[331] Drugs that inhibit the enzyme neuraminidase of influenza A and B, zamanivir and oseltamivir, have been approved for use to treat influenza.[332-335] These agents also look promising for prophylaxis during influenza outbreaks.[336] Influenza viruses that have been responsible for recent outbreaks in the United States have been found to be resistant to amantadine.[427] If vaccine is not administered, antiviral agents should be given for the duration of influenza activity in the community.[328,337] By far, the best control measure in a health care setting is immunization against influenza; however, it is important that institutions have surveillance for early recognition and isolation of possibly infected individuals.[333] HCWs who are suspected to have influenza should not work until symptoms subside.

Measles

Measles is a highly contagious infection of the respiratory system. Measles is infrequent in the United States, as a result of the introduction of vaccine in 1962. However, more than 20% of young adults are seronegative.[338,339] The transmission of measles occurs by droplet and airborne transmission, especially in medical settings.[340,341] Infectious virus can survive at least several hours in the air. The incubation period is 5 to 21 days, and viral shedding begins 9 to 10 days after exposure.

Since the resurgence of measles in the United States in 1989,[259,342] many outbreaks have been documented.[259,343-349] From 1985 through 1991, 2997 reported measles cases (4% of all reported cases) were transmitted in a medical facility with about half acquired in hospital inpatient units.[259,350] Ninety percent of the 2997 reported measles cases were transmitted from patients and the remaining 10% from HCWs. It has been shown that HCWs are at a 13-fold higher risk than the general population for acquiring measles.[351]

In the United States, the measles vaccine is administered in combination with mumps and rubella. It is a live-attenuated vaccine that induces 90% seroconversion with a single dose, and the second dose immunizes most of the remainder.[352,353] Documentation of immunity to measles (physician diagnosis, serologic immunity, documentation of appropriate vaccination or being born during or before 1957) should be required by the health care institution for all health care workers. Health care institutions should serologically test employees for immunity (targeted approach) and vaccinate seronegatives. This approach has shown to be cost-effective, compared with vaccination without prior screening.[354-356] However, the most important intervention to halt an outbreak is prompt administration of the vaccine. Employees with measles should not care for patients until 7 days after the appearance of rash. Exposed HCWs not immune to measles should be restricted from duty from day 5 through day 21 after exposure. People who cannot be vaccinated can be treated with IG up to 6 days after exposure. IG will not prevent measles, but it does make the disease milder.

Mumps

In the United States, mumps incidence has declined steadily since 1967, when the vaccine was licensed. Between 1985 and 1987, there was resurgence of mumps, probably due to suboptimal vaccine coverage. However, a large community-wide epidemic of mumps occurred in the midwestern U.S. in 2006.[428] Although most cases of mumps in HCWs have been community acquired, nosocomial transmission has been documented.[357-360] Transmission occurs through droplet nuclei and direct contact with saliva of infected person. The incubation period is between 12 and 25 days (16 to 18 days average). Viral shedding may occur 6 to 9 days prior to development of parotitis and may persist 9 days after the onset of disease.[257,361]

The ideal strategy for prevention of nosocomial mumps is to have an effective vaccination program and stringent infection control practices. All HCWs should be considered susceptible unless they have documentation of immunity (physician-diagnosed mumps, serologic immunity, documentation of appropriate vaccination, or being born during or before 1957).[362] Exposed, susceptible HCW should be relieved of duty from day 5 through day 26 after exposure or until 9 days after the onset of parotitis.[363]

Pertussis

Pertussis is extremely contagious, with a greater than 80% secondary attack rate among susceptible household contacts.[364,365] Until recently, due to the widespread use of the vaccine, there had been a steady decline in the incidence of the disease. In recent years, the epidemiology of the disease has changed, and the disease now occurs more frequently among young adults and is frequently asymptomatic.[366] Recent studies indicate that HCWs often may be exposed and may develop the infection more frequently than previously appreciated.[367-370] Transmission occurs by contact with respiratory secretions or large aerosol droplets. The incubation period is between 7 and 10 days, and infectivity starts at the onset of the catarrhal stage through 3 weeks after the onset of symptoms.

Nosocomial transmission of *Bordetella pertussis* has been reported with increased frequency.[366-368,371-373] Because the clinical symptoms are less severe in adults than in children, they may go unnoticed. The failure to recognize the disease has resulted in nosocomial transmission.[367]

Although acellular pertussis vaccine has been shown to be immunogenic with lower risk of adverse events,[372,374] it has not been licensed for people older than 7 years of age. Vaccine (usually given at 4 and 6 years) immunity declines over time, with about 50% of those immunized 12 or more years earlier still immune.[375] Thus, HCWs may play an important role in disease transmission.

Prevention strategies for pertussis transmission include early diagnosis and treatment, implementation of droplet precautions, exclusion of HCWs from duties, and postexposure prophylaxis for exposed persons.[257,368,376] Post-exposure prophylaxis with erythromycin (500 mg orally 4 times daily for 14 days) or trimethoprim-sulfamethazole (one tablet twice a day for 14 days) has been shown to prevent the development of clinical disease and may minimize transmission.[366,368,377,378] More recently, newer antibiotics with fewer side effects are being used. Use of the vaccine may help to prevent secondary infections.[373,379] Exposed HCWs should be excluded from duty from the onset of the catarrhal stage through the third week after the onset of paroxysms or until 5 days after initiation of effective antimicrobial therapy.[257]

Rubella

Rubella is highly contagious, but the incidence of the disease has declined steadily since 1969, when the vaccine was licensed in the United States. However, close to 20% of young adults remains susceptible to rubella.[380,381] The disease is transmitted by direct contact with infectious nasopharyngeal secretions and by aerosolized droplets. The incubation period may range from 12 to 23 days, with the rash appearing 14 to 16 days postexposure. Viral shedding may begin 1 week before through 5 to 7 days after the rash onset,[382] although infants with congenital rubella syndrome may shed virus for months. In adults, it is a mild disease, and 30% to 50% of the cases may be subclinical.

Nosocomial transmission has been well documented.[262,383-388] Outbreaks result in serious health and emotional consequences, especially if the exposure occurs during the first trimester of pregnancy. The rate of perinatal transmission is 40–50% overall and 90% during the first 12 weeks of pregnancy. Studies have demonstrated that medical and dental students can be the source of infection in rubella outbreaks.[262,389]

The ideal strategy for prevention of nosocomial rubella is to have an effective vaccination program and stringent infection control practices. Droplet precautions help to prevent transmission, but, for children with congenital rubella, contact precautions should be used for the first year of life unless urine and nasopharyngeal cultures are negative after 3 months of age.[390] All hospital employees, especially those working with pregnant women, should be immune to rubella and should be considered susceptible unless they have documentation of immunity (physician diagnosis, serologic immunity, documentation of appropriate vaccination). Being born during or before 1957 is acceptable evidence for immunity.[351] Also, a past history of rubella should not be accepted as criteria for immunity. Employees of childbearing age should be checked for pregnancy and should not plan a pregnancy for 3 months after vaccine administration. Pregnant employees who are exposed should be referred for follow-up with their obstetrician, and they should be tested for antirubella IgM antibody.

Varicella-Zoster Virus (VZV)

Varicella (chickenpox) and herpes zoster (shingles) are caused by VZV and are extremely communicable. VZV is spread through direct contact with vesicular fluid or droplets from respiratory secretions and via airborne transmission.[391–396] The incubation period is between 10 and 21 days (14 to 16 days average) but may be prolonged to 28 days after receiving postprophylaxis varicella-zoster immunoglobulin (VZIG).[397] In immunocompromised patients, the incubation period may be much shorter.[398] Viral shedding begins in the late incubation phase and can last between 4 days prior to rash development until crusting of lesions.[399]

Nosocomial transmission of VZV is well recognized, and multiple outbreaks have been reported in the literature.[393,394,400–408] Immunocompromised hosts, premature infants born to susceptible mothers, or infants born before 28 weeks of gestation or weighing less than 1000 g, regardless of mother's susceptibility, are at high risk for acquiring the disease.[409] In hospitals, the risk of transmission is related to air distribution patterns, and the index patient should be treated in a negative-pressure room.[394,395,410]

To reduce the risk of transmission, airborne and contact precautions are recommended, and only varicella-immune HCWs should care for patients with VZV. Studies have demonstrated that the history of varicella in adults is 97% to 99% predictive of seropositivity. Serologic testing is likely to be cost-effective in HCWs uncertain of varicella history, because between 71% and 93% will be seropositive.[351,409,411,412]

Exposure workup should include confirmation of diagnosis and extent of disease.[413,414] Exposure requires either household contact or close contact with a patient with varicella or disseminated zoster. For nondisseminated zoster, exposure requires direct contact with exposed or uncovered lesion. Selected exposed individuals without measurable antibody should be considered for prophylaxis within 96 hours with VZIG (125 units/10 kg up to 625 units). All susceptible pregnant women and seronegative immunocompromised contacts should receive VZIG. VZIG does not prevent infection but modifies and attenuates the disease. Exposed HCWs should be furloughed from day 8 to day 21 after exposure and to day 28 if they receive VZIG. Postexposure prophylaxis with VZIG does not necessarily prevent varicella and may extend the incubation period. Thus, it is not generally recommended,[415] except for immunocompromised subjects or premature infants.

In summary, health care institutions should have mandatory, comprehensive immunization programs and should bear responsibility for implementing these programs with careful planning. Success requires education of HCWs on their responsibility to seek appropriate immunization. Successful programs can be highly cost-effective and can reduce the risk of HCW infection and prevent transmission from HCW to high-risk patients, thus improving patient care and reducing HCW absenteeism.

Antimicrobial Control

In recent years, antimicrobial resistance has become a worldwide problem. Intense pressure exerted on microorganisms as a result of excessive antibiotic use in humans, animals, and agriculture has created this problem. The excessive use of antibiotics has also been linked to adverse drug reactions, adding to hospital costs. The use of antibiotics in any dosage over any period of time leads to selective pressure on the microorganism to either adapt by acquiring additional genetic resistance factors or die. In hospital formularies,

TABLE 14-13   Strategies for Optimizing Antimicrobial Use in Hospitals

- Education of prescribers
- Clinical guidelines
- Formulary restrictions
- Preuse approval
- Automatic stop order
- Audit of use

antimicrobials account for the second most commonly used class of drugs. It is estimated that 23–40% of hospitalized patients receive systemic antimicrobial agents at any given time, and about 40–50% of their use is inappropriate.[220–223,416–418]

To control antimicrobial usage, hospitals need an antimicrobial utilization committee. This committee should be composed of individuals from infectious disease, pharmacy, microbiology, infection control, nursing, quality control and assurance, administration, and data management, as well as a representative physician from surgery, internal medicine, pediatrics, and obstetrics/gynecology. The chairman of infectious diseases often will head this committee. Residents should be included because they prescribe most antimicrobials. The strategies for optimizing antimicrobial use in the hospital are given in Table 14-13.

In summary, antimicrobial use is the driving force behind antibiotic resistance. Bacterial pathogens that cause common illnesses are becoming increasingly resistant to the existing antibiotics. These virulent microbes will have serious implications for global epidemics. Reduction in the use of antibiotics may increase the success of treatment. Although difficult and inconvenient, antimicrobial restriction policies may control the emergence of resistant organisms and improve the outcome of treatment of nosocomial infections.

Conclusion

As we enter a new millennium, nosocomial infections are likely to increase in frequency. As our population ages, more people will be encountering the health care system and will acquire these infections, leading to further morbidity and mortality. Increases in antimicrobial resistance will complicate treatment, increasing the importance of prevention (surveillance, outbreak investigation, education, employee health, antibiotic utilization, and other processes of care). Hospital epidemiologists need to apply creative strategies for prevention of nosocomial infections in a rapidly changing health care system. As the struggle to reduce the growth of health care costs continues, hospital epidemiology will play an important role in evaluating patients' outcomes and in improving the quality of their care.

References

1. Emori TG, Gaynes RP. An overview of nosocomial infections, including the role of the microbiology laboratory. *Clin Microbiol Rev.* 1993;6:428–442.

2. Centers for Disease Control and Prevention. Public health focus: surveillance, prevention, and control of nosocomial infections. *MMWR.* 1992;41:783–787.

3. Kollef MH, Sharpless L, Vlasnik J, Pasque C, Murphy D, Fraser VJ. The impact of nosocomial infections on patient outcomes following cardiac surgery. *Chest.* 1997;112:666–675.

4. Perl TM, Golub JE. New approaches to reduce *Staphylococcus aureus* nosocomial infection rated: treating *S. aureus* nasal carriage. *Ann Pharmacother.* 1998;32:7–16.

5. National Nosocomial Infections Surveillance (NNIS) report. Data summary from October 1986–April 1996, issued May 1996. *Am J Infect Control.* 1996;24:380–388.

6. Emori TG, Culver DH, Horan TC, et al. National Nosocomial Infection Surveillance (NNIS) system: description of surveillance methodology. *Am J Infect Control.* 1991;19:19–35.

7. Gaynes RP, Horan TC. Surveillance of nosocomial infections. In: Mayhall CG, ed. *Hospital Epidemiology and Infection Control.* Baltimore, Md: Williams & Wilkins; 1996:1017–1031.

8. Centers for Disease Control and Prevention. National Nosocomial Infection Study report. In: *CDC Annual Summary, 1977.* US Department of Health, Education and Welfare, Public Health Service; Washington, DC; November 1979.

9. Wenzel RP. Instituting health care reform and preserving quality: role of the hospital epidemiologist. *Clin Infect Dis.* 1993;17:831–834.

10. Kislak JW, Eickhoff TC, Finland M. Hospital-acquired infections and antibiotic usage in the Boston City Hospital. *N Engl J Med.* 1964;271:834–835.

11. Anon. *Charaka-Samhita.* (Sanskrit, c. 4th century B.C.). Kavipatna AC, trans. Vol 1. Calcutta: Privately printed; 1888:168–169.

12. Selwyn S. Hospital infection: the first 2500 years. *J Hosp Infect.* 1991;18:5–64.

13. Major RH. *A History of Medicine.* Vol 1. Oxford, England: Blackwell Publishers; 1954:294–321.

14. Stromayr C. Die handschrift des schnidt und augenarztes. Casper Stromayr [Practicia copiosa] 1559. von Brunn W, ed. Berlin: Idra-Verlagsanstalt; 1925.

15. Tenon JR. *Memoires sur les hopitaux de Paris.* Paris: Ph-D Pierres; 1788:138–424.

16. Simpson JY. Some propositions on hospitalism, by the late Sir JY Simpson, Bart. *Lancet.* 1870;2:698–700.

17. Simpson JY. Presidential address on public health. *Trans Natl Assoc Promotion Soc Sci.* 1867:107–123.

18. Cohen IB. Florence Nightingale. *Sci Am.* 1984;250:128–137.

19. Nightingale F. *Notes on Hospitals.* 3rd ed. London: Longman; 1863.

20. Semmelewis IP. The etiology, the concept and the prophylaxis of childbed fever. Pest, Wien, u. Leipzig. C. A. Hartleben, 1861 (reprinted in translation by FP Murphy). *Med Classics.* 5:334–773.

21. Absolon KB, Absolon MJ, Zientek R. From antisepsis to asepsis. Louis Pasteur's publication on "The germ theory and its application to medicine and surgery." *Rev Surg.* 1970;27:245–258.

22. Toledo-Pereyra LH, Toledo MM. A critical study of Lister's work on antiseptic surgery. *Am J Surg.* 1976;131:736–744.

23. Delaunay A. Centennial of the "germ theory and its applications to medicine and surgery," presented by Louis Pasteur in April of 1878. *Gac Med Mex.* 1979;115:145–149.

24. Lister J. On the effects of the antiseptic system of treatment upon the salubrity of a surgical hospital. *Lancet.* 1870;1:40, 400. In: *Collected Papers.* Vol 2. Oxford, 1909. Republished, *Classics of Medicine Library.* Birmingham, England; 1979.

25. Brewer GE. Operative surgery at the City Hospital with preliminary report on the study of wound infection. *New York Med J.* 1896.

26. Brewer GE. Studies in aseptic technique, with a report of some recent infections at the Roosevelt Hospital. *JAMA.* 1915;64:1369–1372.

27. Wise RI, Ossman EA, Littlefield DR. Personal reflections on nosocomial staphylococcal infections and the development of hospital surveillance. *Rev Infect Dis.* 1989;11:1005–1018.

28. Schaberg DR, Culver DH, Gaynes RP. Major trends in the microbial etiology of nosocomial infections. *Am J Med.* 1991;91:72–75.

29. Centers for Disease Control. National Nosocomial Infections Surveillance system. Nosocomial infection rates for interhospital comparison: limitations and possible solutions. *Infect Control Hosp Epidemiol.* 1991;12:609–621.

30. Wenzel K. The role of the infection control nurse. *Nurs Clin North Am.* 1970;5:89–98.

31. Barrett FF, Casey JI, Finland M. Infections and antibiotic usage among patients at Boston City Hospital. *N Engl J Med.* 1968;278:5–9.

32. Haley RW, Culver DH, Hooton TM, et al. Progress report on the evaluation of the efficacy of infection surveillance and control programs. *Am J Med.* 1981;70:971–975.

33. Haley RW, Culver DH, White JW, et al. The efficacy of infection surveillance and control programs in preventing nosocomial infections in US hospitals. *Am J Epidemiol.* 1985;121:182–205.

34. Donowitz LG, Wenzel RP, Hoyt JW. High risk of hospital-acquired infection in the ICU patient. *Crit Care Med.* 1982;10:355–357.

35. Sing-Naz N, Sprague BM, Patel KM, Pollack MM. Risk factors for nosocomial infection in critically ill children: a prospective cohort study. *Crit Care Med.* 1996;24:875–878.

36. National Academy of Sciences, National Research Council. Postoperative wound infections: the influence of ultraviolet irradiation of the operative room and various other factors. *Ann Surg.* 1964;160(suppl 2):1–132.

37. Haley RW, Culver DH, Morgan WM, White JW, Emori TG, Hooton TM. Identifying patients at high risk of surgical wound infection: a simple multivariate index of patient susceptibility and wound contamination. *Am J Epidemiol.* 1985;121:206–215.

38. Culver DH, Horan TC, Gaynes RP, et al. Surgical wound infection rates by wound class, operative procedure, and patient risk index. *Am J Med.* 1991;91(suppl 3B):152S–157S.

39. Roy MC, Herwaldt A, Embrey R, Kuhns K, Wenzel RP, Perl TM. Does the Centers for Disease Control's NNIS risk index stratify patients undergoing cardiothoracic operations by their risk of surgical site infection? *Infect Control Hosp Epidemiol.* 2000;21:186–190.

40. Freeman J, McGowan JE Jr. Day-specific incidence of nosocomial infection estimated from a prevalence survey. *Am J Epidemiol.* 1981;114:888–901.

41. Rhame FS, Sudderth WD. Incidence and prevalence as used in the analysis of the occurrence of nosocomial infections. *Am J Epidemiol.* 1981;113:1-11.

42. Pottinger JM, Herwaldt LA, Perl TM. Basics of surveillance—an overview. *Infect Control Hosp Epidemiol.* 1997;18:513-527.

43. Haley RW, Hooton TM, Schoenfelder JR, et al. Effect of an infection surveillance and control program on the accuracy of retrospective chart review. *Am J Epidemiol.* 1980;111:543-555.

44. Haley RW, Tenney JH, Lindsey JO, Garner JS, Bennett JV. How frequent are outbreaks of nosocomial infection in community hospitals? *Infect Control.* 1985;6:233-236.

45. Givens CD, Wenzel RP. Catheter-associated urinary tract infections in surgical patients: a controlled study on the excess morbidity and costs. *J Urol.* 1980;124:646-648.

46. Coello R, Glenister H, Fereres J, et al. The cost of infection in surgical patients: a case-control study. *J Hosp Infect.* 1993;25:239-250.

47. Eickhoff TC. The Third Decennial International Conference on Nosocomial Infections. Historical perspective: the landmark conference in 1970. *Am J Med.* 1991;91:3-5.

48. Warren JW, Anthony WC, Hoopes JM, Muncie HL Jr. Cephalexin for susceptible bacteriuria in afebrile, long-term catheterized patients. *JAMA.* 1982;248:454-458.

49. Freeman J, McGowan JE Jr. Risk factors for nosocomial infections. *J Infect Dis.* 1978;138:811-819.

50. Stamm WE, Martins SM, Bennett JV. Epidemiology of nosocomial infections due to gram-negative bacilli: aspects relevant to development and use of vaccine. *J Infect Dis.* 1977;136:151-160.

51. Ayliefe GA, Brightwell KM, Collins BJ, Lowbury EJL. Surveys of hospital infections in the Birmingham region. *J Hyg (Cambridge).* 1977;79:299-314.

52. Saviteer SM, Samsa GP, Rutala WA. Nosocomial infections in elderly: increase risk per hospital day. *Am J Med.* 1988;84:661-666.

53. Gross PA, Rapuano C, Adrignolo A, Shaw B. Nosocomial infections: decade-specific risk. *Infect Control.* 1983;4:145-147.

54. Emory TG, Banerjee SN, Culver DH, et al. Nosocomial infection in the elderly patients in the United States, 1986-1990. *Am J Med.* 1991;91:289-293.

55. Velasco E, Thuler LC, Martins CA, Dias LM, Goncalves VM. Nosocomial infections in an oncology intensive care unit. *Am J Infect Control.* 1997;25:458-462.

56. Perl T, Chotani R, Agawala R. Infection control and prevention in bone marrow transplant patients. In Mayhall CG, ed. *Hospital Epidemiology and Infection Control.* 2nd ed. Baltimore, Md: Lippincott Williams & Wilkins; 1999:803-844.

57. Craven DE, Steger KA, Hirschhorn LR. Nosocomial colonization and infection in persons infected with human immunodeficiency virus. *Infect Control Hosp Epidemiol.* 1996;17:304-318.

58. Goetz AM, Squier C, Wagener MM, Muder RR. Nosocomial infections in the human immunodeficiency virus-infected patient: a two-year survey. *Am J Infect Control.* 1994;22:334-339.

59. Stroud L, Srivastava P, Culver D, et al. Nosocomial infections in HIV-infected patients: preliminary results from a multicenter surveillance system (1989-1995). *Infect Control Hosp Epidemiol.* 1997;18:479-485.

60. Barsic B, Beus I, Marton E, Himbele J, Klinar I. Nosocomial infections in critically ill infectious disease patients: results of a 7-year focal surveillance. *Infection.* 1999;27:16–22.
61. Kampf G, Wischnewski N, Schulgen G, Schumacher M, Daschner F. Prevalence and risk factors for nosocomial lower respiratory tract infections in German hospitals. *J Clin Epidemiol.* 1998;51:495–502.
62. Berbari EF, Hanssen AD, Duffy MC, et al. Risk factors for prosthetic joint infection: case-control study. *Clin Infect Dis.* 1998;27:1247–1254.
63. Keita-Perse O, Gaynes RP. Severity of illness scoring system to adjust nosocomial infection rates: a review and commentary. *Am J Infect Control.* 1996;24:429–434.
64. Rhame FS, Streifel AJ, Kersey JH Jr, et al. Extrinsic risk factors for pneumonia in the patient at high risk of infection. *Am J Med.* 1984;76:42–52.
65. Rhame FS. Prevention of nosocomial aspergillosis. *J Hosp Infect.* 1991;18:466–472.
66. Centers for Disease Control and Prevention. Guidelines for prevention on nosocomial pneumonia. *MMWR.* 1997;46:28–34, 54–57, 74–79.
67. Joseph CA, Watson JM, Harrison TG, Bartlett CLR. Nosocomial Legionnaires' disease in England and Wales, 1980–92. *Epidemiol Infect.* 1992;112:329–345.
68. McGowan JE Jr. Environmental factors in nosocomial infection: a selective focus. *Rev Infect Dis.* 1981;3:760–769.
69. Centers for Disease Control and Prevention. Sustained transmission of nosocomial Legionnaires disease—Arizona and Ohio. *MMWR.* 1997;46:416–421.
70. Marks JS, Tasi TF, Martone WJ, et al. Nosocomial Legionnaires' disease in Columbus, Ohio. *Ann Intern Med.* 1997;90:565–569.
71. Astagneau P, Duneton P. Management of epidemics of nosocomial infections. *Pathol Biol (Paris).* 1998;46:272–278.
72. Nishijima S, Sugimachi T, Higashida T, Asada Y, Okuda K, Murata K. An epidemiological study of methicillin-resistant *Staphylococcus aureus* (MRSA) isolated from medical staff, inpatients, and hospital environment in one ward at our hospital. *J Dermatol.* 1992;19:356–361.
73. Vrankova J, Bendova E, Konigova R, Broz L. Bacteriological monitoring in the Prague Burns Center. *Acta Chir Plast.* 1998;4:105–108.
74. Warnick F. Vancomycin-resistant enterococcus. *Clin J Oncol Nurs.* 1997;1:73–77.
75. Graman PS, Hall CB. Nosocomial viral respiratory infections. *Semin Respir Infect.* 1989;4:253–260.
76. Berthelot P, Grattard F, Mahul P, et al. Ventilator temperature sensors: an unusual source of *Pseudomonas cepacia* in nosocomial infection. *J Hosp Infect.* 1993;25:33–43.
77. Vesley D, Norlien KG, Nelson B, Ott B, Streifel AJ. Significant factors in the disinfection and sterilization of flexible endoscopes. *Am J Infect Control.* 1992;20:291–300.
78. Nosocomial infection and pseudoinfection from contaminated endoscopes and bronchoscopes—Wisconsin and Missouri. *MMWR.* 1991;40:675–678.
79. Jawad A, Heritage J, Snelling AM, Gascoyne-Binzi DM, Hawkey PM. Influence of relative humidity and suspending menstrua on survival of

Acinetobacter spp. on dry surfaces. *J Clin Microbiol.* 1996;34: 2881–2887.

80. Craven DE, Steger K. Nosocomial pneumonia in mechanically ventilated adult patients: epidemiology and prevention in 1996. *Semin Respir Infect.* 1996;11:32–53.

81. Carratala J, Fernandez-Sevilla A, Tubau F, Callis M, Gudiol F. Emergence of quinolone-resistant *Escherichia coli* bacteremia in neutropenia patients with cancer who received prophylactic norfloxacin. *Clin Infect Dis.* 1995;20:557–560.

82. Wingard JR, Merz WG, Rinaldi MG, Johnson TR, Karp JE, Saral R. Increase in *Candida krusei* infection among patients with bone marrow transplantation and neutropenia treated prophylactically with fluconazole. *N Engl J Med.* 1991;325:1274–1277.

83. Sherertz RJ, Reagan DR, Hampton KD, et al. A cloud adult: the *Staphylococcus aureus*-virus interaction revisited. *Annals of Intern Med.* 1996;124:539–547.

84. Perl TM. The threat of vancomycin resistance. *Am J Med.* 1999;106:26S–37S.

85. Weber DJ, Rutala WA. Role of environmental contamination in the transmission of vancomycin-resistant enterococci. *Infect Control Hosp Epidemiol.* 1997;18:306–309.

86. Hughes WT, Williams B, Williams B, et al. The nosocomial colonization of teddy bear. *Infect Control.* 1986;7:495–500.

87. Garibaldi RA, Mooney BR, Epstein BJ, Britt MR. An evaluation of daily bacteriologic monitoring to identify preventable episodes of catheter-associated urinary tract infection. *Infect Control.* 1982;3:466–470.

88. Richards MJ, Edwards JR, Culver DH, Gaynes RP. National Nosocomial Infections Surveillance system. Nosocomial infections in coronary care units in the United States. *Am J Cardiol.* 1998;82:789–793.

89. Garibaldi RA, Burke JP, Britt MR, Miller MA, Smith CB. Meatal colonization and catheter-associated bacteriuria. *N Engl J Med.* 1980;303:316–318.

90. Warren JW, Platt R, Thomas RJ, Rosner B, Kass EH. Antibiotic irrigation and catheter-associated urinary-tract infections. *N Engl J Med.* 1978;299:570–573.

91. Thompson RL, Haley CE, Searcy MA, et al. Catheter-associated bacteriuria. Failure to reduce attack rates using periodic instillations of a disinfectant into urinary drainage systems. *JAMA.* 1984;251: 747–751.

92. Gross PA. Epidemiology of hospital-acquired pneumonia. *Semin Respir Infect.* 1987;2:2–7.

93. Horan TC, White JW, Jarvis WR, et al. Nosocomial infection surveillance, 1984. *MMWR.* 1986;35:17–29.

94. Leu H-S, Kaiser DL, Mori M, et al. Hospital acquired pneumonia: attributable mortality and morbidity. *Am J Epidemiol.* 1989;129: 1258–1267.

95. Centers for Disease Control and Prevention. National Nosocomial Infections Study report. Annual summary 1984. *MMWR.* 1986;35: 17–29.

96. Wenzel RP. Hospital-acquired pneumonia: overview of the current state of the art for prevention and control. *Eur J Clin Microbiol Infect Dis.* 1989;70:681–685.

97. Broderic A, Mori M, Netlemann WD, et al. Nosocomial infections: validation of surveillance and computer modeling to identify patients at risk. *Am J Epidemiol.* 1990;131:734–742.

98. Boyce JM, Potter-Bynoe G, Dziobek L, et al. Nosocomial pneumonia in Medicare patients. Hospital costs and reimbursement patterns under the prospective payment system. *Arch Intern Med.* 1991;151:1109–1114.

99. National Nosocomial Infections Surveillance (NNIS) report, data summary from October 1986–April 1997, issued May 1997. A report from the NNIS system. *Am J Infect Control.* May 1997.

100. Celis R, Torres A, Gatell JM, et al. Nosocomial pneumonia: a multivariate analysis of the risk and prognosis. *Chest.* 1988;93:318–324.

101. Bartlett JG, O'Keefe P, Tally FP, et al. Bacteriology of hospital-acquired pneumonia. *Arch Intern Med.* 1986;146:868–871.

102. Fagon JY, Chastre J, Hance AJ, Montravers P, Novara A, Gibert C. Nosocomial pneumonia in ventilated patients: a cohort study evaluating attributable mortality and hospital stay. *Am J Med.* 1993;94:281–288.

103. Gross PA, Van Antwerpen C. Nosocomial infections and hospital deaths. *Am J Med.* 1983;75:658–662.

104. Graybill JR, Marshall LW, Charache P, Wallace CK, Melvin VB. Nosocomial pneumonia: a continuing major problem. *Am Rev Respir Dis.* 1973;108:1130–1140.

105. Stevens RM, Teres D, Skillman JJ, Feingold DS. Pneumonia in an intensive care unit: a 30-month experience. *Arch Intern Med.* 1974;134:106–111.

106. Craig CP, Connelly S. Effect of intensive care unit nosocomial pneumonia on duration of stay and mortality. *Am J Infect Control.* 1984;12:233–238.

107. Craven DE, Kunches LM, Lichtenberg DA, et al. Nosocomial infection and fatality in medical and surgical intensive care unit patients. *Arch Intern Med.* 1988;148:1161–1168.

108. Prodinger WM, Bonatti H, Allerberger F, et al. Legionella pneumonia in transplant recipients: a cluster of cases of three-year duration. *J Hosp Infect.* 1994;26:191–202.

109. Harrington RD, Hooton TM, Hackman RC, et al. An outbreak of respiratory syncytial virus in a bone marrow transplant center. *J Infect Dis.* 1992;165:987–993.

110. Pannuti C, Gingrich R, Pfaller MA, et al. Nosocomial pneumonia in patients having bone marrow transplant: attributable mortality and risk factors. *Cancer.* 1992;69:2653–2662.

111. Hall CB, Douglas RG Jr, Geiman JM, et al. Nosocomial respiratory syncytial virus infections. *N Engl J Med.* 1975;293:1343–1346.

112. Hoffman PC, Dixon RE. Control of influenza in the hospital. *Ann Intern Med.* 1977;87:725–728.

113. Kapila R, Lintz DI, Tecson FT, et al. A nosocomial outbreak of influenza A. *Chest.* 1977;71:576–579.

114. Mosconi P, Langer M, Cigada M, et al. Epidemiology and risk factors of pneumonia in critically ill patients. *Eur J Epidemiol.* 1991;7:320–327.

115. Torres A, Azner R, Gatell J, et al. Incidence, risk, and prognosis factors of nosocomial pneumonia in mechanically ventilated patients. *Am Rev Respir Dis.* 1990;142:523–528.

116. Jimenez P, Torres A, Rodriguez-Roisin R, et al. Incidence and etiology of pneumonia acquired during mechanical ventilation. *Crit Care Med.* 1989;17:882–885.

117. Rodriguez JL, Gibbons KJ, Bitzer, et al. Pneumonia: incidence, risk factors, and outcome in injured patients. *J Trauma.* 1991;31:907–912.

118. Garibaldi RA, Britt MR, Coleman ML, et al. Risk factors for postoperative pneumonia. *Am J Med.* 1981;70:677–680.

119. Hanson LC, Weber DJ, Rutala WA, et al. Risk factors for nosocomial pneumonia in the elderly. *Am J Med.* 1992;92:161–166.

120. Josji N, Localio AR, Hamory BH. A predictive risk index of nosocomial pneumonia in the intensive care unit. *Am J Med.* 1992;93:135–141.

121. Craven DE, Steger KA, Barber TW. Preventing nosocomial pneumonia: state of the art and perspectives for the 1990s. *Am J Med.* 1991;91: 44–53.

122. Cross AS, Roup B. Role of respiratory assistance devices in endemic nosocomial pneumonia. *Am J Med.* 1981;70:681–685.

123. Torres A, el-Ebiary N, Gonzalez J, et al. Gastric and pharyngeal flora in nosocomial pneumonia acquired during mechanical ventilation. *Am Rev Respir Dis.* 1993;148:352–357.

124. Centers for Disease Control and Prevention. Guidelines for prevention of nosocomial pneumonia. *MMWR.* 1997;46:1–9.

125. Wenzel RP. Preoperative antibiotic prophylaxis. *N Engl J Med.* 1992;326:337–339.

126. Leape LL, Brennan TA, Laird N, et al. The nature of adverse events in hospitalized patients: results of the Harvard Medical Practice Study II. *N Engl J Med.* 1991;324:377–384.

127. Haley RW. Surveillance by objective: a new priority-directed approach to the control of nosocomial infections. *Am J Infect Control.* 1985;13:78–89.

128. Martone W, Jarvis W, Culver D, Haley R. Incidence and nature of endemic and epidemic nosocomial infections. In: Bennett J, Brachman P, eds. *Hospital Infections.* 3rd ed. Boston, Mass: Little, Brown and Company; 1992:577–596.

129. Public health focus: surveillance, prevalence, and control of nosocomial infections. *MMWR.* 1992;41:783–787.

130. Mayhall CG. Surgical infections including burns. In: Wenzel RP, ed. *Prevention and Control of Nosocomial Infections.* Baltimore, Md: Williams & Wilkins; 1992:614–664.

131. Manian F, Meyer L. Comprehensive surveillance of surgical wound infection in outpatient and inpatient surgery. *Infect Control Hosp Epidemiol.* 1990;11:515–520.

132. Perl TM, Roy MC. Postoperative wound infections: risk factors and role of *Staphylococcus aureus* nasal carriage. *J Chemother.* 1995;7: 29–35.

133. Society for Hospital Epidemiology of America, Association of Professionals of Infection Control, Centers for Disease Control, Surgical Infection Society. Consensus paper on the surveillance of surgical wound infections. *Infect Control Hosp Epidemiol.* 1992;13: 599–605.

134. Simchen E, Stein H, Sacks TG, Shapiro M, Michel J. Multivariate analysis of determinants of postoperative wound infection in orthopaedic patients. *J Hosp Infect.* 1984;5:137–146.

135. Kurz A, Sessler DI, Lenhardt R. Perioperative normothermia to reduce the incidence of surgical-wound infection and shorten hospitalization. Study of Wound Infection and Temperature Group. *N Engl J Med.* 1996;334:1209–1215.

136. Roy MC, Perl TM. Basics of surgical-site infection surveillance. *Infect Control Hosp Epidemiol.* 1997;18:659–668.

137. Classen DC, Evans RS, Pestotnik SL, Horn SD, Menlove RL, Burke JP. The timing of prophylactic administration of antibiotics and the risk of surgical wound infection. *N Engl J Med.* 1992;326:281–286.

138. Sands K, Vineyard G, Platt R. Surgical site infections occurring after hospital discharge. *J Infect Dis.* 1996;173:963–970.

139. Roy MC, Herwaldt LA, Embrey R, Kuhns K, Perl TM. A three-year wound surveillance study in cardio-thoracic (CT) surgery. Paper presented at: The 34th Interscience Conference on Antimicrobial Agents and Chemotherapy; 1994; Orlando, Florida.

140. Simchen E, Rozin R, Wax Y. The Israeli study of surgical infection of drains and the risk of wound infection in operation for hernia. *Surg Gynecol Obstet.* 1990;170:331–337.

141. Brown R, Bradley S, Opitz E, Cipriani D, Pieczarka, Sands M. Surgical wound infections documented after hospital discharge. *Am J Infect Control.* 1987;15:54–58.

142. Pittet D, Wenzel RP. Nosocomial bloodstream infections. Secular trends in rates, mortality, and contribution to total hospital stay. *Arch Intern Med.* 1995;155:1177–1184.

143. Pittet D. Nosocomial bloodstream infections. In: Wenzel RP, ed. *Prevention and Control of Nosocomial Infections.* 3rd ed. Baltimore, Md: Williams & Wilkins; 1997:711–769.

144. Bryant RE, Hood AF, Hood CE, et al. Endemic bacteremia in Columbia, SC. *Am J Epidemiol.* 1986;123:113–127.

145. Pittet D, Tarara D, Wenzel RP. Nosocomial bloodstream infection in critically ill patients. Excess length of stay, extra costs, and attributable mortality. *JAMA.* 1994;271:1598–1601.

146. Daschner FD, Frey P, Wolff G, Baumann PC, Suter P. Nosocomial infections in intensive care wards: a multicenter prospective study. *Intensive Care Med.* 1982;8:5–9.

147. Banerjee SN, Emory TG, Culver DH, et al. Secular trends in nosocomial primary bloodstream infections in the United States, 1980–89. National Nosocomial Infection Surveillance system. *Am J Med.* 1991;91:86–89.

148. Centers for Disease Control and Prevention. Increase in national hospital discharge survey rates for septicemia—United States. *MMWR.* 1990;39:31–34.

149. Schneider EL. Infectious diseases in the elderly. *Ann Intern Med.* 1983;98:395–400.

150. Garner J, Jarvis W, Emori G, Horan T, Hughes J. Centers for Disease Control and Prevention definitions of nosocomial infections. *Am J Infect Control.* 1988;16:128–140.

151. Maki DG. Infections due to infusion therapy. In: Bennett JV, Brachman PS, eds. *Hospital Infections.* Boston, Mass: Little, Brown and Company; 1992:849–898.

152. Pittet D, Li N, Woolson R, Wenzel R. Microbiological factors influencing the outcome of nosocomial bloodstream infections: a 6-year validation, population based model. *Clin Infect Dis.* 1997;24:1068–1078.

153. Jarvis WR. Epidemiology of nosocomial fungal infections, with emphasis on *Candida* species. *Clin Infect Dis.* 1995;20:1526–1530.

154. Wingard JR. Importance of *Candida* species other than *C. albicans* as pathogens in oncology patients. *Clin Infect Dis.* 1995;20:115–125.

155. Rex JH, Bennett JE, Sugar AM, et al. A random trial comparing fluconazole with amphotericin B for the treatment of candidemia in patients with neutropenia. *N Engl J Med.* 1994;331:1325–1330.

156. Pfaller MA. Nosocomial candidiasis: emerging species, reservoirs, and modes of transmission. *Clin Infect Dis.* 1996;22:89–94.
157. Martin MA, Pfaller MA, Wenzel RP. Coagulase-negative staphylococcal bacteremia. Mortality and hospital stay. *Ann Intern Med.* 1989;110: 9–16.
158. Smith RL, Meixler SM, Simberkoff MS. Excess mortality in critically ill patients with nosocomial bloodstream infections. *Chest.* 1991;100:164–167.
159. Miller PJ, Wenzel RP. Etiologic organisms as independent predictors of death and morbidity associated with bloodstream infections. *J Infect Dis.* 1987;156:471–477.
160. Wey SB, Mori M, Pfaller MA, Woolson RF, Wenzel RP. Hospital-acquired candidemia: the attributable mortality and excess length of stay. *Arch Intern Med.* 1988;148:2642–2645.
161. Pearson ML. Hospital Infection Control Practices Advisory Committee. Centers for Disease Control and Prevention. Guideline for prevention of intravascular device-related infections. *Am J Infect Control.* 1996;24:262–293.
162. Pittet D, Davis CS, Li N, Wenzel RP. Identifying the hospitalized patient at risk for nosocomial bloodstream infections: a population-based study. *Proc Assoc Am Phys.* 1997;109:58–67.
163. Velasco E, Thuler LC, Martins CA, Dias LM, Goncalves VM. Risk factors for bloodstream infections at a cancer center. *Eur J Clin Microbiol Infect Dis.* 1998;17:587–590.
164. Gaynes RP, Edwards JR, Jarvis WR, Culver DH, Tolson JS, Martone WJ. Nosocomial infections among neonates in high-risk nurseries in the United States. National Nosocomial Infections Surveillance system. *Pediatrics.* 1996;98:357–361.
165. MacDonald L, Baker C, Chenoweth C. Risk factors for candidemia in a children's hospital. *Clin Infect Dis.* 1998;26:642–645.
166. Miller JM, Goetz AM, Squier C, Muder RR. Reduction in nosocomial intravenous device-related bacteremias after institution of an intravenous therapy team. *J Intraven Nurs.* 1996;19:103–106.
167. Meier PA, Fredrickson M, Catney M, Nettleman MD. Impact of a dedicated intravenous therapy team on nosocomial bloodstream infection rates. *Am J Infect Control.* 1998;26:388–392.
168. Wenzel RP, Osterman CA, Hunting KJ, et al. Hospital-acquired infections. Surveillance in a university hospital. *Am J Epidemiol.* 1976;103:251–260.
169. Ford-Jones EL, Mindorff CM, Langley JM, et al. Epidemiologic study of 4684 hospital-acquired infections in pediatric patients. *Pediatr Infect Dis J.* 1989;8:668–675.
170. Welliver RC, McLaughlin S. Unique epidemiology of nosocomial infection in a children's hospital. *Am J Dis Child.* 1984;138:131–135.
171. Anderson LJ. Major trends in nosocomial viral infections. *Am J Med.* 1991;91:107–111.
172. Yolken RJ, Bishop CA, Townsend TR, et al. Infectious gastroenteritis in bone marrow transplant recipients. *N Engl J Med.* 1982;306:1009–1012.
173. Stamm WE, Weinstein RA, Dixon RE. Comparison of endemic and epidemic nosocomial infections. *Am J Med.* 1981;70:393–397.
174. DuPont HL. Nosocomial salmonellosis and shigellosis. *Infect Control Hosp Epidemiol.* 1991;12:707–709.

175. Lightfoot NF, Ahmad F, Cowden J. Management of institutional outbreaks of salmonella gastroenteritis. *J Antimicrob Chemother.* 1990:26;37–46.

176. Dwyer DM, Klein EG, Istre GR, Robinson MG, Neumann DA, McCoy GA. *Salmonella newport* infections transmitted by fiberoptic colonoscopy. *Gastrointest Endosc.* 1987;33:84–87.

177. Stephens JL, Peacock JE. Uncommon infections: eye and central nervous system. In: Wenzel RP, ed. *Prevention and Control of Nosocomial Infections.* 2nd ed. Baltimore, Md: Williams & Wilkins; 1993:746–775.

178. Dhaliwal RS, Meredith TA. Endophthalmitis. In: Charlton JF, Weinstein GW, eds. *Ophthalmic Surgery Complications: Prevention and Management.* Philadelphia, Pa: JB Lippincott Co; 1995:409–430.

179. Baum JL. Current concepts in ophthalmology. Ocular infections. *N Engl J Med.* 1978;299:28–31.

180. Syed NA, Hyndiuk RA. Infectious conjunctivitis. *Infect Dis Clin North Am.* 1992;6:789–805.

181. Ford E, Nelson KE, Warren D. Epidemiology of epidemic keratoconjunctivitis. *Epidemiol Review.* 1987;9:244–261.

182. Warren D, Nelson KE, Frorar J, et al. A large outbreak of adenovirus epidemic keratoconjunctivitis: problems in controlling nosocomial spread. *J Infect Dis.* 1989;160:938–943.

183. Gottsch JD. Surveillance and control of epidemic keratoconjunctivitis. *Trans Am Ophthalmol Soc.* 1996;94:539–587.

184. Buckwold FJ, Hand R, Hansebout RR. Hospital-acquired bacterial meningitis in neurosurgical patients. *J Neurosurg.* 1977;46:494–500.

185. Hodges GR, Perkins RL. Hospital-associated bacterial meningitis. *Am J Med Sci.* 1976;271:335–341.

186. Durand ML, Calderwood SB, Weber DJ, et al. Acute bacterial meningitis in adults. A review of 493 episodes. *N Engl J Med.* 1993;328:21–28.

187. Mangi RJ, Quintiliani R, Anmdriole VT. Gram-negative bacillary meningitis. *Am J Med.* 1975;59:829–836.

188. Berk SL, McCabe WR. Meningitis caused by gram-negative bacilli. *Ann Intern Med.* 1980;93:253–260.

189. Mancebo J, Domingo P, Blanch L, Coll P, Net A, Nolla J. Post-neurosurgical and spontaneous gram-negative bacillary meningitis in adults. *Scand J Infect Dis.* 1986;18:533–538.

190. James HE, Bejar R, Gluck L, et al. Ventriculoperitoneal shunts in high-risk newborns weighing under 2000 grams: a clinical report. *Neurosurgery.* 1984;15:198–202.

191. Unhanand M, Mustafa MM, McCracken GH Jr, Nelson JD. Gram-negative enteric bacillary meningitis: a twenty-one-year experience. *J Pediatr.* 1993;122:15–21.

192. Pople IK, Bayston R, Hayward RD. Infection of cerebrospinal fluid shunts in infants: a study of etiological factors. *J Neurosurg.* 1992;77:29–36.

193. Kernodle DS, Kaiser AB. Postoperative infections and antimicrobial prophylaxis. In: Mandell D, Bennett JE eds. *Principles and Practice of Infectious Diseases.* 4th ed. New York, NY: Churchill Livingstone; 1990:2742–2753.

194. Boyce JM, White RL, Spruill EY. Impact of methicillin-resistant *Staphylococcus aureus* on the incidence of nosocomial staphylococcal infections. *J Infect Dis.* 1983;148:763.

195. Nosocomial enterococci resistant to vancomycin–United States, 1989–1993. *MMWR.* 1993;42:597–599.

196. Edmond MB, Wallace SE, McClish DK, Pfaller MA, Jones RN, Wenzel RP. Nosocomial bloodstream infections in United States hospitals: a three-year analysis. *Clin Infect Dis.* 1999;29:239–244.

197. Edmond M, Ober J, Dawson DW, et al. Vancomycin-resistant enterococcal bacteremia: natural history and attributable mortality. *Clin Infect Dis.* 1996;23:1234–1239.

198. Edmond MB, Ober JF, Weinbaum DL, et al. Vancomycin-resistant *Enterococcus faecium* bacteremia: risk factors for infection. *Clin Infect Dis.* 1995;20:1126–1133.

199. Shay DK, Maloney SA, Montecalvo M, et al. Epidemiology and mortality risk of vancomycin-resistant enterococcal bloodstream infections. *J Infect Dis.* 1995;172:993–1000.

200. Montecalvo MA, Horowitz H, Gedris C, et al. Outbreak of vancomycin-, ampicillin-, and aminoglyco-side-resistant *Enterococcus faecium* bacteremia in an adult oncology unit. *Antimicrob Agents Chemother.* 1994;38:1363–1367.

201. Livornese LL Jr, Dias S, Samel C, et al. Hospital-acquired infection with vancomycin-resistant *Enterococcus faecium* transmitted by electronic thermometers. *Ann Intern Med.* 1992;117:112–116.

202. Handwerger S, Raucher B, Altarac D, et al. Nosocomial outbreak due to *Enterococcus faecium* highly resistant to vancomycin, penicillin, and gentamicin. *Clin Infect Dis.* 1993;16:750–755.

203. Tornieporth NG, Roberts RB, John J, Hafner A, Riley LW. Risk factors associated with vancomycin-resistant *Enterococcus faecium* infection or colonization in 145 matched case patients and control patients. *Clin Infect Dis.* 1996;23:767–772.

204. Roghmann M-C, McCarter RJ, Brewrink J, Cross AS, Morris JG. *Clostridium difficile* infection is a risk factor for bacteremia due to vancomycin-resistant enterococcus (VRE) in VRE-colonized patients with acute leukemia. *Clin Infect Dis.* 1997;25:1056–1059.

205. Perl TM, DeLisle S. The emergence and control of vancomycin-resistant enterococci. In: Bartlett JG, ed. *Grand Round in Infectious Disease.* Islip, NY: Scientific Exchange, Inc; 1998:7–32.

206. Smith TL, Pearson ML, Wilcox KR, et al. Emergence of vancomycin resistance in *Staphylococcus aureus. N Engl J Med.* 1999;340:493–501.

207. Centers for Disease Control and Prevention. Update: *Staphylococcus aureus* with reduced susceptibility to vancomycin–United States, 1997. *MMWR.* 1997;46:813–815.

208. Hiramatsu K, Hanaki H, Ino T, Yabuta K, Oguri T, Tenover FC. Methicillin-resistant *Staphylococcus aureus* clinical strain with reduced vancomycin susceptibility. *J Antimicrob Chemother.* 1997;40:135–136.

209. Hiramatsu K, Aritaka N, Hanaki H, et al. Dissemination in Japanese hospitals of strains of *Staphylococcus aureus* heterogeneously resistant to vancomycin. *Lancet.* 1997;350:1670–1673.

210. Waldvogel FA. New resistance in *Staphylococcus aureus. N Engl J Med.* 1999;340:556–557.

211. Sieradzki K, Roberts RB, Haber SW, Tomasz A. The development of vancomycin resistance in a patient with methicillin-resistant *Staphylococcus aureus* infection. *N Engl J Med.* 1999;340:517–523.

212. Butler JC, Hofmann J, Cetron MS, Elliott JA, Facklam RR, Breiman RF. The continued emergence of drug-resistant *Streptococcus pneumoniae* in the United States: an update from the Centers for Disease Control

and Prevention's Pneumococcal Sentinel Surveillance System. *J Infect Dis.* 1996;174:986–993.

213. Pallares R, Gudiol F, Linares J, et al. Risk factors and response to antibiotic therapy in adults with bacteremic pneumonia caused by penicillin-resistant pneumococci. *N Engl J Med.* 1987;317:18–22.

214. Reichler MR, Allphin AA, Breiman RF, et al. The spread of multiply resistant *Streptococcus pneumoniae* at a day care center in Ohio. *J Infect Dis.* 1992;166:1346–1353.

215. Meyer KS, Urban C, Eagan JA, Berger BJ, Rahal JJ. Nosocomial outbreak of *Klebsiella* infection resistant to late-generation cephalosporins. *Ann Intern Med.* 1993;119:353–358.

216. Fridkin SK, Pear SM, Williamson TH, Galgiani JN, Jarvis WR. The role of understaffing in central venous catheter-associated bloodstream infections. *Infect Control Hosp Epidemiol.* 1996;17:150–158.

217. Archibald LK, Manning ML, Bell LM, Banerjee S, Jarvis WR. Patient density, nurse-to-patient ratio and nosocomial infection risk in a pediatric cardiac intensive care unit. *Pediatr Infect Dis J.* 1997;16:1045–1048.

218. American Society of American Pharmacists. ASHP mission statement. *Am J Hosp Pharm.* 1987;44:1869.

219. Craig WA, Sarver KP. Antimicrobial usage in the USA. In: Williams JD, Geddles AM, eds. *Chemo-therapy.* Vol 4. New York: Plenum Publishing; 1976:293–301.

220. Jorgest GJ, Dippe SE. Antibiotic use among medical specialties in community hospitals. *JAMA.* 1981;245:842–846.

221. Maki DG, Schuna AA. A study of antimicrobial misuse in a university hospital. *Am J Med Sci.* 1978:275;271–282.

222. Castle M, Wilfert CM, Cate TR, Osterhout S. Antimicrobial use at a Duke University Medical Center. *JAMA.* 1977;237:2819–2822.

223. Stevens GP, Jacobson JA, Burke JP. Changing pattern of hospital infections and antibiotic use, prevalence survey in a community hospital. *Arch Intern Med.* 1981;141:587–592.

224. Ayleffe GAJ. Nosocomial infections—the irreducible minimum. *Infect Control.* 1986;7:92–95.

225. Steere AC, Mallison GF. Handwashing practices for the prevention of nosocomial infections. *Ann Intern Med.* 1975;83:683–690.

226. Lilly HA, Lowbury EJL. Transient skin flora. *J Clin Pathol.* 1978;31:919–922.

227. Bryan JL, Cohran J, Larson EL. Hand washing: a ritual revisited. *Crit Care Nurs Clin North Am.* 1995;7:617–625.

228. Garner IS, Favero MS. *Guideline for Handwashing and Hospital Environmental Control.* Atlanta, Ga: Centers for Disease Control; 1985.

229. Woodroffe RCS, Shaw DA. Natural control and etiology microbial populations on skin and hair. In: Skinner FA, Carr JG, eds. *The Normal Microbial Flora of Man.* New York, NY: Academic Press; 1974: 3–34.

230. Casewell M, Phillips I. Hands as a route of transmission of *Klebsiella* species. *Br Med J.* 1977;2:1315–1317.

231. Al-Khoja MS, Darrell JH. The skin as a source of *Acinetobacter* and *Moraxella* species occurring in blood cultures. *J Clin Pathol.* 1979;32:497–499.

232. Larson E, McGinley KJ, Grove GL, et al. Physiologic, microbiologic, and seasonal effects of handwashing of the healthcare personnel. *Am J Infect Control.* 1986;14:51–59.

233. Pittet D, Dharan S, Touveneau S, Sauvan V, Perneger TV. Bacterial contamination of the hands of hospital staff during routine patient care. *Arch Intern Med.* 1999;159:821–826.

234. Larson EL. Persistent carriage of gram-negative bacteria on hands. *Am J Infect Control.* 1981;9:112–119.

235. Noble W. Skin as a source for hospital infection. *Infect Control.* 1986;7:111–112.

236. Price PB. New studies in surgical bacteriology and surgical technique. *JAMA.* 1938;111:1993–1996.

237. Ulrich JA. Techniques of skin sampling for microbial contaminants. *Hosp Top.* 1965;43:121–123.

238. Coovadia YM, Johnson AP, Bhana RH, et al. Multiresistant *Klebsiella aerogenes* in a neonatal nursery: the importance of infection control policies and procedures in the prevention of outbreaks. *J Hosp Infect.* 1992;22:197–205.

239. Guiguet M, Rekacewicz C, Leclercq B, et al. Effectiveness of simple measures to control an outbreak of nosocomial methicillin-resistant *Staphylococcus aureus* infections in an intensive care unit. *Infect Control Hosp Epidemiol.* 1990;11:23–26.

240. Issacs D, Dobson SR, Wilkinson AR, et al. Conservative management of echovirus 11 outbreak in a neonatal unit. *Lancet.* 1989;1:543–545.

241. Doebbeling BN, Li N, Wenzel RP. An outbreak of hepatitis A among health care workers: risk factors for transmission. *Am J Public Health.* 1993;83:1679–1684.

242. Widmer AF, Wenzel RP, Trilla A, Bale MJ, Jones RN, Doebbeling BN. Outbreak of *Pseudomonas aeruginosa* infections in a surgical intensive care unit: probable transmission via hands of a health care worker. *Clin Infect Dis.* 1993;16:372–376.

243. Doebbeling BN, Stanley GL, Sheetz CT, et al. Comparative efficacy of alternative hand-washing agents in reducing nosocomial infections in intensive care units. *N Engl J Med.* 1992;327:88–93.

244. Pittet D, Mourouga P, Perneger TV. Compliance with handwashing in a teaching hospital. Infection control program. *Annals Intern Med.* 1999;130:126–130.

245. Donowitz LG. Handwashing techniques in a pediatric intensive care unit. *AJDC.* 1987;141:683–685.

246. Meengs MR, Giles BK, Chisholm CD, Cordell WH, Nelson DR. Hand washing frequency in an emergency department. *J Emerg Nurs.* 1994;20:183–188.

247. Voss A, Widmer AF. No time for handwashing!? Handwashing versus alcoholic rub: can we afford 100% compliance? *Infect Control Hosp Epidemiol.* 1997;18:205–208.

248. Larson E, Killien M. Factors influencing handwashing behavior of patient care personnel. *Am J Infect Control.* 1982;10:93–99.

249. Larson E, Kretzer EK. Compliance with handwashing and barrier precautions. *J Hosp Infect.* 1995;30:88–106.

250. Nystrom B. Impact of handwashing on mortality in intensive care: examination of the evidence. *Infect Control Hosp Epidemiol.* 1994;15:435–436.

251. Cohen HA, Matalon A, Amir J, Paret G, Barzilai A. Handwashing patterns in primary pediatric community clinics. *Infection.* 1998;26:45–47.

252. Heenan A. Handwashing practices. *Nurs Times.* 1992;88:70.

253. Kesavan S, Barodawala S, Mulley GP. Now wash your hands? A survey of hospital handwashing facilities. *J Hosp Infect.* 1998;40:291-293.

254. Zimakoff J, Kjelsberg AB, Larsen SO, Holstein B. A multicenter questionnaire investigation of attitudes toward hand hygiene, assessed by the staff in fifteen hospitals in Denmark and Norway. *Am J Infect Control.* 1992;20:58-64.

255. Beck-Sague C, Jarvis W, Martone W. Outbreak investigation. In: Herwaldt LA, Decker MD, eds. *A Practical Handbook for Hospital Epidemiologists.* Thorofare, NJ: SLACK Incorporated and The Society for Healthcare Epidemiology of America; 1998:135-144.

256. Wendt C, Herwaldt L. Epidemics: identification and management. In: Wenzel RP, ed. *Prevention and Control of Nosocomial Infections.* 3rd ed. Baltimore, Md: Williams & Wilkins; 1997:175-213.

257. Bolyard EA, Tablan OC, Williams WW, Pearson ML, Shapiro CN, Deitchmann SD. Guideline for infection control in healthcare personnel, 1998. Hospital Infection Control Practices Advisory Committee. *Infect Control Hosp Epidemiol.* 1998;19:407-463.

258. Decker MD, Schaffner W. Immunization of hospital personnel and other health care workers. *Infect Dis Clin North Am.* 1990;4:211-221.

259. Atkinson WL, Markowitz LE, Adams NC, Seastrom GR. Transmission of measles in medical settings–United States, 1985-1989. *Am J Med.* 1991;91:320-324.

260. Davis RM, Orenstein WA, Frank JA Jr, et al. Transmission of measles in medical settings. 1980 through 1984. *JAMA.* 1986;255:1295-1298.

261. Poland GA, Nichol KL. Medical schools and immunization policies: missed opportunities for disease prevention. *Ann Intern Med.* 1990;113:628-631.

262. Poland GA, Nichol KL. Medical students as sources of rubella and measles outbreaks. *Arch Intern Med.* 1990;150:44-46.

263. Lane NE, Paul RI, Bratcher DF, Stover BH. A survey of policies at children's hospitals regarding immunity of healthcare workers: are physicians protected? *Infect Control Hosp Epidemiol.* 1997;18:400-404.

264. Anderson GS, Penfold JB. An outbreak of diphtheria in a hospital for the mentally subnormal. *J Clin Pathol.* 1973;26:606-615.

265. Gray RD, James SM. Occult diphtheria infection in a hospital for the mentally subnormal. *Lancet.* 1973;1:1105-1106.

266. Palmer SR, Balfour AH, Jephcott AE. Immunisation of adults during an outbreak of diphtheria. *Br Med J (Clin Res Educ).* 1983;286:624-626.

267. Vitek CR, Brennan MB, Gotway CA, et al. Risk of diphtheria among schoolchildren in the Russian Federation in relation to time since last vaccination. *Lancet.* 1999;353:355-358.

268. Centers for Disease Control and Prevention. Update: diphtheria epidemic–new independent states of the former Soviet Union, January 1995-March 1996. *MMWR.* 1996;45:693-697.

269. Vitek CR, Wharton M. Diphtheria in the former Soviet Union: reemergence of a pandemic disease. *Emerg Infect Dis.* 1998;4:539-550.

270. Centers for Disease Control and Prevention. Toxigenic *Corynebacterium diphtheriae*–Northern Plains Indian Community, August-October 1996. *MMWR.* 1997;46:506-510.

271. Centers for Disease Control and Prevention. Diphtheria, tetanus, and pertussis: recommendations for vaccine use and other preventive measures. Recommendations of the Immunization Practices Advisory Committee (ACIP). *MMWR.* 1991;40:1-28.

272. Vrielink H, Reesink HW. Transfusion-transmissible infections. *Curr Opin Hematol.* 1998;5:396–405.
273. Mosley JW, Nowicki MJ, Kasper CK, et al. Hepatitis A virus transmission by blood products in the United States. Transfusion Safety Study Group. *Vox Sang.* 1994;67:24–28.
274. Lemon SM. Hepatitis A virus and blood products: virus validation studies. *Blood Coagul Fibrinolysis.* 1995;6:20–22.
275. Lemon SM. The natural history of hepatitis A: the potential for transmission by transfusion of blood or blood products. *Vox Sang.* 1994;67:19–23.
276. Noble RC, Kane MA, Reeves SA, Roeckel I. Post-transfusion hepatitis A in a neonatal intensive care unit. *JAMA.* 1984;252:2711–2715.
277. Rosenblum LS, Villarino ME, Nainan OV, et al. Hepatitis A outbreak in a neonatal intensive care unit: risk factors for transmission and evidence of prolonged viral excretion among preterm infants. *J Infect Dis.* 1991;164:476–482.
278. Ebisawa I, Kurosu Y, Hatashita T. Nursery-associated hepatitis A traced to a male nurse. *J Hyg (Lond).* 1984;92:251–254.
279. Watson JC, Fleming DW, Borella AJ, Olcott ES, Conrad RE, Baron RC. Vertical transmission of hepatitis A resulting in an outbreak in a neonatal intensive care unit. *J Infect Dis.* 1993;167:567–571.
280. Goodman RA, Carder CC, Allen JR, Orenstein WA, Finton RJ. Nosocomial hepatitis A transmission by an adult patient with diarrhea. *Am J Med.* 1982;73:220–226.
281. Centers for Disease Control and Prevention. Prevention of hepatitis A through active or passive immunization: recommendations of the Advisory Committee on Immunization Practices. *MMWR.* 1996;45:1–30.
282. Innis BL, Snitbhan R, Kunasol P, et al. Protection against hepatitis A by an inactivated vaccine. *JAMA.* 1994;271:1328–1334.
283. Furesz J, Scheifele DW, Palkonyay L. Safety and effectiveness of the new inactivated hepatitis A virus vaccine. *CMAJ.* 1995;152:343–348.
284. Sandman L, Davidson M, Krugman S. Inactivated hepatitis A vaccine: a safety and immunogenicity study in health professionals. *J Infect Dis.* 1995;171:50–52.
285. Doebbeling BN, Wenzel RP. Nosocomial viral hepatitis and infectious transmission by blood and body products. In: Mandell GL, Bennett JE, Dolin R, eds. *Principles and Practices of Infectious Diseases.* 4th ed. New York, NY: Churchill Livingstone, 1995:2616–2632.
286. Thomas DL, Factor SH, Kelen GD, Washington AS, Taylor E Jr, Quinn TC. Viral hepatitis in health care personnel at the Johns Hopkins Hospital. The seroprevalence of and risk factors for hepatitis B virus and hepatitis C virus infection. *Arch Intern Med.* 1993;153:1705–1712.
287. Hadler SC, Doto IL, Maynard JE, et al. Occupational risk of hepatitis B infection in hospital workers. *Infect Control.* 1985;6:24–31.
288. Levy BS, Harris JC, Smith JL, et al. Hepatitis B in ward and clinical laboratory employees of a general hospital. *Am J Epidemiol.* 1977;106:330–335.
289. Scheiermann N, Kuwert EK, Pieringer E, Dermietzel R. High-risk groups for hepatitis B virus infection in a university hospital staff as determined by detection of HB antigens, antibodies, and Dane particles. *Med Microbiol Immunol (Berl).* 1978;166:241–247.
290. Shapiro CN, Tokars JI, Chamberland ME. Use of the hepatitis-B vaccine and infection with hepatitis B and C among orthopaedic surgeons.

The American Academy of Orthopaedic Surgeons Serosurvey Study Committee. *J Bone Joint Surg Am.* 1996;78:1791–1800.

291. Gibas A, Blewett DR, Schoenfeld DA, Dienstag JL. Prevalence and incidence of viral hepatitis in health workers in the prehepatitis B vaccination era. *Am J Epidemiol.* 1992;136:603–610.

292. Kane M. Epidemiology of hepatitis B infection in North America. *Vaccine.* 1995;13:16–17.

293. Shapiro CN. Occupational risk of infection with hepatitis B and hepatitis C virus. *Surg Clin North Am.* 1995;75:1047–1056.

294. Diekema DJ, Bradley DN. Employee health and infection control. In: Herwaldt LA, Decker MD, eds. *A Practical Handbook for Hospital Epidemiologists.* Thorofare, NJ: SLACK Incorporated and The Society for Healthcare Epidemiology of America; 1998:291–304.

295. Snydman DR, Hindman SH, Wineland MD, Bryan JA, Maynard JE. Nosocomial viral hepatitis B. A cluster among staff with subsequent transmission to patients. *Ann Intern Med.* 1976;85:573–577.

296. Grob PJ, Bischof B, Naeff F. Cluster of hepatitis B transmitted by a physician. *Lancet.* 1981;2:1218–1220.

297. Rimland D, Parkin WE, Miller GB Jr, Schrack WD. Hepatitis B outbreak traced to an oral surgeon. *N Engl J Med.* 1977;296:953–958.

298. Ahtone J, Goodman RA. Hepatitis B and dental personnel: transmission to patients and prevention issues. *J Am Dent Assoc.* 1983;106:219–222.

299. Centers for Disease Control and Prevention. Outbreaks of hepatitis B virus infection among hemodialysis patients—California, Nebraska, and Texas, 1994. *MMWR.* 1996;45:285–289.

300. Drescher J, Wagner D, Haverich A, et al. Nosocomial hepatitis B virus infections in cardiac transplant recipients transmitted during transvenous endomyocardial biopsy. *J Hosp Infect.* 1994;26:81–92.

301. Liang TJ, Hasegawa K, Rimon N, Wands JR, Ben-Porath E. A hepatitis B virus mutant associated with an epidemic of fulminant hepatitis. *N Engl J Med.* 1991;324:1705–1709.

302. Oren I, Hershow RC, Ben-Porath E, et al. A common-source outbreak of fulminant hepatitis B in a hospital. *Ann Intern Med.* 1989;110:691–698.

303. Coutinho RA, Albrecht-van Lent P, Stoutjesdijk L, et al. Hepatitis B from doctors. *Lancet.* 1982;1:345–346.

304. Centers for Disease Control and Prevention. Protection against viral hepatitis. Recommendations of the Immunization Practices Advisory Committee (ACIP). *MMWR.* 1990;39:1–26.

305. Evans ME, Hall KL, Berry SE. Influenza control in acute care hospitals. *Am J Infect Control.* 1997;25:357–362.

306. Adal KA, Flowers RH, Anglim AM, et al. Prevention of nosocomial influenza. *Infect Control Hosp Epidemiol.* 1996;17:641–648.

307. Balkovic ES, Goodman RA, Rose FB, Borel CO. Nosocomial influenza A (H1N1) infection. *Am J Med Technol.* 1980;46:318–320.

308. Serwint JR, Miller RM. Why diagnose influenza infections in hospitalized pediatric patients? *Pediatr Infect Dis J.* 1993;12:200–204.

309. Tanaka Y, Ueda K, Miyazaki C, et al. Trivalent cold recombinant influenza live vaccine in institutionalized children with bronchial asthma and patients with psychomotor retardation. *Pediatr Infect Dis J.* 1993;12:600–605.

310. Serwint JR, Miller RM, Korsch BM. Influenza type A and B infections in hospitalized pediatric patients. Who should be immunized? *Am J Dis Child.* 1991;145:623–626.

311. Glezen WP, Falcao O, Cate TR, Mintz AA. Nosocomial influenza in a general hospital for indigent patients. *Can J Infect Control.* 1991;6:65–67.
312. Whimbey E, Elting LS, Couch RB, et al. Influenza A virus infections among hospitalized adult bone marrow transplant recipients. *Bone Marrow Trans.* 1994;13:437–440.
313. Alford RH, Kasel JA, Gerone PJ, Knight V. Human influenza resulting from aerosol inhalation. *Proc Soc Exp Biol Med.* 1966;122:800–804.
314. Moser MR, Bender TR, Margolis HS, Noble GR, Kendal AP, Ritter DG. An outbreak of influenza aboard a commercial airliner. *Am J Epidemiol.* 1979;110:1–6.
315. Knight V. Airborne transmission and pulmonary deposition of respiratory viruses. In: Mulder J, Hers JFP, eds. *Influenza.* Groningen, Netherlands: Wolters-Noordhoff; 1972:1–9.
316. Loosli CG, Lemon HM, Robertson OH, et al. Experimental air-borne influenza infection. I. Influence of humidity on survival of virus in air. *Proc Soc Exp Biol Med.* 1943;53:205–206.
317. Nabeshima A, Ikematsu H, Yamaga S, Hayashi J, Hara H, Kashiwagi S. An outbreak of influenza A (H3N2) among hospitalized geriatric patients. *Kansenshogaku Zasshi.* 1996;70:801–807.
318. Centers for Disease Control and Prevention. Influenza A in a hospital—Illinois. *MMWR.* 1981;30:79–80.
319. Hall CB, Douglas RG Jr. Nosocomial influenza infection as a cause of intercurrent fevers in infants. *Pediatrics.* 1975;55:673–677.
320. Arden NH, Patriarca PA, Fasano MB, et al. The roles of vaccination and amantadine prophylaxis in controlling an outbreak of influenza A (H3N2) in a nursing home. *Arch Intern Med.* 1988;148:865–868.
321. Arroyo JC, Postic B, Brown A, et al. Influenza A/Philippines/2/82 outbreak in a nursing home: limitations of influenza vaccination in the elderly. *Am J Infect Control.* 1984;12:329–334.
322. Patriarca PA, Weber JA, Parker RA, et al. Efficacy of influenza vaccine in nursing homes: reduction in illness and complications during influenza A (H3N2) epidemic. *JAMA.* 1985;253:1136–1139.
323. Saah AJ, Neufeld R, Rodstein M, et al. Influenza vaccine and pneumonia mortality in a nursing home population. *Arch Intern Med.* 1986;146:2353–2357.
324. Kashiwagi S, Ikematsu H, Hayashi J, Nomura H, Kajiyama W, Kaji M. An outbreak of influenza A (H3N2) in a hospital for the elderly with emphasis on pulmonary complications. *Jpn J Med.* May 1988;27:177–182.
325. Aktas F, Ulutan F, Artuk C, Usta D, Kurtar K, Atalay S. An outbreak of influenza in hospital personnel. *Mikrobiyol Bull.* 1990;24:344–351.
326. Rivera M, Gonzalez N. An influenza outbreak in a hospital. *Am J Nurs.* 1982;82:1836–1838.
327. Malanowicz W, Tyminska K, Czarniak S, Semenicki K. Clinical picture of the 1971 influenza outbreak on the basis of hospital observation of 60 patients. *Wiad Lek.* 1974;27:1049–1054.
328. Centers for Disease Control and Prevention. Prevention and control of influenza: recommendations of the Advisory Committee on Immunization Practices (ACIP). *MMWR.* 1998;47:1–26.
329. Potter J, Stott DJ, Roberts MA, et al. Influenza vaccination of health care workers in long-term-care hospitals reduces the mortality of elderly patients. *J Infect Dis.* 1997;175:1–6.

330. Wilde JA, McMillan JA, Serwint J, Butta J, O'Riordan MA, Steinhoff MC. Effectiveness of influenza vaccine in health care professionals: a randomized trial. *JAMA*. 1999;218:908-913.

331. Mast EE, Harmon MW, Gravenstein S, et al. Emergence and possible transmission of amantadine-resistant viruses during nursing home outbreaks of influenza A (H3N2). *Am J Epidemiol*. 1991;134:988-997.

332. Monto AS, Robinson DP, Herlocher ML, Hinson JM Jr, Elliott MJ, Crisp A. Zanamivir in the prevention of influenza among healthy adults: a randomized controlled trial. *JAMA*. 1999;282:31-35.

333. Monto AS, Fleming DM, Henry D, et al. Efficacy and safety of the neuraminidase inhibitor zanamivirin in the treatment of influenza A and B virus infections. *J Infect Dis*. 1999;180:254-261.

334. Calfee DP, Peng AW, Cass LM, Lobo M, Hayden FG. Safety and efficacy of intravenous zanamivir in preventing experimental human influenza A virus infection. *Antimicrob Agents Chemother*. 1999;43:1616-1620.

335. Hayden FG, Atmar RL, Schilling M, et al. Use of the selective oral neuraminidase inhibitor oseltamivir to prevent influenza. *N Engl J Med*. 1999;341:1336-1342.

336. Schilling M, Povinelli L, Krause P, et al. Efficacy of zanamivir for chemoprophylaxis of nursing home influenza outbreaks. *Vaccine*. 1998;16:1771-1774.

337. Pachucki CT, Pappas SA, Fuller GF, Krause SL, Lentino JR, Schaaff DM. Influenza A among hospital personnel and patients. Implications for recognition, prevention, and control. *Arch Intern Med*. 1989;149:77-80.

338. Krause PJ, Cherry JD, Deseda-Tous J, et al. Epidemic measles in young adults. Clinical, epidemiologic, and serologic studies. *Ann Intern Med*. 1979;90:873-876.

339. Crawford GE, Gremillion DH. Epidemic measles and rubella in Air Force recruits: impact of immunization. *J Infect Dis*. 1981;144:403-410.

340. Remington PL, Hall WN, Davis IH, Herald A, Gunn RA. Airborne transmission of measles in a physician's office. *JAMA*. 1985;253:1574-1577.

341. Bloch AB, Orenstein WA, Ewing WM, et al. Measles outbreak in a pediatric practice: airborne transmission in an office setting. *Pediatrics*. 1985;75:676-683.

342. Fedson DS. Adult immunization. Summary of the National Vaccine Advisory Committee Report. *JAMA*. 1994;272:1133-1137.

343. Raad II, Sherertz RJ, Rains CS, et al. The importance of nosocomial transmission of measles in the propagation of a community outbreak. *Infect Control Hosp Epidemiol*. 1989;10:161-166.

344. Rivera ME, Mason WH, Ross LA, Wright HT Jr. Nosocomial measles infection in a pediatric hospital during a community-wide epidemic. *J Pediatr*. 1991;119:183-186.

345. Gurevich I, Barzarga RA, Cunha BA. Measles: lessons from an outbreak. *Am J Infect Control*. 1992;20:319-325.

346. Enguidanos R, Mascola L, Frederick P. A survey of hospital infection control policies and employee measles cases during Los Angeles County's measles epidemic, 1987 to 1989. *Am J Infect Control*. 1992;20:301-304.

347. Istre GR, McKee PA, West GR, et al. Measles spread in medical settings: an important focus of disease transmission? *Pediatrics*. 1987;79:356-358.

348. Rank EL, Brettman L, Katz-Pollack H, DeHertogh D, Neville D. Chronology of a hospital-wide measles outbreak: lessons learned and shared from an extraordinary week in late March 1989. *Am J Infect Control.* 1992;20:315–318.

349. Sienko DG, Friedman C, McGee HB, et al. A measles outbreak at university medical settings involving health care providers. *Am J Public Health.* 1987;77:1222–1224.

350. Atkinson WL. Measles and healthcare workers. *Infect Control Hosp Epidemiol.* 1994;15:5–7.

351. Centers for Disease Control and Prevention. Immunization of health-care workers: recommendations of the Advisory Committee on Immunization Practices (ACIP) and the Hospital Infection Control Practices Advisory Committee (HICPAC). *MMWR.* 1997;46:1–42.

352. Willy ME, Koziol DE, Fleisher T, et al. Measles immunity in a population of healthcare workers. *Infect Control Hosp Epidemiol.* 1994;15:12–17.

353. Cote TR, Sivertson D, Horan JM, Lindegren ML, Dwyer DM. Evaluation of a two-dose measles, mumps, and rubella vaccination schedule in a cohort of college athletes. *Public Health Rep.* 1993;108:431–435.

354. Stover BH, Adams G, Kuebler CA, Cost KM, Rabalais GP. Measles-mumps-rubella immunization of susceptible hospital employees during a community measles outbreak: cost-effectiveness and protective efficacy. *Infect Control Hosp Epidemiol.* 1994;15:18–21.

355. Subbarao EK, Amin S, Kumar ML. Prevaccination serologic screening for measles in health care workers. *J Infect Dis.* 1991;163:876–878.

356. Sellick JA Jr, Longbine D, Schifeling R, Mylotte JM. Screening hospital employees for measles immunity is more cost effective than blind immunization. *Ann Intern Med.* 1992;116:982–984.

357. Kaplan KM, Marder DC, Cochi SL, Preblud SR. Mumps in the workplace. Further evidence of the changing epidemiology of a childhood vaccine-preventable disease. *JAMA.* 1988;260:1434–1438.

358. Wharton M, Cochi SL, Hutcheson RH, Schaffner W. Mumps transmission in hospitals. *Arch Intern Med.* 1990;150:47–49.

359. Fischer PR, Brunetti C, Welch V, Christenson JC. Nosocomial mumps: report of an outbreak and its control. *Am J Infect Control.* 1996;24:13–18.

360. American Academy of Pediatrics. Summaries of infectious diseases: mumps. In: Peter G, ed. *1997 Red Book: Report of the Committee on Infectious Diseases.* 24th ed. Elk Grove Village, Ill: American Academy of Pediatrics; 1997:366–369.

361. Brunell PA, Brickman A, O'Hare D, Steinberg S. Ineffectiveness of isolation of patients as a method of preventing the spread of mumps. Failure of the mumps skin-test antigen to predict immune status. *N Engl J Med.* 1968;279:1357–1361.

362. Centers for Disease Control and Prevention. Mumps prevention. *MMWR.* 1989;38:388–392, 397–400.

363. Polder JA, Tablan OC, Williams WW. Personnel health services. In: Bennett JV, Brachman PS, eds. *Hospital Infections.* 3rd ed. Boston, Mass: Little, Brown and Company; 1992:31–61.

364. Deen JL, Mink CA, Cherry JD, et al. Household contact study of *Bordetella pertussis* infections. *Clin Infect Dis.* 1995;21:1211–1219.

365. Mortimer EA Jr. Pertussis and its prevention: a family affair. *J Infect Dis.* 1990;161:473–479.

366. Weber DJ, Rutala WA. Management of healthcare workers exposed to pertussis. *Infect Control Hosp Epidemiol.* 1994;15:411–415.

367. Valenti WM, Pincus PH, Messner MK. Nosocomial pertussis: possible spread by a hospital visitor. *Am J Dis Child.* 1980;134:520–521.
368. Christie CD, Glover AM, Willke MJ, Marx ML, Reising SF, Hutchinson NM. Containment of pertussis in the regional pediatric hospital during the Greater Cincinnati epidemic of 1993. *Infect Control Hosp Epidemiol.* 1995;16:556–563.
369. Deville JG, Cherry JD, Christenson PD, et al. Frequency of unrecognized *Bordetella pertussis* infections in adults. *Clin Infect Dis.* 1995;21:639–642.
370. Nennig ME, Shinefield HR, Edwards KM, Black SB, Fireman BH. Prevalence and incidence of adult pertussis in an urban population. *JAMA.* 1996;275:1672–1674.
371. Kurt TL, Yeager AS, Guenette S, Dunlop S. Spread of pertussis by hospital staff. *JAMA.* 1972;221:264–267.
372. Shefer A, Dales L, Nelson M, Werner B, Baron R, Jackson R. Use and safety of acellular pertussis vaccine among adult hospital staff during an outbreak of pertussis. *J Infect Dis.* 1995;171:1053–1056.
373. Linnemann CC Jr, Ramundo N, Perlstein PH, Minton SD, Englender GS. Use of pertussis vaccine in an epidemic involving hospital staff. *Lancet.* 1975;2:540–543.
374. Edwards KM, Decker MD, Graham BS, Mezzatesta J, Scott J, Hackell J. Adult immunization with acellular pertussis vaccine. *JAMA.* 1993;269:53–56.
375. Lambert HJ. Epidemiology of a small pertussis outbreak in Kent County, Mich. *Public Health Rep.* 1965;80:365–369.
376. Garner JS. Guideline for isolation precautions in hospitals. I. Evolution of isolation practices, Hospital Infection Control Practices Advisory Committee. *Am J Infect Control.* 1996;24:24–31.
377. Management of people exposed to pertussis and control of pertussis outbreaks. *CMAJ.* 1990;143:751–753.
378. Halsey NA, Welling MA, Lehman RM. Nosocomial pertussis: a failure of erythromycin treatment and prophylaxis. *Am J Dis Child.* 1980;134:521–522.
379. Steketee RW, Wassilak SG, Adkins WN Jr, et al. Evidence for a high attack rate and efficacy of erythromycin prophylaxis in a pertussis outbreak in a facility for the developmentally disabled. *J Infect Dis.* 1988;157:434–440.
380. Fliegel PE, Weinstein WM. Rubella outbreak in a prenatal clinic: management and prevention. *Am J Infect Control.* 1982;10:29–33.
381. McLaughlin MC, Gold LH. The New York rubella incident: a case for changing hospital policy regarding rubella testing and immunization. *Am J Public Health.* 1979;69:287–289.
382. American Academy of Pediatrics. Summaries of infectious diseases: rubella. In: Peter G, ed. *1997 Red Book: Report of the Committee on Infectious Diseases.* 24th ed. Elk Grove Village, Ill: American Academy of Pediatrics; 1997:456–462.
383. Polk BF, White JA, DeGirolami PC, Modlin JF. An outbreak of rubella among hospital personnel. *N Engl J Med.* 1980;303:541–545.
384. Reves RR, Pickering LK. Impact of child day care on infectious diseases in adults. *Infect Dis Clin North Am.* 1992;6:239–250.
385. Greaves WL, Orenstein WA, Stetler HC, Preblud SR, Hinman AR, Bart KJ. Prevention of rubella transmission in medical facilities. *JAMA.* 1982;248:861–864.
386. Strassburg MA, Imagawa DT, Fannin SL, et al. Rubella outbreak among hospital employees. *Obstet Gynecol.* 1981;57:283–288.

387. Gladstone JL, Millian SJ. Rubella exposure in an obstetric clinic. *Obstet Gynecol*. 1981;57:182–186.
388. Centers for Disease Control and Prevention. Rubella in hospitals—California. *MMWR*. 1983;32:37–39.
389. Storch GA, Gruber C, Benz B, Beaudoin J, Hayes J. A rubella outbreak among dental students: description of the outbreak and analysis of control measures. *Infect Control*. 1985;6:150–156.
390. Immunization Practices Advisory Committee. Recommendation of the Immunization Practices Advisory Committee (ACIP): rubella prevention. *MMWR*. 1984;33(22):301–310, 315–318.
391. Sawyer MH, Chamberlin CJ, Wu YN, Aintablian N, Wallace MR. Detection of varicella-zoster virus DNA in air samples from hospital rooms. *J Infect Dis*. 1994;169:91–94.
392. Eickhoff TC. Airborne nosocomial infection: a contemporary perspective. *Infect Control Hosp Epidemiol*. 1994;15:663–672.
393. Josephson A, Gombert ME. Airborne transmission of nosocomial varicella from localized zoster. *J Infect Dis*. 1988;158:238–241.
394. Gustafson TL, Lavely GB, Brawner ER Jr, Hutcheson RH Jr, Wright PF, Schaffner W. An outbreak of airborne nosocomial varicella. *Pediatrics*. 1982;70:550–556.
395. Leclair JM, Zaia JA, Levin MJ, Congdon RG, Goldmann DA. Airborne transmission of chickenpox in a hospital. *N Engl J Med*. 1980;302:450–453.
396. Asano Y, Iwayama S, Miyata T, et al. Spread of varicella in hospitalized children having no direct contact with an indicator zoster case and its prevention by a live vaccine. *Biken J*. 1980;2:157–161.
397. Gordon JE, Meader FM. The period of infectivity and serum prevention of chickenpox. *JAMA*. 1929;93:2013–2015.
398. American Academy of Pediatrics. Summaries of infectious diseases: varicella-zoster infections. In: Peter G, ed. *1997 Red Book: Report of the Committee on Infectious Diseases*. 24th ed. Elk Grove Village, Ill: American Academy of Pediatrics; 1997:573–585.
399. Brunell PA. Transmission of chickenpox in a school setting prior to the observed exanthem. *Am J Dis Child*. 1989;143:1451–1452.
400. Williams WW. CDC guidelines for the prevention and control of nosocomial infections. Guideline for infection control in hospital personnel. *Am J Infect Control*. 1984;12:34–63.
401. Hyams PJ, Stuewe MC, Heitzer V. Herpes zoster causing varicella (chickenpox) in hospital employees: cost of a casual attitude. *Am J Infect Control*. 1984;12:2–5.
402. Berlin BS, Campbell T. Hospital-acquired herpes zoster following exposure to chickenpox. *JAMA*. 1970;211:1831–1833.
403. Weintraub WH, Lilly JR, Randolph JG. A chickenpox epidemic in a pediatric burn unit. *Surgery*. 1974;76:490–494.
404. Morens DM, Bregman DJ, West CM, et al. An outbreak of varicella-zoster virus infection among cancer patients. *Ann Intern Med*. 1980;93:414–419.
405. Meyers JD, MacQuarrie MB, Merigan TC, Jennison MH. Nosocomial varicella. Part I: outbreak in oncology patients at a children's hospital. *West J Med*. 1979;130:196–199.
406. Alter SJ, Hammond JA, McVey CJ, Myers MG. Susceptibility to varicella-zoster virus among adults at high risk for exposure. *Infect Control*. 1986;7:448–451.

407. Weber DJ, Rutala WA, Parham C. Impact and costs of varicella prevention in a university hospital. *Am J Public Health.* 1988;78:19–23.

408. Weber DJ, Rutala WA, Hamilton H. Prevention and control of varicella-zoster infections in healthcare facilities. *Infect Control Hosp Epidemiol.* 1996;17:694–705.

409. Centers for Disease Control and Prevention. Prevention of varicella: recommendations of the Advisory Committee on Immunization Practices (ACIP). *MMWR.* 1996;45:1–36.

410. Anderson JD, Bonner M, Scheifele DW, Schneider BC. Lack of nosocomial spread of varicella in a pediatric hospital with negative pressure ventilated patient rooms. *Infect Control.* 1985;6:120–121.

411. Steele RW, Coleman MA, Fiser M, Bradsher RW. Varicella zoster in hospital personnel: skin test reactivity to monitor susceptibility. *Pediatrics.* 1982;70:604–608.

412. Shehab ZM, Brunell PA. Susceptibility of hospital personnel to varicella-zoster virus. *J Infect Dis.* 1984;150:786.

413. Haiduven DJ, Hench CP, Stevens DA. Postexposure varicella management of nonimmune personnel: an alternative approach. *Infect Control Hosp Epidemiol.* 1994;15:329–334.

414. Josephson A, Karanfil L, Gombert ME. Strategies for the management of varicella-susceptible healthcare workers after a known exposure. *Infect Control Hosp Epidemiol.* 1990;11:309–313.

415. Advisory Committee on Immunization. Prevention of varicella: recommendations of the Advisory Committee on Immunization Practices (ACIP). *MMWR.* 1996;45(RR11):1–25.

416. Buckwold FJ, Ronald AR. Antimicrobial misuse—effects and suggestions for control. *J Antimicrob Chemother.* 1979;5:129–136.

417. Kunin CM, Tupasi T, Craig WA. Use of antibiotics. A brief exposition of the problem and some tentative solutions. *Ann Intern Med.* 1973;79:555–560.

418. Pallares R, Dick R, Wenzel RP, Adams JR, Nettleman MD. Trends in antimicrobial utilization at a tertiary teaching hospital during a 15-year period (1978–1992). *Infect Control Hosp Epidemiol.* 1993;14:376–382.

419. Simchen E, Wax Y, Galai N, Israeli A. Discharge from hospital and its effect on surgical wound infections. The Israeli Study of Surgical Infections (ISSI). *J Clin Epidemiol.* 1992;45:1155–1163.

420. Hulton LJ, Olmsted RN, Treston-Aurand J, Craig CP. Effect of postdischarge surveillance on rates of infectious complications after cesarean section. *Am J Infect Control.* 1992;20:198–201.

421. Weigelt JA, Dryer D, Haley RW. The necessity and efficiency of wound surveillance after discharge. *Arch Surg.* 1992;127:77–81.

422. Law DJ, Mishriki SF, Jeffery PJ. The importance of surveillance after discharge from hospital in the diagnosis of postoperative wound infection. *Ann R Coll Surg Engl.* 1990;72:207–209.

423. Olson MM, Lee JT Jr. Continuous, 10-year wound infection surveillance. Results, advantages, and unanswered questions. *Arch Surg.* 1990;125:794–803.

424. Krukowski ZH, Irwin ST, Denholm S, Matheson NA. Preventing wound infection after appendectomy: a review. *Br J Surg.* 1988;75:1023–1033.

425. Reimer K, Gleed C, Nicolle LE. The impact of post-discharge infection on surgical wound infection rates. *Infect Control.* 1987;8:237–240.

426. Brown RB, Bradley S, Opitz E, Cipriani D, Pieczarka R, Sands M. Surgical wound infections documented after hospital discharge. *Am J Infect Control.* 1987;15:54–58.

427. Bright RA, Shay DK, Shu B, Cox NJ, Kliamov AI. Adamantane resistance among Influenza A viruses isolated early during the 2005–2006 Influenza season in the United States. *JAMA.* 2006;295:891–894.

428. Centers for Disease Control and Prevention. Update: Multistate outbreak of Mumps–United States. *MMWR.* 2006;55:559–563.

PART II

AIRBORNE TRANSMISSION

EPIDEMIOLOGY AND PREVENTION OF INFLUENZA

Mark C. Steinhoff

Introduction

Influenza virus has a unique epidemiology with two aspects: (1) annual epidemics of respiratory disease with attack rates of 10% to 30% in all regions of the world, and (2) the classical emerging infection, causing global pandemics when new antigenic variants emerge. Influenza viruses are epizootic in avian and animal species, and analyses of nucleic acid sequences suggest that human influenza A viruses derive from avian influenza viruses. The antigenic variation of this virus is the key to its ability to cause annual epidemics and periodic pandemics. The genetic and molecular aspects of antigenic variation will be described in relation to the unique epidemiology of this virus. Because antigenic change is random and not predictable, the influenza virus will continue to cause widespread epidemics, although many aspects of the epidemiology and variability of this virus are understood and effective antivirals and vaccines are available. Current control strategies require reevaluation to achieve a true reduction in the toll of influenza morbidity and mortality, and enhanced pandemic preparedness is essential.

Clinical Features of Influenza

The word *influenza* is from the Italian (derived from Latin *influentia*), referring to the influence of the stars, reflecting ancient concepts of the causation of influenza epidemics. The clinical disease influenza is familiar, because everyone has been infected. It is characterized by an abrupt onset of fever and respiratory symptoms, including rhinorrhea, cough, and sore throat. Myalgia and headache are more common with influenza than with other respiratory viral infections, and the malaise and prostration of this disease are well known. Gastrointestinal symptoms are not common in adults, but 50%

of infants and children may have vomiting, abdominal pain, and diarrhea with influenza. Influenza disease is usually self-limited, lasting for 3 to 5 days, but complications, which are more frequent in the elderly and persons with chronic illnesses, can prolong illness. Some patients may develop a primary influenza viral pneumonia, which can be fatal. More commonly, a secondary bacterial pneumonia may occur up to 2 weeks after the acute viral infection.[3a,3b] In infants and children, otitis media and croup are common complications. Other less frequent complications include myocarditis, myositis, and encephalitis. Reye's syndrome, a hepatic and CNS complication seen in children, is associated with the use of aspirin and other salicylates.

Transmission

Influenza virus spreads through respiratory secretions of infected persons, which may contain up to 10^5 virus particles/mL. An infected person generates infectious aerosols of secretions during coughing, sneezing, and talking. In addition, infectious secretions are spread by direct (by kissing) or indirect (by nose-finger-doorknob) contact with respiratory mucosa. The inhaled virus attaches to columnar epithelial cells of the upper respiratory tract and initiates a new infection in the host. The incubation period is from 1 to 4 days, and infected hosts are capable of transmitting the virus from shortly before the onset of clinical disease up to the fourth or fifth day of illness.

Diagnosis

Because of the clinical similarity of influenza virus infection to the manifestations of other respiratory viral infections, influenza virus infection cannot be reliably diagnosed from clinical signs and minor symptoms.[4] Although some clinicians and many laypersons use the term *flu* or *influenza* to describe respiratory illness, only viral culture or serology can prove the presence of influenza virus. Culture requires nasal or throat secretions obtained within 3 days of onset, which are then cultured in embryonated hens' eggs or tissue culture. Viral growth occurs in 2 to 3 days, after which the virus is identified using reagents for type and subtype. Influenza virus can also be identified rapidly within several hours in clinic settings using rapid antigen detection methods, such as immunofluorescence or enzyme-linked immunosorbent assay (ELISA) and other techniques. Infection is proven by serology to show a four-fold increase in antibodies to influenza virus and requires acute and convalescent blood specimens obtained approximately 3 weeks apart. Standard techniques for detection of influenza antibodies include hemagglutination inhibition (HI), complement fixation (CF), and ELISA techniques.

The Virus

Influenza virus was one of the first human viruses to be cultured and studied. In 1933, Wilson Smith, Andrews, and Laidlaw in the United Kingdom first isolated human influenza A virus from a ferret (infected by secretions from an ill Andrews).[1] Burnet developed the technique of culture in hens' eggs in 1936, which enabled study of the viruses and the development of vaccines. Influenza B virus was isolated in 1940, and type C virus in 1947.[2]

Influenza type A and B viruses contain eight segments of single-stranded RNA that code for 10 separate proteins. Influenza type C has seven RNA segments and a single surface glycoprotein. Table 15-1 summarizes the gene segments and their associated proteins. The hemagglutinin (HA) and neuraminidase (NA) are surface glycoproteins that are important in both pathogenesis and immune protection from infection. The HA functions as the attachment protein, mediating attachment to sialic acid-containing glycoproteins on columnar epithelial cells of the respiratory tract. HA has a binding site that is highly conserved and surrounded by five specific antigenic epitopes that manifest rapid changes. Specific antibody to these HA epitopes prevents attachment and entry of influenza viruses into host cells. HA specificity for receptor binding is a determinant of which species can be infected, or host range.[3,3a,3b] The HA is also a virulence determinant. The HA protein must be cleaved into H1 and H2 proteins by host proteases to create a hydrophobic tail necessary for fusion of viral and host cell membranes. The host proteases are found in human respiratory and avian enteric tissues. In avian viruses, the introduction of basic amino acids near the HA cleavage site permits cleavage by proteases of other tissues, which allows viral infection of vascular, central nervous system, and other tissues (pantropism) and a dramatic increase in virulence. The NA cleaves sialic acid residues to allow virus release from the host epithelial cell; specific anti-NA antibody presumably diminishes release of virons from host cells.

The subtypes of influenza A virus are determined by these two surface antigens. Among influenza A viruses that infect humans, three different HA subtypes have classically been described—H1, H2, and H3. H5, H7, and H9 have also recently been shown to infect humans.

TABLE 15-1   The Genes of Influenza A Virus and Their Protein Products

RNA Segment Number	Gene Product	Protein	Proposed Functions of Protein
1	PB1	Polymerase	RNA transcriptase
2	PB2	Polymerase	RNA transcriptase (host range determinant)
3	PA	Polymerase	RNA transcriptase
4	HA	Hemagglutinin	Viral attachment to cell membranes; major antigenic and virulence determinant
5	NA	Neuraminidase	Release from membranes; major antigenic determinant
6	NP	Nucleoprotein	Encapsidates RNA, type-specific antigen
7	M1	Matrix	Surrounds viral core; involved in assembly and budding
	M2	Ion channel	
8	NS1	Nonstructural	RNA binding, anti-interferon
	NS2	Nonstructural	Unknown

Nomenclature

The nomenclature of influenza viruses is necessarily somewhat complex because of the need to name all new strains. Virus strains are named with (1) the virus type, (2) the geographic site of first identification of the specific virus, (3) the strain number from the isolating laboratory, (4) the year of virus isolation, and (5) the virus subtype (for influenza A). For example, one of the viruses in the influenza vaccine that was recently recommended for 2004–2005 is A California/7/2004(H3N2). This refers to a type A virus first isolated in California in 2004, as laboratory strain number 7, which is subtype H3N2. The early isolate of influenza is A/WS(WilsonSmith)/33/H1N1.

Epidemiology

Epidemics and Pandemics

The influenza virus causes annual epidemics of disease, and it caused three global pandemics in the 20th century (*pandemic* from the Greek: *pan* = all, *demos* = people). Pandemics of febrile respiratory disease that resemble influenza have been described since the days of Hippocrates (Table 15-2). The characteristic pattern of an influenza pandemic is initiation from a single geographic focus (often in Asia) and rapid spread, often along routes of travel. High attack rates of all age groups are observed. Although case fatality rates are usually not increased substantially, because of the very large number of infections and cases, the number of hospitalizations and deaths are unusually high. In a pandemic, multiple waves of infections can sweep through a community, each wave infecting sectors of the population different from those affected in the initial pandemic episode.

TABLE 15-2 A Century of Antigenic Shifts of Influenza A Virus

Years	Virus Description	Antigenic Change (Source)	Pandemic
1889	H3N2*	Not known	Severe
1900	H3N8*	Not known	Moderate
1918→1956	H1N1 "Spanish"*	HA, NA (? avian)	Major; 50 million deaths in first year
1957→1968	H2N2 "Asian"	New HA, NA, PB1 (avian)	Severe
1968→	H3N2 "Hong Kong"	New HA,[†] PB1 (avian)	Moderate
1977→	H1N1 "Russian"	Apparently identical with 1956 H1N1[‡]	Relatively mild[§]

Notes: *Data derived from serology; pandemic virus not available for study because influenza virus was first cultured in 1933.
[†]New human H3HA varied by only six amino acids from parent avian H3HA, with all changes at sites important for receptor binding and antigenicity.
[‡]May have escaped from a laboratory.
[§]Those aged more than 22 years had antibody from 1918–1956 H1N1 strain.

The 1918 Spanish influenza pandemic had an attack rate of 20% to 30% in adults, and 30% to 45% in children. The case fatality rate in adults was as high as 15% to 50%, with an unusual occurrence of deaths in young adults (Figure 15-1). It is estimated that at least 20 to 50 million persons died in a single year in this global pandemic, many of them young adults (see text box, "1918 Pandemic Flo").

Annual local epidemics follow a fairly predictable pattern.[5] In North America, epidemics usually occur between November and March, manifested first by high rates of school and industrial absenteeism, followed by an increase in visits to health care facilities, an increase in pneumonia and influenza hospital admissions, and finally an increase in deaths from pneumonia or influenza.[5] In any single locality, epidemic influenza often begins abruptly, reaches a peak within 3 weeks, and usually ends by 8 weeks. A city or region can experience two sequential or overlapping epidemics with different strains of viruses in a single winter. Epidemics in the Southern Hemisphere usually occur in the May to September winter season; in some cases, they are caused by the new strain of epidemic virus that will cause epidemics in the Northern Hemisphere the following winter. In the tropics, disease seasonality can be associated with monsoons, or a year-round isolation of influenza virus may be observed.[6,6a,6b] Virus spread during the winter season is said to be favored by the fact that virus survives better in environments of lower temperature and humidity. In tropical areas, spread during the monsoon suggests that indoor crowding caused by weather may be a more important factor.

In general, rates of infection in infants and children are higher than those of adults, and the rates of hospitalization are highest in infants and lower in children and high in the elderly.[6c,6d] Families with school-aged children have

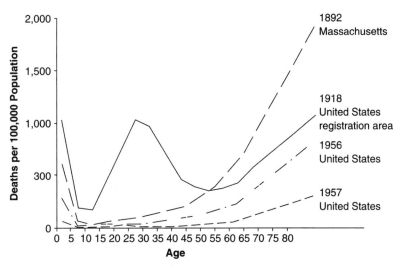

FIGURE 15-1 Age distribution of mortality of selected influenza epidemics in the United States. Note the difference between the 1918 pandemic with high young adult mortality rates and other epidemics with higher mortality at the extremes of the age spectrum.
Source: C.C. Dauer and R.E. Sterling, 1961, Mortality from Influenza, *American Review of Respiratory Diseases*, Vol. 82, Supplement, pp. 15–26. Official Journal of the American Thoracic Society, © American Lung Association.

the highest rates of infection.[6b] These observations suggest that relatively immunologically naive children are important in the spread of epidemic strains. Table 15-3 summarizes recent US data on rates for hospitalization for influenza.

Each epidemic and pandemic varies in size and impact, determined by the degree of the antigenic variation of the new virus, its virulence, and the level of existing protective immunity in the infected population. (See Table 15-2, noting the association between the degree of antigenic difference and the size of the pandemic.) During average epidemics in North America, attack rates are often 10% to 20% in large populations, although certain population groups (e.g., school children or nursing home residents) and local outbreaks can have attack rates of 40% to 50%. More than 20,000 influenza-associated excess deaths occurred in the United States during each of nine epidemics between 1972 and 1991, and more than 40,000 deaths occurred during three of them. Recent analyses suggest the annual winter increase in all mortality is substantially due to influenza.[7] Persons aged more than 65 years account for 90% of the excess deaths associated with annual epidemics. Although pandemics cause many deaths over one or two winters, mortality from an emergent influenza strain is by no means restricted to the first two years after a new strain emerges. The cumulative deaths during successive annual epidemics of an interpandemic period often exceed the death in the pandemic period. For example, it has been estimated that the H3N2 virus in its first pandemic in 1968–1969 caused 34,000 deaths in the United States, but it has caused more than 300,000 deaths in the annual epidemics in the subsequent 21 years during which it has circulated (from 1969 until the early 1990s). Not only does influenza have a large impact on mortality, morbidity from influenza is significant. Since the 1990s, annual influenza has been associated with an average of 226,000 hospitalizations per year in the United States.[7a]

Surveillance for influenza disease and for specific influenza viruses is necessary to track epidemic disease, to detect pandemics, and to determine virus serotypes for vaccine policy. In the United States, the Centers for Disease Control and Prevention (CDC) uses several surveillance systems.

TABLE 15-3   Influenza Disease by Age Group

Age (years)	Rate of Hospitalization/100,000	
	Normal	High Risk
0–11 mo	496–1038	1900
1–2	186	800
3–4	86	320
5–14	8–41	92
15–44	20–30	56–110
45–64	13–23	392–635
≥65	125–228	399–518

Source: MMWR, Vol. 52, RR06-, 2004; 1-40. Centers for Disease Control and Prevention.

1. A sentinel physician surveillance network, utilizing a simple clinical definition of influenza-like illness (ILI); a fever greater than 100°F, plus cough or sore throat. Approximately 1000 physicians each week from October through May record the total number of patient visits for the week, and the number of patients examined for influenza-like illness by age group.
2. The collaborating laboratory surveillance system of 75 World Health Organization (WHO) collaborating laboratories and 50 other laboratories in the United States from October through May report the total number of specimens received for respiratory virus testing and the number of positive isolates of influenza virus.
3. The 122-city mortality reporting system includes selected cities with a population of more than 100,000 that provide data on the percentage of deaths listed with pneumonia or influenza as the underlying cause or as being associated with influenza.
4. State and territorial epidemiologists' report influenza activity levels. Each state epidemiologist reports the estimated level of influenza activity as no activity or sporadic (sporadically occurring cases of ILI or culture-confirmed influenza [CCI] without school or institutional outbreaks), regional (outbreaks of ILI or CCI in counties that total less than 50% of the state population), or widespread activity (outbreaks of ILI or CCI in counties that are larger than 50% of the total state population).
5. Influenza pediatric mortality and morbidity are reported; deaths in children younger than 18 years is a new reportable death category.
6. In 10 states admissions related to influenza in children are reported.
7. Reports of influenza child hospitalization in single counties in three states provide true incidence data.[17] These data are summarized in the *Morbidity and Mortality Weekly Report* (*MMWR*) from the CDC and are found on its Web site.

Mechanisms of Antigenic Variation

Because most epidemic and all 20th-century pandemic infections by influenza virus are type A, the following discussion will focus on type A influenza. Although indistinguishable from type A in an individual patient, type B influenza disease is usually less severe, and it does not appear to cause pandemics. Type C disease is generally mild and not associated with widespread epidemics or pandemics.

The mutability or antigenic variation of influenza virus has been described by the term *antigenic drift*, denoting minor antigen changes through mutations, and *antigenic shift* describes major genetic and antigenic changes through reassortment.

Antigenic drift describes the frequent minor antigenic changes in the HA and NA surface antigens that account for the annual epidemics. Antigenic drift is ascribed to the relatively high rate of spontaneous mutation in RNA viruses. RNA polymerase is a low-fidelity transcription enzyme without a proofreading function. The high rate of replication of these viruses with low fidelity generates many new amino acid substitutions in surface glycoproteins, some of which will be advantageous to the virus, allowing it to become an epidemic strain. Studies have shown that from 1968 to 1979, 7.9 nucleotide and 3.4 amino acid changes occurred per year, equivalent to an approximate annual 1% change in the amino acid composition of the HA. High rates of antigenic change are observed in the five specific epitopes of HA that surround the binding site; as noted previously, the binding site itself demonstrates little sequence variation. It is assumed that antibody to these epitopes sterically block access to the specific binding site, preventing attachment to and infection of host cells. Amino acid sequencing has shown that drift variants are sequential, suggesting selective pressure. For example, H3 sequential drift variants from 1968 to 1988 had four or more amino acid differences in at least two antigenic sites. The 1930s H1N1 virus strain (which was the first cultured influenza) shows substantial genetic drift from the ancestral 1918 H1N1 pandemic strain. It is also possible that changes in nonsurface proteins may influence replication, transmission, or tissue tropism (virulence), conferring a selective advantage to a specific strain. It is thought that after 10 to 30 years of circulation of a specific subtype most members of the population will have antibody to that subtype, increasing the selection pressure for a new shift variant.

Antigenic shift describes the major changes of HA, NA, or both of these surface antigens that create a new subtype. If the HA and NA determinants are novel, no antibody protection is present in human populations, and the stage may be set for a pandemic.

Viruses with segmented genomes can generate new variants rapidly by the random reassortment of the RNA segments. Coinfection of a single host cell by two influenza strains, each with a different eight-segmented genome, theoretically can generate 2^8 or 254 variants. It is thought that the "mixing vessel" host for influenza is likely swine, which are in contact with birds and humans, although humans can also serve this role. Most new variants do not have a survival advantage and die out. However, if a shift variant (1) retains the ability to replicate well in humans, (2) is efficiently transmissible between humans, and (3) has new surface HA or NA determinants that evade existing influenza antibody profiles in the human population, a pandemic may ensue. Historically, serology and virology reveal that three antigenic shifts occurred during the 20th century, leading to three pandemics. Table 15-2 summarizes antigenic shifts of influenza A virus over the last century. Figure 15-2 demonstrates details of the antigenic shift of 1968, and Figure 15-3 shows all pandemics.

Four pandemics have occurred in the 20th century: in 1918, the pandemic of influenza A H1N1 Spanish flu killed at least 50 million people in the first year; 500,000 died in the United States alone. In 1957, a major shift occurred with both new avian HA and NA (H1N1 to H2N2). In 1968, a new HA (H2N2 to H3N2) from an avian source was introduced, leading to a moderately severe pandemic. In 1977, the old 1951 H1N1 strain reappeared (likely having escaped from a laboratory), causing attack rates of more than 50% in younger members of the population who had been born after 1956 and, therefore, had no antibody to the earlier H1N1 subtype present from 1918 to 1957. Since 1977, both H1N1 and H3N2 subtypes cocirculate worldwide (Figure 15-2 and Figure 15-3).

To summarize, influenza viruses with new surface antigens emerge, cause a pandemic, and become established in human populations. As the proportion

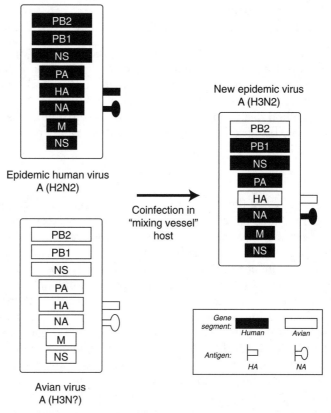

FIGURE 15-2   Diagram showing the last antigenic shift in 1968, when a new avian gene was acquired. Gene segments represent avian or human species origin and their associated surface proteins.
Source: Copyright © Mark C. Steinhoff.

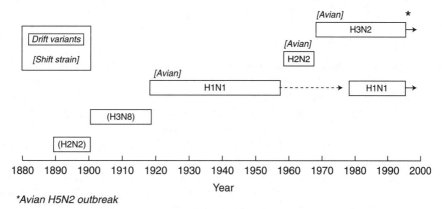

*Avian H5N2 outbreak

FIGURE 15-3   Twentieth-century history of influenza antigenic shifts and pandemics, and interpandemic antigenic drift.
Source: Centers for Disease Control and Prevention.

BOX 15-1   1918 Pandemic Flu

The influenza pandemic of 1918–1919, referred to as the "Spanish flu," caused more deaths globally than any pandemic since the Black Death (bubonic plague) of the 14th century. Estimates of the total number of deaths worldwide vary, but most sources estimate the pandemic caused at least 20 to 50 million deaths in the first 12 months. This estimate is an obvious underestimate because deaths in Asia and Africa were crudely estimated by colonial authorities.

First Wave

It appears influenza illness was first reported among American troops in the midwestern United States, from where it seems to have spread across the Atlantic with the movement of 1.5 million US forces to the Western front. Influenza was reported in March 1918 from Ft. Riley, Kansas. In April, relatively mild influenza disease with low mortality was reported in troops on the East Coast. By the 15th of April, US troops in France were reporting influenza illnesses, as were troops in Britain. It is likely that crowding increased attack rates and mortality in the military; the U.S. Navy estimated that 40% of its seamen became ill. There were 54,000 battle deaths among US forces in Europe and 43,000 influenza and pneumonia deaths. Battle lines were no barrier; German troops reported *blitzkatarrh* shortly after US troops reported influenza, and German commanders complained that the disease disrupted their attack plans. By May and June 1918, most of Europe was experiencing the epidemic. Disease was reported in Africa in May, in India and China in July and August—influenza had circled the world in 5 months. During the summer, the character of the disease changed, showing higher rates of pneumonia in young adults with case fatality rates of 50%. Some authorities suggest that the virus had mutated into a more virulent form. Isolated island populations suffered greatly. For example, in Tahiti 10% of the population died within 25 days of the onset of the epidemic. Similarly, in Western Samoa in November 1918, 20% of the population of 38,000 died within a 2-month period. On the other hand, the Tristan da Cunha islands, isolated in the South Atlantic, did not experience the pandemic.

Second Wave

Beginning in August 1918, a second wave of severe disease which was called "Spanish flu" swept the East Coast of the United States, following the European outbreaks. (Because of wartime censorship, British, French, German, and US authorities did not report epidemic disease; Spain was neutral, and reported the epidemic awarded the name.) This time the United States experienced the severe influenza disease with higher case fatality rates seen in the European Western Front. A common description is of cyanosis and death from pneumonia within 2 to 3 days of illness onset.[17a] Surveys in the United States showed that 280/1000 persons had clinical influenza symptoms. An estimated 550,000 excess deaths occurred in the United States, meaning approximately 1 of 200 persons died of influenza during the winter of 1918–1919. Philadelphia reported the highest mortality rate: 12,897 influenza and pneumonia deaths in October and November of 1918, with a peak of 700 deaths/day in late October, a 2-month mortality rate of 0.77%, leading to disruption of civic life, including a shortage of coffins. Desperate medical and public health authorities recommended many remedies and preventive actions now regarded as ineffective, including the use of gauze face masks, aerosol sprays, garlic or camphor necklaces, and legislation against public spitting. Mortality rates were lower in military and civilian African-Americans than in whites, but approximately 2% of all Native Americans died during the epidemic. The Spanish influenza epidemic of 1918 has been substantially ignored by historians until recently, perhaps because it occurred at the end of World War I. Katherine Anne Porter's novel, *Pale Horse, Pale Rider*, describes the experiences of young Americans during the pandemic.

1976 Swine Flu

When in January 1976 a similar swine H1N1 strain (A/New Jersey/76) was isolated in an ill soldier who died at Fort Dix, New Jersey, some United States public health authorities feared another pandemic and advised expanded immunization. Although not supported by all experts, a decision was reached to initiate mass immunization against swine flu, and the Swine Flu Program was announced in March 1976. A new national surveillance program for influenza disease and for vaccine adverse events was implemented. When liability issues were raised by the manufacturers, a special Swine Flu Tort Claims bill was passed by Congress, which specified that any claim arising from the swine flu program should be filed against the federal government. Vaccination started in October 1976, although no cases of swine flu disease had been reported. When, in December 1976, hundreds of cases of Guillain-Barré disease were reported following swine flu immunization, the vaccination program was suspended.[9]

The two major architects of the program, the Director of the CDC and the Assistant Secretary for Health of HEW, resigned. A total of 48 million Americans received the swine flu vaccine, but only six cases of swine flu H1N1 disease were recorded, which suggests that the A/New Jersey/76 strain was not transmitted efficiently. More than 500 cases of Guillain-Barré syndrome were reported, apparently associated with influenza vaccine, for which the federal government assumed liability and paid damages. Analysis suggested the risk of Guillain-Barré syndrome in 1976 vaccinees was 7 to 10 times increased over background risk, to about 10 cases for every million vaccine recipients. A recent evaluation of Guillain-Barré syndrome associated with current influenza vaccine suggests a relative risk of 1.7, approximately 1 case per million vaccinees.[10] This suggests the 1976 H1N1 vaccine had a unique association with Guillain-Barré syndrome.[10]

1918 Virus Resurrected

The 1918 pandemic virus was unique in its disease syndrome and epidemiology, but it was not available for study as virology techniques did not exist at that time. In late 2005, the 1918 pandemic virus was re-created from viral RNA from a victim buried in permafrost and from autopsy material from two soldiers. Genomic viral RNA was obtained from these three sources and sequenced to generate a complete 1918 genomic sequence. These sequences show the avian heritage of the virus. Using plasmid-mediated reverse genetics, the 1918 pandemic virus was generated and studied in a high-containment laboratory. In comparison to current epidemic H1N1 viruses, the 1918 virus displayed high growth characteristics in human bronchial epithelial cells in culture. It caused death in 100% of mice within 4 days, whereas the control viruses killed none. In summary, the biologic tour de force of resurrecting the 1918 virus will allow detailed assessment of the molecular basis of its high pathogenicity and unique transmission patterns.[11,12]

of persons with antibodies against the specific pandemic strain increases within the population, the circulating influenza virus subtype must change or die out. Antigenic drift allows a specific influenza subtype to persist in the human population. It is assumed that annual epidemics occur in the interpandemic period because drift variant viruses with new minor antigenic changes can infect some members of the population.

A new pandemic occurs after an antigenic shift. The shift can result from genetic reassortment between human and animal influenza viruses or from direct transmission of an animal strain to humans, as was documented with influenza A (H5N1) in Hong Kong in the winter of 1997–1998 and again in Southeast Asia in 2002–2004.[13] This virus when isolated from humans had only avian genes, with no evidence of reassortment with human viruses. It is apparent that the novel avian influenza A (H5N1) virus did cause disease in at least 18 humans in Hong Kong (6 of whom died), but did not efficiently transmit from human to human, hence did not become pandemic. H5N1 has reappeared in humans in 2003 in Hong Kong, and in 2004–2005 in Vietnam, Thailand, Cambodia, and Indonesia with evidence of rapid mutation.[10] This avian virus may at any time reassort with human-adapted viruses and acquire efficient transmissibility and could cause a pandemic in the near future. For this reason, public health authorities have begun development of H5 vaccines. H9N2 avian strains caused mild disease in Hong Kong in 1999 and 2003. Avian H7N7 caused poultry and human illness in Netherlands in 2003.[10]

The 1998 Hong Kong experience and the 1976 swine influenza episode show that surface antigens, virulence, and transmissibility all vary independently and unpredictably. Not all new shift viruses with novel antigens will cause a pandemic; the criteria of transmissibility and human infectivity must also be met.

Genetic reassortment also occurs frequently in egg or tissue culture. The vaccine manufacturers use this viral characteristic to rapidly develop new vaccine strains. Two viruses are selected: a wild virus with the epidemic NA and HA antigens, and an egg-adapted virus (A/Puerto Rico/8/34) with the characteristics of vigorous growth in egg culture. Eggs are infected simultaneously with both viruses and the reassortant progeny virus that exhibits both the epidemic HA and NA and the property of good growth in eggs is selected as the vaccine strain for production.

Epizootic Infections and Evolutionary History

The current working hypothesis developed by Webster and others is that avian influenza strains are the source for all influenza viruses seen in birds and mammals.[11-13] Analysis of molecular relationships suggests that all A subtypes are descended from a primordial avian influenza virus. All the known 15 HA and 9 NA influenza subtypes have been isolated from aquatic avian sources, which is likely their natural habitat, but only certain subtypes are found in mammalian species including swine, horses, seals, whales, and mink. Infection of feral (ducks, geese, gulls, terns, and shearwaters) or domestic (turkeys, chickens, geese, ducks, quail, and pheasants) avian species is usually asymptomatic, but occasionally has resulted in epidemics of avian disease, or "fowl plague." Ducks excrete up to $10^{8,7}$ virus particles per gram of feces, and influenza virus is found in waters where ducks reside. The rate of antigenic drift is low in birds, suggesting stable adaptation between virus and avian host. It has been found that pigs have epithelial cell receptors for both human and avian HA. Pigs are thought to be the mixing vessels or intermediate hosts of avian and mammalian influenza virus, providing an opportunity for reassortment and antigenic shift.

Although the virus of the 1918 pandemic has not been cultured, pandemic H1N1 viral RNA from bodies buried in permafrost in Alaska and from WWI autopsy material from the military has been analyzed and shows that the pandemic strain was unique and related to avian strains. Further analysis of the RNA sequence is being carried out to determine if a genetic explanation for its high virulence can be obtained.[14,16,16a] It is of note that the avian equivalent of H1N1 is still circulating in avian species. The role of avian carriage of virus during annual waterfowl migration from the Northern to the Southern Hemisphere in the spread of new influenza variants is being investigated.

Prevention Strategies and Treatment

Vaccines to prevent infection and use of antiviral drugs either prophylactically or for treatment are the currently available strategies to reduce influenza disease. This section will describe the recommended use of inactivated and live attenuated influenza vaccines, and of antiviral drugs.

Vaccines

Vaccines were developed soon after influenza virus was shown to grow in embryonated hens' eggs. An early vaccine trial in 1943 showed that a killed virus vaccine was effective in young adults. The current inactivated vaccine is derived from virus grown on chorioallantoic membranes of embryonated eggs. The allantoic fluids are ultracentrifuged to purify the virus particles, and the viruses are inactivated by formaldehyde or beta-propriolactone. Some manufacturers disrupt the virus particles to produce a "split virus vaccine" using detergents or ether. The potency is assessed by measuring HA antigen, and vaccines are standardized to contain 15 to 20 μg of HA antigen per dose. Egg-grown influenza viruses have been shown to have antigenic variation from the parent human strain, which may account for the variable protection of inactivated vaccines. Some workers have shown that growth of human-derived influenza virus in human cell lines produces HA antigens with identical amino acid sequences to the parent strain. In general, vaccines are immunogenic in adults after a single dose, but require two doses in infants and children who are immunologically naive. Current inactivated vaccines are 50% to 80% effective in preventing disease when the epidemic influenza virus matches the vaccine strains.[17]

The current vaccine strategy in the United States has evolved from protection for persons at high risk for adverse outcomes from influenza virus infection,[17a,17b] to now also vaccinating healthy persons who may transmit virus to high-risk persons.[18-22] In brief, these groups include those at increased risk for influenza complications (see Table 15-4), persons who can transmit influenza to those at high risk, as well as other special groups including persons infected with HIV,[23] travelers, and members of the population who wish to avoid influenza infection. Cost-effectiveness analyses mostly support immunization of healthy subjects.[20,21] Table 15-4 summarizes 2004 influenza vaccine recommendations for the United States (see CDC Web site for updates). Over the past few years infants and others have been added to the high-risk group.[24-26] Pregnancy was associated with excess mortality in the 1918 influenza pandemic. Recent evaluations have shown a relative risk of 4.7 for influenza-related hospitalization of pregnant women in the third trimester, compared with postpartum controls.[27]

Virus mutability with antigenic shift and drift means a new vaccine must be produced each year to counter the new antigenic variants that continually arise. Each year in January a review of circulating viruses in the Northern and Southern Hemispheres is undertaken by WHO, using data from a global network of surveillance laboratories, and the most likely epidemic influenza A (H1N1, H3N2) and a B strain are selected. The vaccine seed viruses are produced and distributed to manufacturers for production in eggs, clinical testing, licensing,[28,29] packaging, and distribution by October before the winter influenza season. The US vaccine manufacturers produce up to 100 million doses each year between February and October. Globally, nine manufacturers produce about 250 million doses annually.[30,31] This complex process is repeated annually and is usually effective, though in some years manufacturing problems have lead to late or nondelivery of vaccine.[56]

Usually this vaccine strategy is relatively effective in preventing disease and mortality in vaccinated persons in those years in which the vaccine composition closely matches the epidemic virus. It is unlikely to have any impact on the overall epidemic pattern, however, because only a small proportion of the susceptible population (i.e., those at high risk) is vaccinated. Recent studies suggest that influenza immunization of healthy children will reduce all otitis media episodes by 40%, and immunization of day-care children reduces illness in their families.[33-34] Immunization of healthy adults will reduce reported respiratory illness by 20% and absenteeism by 36%.[20] The vaccine strategy to vaccinate healthy persons, especially children, is increasingly used and had been used in Japan until the early 1990s.[32] Strategies to vaccinate a proportion of the children have the potential to disrupt epidemic transmission and protect adults.[35]

The inactivated influenza vaccines that are currently recommended and commercially available do not contain live viruses and cannot cause influenza

TABLE 15-4   Target Groups for Vaccination, CDC/ACIP 2005–2006 (see www.CDC. GOV/flu for latest recommendations)

A. Persons at Increased Risk for Complications

Vaccination with inactivated influenza vaccine is recommended for the following persons who are at increased risk for complications from influenza:

- Persons aged ≥65 years;
- Residents of nursing homes and other chronic-care facilities that house persons of any age who have chronic medical conditions;
- Adults and children who have chronic disorders of the pulmonary or cardiovascular systems, including asthma (hypertension is not considered a high-risk condition);
- Adults and children who have required regular medical follow-up or hospitalization during the preceding year because of chronic metabolic diseases (including diabetes mellitus), renal dysfunction, hemoglobinopathies, or immunosuppression (including immunosuppression caused by medications or by human immunodeficiency virus [HIV]);
- Adults and children who have any condition (e.g., cognitive dysfunction, spinal cord injuries, seizure disorders, or other neuromuscular disorders) that can compromise respiratory function or the handling of respiratory secretions or that can increase the risk for aspiration;
- Children and adolescents (aged 6 months–18 years) who are receiving long-term aspirin therapy and, therefore, might be at risk for experiencing Reye syndrome after influenza infection;
- Women who will be pregnant during the influenza season; and
- Children aged 6–23 months.

B. Persons Aged 50–64 Years

C. Persons Who Can Transmit Influenza to Those at High Risk

- Employees of assisted living and other residences for persons in groups at high risk;
- Persons who provide home care to persons in groups at high risk; and
- Household contacts (including children) of persons in groups at high risk.

D. Health-Care Workers

E. Pregnant Women

Because of the increased risk for influenza-related complications, women who will be pregnant during the influenza season should be vaccinated. Vaccination can occur in any trimester.

F. Persons Infected with HIV

Because influenza can result in serious illness and because vaccination with inactivated influenza vaccine can result in the production of protective antibody titers, vaccination will benefit HIV-infected persons, including HIV-infected pregnant women.

G. Breastfeeding Mothers, to Protect Young Infants

H. Travelers

- Travel to the tropics,
- Travel with organized tourist groups at any time of year, or
- Travel to the Southern Hemisphere during April–September.

I. General Population

Physicians should administer influenza vaccine to any person who wishes to reduce the likelihood of becoming ill with influenza or transmitting influenza to others should they become infected.

Source: Centers for Disease Control and Prevention.[17,17a,17b,17c]

disease. The most frequent side effect of vaccination is local soreness at the vaccination site, which can last for 1 or 2 days. Symptoms of fever, malaise, and myalgia have been infrequently reported, most often in persons who have had no exposure to influenza vaccine (e.g., young children). Allergic anaphylactic reactions, which can occur rarely after influenza vaccination, are related to hypersensitivity to residual egg protein in these vaccines or to thimerosal. The 1976 swine influenza vaccine was associated with an increased frequency of Guillain-Barré syndrome of ascending paralysis.[36] Recently, the association has been evaluated with current vaccines, and it is estimated to occur in approximately one case per million vaccinees—far less than the risk of severe influenza complications if not vaccinated.[37]

Live Influenza Vaccine

Live attenuated influenza viruses (LAIV) have been shown to be as effective as the inactivated virus vaccines.[20] The cold-adapted virus does not replicate effectively at 37°C, hence it can infect humans, but does not cause disease.[38] The cold-adapted attenuated influenza virus is derived from an epidemic strain and an attenuated cold-adapted virus. After reassortment of the two viruses, progeny with the epidemic surface antigens and the characteristic of attenuated growth in humans are selected and produced. These vaccine strains have been extensively tested in adults and children, and demonstrate protective efficacy of 92% against confirmed influenza infection and excellent safety characteristics.[19,39,40] Their chief advantage is that they can be administered as nose drops or aerosol, and, therefore, are more acceptable to patients and do not require medical personnel for administration. The cold-adapted influenza vaccine (FluMist®) was licensed in 2004 for use in people aged 5 years to 55 years in the United States with important exceptions (Table 15-5).[41] The ease of administration of LAIV vaccines and their ready acceptance may allow strategies of population vaccination to avert an epidemic.

Vaccine Production Issues

Production of influenza vaccine is a complex process nearly 50 years old that involves production, licensing, and delivery of a trivalent vaccine every

---

TABLE 15-5   Persons Who Should Not Be Vaccinated with LAIV

The following populations should not be vaccinated with LAIV:

- Persons younger than 5 years or those *older than* 50 years
- Persons with asthma, reactive airways disease, or other chronic disorders of the pulmonary or cardiovascular systems; persons with other underlying medical conditions, including such metabolic diseases as diabetes, renal dysfunction, and hemoglobinopathies; or persons with known or suspected immunodeficiency diseases or who are receiving immunosuppressive therapies
- Children or adolescents receiving aspirin or other salicylates (because of the association of Reye syndrome with wild-type influenza infection)
- Persons with a history of GBS
- Pregnant women
- Persons with a history of hypersensitivity, including anaphylaxis, to any of the components of LAIV or to eggs

---

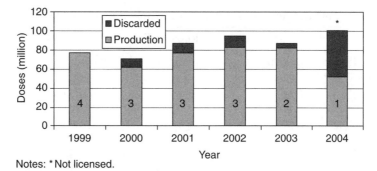

FIGURE 15-4   Influenza vaccine doses.
Source: Data from Centers for Disease Control and Prevention, Figure © Mark C. Steinhoff.

year. The current licensed vaccines are made in embryonated hens' eggs, and approximately 80 to 100 million doses are produced in the United States each year reguiring 300 million eggs. Because of increased information regarding high-risk groups, policy decisions have gradually increased the number of people who are recommended to receive the vaccine annually. In 1997, pregnant women were added, persons aged 50 to 64 were added in 2000, and young children from 6 to 24 months were added in 2004[40a] bringing the total number to 180 million. At the same time, the number of vaccine producers in the United States declined from four to two. Figure 15-4 shows the total production of doses each year and the number of doses discarded unsold at the end of the season. In 2004, there were only two producers who between them produced a 100 million doses. However, one of the producers was not able to distribute approximately 48 million doses because of production problems and withdrawal of its license by FDA. The resulting shortfall of vaccine required revision of priority groups for immunization by authorities and redistribution of vaccine doses as well as importation of vaccine as investigational drugs from producers who are not licensed in the United States.

The combination of complex manufacture process, reduction of producers, and the complexities of annual vaccine production conspired to produce a disruption of the vaccine supply. These events and increased concern about new pandemic strains prompted the US government in 2005 to a series of actions including (1) funding support to maintain the chicken flocks so that large numbers of embryonated eggs can be made available for vaccine production with a short lead time. In addition, (2) encouragement of new manufacturers to apply for US licensure to increase vaccine production sources, and (3) initiation of the process to produce influenza vaccine from cell culture rather than from hens' eggs.

Antiviral Drugs

The older antiviral agents, amantadine and rimantadine, inhibit the replication of type A influenza viruses (but have no effect on type B) by interfering with the M2 protein, which forms an ion channel. When taken prophylactically, these drugs have been shown to be 70% to 90% effective in preventing illness during influenza A epidemics. In addition, if begun within 48

TABLE 15-6 Antiviral Agents for Influenza Treatment and Prophylaxis

	Amantadine	Rimantadine	Zanamivir	Oseltamivir
Types of influenza viruses inhibited	Influenza A	Influenza A	Influenza A and B	Influenza A and B
Route of administration	Oral (tablet, capsule, syrup)	Oral (tablet, syrup)	Oral inhalation*	Oral (capsule)
Ages for which treatment is approved	≥1 year	≥14 years	≥1 year	≥7 years
Ages for which prophylaxis is approved	≥1 year	≥1 year	Not approved for prophylaxis	≥1 year

*Zanamivir is administered by a plastic oral inhalation device.
Source: Adapted from MMWR, Vol. 48, RR14, 1999, Centers for Disease Control and Prevention.

hours of illness onset in healthy adults, these drugs can reduce the severity and duration of influenza A illness. Both drugs have CNS side effects of nervousness, anxiety, difficulty in concentrating, and light-headedness. These drugs are advised for children only above the age of 1 year (Table 15-6) and are not effective against H5N1.[41,42]

New drugs have been designed to inhibit NA activity.[43,44] An NA inhibitor, zanamivir (a sialic acid analogue), reduces disease duration by 1 or more days and prevents both type A and B disease with 67% to 82% effectiveness when taken prophylactically.[45] Zanamivir (or Relenza) was licensed in the United States in July 1999 as inhalation therapy for persons older than 7 years. An oral NA inhibitor, oseltamivir (Tamiflu), is equally effective for prophylaxis and treatment for influenza in children older than 1 year.[46]

Preparing for the Pandemic [as of June, 2006]

Many experts predict that a new pandemic with a unique influenza shift virus is inevitable. The ceaseless random variation of influenza virus will eventually result in the development of a pandemic strain.

The increasing cases of avian H5N1 virus in humans in Asia since 2003 has led to a reassessment of pandemic planning in the United States and globally.

Avian Influenza Virus

The H5N1 avian influenza strain has been causing disease and outbreaks in birds and humans in Asia since 1997. As of late May 2006, 225 human cases of laboratory-confirmed avian influenza A/H5N1 had been reported to WHO since 2003. The majority of cases were from Asia, including the countries of Cambodia, China, Indonesia, Thailand and Vietnam; with fewer cases from Africa in Egypt, and Djibouti, and several cases from Europe and the Middle East, in Iraq, Turkey and Azerbaijan. Overall mortality in these reported cases was 57%. Analysis of recent strains of H5N1 show that it has mutated substantially from the strain first seen in 1997.[47,47A] There is increasing concern regarding this avian virus that exhibits new surface antigen, has virulence in humans, but does not yet have efficient transmissibility between humans.[47b,47c]

The virus may acquire the human transmission phenotype properties needed to become the next pandemic strain.[9]

In its review of preparedness, the CDC has estimated that a new virus would arrive in the United States within 1 to 6 months of its appearance elsewhere, and would likely initiate the pandemic at many cities with international airports. It is unlikely that any existing vaccine would be useful, and stocks of antivirals would not be adequate to treat the large number of cases expected in a naive population. As in previous pandemics, health care workers will likely be at increased risk of illness, affecting the care of the ill. Current estimates are that the United States would have 200 million cases, up to 800,000 hospitalizations, and as many as 300,000 influenza deaths within the 3- to 4-month period of the first sweep of the pandemic. (See www.cdc.gov/vd/nvpo/pandemicflu.htm for the current planning guide.) Current plans include improved surveillance and monitoring of the emergence of new viruses,[48] stockpiling of antiviral drugs,[49] development of a drug distribution system, strategic planning to develop and distribute new vaccines, and improved communications between WHO and national and local authorities.[50,51,51a] Priority groups to receive vaccine and hospital care have been described and debated.[51b–51f]

The WHO has strengthened the FluNet, a global surveillance system with laboratories in 83 countries and has sped up the process of identifying possible new shift viruses (those that are not typed with existing antisera). The FluNet showed its effectiveness in identifying the new coronavirus agent of SARS, not influenza, as the cause of an outbreak of severe febrile respiratory illness in Hong Kong in 2003. FluNet was used to rapidly identify human cases of avian influenza in 1997. Some experts have suggested that closer monitoring of avian and swine influenza viruses and epidemic diseases may assist in prediction of new pandemic human influenza strains.[52] Virologists are working on techniques to adapt a newly arising influenza virus for rapid production of a vaccine.[53] Because the onset of a new pandemic or the characteristics of a new pandemic virus cannot be predicted reliably, preparation to speed the response to the pandemic may be the best approach.[54,55]

If a pandemic should occur before sufficient antiviral drugs are available, and few or no doses of specific vaccines are available,[56,57] epidemic control will have to rely on public health strategies that are centuries old, namely physical restrictions of citizens. This includes (1) isolation of those with influenza illness, (2) quarantine of all their contacts, and (3) banning of all public gatherings including schools, workplaces, shopping centers, churches, and bars. A presidential executive order was signed on April 2, 2004, permitting the use of quarantine if an avian influenza outbreak should occur.

References

1. Smith W, Andrews CH, Laidlaw PP. A virus isolated from influenza patients. *Lancet*. 1933;2:66–68.
2. Murphy BR, Webster RG. "Orthomyxovirus." In: Fields BN, Knipe DM, Howley PM, et al., eds. *Virology*. 3rd ed. Philadelphia, Pa: Lippincott-Raven Publishers; 1996:1409–1432.
3. Matrosovich MN, Gambaryan AS, Teneberg S, et al. Avian influenza A viruses differ from human viruses by recognition of

sialyloligosaccharides and gangliosides and by a higher conservation of the HA receptor-binding site. *Virology.* 1997;233:224–234.

3a. Brundage JF. Interactions between influenza and bacterial respiratory pathogens: implications for pandemic preparedness. *Lancet Infect Dis.* 2006;6:303–312.

3b. O'Brien KL, Walters MI, Sellman J, Quinlisk P, Regnery H, Schwartz B, Dowell SF. Severe pneumococcal pneumonia in previously healthy children: the role of preceding influenza infections. *Clin Infect Dis.* 2000;30:784–789.

4. Monto AS, Gravenstein S, Elliott M, Colopy M, Schweinle J. Clinical signs and symptoms predicting influenza infection. *Arch Intern Med.* 2000;160:3243–3247.

5. Couch RB, Kasel WP, Glezen TR, et al. Influenza: its control and person and populations. *J Infect Dis.* 1986;153:431–440.

6. Rao BL, Banerjee K. Influenza surveillance in Pune, India, 1978–90. *Bull World Health Organ.* 1993.

6a. Viboud C, Alonso WJ, Simonsen L. Influenza in tropical regions. PLoS Medicine Vol. 3 , No. 4, DOI: 10.1371/journal.pmed.0030089.

6b. Chiu SS, Lau YL, Chan KH, Wong WHS, Peiris JSM. Influenza-related hospitalizations among children in Hong Kong. *N Engl J Med.* 2002;347:2097–2103.

6c. Neuzil KM, Zhu Y, Griffin MR, et al. Burden of interpandemic influenza in children young than 5 years: a 25 year prospective study. *J Infect Dis.* 2002;185:147–152.

6d. Bhat N, Wright JG, Broder KR, et al. Influenza-associated deaths among children in the United States, 2003-2004. *N Engl J Med.* 2005;353(24):2559–2567.

7. Reichert TA, Simonsen L, Sharma A, Pardo SA, Fedson DS, Miller MA. Influenza and the winter increase in mortality in the United States, 1959-1999. *Am J Epidemiol.* 2004;160:492–502.

7a. Thompson WW, Shay DK, Weintraub E, Brammer L, Bridges CB, Cox NJ, Fukuda K. Influenza-associated hospitalizations in the United States. *JAMA.* 2004 15;292(11):1333–1340.

8. Subbarao K, Klimov A, Katz J, et al. Characterization of an avian influenza A (H5N1) virus isolated from a child with fatal respiratory illness. *Science.* 1998;279:393–396.

9. Stöhr K. Avian influenza and pandemics—research needs and opportunities. *N Engl J Med.* 2005;352;405–407.

10. Koopmans M, Wilbrink B, Conyn M, et al. Transmission of H7N7 avian influenza A virus to human beings during a large outbreak in commercial poultry farms in the Netherlands. *Lancet.* 2004;363: 587–593.

11. Webster RG. Influenza: an emerging microbial pathogen. In: Krause RM, ed. *Emerging Infections.* New York, NY: Academic Press; 1998:275–300.

12. Hay AJ, Gregory V, Douglas AR, Lin YP. The evolution of human influenza viruses. *Phil Trans R Soc Lond B.* 2001;356:1861–1870.

12a. Tumpey TM, Garcia-Sastre A, Taubenberger, et al. Pathogenicity of influenza viruses with genes from the 1918 pandemic virus: functional roles of alveolar macrophages and neutrophils in limiting virus replication and mortality in mice. *J Virol.* 2005;79(23):14933–14944.

13. Webby R, Hoffmann E, Webster R. Molecular constraints to interspecies transmission of viral pathogens. *Nature Med.* 2004;10: S77-S81.

14. Reid AH, Fanning TG, Hultin JV, Taubenberger JK. Origin and evolution of the 1918 "Spanish" influenza virus hemagglutinin gene [comment]. *Proc Natl Acad Sci U S A*. 1999;96:1164–1166.

15. Tumpey TM, Basler CF, Aguilar PV, et al. Characterization of the reconstructed 1918 Spanish influenza pandemic virus. *Science*. 2005;310:77–80.

16. Taubenberger JK, Reid AH, Lourens RM, et al. Characterization of the 1918 influenza virus polymerase genes [letter]. *Nature*. 2005;437: 889–892.

17. Recommendations of the Advisory Committee on Immunization Practices (ACIP). Prevention and Control of Influenza. *MMWR*. 2005;54(RR08):1–40.

17a. Recommendations of the Healthcare Infection Control Practices Advisory Committee (HICPAC) and the Advisory Committee on Immunization Practices (ACIP). Influenza Vaccination of Health-Care Personnel. *MMWR*. 2006;55(RR02);1–16.

17b. Poland GA, Tosh P, Jacobson RM. Requiring influenza vaccination for health care workers: seven truths we must accept. *Vaccine*. 2005;23(17–18):2251–2255.

17c. American Academy of Pediatrics. Influenza. In: Pickering LK, Baker CJ, Long SS, McMillan JA, eds. *Red Book: 2006 Report of the Committee on Infectious Diseases*. 27th ed. Elk Grove Village, IL: American Academy of Pediatrics; 2006:401–410.

18. Nichol KL, Lind A, Margolis KL, et al. The effectiveness of vaccination against influenza in healthy, working adults. *N Engl J Med*. 1995;333:889–893.

19. Nichol KL, Mendelman PM, Mallon KP, et al. Effectiveness of live, attenuated intranasal influenza virus vaccine in healthy, working adults. A randomized controlled trial. *JAMA*. 1999;282:137–144.

20. Nichol KL. The efficacy, effectiveness and cost-effectiveness of inactivated influenza virus vaccines. *Vaccine*. 2003;21:1769–1775.

21. Bridges CB, Thompson WW, Meltzer MI, et al. Effectiveness and cost-benefit of influenza vaccination of healthy working adults. *JAMA*. 2000;284:1655–1663.

22. Wilde JA, McMillan J, Serwint J, Butta J, O'Riordan MA, Steinhoff MC. Effectiveness of influenza vaccine in health care professionals: a randomized controlled trial. *JAMA*. 1999;281:908–913.

23. Tasker SA, Treanor JJ, Paxton WB, Wallace MR. Efficacy of influenza vaccination in HIV-infected persons. A randomized, double-blind, placebo-controlled trial. *Ann Intern Med*. 1999;131:430–433.

24. Hurwitz ES, Haber M, Chang A, et al. Effectiveness of influenza vaccination of day care children in reducing influenza-related morbidity among household contacts. *JAMA*. 2000;284:1677–1682.

25. Izurieta HS, Thompson WW, Kramarz P, et al. Influenza and the rates of hospitalization for respiratory disease among infants and young children. *N Engl J Med*. 2000;232:232–239.

26. Neuzil KM, Mellen BG, Wright PF, Mitchel EF, Griffin MR. The effect of influenza on hospitalizations, outpatient visits, and courses of antibiotics in children. *N Engl J Med*. 2000;342:225–231.

27. Neuzil KM, Reed GW, Mitchel EF, Simonsen L, Griffin MR. Impact of influenza on acute cardiopulmonary hospitalizations in pregnant women. *Am J Epidemiol*. 1998;148:1094–1102.

28. Gerdil C. The annual production cycle for influenza vaccine. *Vaccine*. 2003;21:1776–1779.

29. Wood JM, Levandowski RA. The influenza vaccine licensing process. *Vaccine.* 2003;21:1786–1788.

30. Fedson DS, Hirota Y, Shin H-K, et al. Influenza vaccination in 22 developed countries: an update to 1995. *Vaccine.* 1997;15:1506–1511.

31. van Essen GA, Palache AM, Forleo E, Fedson DS. Influenza vaccination in 2000: recommendations and vaccine use in 50 developed and rapidly developing countries. *Vaccine.* 2003;21:1780–1785.

32. Reichert TA, Sugaya, Fedson DS, Glezen WP, Simonsen L, Tashiro M. The Japanese experience with vaccinating school children against influenza. *N Engl J Med.* 2001;344:889–896.

33. Heikkinen T, Ruuskanen O, Waris M, Ziegler T, Arola M, Halonen P. Influenza vaccination in the prevention of acute otitis media in children. *Am J Dis Child.* 1991;145:445–448.

34. Clements DA, Langdon L, Bland C, Walter E. Influenza A vaccine decreases the incidence of otitis media in 6- to 30-month-old children in day care. *Arch Pediatr Adolesc Med.* 1995;1490:1113–1117.

35. Piedra PA, Gaglani MJ, Kozinetz CA, et al. Herd immunity in adults against influenza-related illnesses with use of the trivalent-live attenuated influenza vaccine (CAIV-T) in children. *Vaccine.* 2005;23:1540–1548.

36. Langmuir AD, Bregman DJ, Kurland LT, Nathanson N, Victor M. An epidemiologic and clinical evaluation of Guillain-Barré syndrome reported in association with the administration of swine influenza vaccines. *Am J Epidemiol.* 1984;119:841–879.

37. Lasky T, Terracciano GJ, Magder L, et al. The Guillain-Barré Syndrome and the 1992–1993 and 1993–1994 influenza vaccines. *N Engl J Med.* 1998;339:1797–1802.

38. Steinhoff MC, Halsey NA, Fries LF, et al. The A/Mallard/6750/78 avian-human, but not the A/Ann Arbor/6/60 cold-adapted, Influenza A/Kawasaki/86 (H1N1) reassortant virus vaccine retains partial virulence for infants and children. *J Infect Dis.* 1991;163:1023–1028.

39. Belshe RB, Mendelman PM, Treanor J, et al.The efficacy of live attenuated, cold-adapted, trivalent, intranasal influenza virus vaccine in children. *N Engl J Med.* 1998;338:1405–1412.

40. Belshe RB, Nichol KL, Black SB, et al. Safety, efficacy, and effectiveness of live, attenuated, cold-adapted influenza vaccine in an indicated population aged 5–49 years. *CID.* 2004;39:920–927.

40a. http://www.cdc.gov/flu/professionals/vaccination/pdf/targetpopchart. pdf accessed 16 June, 2006.

41. Cooper NJ, Sutton AJ, Abrams KR, Wailoo A, Turner D, Nicholson KG. Effectiveness of neuraminidase inhibitors in treatment and prevention of influenza A and B: systematic review and meta-analyses of randomised controlled trials. *BMJ.* 2003;326:1235.

42. American Academy of Pediatrics. In: Pickering LK, ed. *Red Book: 2003 Report of the Committee on Infectious Diseases.* 26th ed. Elk Grove Village, Ill: American Academy of Pediatrics; 2003.

43. Hayden FG, Osterhaus ADME, Treanor JJ, et al, for the GG167 Influenza Study Group. Efficacy and safety of the neuraminidase inhibitor zanamivir in the treatment of influenzavirus infections. *N Engl J Med.* 1997;337:874–880.

44. Monto AS, Robinson DP, Herlocher ML, Hinson JM Jr, Elliott MJ, Crisp A. Zanamivir in the prevention of influenza among healthy adults. A randomized controlled trial. *JAMA.* 1999;282:31–35.

45. Monto AS, Pichichero ME, Blanckenberg SJ, et al. Zanamivir prophylaxis: an effective strategy for the prevention of influenza types A and B within households. *J Infect Dis.* 2002;186:1582–1588.

46. Welliver R, Monto AS, Carewicz O, et al. Effectiveness of oseltamivir in preventing influenza in household contacts: a randomized controlled trial. *JAMA.* 2001;285:748-754.
47. Webby RJ, Webster RG. Are we ready for pandemic influenza? *Science.* 2003;302:1519-1522.
47a. Chen H, Deng G, Li Z, et al. The evolution of H5N1 influenza viruses in ducks in southern China. *PNAS.* 2004;101:10452-10457.
47b. Beigel JH, Farrar J, Han AM, et al, Writing Committee of the World Health Organization (WHO) Consultation on Human Influenza A/H5. Avian influenza A (H5N1) infection in humans. *N Engl J Med.* 2005;353:1374-1385.
47c. Peltola VT, Murti KG, McCullers JA. Influenza virus neuraminidase contributes to secondary bacterial pneumonia. *J Infect Dis.* 2005;192:249-257.
48. Stöhr K. Asian influenza and pandemics. *N Engl J M* ed. 2005;352:405-407.
49. Longini IM Jr, Halloran E, Nizam A, Yang Y. Containing pandemic influenza with antiviral agents. *Am J Epidemiol.* 2004;159:623-633.
50. Fedson DS. Preparing for pandemic vaccination: an international policy agenda for vaccine development. *J Public Health Policy.* 2005;26:4-29.
51. World Health Organization. Department of Communicable Disease. Surveillance and Response Global Influenza Programme. WHO checklist for influenza pandemic preparedness planning. *WHO/CDS/CSR/GIP/2005.4, WHO/CDS/CSR/GIP/2005.5.*
51a. Osterholm MT. Preparing for the next pandemic. *N Engl J Med.* 2005;352:1839-1842.
51b. Emanuel EJ, Wertheimer A. Public health. Who should get influenza vaccine when not all can? *Science.* 2006;312(5775):854-855.
51c. Centers for Disease Control and Prevention (CDC). Update: influenza vaccine supply and recommendations for prioritization during the 2005-06 influenza season. *MMWR Morb Mortal Wkly Rep.* 2005;54(34):850.
51d. Daniel J. Barnett, Ran D. Balicer, Daniel R. Lucey, George S. Everly Jr., Saad B. Omer, Mark C. Steinhoff, Itamar Grotto. A Systematic Analytic Approach to Pandemic Influenza Preparedness Planning.
51e. Ferguson NM, Cummings DAT, Fraser C, Cajka JC, Cooley PC, Burke DS. Strategies for mitigating an influenza pandemic. Nature 2006;doi:10.1038/nature04795 http://www.nature.com/nature.
51f. World Health Organization Writing Group. Nonpharmaceutical interventions for pandemic influenza, international measures. Emerg Infect Dis 2006;12:81-87.
52. Lipatov AS, Govorkova EA, Webby RJ, et al. Influenza: emergence and control. *J Virol.* 2004;78:8951-8959.
53. Stephenson I, Nicholson KG, Wood JM, Zambon MC, Katz JM. Confronting the avian influenza threat: vaccine development for a potential pandemic. *Lancet Infect Dis.* 2004;4:499-509.
54. Ferguson NM, Cummings DAT, Cauchemez S, et al. Strategies for containing an emerging influenza pandemic in Southeast Asia. *Nature.* 2005;437:209-214.
55. Longini IM Jr, Nizam A, Xu S, et al. Containing pandemic influenza at the source. *Science.* 2005;309:1083-1087.
56. Sloan FA, Berman S, Rosenbaum S, Chalk RA, Griffin RB. The fragility of the U.S. vaccine supply. *N Engl J Med.* 2004;351:2443-2447.
56. Treanor J. Weathering the influenza vaccine crisis. *N Engl J Med.* 2004;351:2037-2040.

57. Dale RC, Church AJ, Surtees RAH, et al. Encephalitis lethargica syndrome: 20 new cases and evidence of basal ganglia autoimmunity. *Brain.* 2004;127:21–33.

Internet Resources

- CDC influenza Web site: http://www.cdc.gov/flu.
- WHO influenza Web site: http://who.int/emc/diseases/flu/index.html.
- Interactive maps of global flu data: http://oms/b3e/jussieu/fr/flunet.
- Weekly report, influenza summary update: http://www.cdc.gov/flu/weekly/
- US pandemic plan: http://www.hhs.gov/nvpo/pandemicplan/index.html.
- Good summaries and updates from Center for Infectious Disease Research and Policy: www.CIDRAP/imn.edu
- CDC's flu activity report: http://www.cdc.gov/flu/weekly/fluactivity.htm
- US Government pandemic flu web page: www.pandemicflu.gov
- Nature's avian flu mapping on Google Earth: http://www.nature.com/nature/googleearth/avianflu1.kml
- US HHS flu pandemic planning update March 2006: http://pandemicflu.gov/plan/pdf/panflu20060313.pdf
- US National Strategy Pandemic Influenza plan document, May 2006.
- Homeland Security Council: http://www.whitehouse.gov/homeland/nspi_implementation.
- W.H.O. New International Health regulations for influenza: http://www.who.int/gb/ebwha/pdf_files/WHA59/A59_47-en.pdf
- W H O influenza web site: http://www.who.int/csr/disease/influenza/en/
- WHO global influenza preparedness plan: http://www.who.int/csr/resources/publications/influenza/WHO_CDS_CSR_GIP_2005_5.pdf
- WHO avian influenza page: http://www.who.int/csr/disease/avian_influenza/en/
- Cumulative number of confirmed human cases of avian influenza a/(H5N1) reported to WHO: http://www.who.int/csr/disease/avian_influenza/country/cases_table_2006_06_06/en/print.html

Bibliography

Barry JM. *The Great Influenza: The Epic Story of the Deadliest Plague in History.* New York, NY: Viking; 2004.

Crosby AW. *America's Forgotten Pandemic: The Influenza of 1918.* New York, NY: Cambridge University Press; 1989.

Getz D. *Purple Death: The Mysterious Flu of 1918.* New York, NY: Henry Holt & Company; 2000.

Kolata G. *Flu: The Story of the Great Influenza Pandemic of 1918 and the Search for the Virus That Caused It.* New York, NY: Farrar, Straus and Giroux; 1999.

Neustadt RE, Fineberg HV. *The Swine Flu Affair: Decision-Making on a Slippery Disease.* Washington, DC: US Dept of Health, Education, and Welfare; 1978.

CHAPTER SIXTEEN

MEASLES

William J. Moss and Martin O. Ota

Introduction

Measles virus infection is one of the most important infectious diseases of humans and has caused millions of deaths since its emergence as a zoonotic disease thousands of years ago. For infectious disease epidemiologists, measles has served as a model of an acute infectious disease, particularly for understanding the nature of epidemics. Kenneth Maxcy, the second chair of the Department of Epidemiology at the Johns Hopkins University School of Public Health, wrote in 1948, "The simplest of all infectious diseases is measles."[1] Despite the apparent simplicity, much has been learned about measles in the half century since Maxcy's chapter on the epidemiology of infectious diseases. Detailed investigations of the virology, immunology, and transmission dynamics have shown measles to be a much more complex disease than Maxcy's statement indicates, and many questions remain unanswered. But this ignorance has not impeded enormous progress in global measles control.

Biologic Characteristics of the Measles Virus

Measles virus is the causative agent of measles and was first isolated from the blood of David Edmonston in 1954 by John Enders and Thomas Peebles.[2] The development of vaccines against measles soon followed. Measles virus is a spherical, nonsegmented, single-stranded, negative-sense RNA virus and a member of the *Morbillivirus* genus in the family of Paramyxoviridae. Other members of the *Morbillivirus* genus, although not pathogenic to humans, are rinderpest virus and canine distemper virus. Rinderpest virus causes an important disease of cattle and swine and is the morbillivirus most closely related to measles virus. Measles was originally a zoonotic infection, arising

601

from cross-species transmission from animals to humans by an ancestor morbillivirus. Although RNA viruses have high mutation rates, measles virus is considered to be an antigenically monotypic virus, meaning that the surface proteins responsible for inducing protective immunity have retained their antigenic structure across time and space. The public health significance is that measles vaccines developed decades ago from a single measles virus strain remain protective worldwide. Measles virus is killed by ultraviolet light and heat. Attenuated measles vaccine viruses retain these characteristics, necessitating a cold chain for transporting and storing measles vaccines.

Measles Virus Genes and Proteins

The measles virus RNA genome consists of approximately 16,000 nucleotides and is enclosed in a lipid-containing envelope derived from the host cell. The genome encodes eight proteins, two of which (V and C) are nonstructural proteins and are expressed from the phosphoprotein (P) gene. Of the six structural proteins, P, large protein (L), and nucleoprotein (N) form the nucleocapsid housing the viral RNA. The hemagglutinin protein (H), fusion protein (F), and matrix protein (M), together with lipids from the host cell membrane, form the viral envelope. This relatively simple combination of proteins and ribonucleic acid has evolved to be one of the most highly infectious agents known and the cause of millions of deaths.

In terms of understanding the epidemiology and control of measles, the two surface proteins F and H are most important. The H protein interacts with F to mediate fusion of the viral envelope with the host cell membrane.[3] The primary function of the H protein is to bind to the host cellular receptors for measles virus, CD46 and CD150 (SLAM). CD46 is a complement regulatory molecule expressed on all nucleated cells in humans. SLAM, an acronym for signaling lymphocyte activation molecule, is expressed on activated T and B lymphocytes and antigen-presenting cells. The distribution of these host proteins determines the cell types, or tissue tropism, infected by measles virus. Wild-type measles virus enters cells primarily through the cellular receptor SLAM, and most vaccine strains bind to CD46, although wild-type measles virus may use both CD46 and SLAM as receptors during acute infection.[4] Additional, as yet unidentified receptors for measles virus exist on human endothelial and epithelial cells.[5] The H protein elicits strong immune responses, and the lifelong immunity that follows infection is attributed to neutralizing antibodies against H.

Other measles virus proteins are involved in viral replication. The P protein regulates transcription, replication, and the efficiency with which the nucleoprotein assembles into nucleocapsids.[6] The M protein links ribonucleoproteins with envelope proteins during virion assembly. The functions of V and C proteins have not been clearly defined, but both proteins appear to contribute to the virulence of measles virus by blocking signal transduction in response to the antiviral proteins interferon-α and interferon-γ.[7,8]

Pathogenesis

Respiratory droplets from infected persons serve as vehicles of transmission by carrying infectious virus to epithelial cells of the respiratory tract of susceptible hosts. During the 10- to 14-day incubation period between infection and the onset of clinical signs and symptoms, measles virus replicates and spreads within the infected host (Figure 16-1). Initial viral replication occurs in epithelial cells at the portal of entry in the upper respiratory tract, and the virus then spreads to local lymphatic tissue. Replication in local lymph nodes is followed by viremia (the presence of virus in the blood) and the dissemination of measles virus to many organs, including lymph nodes, skin, kidney, gastrointestinal tract, and liver, where the virus replicates in epithelial and endothelial cells as well as monocytes and macrophages.

Although measles virus infection is clinically inapparent during the incubation period, the virus is actively replicating, and the host immune responses are developing. Evidence of these processes can be detected. During the incubation period, the number of circulating lymphocytes is reduced (lymphopenia).[9] Measles virus can be isolated from the nasopharynx and blood during the later part of the incubation period and in the several-day prodromal period prior to the onset of rash when levels of viremia are highest. The prodrome ends with the appearance of the measles rash. The rash results from

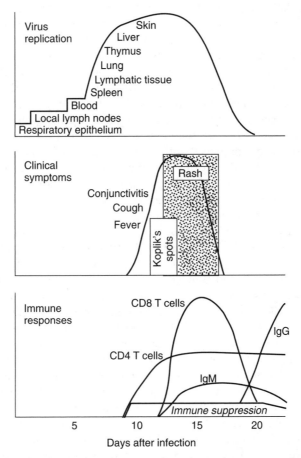

FIGURE 16-1 Measles virus replication, clinical manifestations, and immune responses following infection.
Source: Knipe DM et al., Eds, Fields Virology. 2001. 4th Edition. Lippincott Williams and Wilkins.

measles virus-specific cellular immune responses and marks the beginning of viral clearance from blood and tissue. Histologic examination of the rash reveals infected capillary endothelial cells and a mononuclear cell infiltrate.[10] Clearance of infectious virus from the blood and other tissues occurs within the first week after the appearance of the rash, although measles virus RNA can be detected in body fluids of some children for at least one month using a polymerase chain reaction (PCR)-based assay.[11]

Immune Responses to Measles Virus

Host immune responses to measles virus are essential for viral clearance, clinical recovery, and the establishment of long-term immunity (Figure 16-1). The early nonspecific (innate) immune responses that occur during the prodromal phase of the illness include activation of natural killer (NK) cells and increased production of the antiviral proteins interferon (IFN)-α and IFN-γ. These innate immune responses contribute to the control of measles virus replication before the onset of more specific (adaptive) immune responses. The adaptive immune responses consist of measles virus-specific humoral (antibody) and cellular responses. The protective efficacy of antibodies to measles virus is illustrated by the immunity conferred to infants from passively acquired maternal antibodies and the protection of exposed, susceptible individuals following administration of antimeasles virus immune globulin.[12] The first measles virus-specific antibodies produced after infection are of the IgM subtype, followed by a switch to predominantly IgG1 and IgG4 isotypes.[13] The IgM antibody response is typically absent following reexposure or revaccination and serves as a marker of primary infection. IgA antibodies to measles virus are found in mucosal secretions. The most abundant and most rapidly produced antibodies are against the nucleoprotein (N), and the absence of antibodies to N is the most accurate indicator of seronegativity to measles virus. Although not as abundant, antibodies to H and F proteins contribute to virus neutralization and are sufficient to provide protection against measles virus infection.

Evidence for the importance of cellular immunity to measles virus is demonstrated by the ability of children with agammaglobulinemia (congenital inability to produce antibodies) to fully recover from measles, whereas children with severe defects in T-lymphocyte function often develop severe or fatal disease.[14] Monkeys depleted of CD8+ T lymphocytes and challenged with wild-type measles virus had a more extensive rash, higher measles virus loads, and longer duration of viremia than control animals, further confirming the importance of cellular immunity in measles virus clearance.[15] CD4+ T lymphocytes also are activated in response to measles virus infection and secrete cytokines capable of modulating the humoral and cellular immune responses. Plasma cytokine profiles show increased levels of IFN-γ during the acute phase, followed by a shift to high levels of interleukin (IL)-4 and IL-10 during convalescence.[16] The initial predominant Th1 response (characterized by IFN-γ) is essential for viral clearance, and the later Th2 response (characterized by IL-4) promotes the development of measles virus-specific antibodies.

The duration of protective immunity following wild-type measles virus infection is generally thought to be lifelong. The immunologic mechanisms involved in sustaining high levels of neutralizing antibody to measles virus are not completely understood, although general principles of immunologic memory probably govern this process. Immunologic memory to measles virus includes both continued production of measles virus-specific antibodies and the circulation of measles virus-specific CD4+ and CD8+ T lymphocytes.[17] Although immune protection is determined by measurement of antimeasles virus antibodies, long-lasting cellular immune response almost certainly plays an important role in protection from infection. Observations of the measles epidemic on the isolated Faroe Islands in 1846 demonstrated the long-term protective immunity conferred by measles. In this population a measles epidemic occurred decades after the last exposure. Adults who had been exposed earlier were protected despite having no exposures to measles between epidemics. Thus, reexposure to measles virus was not necessary to maintain this long-term protection.[18]

Measles vaccine also induces both humoral and cellular immune responses. Antibodies first appear between 12 and 15 days after vaccination and peak at 21 to 28 days. IgM antibodies appear transiently in blood, IgA antibodies are predominant in mucosal secretions, and IgG antibodies persist in blood for years. Vaccination also induces measles virus-specific T lymphocytes.[17,19] Although both humoral and cellular responses can be induced by measles vaccine, they are of lower magnitude and shorter duration compared to those following wild-type measles virus infection.[20]

Measles Virus-Associated Immune Suppression

The intense immune responses induced by measles virus infection are paradoxically associated with depressed responses to unrelated (nonmeasles virus) antigens, lasting for several weeks to months beyond resolution of the acute illness. This state of immune suppression enhances susceptibility to secondary bacterial and viral infections causing pneumonia and diarrhea, and is responsible for much of the measles-related morbidity and mortality.[21,22] Delayed-type hypersensitivity (DTH) responses to recall antigens, such as tuberculin, are suppressed[23] and cellular and humoral responses to new antigens are impaired following measles virus infection.[24] Reactivation of tuberculosis and remission of autoimmune diseases have been described after measles and are attributed to this state of immune suppression.

Abnormalities of both the innate and adaptive immune responses have been described following measles virus infection. Transient lymphopenia with a reduction in CD4+ and CD8+ T lymphocytes occurs in children following measles virus infection. Functional abnormalities of immune cells have also been detected, including decreased lymphocyte proliferative responses.[25] Dendritic cells, major antigen-presenting cells, mature poorly, lose the ability to stimulate proliferative responses in lymphocytes, and undergo cell death when infected with measles virus in vitro.[26] The dominant Th2 response in children recovering from measles can inhibit Th1 responses and increase susceptibility to intracellular pathogens.[27,28] The production of IL-12, important for the generation of Th1-type immune response, decreases following binding of the CD46 receptor[29] and was low for several weeks in children with measles.[30] This diminished ability to produce IL-12 could further result in a limited Th1 immune response to other pathogens. Furthermore, engagement of CD46 and CD3 on monocytes induced production of high levels of IL-10 and transforming growth factor (TGF)-β, an immunomodulatory and immunosuppressive cytokine profile characteristic of regulatory T cells.[31] The role of these cytokines in the immune suppression following measles is supported by in vivo evidence of elevated levels of IL-10 in the plasma of children after measles virus infection.[16]

Clinical Disease and Complications

Clinically apparent measles begins with a prodrome characterized by fever, cough, coryza (runny nose), and conjunctivitis (Figure 16-1). Koplik's spots, small white lesions on the buccal mucosa inside the mouth, may be visible during the prodrome and allow the astute clinician to diagnose measles prior to the onset of rash. The prodromal symptoms intensify several days before the onset of rash. The characteristic erythematous and maculopapular rash appears first on the face and behind the ears, and then spreads in a centrifugal fashion to the trunk and extremities (Figure 16-2). The rash lasts for 3 to 4 days and fades in the same manner as it appeared. Malnourished children may develop a deeply pigmented rash that desquamates or peels during recovery.

In uncomplicated measles, clinical recovery begins soon after appearance of the rash. Unfortunately, complications occur in up to 40% of measles cases, and the risk of complication is increased by extremes of age and malnutrition.[32] Complications of measles have been described in almost every organ system. The respiratory tract is a frequent site of complication, with pneumonia accounting for most measles-associated deaths.[33] Pneumonia is caused by secondary viral or bacterial infections or by measles virus itself. Pathologically, measles virus infection of the lung is characterized by multinucleated giant cells, formed when measles virus proteins on the cell surface allow cells to fuse together. Other respiratory complications include laryngotracheobronchitis (croup) and otitis media (ear infection). Mouth ulcers, or stomatitis, may hinder children from eating or drinking. Many children with measles develop diarrhea, which further contributes to malnutrition. Eye disease (keratoconjunctivitis) is common after measles, particularly in children with vitamin A deficiency, and is a frequent cause of blindness.

Because the rash of measles is a consequence of the cellular immune response, persons with impaired cellular immunity, such as those with the acquired immunodeficiency syndrome (AIDS), may not develop the characteristic measles rash. These persons have a high case fatality and frequently develop a giant cell pneumonitis caused by measles virus. T-lymphocyte defects due to causes other than human immunodeficiency virus type 1 (HIV-1) infection, such as cancer chemotherapy, also are associated with increased severity of measles.

Rare but serious complications of measles involve the central nervous system. Postmeasles encephalomyelitis complicates approximately 1 in 1000 cases, mainly older children and adults. Encephalomyelitis occurs within two weeks of the onset of rash and is characterized by fever, seizures, and a variety of neurologic abnormalities. The finding of periventricular demyelination, the induction of immune responses to myelin basic protein, and the absence of measles virus in the brain suggest that postmeasles

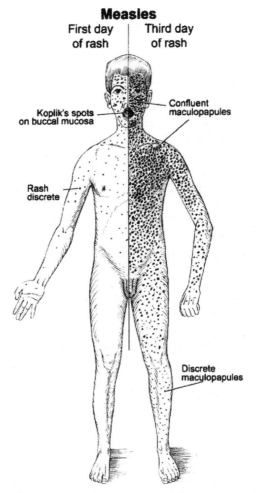

FIGURE 16-2   Development and distribution of measles rash.
Source: Perry RT et al. The Clinical Significance of Measles: A Review, The Journal
of Infectious Diseases. 2004;189:S4–S16. Copyright University of Chicago Press.

encephalomyelitis is an autoimmune disorder triggered by measles virus
infection. Other central nervous system complications that occur months to
years after acute infection are measles inclusion body encephalitis (MIBE)
and subacute sclerosing panencephalitis (SSPE). In contrast to postmeasles
encephalomyelitis, MIBE and SSPE are caused by persistent measles virus
infection. MIBE is a rare but fatal complication that affects individuals with
defective cellular immunity; it typically occurs months after infection. SSPE
is a slowly progressive disease characterized by seizures, progressive deterioration of cognitive and motor functions, followed by death that occurs 5–15
years after measles virus infection. It most often occurs in persons infected
with measles virus before 2 years of age.

There are conflicting and inconclusive data suggesting that measles
virus infection causes or contributes to the development of chronic diseases,
including multiple sclerosis, Paget's disease, inflammatory bowel disease, and

otosclerosis.[34] However, no causal association has been established between measles and these conditions.

Laboratory Diagnosis of Measles

The characteristic clinical features of measles are of sufficient sensitivity and specificity to have high predictive value in regions where measles is endemic. However, laboratory diagnosis is necessary where measles virus transmission rates are low or in immunocompromised persons who may not have the characteristic clinical manifestations. Infection with rubella, parvovirus B19, human herpes virus 6, and dengue viruses may mimic measles. Detection of IgM antibodies to measles virus by enzyme immunoassay (EIA) is the standard method of diagnosing acute measles (Figure 16-1).[35] Alternatively, seroconversion using IgG-specific EIA, hemagglutinin inhibition, complement fixation, or virus neutralization assays can be used to diagnose acute measles based on testing serum or plasma obtained during the acute and convalescent phases.

Measles virus can be isolated in tissue culture from white blood cells, respiratory tract secretions and urine, although the ability to isolate measles virus diminishes quickly after rash onset. Amplification and detection of measles virus RNA by reverse transcription-polymerase chain reaction (RT-PCR) from blood, urine, and nasal discharge is highly sensitive in detecting measles virus RNA and allows sequencing of the measles virus genome for molecular epidemiologic studies.

Disease Burden

The disease burden caused by measles has decreased over the past decades because of a number of factors. Measles mortality declined in developed countries in association with economic development, improved nutritional status, and supportive care, particularly antibiotic therapy for secondary bacterial pneumonia. Remarkable progress in reducing measles incidence and mortality has been, and continues to be, made in resource-poor countries as a consequence of increasing measles vaccine coverage (Figure 16-3), provision of a second opportunity for measles vaccination through supplementary immunization activities (SIA), and efforts by the World Health Organization, the United Nations Children's Fund (UNICEF), and their partners to target 45 countries for accelerated and sustained measles mortality reduction. Specifically, this targeted strategy aims to achieve greater than 90% measles vaccination coverage in every district of the 45 countries and to ensure that all children receive a second opportunity for measles immunization.[36] Provision of vitamin A through polio and measles SIA has contributed further to the reduction in measles mortality.[37]

In 2003, the World Health Assembly endorsed a resolution urging member countries to reduce the number of deaths attributed to measles by 50% by the end of 2005 compared with 1999 estimates. Overall global measles mortality in 2003 was estimated to be 530,000 deaths (uncertainty bounds 383,000 and 731,000 deaths).[37] This estimate represents a 39% decrease from 1999,

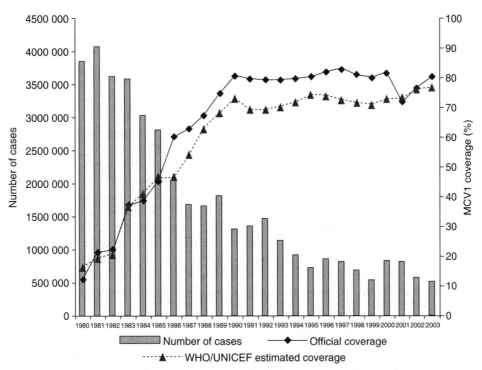

FIGURE 16-3 Global annual reported measles incidence and measles vaccine coverage, 1980–2003.
Source: WHO website (http://www.who.int/vaccines-surveillance/graphics/htmls/measlescascov.htm)

when the global number of measles deaths was estimated to be 873,000 (uncertainty bounds 645,000 and 1,196,000 deaths). The largest decrease in measles mortality was in Africa, where measles mortality decreased 46% from 1999 to 2003. Prior to this, an estimated 30 million cases of measles were estimated to occur each year, with more than 1 million deaths. Despite the progress in reducing measles mortality, measles remains a frequent cause of vaccine-preventable death and an important cause of morbidity and mortality in children, particularly in sub-Saharan Africa.[38]

Estimating Measles Mortality

Accurate assessment of the number of deaths attributable to measles is important in assessing progress in measles control. In the prevaccine era, almost all persons acquired measles, and the number of measles cases could be approximated by the number of births. Deaths due to measles could be estimated by multiplying the number of cases by age-specific case fatality proportions. This relatively simple method of counting measles cases and deaths (assuming the number of births and the case fatality proportion could be accurately estimated) was no longer of use after the introduction of measles vaccination. More sophisticated methods of estimating measles mortality were needed.

The first obstacle in estimating the global number of measles deaths is defining those deaths attributable to measles. The difficulty arises from the fact that much of measles mortality is delayed until after resolution of the rash and is due to secondary infections that arise as a consequence of the prolonged state of immune suppression. Most commonly, death is attributed to measles if it occurs within one month of the onset of rash.

The ideal method for estimating measles mortality is through accurate disease surveillance and registration of deaths. In the absence of accurate disease surveillance, measles mortality models have been developed to estimate the global burden of measles and to monitor the progress of control programs. The World Health Organization used two different methods to estimate the global burden of measles in 2000.[39] In countries with an estimated measles vaccine coverage of greater than 80% and intensive case-based surveillance, measles incidence was estimated by adjusting the reported number of cases by a factor to correct for underreporting. This correction factor reflects the notification efficiency and was estimated to be between 5% and 40%. For countries with moderate to poor measles control, the number of children immune to measles in each country was estimated by multiplying the number of births, the estimated measles vaccine coverage, and the estimated vaccine effectiveness (the proportion of vaccinated children who develop protective immunity). All remaining susceptible children were assumed to develop measles, thus providing an estimate of measles incidence. For both methods, the number of measles deaths was determined by multiplying the number of measles cases by a country- and age-specific case fatality proportion. An advantage of this approach is that adjustments can be made for changes in vaccine coverage. A major weakness is the absence of reliable data to estimate several parameters, particularly the case fatality proportions. Most published data on the case fatality proportion for measles are derived from hospital-based studies and are biased toward more severe disease.

Using a different approach, the proportional mortality caused by measles (and other major causes of child mortality) was derived from community-based studies of mortality of children under 5 years of age by cause in a subset of countries with the highest mortality rates for children under 5 years.[40] A metaregression model was used to relate characteristics of the study population to the proportional mortality outcomes. From this model, the proportional distribution of child deaths by major cause, including measles, was estimated for the selected countries. The number of measles deaths was then calculated by multiplying the total number of deaths in children less than 5 years of age (approximately 10 million) by the measles-specific proportional mortality. Using this method, measles was estimated to cause 1% of deaths in children less than 5 years of age (uncertainty bounds 1% and 9%), compared to 5% of deaths estimated by the World Health Organization.[41] These methods highlight the difficulties in accurately estimating measles mortality and in tracking the progress of control programs.

Epidemiologic Characteristics

Mode of Transmission

Measles virus is transmitted primarily by respiratory droplets small enough to traverse several feet but too large to remain suspended in the air for long periods of time. The symptoms induced during the prodrome, particularly sneezing and coughing, enhance transmission. Measles virus also may be transmitted by the airborne route, suspended on small particles for a prolonged time. Direct contact with infected secretions can transmit measles virus, but the virus does not survive long on fomites as it is quickly killed by heat and ultraviolet radiation. Measles virus is excreted in the urine for several days longer than from the respiratory tract, but this is not a major mode of transmission.

Reservoir

Humans are the only reservoir for measles virus, a fact important for the potential eradication of measles. Nonhuman primates may be infected with measles virus and develop an illness similar to measles in humans, with rash, coryza, and conjunctivitis. However, populations of wild monkeys are not of sufficient size to maintain measles virus transmission.

Incubation Period

The incubation period for measles, the time from infection to clinical disease, is approximately 10 days to the onset of fever and 14 days to the onset of rash. The incubation period may be shorter in infants or following a large inoculum of virus, and it may be longer in adults. During this seemingly quiescent period, the virus is rapidly replicating and infecting target tissues as described above. The incubation period is best measured during outbreaks in which the time of exposure to the index case can be precisely determined. The first accurate measurement of the incubation period for measles was by the Danish physician Peter Panum during the measles outbreak on the sparsely populated Faroe Islands in 1846.

Infectious Period

The infectious period is more difficult to measure than the incubation period as it requires careful observation of the contacts of exposed persons prior to the onset of rash. Generally, persons with measles are infectious for several days before and after the onset of rash, when titers of measles virus in the blood and body fluids are highest (Figure 16-1). As with many other acute viral infections (SARS-coronavirus being a notable exception), the fact that measles virus is contagious prior to the onset of recognizable disease hinders the effectiveness of quarantine measures. Measles virus can be isolated in tissue culture from the urine as late as one week after rash onset. Detection of measles virus in body fluids by a variety of means, including identification of multinucleated giant cells in nasal secretions or the use of RT-PCR, suggests the potential for prolonged infectious periods in persons immunocompromised by severe malnutrition or human immunodeficiency virus type 1 (HIV-1) infection.[11,42] However, whether detection of measles virus by these methods indicates prolonged contagiousness is unclear.

Infectivity

Measles virus is one of the most highly contagious infectious agents and outbreaks can occur in populations in which less than 10% of persons are susceptible. Chains of transmission commonly occur among household contacts, school-age children, and health care workers. The contagiousness of measles virus is best expressed by the basic reproductive number R_0, which represents the mean number of secondary cases that arise if an infectious agent is introduced into a completely susceptible population. R_0 can be empirically measured, although the introduction of measles virus into a completely susceptible population is rare. In the 1951 measles epidemic in Greenland, the index case attended a community dance during the infectious period resulting in a R_0 of 200.[43] R_0 may also be estimated from the average age of infection (A), the life expectancy (L), and the duration of protection from maternally acquired antibodies (M) using the following equation:

$$R_0 = (L - M)/(A - M)$$

The estimated R_0 for measles virus is 12–18, compared to only 5–7 for smallpox virus and 2–3 for SARS-coronavirus. The high infectivity of measles virus implies that a high level of population immunity is required to interrupt measles virus transmission, as described below. Previously vaccinated children who acquire measles are less infectious than unvaccinated index cases.

Maternally Acquired Antimeasles Antibodies

Young infants in the first months of life are protected against measles by maternally acquired IgG antibodies. An active transport mechanism in the placenta is responsible for the transfer of IgG antibodies from the maternal circulation to the fetus starting at about 28 weeks gestation and continuing until birth.[44] Three factors determine the degree and duration of protection in the newborn: (1) the level of maternal antimeasles antibodies; (2) the efficiency of placental transfer; and (3) the rate of catabolism in the child. Although providing passive immunity to young infants, maternally acquired antibodies can interfere with the immune responses to the attenuated measles vaccine by inhibiting replication of vaccine virus. In general, maternally acquired antibodies are no longer present in the majority of children by 9 months of age, the time of routine measles vaccination in many countries. The half-life of antimeasles antibodies was estimated to be 48 days in the United States and Finland, but it is shorter in developing countries. Women with vaccine-induced immunity tend to have lower antimeasles virus antibody titers than women with naturally acquired immunity, and their children may be susceptible to measles at an earlier age. Infants born to HIV-infected women may have lower levels of protective maternal antibodies independent of their own HIV infection status and may thus be susceptible to measles at a younger age.[7]

Average Age of Infection

The average age of measles virus infection depends upon the rate of contact with infected persons, the rate of decline of protective maternal antibodies, and the vaccine coverage rate. Infants in the first few months of life are protected by passively acquired maternal antibodies, and measles is rare in this age group.

In densely populated urban settings with low vaccination coverage rates, measles is a disease of young children. The cumulative distribution can reach 50% by 1 year of age, with a significant proportion of children acquiring measles virus infection before 9 months, the age of routine vaccination. As measles vaccine coverage increases, or population density decreases, the age distribution shifts toward older children. In such situations, measles cases predominate in school-age children. Infants and younger children, although susceptible if not protected by immunization, are not exposed to measles virus at a rate sufficient to cause a large disease burden in this age group. As vaccination coverage increases further, the age distribution of cases may be shifted into adolescence and young adulthood, as seen in measles outbreaks in the United States, Brazil, and Australia,[45-47] and necessitating targeted measles vaccination programs for these older age groups.

Geographic Distribution

Measles is a global disease but may have been absent from the Americas prior to contact with Europeans. Measles, in combination with smallpox, likely was responsible for large numbers of deaths of Native Americans, facilitating European conquest.[48] Progress in measles elimination efforts has resulted in the interruption of measles virus transmission in large geographic regions, including the Americas. Because of its mode of transmission and high infectivity, measles virus is most readily maintained in densely populated urban settings. Migration of infected persons to rural areas results in outbreaks in susceptible rural populations too small to maintain measles virus transmission. An extreme example occurs in isolated island populations where periodic introduction of measles virus results in widespread but self-limiting outbreaks.

Population Size and Measles Virus Transmission

To provide a sufficient number of new susceptibles through births to maintain measles virus transmission, a population size of several hundred thousand persons with 5000–10,000 births per year is required.[49] Measles virus is believed to have become established in human populations about 5000 to 10,000 years ago when human populations achieved sufficient size in the Middle Eastern river valley civilizations to maintain virus transmission. Measles virus presumably was a zoonotic infection, resulting from the cross-species transmission of an ancestral morbillivirus, likely from domesticated cattle.

Transmission Dynamics

Measles incidence has a typical temporal pattern characterized by yearly seasonal epidemics superimposed upon longer epidemic cycles of 2 to 5 years or more (Figure 16-4). These epidemic cycles have been well documented over many decades in different geographic locations and have been characterized analytically in both simple and sophisticated mathematic models. In

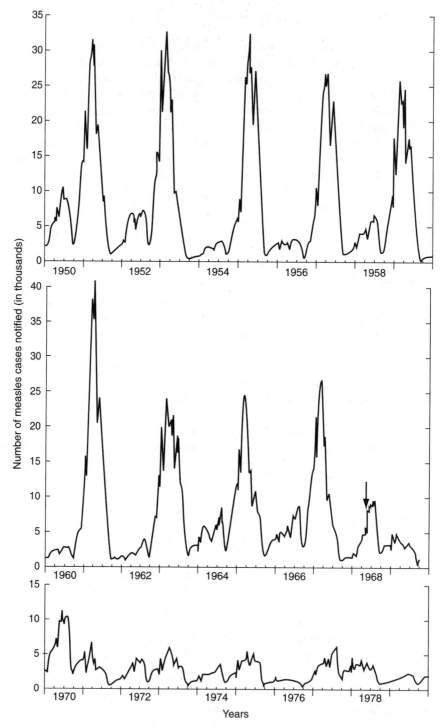

FIGURE 16-4 Measles notifications in England and Wales, by week, 1950–79. The arrow indicates the beginning of the national measles vaccination programme in 1968.
Source: Fine PE and Clarkson JA. Measles in England and Wales—I. An analysis of factors underlying seasonal patterns. Int J Epidemiol 1982;11:5–14, by permission of The Oxford University Press.

temperate climates, annual measles outbreaks typically occur in the late winter and early spring. These annual outbreaks are likely the result of social networks facilitating transmission (e.g., congregation of children at school) and environmental factors favoring the viability and transmission of measles virus.[50] Measles cases continue to occur during the interepidemic period in large populations but at low incidence. The longer cycles occurring every several years result from the accumulation of susceptible persons over successive birth cohorts and the subsequent decline in the number of susceptibles following an outbreak. In the absence of a vaccination program these longer epidemic cycles tend to occur every 2 to 4 years. Measles vaccination programs that achieve coverage rates in excess of 80% extend the interepidemic period to 4–8 years by reducing the number of susceptibles.

Modeling Measles Virus Transmission Dynamics

Because of characteristic epidemic cycles, measles has served as a model for understanding the transmission dynamics of an acute infectious disease and the impact of different vaccination strategies. Mathematic modeling of measles dynamics was first attempted 100 years ago by Sir William Hamer.[51] The basic principle underlying early models was the law of mass action, in which the periodicity of measles incidence was described as a function of the changing number of infectious and susceptible persons as they contact one another. The number of susceptible persons, in turn, was determined by the introduction of new susceptibles through birth and the removal of susceptibles through the acquisition of protective immunity following infection. However, the epidemic cycles generated by these simple deterministic models approached a steady state, losing their periodicity. The introduction of stochastic (chance) and seasonal processes resulted in models of measles epidemics that closely resembled observed data. Further development of these models allowed for predictions of the impact of vaccination strategies on various epidemiologic characteristics of measles virus transmission, including the increase in the average age of infection and the interepidemic period.[52] More sophisticated models of measles virus transmission dynamics have investigated the role of nonlinear dynamics in temporal and spatial patterns of measles incidence,[53] traveling waves of infection originating in large cities and spreading to small towns,[54] and the loss of spatial synchrony in measles epidemics following the introduction of measles vaccination.[55]

Measles Mortality

Case Fatality

Measles case fatality proportions vary widely, depending upon the average age of infection, nutritional status of the population, measles vaccine coverage, and access to health care. In developed countries, such at the United States, less than 1 in 1000 children with measles die. In endemic areas in sub-Saharan Africa, the measles case fatality proportion may be 5%. Measles is a major cause of child deaths in refugee camps and in internally displaced populations. Measles case fatality proportions in children in complex emergencies have been as high as 20–30%. During a famine in Ethiopia, measles alone or in combination with wasting accounted for 22% of 159 deaths among children younger than 5 years of age, and 17% of 72 deaths among children aged 5 to 14 years.[56]

The measles case fatality proportion is highest at extremes of age. Exposure to an index case within the household may result in more severe disease, perhaps because of transmission of a larger inoculum of virus.[57] Vaccinated children, should they develop disease after exposure, have less severe disease and significantly lower mortality rates. Vaccination programs, by increasing the average age of infection, shift the burden of disease out of the age group with the highest case fatality (infancy), further reducing measles mortality.

Nutritional Status

Measles and malnutrition have important bidirectional interactions. Measles is more severe in malnourished children, although separating the independent effects of nutritional and socioeconomic factors is often difficult. Children with severe malnutrition, such as those with marasmus or kwashiorkor, are at particular risk of death following measles. Measles, in turn, can exacerbate malnutrition by decreasing intake (particularly in children with mouth ulcers), increasing metabolic demands, and enhancing gastrointestinal loss of nutrients as a consequence of a protein-losing enteropathy.[58] Measles in persons with vitamin A deficiency leads to severe keratitis, corneal scarring, and blindness.[59]

Sex Differences

Interestingly, data suggest that measles mortality may be higher in girls. Among persons of different ages and across different regions, measles mortality in girls was estimated to be 5% higher than in boys.[60] Although older historical data and recent surveillance data from the United States do not support this conclusion,[34] if true, the higher mortality in girls is in contrast to most infectious diseases in which disease severity and mortality is highest in males. Supporting the hypothesis of biologic differences in the response to measles virus was the observation that girls were more likely than boys to have delayed mortality following receipt of high-titer measles vaccine.[61] The underlying mechanisms are likely differences in immune responses to measles virus between girls and boys, although no cogent theory has been developed.

Host Genetics

All persons without preexisting protective immunity are believed to be susceptible to infection with measles virus, and geographic differences in disease severity and mortality are likely due to environmental and nutritional factors rather than genetic differences. Nevertheless, genetic factors (e.g., genes regulating cytokine production) may explain some of the differences in response to measles virus between individuals. The host genetics underlying immune responses to measles vaccine have been more extensively studied and suggest that polymorphisms in human leukocyte antigen (HLA) genes are associated with differences in antibody responses.[62]

Measles Vaccine

Attenuation of measles virus is commonly achieved by serial passage in chick embryo cells. The first attenuated measles vaccine licensed in the United States was called Edmonston B. This vaccine was safe and immunogenic but frequently was associated with fever and rash. The Schwarz and Moraten ("more attenuated") strains were derived from the original Edmonston strain but further attenuated through passage in chick embryo fibroblasts. Despite differences in their passage history, these vaccine strains have identical genomic sequences.[63] The Moraten vaccine (Merck) is the only measles vaccine used in the United States, whereas the Schwarz vaccine is used in many countries throughout the world. Other attenuated measles vaccines have been produced from locally derived wild-type strains, particularly in Russia, China, and Japan. One vaccine strain, the Edmonston-Zagreb vaccine, was passaged in human diploid cells rather than chick embryo fibroblasts, which may be responsible for its increased immunogenicity and reactogenicity. Measles vaccines are relatively heat stable in the lyophilized (dry) form, but rapidly lose potency when exposed to heat after reconstitution.

Measles vaccines are administered by subcutaneous injection, necessitating needles, syringes, and trained health care workers. Proper disposal of used needles and syringes can be a major logistic problem, particularly after mass vaccination campaigns. Autodestruct syringes are widely used in mass measles vaccination campaigns to prevent reuse. Aerosol administration of measles vaccine was first evaluated in the early 1960s in several countries, including the former Soviet Union and the United States. More recent studies in South Africa and Mexico have shown that aerosol administration of measles vaccine is highly effective in boosting antibody titers, although the primary immune response to aerosol measles vaccine is lower than following subcutaneous administration.[19,64,65] Administration of measles vaccine by aerosol has the potential to greatly facilitate measles vaccination during mass campaigns, and the World Health Organization plans to test and bring to licensure an aerosol measles vaccine by 2009.

Formalin-Inactivated Measles Vaccine and Atypical Measles

In the 1960s, a formalin-inactivated, alum-precipitated measles vaccine (FIMV) was licensed and administered to children in the United States. Three doses of inactivated vaccine elicited a protective antibody response that waned within months.[66] Up to 60% of immunized children exposed to measles developed atypical measles, characterized by high fever, pneumonitis, and a petechial rash on the extremities,[67,68] leading to withdrawal of the FIMV in 1967. In a rhesus macaque model, atypical measles was shown to be associated with immune complex deposition in affected tissues and a systemic and pulmonary eosinophilia.[69] The antibody response consisted of high levels of complement fixing antibodies with low avidity for measles virus, characteristics that may have promoted exaggerated immune complex formation and disease.

High-Titer Measles Vaccines

Seroconversion rates with attenuated measles vaccines in young infants are low because of immunologic immaturity and the interference of transplacentally acquired maternal antibodies with replication of vaccine virus.[70] To protect young infants against measles, high-titer preparations containing 10–100 times the standard dose of vaccine virus were evaluated in several countries. Seroconversion rates in 4 to 6-month-old infants immunized with high-titer measles vaccine were comparable to those of 9- to 15-month-old children vaccinated with standard-titer measles vaccine, and the protective antibody response persisted for over 2 years. But high-titer measles vaccine resulted in a poorly understood increase in mortality in immunized girls 1 to 2 years after vaccination compared to girls immunized with standard-titer vaccine at 9 months of age.[71,72] The increased mortality was attributable to secondary infections commonly associated with measles, such as diarrhea and pneumonia. Although these studies were carried out in countries with different levels of socioeconomic development, excess mortality was observed only in countries with poor socioeconomic conditions and frequent malnutrition (Senegal, Haiti, and Guinea Bissau). The basis for the increased mortality in girls is not understood.

Measures of Protection

Measles vaccine efficacy under study conditions, or effectiveness under field conditions, is measured as 1 minus a measure of the relative risk in the vaccinated group compared to the unvaccinated group (VE = 1 − RR). A number of field methods and study designs can be used to measure measles vaccine efficacy.[73,74] For example, measles vaccine efficacy can be estimated by measuring the proportion of measles cases occurring in vaccinated persons and the proportion of the population that is vaccinated. Measles vaccine efficacy (VE) then can be calculated using the following equation:

$$VE = \frac{PPV - PCV}{PPV - (PCV \times PPV)}$$

where PPV is the proportion of the population that is vaccinated against measles and PCV is the proportion of measles cases that are vaccinated.

More commonly, immunologic markers of protective immunity are used to assess measles vaccines. Measurement of antibodies to measles virus by the plaque reduction neutralization assay is best correlated with protection from infection and remains the gold standard for determination of protective antibody titers. Neutralizing antibody levels of 120 mIU/mL (or 200 mIU/mL depending upon the WHO reference serum used) are considered protective following vaccination.[75]

Determinants and Duration of Protection

The proportion of children who develop protective antibody titers following measles vaccination depends on the presence of inhibitory maternal antibodies and the immunologic maturity of the vaccine recipient, as well as dose and strain of vaccine virus. Frequently cited figures are that approximately 85% of children develop protective antibody titers when given measles vaccine at 9 months of age and 90–95% respond when vaccinated at 12 months of age.[76] Concurrent acute infections may interfere with the immune response to measles vaccine, although this is probably uncommon.[77] Polymorphisms in human immune response genes also determine immune responses to measles vaccine.[62]

The duration of immunity following measles vaccination is more variable and shorter than following wild-type measles virus infection, with an estimated 5% of children developing secondary vaccine failure at 10 to 15 years after vaccination.[78] Immunologic boosting from repeated exposure to measles virus may play a role in maintaining protective antibody levels in communities with measles virus transmission.[79]

Optimal Age of Vaccination

The optimal age of measles vaccination is determined by consideration of the age-dependent increase in seroconversion following measles vaccination and the average age of infection (Figure 16-5). In regions of intense measles virus transmission, the average age of infection is low and the optimal strategy is to vaccinate against measles as young as possible. However, both maternally acquired antibodies and immunologic immaturity reduce the protective efficacy of measles vaccination in early infancy.[70] In many parts of the world, 9 months is considered the optimal age of measles vaccination and is the age recommended by the Expanded Programme on Immunization (EPI).[80] Most countries following the EPI schedule administer measles vaccine alone, although more countries are introducing combined measles and rubella vaccines as rubella control programs expand. In

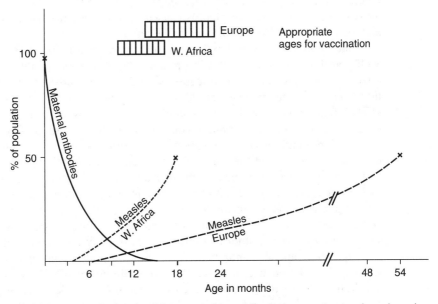

FIGURE 16-5   Estimation of the optimal age of measles vaccination based on the rate of loss of maternal antibodies and the age of measles virus infection. *Source:* Walsh JA. Rev Infect Dis 1983;5:330–340.

communities with intense measles virus transmission, a significant proportion of children may acquire measles before 9 months of age. For example,
in Lusaka, Zambia, one quarter of HIV-uninfected and one third of HIV-
infected children hospitalized with measles were less than 9 months of age.[81]
Under some circumstances, provision of an early dose of measles vaccine at 6
months of age (e.g., in outbreaks or to HIV-infected children) is appropriate.
In contrast, in regions that have achieved measles control or elimination and
where the risk of measles in infants is low, the age of measles vaccination
is increased to ensure that a higher proportion of children develop protective immunity. For example, in the United States the first dose of measles
vaccine is administered at 12–15 months of age, as a combined measles,
mumps, and rubella (MMR) vaccine.

Adverse Events Associated with Measles Vaccine

Fever occurs in approximately 5% to 15% of recipients 6 to 12 days following
measles vaccination, and a rash occurs in approximately 5% of recipients.
These signs and symptoms are a consequence of the host immune response
to replicating measles vaccine virus but do not result in serious morbidity or
mortality. Rarely, thrombocytopenia (low platelets) may occur.

Although assumed to be rare, the risk of disease caused by attenuated
measles vaccine virus in HIV-infected persons is unknown. The only documented case of disease induced by vaccine virus in an HIV-infected person
was in a 20-year-old man who died 15 months after receiving his second
dose of measles vaccine.[82] He had a very low CD4+ T-lymphocyte cell count
but no HIV-related symptoms at the time of vaccination. Ten months later he
developed a giant cell pneumonitis, and measles vaccine virus was identified
in his lung. Fatal, disseminated infection with measles vaccine virus has been
reported rarely in persons with other impairments of immune function,[83] and
measles inclusion body encephalitis caused by vaccine virus was reported in
a child with an uncharacterized immune deficiency.[84]

Much public attention has focused on a purported association between
MMR vaccine and autism following publication of a report in 1998 hypoth-
esizing that MMR vaccine may cause a syndrome of autism and intestinal
inflammation.[85] The events that followed, and the public concern over the
safety of MMR vaccine, led to diminished vaccine coverage in the United
Kingdom and provide important lessons in the misinterpretation of epidemiologic evidence and the communication of scientific results to the public.[86] The
publication that incited the concern was a case series describing 12 children
with a regressive developmental disorder and chronic enterocolitis. Nine of
the children had autism. Onset of the developmental delay was associated by
the parents with MMR vaccination in 8 children. This simple temporal association was misinterpreted and misrepresented as a possible causal relationship, first by the lead author of the study and then by the media and public.
Subsequently, several comprehensive reviews and additional epidemiologic
studies rejected evidence of a causal relationship between MMR vaccination
and autism.[87] One of the most conclusive studies was a large retrospective
cohort study of over half a million Danish children that found the relative
risk of MMR vaccine to be 0.92 (95% confidence interval, 0.68–1.24) for
autistic disorder.[88]

Potential Nonspecific Benefits of Measles Vaccination on Child Health

A group of investigators has suggested that vaccination with standard-titer measles vaccine, or mild infection with wild-type measles virus, may have nonspecific beneficial effects resulting in reduced child mortality in excess of deaths attributable to measles.[89-91] Evidence for a nonspecific beneficial effect of standard-titer measles vaccine includes: (1) the protective efficacy against death after measles vaccination (30% to 86%) exceeds the expected efficacy attributable to a reduction in measles deaths (10%);[89] (2) in the absence of a history of measles, children vaccinated against measles have a lower mortality rate than children who did not receive measles vaccine;[89] and (3) measles vaccination at 6 months of age results in a lower overall mortality than vaccination at 9 months of age despite a reduction in seroconversion rates, presumably due to a reduction in nonmeasles deaths.[92] If true, these findings would imply a reevaluation of the age of administration and number of doses of measles vaccine, and the possible need to continue measles vaccination even after measles elimination or eradication. A study in Bangladesh by another group of investigators appeared to support the hypothesis of a nonspecific beneficial effect of measles vaccination on child survival.[93] However, the hypothesis that measles vaccination results in a nonspecific reduction in childhood mortality remains controversial and unproven and is based on potentially biased or confounded data.[94,95] For example, access to the vaccine may indicate a higher level of health care than for those children who were not vaccinated.

Measles Control, Elimination, and Eradication

Different goals for measles control have been established, necessitating different vaccination strategies. Three broad goals can be defined: mortality reduction, regional elimination, and global eradication.

Mortality Reduction

Mortality reduction, the least demanding of the three goals, calls for a reduction in measles mortality from a predetermined level through reductions in incidence, case fatality, or both. Although a reduction in case fatality using appropriate case management (see below) is an important component, measles mortality reduction is achieved largely through a reduction in incidence. To reduce incidence, measles vaccine is administered as a single dose through routine immunization services in child health clinics, with the optimal age of immunization determined by the transmission intensity and rate of decline of maternal antibodies. The Expanded Programme on Immunization recommends a single dose of measles vaccine at 9 months of age. If vaccination coverage is sufficiently high, substantial reductions in incidence and mortality occur, the interepidemic period lengthens, and the age distribution shifts toward older children, further contributing to a reduction in case fatality.

Regional Elimination

Measles elimination is the interruption of measles virus transmission within a defined geographic area, such as country, continent, or World Health Organization region. Small outbreaks of primary and secondary cases may still occur following importation from outside the region, but sustained transmission does not occur. Because of the high infectivity of measles virus and the fact that not all persons develop protective immunity following vaccination, a single-dose of measles vaccine does not achieve a sufficient level of population immunity to eliminate measles. A second opportunity for measles immunization is necessary to eliminate measles by providing protective immunity to children who failed to respond to the first dose and to those who were not previously vaccinated. Two broad strategies to administer the second dose have been used. In countries with sufficient infrastructure, the second dose of measles vaccine is administered through routine immunization services, typically prior to the start of school (4–6 years of age). High coverage levels are ensured by school entry requirements. A second approach, first developed by the Pan American Health Organization (PAHO) for South and Central America,[96] involves mass immunization campaigns (called supplementary immunization activities, or SIA) to deliver the second dose of measles vaccine. This strategy was very successful in eliminating measles in South and Central America and has resulted in a marked reduction in measles incidence and mortality in parts of sub-Saharan Africa.[97]

The PAHO strategy consists of four subprograms: catch-up, keep-up, follow-up, and mop-up (Figure 16-6).[96] The catch-up phase is a one-time, mass immunization campaign that targets all children within a broad age group regardless of whether they have previously had wild-type measles virus infection or measles vaccination. The goal is to rapidly achieve a high level of population immunity and interrupt measles virus transmission. These campaigns are conducted over a short period of time, usually over several weeks, and during a low transmission season. Under the PAHO strategy, children 9 months to 14 years of age were targeted for vaccination. In many countries, this is a substantial proportion of the total population. The appropriate target age range depends upon the age distribution of measles seropositivity. In regions endemic for measles, the vast majority of older children are likely to be immune. Nevertheless, seroprevalence studies usually are not conducted prior to catch-up campaigns, and this broad age range first adopted by PAHO has been widely used in sub-Saharan Africa. These campaigns require large investments of financial resources and personnel; extensive logistical planning to transport and store vaccines, maintain cold chains, and dispose of syringes and needles; and community mobilization to ensure participation. But if successful, supplementary immunization activities are cost effective and can abruptly interrupt measles virus transmission with dramatic declines in incidence and mortality.[98,99]

Keep-up refers to the need to maintain greater than 90% routine measles vaccine coverage through improved access to measles vaccination and a reduction in missed opportunities (e.g., because of false contraindications to vaccination). Follow-up refers to periodic mass campaigns to prevent the accumulation of susceptible children. Follow-up campaigns typically target children 1 to 4 years of age, a narrower age group than targeted in catch-up

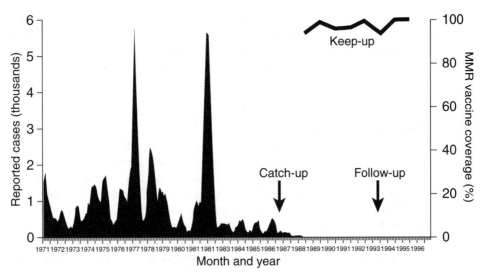

Month and year

Note: Measles cases reported through 31 December 1996.

FIGURE 16-6   Measles vaccination campaign impact on morbidity: Cuba, 1971–1996.
Source: Measles Eradication Field Guide. Pan American Health Organization. Technical
Paper No. 41. Washington DC, 1999.

campaigns. Follow-up campaigns should be conducted when the estimated
number of susceptible children reaches the size of one birth cohort, generally every 3 to 5 years after the catch-up campaign. Mop-up campaigns
target difficult to reach children in sites of measles outbreaks or low vaccine
coverage. Difficult to reach children include those living on the street or in
areas of conflict.

Two doses of measles vaccine are recommended in two situations apart
from an elimination strategy. In communities where measles occurs in a significant proportion of children less than 9 months of age, measles vaccine
should be administered at 6 months of age and repeated at 9 months of age.
Such a situation may arise in a refugee camp or densely populated urban slum
area with intense measles virus transmission. Two doses of measles vaccine
also are recommended for HIV-infected children. Although there is limited
data at present to support this recommendation, HIV-infected children are
at risk of severe and fatal measles and likely are less immunocompromised
at 6 months of age. However, in much of sub-Saharan Africa where HIV
prevalence rates are highest, most HIV-infected children are not diagnosed
until later in life when they present with severe illness. This may change with
increased access to antiretroviral drugs.

Global Eradication

Eradication refers to the global interruption of transmission of an infectious
agent. The pathogen need not be extinct (e.g., laboratory isolates of smallpox
exist), but human infection and disease have ceased. Following eradication,
control efforts such as vaccination programs and disease surveillance can

cease. The possibility of measles eradication has been discussed for almost 40 years.[100] Serious discussion of measles eradication began in the late 1960s as smallpox eradication was nearing completion and the effective, long-term immunity induced by measles vaccine became apparent. Measles virus meets many of the biologic criteria for disease eradication. Measles virus has no nonhuman reservoir, is accurately diagnosed, and measles vaccination is a highly effective intervention. Although measles virus displays sufficient genetic variability to conduct molecular epidemiologic analyses, the antigenic epitopes against which protective antibodies develop have remained stable. In this sense, measles virus is a monotypic virus: vaccines derived from a measles virus isolate from the United States in the 1950s remains protective across space and time. The reason measles virus has not mutated significantly is not fully known, but presumably the antigenic epitopes that confer protective immunity are critical to viral entry and replication. Where measles virus differs from smallpox and polio viruses is that it is more highly infectious, necessitating much higher levels of population immunity to interrupt transmission (see below).

The vaccination strategy necessary for measles eradication is not different from that of elimination, only that the target population is global. The success of measles elimination in large geographic regions suggests that measles eradication is possible. Two doses of measles vaccine, administered through routine immunization services or via supplementary immunization activities, would need to be administered to the children of the world. Many believe this to be a realistic and morally imperative goal, but, as polio eradication efforts have shown, the endgame may be full of challenges.

Case Management

Although the most important strategy to reduce the number of measles deaths is primary prevention through vaccination, secondary prevention of deaths also is important. No specific antiviral drug is used routinely to treat measles virus infection, although the broad antiviral agent ribavirin has been used to treat immunocompromised persons or persons with SSPE, alone or in combination with interferon-γ or intravenous immunoglobulin.[101,102] Intravenous immunoglobulin also has been used to prevent severe measles in high-risk individuals following exposure, but as with ribavirin, the high cost precludes its use in most regions where measles is endemic.

The major components of case management include provision of vitamin A, prompt treatment of secondary bacterial infections, and nutritional support. Several placebo-controlled trials have demonstrated marked reductions in morbidity and mortality in hospitalized children with measles treated with vitamin A. The World Health Organization recommends administration of two daily doses of 200,000 IU of vitamin A to all children with measles 12 months of age or older. Lower doses (100,000 IU) are recommended for children less than 12 months of age. Overall, this regimen results in a 64% reduction in the risk of mortality (RR = 0.36, 95% CI, 0.14–0.82).[103] Pneumonia-specific mortality is reduced, and the impact is greatest in children less than 2 years of age.[103] The mechanisms by which vitamin A reduces measles morbidity and mortality are not known, but likely these effects are mediated through beneficial effects on epithelial cells and host immune responses.

Secondary bacterial infections are a major cause of morbidity and mortality following measles,[33] and effective case management involves prompt treatment with antibiotics. Various strategies have been used to guide antibiotic therapy in children with measles. Antibiotics are indicated for children with measles who have clinical evidence of bacterial infection, including pneumonia, otitis media, skin infection, eye infection, or severe mouth ulcers. *Streptococcus pneumoniae* and *Haemophilus influenzae* type b are the most common causes of bacterial pneumonia following measles, and antibiotic therapy should be directed against these pathogens. Whether all children with measles, or all hospitalized children with measles, should be given prophylactic antibiotics remains controversial. Limited evidence suggests that antibiotics administered as prophylaxis to all children presenting with measles may reduce the incidence of pneumonia but not mortality.[33] The potential benefits of antibiotic prophylaxis need to be weighed against the risks of accelerating antibiotic resistance.

Vitamin A Prophylaxis

Vitamin A has been widely distributed through polio and measles SIAs as well as through routine child health services. Pooled analysis of community-based studies of vitamin A supplementation of apparently healthy children resulted in a 39% reduction in measles-associated mortality.[104] Thus, vitamin A is not only effective in reducing mortality when used to treat hospitalized children with measles, but community-based supplementation programs can result in measles mortality reduction.

Surveillance and Outbreak Investigation

Disease surveillance is an important component of measles elimination programs, providing estimates of measles incidence and mortality, the effectiveness of the control program, and information to support targeted interventions. Case-based surveillance with laboratory confirmation of suspected cases should be the gold standard. Not all suspected cases in an outbreak need to be laboratory confirmed if they can be epidemiologically linked to a confirmed case. As the incidence of measles declines, other viral causes of fever and rash may be mistaken for measles. Other viral infections that can mimic measles are rubella, parvovirus B19, human herpes virus 6, and dengue virus, and many surveillance programs test specimens for rubella virus-specific IgM antibodies. Although confirmation typically requires detection of antimeasles virus IgM antibodies in plasma or serum, less invasive specimen collection methods, including oral fluid swabs and dried blood spots collected on filter paper, may be more acceptable.[35]

Molecular Epidemiology

Although measles virus is considered to be monotypic, variability within the genome is sufficient to allow for molecular epidemiologic investigation. Genetic characterization of wild-type measles viruses is based on sequence analysis of the genes coding for the N and H proteins. One of the most variable regions of the measles virus genome is the 450-nucleotide sequence at the carboxy-terminal of the N protein, with up to 12% variability between wild-type viruses. The World Health Organization recognizes eight clades of measles virus (designated A through H) and 23 genotypes (Figure 16-7).[105] New genotypes will likely be identified with enhanced surveillance and molecular characterization. As measles control efforts intensify, molecular surveillance of circulating measles virus strains can be used to document interruption of measles virus transmission and to identify the source and transmission pathways of measles virus outbreaks.[106]

Obstacles to Measles Control and Prospects for Eradication

The build-up of susceptible children over time in a population is the most serious obstacle to measles eradication.

—PAHO Measles Eradication Field Guide[96]

Herd Immunity Threshold

Interruption of measles virus transmission does not require that all persons be immunized and protected. If a sufficient proportion of the population is immune, the chance that an unprotected person will encounter an infectious individual is reduced to almost zero. Protection of unvaccinated persons by a reduction in the risk of exposure is referred to as herd immunity,[107] and the level of population immunity necessary to interrupt transmission is known as the herd immunity threshold (H). The herd immunity threshold can be derived using analytical models of infectious disease dynamics from the equation:

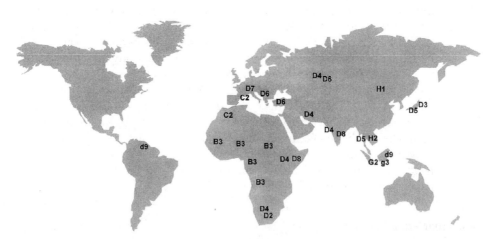

FIGURE 16-7   Distribution of measles genotypes associated with endemic transmission in various areas of the world based on information available in 2002. Genotype designations are shown for each measles-endemic area where virologic surveillance has been conducted. *Source:* Bellini WJ et al. Update on the Global Distribution of Genotypes of Wild Type Measles Viruses, *Journal of Infectious Diseases* 2003;187(Suppl 1):S274. Copyright University of Chicago Press.

$$H = 1 - 1/R_o$$

where R_o is the basic reproductive number.[52] A number of assumptions are made in deriving this formula, including the unrealistic assumption of homogenous mixing of the population (i.e., an individual has an equal chance of coming into contact with any other individual). Nevertheless, this simple equation provides a means of assessing the level of population immunity required to interrupt transmission based upon a measure of infectivity (R_o). For measles, with an R_o of 12–18, the herd immunity threshold is 93–95%. This does not represent vaccine coverage but the proportion of the population protected against measles. As we have seen, this level of population immunity cannot be achieved with a single dose of measles vaccine in which the primary vaccine failure rate is about 15% when administered at 9 months of age. In contrast, for smallpox and polio viruses, each with an R_o of 5–7, the herd immunity threshold is estimated to be 80–85%. Clearly, much higher levels of population immunity are required to interrupt transmission of measles virus than for smallpox or polio viruses.

Measles Outbreaks in Highly Vaccinated Populations

Measles outbreaks have been reported in highly vaccinated populations,[108–110] demonstrating the highly contagious nature of measles and the inability of a single dose of measles vaccine to provide sufficient levels of population immunity to prevent measles virus transmission. Furthermore, in several carefully investigated measles outbreaks in highly vaccinated persons, mild or asymptomatic measles virus infection was demonstrated by a boosting of antimeasles virus antibodies in vaccinated persons, evidence that prior immunity can prevent disease manifestations but not necessarily infection.[111–113]

Failure to Vaccinate

The most important reason for not achieving high levels of population immunity is the failure to vaccinate susceptible persons. Underlying this failure are several causes, including insufficient resources, lack of political will, populations that are difficult to reach (e.g., street children, nomadic persons), fear of real or perceived adverse events, and religious or philosophical objections to vaccination.

The problem of limited resources remains an important one for many countries with a high burden of disease caused by measles, particularly in parts of sub-Saharan Africa. Many of these countries have high child and adult mortality rates, and are attempting to deal with epidemics of tuberculosis, HIV, and malaria in addition to the common causes of child mortality from pneumonia, diarrhea, and undernutrition. However, successful efforts to generate funds to support measles control efforts have been made. Of particular importance has been the Africa Measles Initiative. Led by the American Red Cross, Centers for Disease Control and Prevention, UNICEF, WHO, and the United Nations Foundation, by early 2005 this initiative had mobilized $144 million to support African countries in their measles mortality reduction efforts and the vaccination of 150 million children against measles.

The political commitment to control measles is high in much of sub-Saharan Africa and Asia where measles is known to be a major cause of child mortality, but low in some industrialized countries, including Japan, Italy, France, and Germany, where measles vaccine coverage is low.[114] Measles eradication requires the full political commitment of all countries.

Following the public scare surrounding the alleged association between MMR vaccine and autism, measles vaccine coverage in the United Kingdom declined from 91% in 1998 to only 79% in 2003. The decline in measles vaccine coverage coincided with several large measles outbreaks and the potential for the basic reproductive number to exceed 1 and the reestablishment of endemic measles.[115] Measles outbreaks have been reported in religious communities with low vaccine coverage,[116] further highlighting the ability of measles virus to cause disease and death in pockets of susceptible persons. A measles outbreak in the Netherlands began in a community with religious objections to measles vaccination and subsequently spread to involve almost 3000 persons, with 5 deaths.[117]

Vaccine Failure

A less common cause for not achieving high levels of population immunity is vaccine failure. As described above, primary vaccine failure occurs in approximately 15% of children vaccinated at 9 months of age and 5–10% of children vaccinated at 1 year of age.[76] Improper administration of measles vaccine and loss of immunogenicity because of inadequate storage are less common causes of measles vaccine failure. It is important to recognize that as measles vaccine coverage increases, the proportion of cases in vaccinated children also increases. This is sometimes misinterpreted as a loss of vaccine potency (e.g., because of inadequate vaccine storage), but merely reflects the fact that with sufficiently high vaccination coverage rates, a greater proportion of cases will occur in children who did not respond to the first dose of measles vaccine than in children who were never vaccinated.

Subclinical Measles

Subclinical measles is defined as a fourfold rise in measles virus-specific IgG antibodies following exposure to wild-type measles virus in an asymptomatic individual with some prior measles immunity. Subclinical infection may be important in boosting protective antibody levels in children with waning immunity,[79] but it raises the concern that persons with incomplete immunity and subclinical infection may be capable of transmitting measles virus. Whether partially immune individuals with subclinical infection can sustain measles virus transmission is unknown. Measles virus has been isolated from a naturally immune, asymptomatically reinfected individual,[118] and extensive epidemiologic investigation of a person with measles in the Netherlands failed to identify a contact with clinically apparent measles, implying transmission from a person with subclinical infection.[119]

HIV Epidemic

In regions of high HIV prevalence and crowding, such as urban centers in sub-Saharan Africa, HIV-infected children could play a role in the sustained transmission of measles virus.[120] HIV-infected mothers may have defective transfer of IgG antibody across the placenta, resulting in lower titers of protective antibodies in the infant and enlarging the period of susceptibility to measles virus infection prior to routine immunization. HIV-infected children may not have an adequate primary response to measles immunization and may lose immunity with progressive immunosuppression, thus remaining susceptible to measles virus despite immunization. Children with defective cell-mediated immunity may not develop the characteristic measles rash, and infection may go unrecognized, with the potential for widespread transmission of measles virus, particularly in health care settings. Finally, HIV-infected children may have prolonged shedding of measles virus,[11] increasing the period of infectivity and the spread of measles virus to secondary contacts. Counteracting the increased susceptibility of HIV-infected children to measles is the high mortality rate of HIV-infected children, particularly in sub-Saharan Africa, such that these children do not live long enough to build up a sizeable pool of susceptible children.[121] This may change with increased access to antiretroviral drugs. The good news is that successful control of measles in southern Africa suggests the HIV epidemic is not a major barrier to measles control.[97]

New Tools for Measles Eradication

The ideal measles vaccine would be inexpensive, safe, heat-stable, immunogenic in neonates or very young infants, and administered as a single dose without needle or syringe. The age at vaccination should coincide with the schedule of the Expanded Programme on Immunization (EPI) to maximize compliance and share resources. Finally, a new vaccine should not elicit atypical measles upon exposure of immunized individuals to wild-type measles virus and should not be associated with prolonged immunosuppression, adversely affecting immune responses to subsequent infections.

A number of vaccine candidates with some of these characteristics are undergoing preclinical studies. Naked cDNA vaccines are thermostable, inexpensive, and could theoretically elicit antibody responses in the presence of passively acquired maternal antibody. DNA vaccines encoding either or both the measles hemagglutinin and fusion proteins are safe, immunogenic, and protective against measles challenge in naive, juvenile rhesus macaques.[122] Alternative techniques for administering measles DNA, such as alphavirus, parainfluenza virus, or enteric bacterial vectors, also are under investigation.

Measles Eradication

The elimination of measles in large geographic areas, such as the Americas, suggest that global eradication is feasible with current vaccination strategies.[123] As discussed above, potential barriers to eradication include: (1) lack of political will; (2) difficulties of measles control in densely populated urban environments; (3) the HIV epidemic; (4) waning immunity and the potential transmission from subclinical cases; (5) transmission among susceptible adults; (6) the risk of unsafe injections; and (7) unfounded fears of disease caused by measles vaccine.[124] Whether the threat from bioterrorism precludes stopping measles vaccination after eradication is a topic of debate, but, at the least, a single-dose rather than a two-dose measles vaccination strategy could be adopted.[125] Serious discussion of measles eradication likely will take place after polio eradication is achieved and will be a focus of infectious disease epidemiologists in the years to come.

Acknowledgments

We thank Dr. Diane E. Griffin for helpful comments.

References

1. Maxcy KF. Epidemiology. In: Rivers TM, ed. *Viral and Rickettsial Infections of Man*. Philadelphia, Pa: Lippincott; 1948:128–146.
2. Enders JF, Peebles TC. Propagation in tissue cultures of cytopathic agents from patients with measles. *Proc Soc Exp Biol Med*. 1954;86:277–286.
3. Malvoisin E, Wild TF. Measles virus glycoproteins: studies on the structure and interaction of the haemagglutinin and fusion proteins. *J Gen Virol*. 1993;74:2365–2372.
4. Schneider U, von Messling V, Devaux P, Cattaneo R. Efficiency of measles virus entry and dissemination through different receptors. *J Virol*. 2002;76:7460–7467.
5. Andres O, Obojes K, Kim KS, ter Meulen V, Schneider-Schaulies J. CD46- and CD150-independent endothelial cell infection with wild-type measles viruses. *J Gen Virol*. 2003;84:1189–1197.
6. Spehner D, Drillien R, Howley PM. The assembly of the measles virus nucleoprotein into nucleocapsid-like particles is modulated by the phosphoprotein. *Virology*. 1997;232:260–268.
7. Valsamakis A, Schneider H, Auwaerter PG, Kaneshima H, Billeter MA, Griffin DE. Recombinant measles viruses with mutations in the C, V, or F gene have altered growth phenotypes in vivo. *J Virol*. 1998;72:7754–7761.
8. Patterson JB, Thomas D, Lewicki H, Billeter MA, Oldstone MB. V and C proteins of measles virus function as virulence factors in vivo. *Virology*. 2000;267:80–89.
9. Auwaerter PG, Rota PA, Elkins WR, et al. Measles virus infection in rhesus macaques: altered immune responses and comparison of the virulence of six different virus strains. *J Infect Dis*. 1999;180:950–958.
10. Kimura A, Tosaka K, Nakao T. Measles rash. I. Light and electron microscopic study of skin eruptions. *Arch Virol*. 1975;47:295–307.
11. Permar SR, Moss WJ, Ryon JJ, et al. Prolonged measles virus shedding in human immunodeficiency virus-infected children detected by reverse transcriptase-polymerase chain reaction. *J Infect Dis*. 2001;183:532–538.
12. Black FL, Yannet H. Inapparent measles after gamma globulin administration. *JAMA*. 1960;173:1183–1188.
13. Isa MB, Martinez L, Giordano M, Passeggi C, de Wolff MC, Nates S. Comparison of immunoglobulin G subclass profiles induced by measles virus in vaccinated and naturally infected individuals. *Clin Diagn Lab Immunol*. 2002;9:693–697.

14. Good RA, Zak SJ. Disturbances in gamma globulin synthesis as "experiments of nature." *Pediatrics.* 1956;18(1):109–149.

15. Permar SR, Klumpp SA, Mansfield KG, Lifton MA et al. Role of CD8(+) lymphocytes in control and clearance of measles virus infection of rhesus monkeys. *J Virol.* 2003;77:4396–4400.

16. Moss WJ, Ryon JJ, Monze M, Griffin DE. Differential regulation of interleukin (IL)-4, IL-5, and IL-10 during measles in Zambian children. *J Infect Dis.* 2002;186:879–887.

17. Ovsyannikova IG, Dhiman N, Jacobson RM, Vierkant RA, Poland GA. Frequency of measles virus-specific CD4+ and CD8+ T cells in subjects seronegative or highly seropositive for measles vaccine. *Clin Diagn Lab Immunol.* 2003;10:411–416.

18. Panum P. Observations made during the epidemic of measles on the Faroe Islands in the year 1846. *Med Classics.* 1938;3:829–886.

19. Wong-Chew RM, Islas-Romero R, Garcia-Garcia M de L, et al. Induction of cellular and humoral immunity after aerosol or subcutaneous administration of Edmonston-Zagreb measles vaccine as a primary dose to 12-month-old children. *J Infect Dis.* 2004;189: 254–257.

20. Ward B, Boulianne N, Ratnam S, Guiot MC, Couilard M, De Serres G. Cellular immunity in measles vaccine failure: demonstration of measles antigen-specific lymphoproliferative responses despite limited serum antibody production after revaccination. *J Infect Dis.* 1995;172: 1591–1595.

21. Beckford AP, Kaschula RO, Stephen C. Factors associated with fatal cases of measles. A retrospective autopsy study. *S Afr Med J.* 1985;68:858–863.

22. Greenberg BL, Sack RB, Salazar-Lindo E, et al. Measles-associated diarrhea in hospitalized children in Lima, Peru: pathogenic agents and impact on growth. *J Infect Dis.* 1991;163:495–502.

23. Tamashiro VG, Perez HH, Griffin DE. Prospective study of the magnitude and duration of changes in tuberculin reactivity during uncomplicated and complicated measles. *Pediatr Infect Dis J.* 1987;6:451–454.

24. Coovadia HM, Wesley A, Henderson LG, Brain P, Vos GH, Hallett AF. Alterations in immune responsiveness in acute measles and chronic post-measles chest disease. *Int Arch Allergy Appl Immunol.* 1978;56: 14–23.

25. Hirsch RL, Griffin DE, Johnson RT, et al. Cellular immune responses during complicated and uncomplicated measles virus infections of man. *Clin Immunol Immunopathol.* 1984;31:1–12.

26. Servet-Delprat C, Vidalain PO, Azocar O, Le Deist F, Fischer A, Rabourdin-Combe C. Consequences of Fas-mediated human dendritic cell apoptosis induced by measles virus. *J Virol.* 2000;74:4387–4393.

27. Griffin DE, Cooper SJ, Hirsch RL, et al. Changes in plasma IgE levels during complicated and uncomplicated measles virus infections. *J Allergy Clin Immunol.* 1985;76:206–213.

28. Griffin DE, Ward BJ. Differential CD4 T cell activation in measles. *J Infect Dis.* 1993;168:275–281.

29. Karp CL, Wysocka M, Wahl LM, et al. Mechanism of suppression of cell-mediated immunity by measles virus. *Science.* 1996;273: 228–231.

30. Atabani SF, Byrnes AA, Jaye A, et al. Natural measles causes prolonged suppression of interleukin-12 production. *J Infect Dis.* 2001;184:1–9.

31. Kemper C, Chan AC, Green JM, Brett KA, Murphy KM, Atkinson JP. Activation of human CD4+ cells with CD3 and CD46 induces a T-regulatory cell 1 phenotype. *Nature*. 2003;421:388–392.

32. Morley D. Severe measles in the tropics. *Brit Med J*. 1969;1:297–300.

33. Duke T, Mgone CS. Measles: not just another viral exanthem. *Lancet*. 2003;361:763–773.

34. Perry RT, Halsey NA. The clinical significance of measles: a review. *J Infect Dis*. 2004;189(suppl 1):S4–S16.

35. Bellini WJ, Helfand RF. The challenges and strategies for laboratory diagnosis of measles in an international setting. *J Infect Dis*. 2003;187(suppl 1):S283–S290.

36. World Health Organization, United Nations Children's Fund. *Measles Mortality Reduction and Regional Elimination Strategic Plan 2001–2005*. Geneva, Switzerland; World Health Organization; 2001.

37. World Health Organization. Progress in reducing measles mortality—worldwide 1999–2003. *Weekly Epidemiol Rec*. 2005;80(9):78–81.

38. Henao-Restrepo AM, Strebel P, Hoekstra EJ, Birmingham M, Bilous J. Experience in global measles control, 1990–2001. *J Infect Dis*. 2003;187(suppl 1):S15–S21.

39. Stein CE, Birmingham M, Kurian M, Duclos P, Strebel P. The global burden of measles in the year 2000: a model that uses country-specific indicators. *J Infect Dis*. 2003;187(suppl 1):S8–S14.

40. Morris SS, Black RE, Tomaskovic L. Predicting the distribution of under-five deaths by cause in countries without adequate vital registration systems. *Int J Epidemiol*. 2003;32:1041–1051.

41. Black RE, Morris SS, Bryce J. Where and why are 10 million children dying every year? *Lancet*. 2003;361:2226–2234.

42. Dossetor J, Whittle HC, Greenwood BM. Persistent measles infection in malnourished children. *BMJ*. 1977;1:1633–1635.

43. Christensen PE, Schmidt H, Bang HO, Andersen V, Jordal B, Jensen O. An epidemic of measles in southern Greenland, 1951. Measles in virgin soil. II. The epidemic proper. *Acta Med Scand*. 1953;144:430–449.

44. Crowe JE. Influence of maternal antibodies on neonatal immunization against respiratory viruses. *Clin Infect Dis*. 2001;33:1720–1727.

45. Hutchins S, Markowitz L, Atkinson W, Swint E, Hadler S. Measles outbreaks in the United States, 1987 through 1990. *Pediatr Infect Dis J*. 1996;15:31–38.

46. de Quadros CA, Hersh BS, Nogueira AC, Carrasco PA, da Silveira CM. Measles eradication: experience in the Americas. *Bull World Health Organ*. 1998;76(suppl 2):47–52.

47. Lambert SB, Morgan ML, Riddell MA, et al. Measles outbreak in young adults in Victoria, 1999. *Med J Aust*. 2000;173:467–471.

48. McNeill WH. *Plagues and Peoples*. London, UK: Penguin; 1976.

49. Black FL. Measles endemicity in insular populations: critical community size and its evolutionary implication. *J Theor Biol*. 1966;11:207–211.

50. Fine PE, Clarkson JA. Measles in England and Wales–I: An analysis of factors underlying seasonal patterns. *Int J Epidemiol*. 1982;11:5–14.

51. Hamer WH. The Milroy lectures on epidemic disease in England–the evidence of variability and persistence of type. *Lancet*. 1906;1:733–739.

52. Anderson RM, May RM. *Infectious Diseases of Humans. Dynamics and Control*. Oxford, UK: Oxford University Press; 1992.

53. Earn DJ, Rohani P, Bolker BM, Grenfell BT. A simple model for complex dynamical transitions in epidemics. *Science.* 2000;287: 667–670.

54. Grenfell BT, Bjornstad ON, Kappey J. Travelling waves and spatial hierarchies in measles epidemics. *Nature.* 2001;414:716–723.

55. Rohani P, Earn DJ, Grenfell BT. Opposite patterns of synchrony in sympatric disease metapopulations. *Science.* 1999;286:968–971.

56. Salama P, Assefa F, Talley L, Spiegel P, van Der V, Gotway CA. Malnutrition, measles, mortality, and the humanitarian response during a famine in Ethiopia. *JAMA.* 2001;286:563–571.

57. Aaby P, Bukh J, Lisse IM, Smits AJ. Overcrowding and intensive exposure as determinants of measles mortality. *Am J Epidemiol.* 1984;120:49–63.

58. Dossetor JF, Whittle HC. Protein-losing enteropathy and malabsorption in acute measles enteritis. *Br Med J.* 1975;2:592–593.

59. Semba RD, Bloem MW. Measles blindness. *Surv Ophthalmol.* 2004;49:243–255.

60. Garenne M. Sex differences in measles mortality: a world review. *Int J Epidemiol.* 1994;23:632–642.

61. Halsey NA. Increased mortality after high-titre measles vaccines: too much of a good thing. *Pediatr Infect Dis J.* 1993;12:462–465.

62. Ovsyannikova IG, Jacobson RM, Poland GA. Variation in vaccine response in normal populations. *Pharmacogenomics.* 2004;5: 417–427.

63. Parks CL, Lerch RA, Walpita P, Wang HP, Sidhu MS, Udem SA. Comparison of predicted amino acid sequences of measles virus strains in the Edmonston vaccine lineage. *J Virol.* 2001;75:910–920.

64. Dilraj A, Cutts FT, de Castro JF, et al. Response to different measles vaccine strains given by aerosol and subcutaneous routes to schoolchildren: a randomised trial. *Lancet.* 2000;355:798–803.

65. Bennett JV, Fernandez de Castro J, Valdespino-Gomez JL, et al. Aerosolized measles and measles-rubella vaccines induce better measles antibody booster responses than injected vaccines: randomized trials in Mexican schoolchildren. *Bull WHO.* 2002;80:806–812.

66. Carter CH, Conway TJ, Cornfeld D, et al. Serologic response of children to inactivated measles vaccine. *JAMA.* 1962;179:848–853.

67. Fulginiti VA, Eller JJ, Downie AW, Kempe CH. Altered reactivity to measles virus: atypical measles in children previously immunized with inactivated measles virus vaccines. *JAMA.* 1967;202:1075.

68. Nader RR, Horwitz MS, Rousseau J. Atypical exanthem following exposure to natural measles: eleven cases in children previously inoculated with killed vaccine. *J Pediatr.* 1968;72:22–28.

69. Polack FP, Auwaerter PG, Lee SH, et al. Production of atypical measles in rhesus macaques: evidence for disease mediated by immune complex formation and eosinophils in the presence of fusion-inhibiting antibody. *Nat Med.* 1999;5:629–634.

70. Gans HA, Arvin AM, Galinus J, Logan L, DeHovitz R, Maldonado Y. Deficiency of the humoral immune response to measles vaccine in infants immunized at age 6 months. *JAMA.* 1998;280:527–532.

71. Holt EA, Moulton LH, Siberry GK, Halsey NA. Differential mortality by measles vaccine titer and sex. *J Infect Dis.* 1993;168:1087–1096.

72. Aaby P, Samb B, Simondon F, et al. A comparison of vaccine efficacy and mortality during routine use of high-titre Edmonston-Zagreb and

Schwarz standard measles vaccines in rural Senegal. *Trans Roy Soc Trop Med Hyg.* 1996;90:326–330.

73. Orenstein WA, Bernier RH, Hinman AR. Assessing vaccine efficacy in the field. Further observations. *Epidemiol Rev.* 1988;10:212–241.

74. Halloran ME, Struchiner CJ, Longini IMJ. Study designs for evaluating different efficacy and effectiveness aspects of vaccines. *Am J Epidemiol.* 1997;146:789–803.

75. Chen RT, Markowitz LE, Albrecht P, et al. Measles antibody: reevaluation of protective titers. *J Infect Dis.* 1990;162:1036–1042.

76. Cutts FT, Grabowsky M, Markowitz LE. The effect of dose and strain of live attenuated measles vaccines on serological responses in young infants. *Biologicals.* 1995;23:95–106.

77. Scott S, Cutts FT, Nyandu B. Mild illness at or after measles vaccination does not reduce seroresponse in young children. *Vaccine.* 1999;17:837–843.

78. Anders JF, Jacobson RM, Poland GA, Jacobsen SJ, Wollan PC. Secondary failure rates of measles vaccines: a meta-analysis of published studies. *Pediatr Infect Dis J.* 1996;15:62–66.

79. Whittle HC, Aaby P, Samb B, Jensen H, Bennett J, Simondon F. Effect of subclinical infection on maintaining immunity against measles in vaccinated children in West Africa. *Lancet.* 1999;353: 98–101.

80. Halsey NA. The optimal age for administering measles vaccine in developing countries. In: Halsey NA, de Quadros CA, eds. *Recent Advances in Immunization: A Bibliographic Review.* Washington, DC: Pan American Health Organization, 1983; PAHO publication no. 451:4–17.

81. Moss WJ, Monze M, Ryon JJ, Quinn TC, Griffin DE, Cutts F. Prospective study of measles in hospitalized human immunodeficiency virus (HIV)-infected and HIV-uninfected children in Zambia. *Clin Infect Dis.* 2002;35:189–196.

82. Angel JB, Walpita P, Lerch RA, et al. Vaccine-associated measles pneumonitis in an adult with AIDS. *Ann Intern Med.* 1998;129: 104–106.

83. Monafo WJ, Haslam DB, Roberts RL, Zaki SR, Bellini WJ, Coffin CM. Disseminated measles infection after vaccination in a child with a congenital immunodeficiency. *J Pediatr.* 1994;124:273–276.

84. Bitnun A, Shannon P, Durward A, et al. Measles inclusion-body encephalitis caused by the vaccine strain of measles virus. *Clin Infect Dis.* 1999;29:855–861.

85. Wakefield AJ, Murch SH, Anthony A, et al. Ileal-lymphoid-nodular hyperplasia, nonspecific colitis, and pervasive developmental disorder in children. *Lancet.* 1998;351:637–641.

86. Offit PA, Coffin SE. Communicating science to the public: MMR vaccine and autism. *Vaccine.* 2003;22:1–6.

87. DeStefano F, Thompson WW. MMR vaccine and autism: an update of the scientific evidence. *Expert Rev Vaccines.* 2004;3:19–22.

88. Madsen KM, Hviid A, Vestergaard M, et al. A population-based study of measles, mumps, and rubella vaccination and autism. *N Engl J Med.* 2002;347:1477–1482.

89. Aaby P, Samb B, Simondon F, Seck AMC, Knudsen K, Whittle H. Non-specific beneficial effect of measles immunisation: analysis of mortality studies from developing countries. *Brit Med J.* 1995;311:481–485.

90. Kristensen I, Aaby P, Jensen H. Routine vaccinations and child survival: follow up study in Guinea-Bissau, West Africa. *BMJ.* 2000;321:1–7.

91. Shann F. Non-specific effects of vaccines in developing countries. *BMJ.* 2000;321:1423–1424.

92. Aaby P, Andersen M, Sodemann M, Jakobsen M, Gomes J, Fernandes M. Reduced childhood mortality following standard measles vaccination at 4–8 months compared to 9–11 months of age. *BMJ.* 1993;307:1308–1311.

93. Breiman RF, Streatfield PK, Phelan M, Shifa N, Rashid M, Yunus M. Effect of infant immunisation on childhood mortality in rural Bangladesh: analysis of health and demographic surveillance data. *Lancet.* 2004;364:2204–2211.

94. Fine P. Commentary: an unexpected finding that needs confirmation or rejection. *BMJ.* 2000;321:7–8.

95. Cooper WO, Boyce TG, Wright PF, Griffin MR. Do childhood vaccines have non-specific effects on mortality? *Bull WHO.* 2003;81:821–826.

96. Pan American Health Organization. *Measles Eradication. Field Guide.* Washington, DC: Pan American Health Organization; 1999.

97. Biellik R, Madema S, Taole A, et al. First 5 years of measles elimination in southern Africa: 1996–2000. *Lancet.* 2002;359:1564–1568.

98. Dayan GH, Cairns L, Sangrujee N, Mtonga A, Nguyen V, Strebel P. Cost-effectiveness of three different vaccination strategies against measles in Zambian children. *Vaccine.* 2004;22:475–484.

99. Uzicanin A, Zhou F, Eggers R, Webb E, Strebel P. Economic analysis of the 1996–1997 mass measles immunization campaigns in South Africa. *Vaccine.* 2004;22:3419–3426.

100. Sencer DJ, Dull HB, Langmuir AD. Epidemiologic basis for eradication of measles in 1967. *Public Health Rep.* 1967;82:253–256.

101. Forni AL, Schluger NW, Roberts RB. Severe measles pneumonitis in adults: evaluation of clinical characteristics and therapy with intravenous ribavirin. *Clin Infect Dis.* 1994;19:454–462.

102. Solomon T, Hart CA, Vinjamuri S, Beeching NJ, Malucci C, Humphrey P. Treatment of subacute sclerosing panencephalitis with interferon-alpha, ribavirin, and inosiplex. *J Child Neurol.* 2002;17:703–705.

103. D'Souza RM, D'Souza R. Vitamin A for the treatment of children with measles—a systematic review. *J Trop Pediatr.* 2002;48:323–327.

104. Villamor E, Fawzi WW. Vitamin A supplementation: implications for morbidity and mortality in children. *J Infect Dis.* 2000;182(suppl 1):S122–S133.

105. World Health Organization. Update of the nomenclature for describing the genetic characteristics of wild-type measles viruses: new genotypes and reference strains. *Weekly Epidemiol Rec.* 2003;78:229–232.

106. Rota PA, Bellini WJ. Update on the global distribution of genotypes of wild type measles viruses. *J Infect Dis.* 2003;187(suppl 1):S270–S276.

107. Fine PEM. Herd immunity: history, theory, practice. *Epidemiologic Rev.* 1993;15:265–302.

108. Shasby DM, Shope TC, Downs H, Herrmann KL, Polkowski J. Epidemic measles in a highly vaccinated population. *N Engl J Med.* 1977;296:585–589.

109. Nkowane BM, Bart SW, Orenstein WA, Baltier M. Measles outbreak in a vaccinated school population: epidemiology, chains of transmission and the role of vaccine failures. *Am J Public Health.* 1987;77:434–438.

110. Chen RT, Goldbaum GM, Wassilak SG, Markowitz LE, Orenstein WA. An explosive point-source measles outbreak in a highly vaccinated population. Modes of transmission and risk factors for disease. *Am J Epidemiol.* 1989;129:173–182.

111. Pedersen IR, Mordhorst CH, Glikmann G, von Magnus H. Subclinical measles infection in vaccinated seropositive individuals in arctic Greenland. *Vaccine.* 1989;7:345–348.

112. Edmonson MB, Addiss DG, McPherson JT, Berg JL, Circo SR, Davis JP. Mild measles and secondary vaccine failure during a sustained outbreak in a highly vaccinated population. *JAMA.* 1990;263: 2467–2471.

113. Helfand RF, Kim DK, Gary HE Jr, et al. Nonclassic measles infections in an immune population exposed to measles during a college bus trip. *J Med Virol.* 1998;56:337–341.

114. Strebel P, Cochi S, Grabowsky M, et al. The unfinished measles immunization agenda. *J Infect Dis.* 2003;187(suppl 1):S1–S7.

115. Jansen VA, Stollenwerk N, Jensen HJ, Ramsay ME, Edmunds WJ, Rhodes CJ. Measles outbreaks in a population with declining vaccine uptake. *Science.* 2003;301:804.

116. Rodgers DV, Gindler JS, Atkinson WL, Markowitz LE. High attack rates and case fatality during a measles outbreak in groups with religious exemption to vaccination. *Pediatr Infect Dis J.* 1993;12:288–292.

117. Centers for Disease Control. Measles outbreak—Netherlands, April 1999–January 2000. *MMWR.* 2000;49:299–303.

118. Vardas E, Kreis S. Isolation of measles virus from a naturally immune asymptomatically re-infected individual. *J Clin Virol.* 1999;13: 173–179.

119. World Health Organization. Strategies for reducing global measles mortality. *Wkly Epidem Rec.* 2000;75:411–416.

120. Moss WJ, Cutts F, Griffin DE. Implications of the human immunodeficiency virus epidemic for control and eradication of measles. *Clin Infect Dis.* 1999;29:106–112.

121. Helfand RF, Moss WJ, Harpaz R, Scott S, Cutts F. Evaluating the impact of the HIV pandemic on measles control and elimination. *Bull World Health Organ.* 2005;83:329–337.

122. Polack FP, Lee SH, Permar S, et al. Successful DNA immunization against measles: neutralizing antibody against either the hemagglutinin or fusion glycoprotein protects rhesus macaques without evidence of atypical measles. *Nat Med.* 2000;6:776–781.

123. de Quadros CA. Can measles be eradicated globally? *Bull World Health Organ.* 2004;82:134–138.

124. Orenstein WA, Strebel PM, Papania M, Sutter RW, Bellini WJ, Cochi SL. Measles eradication: is it in our future? *Am J Public Health.* 2000;90:1521–1525.

125. Meissner HC, Strebel PM, Orenstein WA. Measles vaccines and the potential for worldwide eradication of measles. *Pediatrics.* 2004;114:1065–1069.

CHAPTER SEVENTEEN

GLOBAL EPIDEMIOLOGY OF MENINGOCOCCAL INFECTIONS

Mark C. Steinhoff

Introduction

Meningococcal disease is a global problem, with disease patterns that vary widely by region. The meningococcus bacteria cause severe disease with rapid onset and poor outcomes, even with treatment. The endemic disease is rare, but epidemic meningococcal disease can also occur in outbreaks characteristically in the "meningitis belt" in sub-Saharan Africa. Because of the varied epidemiologic pattern of disease, control strategies are substantially different between geographic regions.

This description will compare meningococcal disease and control strategies in both industrial and developing regions. Because of the potential for epidemics and the continuing endemic illnesses, vaccines are a mainstay of control. Recent development and licensure of new vaccines in Europe and the United States, and the development of a vaccine tailored for the African meningitis belt, suggest better control can be expected.

The Organism

Epidemic meningitis was described in Switzerland in 1805 and in the United States in 1806.[1] The bacterium *Neisseria meningitidis*, also called meningococcus, was first isolated in 1887 at the beginning of the era of discovery of infectious organisms.[2] Reviews of historical data from sub-Saharan Africa have shown large epidemics in that setting since the early 1900s,[3] but likely not before then.

Worldwide there are approximately 500,000 cases a year, and in the United States approximately 3000 cases.[4] Because of the success of vaccines against *Haemophilus* and pneumococcal meningitis, meningococcal meningitis is now the most important cause of endemic bacterial meningitis in children in the United States.[5]

The meningococcus is a gram-negative encapsulated aerobic bacterium. The capsular polysaccharide defines the 14 serogroups, among which groups A, B, C, W135, and Y are the most common. In addition to the *serogroups*, meningococci are also classified two ways: by *serotypes*, defined by the PorB outer membrane proteins, and by *serosubtype*, defined by the PorA proteins. In addition, immunotypes related to lipopolysaccharides are also used to classify strains. The genomes for isolates of group A and group B have been published,[6,7] and a group C genome is currently being sequenced. For epidemiologic purposes, many other strain classifications are used, including electropherotyping, and MLST.[8]

The meningococcus colonizes and infects humans, and there are no other hosts. It usually resides as a harmless commensal in the nasopharynx in 10–20% of adults. Transmission from person to person is either by direct contact with respiratory secretions (kissing), indirect contact (sharing of eating utensils), or by aerosol droplets (coughing, sneezing). Only a small proportion of persons who are colonized in the nasopharynx develop invasive disease. Invasive disease is related both to virulence characteristics of the particular strain and to host factors.

Meningococci are similar to pneumococci, because they are transformable, meaning they can acquire DNA from other organisms; capsular switching and other genetic variance occurs to generate new epidemic strains.[9] Genetic sequence data suggest that genes have been acquired from other meningococci and other respiratory commensals such as *H. influenzae*, and the presence of many repeating sequences of DNA specifying surface proteins allows substantial antigenic variations.

The major unknowns regarding meningococcal disease are the factors determining: (1) acquisition and transmission of organisms, (2) the development of invasive disease in a small proportion of all persons who have nasopharyngeal colonization, (3) the development of epidemics, and (4) the shifting serogroups, subtypes, and clones that cause epidemics in various geographic settings. A summary of the processes and stages of meningococcal infection and epidemics is shown in Figure 17-1. Recent genomic analyses of invasive strains compared to colonizing strains in a large collection in

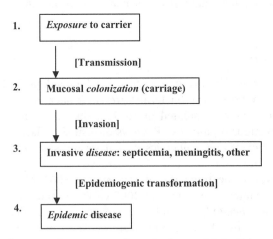

FIGURE 17-1 Stages and processes of meningococcal infection and disease.

the Czech Republic showed that the invasive strains all had a specific phage DNA gene cluster, compared to only 10% of the carried strains. This suggests that this phage DNA mediates invasiveness and possibly determines epidemic clones.[10]

Acquisition and Carriage

Rates of carriage in European children are generally less than 3%, increasing to 20% to 30% in the 15- to 24-year age group. Carriage rates among military recruits and contacts of cases are generally much higher, ranging from 20% to 70%. Respiratory infections by some viruses and exposure to tobacco smoke are associated with increased carriage.[11] The heterogeneity of subtypes and immunotypes is greater among carriers than among patients with invasive disease during epidemics. Colonization of the nasopharynx by meningococci usually produces an antibody response several weeks after acquisition of the organism. Because carriage of meningococcus and related nonpathogenic *N. lactamica* results in natural bactericidal antibody, 65% to 85% of adult individuals have naturally acquired protective bactericidal serum antibody titers.[12-15]

Disease

Invasive disease usually occurs within 1 to 4 days of acquisition. Approximately 60% of all acute cases of meningococcal disease have less than 24 hours of illness before hospitalization. In endemic pattern disease, 30% of meningococcal disease is meningitis, which, even with therapy, has a mortality rate of 10% to 15% and neurologic sequelae in a high proportion of survivors. Septicemia without meningitis (meningococcemia) occurs in 10–20% and can lead to loss of limbs and death. Pneumonia (5–10% of all meningococcal disease) and other syndromes including arthritis, pericarditis, endocarditis, pharyngitis, urethritis, and cervicitis have been described.[5,16]

Treatment

Before the use of antibiotics, mortality from meningococcal disease was as high as 85%. Flexner and others showed that passive antibody treatment with specific animal sera was effective in reducing mortality.[17] Treatment with penicillin is effective, because resistance to penicillin among meningococcal isolates is rare. Antibiotic treatment with broader spectrum drugs including ceftriaxone to cover additional bacteria is often used for empirical treatment of bacterial meningitis and is effective. Chloremphenicol is also still effective treatment in many settings, though resistance has been reported.[18] In addition to antibiotic treatment, good supportive care to treat shock and disseminated intravascular coagulation reduces mortality, which still is between 10% and 15% in wealthy countries.[19]

In the setting of endemic disease *chemoprophylaxis* can be effective to prevent illness in family members and other close contacts. In the United

States chemoprophylaxis of close contacts is recommended for prevention of sporadic meningococcal disease. Close contacts are defined as household members, day-care center contacts, and anyone directly exposed to the oral secretions of the index case. Antimicrobial chemoprophylaxis should be administered to these contacts as soon as possible, because the risk of invasive disease is greatest within a few days of the index case. See the CDC Web site for information on the dose and duration of the recommended drugs, which include rifampin, ciprofloxacin, and ceftriaxone.[20]

Risk Factors

Important host factors are the absence of bactericidal antibodies in serum, absence of a normal complement cascade, as well as the presence of certain mannose-binding lectins.[21] A variety of human genetic polymorphisms is associated with severity of disease without apparently effecting the risk of acquisition.[22] Other biological risk factors include complement deficiencies, anatomic or functional asplenia, and chronic disease. For meningococcal disease in the United States, risk factors include age under 11 months, household crowding, viral infection,[11] active and passive smoking,[23] and chronic underlying illnesses. During outbreaks in the United States, bar or nightclub patronage and alcohol use have been associated with increased risk of acquisition.[24] In the African settings, risk factors include exposure to cooking fire smoke and sharing a bedroom with a case.[25] During World War I, the importance of spacing of beds in sleeping quarters to reduce transmission and carriage of meningococci was understood and led to bed spacing regulations in military barracks (see Figure 17-2).

Feet (Scale t)			1					2				3
Inches 3	6	9	0	3	6	9	0	3	6	9	0	

Beds less than 9″ apart Carrier Rate = 30% or more.

Beds less than one foot apart. Carrier Rate = 20% or more.

Beds 1′4″ apart (The usual distance in mobilisation standard strictly observed) Carrier Rate = 9%

Beds 2′6″ apart (as in "spacing out" Caterham) Carrier Rate = under 5%

Beds 3 feet apart. Carrier Rate = under 2%

FIGURE 17-2 Glover in 1920 reported on the effect of crowding in the British Army Guards Depot at Caterham in 1916. These barracks were designed for 800 men, but with World War I mobilization up to 13,000 were housed in the barracks and in huts and tents around it. The normal military rule for bed separation was 3 feet, but "there were great temptations to hygienically unprincipled authorities . . . to put in more beds." Glover was able to show that decreased distance between beds (crowding) was correlated with increased carriage rates of meningococcus A, and eventually with an outbreak of meningococcal disease in the barracks. The figure shows his graph of data relating bed separation with carriage rates in the recruits.
Source: Glover JA. Observation of the meningococcus carrier rate, and their application to the prevention of cerebrospinal fever. In: Medical Research Council. Cerebrospinal fever. Special Report Series no. 50. London: His Majesty's Stationery Office, 1920:133–65.

Epidemiology

In the past, meningococcus caused large epidemics in North America and Europe, but these have not occurred in industrial countries (except for Norway and New Zealand) for the last 60 years. Rates of endemic meningococcal disease of all groups in the United States recently ranged from 1 to 1.5/100,000 population.[20] In Europe, rates have been higher,[26-28] and rates of 5/100,000 in Great Britain prompted universal use of vaccine.[29] Table 17-1 contrasts the characteristics of meningococcal disease in wealthier countries and countries with limited resources.

The epidemiology of meningococcal disease varies by the major serogroups and geography. Group A historically has been the cause of large epidemic outbreaks and causes endemic and epidemic outbreaks in the meningitis belt of Africa. Currently group A disease is rare in the United States and Europe.

Group B disease currently is the most important cause of endemic disease in developed countries, causing approximately 30% to 40% in the United States and up to 80% in European countries. Norway, Cuba, and New Zealand have experienced epidemic group B disease in the recent past.

Meningococcal group C disease has variable rates of endemic disease, and currently accounts for about 30% of disease in the United States and in Europe. Group Y has become more frequent in the United States. Group W135 disease has become increasingly important and has been related to the Hajj pilgrimage since the late 1990s.[30]

In the United States, in recent years serogroup Y causes 39% of disease, serogroup C 31%, serogroup B 23%, W135 2%, and group A is absent (Figure 17-3). In Canada and Europe, serogroups B and C predominate, but in Africa serogroups A and W135 are most common. The distribution of serogroups in the United States changed during the 1990s.[31] For example, group Y represented 9% of all cases between 1990 and 1992, but from 1997 to 2003, group Y represented 28% of all cases. Group B ranged from 43% to 34%.[32]

Epidemic meningitis was a feature in the North American and European countries until the middle of the last century (Figure 17-4). During the last decades large epidemics have occurred in the African meningitis belt and within China.[33]

Serogroup A, subgroup III has caused two large global pandemics. The first occurred from the 1960s to 1970s in China, Russia, Scandinavia, and Brazil.

TABLE 17-1   Comparison of Meningococcal Disease Epidemiology

Characteristic	High-Income Regions	Low Income; Meningitis belt
Serogroups	B,C	A, C, now W135
Epidemiology	Endemic, winter	Endemic/epidemic, dry season
Incidence (per 100,000)	1–5	20/600
Peak Age	College age	School age
Case Fatality	5–15%	>15%

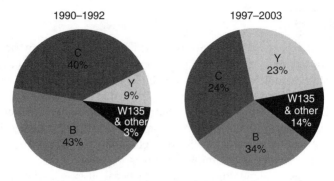

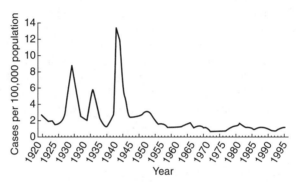

FIGURE 17-3 N meningitides serogroup disributions in the US (all age groups). *Source:* Centers for Disease Control and Prevention.

FIGURE 17-4 Incidence of meningococcal disease in the USA. *Source:* Wegner JD and Perkins BA. Patterns in the emergence of epidemic meningoccocal disease. In Scheld WM. Armstong and Hughes (eds). Emerging Infections 1. Washington DC. American Society for Microbiology Press. 1998. pp. 125–136.

A second group A pandemic was associated with epidemics in the 1980s in China and an outbreak from 1982 to 1984 in Kathmandu, Nepal, with approximately 1500 cases.[33,34] In 1985, 6000 cases occurred in New Delhi, India. During the 1987 Hajj in Mecca, Saudi Arabia, the same strain caused an outbreak among pilgrims and later was found in epidemics in the meningitis belt in Africa. This strain caused epidemic disease in areas not historically in the belt including Kenya, Tanzania, Zambia, and South Africa.[35,36]

It is possible the use of group A/C vaccine among pilgrims has modified the transmission of these serogroups during the Hajj. In 2001, serogroup W135 caused 400 cases in Hajj pilgrims and their contacts. This W135 clone has been spread likely through returning Hajj pilgrims, and has been described in the meningitis belt and in many other countries ranging from North America and Europe through the Far East.[30,37,38] Saudi authorities have modified the immunization regulations for Hajj pilgrims, who must now show evidence of immunization with A, C, Y, W135 vaccine.[39]

Meningococcal Belt

The meningitis belt in Africa was defined by Lapeyssonie in 1963 when he described a sub-Saharan region, stretching from Ethiopia to Senegal, characterized by periodic large epidemics of meningococcal meningitis.[40] (Figure 17-6.) The belt is dry grassland and scrub with subsistence farming, stretching across 16 sub-Saharan Sahel countries with 170 million affected people with a GNP per capita between $100 and $800 per person, the least developed category. The region is characterized by a northern boundary of the Sahara Desert and a southern boundary of humid savannah and rainforest. This region has limited rainfall, mostly confined to May to November of the year. There are few epidemics in regions within the rainfall isohyet of 300–1000 millimeters or with mean humidity greater than 10 grams/m^3.[41-43] The characteristic epidemics occur during the dry season.[41] The endemic incidence is from 3 to 60/100,000 (rates that would be considered epidemics elsewhere), increasing to 200 to 600/100,000 during the epidemics. In the 1996–1997 epidemic there were more than 214,000 cases and 21,800 deaths reported.[39] In this region, it estimated that during the decade of the 1990s, there were approximately 700,000 cases and at least 100,000 deaths. In contrast, in the United States during this same time period there were 22,000 cases and approximately 2000 deaths. Historically groups A and C have caused epidemics in this region; group W135 is now also seen.

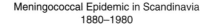

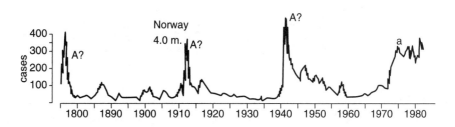

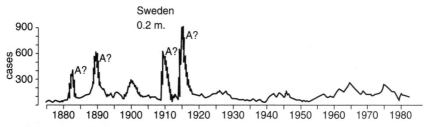

FIGURE 17-5 Meningococcal Epidemic in Scandinavia, 1880–1980.
Source: Wegner JD and Perkins BA. Patterns in the emergence of epidemic meningoccocol disease. In Scheld WM. Armstong and Hughes (eds). Emerging Infections 1. Washington DC. American Society for Microbiology Press. 1998. pp.125–136.

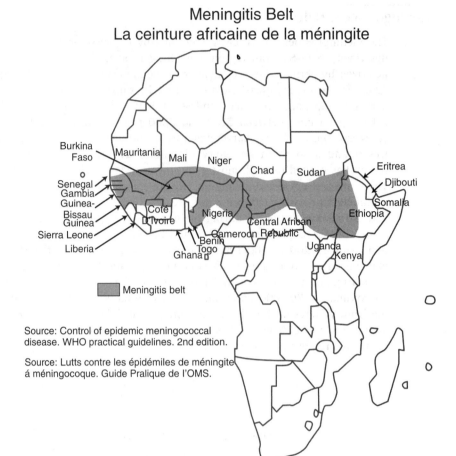

Meningitis Belt
La ceinture africaine de la méningite

Meningitis belt

Source: Control of epidemic meningococcal
disease. WHO practical guidelines. 2nd edition.

Source: Lutts contre les épidémiles de méningite
á méningocoque. Guide Pralique de l'OMS.

FIGURE 17-6 The African meningitis belt. The hatched area indicates the belt as
originally defined by Lepeyssonnie (1963); the speckled areas indicate the regions
in which characteristic African epidemics have been described.
Source: Modified from http://www.who.int/csr/disease/meningococcal/impact/en/

Vaccines

Polysaccharide capsules of serogroups A, C, Y, and W135 elicit bactericidal
antibodies that are serogroup specific. These antibodies have been shown
to correlate with protection from disease. Studies in the 1960s showed the
serum bactericidal antibodies are important in protection of military recruits
from epidemic disease. Recruits who arrived in camp with detectable bactericidal serum antibody levels did not develop disease even though colonized,
whereas recruits who did not have antibody had attack rates as high as 38%.
In contrast, serogroup B polysaccharide capsule is poorly immunogenic, likely
because of its similarity to sialic glycopeptides expressed on the surface
of developing neural cells. For this reason, vaccines against serogroups B
meningococci utilize noncapsular antigens, often surface proteins that have
a high level of diversity.[45]

A number of meningococcal vaccines have been available since at least
the 1960s.[46,47] The vaccines consist of the purified polysaccharide capsule

and vary by the number of serogroups they contain and whether they are polysaccharide alone or polysaccharide conjugated to a protein. As with other capsular polysaccharide vaccines, the meningococcal polysaccharide is less immunogenic in children and does not appear to stimulate long-term immunologic memory. Also similar to developments for other bacterial capsular polysaccharides, it has been shown that the chemical conjugation of protein to polysaccharides results in improved immunogenicity, enhanced immunologic memory, and longer-term protection, especially in infants and children. The enhanced immunogenicity and high effectiveness of polysaccharide conjugate vaccines in young infants has allowed effective vaccines for infants to be made available in the United States and the United Kingdom.

Conjugation does not improve the poor immunogenicity of the group B polysaccharide, so the outer membrane protein (OMP) and outer membrane vesicle remain the optimal vaccine antigens.

The efficacy of the polysaccharide vaccines varies from 80% to 100% in military recruits and epidemic situations. The conjugate group C vaccine as used in Britain has an overall efficacy greater than 90% for all vaccinated age groups.[48] The use of this vaccine has also resulted in reduction of carriage of group C strains in the entire population, suggesting a herd effect.

A summary table of the availability of vaccines for meningococcal disease is shown in Table 17-2. The quadravalent (groups A, C, Y, and W135) conjugate vaccine was licensed by the FDA for use in United States in February 2005 and was recommended for children 11 or older, students entering high school, and college freshmen living in dormitories. The quadravalent PS vaccine in the United States is sold for approximately $60; the PS vaccine for Hajj pilgrims is sold for around $5. The trivalent PS vaccine used only in Africa in 2002 cost approximately $1.50.

Because group B now causes a substantial proportion of disease in the United States and has caused outbreaks elsewhere, development of noncapsular vaccine has been of recent interest. Currently, vaccines have been produced using outer membrane proteins from epidemic strains in Norway

TABLE 17-2　Current Meningococcal Vaccines

Serogroup Polysaccharide Vaccines	Protein	Producer Vaccines	Licensed in	Licensed
A/C	—	Sanofi (Aventis)	Europe, Asia, Africa	1978
A, C, Y, W135	—	Sanofi (Aventis)	Widely used, but not in the United States	1981
A, C, Y, W135	—	GSK		
A, C, W135	—	GSK	Africa only	2002
Conjugate Vaccines				
C	Variable	Wyeth, Chiron, Baxter	United Kingdom, Europe, Canada	2001
A, B, C, W135	DT	Sanofi Pasteur (Aventis)	United States	2005
A	TT	MVP	pending	NA

Notes: DT, diphtheria toxoid; TT, tetanus toxoid; MVP, Meningococcal Vaccine Program.

and Cuba. These vaccines were relatively effective in reducing disease in those epidemics.[49-51] New Zealand has experienced an outbreak of group B since 2001 and will use an epidemic-specific OMP vaccine. Because of the heterogeneity of OMP antigens there is interest in additional strategies. The genome sequence of a group B strain has been analyzed and an assessment of the open reading frames yielded 570 surface exposed proteins, of which 5 were expressed as recombinant proteins and were able to prevent disease in a rodent model, and 2 induced bactericidal antibody when used as vaccines in mice.[52] This identification of potential vaccine antigens from genome sequencing has been termed *reverse vaccinology* because it identifies potentially protective surface proteins from genome sequence data directly, rather than from the classical sequence of detection, and isolation of the surface proteins and testing for natural antibody.[6,50]

Vaccine Strategies

There are three strategies for utilization of meningococcal vaccines: (1) immunization of high-risk population, (2) universal immunization, usually as part of infant immunization, and (3) epidemic response, or mass immunization of an affected population to curtail an epidemic (Table 17-3). Because disease patterns vary widely by regions and through time, these strategies and their adoption/relation to local disease patterns will be discussed below.

High-Risk Populations

The experience of the epidemics in the US military recruits in 1960s and 1970s resulted in the development of the quadravalent polysaccharide vaccine, which is still received by all recruits in the United States and many other militaries.

In the United States, college freshmen have been identified as a high-risk group, and immunization with polysaccharide quadravalent PS vaccine has been recommended since 2000.[53] Recently the licensure of a quadravalent conjugate polysaccharide vaccine has led to the recommendation of the use of this vaccine in children older than 11, those starting high school, or those living in dormitories in a university.[54,55]

The use of conjugate quadravalent A, C, Y, and W135 vaccine in older children and college populations in the United States suggests it may eventually be feasible to use this vaccine in infants, who have the highest incidence rates in the United States. If the conjugate vaccine is licensed for the infant age group, universal immunization may be a policy option. Reduction of disease due to these serotypes will increase interest in a vaccine for group B disease.

In 1992, the Egyptian Ministry of Health initiated a vaccination program for all school children using a bivalent A/C polysaccharide vaccine, which is immunogenic in older children. This strategy disrupted a previously observed pattern of outbreaks of illness approximately every 8 years with incidences of 20/100,000.[56]

Universal immunization through infant immunization was adopted by Great Britain in response to high rates of group C disease among infants and adolescents in that country. This program has been successful in curtailing

TABLE 17-3   National Immunization Policies: Examples in Four Countries

Country	Income (GNP per capita)	Incidence per 100,000	Vaccine Policy	Vaccine Used	Groups
United States	$25,850	1.1	High risk College age	PS, now Cj	A, C, Y, W135
United Kingdom	$16,561	5	Universal infant	Cj	C
Egypt	$1,200	20	High risk School age	PS	A/C
Benin	$380	65.9	Epidemic response	PS	A/C or A, C, W135

Notes: PS, polysaccharide; Cj, conjugate polysaccharide.

the epidemic of group C disease in Britain and has now been adopted by other European countries and several provinces in Canada.[57,58]

Both Norway and Cuba adopted a strategy of mass immunization for their group B epidemics. Each developed a protein vaccine with the specific protein of their own epidemic.

The vaccine strategy of *epidemic response* in the meningitis belt has been the subject of much discussion.[59-63] Currently the WHO strategy suggests enhanced surveillance for meningococcal disease to detect the onset of meningococcal epidemic, followed by mass vaccination in the affected regions. It is claimed that epidemic response of mass immunization can curtail epidemics.[64] This approach means that vaccine control procedures start some weeks after epidemics begin and has been criticized by some. A strategy of using the available and low-cost polysaccharide vaccine in young children and school children as part of routine immunization in this region is controversial.[61] The strengthening of both surveillance and routine EPI immunization systems to achieve high coverage of immunization among young children has made preventative immunization a more attractive strategy. WHO currently proposes a threshold for epidemics of 10/100,000 inhabitants per week. A lower alert threshold of 5/100,000 inhabitants allows time to prepare for an epidemic and initiate mass vaccination if appropriate. For populations under 30,000 the alert threshold is 2 cases a week.[65,66] The CDC defines an outbreak of serogroup C meningococcus as 3 or more confirmed or probable cases during a period of less than 3 months, a primary attack rate of at least 10/100,000 population.[20]

The availability of an affordable conjugate polysaccharide vaccine would enable universal infant immunization in the meningitis belt. The Meningococcal Vaccine Project (MVP) has undertaken the development of a group A conjugate vaccine, specifically for use in the meningococcal belt, where conjugate vaccine is not available. MVP has arranged delivery of 25 million doses a year at a cost affordable by local governments.[67] A strategy of preventive immunization with a conjugate polysaccharide vaccine, including routine immunization of infants and a single mass immunization of adults has a high probability of eliminating group A epidemics in the meningococcal belt.[68]

The recent development of local epidemics with group W135 disease has prompted a short-term solution of a low-cost, specially formulated trivalent vaccine containing A, C, and W135 for use in the meningococcal belt. Should the group W135 become more prevalent in the meningococcal belt, the MVP program will consider making a bivalent conjugate polysaccharide vaccine available in its program.[69]

References

1. Vieusseux M. Mep1moire sur la maladie qui a regné a Genêve au printemps de 1805. *J Med Chir Pharmacol.* 1805;11:163.
2. Weichselbaum A. Ueber die aetiologie der akuten meningitis cerebro-spinalis. *Fortschr Med.* 1887;5:573–583.
3. Greenwood B. Manson lecture. Meningococcal meningitis in Africa. *Trans R Soc Trop Med Hyg.* 1999;93:341–353.
4. Sharip A, Sorvillo F, Redelings MD, Mascola L, Wise M, Nguyen DM. Population-based analysis of meningococcal disease mortality in the United States 1990–2002. *Pediatr Infects Dis J.* 2006;25:191–194.
5. Rosenstein NE, Perkins BA, Stephens DS, Popovic T, Hughes JM. Meningococcal disease. *N Engl J Med.* 2001;344:1378–1388.
6. Pizza M, Scarlato V, Masignani V, et al. Identification of vaccine candidates against serogroups B meningococcus by whole-genome sequencing. *Science.* 2000;287:1816–1820.
7. Parkhill J, Achtman M, James KD, et al. Complete DNA sequence of a serogroup A strain of *Neisseria meningitidis* Z2491. *Nature.* 2000;404:502–506.
8. Maiden MC, Bygraves JA, Feil E, et al. Multilocus sequence typing: a portable approach to the identification of clones within populations of pathogenic microorganisms. *Proc Natl Acad Sci USA.* 1998;95: 3140–3145.
9. Swartley JS, Marfin AA, Edupuganti S, et al. Capsule switching of *Neisseria meningitidis. Proc Natl Acad Sci USA.* 1997;94:271–276.
10. Bille E, Zahar J-R, Perrin A, et al. A chromosomally integrated bacteriophage in invasive meningococci. *J Exp Med.* 2005;201: 1905–1913.
11. Moore PS, Hierholzer J, DeWitt W, et al. Respiratory viruses and mycoplasma as cofactors for epidemic group A meningococcal meningitis. *JAMA.* 1990;264:1271–1275.
12. Yazdankhah SP, Caugant DA. *Neisseria meningitidis*: an overview of the carriage state. *J Med Microbiol.* 2004;53:821–832.
13. Broome CV. The carrier state. *Neisseria meningitidis. J Antimicrob Chemother.* 1986;18(suppl A):25–34.
14. Maiden MC. Dynamics of bacterial carriage and disease: lessons from the meningococcus. *Adv Exp Med Biol.* 2004;549:23–29.
15. Caugant DA, Hoiby EA, Magnus P, et al. Asymptomatic carriage of *Neisseria meningitidis* in a randomly sampled population. *J Clin Microbiol.* 1994;32:323–330.
16. Apicella MA. *N. meningitidis.* In: Mandell GL, Bennet JE, Livingston RDC, eds. *Principles and Practice of Infectious Disease.* Philadelphia, Pa: Churchill, Livingston; 2000:2228–2241.
17. Flexner S. The results of serum treatment in thirteen hundred cases of epidemic meningitis. *J Exp Med.* 1913;17:553–576.
18. Tondella ML, Rosenstein NE, Mayer LW, et al. Lack of evidence for chloramphenicol resistance in *Neisseria meningitidis*, Africa. *Emerg Infect Dis.* 2001;7:163–164.

19. Kirsch EA, Barton RP, Kitchen L, Giroir BP. Pathophysiology, treatment and outcome of meningococcemia: a review and recent experience. *Pediatr Infect Dis J.* 1996;15:967–978; quiz 979. Comment in: *Pediatr Infect Dis J.* 1997;16:540–542.

20. Centers for Disease Control and Prevention. Prevention and control of meningococcal disease and meningococcal disease and college students: recommendation of the Advisory Committee on Immunization Practices (ACIP). *MMWR.* 2000;49(No. RR-7):1–22.

21. Hibberd ML, Sumiya M, Summerfield JA, Booy R, Levin M. Association of variants of the gene for mannose-binding lectin with susceptibility to meningococcal disease. *Lancet.* 1999;353:1049–1053.

22. Emonts M, Hazelzet JA, de Groot R, Hermans PW. Host genetic determinants of *Neisseria meningitidis* infections. *Lancet Infect Dis.* 2003;3:565–577.

23. Stuart JM, Cartwright KA, Robinson PM, Noah ND. Effect of smoking on meningococcal carriage. *Lancet.* 1989;2:723–725.

24. Harrison LH, Dwyer DM, Maples CT, Billmann L. Risk of meningococcal infection in college students. *JAMA.* 1999;281:1906–1910.

25. Hodgson A, Smith T, Gagneux S, et al. Risk factors for meningococcal meningitis in northern Ghana. *Trans R Soc Trop Med Hyg.* 2001;95: 477–480.

26. Cartwright K, Noah N, Peltola H, Meningococcal Disease Advisory Board. Meningococcal disease in Europe: epidemiology, mortality, and prevention with conjugate vaccines. Report of a European advisory board meeting Vienna, Austria, 6–8 October 2000. *Vaccine.* 2001;19:4347–4356.

27. Greenwood BM, Greenwood AM, Bradley AK, et al. Factors influencing susceptibility to meningococcal disease during an epidemic in the Gambia, West Africa. *J Infect.* 1987;14:167–184.

28. Noah N, Henderson B. *Surveillance of Bacterial Meningitis in Europe 1999/2000.* London, UK: PHLS; 2002:1–47. Available at: http://www.phls.org.uk/topics_az/meningo/m_surveillance9900.pdf. Accessed April 25, 2005.

29. Ramsay ME, Andrews N, Kaczmarski EB, Miller E. Efficacy of meningococcal serogroup C conjugate vaccine in teenagers and toddlers in England. *Lancet.* 2001;357:195–196.

30. Lingappa JR, Al-Rabeah AM, Hajjeh R, et al. Serogroup W-135 meningococcal disease during the Hajj, 2000. *Emerg Infect Dis.* 2003;9:665–671.

31. Rosenstein NE, Perkins BA, Stephens DS, et al. The changing epidemiology of meningococcal disease in the United States, 1992–1996. *J Infect Dis.* 1999;180:1894–1901.

32. Tondella MLC, Popovic T, Rosenstein NE, et al. Distribution of *Neisseria meningitidis* serogroup B serosubtypes and serotypes circulating in the United States. *J Clin Microbiol.* 2000;38:3323–3328.

33. Wang J-F, Caugant DA, Li X, et al. Clonal and antigenic analysis of serogroup A *Neisseria meningitidis* with particular reference to epidemiological features of epidemic meningitis in the People's Republic of China. *Infect Immun.* 1992;60:5267–5282.

34. Zhu P, van der Ende A, Falush D, et al. Fit genotypes and escape variants of subgroup III *Neisseria meningitidis* during three pandemics of epidemic meningitis. *Proc Natl Acad Sci.* 2001;98:5234–5239.

35. Moore PS. Meningococcal meningitis in sub-Saharan Africa: a model for the epidemic process. *Clin Infect Dis.* 1992;14:515–525.

36. Riou JY, Djibo S, Sangare L, et al. A predictable comeback: the second pandemic of infections caused by *Neisseria meningitidis* serogroup A subgroup III in Africa, 1995. *Bull WHO.* 1996;74:181–187.

37. Dull PM, Abdelwahab J, Sacchi CT, et al. *Neisseria meningitidis* serogroup W-135 carriage among US travelers to the 2001 Hajj. *J Infect Dis.* 2005;191:33–39.

38. Wilder-Smith A, Goh KT, Barkham T, Paton NI. Hajj-associated outbreak strain of *Neisseria meningitidis* serogroup W135: estimates of the attack rate in a defined population and the risk of invasive disease developing in carriers. *Clin Infect Dis.* 2003;36:679–683.

39. Tikhomirov E, Santamaria M, Esteves K. Meningococcal disease: public health burden and control. *World Health Stat Q.* 1997;50:170–177.

40. Lepeyssonnie L. La méningite cérébrospinale en Afrique. *Bull WHO.* 1963;28(suppl):53–114.

41. Cheesbrough JS, Morse AP, Green DR. Meningococcal meningitis and carriage in western Zaire: a hypoendemic zone related to climate? *Epidemiol Infect.* 1995;114:75–92.

42. Sultan B, Labadi K, Guégan JF, Janicot S. Climate drives the meningitis epidemics onset in West Africa. *PLoS Med.* 2005;2:0045–0049.

43. Molesworth AM, Cuevas LE, Connor SJ, Morse AP, Thomson MC. Environmental risk and meningitis epidemics in Africa. *Emerg Infect Dis.* 2003;9:1287–1293.

44. Greenwood BM, Bradley AK, Wall RA. Meningococcal disease and season in sub-Saharan Africa. *Lancet.* 1985;2:829–830.

45. Sacchi CT, Whitney AM, Popovic T, et al. Diversity and prevalence of PorA types in *Neisseria meningitidis* serogroup B in the United States, 1992–1998. *J Infect Dis.* 2000;182:1169–1176.

46. Danzig L. Meningococcal vaccines. *Pediatr Infect Dis J.* 2004;23:S285–S292.

47. Jódar L, Feavers IM, Salisbury D, Granoff DM. Development of vaccines against meningococcal disease. *Lancet.* 2002;359:1499–1508.

48. Balmer P, Borrow R, Miller E. Impact of meningococcal C conjugate vaccine in the UK. *J Med Microbiol.* 2002;51:717–722.

49. Sierra GVG, Campa HC, Varcacel NM, et al. Vaccine against group B *Neisseria meningitidis*: protection trial and mass vaccination results in Cuba. *NIPH Ann.* 1991;14:195–210.

50. Bjune G, Hoiby EA, Gronnesby JK, et al. Effect of outer membrane vesicle vaccine against group B meningococcal disease in Norway. *Lancet.* 1991;338:1093–1096.

51. Holst J, Feiring B, Fuglesang JE, et al. Serum bactericidal activity correlates with the vaccine efficacy of outer membrane vesicle vaccines against *Neisseria meningitidis* serogroup B disease. *Vaccine.* 2003;21:734–737.

52. Rappuoli R. Reverse vaccinology, a genome-based approach to vaccine development. *Vaccine.* 2001;19:2688–2691.

53. Centers for Disease Control and Prevention. Prevention and control of meningococcal disease recommendations of the Advisory Committee on Immunization Practices (ACIP). *MMWR.* 2005;54(No. RR-7):1–21.

54. Raghunathan PL, Bernhardt SA, Rosenstein NE. Opportunities for control of meningococcal disease in the United States. *Annu Rev Med.* 2004;55:333–353.

55. Committee on Infectious Diseases. Prevention and control of meningococcal disease: recommendations for use of meningococcal vaccines in pediatric patients. *Pediatrics.* 2005;116:496–505.

56. Nakhla I, Frenck RW Jr, Teleb NA, et al. The changing epidemiology of meningococcal meningitis after introduction of bivalent A/C polysaccharide vaccine into school-based vaccination programs in Egypt. *Vaccine.* 2005;23;3288–3293.
57. Trotter CL, Andrews NJ, Kaczmarski EB, Miller E, Ramsay ME. Effectiveness of meningococcal serogroup C conjugate vaccine 4 years after introduction. *Lancet.* 2004;364:365–367.
58. Snape MD, Pollard AJ. Meningococcal polysaccharide-protein conjugate vaccines. *Lancet Infect Dis.* 2005;5:21–30.
59. World Health Organization. Detecting meningococcal meningitis epidemics in highly endemic African countries. *Wkly Epidemiol Rec.* 2000;38:306–309.
60. Robbins JB, Towne DW, Gotschlich EC, Schneerson R. "Love's labours lost": failure to implement mass vaccination against group A meningococcal meningitis in sub-Saharan Africa. *Lancet.* 1997;350:819,880–882.
61. Robbins JB, Schneerson R, Gotschlich EC. A rebuttal: epidemic and endemic meningococcal meningitis in sub-Saharan Africa can be prevented now by routine immunization with group A meningococcal capsular polysaccharide vaccine. *Pediatr Infect Dis J.* 2000;19:945–953.
62. Robbins JB, Schneerson R, Gotschlich EC, et al. Meningococcal meningitis in sub-Saharan Africa: the case for mass and routine vaccination with available polysaccharide vaccines. *Bull WHO.* 2003;81:745–750.
63. See responses to 57 in *Bull WHO* 2003;81:751–755.
64. Miller MA, Wenger J, Rosenstein N, Perkins B. Evaluation of meningococcal meningitis vaccination strategies for the meningitis belt in Africa. *Pediatr Infect Dis J.* 1999;18:1051–1059.
65. Lewis R, Nathan N, Diarra L, Belanger F, Paquet C. Timely detection of meningococcal meningitis epidemics in Africa. *Lancet.* 2001;358: 287–293.
66. Leake JA, Kone ML, Yada AA, et al. Early detection and response to meningococcal disease epidemics in sub-Saharan Africa: appraisal of the WHO strategy. *Bull WHO.* 2002;80:342–349.
67. www.menigvax.org/about-mvp.htm, accessed January 2006.
68. Jódar L, LaForce FM, Ceccarini C, Aguado T, Granoff DM. Meningococcal conjugate vaccine for Africa: a model for development of new vaccines for the poorest countries. *Lancet.* 2003;361: 1902–1904.
69. Leach A, Twumasi PA, Kumah S, et al. Induction of immunologic memory in Gambian children by vaccination in infancy with a group A plus group C meningococcal polysaccharide-protein conjugate vaccine. *J Infect Dis.* 1997;175:200–204.

For Your Reference

WHO Web site for reports of meningococcal disease in Africa. Available at: http://www.who.int/csr/disease/meningococcal/epidemiological/en/.

CHAPTER EIGHTEEN

TUBERCULOSIS

Jacqueline S. Coberly and Richard E. Chaisson

Introduction

The ancient Greeks called it *phthisis*, the Romans *tabes*, the Hindus *rajay-akshma*, and in Victorian England it was *consumption*.[1] All these names referred to the wasting illness that is characteristic of the disease we now call *tuberculosis*. Tuberculosis is a complex communicable disease of humans caused by the tubercle bacilli, a group of genetically related mycobacteria also known collectively as the *Mycobacterium tuberculosis* complex. The tubercle bacilli are a group of slow-growing mycobacteria that includes *M. tuberculosis, M. africanum, M. canettii, M. bovis,* and *M. microti.* The first three members of this group are, at least to date, strictly human pathogens. *M. bovis* causes illness in a variety of animals as well as in man.[2-4] Similarly *M. microti* generally causes disease in rodents, but has been linked retrospectively to infections in llamas, ferrets, and cats. It has also been implicated as the cause of pulmonary tuberculosis in a small number of humans.[5] With the advent of effective drug treatment in the 1950s and preventive therapy, or chemoprophylaxis as it was then called, in the 1960s, many in the medical and public health communities, particularly in the industrialized countries, assumed tuberculosis was conquered. This hubris led to several decades of neglect by the biomedical community, during which control efforts were ignored or deliberately weakened.[6] Unfortunately, the economic, social, and public health factors that foster the propagation of tuberculosis had not been eliminated, not even from the industrialized nations. So in the 1980s and 1990s, as the deterioration of control programs coincided with the burgeoning epidemic of human immunodeficiency virus (HIV), tuberculosis rebounded. Numerous outbreaks were seen in the larger cities of the United States that had the highest incidence of HIV.[7] More serious, however, was that in some areas of the developing world where tuberculosis and HIV are both endemic, the incidence of tuberculosis doubled, and health care facilities were over-whelmed by the dual epidemic.[6]

The World Health Organization (WHO) declared tuberculosis to be a global emergency in 1993.[6] Twelve years later, considerable progress has been made, but tuberculosis remains a leading cause of premature death in young adults around the world.[8] Roughly one third of the world's inhabitants are latently infected with *M. tuberculosis*, and in 2003, the most recent year for which statistics are available, WHO estimated that 8.8 million people developed tuberculosis and 1.7 million died from it.[9,10] Efforts to promote tuberculosis control have more than doubled since 1993, and although the tuberculosis incidence continued to increase in 2003, incidence, prevalence, and mortality rates were stable or dropped in seven of WHO's nine health regions. Unfortunately the situation is not as promising in Africa and Eastern Europe. The high prevalence of latent infection and HIV infection, developing drug resistance, and the complex epidemiology and natural history of tuberculosis continues to make tuberculosis control in these areas particularly challenging.[11]

The Organism

The family Mycobacteriaceae, of the order Actinomycetales, is composed of a number of slow-growing, acid-fast bacilli. Most are saprophytes—useful inhabitants of soil and water that fix nitrogen and help degrade organic material. Some are pathogens in animals and occasionally cause opportunistic infection in man.[12,13] Only four species are highly pathogenic in humans: *Mycobacterium leprae* which causes leprosy, and three of the tubercle bacilli. The tubercle bacilli, or *Mycobacterium tuberculosis* complex, are a group of five closely related mycobacteria that cause tuberculosis. *M. tuberculosis*, *M. africanum*, and *M. bovis* are the most common cause of human tuberculosis, although *M. bovis* is also known to cause disease in a variety of animal species. The other two members of the complex, *M. canettii* and *M. microti*, do cause tuberculosis in humans but infrequently.[1,3–5,13] In fact, *M. microti* has only been identified as a human pathogen relatively recently.[5] Although they vary widely by favored host, phenotype, and pathogenicity, the bacteria that make up the *M. tuberculosis* complex share more than 90% of their genome and have identical 16S rRNA sequences.[2,14] With the advent of the HIV epidemic, several other mycobacteria, most notably *M. avium* complex (MAC), have become common opportunistic pathogens and, in people infected with HIV, cause illness that is clinically similar to disseminated tuberculosis.[1,12] See Table 18-1.

The bacteria that make up the *M. tuberculosis* complex are slender, slightly curved, rod-shaped bacteria averaging 4 by 0.3 μm.[1,3,13] *M. tuberculosis* is strictly aerobic; *M. bovis* is microaerophilic and adapts more easily to nonpulmonary sites of infection. As with other mycobacteria, the tubercle bacilli have an unusual concentration of high molecular weight lipids in their cell wall, accounting for approximately 50% of dry weight. This high lipid content makes these organisms hydrophobic and resistant to aqueous bactericidal agents and drying. It is also responsible for their acid-fast nature, a characteristic that is essentially synonymous with mycobacteria.[3,12]

TABLE 18-1   Species of *Mycobacteria*

	Microbe	Reservoir	Clinical Manifestation
Always pathogenic in man	*M. tuberculosis*	Man	Pulmonary and disseminated TB
	M. bovis	Cattle, man	TB-like disease
	M. leprae	Man	Leprosy
	M. africanum	Man, monkey	Rarely TB-like pulmonary disease
Potentially pathogenic in man	*M. avium* complex	Soil, water, birds, fowl, swine, cattle, and environment	Disseminated and pulmonary TB-like disease
	M. canettii	Man, possibly others	Rarely TB-like pulmonary disease
	M. microti	Rodents, llamas, cats, ferrets, and possibly man	Rarely TB-like pulmonary disease
	M. kansasii	Water, cattle	TB-like disease
Uncommon or rarely pathogenic in man	*M. genavense*	Possibly man and pet birds	Blood-borne disease with AIDS
	M. haemophilum	Unknown	Subcutaneous nodules and ulcers primarily with AIDS
	M. malmoense	Environment, possibly others	Adults: TB-like pulmonary Children: Lymphadenitis
	M. marinum	Fish, water	Skin infections
	M. scrofulaceum	Soil, water	Cervical lymphadenitis
	M. simiae	Monkey, water	TB-like pulmonary and disseminated disease with AIDS
	M. szulgai	Unknown	TB-like pulmonary disease
	M. ulcerans	Man, environment	Skin infections (Buruli ulcer)
	M. xenopi	Water, birds	TB-like pulmonary disease

Source: Adapted from: Brooks GF, Butel JS, Morse SA, editors. Jawetz, Melnick & Adelberg's Medical Microbiology, 21st Edition. Stamford: Appleton & Lange; 1998. And Niemann, S, E Richter, H Dalugge-Tamm, H Schlesinger, D Graupner, B Koniegstein, G Gurath, U Greinert, S Rusch-Gerdes (2000). "Two cases of *Mycobacterium microti*-derived tuberculosis in HIV-negative immunocompetent patients." *Emerging Infectious Diseases* 6(5): 539–42. And Pfyffer, G, R Auckenthaler, JDA van Embden, D van Soolingen (1998). "*Mycobacterium canettii*, the smooth variant of *M. tuberculosis*, isolated from a Swiss patient exposed in Africa." *Emerging Infectious Diseases* 4(4): 631–4.

Mycobacteria are slow-growing and fastidious in culture, and because *M. tuberculosis* has a very long generation time (approximately 24 hours), culture is a slow process, often resulting in diagnostic delays and sometimes misdiagnosis.[5] Traditionally mycobacteria are grown on solid, enriched media where colonies generally appear 4 to 6 weeks after inoculation. They can also be grown in liquid culture where they form characteristic strings that can be seen by light microscopy. Rapid liquid culture systems (e.g., BACTEC) have been adapted for use with mycobacteria and allow identification of organisms in as little as 9–16 days, depending on the concentration of microbes in the specimen being tested.[3,15] DNA probes speed speciation of organisms following growth. Alternatively a number of biochemical tests can be used to speciate mycobacteria, though these are time consuming.[3,16]

In 1998 a consortium of scientists deciphered and published the genome map of the H37Rv strain of *M. tuberculosis* (Figure 18-1). The complete genome is 4,411,529 base pairs long and contains approximately 4000 genes.[17] Since then, advances in genotyping technology have been rapidly applied to studies of the molecular epidemiology of the tubercle bacilli. Genotyping methods including restriction fragment-length polymorphism (RFLP), polymerase chain reaction (PCR)-based spoligotyping, and profiling of the mycobacterial interspersed repetitive units by the number and size of the variable number tandem repeats in the genome (MIRU-VNTR) have been rapidly adopted. These methods vary in sensitivity and specificity, so some caution is needed when interpreting results.[18] Genotyping studies are providing some interesting insights into the epidemiology of tuberculosis. For example, 10 years ago it was dogma that *M. tuberculosis* was a mutated form of *M. bovis*; the assumption being that around 7000–4000 BCE when man began domesticating animals he was exposed to *M. bovis*, which, over time, mutated into a human pathogen.[19] In a recent fingerprinting study, however, the genomes of 100 strains of *M. tuberculosis* complex were mapped and compared. The genetic lineage developed from these analyses provides evidence that *M. tuberculosis* is not a mutation of *M. bovis*; rather both bacteria diverged from a common ancestor long before either infected humans.[2,14] See Figure 18-2. DNA fingerprinting is also being used with traditional field epidemiology to help link index and secondary cases and distinguish active disease resulting from reactivation versus recent transmission. When distinguishing between reactivation and recent transmission, the presumption is that the genotype of cases due to reactivation will not match the genotype of other cases in the community because infection was acquired at some distant point in the past. Whereas in cases due to recent infection the genotype of the organism should be shared with at least the index case and probably other cases in the community resulting from the same index case. Note, however, that these "orphan" isolates that do not share a genotype with any other organism from the community could still be related to other cases in the community, but the link cannot be identified with traditional epidemiology; this can happen when the index case is sputum negative, or the DNA fingerprint of the index is obtained for other reasons. In general, however, cluster analysis is fairly reliable and has provided new and interesting epidemiologic information about tuberculosis.

Before fingerprinting was commonly available it was dogma that most infections in immunosuppressed people in low prevalence areas were due to

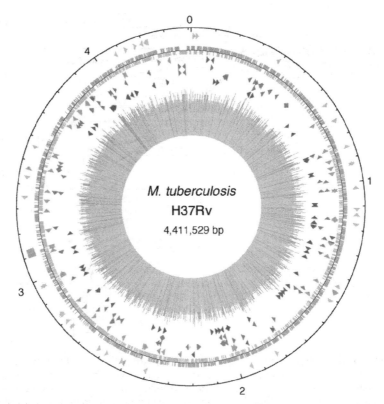

FIGURE 18-1 Circular map of the chromosome of *M. tuberculosis* H37Rv. The outer circle shows the scale in Mb, with 0 representing the origin of replication. The first ring from the exterior denotes the positions of stable RNA genes and the direct repeat region; the second ring inward shows the coding sequence by strand; the third ring depicts repetitive DNA; the fourth ring shows the positions of the PPE family members; the fifth ring shows the PE family members; and the sixth ring shows the positions of the PGRS sequences. The figure was generated with software from DNASTAR.
Source: Cole, ST et al. Deciphering the biology of *Mycobacterium tuberculosis* from the complete genome sequence. Nature 1998 Jun 11; 393(6685):537–44. Reprinted by permission from Macmillan Publishers, Ltd.

reactivation. The populations at risk were often transient, and linking cases epidemiologically was difficult. DNA fingerprinting studies of community cohorts have identified some surprising clusters and helped guide the shoe-leather epidemiology needed to confirm the linkages suggested by fingerprint evidence.[20] Fingerprinting studies have also helped characterize the global distribution of genotypes, clarify patterns of transmission in communities, and prioritize control activities.[21-26] DNA fingerprinting is also being used to investigate the origins of susceptibility to the tuberculosis bacilli and innate host immunity to it.[18,27,28]

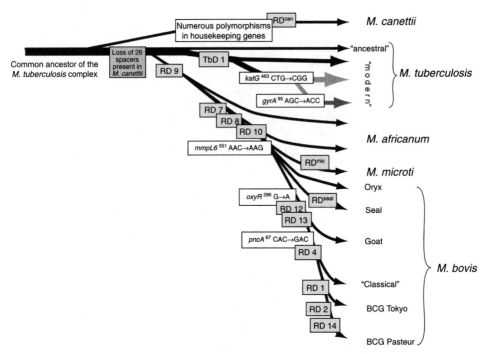

FIGURE 18-2   Scheme of the proposed evolutionary pathway of the tubercle bacilli illustrating successive loss of DNA in certain lineages (gray boxes). The scheme is based on the presence or absence of conserved deleted regions and on sequence polymorphisms in five selected genes. Note that the distances between certain branches may not correspond to actual phylogenetic differences calculated by other methods. The Top five dark arrows indicate that strains are characterized by *katG*463. CTG (Leu), *gyrA*95 ACC (Thr), typical for group 1 organisms. The bottom seven arrows indicate that strains belong to group 2 characterized by *katG*463 CGG (Arg), *gyrA*95 ACC (Thr). The light gray arrow indicates that strains belong to group 3, characterized by *katG*463 CGG (Arg), *gyrA*95 AGC(Ser), as defined by Sreevatsan *et al.* (2).
Source: Brosch, R, AS Pym, SV Gordon, ST Cole (2001), "The evolution of mycobacterial pathogenicity: clues from comparative genomics." *Trends in Microbiology* 9(9):452–8.

History

Evolution of the Tubercle Bacilli

Mycobacteria are ancient organisms that probably first appeared more than a million years ago in soil and water and gradually adapted to animal hosts during the Paleolithic period.[19,29] Until recently, it was hypothesized that when humans began domesticating cattle they began to be exposed to *M. bovis*, which eventually mutated into the human pathogen *M. tuberculosis*. A recent comparison of the genotype of 100 tubercle bacilli showed, however, that *M. bovis*, *M. tuberculosis*, and the other members of the *M. tuberculosis* complex all diverged from a common ancestor through successive loss of DNA (Figure 18-2).[2]

Regardless of the evolutionary path of the tubercle bacilli, at some point in early prehistory tuberculosis became pathogenic for humans. Skeletal remains of Neolithic man with deformities suggestive of tuberculosis have been found in Germany, France, Italy, Denmark, and Jordan and are dated from 8000 to 5000 BCE.[1,30] It cannot be conclusively proved that these defor-mities are the result of infection with the tubercle bacillus as the organism cannot be cultured from the bone. The deformities themselves are strongly suggestive of spinal tuberculosis or Pott's disease, however.[1,19]

Traces of tuberculosis-like disease have also been identified in Egyptian mummies dating from 3500 to 400 BCE.[3,29] One particularly well-preserved mummy of a 5-year-old boy from about 1000 BCE was discovered with the lungs intact. Again, the causative organism could not be conclusively identi-fied, but a diagnosis of tuberculosis was made based on the observation of pleural adhesion, blood in the trachea, and the presence of acid-fast bacilli in the lung tissue.[3] Egyptian artifacts from this period also begin to show people with the spinal deformities characteristic of Pott's disease.[3]

Based on available evidence, tuberculosis appears to have initially been a sporadic disease in humans. This is difficult to verify, however, because relatively few large collections of skeletal remains of prehistoric man are available for examination. What is known with certainty is that as civilization developed and people began to gather together in ever increasing numbers, reports of tuberculosis became more numerous, leading to the establishment of tuberculosis as an endemic disease of humans by the beginning of the first millennium.[1,19]

Global Evolution of the Epidemic

By AD 100, tuberculosis was well established in the Mediterranean states and Western Europe. It remained relatively sporadic for centuries, until people began settling in larger communities.[19] The advent of the Industrial Revolu-tion and the great migrations to the cities that followed created an ideal environment for the spread of tuberculosis.[29,31] In 1662, 1 of every 6 north-ern Europeans had tuberculosis; a 100 years later the figure had doubled.[3] Tuberculosis was so common that most of the population became infected, and 25% of all deaths were attributed to tuberculosis.[19] Thomas Sydenham was quoted in 1682 as saying, "Two thirds of those who die of chronic diseases . . . (are) . . . killed by phthisis."[31] The epidemic peaked in England in 1780s and in Western Europe by 1800.[29]

Although sporadic, *M. bovis* infections were not uncommon in the largely agrarian societies of the New World; but the English and European colonists are probably responsible for spreading *M. tuberculosis* throughout the world. Tuberculosis came to North America on the *Mayflower* and was well estab-lished in the colonies by the early 1700s.[1,29] The epidemic passed through the United States in a wave pushing south and west with the spread of industrialization, and by the early 1900s it was endemic in North America.[29] Tuberculosis was also spread to South America by colonists, but because the Spanish quarantined consumptives in the 1600s and 1700s, the disease was introduced there somewhat later.[1] Tuberculosis also spread into Eastern Europe, Asia, and Africa from Western Europe. The epidemics in Russia came in the late 1800s and in Asia in the early 1900s. Tuberculosis was still largely unknown in Africa at the beginning of the 1900s and spread slowly through the interior with the colonizing Europeans.[1,19] Herd immunity to tuberculosis develops slowly because of the long incubation period of the organism. Dif-ferences in the epidemiology in different parts of the world may be related to when tuberculosis was introduced to the population, with the most serious disease present in Africa where tuberculosis was introduced latest leaving the least amount of time for herd immunity to develop.[19,32]

Clinical Manifestations

As discussed in more detail later, tuberculosis begins with latent infection that can progress to active disease. Latent tuberculosis infection (LTBI) causes no symptoms, and most latently infected people are unaware that they harbor tubercle bacilli. Tuberculosis disease generally affects the lungs and respiratory tract, but can strike nearly any organ system in the body. Both primary and reactivation tuberculosis disease can result in pulmonary or extrapulmonary manifestations. In immunocompetent people, about 80% of tuberculosis is pulmonary, and extrapulmonary disease is less common. Extrapulmonary disease is, however, much more common in immunodeficient individuals and children.[33,34] A small percentage of immunocompetent patients and many more immunodeficient ones develop both pulmonary and extrapulmonary tuberculosis.[34]

The onset of active tuberculosis is insidious, and the symptoms can be nonspecific. Pulmonary disease causes symptoms ranging from very mild to severe and can present with productive cough with or without bloody sputum, fatigue, anorexia, weight loss, fever, sweating and/or chills, and chest pain.[13,33,34] Extrapulmonary tuberculosis also causes fatigue and night sweats, but generally other symptoms specifically related to the affected organ system will be prominent.[13,33-35] More frequent sites of extrapulmonary infection include the pleura, pericardium, larynx, lymph nodes, skeleton (particularly the spine), genitourinary tract, eyes, meninges, gastrointestinal tract, adrenal glands, and skin.[3,36-38] Systemic infection with tubercle bacilli occurs when hematogenous or lymphatic dissemination spreads the organism throughout the body, producing small nodules of infection in essentially every organ. Early researchers named disseminated disease *miliary tuberculosis* because they thought the tiny nodules resembled grains of millet, particularly when seen by chest radiography.[13,34,39] Miliary tuberculosis is especially common in children and in people with immunosuppression.[7,33,40]

Diagnosis

Latent Tuberculosis Infection

Latent tuberculosis infection (LTBI) is asymptomatic; therefore, diagnosis is based on clinical tests that identify signs of infection or immunologic responses to tuberculosis antigens. In the past, tuberculosis infection was often diagnosed radiographically, with calcified lesions interpreted as evidence of infection.[3,41] This technique has been shown to lack both sensitivity and specificity and has been abandoned. Serologic diagnosis of tuberculosis infection has been extensively investigated but also lacks sensitivity because the number of tubercle bacilli in latent tuberculosis is very low, and antibody responses are limited.[42] Identification of specific cellular immune responses through the induction of delayed-type hypersensitivity with a tuberculin skin test (TST) is still the most widely used method for diagnosing latent infection.[42,43]

Purified protein derivative (PPD) of tuberculin is a solution prepared from cultures of tubercle bacilli.[44,45] It was developed by Robert Koch in 1890 and touted as a cure for tuberculosis. The curative value of tuberculin was soon disproved, but further studies showed that it could be used to identify people with tuberculosis infection.[41,45,46] The Mantoux method of intracutaneous injection of a standardized dose of PPD has been widely validated, while other methods (e.g., the Tine test) have not. Individuals with LTBI develop a zone of induration when a standardized amount of tuberculin is injected intracutaneously, whereas uninfected people react minimally or not at all. The TST result is reported as the width of induration that surrounds the test site a minimum of 48–72 hours following injection.[47] The test is usually applied to the volar surface of the forearm and read by a trained observer, who measures induration by marking the edge of the hardened area of skin, either visually or manually, to demarcate the border, and recording the distance across in millimeters. Induration of the injection site is the result of a delayed-type hypersensitivity response in which activated T cells and macrophages migrate to the site of antigen injection and mount a localized cellular immune response. It is essential that at least 48 hours be allowed for this process to mature; earlier readings may produce falsely negative or positive results. Erythema of the site is nonspecific and with the exception of Japan is not used to determine test results. Positive results remain measurable for more than one week in most instances.[48]

The performance characteristics of the tuberculin test were standardized in the 1940s in an important study by Dr. Carroll Palmer, where varying concentrations of tuberculin were administered to a group of patients with active tuberculosis and to controls who were unlikely to have ever encountered tuberculosis.[49] The currently used standard dose of 5 tuberculin units of PPD-S was found to elicit a reaction of greater than 10 mm of induration in almost 98% of tuberculosis patients and in less than 5% of controls. A smaller dose, 2 tuberculin units, of another preparation, RT-23 tuberculin, produces similar results.

Exposure to nontuberculous mycobacteria may induce cross-reactivity to the tuberculin, which can result in a falsely positive reaction.[45] Similarly, vaccination against tuberculosis with BCG vaccine can induce a response. The strength and durability of the reaction produced by BCG is less than with tuberculosis infection, and after three to five years it does not generally interfere with PPD testing.[33,50,51] Skin test results can also be falsely negative when the cellular immune system is impaired. People with active tuberculosis who are coinfected with HIV or have cancer or other immunosuppressive illnesses are frequently unable to mount a response to any skin test antigen, so tuberculin results in these people should be interpreted with some care.[35,36,45,49] Malnutrition and micronutrient deficiencies also interfere with immunity and can inhibit response to tuberculin as can acute viral infections such as measles.[13,33,41,52–55] In addition, between 10% and 25% of people with active tuberculosis fail to respond to tuberculin.[45,56] The size of the tuberculin response is not, however, associated with the patient's stage of disease as the size of reaction in active cases and their close contacts is similar.[36,45]

Thus the size of the reaction to tuberculin varies considerably depending on the individual's exposure to the tubercle bacilli and other nontuberculous mycobacteria, BCG vaccination history, and immune status.[45]

Although the sensitivity and specificity of tuberculin testing can be evaluated in people with active tuberculosis, determining the accuracy of the test in people with latent infection is more difficult, as no gold standard for diagnosis exists. In studies of US Navy recruits undertaken in the 1950s and 1960s, a tuberculin reaction of greater than 10 mm was strongly associated with the subsequent risk of tuberculosis. Nonetheless, because some people with negative tests develop tuberculosis and many people with positive tests do not, the interpretation of test results must be modified on the basis of clinical and epidemiologic knowledge. Perhaps more so than with most clinical tests, interpretation of the tuberculin test is highly dependent on prior probability of tuberculosis infection and clinical consequences of misreading the result. As shown in Table 18-2, the reaction size that is considered positive varies by the clinical status of the person being tested.[47] For example, people likely to have been recently exposed to tuberculosis such as household contacts of an active infectious case have a high prior probability of infection and the cut-point for a positive test is reduced to 5 mm. Similarly, an HIV-infected person has a very high risk of developing active tuberculosis if infected, so a 5-mm reaction is considered positive because the consequences of misinterpreting the result are severe and because HIV infection suppresses the cellular immune response and can diminish the size of the reaction to

TABLE 18-2   Cut-Points for Positive Tuberculin Skin Test (TST)

Category	Induration = TST Positive
• Coinfected with HIV	≥5 mm
• Close contacts of known active case	
• People with fibrotic changes consistent with prior tuberculosis	
• People with organ transplants or other immunosuppression	
• Recent immigrants (<5 yrs)	≥10 mm
• Injection drug users (IDUs)	
• Prolonged exposure to high-risk congregate settings	
• Mycobacterial laboratory personnel	
• People with clinical conditions that put them at increased risk	
• Infant, children, and adolescent contacts exposed to adults in high-risk categories	
• People with no known risk factors for TB, but recommend only targeted skin testing	≥15 mm

Source: Adapted from Centers for Disease Control and Prevention, D. o. T. E. (2005). Tuberculin skin testing, document #250140.

PPD.[48] People who come from an area where tuberculosis is prevalent have a lower risk than household contacts but higher than someone who lives in a low incidence country; therefore, a 10-mm response is considered positive. For people with a low prior probability of tuberculosis exposure the cut-point for a positive test is 15 mm of induration.[47]

In recent years, attempts to modernize the diagnosis of latent tuberculosis have focused on assays that detect the production of interferon-gamma by T cells in response to stimulation with mycobacterial antigens.[57-61] Such immunodiagnostic assays promise to improve on the tuberculin test by eliminating skin test placement and reading errors, obviating the need for patients to return for interpretation of results and standardizing the assessment of results with objective measurements in a laboratory. Cells obtained from individuals who have been infected with *M. tuberculosis* will produce interferon-gamma when cocultivated with tuberculous antigens, whereas cells from uninfected individuals will not. Detection of the elaborated interferon-gamma is possible with either an ELISA that measures soluble cytokines or an enzyme-linked immunospot assay (ELISPOT) that stains intracellular interferon-gamma in T cells. Two commercial applications of this approach have been developed: an ELISA-based method called Quantiferon-Gold and an ELISPOT assay called T SPOT TB. Early versions of these assays relied on PPD-S as the antigen, and therefore were associated with false positive results in people who had been vaccinated with BCG or who had nontuberculous mycobacterial infections.[58] Second- and third-generation assays, now commercially available in a number of countries, rely on *M. tuberculosis*-specific antigens from a region of the mycobacterial genome known as RD-1 that is absent in BCG and most nontuberculous mycobacteria.[59] Studies of these tests show that they have excellent agreement with the tuberculin skin test, but appear to be more specific, as they are less likely to be positive in individuals with a history of BCG vaccination who are otherwise at low risk for tuberculosis infection.[59,60] These tests represent an enormous step forward in diagnosing latent TB, but they are limited by high cost, exacting technical requirements (fresh blood must be put into cell culture within several hours of being collected), and lack of prospective validation. Nonetheless, they are a welcome addition to the diagnostic arsenal and will play a valuable role in both clinical practice and epidemiologic research in the coming years.

Active Tuberculosis Disease

In active tuberculosis, clinical signs and symptoms result from the replication of large numbers of tubercle bacilli and the ensuing inflammatory host response. Diagnosis of active tuberculosis is based on evaluation of epidemiologic assessment of tuberculosis risk, clinical findings and symptoms, and laboratory tests including chest radiographs, tuberculin skin tests, microscopic examination, and culture of tissues such as sputum or biopsy specimens.

The signs and symptoms of active tuberculosis are nonspecific and overlap with a number of other pulmonary and systemic diseases. Fever, sweats, and weight loss are prominent systemic findings and are usually of several weeks or months duration. Cough is a principal feature of pulmonary tuberculosis and can be associated with sputum production or hemoptysis. The symptoms of extrapulmonary tuberculosis are highly variable and depend on the specific organ involved.

Chest radiographs are critically important in diagnosing pulmonary tuberculosis. Classically, patients with reactivation tuberculosis have upper-lobe cavitary infiltrates or involvement of the superior segments of the lower lobes, whereas patients with primary tuberculosis have mostly lower or midlung infiltrates and hilar adenopathy. Recent studies using molecular epidemiologic techniques, however, have shown that both primary and reactivation tuberculosis can present with chest X-ray findings that are classic for the other form of disease. In the setting of clinical symptoms consistent with tuberculosis and an abnormal chest radiograph, specific diagnostic tests for tuberculosis should be undertaken. With HIV infection and tuberculosis, however, the chest X-ray in some patients may be normal.

Diagnosis of tuberculosis is confirmed by identification of acid-fast bacilli by smear or by isolation of *M. tuberculosis* in cultures of sputum or other tissues. Zeihl-Nielsen staining is the standard method used globally for microscopic identification of acid-fast bacilli. In this process a fixed smear is exposed to hot carbol fushin dye for 2 to 3 minutes, rinsed, and decolorized with a dilute acid-alcohol solution. Mycobacteria absorb the carbol fushin dye but resist decolorization, because of the high lipid content in their cell walls, hence the name acid-fast bacilli.[15] Fluorescent staining with auramine-rhodamine is a more sensitive but more expensive technique. Unfortunately the number of tubercle bacilli present in sputum may be very low, particularly in noncavitary disease, so direct microscopic observation is a fairly insensitive way to diagnose tuberculosis. Only about 60% of culture-confirmed cases of tuberculosis are smear positive. Also, positive microscopy only proves the presence of acid-fast bacilli, which could include nonpathogenic species of mycobacteria or other acid-fast bacteria such as *Nocardia*.[35,36]

Several types of tests, including nucleic acid amplification assays (e.g., polymerase chain reaction), mass spectrometry, or gas-liquid chromatography for tuberculostearic acid, and immunoassays for mycobacterial antigens and antibodies, have been evaluated, with mixed results. Nucleic acid amplification tests have been approved in the United States for the diagnosis of tuberculosis in patients with positive sputum smears. Both the positive and negative predictive value of these tests are high if the sputum smear is positive, but in sputum smear negative patients the positive predictive value of nucleic acid amplification is only about 50%. In many parts of the world where tuberculosis is endemic, culture and radiography are unavailable or extremely limited. In these areas diagnosis relies primarily on clinical history and microscopic examination of sputum. New, simple, rapid diagnostic techniques are desperately needed in these areas and would also be valuable in more industrialized areas. Research in this area is ongoing but has been disappointing to date.

Ultimately, the diagnosis of tuberculosis involves a synthesis of clinical and laboratory findings. The case definition of tuberculosis used for surveillance purposes accepts the diagnosis if there is a positive culture, a positive acid-fast smear with compatible clinical findings, or a characteristic illness with other evidence suggestive of tuberculosis and an appropriate response to antituberculosis therapy.

Therapy

History of Therapy

The history of tuberculosis therapy is divided into three eras: the presanatorium, the sanatorium, and chemotherapeutic eras. From earliest recognition of tuberculosis as a disease until the middle of the 1800s, therapy for tuberculosis was based on the prevailing medical dogma.[62] When ill airs were thought to cause tuberculosis, patients were told to move to mild, mountain, or seaside climates. When imbalance of bodily humors was thought to be the cause of all disease, bloodletting was recommended for tuberculosis. Rest or mild exercise and different variations in diet were also recommended at various times. Although most of these treatments did the patient no harm, they also did little to deter the progress of the infection.

In the 1850s a number of physicians observed that a prolonged rest in quiet, mountainous, rural areas had cured their patients of tuberculosis, and the sanatorium movement was born. The premise was that clean air combined with rest or mild exercise and good food would stimulate the body to heal itself. Therefore patients were isolated in rural institutions built solely for the treatment of tuberculosis.[41,62] The first sanatorium was established by Brehmer in 1854 in the mountains of Germany, and as the idea took hold, sanatoria were built throughout Europe, the United States, and England.[41,62] Isolation of tuberculosis cases in sanatoria, although perhaps no more beneficial to patients than extended rest at home, decreased the spread of tuberculosis in the community, contributing to the large decline in tuberculosis incidence seen in the late 1800s and early 1900s in Europe and the United States.[62] Developments in the basic sciences during the sanatoria movement also contributed to this decline. During this time Koch discovered the causative agent of tuberculosis, and radiographic technology and surgical techniques were developed that greatly enhanced physicians' ability to diagnose and treat tuberculosis.

Unfortunately sanatorium care had its limitations, and in the early 1900s tuberculosis was still a major cause of death. In 1938 Rich and Follis showed that sulfanilamide inhibited the growth of *M. tuberculosis* in guinea pigs, and the search for effective chemotherapeutic agents for tuberculosis began. Dapsone was tested against tuberculosis in 1940, and in 1943 streptomycin was found to have antituberculosis action. The identification of other antituberculosis drugs, including para-aminosalicylic acid (PAS) and isoniazid (INH), soon followed.[62] The tradition of randomized clinical trials has a prominent place in the history of tuberculosis research. The scarcity of streptomycin in the early 1940s led the British Medical Research Council to perform the first multicenter, randomized, controlled clinical trial to estimate the efficacy of streptomycin against a placebo.[63] This elegant trial showed the profound efficacy of streptomycin against the tubercle bacilli and the limitations of single drug therapy in the treatment of tuberculosis. More trials followed the first rapidly as new drugs were identified, each building on the information provided by earlier work. A series of trials over several decades proved the value of combination therapy for curing tuberculosis and preventing drug resistance: the efficacy of dual therapy with streptomycin and PAS[64,65]; the efficacy of combined therapy using isoniazid[64]; the utility of multidrug therapy in shortening the duration of tuberculosis treatment[65]; the minimum treatment time needed for effective cure of tuberculosis[61-64]; the optimum drug combination for therapy[66-69]; the efficacy of intermittent (twice or thrice weekly) treatment[68,72-74]; and the efficacy of treatment for tuberculosis in HIV-infected people.[75-78]

Current Therapy

The drugs most commonly used in treatment of tuberculosis today and their mode of action are shown in Table 18-3. Because the bacillary population in an infected person consists of actively growing, semidormant, and dormant mycobacteria,[79] effective chemotherapy is complex. Some drugs that kill actively growing bacilli cannot kill those in the latent, resting phase. Drug treatment must, therefore, continue for a minimum of six months in order to allow the majority of latent organisms to be exposed to the drugs during periods of metabolic activity and to be killed. Unfortunately this long period of treatment also allows sufficient time for mutant bacilli to emerge that are resistant to the drug being used for treatment. When a single drug is used for treatment of tuberculosis, mutants resistant to that drug rapidly emerge, eventually become the predominant bacilli, and therapy fails. Use of at least two drugs to which the organisms are susceptible reduces the probability of developing drug-resistant microbes to essentially zero.

Key to treatment success is adherence with the full drug regimen, which reduces the risk of treatment failure and the emergence of drug resistance.[80] The CDC and other authorities recommend that directly observed therapy (DOT) be used for tuberculosis therapy. DOT implies that a health care worker monitors each tuberculosis patient closely and observes the patient take each dose of antituberculosis medication. Historical analysis suggests that use of DOT contributes to reductions in tuberculosis incidence and dramatically reduces the incidence of drug-resistant tuberculosis.[81] One randomized trial that compared DOT with self-administered therapy found no advantage to DOT; however, treatment outcomes in both groups were poor and the study was flawed in other aspects.[82] DOT is generally accepted as a highly effective tuberculosis control strategy.

TABLE 18-3   First-Line Antituberculosis Drugs and Their Modes of Action

Drug (Abbreviation)	Mode of Action	Effect
Isoniazid (H)	Bactericidal	Kills metabolically active mycobacteria
Rifampicin (R)	Bactericidal	Kills metabolically active and inactive mycobacteria
Pyrazinamide (Z)	Bactericidal	Kills mycobacteria at acid pH (within cells)
Streptomycin (S)	Bacteriostatic	Halts growth and reproduction; does not kill
Ethambutol (E)	Bacteriostatic	Halts growth and reproduction; does not kill
Thiacetazone (T)	Bacteriostatic	Halts growth and reproduction; does not kill

Source: A.D. Harries and A.D. Maher, TB/HIV: A Clinical Manual, Copyright 1996, World Health Organization, and R.H. Alford, Antimycobacterial Agents, in Principles and Practice of Infectious Diseases, 3rd ed., pp. 350–360, G.L. Mandell, R.G. Douglas, Jr., and J.E. Bennett, eds., © 1990, Churchill Livingstone.

The World Health Organization currently recommends a short-course DOT drug regimen (DOTS) for treatment of tuberculosis that includes treatment with four drugs, generally isoniazid, rifampin, pyrazinamide, and ethambutol, for two months, followed by four months treatment with isoniazid and rifampin.[79] (see Table 18-4.) Review of many studies showed that less than six months of drug therapy results in unacceptably high treatment failure or relapse rates, while longer treatment regimens do not yield substantially better outcomes, with relapse rates of 5% or less.[66]

Epidemiology

Global Prevalence and Incidence

The magnitude of the global tuberculosis epidemic is staggering. One third of the world population, roughly 1.9 billion people, are infected with *M. tuberculosis*.[10,79,83] It is the eighth leading cause of death in the world and causes more deaths each year (approximately 1.8 million in 2003) than all other infectious agents except HIV.[84-86]

Although tuberculosis reemerged in the 1980s as a public health problem in the United States and other industrialized nations, the majority of all tuberculosis cases occur in the developing world.[83] See Figure 18-3. Tuberculosis causes 25% of preventable adult deaths in the developing world,[82] and 75% of cases and 80% of deaths in these areas occur in adults aged 15–55, the most productive members of society.[53,82]

Global Variation in Disease

The World Health Organization (WHO) collects and reports global tuberculosis incidence data annually. Although reporting to WHO is voluntary, nearly all countries in the world comply. Types of data include the number of new tuberculosis cases of all types, the number of new smear positive cases, age and sex information for smear positive cases, the number of cases coinfected with HIV, and information on the status of their tuberculosis control program.[83] The quality of the data reported to WHO varies. To compensate for these differences, WHO reports both the number of cases reported by each country (case notifications) as well as an estimated number of tuberculosis cases that is a standardized

---

TABLE 18-4 Components of an Effective WHO DOTS Program

- A governmental commitment to tuberculosis control
- Case detection by microscopy, focusing on symptomatic patients who seek care
- Short-course therapy with at least the first two months of treatment supervised
- An administrative system for recording cases and assessing outcomes
- A reliable supply of antituberculosis drugs

Source: Adapted from Harries AD, Maher D. TB/HIV A Clinical Manual. Geneva: World Health Organization; 1996. http://www.who.int.

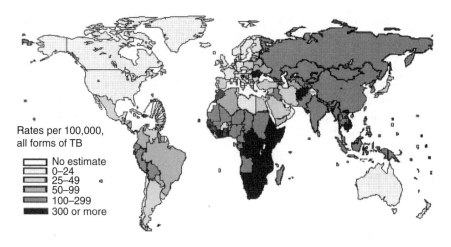

Rates per 100,000,
all forms of TB

- No estimate
- 0–24
- 25–49
- 50–99
- 100–299
- 300 or more

The designations employed and the presentation of material on this map do not imply the expression of any opinion whatsoever on the part of the World Heath Organization concerning the legal status of any country, territory, city or area or of its authorities, or concerning the delimitation of its fronteirs or boundaries. While illnes on maps represent approximate border lines for which there may not yet be full agreement.

FIGURE 18-3   Estimated TB incidence rate, 2003.
Source: World Health Organization, G. T. P. (2005). Global Tuberculosis Control, WHO Report 2005. Geneva, World Health Organization. http://www.who.int.

adjustment of the case notifications based on country-specific information.[87] There are considerable differences between the number of case notifications and number of estimated cases in some instances (Table 18-5), generally due to undercounting incident disease. For comparison across countries or between WHO world regions, therefore, the estimated incidence is preferable.

WHO presents data annually by geographic regions of the world. Although convenient and logical, in some of the six regions there are countries with very different risks of tuberculosis. This confuses the epidemiologic picture somewhat, but the WHO regions are the only available source of standardized global information. As shown in Figure 18-3, the incidence and prevalence of tuberculosis varies greatly around the world.[83]

The SE Asia Region (SEAR) has the highest number of cases of any of the regions (WHO estimate 3,061,657 in 2003). The per capita rate of disease is highest in the Africa region (AFR) however; 345/100,000 in 2003 versus 190/100,000 for SEAR. Either way, the SEAR and AFR together account for roughly 60% of all tuberculosis in the world, and as many as 60% to 70% of adults in these regions are latently infected. Incidence and mortality curves show two peaks, first in infancy when rates are higher in boys than girls. This differential equalizes later in childhood. In late adolescence, the curves again rise sharply, with the rates in women exceeding those in men. After about age 60 the rates flip once more, and the incidence in men exceeds that in women for the remainder of life.[29,83,84] The rates of disease in the E. Mediterranean region (EMR) and the W. Pacific Region (WPR) are also high but only about one third of the rate seen in AFR.

The number of cases and rate of disease are lowest in the Americas (AMR) and European (EUR) regions, although there is fairly wide variation by country within these regions. Incidence and mortality curves show two peaks in these regions also. The first is in infancy, and males predominate. The second peak is at

TABLE 18-5   Number of Notified and Estimated Tuberculosis Cases (all types), Cumulative Incidence, and Estimated Rate of Tuberculosis (all types), Worldwide and by WHO Region, 2003

WHO Region	Number of Cases				Estimated Annual Incidence Rate (per 100,000)
	Notified	Estimated Incident	Estimated Prevalent	Estimated Deaths	
Africa (AFR)	1,072,671	2,371,745	3,486,914	438,212	345
Americas (AMR)	227,551	370,107	502,605	53,803	43
E. Mediterranean (EMR)	209,941	634,112	1,119,950	143,937	122
European (EUR)	338,433	438,960	577,371	67,217	50
SE Asia (SEAR)	1,552,625	3,061,657	5,661,702	617,211	190
W. Pacific (WPR)	987,927	1,933,054	4,081,005	326,862	112
GLOBAL TOTAL					

Source: Adapted from WHO Global Tuberculosis Report, 2005. http://www.who.int.

adolescence and early adulthood, and females predominate. As rates decline after the second peak, the incidence and mortality in males surpasses that in females at about 35 years of age (lower than in AFR and SER) and remains higher until death.[29,83]

Figures 18-4 and 18-5 show trends in WHO case notification rates for 1982–2002 for different world populations. The notification rates in the figures are expressed relative to an arbitrary standard of 100 in 1990 to emphasize time trends, and the 95% confidence interval for each year is shown by the error bar. Countries represented in the graphs are representative of their WHO region for that time period. Increases observed in notification rates in the late 1990s in some areas may be due to improvements in tuberculosis control programs rather than true increases in disease rates, but in general the standardized notification rates shown accurately reflect changes in disease trends in the populations.[84]

In the established market economies and central Europe, notification rates dropped fairly steadily except for 1985–1992, the period mentioned earlier that is visible in Figure 18-5 as a flattening of the trend line around 1990. Similarly, rates in the EMR and Latin America have been dropping steadily. In the SEAR the trend is less clear, but since 1996 notification rates have been dropping steadily. Declines seen prior to 1996 have been lost in the WPR, and the trend in notification rates has flattened. In Eastern European countries, case and death rates from tuberculosis have historically been higher than in Western Europe, but were declining in most of the countries through 1992.[88] Unfortunately, notification rates have climbed steadily since then, and in 2002 were roughly twice what they were 20 years earlier. Increases are probably due to increases in HIV infection, MDR-TB, and a general breakdown in the health infrastructure following recent political instability.

Disease trends in Africa vary by HIV prevalence. In high-prevalence areas notification rates continue to increase as they have since the mid-1980s, although the increase in some countries has been mitigated by effective tuberculosis control

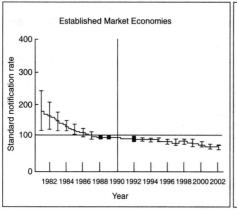

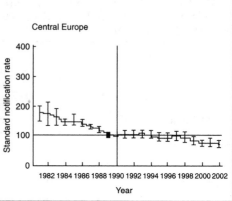

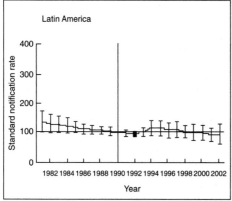

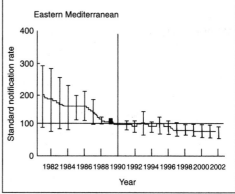

FIGURE 18-4　Trends in tuberculosis case notification rates, all types, for selected countries and world regions, 1981–2002.
Source: WHO (2004). Global Tuberculosis Control: Surveillance, Planning, Financing. WHO. Geneva, Switzerland, WHO. http://www.who.int.

activities. In low-prevalence countries a previously flat trend began increasing in 2000, perhaps due to HIV infection and political instability.

Natural History

The tubercle bacilli are only moderately infectious; about 20–30% of people exposed to an active case become infected.[88] As with most other infectious diseases, development of clinical tuberculosis is a two-step process: infection of the host with the microorganism, and then development of active disease caused by unchecked microbial replication and the body's immune response. What is different about the tubercle bacillus is that after it infects tissues, it can remain dormant for 20 to 30 years before active disease develops.

In a classic infection, *M. tuberculosis* enters the body via minute droplet nuclei deposited in the air when a person with active tuberculosis coughs, talks, or sneezes.[13,88] The droplet nuclei travel through the airways and are deposited on the alveolar surface, where the microbe is ingested by alveolar macrophages and begins replication. Activated macrophages release cytokines,

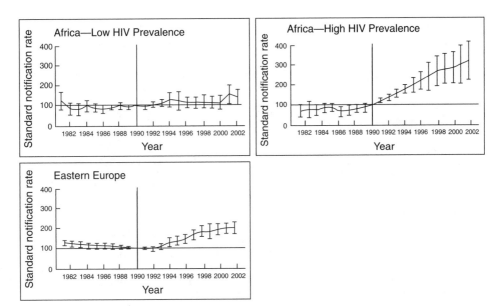

FIGURE 18-5 Trends in tuberculosis case notification rates, all types, for Africa and Eastern Europe, 1981–2002.
Source: WHO (2004). Global Tuberculosis Control: Surveillance, Planning, Financing. WHO. Geneva, Switzerland, WHO. http://www.who.int.

which in turn recruit more macrophages and activated T cells in an effort to control the infection.[12,13,34] At this point either the inflammation-infection cycle continues and active primary tuberculosis develops (5–10% of people[62,86]), or the immune system contains the primary infection. A sizeable, but unknown, proportion of the 90–95% of people whose immune system contains the primary infection develop latent infection.[13,62] In these people the microbe can remain in macrophages and other cells for decades in a quiescent yet viable state. In 5–10% of people with a latent infection, some later waning of cellular immunity allows these dormant bacilli to begin growing again, resulting in an active infection that is referred to as *reactivation tuberculosis*.[12,13,15]

The propagation of tuberculosis within a population can be viewed as a series of steps related to the natural history of tuberculosis infection in individuals, as illustrated in Figure 18-6.[89] Within a population, a reservoir of tuberculosis exists within people with latent tuberculosis infection (Stage 1). Each year a proportion of latently infected individuals develops active tuberculosis (Stage 2). Reactivation of latent tuberculosis is facilitated by recency of infection, malnutrition, immunosuppression, and other medical conditions that affect cellular immunity. Thus, in a population with a high prevalence of HIV infection, a large proportion of tuberculosis cases will be HIV-infected (Figure 18-6, shaded area). People with reactivation tuberculosis transmit infection to their contacts, causing tuberculosis infection (Stage 3). Rapid diagnosis of infectious cases and effective therapy reduce the number of contacts who are infected, but even in the best of circumstances an average of 10 contacts are infected before the case is sterilized with appropriate chemotherapy. Five percent to 10% of these contacts will develop active tuberculosis within the next year or two (Stage 4), and then will pass

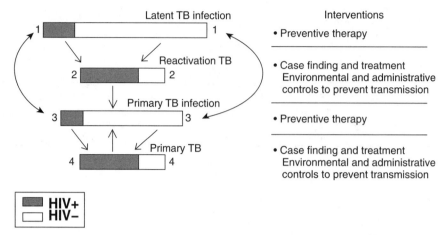

FIGURE 18-6   Dynamics of TB in a population with high HIV prevalence.
Source: K.M. De Cock and R.E. Chaisson, Tuberculosis Control in Countries with High Rates of HIV Infection, *International Journal of Tuberculosis and Lung Disease,* Vol. 3, pp. 457–465, © 1999, Churchill Livingstone.

active tuberculosis infection on to a number of their contacts (Stage 3). The remainder of the newly infected will enlarge the pool of latently infected individuals (Stage 1).

Mechanism of Transmission

Airborne transmission via the respiratory tract is the primary and most efficient mode of transmitting tuberculosis. People with active pulmonary or laryngeal tuberculosis discharge minute particles of sputum into the air when coughing, talking, sneezing, or singing.[42,90–92] The liquid in these sputum droplets evaporates, leaving droplet nuclei that contain the solid parts of the droplet and sometimes a few mycobacteria.[93] The speed of evaporation depends primarily on the size of the droplet, although environmental factors, such as humidity, also affect the process. Large droplets evaporate more slowly, and so they quickly drop out of the air. Smaller droplets, 1 to 10 μm in diameter, dry more quickly and can be in the air for long periods of time.[93] It is the floating droplet nuclei that cause infection. They are inhaled by uninfected people and lodge in the alveoli or terminal bronchioles to form the nidus of infection.[29] The size of the droplet nuclei is critical as larger ones lodge in the lining of the nose and trachea, and very tiny ones can be expired before they lodge in the respiratory tract.[94]

The infectivity of an individual with pulmonary tuberculosis is a function of the virulence of the bacteria, the frequency of their cough, and the degree of pulmonary cavitation. Loudon and colleagues showed that coughing, talking, and singing produced both different quantities and different sizes of droplet nuclei and that both properties are important components of infectivity.[90,92] The degree of pulmonary cavitation is important because it correlates with the bacterial load in the sputum. Logically, the more open lesions, or cavities, in the lung, the greater the probability that bacteria will be expired. Similarly, laryngeal tuberculosis is particularly infectious as all exhalations are forced through infected tissue.[29,36,95–97]

M. tuberculosis can also enter the body through mucous membranes in the gut, genitourinary tract, and conjunctiva, or through abrasions or breaks in the skin. Infection via these routes produces an infection at the site of entry that may remain localized or may spread to other organs and tissues via the lymphatic or blood system.[15,37,38] Transmission through these portals is relatively rare, especially in industrialized areas where the incidence of tuberculosis is low. These routes of infection are more common in developing countries where the prevalence of tuberculosis is higher. The respiratory route is still the most efficient and common mode of tuberculosis transmission in all parts of the world.

Risk Factors Associated with Infection

The risk of infection is a function of exposure to the tubercle bacilli, which in turn is controlled by the infectivity of the patient, and the probability of contact with infectious organisms. Characteristics of the infectious case, such as severity of disease,[97,98] frequency of cough and other vocal activities,[85,87] consistency of sputum, and initiation of chemotherapy[99] all affect the number and viability of the microbes expelled into the environment. Factors in the environment that increase the probability of contact with infected air, such as decreased ventilation, increased duration or intimacy of contact with the case, amount of ultraviolet light available, and crowding, increase the risk of acquiring infection.[41,96,100]

The risk of exposure refers to the probability that a susceptible person will come in contact with the tubercle bacilli. Factors associated with exposure are external to the host and include the prevalence of infectious tuberculosis in the population, population density, living conditions, and, sometimes, cultural practices. In areas where tuberculosis is endemic, the risk of exposure to the bacteria is higher simply because more people are infectious at any given time. Similarly, crowding forces people into more frequent contact with one another and increases the risk of exposure to an infectious case. Poverty has been associated with exposure, but it is so closely linked to crowding that it is difficult to tell if it is a surrogate for crowding or a true risk factor for exposure. Chapman and Dyerly noted the association between poverty and tuberculosis but concluded that poverty was probably a surrogate for crowding and increased prevalence.[98] Studies in New York City and Washington County, Maryland, tend to disagree, however.[101,102] These studies examined factors associated with the prevalence of latent tuberculosis as measured by a positive tuberculin skin test reaction and showed that LTBI was more common in impoverished areas, even after adjustment for age and, in New York, for race. When control measures in a population are inadequate, the average duration of infectivity of a case lengthens, and the risk of exposure increases because more susceptible people can be exposed even if crowding is minimal. Cultural factors that control exposure to the public or otherwise modify exposure to an infectious case, such as sequestering women, can also affect the risk of exposure, both positively and negatively.

Risk of infection, given that exposure has occurred, is more difficult to study. Several studies have shown that people with severe tuberculosis, as defined by cavitation or smear positivity, are more infectious than those with milder disease, presumably because they excrete more bacilli. One classic study examined the environmental and social factors associated with acquisition of infection by children living in a household with one or more tuberculous adults. They found that the severity of disease in the index case was the strongest predictor of infection in the children.[98] Another study done in British Columbia and Saskatchewan found that children exposed to smear-positive cases were more likely to become infected than those exposed to smear-negative cases, regardless of duration of contact.[97]

The way in which the index case expels bacteria also affects the number of mycobacteria expelled during exhalation and the risk of acquiring infection given exposure. Coughing is the best way for an index case to spread tuberculosis. A cough produces roughly four to seven times as many droplet nuclei as talking or singing, although singing produces a slightly greater proportion of small droplet nuclei that may be more infectious.[90,92] It is also clear that effective treatment of tuberculosis rapidly eliminates mycobacteria in the lungs and decreases the risk of transmission.[99,100]

It seems, therefore, that the risk of infection is a function of exposure to the tubercle bacilli, which in turn, is controlled by the infectivity of the patient and the probability of contact with infectious organisms. Factors in the patient, such as severity of disease, frequency of cough, consistency of sputum, and initiation of chemotherapy, all affect the number and viability of the microbes expelled into the environment. Factors in the environment that increase the probability of contact with infected air, such as decreased ventilation, increased duration or intimacy of contact with the case, amount of ultraviolet light available, and crowding, increase the risk of acquiring infection.[41,96,100] Fortunately, under normal household circumstances tuberculosis is not highly infectious. The secondary attack rate for tuberculosis in 5- to 9-year-old household contacts was about 48%, two thirds lower than that for measles, mumps, or pertussis.[98] The risk of infection increases dramatically in crowded conditions, such as prisons,[103] naval vessels,[104] and nursing homes,[105] and spread can be explosive in this type of confined setting.

Risk Factors Associated with Development of Disease

In the general population only 5–10% of people infected with the tubercle bacillus develop active, clinical disease.[106] The risk factors that control progression from infection to disease are complex and intertwined, but are different from those that control infection. Logically these factors tend to be intrinsic because the time between infection and development of disease can vary significantly.[88]

Time Since Infection

Most cases of active tuberculosis develop within the first 2 years after infection, although the risk of infection is elevated through the 5th year after exposure.[88,91] In a public health study of tuberculin-positive contacts of tuberculosis cases in the United States, the risk of developing tuberculosis was 1% in the first year after exposure versus 0.07% 8 to 10 years later.[88] Similarly in a cohort of tuberculin-negative, adult Norwegians followed longitudinally for tuberculin conversion and development of tuberculosis, radiographic changes associated with tuberculosis were observed in 130/272 (48%) of tuberculin converters, all within the first year after converting to a positive tuberculin reaction.[46] The question, however, is whether the time since infection is a true risk factor or a marker for another risk factor. Most likely this is a marker for the true risk factors, which may include the virulence of the infecting strain of tuberculosis and the person's inherent susceptibility to developing active disease.

Fibrotic Lesions

The presence of healed fibrotic lesions increases the risk of tuberculosis, presumably from reactivation disease, although this is nearly impossible to prove. In studies of individuals with healed fibrotic lesions the incidence of tuberculosis ranged from 2 to 4 cases per 1000 person-years.[91,107] In a Danish study reactors with calcified lesions were twice as likely to develop tuberculosis as reactors without calcifications.[29]

Age

The main question to be answered is whether the risk of developing active disease varies with age. It may seem logical to tackle this question by examining graphs plotting tuberculosis incidence and mortality by age (Figure 18-7). Such graphs are cross-sectional, however, showing the rates of disease in many different birth cohorts at a particular instant in time, and the risk of tuberculosis can vary drastically for different birth cohorts. To clarify this issue birth cohort analyses have been done in different populations to examine the risk of disease throughout life in cohorts of people born at the same time.[46,91,101] Figure 18-8 shows a cohort analysis done by Comstock from data collected and reported by the United States Public Health Service.[88,108] It shows that as a birth cohort ages, people susceptible to tuberculosis are eliminated by disease or mortality, eventually leaving a cohort that is more resistant to disease. Thus the incidence of tuberculosis actually declines as a specific birth cohort ages. This elimination of susceptible people also has an effect on the overall susceptibility to tuberculosis in the community, eventually producing a community that is more resistant to disease. Thus, the risk of infection, and consequently disease, is lower for each successive birth cohort in the community. If you view the disease incidence cross-sectionally by age, the oldest birth cohorts (i.e., the oldest ages) have the highest incidence of infection. This is because their risk of infection has been higher since birth, not because the incidence of tuberculosis increases with age. If you look instead at the tuberculosis incidence curve for each birth cohort, you see that the risk of tuberculosis declines steadily with age within each cohort.

Sex

Numerous studies, both cross-sectional and longitudinal, have shown that the development of active tuberculosis varies by sex. In a prospective study in Puerto Rico, tuberculin-positive, tuberculosis-free people aged 1 to 19 years at enrollment were followed for over 18 years for the development of active

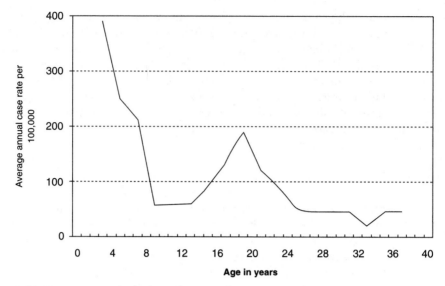

FIGURE 18-7   Standard tuberculosis incidence or mortality by age.
Source: G.W. Comstock, Frost Revisited: The Modern Epidemiology of
Tuberculosis, *American Journal of Epidemiology*, Vol. 101, pp. 363–382, Copyright
1975, by permission of the Oxford University Press.

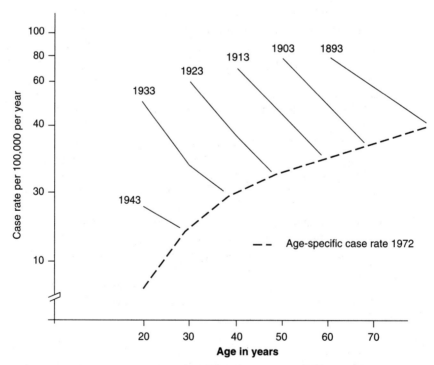

FIGURE 18-8   Cohort analysis of effect of age on tuberculosis incidence.
Source: G.W. Comstock, Frost Revisited: The Modern Epidemiology of
Tuberculosis, *American Journal of Epidemiology*, Vol. 101, pp. 363–382, Copyright
1975, by permission of the Oxford University Press.

disease. In young children aged 1 to 6 years, the incidence of tuberculosis was higher in males than in females of the same age. After 6 years of age, however, the incidence was higher in females at all ages. This cohort was only followed until the oldest members were 40 years of age, however, so the authors could not comment on the risk of disease in older adults. In a similar prospective study conducted in Bangalore, India, a cohort of people was actively screened for tuberculosis annually for 8 years. The authors found that women aged 10 to 44 years had a 130% higher risk of developing tuberculosis than men the same age, but that after age 44 the risk in men was as much as 250% higher than in women.[53] In a similar study in Gedde-Dahl, Norway, a cohort of tuberculin-negative adults was followed for tuberculin conversion and development of tuberculosis. The observed incidence of tuberculosis was equal in males and females under 19 years; 25% to 30% higher in women at age 20 to 29; and 17% to 25% higher in males than females after age 40. In the mass screening campaign in Denmark, investigators found that the incidence of tuberculosis was 71% higher in females than males at 24 to 34 years of age; 22% higher in females aged 35 to 44; and 67% higher in males over 45.[46,53,109] The effect of sex on development of disease was also studied in a population of Alaskan Inuits. Essentially everyone in the population was tuberculin positive by age 15. The investigators found that the incidence of tuberculosis was similar in males and females until about age 10; 25% higher in females from age 10 to 39; and similar in males and females 40 years of age and older.[53,110]

In summary, the risk of developing tuberculosis, given infection, appears to be higher in males than females during infancy and again after about age 45 to 60, and higher in females than males during adolescence and early adulthood. The reason for this divergence is not clear. The peak in women during reproductive years suggests that hormonal factors may be involved, although pregnancy in itself does not seem to affect the risk of developing tuberculosis.[111] It has also been suggested that the excess in men at older ages is due to increased immune suppression related to increased smoking and drinking, but the evidence for this is sketchy.[53]

Genetics

Genetic factors clearly play some role in the development of tuberculosis in humans, but the extent of the role is unclear. Lurie has shown there is some genetic basis for resistance to tuberculosis in rabbits,[112] and a variety of evidence suggests the same is true for humans. In a tragic accident in 1926, 249 infants in Lubeck, Germany, were vaccinated with live *M. tuberculosis* instead of bacilli Calmette-Guerin vaccine (BCG). Seventy-six of the infants died and 173 survived after suffering various levels of illness. None of the infants had been previously vaccinated with BCG, none were old enough to have acquired immunity from natural exposure to tuberculosis, and all infants received the same dose of mycobacteria. The variation in their response to the infection may be partially due to nutritional status and other factors, but some must have been due to differences in innate susceptibility to tuberculosis.[32,62]

It has also been suggested that some of the racial and geographic differences observed in tuberculosis incidence result from differences in population resistance to tuberculosis.[19,113] Population resistance to a specific microbe presumably develops over time as natural selection favors hosts better able to resist or cope with infection. This phenomenon was observed when tuberculosis was introduced for the first time in the Qu'Appelle Indians in the late 1800s. Initially 10% of the population died annually from tuberculosis. Half of the families in the community died out within two generations, but the annual tuberculosis death rate in the remaining population was only 0.2%.[114] A similar scenario occurred when tuberculosis was introduced to the Yanomami Indians in the Amazon.[56] Epidemic tuberculosis arrived in Europe in the 1300s and 1400s and was a major cause of premature death from the Industrial Revolution through the middle of the 1900s. European colonists brought tuberculosis with them to Asia and Africa where epidemic tuberculosis was essentially unknown before 1900. If the notion of population resistance, as seen in the Qu'Appelle and Yanomami Indians, is correct, then present-day people of European ancestry should have more resistance to tuberculosis than people of African origin. In the United States, African-Americans have historically had much higher rates of tuberculosis than Caucasians, but they have also traditionally had higher rates of poverty, crowding, and malnutrition, all of which are strongly associated with exposure to tuberculosis. It is, therefore, difficult to determine whether the difference in incidence is due to exposure or genetics. A study of tuberculin sensitivity in New York City showed that at every socioeconomic level, African-American and Puerto Rican residents were more likely to have evidence of LTBI than Caucasian residents.[101] In another study, African-American nursing home residents were twice as likely to become infected with *M. tuberculosis* as white residents in the same nursing homes. Again the difference remained after correction for socioeconomic and environmental factors.[115] None of these studies are conclusive, but they suggest that genetics have some effect on population-level resistance to tuberculosis.

Perhaps the strongest evidence that genetics plays a role in susceptibility to tuberculosis comes from twin studies, which examine the incidence of disease in pairs of twins. When both twins in a pair develop a disease they are called concordant; they are discordant when only one of the twins is diseased. If genetics plays no role in a disease, the concordance rate should be the same in monozygotic twins and dizygotic twin pairs. If genetics is important, then concordance should be higher in monozygotic twins because they have identical genomes. Several twin studies have shown that the concordance for tuberculosis is roughly twice as high in monozygotic as dizygotic twins.[116-118] Many of these studies were done before multiple regression was widely available, but Comstock reanalyzed the Prophit twin study data using multiple logistic regression. He found that concordance remained more than twice as high in monozygotic twins even after adjustment for sex, age, infectivity of the index, type of tuberculosis, and years of contact.[116] Although environment must play a role in the development of disease in twin pairs, it seems clear that monozygotic twins are at greater risk of disease.

There have been other types of studies suggesting a genetic component in tuberculosis. Edwards and colleagues examined US Navy recruits who had been exposed to tuberculosis.[108] They found that men who had close, generally family, contact with a tuberculosis case were taller and thinner than those without such exposure regardless of their tuberculin status. This suggests that lean body build may be a marker for a familial risk for tuberculosis.[88,108] In a well-executed study by Overfield and Klauber, the prevalence of a positive tuberculin response and active tuberculosis was correlated with ABO and MN blood types in a random sample of Alaskan Eskimos with a very high tuberculosis infection rate. The authors reported that people with blood type AB and B were three times more likely to have moderate to severe tuberculosis compared to people with blood type O and A.[119] There also appears to be some correlation between development of tuberculosis and histocompatibility types.[29] Several studies have also shown that genetic polymorphisms may be associated with tuberculosis risk. A case-control study in the Gambia found that allelic variation in the gene *nramp-1* was associated with tuberculosis risk, though wild-type alleles were present in the majority of cases and polymorphisms in a large proportion of controls.[120] Another study from Cambodia identified a specific HLA-DQ haplotype associated with tuberculosis.[120] Interferon-γR1 deficiency has also been shown to be associated with increased susceptibility to tuberculosis. In a study of French children who developed disseminated BCG after vaccination, a small proportion of children with no other underlying immune defect had a specific autosomal recessively inherited mutation in the gene coding for interferon-γR1.[32,122,123] Studies have also suggested that several other genes or chromosome regions may affect susceptibility to tuberculosis, and research continues in this area.[32]

Stress

It has long been suggested that stress may affect the development of tuberculosis,[18,100] probably by weakening the cell-mediated immune response that holds latent disease in check and prevents new infection. A study in Denmark showed that among tuberculin reactors, the risk of developing active tuberculosis was lowest in married men, who presumably had the highest level of social support, intermediate in single and widowed men, and highest in divorced men who had the least social support. A similar but less dramatic trend was seen in women. In addition, married people who developed tuberculosis had less severe disease than did unmarried people.[29,109] A study of tuberculosis incidence in the US Navy shortly after WWII showed that rates were especially high in personnel from the Philippines. The difference in rates has been attributed to psychosocial stress caused by social isolation and separation from family and other support structures.[100]

Tuberculosis has long been associated with poverty,[62,98,102] even after adjustment for other pertinent factors.[99] Some evidence suggests that poverty is probably a marker for increased risk of infection with tuberculosis,[98] but it is possible that poverty imposes a psychological stress on the body that reduces immune capacity and increases the risk of reactivation or of development of disease given exposure.

Nutrition

The association between poverty, crowding, and malnutrition is well established. It is no surprise, therefore, that tuberculosis, which is strongly associated with crowding and poverty, has also been associated with malnutrition.[41,62] A number of studies have examined the association of specific micronutrients with the development of tuberculosis. In one study, mean plasma vitamin

A levels were lower in children with pulmonary tuberculosis than in those without it. More extensive or more severe disease was also associated with low vitamin A levels. High dose treatment with vitamin A had no effect on the course of the tuberculosis, however.[54] Low vitamin A and selenium levels have also been associated with an increased risk of developing tuberculosis in a cohort of HIV-infected, adult reactors in Haiti.[124]

A study in tuberculin reactors found that reaction size increased as nutritional status improved, and severe malnutrition has also been associated with anergy to tuberculin skin test following BCG vaccine.[52] In times of war, food deprivation has also been associated with increased tuberculosis incidence and mortality; incidence decreased when food became available again. This suggests that the deprivation caused an increase in reactivation disease probably by inhibiting cell-mediated immunity.[41,46] There is also a considerable body of literature suggesting that tall, thin men are more likely to develop tuberculosis than are shorter, heavier men.[108] Similarly a study in Muscogee County, Georgia, measured the thickness of subcutaneous fat over the trapezius ridges in baseline photofluorograms of tuberculosis-free people. The investigators found that people with less than 5 mm of fat over the ridge were twice as likely to develop tuberculosis over the next 14 years than people with 10 mm or more of fat.[88] It seems clear, therefore, that the risk of tuberculosis is higher in thinner people. What is not clear is whether thinness is the risk factor for disease or a marker of genetic susceptibility as suggested by Edwards's studies in navy recruits. [88,108]

Occupation

Few studies have examined occupation as a risk factor for tuberculosis. The notable exception is studies of people exposed to silica in the work site. Silicosis has been shown to lower resistance to tuberculosis infection in animals, and tuberculosis is more common among people exposed to silica on the job than to those who are unexposed.[41] There also appears to be an interaction between silicosis, HIV infection, and tuberculosis in South African miners. Those with both silicosis and HIV are more likely to develop tuberculosis than those with only one of the two risk factors. Inhalation therapists and funeral home workers have been found to have increased risk for tuberculosis infection and disease.[125-127] Health care workers, in general, however, appear to have varying rates of tuberculosis. In some settings the incidence is similar to or lower than rates in other occupational groups,[126] while in other cases, rates are actually increased.[128]

Smoking

Although a link between smoking and tuberculosis seems obvious the evidence supporting the association has been lacking until recently when studies in Kuwait, Hong Kong, and India were published. A study in India showed that male smokers were three times more likely to report a history of tuberculosis than nonsmokers.[129] A prospective study in Hong Kong examined the incidence of tuberculosis in smokers and nonsmokers and found that incidence was highest in current smokers (735/100,000), lowest in never smokers (174/100,000), and intermediate in ex-smokers (427/100,000). The trend was significant ($P < .001$) and persisted after adjustment for multiple factors. In addition, current smokers who developed tuberculosis smoked more cigarettes than those who did not (13.43 cigarettes per day versus 7.87, $P = .01$), and a significant dose response was observed.[130] A study of response to treatment in patients diagnosed with tuberculosis in Kuwait suggests that smoking may delay sputum conversion in some people.[131] How smoking worsens tuberculosis is unclear, but it has been suggested that iron-loading of pulmonary macrophages secondary to smoking may damage the cells and make them more susceptible to infection with *M. tuberculosis*.[132]

HIV Infection and AIDS

Infection with HIV has been identified as the most potent biologic risk factor for developing tuberculosis. In HIV-infected people with evidence of prior tuberculosis infection, the annual risk of reactivation is between 3% and 14%.[133] Among people already infected with HIV, newly acquired tuberculosis infection progresses to active disease within several months in a high proportion (approximately 40%).[134] In areas where tuberculosis infection is common and HIV becomes prevalent, rapidly escalating rates of tuberculosis occur (Figure 18-9). In northern Thailand, for example, the incidence of tuberculosis doubled in one province over a 2-year period after HIV infection was introduced.[135] See Figure 18-10. HIV-related immune deficiency compromises host response to tubercle bacilli, thereby raising the likelihood of reactivation of latent infection. Among HIV-infected people, the most important risk factors for reactivation of tuberculosis are a positive tuberculin skin test and a low CD4 lymphocyte count.[136] Although HIV infection can cause anergy to antigens such as tuberculin, a high proportion of HIV-infected patients with tuberculosis have a positive skin test, and the presence of a

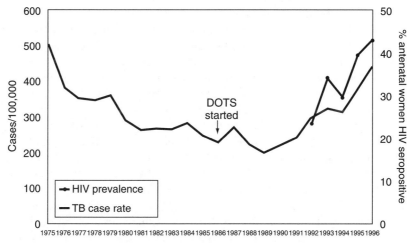

FIGURE 18-9 Despite a well-functioning DOTS program and low levels of anti-TB resistance in Botswana the epidemic of tuberculosis has continued to grow due to the severe epidemic of HIV.
Source: Kenyon, TA et al. Low levels of drug resistance amidst rapidly increasing tuberculosis and human immunodeficiency virus co-epidemics in Botswana. Int J Tuberc Lung Dis. 1999 Jan; 3(1):4–11.

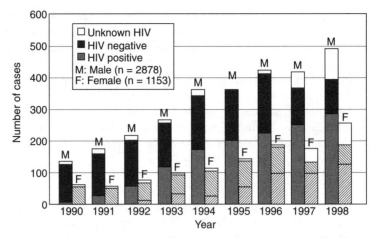

FIGURE 18-10   Despite a success full HIV control program in Thailand the incidence of tuberculosis has continued to grow in northern Thailand—number of new TB cases in Chiang Rai Hospital from 1990 to 1998, classified by sex and HIV serostatus.
Source: Siriarayapon, P et al. The evolving epidemiology of HIV infection and tuberculosis in northern Thailand. J Acquir Immune Defic Syndr. 2002 Sep 1; 31(1):80–9.

positive test is a powerful predictor of subsequent tuberculosis risk. Several early studies suggested that anergy was associated with a very high risk of developing tuberculosis, and it was hypothesized that the lack of response to tuberculin indicated an inability of host immune response to contain tubercle bacilli.[137,138] Subsequent studies have failed to confirm an association between anergy and reactivation tuberculosis,[139] and it has been suggested that anergy is a marker for severe immune deficiency that increases the risk of *primary* tuberculosis in areas where transmission of infection is common. As the CD4 count falls, the incidence of reactivation and primary tuberculosis rises, and extrapulmonary sites of disease become more frequent.[78] Unlike most other opportunistic infections in HIV disease, however, tuberculosis can occur at a relatively high CD4 level and may be a first manifestation of HIV in many patients.[140] In addition, active tuberculosis can be transmitted by the airborne route between HIV-infected people, contributing to microepidemics of institutional and community outbreaks of disease.

The growth of the HIV epidemic over the past two decades has occurred largely in areas of the world where tuberculosis infection is endemic. As a result, tuberculosis has become one of the major opportunistic diseases associated with HIV infection and a leading cause of death in developing countries.[141] As discussed later, the HIV epidemic now seriously undermines tuberculosis control in many developing countries, and new and more aggressive strategies are needed to reduce the high incidence of tuberculosis seen in populations with high levels of HIV infection.

Other Factors

A variety of other factors, most of which have a negative impact on the immune system, is also known to increase the risk of developing tuberculosis. Those factors include malignancies, renal failure, gastrectomy, diabetes, jejunoileal bypass, corticosteroid treatment, and measles.[91,96]

Bacillus Calmette-Guérin

Tuberculosis was one of the first diseases for which a vaccine was developed. In 1921, Albert Calmette and Camille Guérin attenuated a virulent strain of *M. bovis* through serial passage on glycerinated bile potato media.[39,142,143] The final product, BCG, was tested in a human subject later that year and put into common use in France in 1924 to protect child contacts of active cases.[81,144,145]

Use of BCG in Europe soon became fairly common, but its efficacy was questioned by some, particularly in the United States. In 1930, more than 50% of a cohort of children vaccinated with BCG in Lubeck, Germany, contracted tuberculosis and many died. It was subsequently shown that the children had accidentally been vaccinated with virulent tubercle bacilli from a culture stored in the same incubator as the BCG culture.[62,143] The Lubeck disaster, combined with the disruption of Europe during World War II, discouraged the use of BCG for a time. Tuberculosis morbidity and mortality increased markedly during WWII,[46] however, and after the war, vaccination was quickly reinstituted in Europe and became the norm.[39] Today BCG vaccine is one of the standard vaccines in the WHO Expanded Programme on Immunization[33] and is used in nearly every country in the world, with the notable exceptions of the United States and the Netherlands.[42]

Bacillus Calmette-Guérin is one of the safest vaccines in use.[143] It is given at birth to infants in more than 100 countries throughout the world and is recommended for some health care workers at risk of exposure to tuberculosis. The BCG vaccine is rarely given to healthy adult populations because the efficacy in this group is uncertain. It is administered intradermally or percutaneously and generally causes a superficial, crusted ulcer at the site of administration. This heals in 2 to 3 months, generally leaving a 4- to 8-mm concave scar.[42] A small proportion of vaccinees get suppurative axillary or cervical lymphadenopathy, which generally heals best without treatment. Persistent or disseminated BCG is a rare complication of vaccination that occurs in 3 to 6 infants per million vaccinations and in 1 to 14 cases per million vaccinations in people aged 1 to 20 years.[33,51] The risk is higher in immunocompromised individuals, such as those with HIV infection. Although the precise risk of disseminated BCG in HIV-infected individuals is unknown, BCG is contraindicated if HIV infection is present[51] as well as in people with other forms of immune compromise and in those with skin infections or burns.[33,51]

Controlled studies to measure the efficacy of BCG have been ongoing since 1926 and have included observational and case-control studies and clinical trials. Case-control studies have been used to measure the efficacy of BCG vaccine in specific geographic regions. In these studies, the reported cases of tuberculosis in an area are matched to controls, and the efficacy is estimated from the tuberculosis incidence rate in vaccinated and unvaccinated cases and controls where[146]:

$$\% \text{ Efficacy} = (1 - (R)) \times 100, \text{ and}$$

$$R = \frac{\text{Incidence in vaccinated}}{\text{Incidence in the unvaccinated}}$$

The underlying assumption is that fewer than 80% of people have received vaccine; otherwise, there are too few unvaccinated cases and controls to reliably estimate efficacy.

Case-control studies have also been used to measure the relative efficacy of two different BCG vaccines given to the same population.[147,148] In these studies it was possible to determine the relative efficacy of the different vaccines because they were given one after the other to the same population using the same delivery methods. The efficacy for the time period covering each vaccine was estimated separately. Case-control studies are observational, and the lack of randomization means there is a potential for bias. The assumption in a case-control study is that, apart from the effect of the vaccine, the risk of developing tuberculosis is equal in the vaccinated and unvaccinated groups. If this is not true, then the estimated efficacy may be incorrect.

In contact studies, cohorts of children living with newly diagnosed tuberculosis cases are followed for the development of tuberculosis. The incidence of tuberculosis is estimated in vaccinated and unvaccinated children, and vaccine efficacy is computed as in a case-control study.[39] As with the case-control studies, these cohort studies are not randomized, and results are questionable if the probability of vaccination varies with the risk of developing tuberculosis.

Many clinical trials, some randomized and some not, have also been done to determine the efficacy of BCG vaccine. At first glance, the results of these studies are confusing. The efficacy of BCG as estimated in the different studies ranges from −22% to +85%. The difficulty is that the studies have measured different products in different populations. BCG was developed in 1921, during the infancy of microbiology. It came not from a single colony, but from a culture of mycobacteria and, thus, is not a strain in the strictest sense of the word. In addition, the original BCG "strain" was distributed to and subcultured in laboratories around the world, producing a large number of daughter strains, some of them with very different characteristics from the original.[39] Thus, the organism used in the many BCG vaccine studies has varied markedly. The route of administration and the dose of vaccine have also varied in different studies, and the effect these differences have had on efficacy is difficult to predict. Furthermore several studies have shown that exposure to nontuberculous mycobacterium provides some protection against infection with *M. tuberculosis* and may reduce the efficacy of BCG.[106] To summarize, it appears that BCG provides some protection in infants against miliary disease and tuberculosis meningitis, but a good estimate of the efficacy is not available. It does not appear to confer good protection in adults and should probably be used only in extreme circumstances.

New, effective vaccines against tuberculosis are needed badly. Research in the field is expanding, and some new candidate vaccines are beginning clinical trials. Testing the new vaccines will be challenging. BCG vaccination is entrenched in developing countries where the risk of tuberculosis is highest and the need for new tuberculosis vaccines is greatest. WHO has made a determined effort to ensure high coverage rates in infants in areas where tuberculosis is endemic. In these areas, where preventive therapy is rare and treatment for tuberculosis can be problematic, it would be unethical to deprive infants of an available vaccine that provides even minimal protection against disseminated disease. Therefore, it is improbable that the new vaccine(s) will be tested in placebo-controlled efficacy trials; studies will have to measure some as yet unknown biologic marker of protection, or compare the efficacy of the new vaccine against the efficacy of BCG and infer the relative efficacy of the two vaccines from those measurements.

Tuberculosis Control Strategies

Case Finding and Treatment

In 1994, WHO declared tuberculosis a global emergency and developed the DOTS program to combat disease globally. Although short-course directly observed therapy (DOTs) is the cornerstone of the strategy, the WHO DOTS program is really a series of policies that are meant to result in effective tuberculosis control (Table 18-4). The program aims to encourage governments to develop the political will to support tuberculosis control, a strong surveillance system that records and monitors cases, sufficient laboratory components to ensure diagnosis, effective short-course treatments that are at least partially observed, and a reliable supply of antituberculosis drugs.

The DOTS strategy called for country programs to detect 70% of smear-positive tuberculosis cases and to treat 85% of those successfully. It is assumed that implementation of the DOTS strategy and achievement of these goals would make a substantial impact on tuberculosis incidence and contribute to effective tuberculosis control. Indeed, when DOTS is implemented well in a country, large proportions of active tuberculosis cases can be treated and cured, and drug resistance can be prevented.[149] Implementation of a DOTS program requires the establishment of a registration system, microscopy services, a stable drug supply, and adequate staffing to permit supervision of therapy for at least 2 months, but many countries with the greatest tuberculosis burden are the least able to undertake this kind of commitment. Although the per capita cost of effective tuberculosis treatment services is relatively low (e.g., $0.23 per year in Peru), mobilization of resources to create an integrated national program is understandably difficult. A larger problem, however, is the generation of political will to support tuberculosis control. Even in countries where substantial foreign assistance has been provided for tuberculosis services, control efforts frequently lag for many reasons, including governmental disorganization and disruption, competing needs, and lack of interest or commitment in tuberculosis as a public health problem.

Progress is being made however. As of 2003, 182 countries had implemented DOTS, 77% of the world's population lived in countries or regions covered by DOTS and, on average, 82% of newly identified cases completed treatment. Case detection rates have improved in some areas, but this remains a difficult task. WHO estimates that globally about 45% of new cases are being identified. WHO estimated that in 2003, tuberculosis incidence was still increasing globally, but that the rate of increase was slowing and could be reversed.[11,83] In 2000 the United Nations Millennium Development Goals (MDGs) provided a framework to evaluate the implementation and impact of disease control programs, including tuberculosis. The targets for tuberculosis are to detect 70% of new sputum-smear-positive cases and successfully treat 85% of them by 2005, to reduce tuberculosis incidence, and halve tuberculosis prevalence and mortality by 2015. A recent analysis suggests that in much of the world this goal can be met by 2015 through expansion of the current DOTS strategies, but the HIV and MDR-TB epidemics will make it very difficult to meet those goals in Africa and Eastern Europe. Dye et al.[11] suggest that the next phase of DOTS expansion must build on the basic package to address the needs of specific areas, using new technology and methodology designed to address specific deficiencies. They maintain that the MDGs can be met but only with renewed and innovative control measures.

In areas with generalized HIV epidemics, in particular, it is clear that the DOTS strategy is insufficient to control tuberculosis. Sub-Saharan Africa is experiencing devastating increases in tuberculosis rates as a consequence of high levels of HIV infection in the general population. Countries such as South Africa, Botswana, Zambia, Malawi, and others have seen three- to fivefold increases in TB incidence over the past 10–15 years as HIV prevalence has increased.[149] See Figure 18-5. Botswana, a country with a well-functioning and highly efficient DOTS program in place since 1985, has rates of TB that are now well above 500/100,000, illustrating the limitations of the DOTS strategy in holding down tuberculosis incidence in the face of an extensive HIV epidemic.[149] (See Figure 18-9.) In places such as Uganda or Chiang Rai Province, Thailand, where HIV prevalence has fallen over the past decade, tuberculosis incidence rates have continued to climb, presumably as a result of large numbers of individuals with HIV and latent tuberculosis infection who remain at high risk for progressing to active tuberculosis disease.[135] See Figure 18-10. Aggressive public health strategies that extend beyond DOTS, such as active tuberculosis case finding, widespread use of preventive therapy, and other novel approaches are required to contain tuberculosis in these settings.

Epidemiologic Basis of Tuberculosis Control

Control of tuberculosis implies a reduction in the number of cases that occur each year within a community or population. In mathematical terms, tuberculosis control means that the reproductive rate of the disease must be less than 1.0, meaning each case of tuberculosis must produce less than one secondary case. This simple and necessary goal of control has been largely overlooked in most international tuberculosis programming until recently. Programs were largely focused on intermediary goals such as case detection and cure rates. Although there is great medical and humanitarian value in finding, treating, and curing cases of tuberculosis, the perspective of public health requires that the principal aim of tuberculosis control be that the incidence of the disease is reduced.

The propagation of tuberculosis within a population can be viewed as a series of steps related to the natural history of tuberculosis infection in individuals, as illustrated in Figure 18-6.[89] The reservoir of tuberculosis in a community is the group of latently infected people at risk of developing tuberculosis (Stage 1). Some change in immunity in the latently infected allows the tubercle bacillus to begin active growth and reactivation tuberculosis develops (Stage 2). These new cases are infectious, and each will infect a minimum of 8 to 15 contacts (Stage 3) before their infection is sterilized by appropriate chemotherapy. Rapid diagnosis and treatment of the new infectious cases reduces the number of infected contacts. Five to ten percent of these infected contacts will develop primary tuberculosis within 2 years (Stage 4), and the remainder will fuel the pool of latently infected people (Stage 1).

A variety of factors moderates the dynamics of this model in a community. The most obvious is HIV infection. People coinfected with HIV and the tubercle bacillus have a dramatically increased risk of developing tuberculosis and contribute disproportionately to reactivation and new tuberculosis infections (Stages 2 and 3). In areas where HIV and tuberculosis are endemic, this increased risk of disease from reactivation and primary infection substantially increases the case rate (Stages 2 and 4). Other factors that prolong infectivity, such as poor case detection, lack of effective treatment, and drug resistance, also increase case rates.

Current Tuberculosis Control Strategies

On a community level, tuberculosis can be controlled through the use of an effective vaccine, detection and treatment of infectious cases, and screening for and treatment of latent tuberculosis infection.[150] In developing countries, control measures have emphasized BCG vaccination and case detection and treatment.[150] BCG vaccination of uninfected individuals is intended to provide protection against active tuberculosis infection and does not necessarily protect against latent infection (Figure 18-6, Stage 3). Even when BCG vaccine is highly efficacious, new cases of tuberculosis continue to arise from the latently infected pool until all at-risk individuals die. There is also increasing evidence that the efficacy of current BCG vaccines is attenuated. Thus, while BCG vaccination is widespread, the epidemiologic benefit gained from this intervention is limited.

Detection of tuberculosis cases and institution of effective chemotherapy are widely held to be the most important strategies for controlling tuberculosis and are the backbone of tuberculosis control. Rapid identification of cases and institution of effective treatment eliminate ongoing transmission of infection and limit the number of secondary cases, although an average of 8 to 15 contacts are infected before a newly identified infection can be sterilized with chemotherapy. It is, therefore, more accurate to state that case detection and treatment reduce, but do not eliminate, transmission of infection to susceptible individuals.

Treatment of latent tuberculosis infection with isoniazid (INH) or other antituberculosis medications reduces the risk of subsequent tuberculosis by 60% to 90%.[151] Provision of treatment for latent infection to people at high risk of developing tuberculosis is an important adjunct to case identification and treatment in reducing tuberculosis incidence in a community and has been used extensively in the United States and Europe. In the United States, INH preventive therapy is targeted at close contacts of infectious cases, individuals with HIV and latent tuberculosis infection, recent tuberculin converters, and other tuberculin-positive people at high risk of developing active tuberculosis.[47] The use of treatment for latent infection is very limited in resource-poor areas, however, and is usually directed only at young children living in households with smear-positive cases. Unfortunately the HIV epidemic has changed the dynamics of tuberculosis in many resource-poor areas, and some suggest that effective control of tuberculosis in these areas requires treatment of latent infection for people at high-risk of developing tuberculosis.

An additional problem limiting tuberculosis control efforts is the growing prevalence of drug-resistant disease. Between 1994 and 1997, a comprehensive global survey including 50,000 tuberculosis patients showed that the median prevalence of any drug resistance was 9.9% for patients who had not had any prior therapy (primary resistance) and 35.6% for those with a history of previous therapy (acquired resistance).[152] Dramatic outbreaks of multi-drug-resistant tuberculosis (MDR-TB) in HIV-infected patients and among health care workers in the United States in the early 1990s focused international attention on the emergence of strains of *M. tuberculosis* resistant to antimycobacterial drugs. Patients infected with strains resistant to multiple drugs are difficult to cure, and the necessary treatment is much more toxic and expensive. As noted previously, good tuberculosis control programs prevent emergence of drug-resistant tuberculosis in patients with susceptible strains but may fail to cure and prevent secondary cases in individuals with resistant strains, whether previously treated or not.

Currently there are a number of "hot spots" around the world where MDR-TB prevalence is high. In particular, prisoners in Russia have high rates of MDR-TB, and transmission within penal colonies is high.[153] Other areas with high levels of MDR-TB include former Soviet satellite states (particularly in the Baltic), Peru, parts of China, and Thailand.

Aggressive tuberculosis control measures that include prevention of institutional transmission of infection, DOTS, screening, and treatment of latent infection can dramatically reduce the prevalence of MDR-TB.[154] In New York City, for example, such an approach was extremely successful in reversing a disastrous epidemic of MDR-TB that affected that city in the early 1990s.[157] However, in other areas of the world, mobilization of resources to combat drug-resistant disease is more difficult, and community and institutional transmission of MDR strains continues, resulting in escalating levels of resistant cases and more treatment failures and deaths. An important approach to dealing with the growing problem of MDR-TB has been dubbed "DOTS-Plus," and involves the provision of second-line antituberculosis agents to patients with MDR-TB in resource-poor settings. Through extensive advocacy, the developers of DOTS-Plus at Partners in Health, a Harvard-based health advocacy group, have managed to obtain drastic price reductions for second-line drugs, which are now purchased by the Global Drug Facility of the World Health Organization and the STOP-TB Partnership. These groups have formed the Green Light Committee to review and approve applications from countries wishing to initiate DOTS-Plus programs to manage MDR-TB. Basic requirements for starting DOTS-Plus with support from the Green Light Committee and the Global Drug Facility include a well-functioning DOTS program, high treatment-completion rates, and a high case-detection rate.

Preliminary results from a number of DOTS-Plus programs show treatment success rates from 40% to 70%, an impressive accomplishment.

Conclusion

Tuberculosis is one of the most prevalent and deadly infections on Earth. Because humans are the primary reservoir of infection and transmission is via the aerosol route, elimination of tuberculosis is theoretically possible. Although recent advances in molecular epidemiology have improved our understanding of tuberculosis dynamics, the fundamental measures for controlling the disease have been known and available for decades. Despite this, tuberculosis continues to threaten humanity. Aggressive, comprehensive global efforts to control tuberculosis must expand and adapt to meet this threat.

References

1. Haas F, Haas SS. The origins of Mycobacterium tuberculosis and the notion of its contagiousness. In: Rom W, Garay SM, eds. *Tuberculosis.* New York, NY: Little, Brown and Company; 1996:3–19.
2. Brosch R, Pym AS, Gordon SV, Cole ST. The evolution of mycobacterial pathogenicity: clues from comparative genomics. *Trends Microbiol.* 2001;9:452–458.
3. Haas D, des Prez RM. *Mycobacterium tuberculosis.* In: Mandell G, Bennett JE, Dolin R, eds. *Mandell, Douglas and Bennett's Principles and Practice of Infectious Diseases.* New York, NY: Churchill Livingstone; 1995:2213–2243.
4. Pfyffer G, Auckenthaler R, van Embden JDA, van Soolingen D. *Mycobacterium canettii*, the smooth variant of *M. tuberculosis*, isolated from a Swiss patient exposed in Africa. *Emerg Infect Dis.* 1998;4: 631–634.
5. Niemann S, Richter E, Dalugge-Tamm H, et al. Two cases of *Mycobacterium microti*-derived tuberculosis in HIV-negative immunocompetent patients. *Emerg Infect Dis.* 2000;6:539–542.
6. WHO, GTP. *Global Tuberculosis Control, WHO Report 1998.* Geneva, Switzerland: World Health Organization; 1998.
7. Pitchenik A, Cole C, Russell BW, Fischl MA, Spira TJ, Snider DE. Tuberculosis, atypical mycobacteriosis, and the acquired immunodeficiency syndrome among Haitian and non-Haitian patients in south Florida. *Ann Intern Med.* 1984;101:641–645.
8. Bleed D, Dye C, Raviglione MC. Dynamics and control of the global tuberculosis epidemic. *Curr Opin Pulm Med.* 2000;6:174–179.
9. Jabado N, Gros P. Tuberculosis: the genetics of vulnerability. *Nature.* 2005;434:709–711.
10. WHO. *WHO Tuberculosis Factsheet #104.* 2005.
11. Dye C, Watt CJ, Bleed DM, Hosseini SM, Raviglione MC. Evolution of tuberculosis control and prospects for reducing tuberculosis incidence, prevalence, and deaths globally. *JAMA.* 2005;293:2767–2775.
12. Brooks G, Butel JS, Morse SA, eds. *Jawetz, Melnick and Adelberg's Medical Microbiology.* 21st ed. Stanford, Calif: Appleton and Lange; 1998.
13. Robbins S, Angell M, Kumar V, eds. *Basic Pathology.* 3rd ed. Philadelphia, Pa: WB Saunders Company; 1981.

14. Brosch R, Gordon V, Marmiesse M, et al. A new evolutionary scenario for the *Mycobacterium tuberculosis* complex. *PNAS*. 2002;99: 3684–3689.

15. Freeman B. *Burrows Textbook of Microbiology*. 22nd ed. Philadelphia, Pa: WB Saunders Company; 1985.

16. Pediatrics, tuberculosis. In: Peter G, ed. *1997 Red Book: Report of the Committee on Infectious Diseases*. Elk Grove Village, IL: American Academy of Pediatrics; 1997:541–567.

17. Cole S, Brosch R, Parkhill J, et al. Deciphering the biology of *Mycobacterium tuberculosis* from the complete genome sequence. *Nature*. 1998;393:537–544.

18. Daley C. Molecular epidemiology: a tool for understanding control of tuberculosis transmission. *Clin Chest Med*. 2005;26:217–231.

19. Stead W, Bates JH. Geographic and evolutionary epidemiology of tuberculosis. In: Rom W, Garay SM, eds. *Tuberculosis*. New York, NY: Little, Brown and Company; 1996:77–83.

20. Daley C. Tuberculosis contact investigations, please don't fail me now. *Am J Resp Crit Care Med*. 2004;169:779–781.

21. Easterbrook P, Gibson A, Murad S, et al. High rates of clustering of strains causing tuberculosis in Harare, Zimbabwe: a molecular epidemiological study. *J Clin Micro*. 2004;42:4536–4544.

22. Borgdorff M, van der Werf MJ, de Haas PEW, Kremer K, van Soolingen D. Tuberculosis elimination in the Netherlands. *Emerg Infect Dis*. 2005;11:597–602.

23. Bennett D, Onorato IM, Ellis BA, et al. DNA fingerprinting of *Mycobacterium tuberculosis* isolates from epidemiologically linked case pairs. *Emerg Infect Dis*. 2002;8:1224–1229.

24. Ellis B, Crawford JT, Braden CR, McNabb SJN, Moore M, Kammerer S, the National TB Genotyping & Surveillance Network Work Group. Molecular epidemiology of tuberculosis in a sentinel surveillance population. *Emerg Infect Dis*. 2002;8:1197–1209.

25. Centers for Disease Control and Prevention. Human tuberculosis caused by *Mycobacterium bovis*—New York City, 2001–2004. *MMWR*. 2005;54:605–608.

26. van Deutekom H, Hoijng SP, de Haas PEW, et al. Clustered tuberculosis cases: do they represent recent transmission and can they be detected earlier? *Am J Resp Crit Care Med*. 2004;169:806–810.

27. Pan H, Yan B-S Rojas, M, et al. Ipr1 gene mediates innate immunity to tuberculosis. *Nature*. 2005;434:767–772.

28. Narvskaya O, Mokrousov I, Limeschenko E, et al. Molecular characterization of *Mycobacterium tuberculosis* strains from the northwest region of Russia. *EpiNorth J*. 2005;11:18.

29. Stead W, Dutt AK. Epidemiology and host factors. In: Schlossberg D, ed. *Tuberculosis*. New York, NY: Springer-Verlag; 1994:1–16.

30. Formicola V, Milanesi Q, Scarsini C. Evidence of spinal tuberculosis at the beginning of the fourth millennium BC from Arene Candide Cave (Liguria, Italy). *Am J Phys Anthropol*. 1987;72:1–6.

31. Pesanti E. *A history of tuberculosis*. In: Lutwick L, ed *Tuberculosis*. New York, NY: Chapman and Hall Medical; 1995.

32. Bellamy R. Genetic susceptibility to tuberculosis. *Clin Chest Med*. 2005;26:233–246.

33. Tuberculosis. In: Peter G, ed. *1997 Red Book: Report of the Committee on Infectious Diseases*. Elk Grove Village, IL: American Academy of Pediatrics; 1997:541–567.

34. Pitchenik A, Fertel D, Block AB. Mycobacterial disease epidemiology, diagnosis, treatment and prevention. *Clin Chest Med.* 1988;9:425–441.

35. Cohen FJD, ed. *Tuberculosis: A Sourcebook for Nursing Practice.* New York, NY: Springer Publishing; 1995.

36. Isselbacher K, Braunwald E, Wilson JD, Martin JB, Fauci AS, Kasper DL. *Harrison's Principles of Internal Medicine Companion Handbook.* 13th ed. New York, NY: McGraw-Hill; 1995.

37. Abebe M, Lakew M, Kidane D, Lakew Z, Kiros K, Harboe M. Female genital tuberculosis in Ethiopia. *Int J Gyn Obstet.* 2004;84:241–246.

38. Wong H, Tay YK, Sim CS. Papular eruption on a tattoo: a case of primary inoculation tuberculosis. *Australasian J Dermatol.* 2005; 46:84.

39. ten Dam H. BCG vaccination. In: Reichman L, Hershfield ES, eds. *Tuberculosis: A Comprehensive International Approach.* New York, NY: Marcel Dekker Inc; 1993:251–274.

40. Raviglione M, Snider DE, Kochi A. Global epidemiology of tuberculosis: morbidity and mortality of a worldwide epidemic. *JAMA.* 1995;273:220–226.

41. Comstock G, O'Brien RJ. Tuberculosis. In: Evans A, Brachman PS, eds. *Bacterial Infections of Humans, Epidemiology and Control.* New York, NY: Plenum Medical Book Co; 1991:745–772.

42. Starke J. Tuberculosis in children. *Curr Opin Pediatr.* 1995;7:268–277.

43. ATS/CDC. Control of tuberculosis in the United States. *Am Rev Respir Dis.* 1992;146:1623–1633.

44. Thomas C, ed. *Taber's Cyclopedic Medical Dictionary.* Philadelphia, Pa: FA Davis Company; 1977.

45. Schein M, Huebner RE. Tuberculin skin testing. In: Rossman M, MacGregor RR, eds. *Tuberculosis Clinical Management and New Challenges.* New York, NY: McGraw-Hill; 1995:73–88.

46. Sutherland I. Recent studies in the epidemiology of tuberculosis based on the risk of being infected with tubercle bacilli. *Adv Tuberc Res.* 1976;19:1–63.

47. ATS/CDC. Targeted tuberculin testing and treatment of latent tuberculosis in latent tuberculosis infection. *MMWR.* 2000;49(RR06): 1–54.

48. Johnson M, Coberly J, Clermont H, et al. Tuberculin skin test reactivity among adults infected with human immunodeficiency virus. *J Infect Dis.* 1992;166:194–198.

49. Furcolow M, Hewell B, Nelson WE, Palmer CE. I. Titration of tuberculin sensitivity and its relation to tuberculosis infection. *Public Health Reports.* 1941;56:1082–1100.

50. Enarson D. Use of the tuberculin skin test in children. *Paediatr Respir Rev.* 2004;5:S135–S137.

51. Brewer T, Wilson ME, Nardell EA. BCG immunization: review of past experience, current use, and future prospects. *Curr Clin Top Infect Dis.* 1995;15:253–270.

52. Kielmann A, Oberoi IS, Chandra RK, Mehra VL. The effect of nutritional status on immune capacity and immune responses in preschool children in a rural community in India. *Bull WHO.* 1976;54:477–483.

53. Holmes C, Hausler H, Nunn P. A review of sex differences in the epidemiology of tuberculosis. *Int J Tuberc Lung Dis.* 1998;2:96–104.

54. Hanekom W, Potgieter S, Hughes EJ, Malan H, Kessow G, Hussey GD. Vitamin A status and therapy in childhood pulmonary tuberculosis. *J Pediatr.* 1997;131:925–927.

55. Cuevas L, Almeida LMD, Mazunder P, et al. Effect of zinc on the tuberculin response of children exposed to adults with smear-positive tuberculosis. *Ann Trop Pediatr.* 2002;22:313–319.

56. Sousa A, Salem JI, Lee FK, et al. An epidemic of tuberculosis with a high rate of tuberculin anergy among a population previously unexposed to tuberculosis, the Yanomami Indians of the Brazilian Amazon. *Proc Natl Acad Sci.* 1997;94:13227–13232.

57. Frieden T, Fujiwara PI, Washko RM, Hamburg PA. Tuberculosis in New York City: turning the tide. *N Engl J Med.* 1995;333:229–233.

58. Bellete B, Coberly JS, Barnes GL, et al. Evaluation of a whole-blood interferon-gamma release assay for the detection of *Mycobacterium tuberculosis* infection in 2 study populations. *Clin Infect Dis.* 2002;34:1449–1456.

59. Pai M, Riley LW, Colford JM Jr. Interferon-gamma assays in the immunodiagnosis of tuberculosis: a systematic review. *Lancet Infectious Disease.* 2004;4:761–776.

60. Kang YA, Lee HW, Yoon HI, et al. Discrepancy between the tuberculin skin test and the whole-blood interferon-gamma assay for the diagnosis of latent tuberculosis infection in an intermediate tuberculosis-burden county. *JAMA.* 2005; 293:2756–2761.

61. Siriarayapon P, Yanai H, Glynn JR, Yanpaisarn S, Uthaivoravit W. The evolving epidemiology of HIV infection and tuberculosis in northern Thailand. *J AIDS.* 2002;31:80–89.

62. Dubos R, Dubos J. *The White Plague: Tuberculosis, Man and Society.* Boston, Mass: Little, Brown and Co; 1952.

63. BMRC. Streptomycin treatment of pulmonary tuberculosis. *BMJ.* 1948;2:769–782.

64. BMRC, Hong Kong Chest Service. Controlled trial of 4 three-times-weekly regimens and a daily regimen all given for 6 months for pulmonary tuberculosis; second report: the results up to 24 months. *Tubercle.* 1982;63:89–98.

65. BMRC Treatment of pulmonary tuberculosis with streptomycin and p-aminosalicylic acid. *BMJ.* 1950;2:1073–1108.

66. Hong Kong Chest Service/Tuberculosis Research Centre, M.B. A controlled trial of 3-month, 4-month and 6-month regimens of chemotherapy for sputum-smear-negative pulmonary tuberculosis, results at 5 years. *Am Rev Respir Dis.* 1989;139:871–876.

67. Hong Kong Chest Service, B. Five-year follow-up of a controlled trial of five 6-month regimes of chemotherapy for pulmonary tuberculosis. *Am Rev Respir Dis.* 1987;136:1339–1342.

68. Singapore Tuberculosis Service, B. Long-term follow-up of a clinical trial of six-month and four-month regimens of chemotherapy in the treatment of pulmonary tuberculosis. *Am Rev Respir Dis.* 1986;133:779–783.

69. Singapore Tuberculosis Service, B. Five-year follow-up of a clinical trial of three 6-month regimens of chemotherapy given intermittently in the continuation phase in the treatment of pulmonary tuberculosis. *Am Rev Respir Dis.* 1988;137:1147–1150.

70. Azia A, Ishaq M, Jaffer NA, Akhwand R, Bhatti AH. Clinical trial of two short-course (6-month) regimes and a standard regimen (12-month) chemotherapy in retreatment of pulmonary tuberculosis in Pakistan. *Am Rev Respir Dis.* 1986;134:1056–1061.

71. Hong Kong Chest Service, B. Five-year follow-up of a controlled trial of five 6-month regimens of chemotherapy for pulmonary tuberculosis. *Am Rev Respir Dis.* 1987;136:1339–1342.

72. Hong Kong Chest Service, B. Controlled trial of 6-month and 8-month regimens in the treatment of pulmonary tuberculosis: the results up to 24 months. *Tubercle.* 1979;60:201–210.

73. East African, B. Controlled clinical trial of five short-course (4-month) chemotherapy regimens in pulmonary tuberculosis, second report of the 4th study. *Am Rev Respir Dis.* 1981;123:165–170.

74. Castelo A, Jardim JRB, Goihman S, et al. Comparison of daily and twice-weekly regimens to treat pulmonary tuberculosis. *Lancet.* 1989;2:1173–1176.

75. Okwere A, Whalen C, Byckwaso F, et al. Makerene University- Case Western Reserve University research collaboration. *Lancet.* 1994;344:1323–1328.

76. Perriens J, St. Louis ME, Mukadi YB, et al. Pulmonary tuberculosis in HIV-infected patients in Zaire: a controlled trial of treatment for either 6 or 12 months. *N Engl J Med.* 1995;332:779–784.

77. Chaisson R, Clermont HC, Holt EA, et al., JHU-CDS Research Team. Six-month supervised intermittent tuberculosis therapy in Haitian patients with and without HIV infections. *Am J Respir Crit Care Med.* 1996;154:1034–1038.

78. Alwood K, Keruly JC, Moore-Rice K, et al. Effectiveness of supervised, intermittent therapy for tuberculosis in HIV infected patients. *AIDS.* 1994;8:1103–1108.

79. Harries A, Maher D. *TB/HIV: A Clinical Manual.* Geneva, Switzerland: World Health Organization; 1996.

80. ATS/CDC. Treatment of tuberculosis: Official Joint Statement of the American Thoracic Society, CDC, and the Infectious Diseases Society of America. *Am J Resp Crit Care Med.* 2003;167:602–662.

81. Chaisson R, Coberly JS, DeCock KM. DOTS and drug resistance: a silver lining to a darkening cloud. *IJTBLD.* 1999;3:1–3.

82. Zwarenstein M, Schoeman JH, Vundule C, et al. Randomized controlled trial of self supervised and directly observed treatment of tuberculosis. *Lancet.* 1998;352:1340–1343.

83. WHO, GTP. *Global Tuberculosis Control, WHO Report 2005.* Geneva, Switzerland: World Health Organization; 2005.

84. WHO. *Global Tuberculosis Control: Surveillance, Planning, Financing.* Geneva, Switzerland: WHO; 2004.

85. WHO. *What Is the Deadliest Disease in the World?* 2005.

86. Murray C, Styblo K, Rouillon A. Tuberculosis in developing countries: burden, intervention and cost. *Bull Int Union Against Tuberc Lung Dis.* 1990;65:1–20.

87. Dye C, Scheele S, Dolin P, Pathania V, Raviglione MC. Global burden of tuberculosis estimated incidence, prevalence and mortality by country. *JAMA.* 1999;282:677–686.

88. Comstock G. Frost revisited: the modern epidemiology of tuberculosis. *Am J Epidemiol.* 1975;101:363–382.

89. De Cock K, Chaisson RE. Will DOTS do it? A reappraisal of tuberculosis in countries with high rates of HIV infection. *Int J Tuberc Lung Dis.* 1999;3:457–465.

90. Loudon R, Roberts RM. Singing and the dissemination of tuberculosis. *Am Rev Respir Dis.* 1968;98:297–300.

91. Rieder H. Epidemiology of tuberculosis in Europe. *Europ Respir J.* 1995;20(suppl):620–632.

92. Loudon R, Roberts RM. Droplet expulsion from the respiratory tract. *Am Rev Respir Dis.* 1966;95:435–442.

93. Wells W. On air-borne infection. Study II. Droplets and droplet nuclei. *Am J Hyg.* 1934;20:611–618.

94. Sonkin LS. The role of particle size in experimental air-borne infection. *Am J Hyg.* 1951;53:337–354.

95. Rieder H, Cauthen GM, Comstock GW. Epidemiology of tuberculosis in the United States. *Epidemiol Rev.* 1989;11:79–98.

96. Rieder H. *Epidemiologic Basis of Tuberculosis Control.* 1st ed. Paris, France: International Union Against Tuberculosis and Lung Disease; 1999.

97. Grzybowski S, Barnett GD, Styblo K. Contacts of cases of active pulmonary tuberculosis. *Bull Int Union Tuberc.* 1975;50: 107–121.

98. Chapman J, Dyerly MD, Powell DR. Social and other factors in intrafamilial transmission of tuberculosis. *Am Rev Respir Dis.* 1964;90:48–60.

99. Kamat S, Dawson JJY, Devadatta S, et al. A controlled study of the influence of segregation of tuberculosis patients for one year on the attack rate of tuberculosis in a 5-year period in close family contacts in south India. *Bull WHO.* 1966;34:517–532.

100. Comstock G. Epidemiology of tuberculosis. *Am Rev Respir Dis.* 1982;125(suppl):8–15.

101. Reichman L, O'Day R. Tuberculous infection in a large urban population. *Am Rev Respir Dis.* 1978;117:705–712.

102. Kuemmerer J, Comstock GW. Sociologic concomitants of tuberculin sensitivity. *Am Rev Respir Dis.* 1967;96:885–892.

103. Stead W. Undetected tuberculosis in prison. *JAMA.* 1978;240: 2544–2547.

104. Houk V, Baker JH, Sorensen K, Kent DC. The epidemiology of tuberculosis infection in a closed environment. *Arch Environ Health.* 1968;16:26–35.

105. Stead W, Lofgren JP, Warren E, Thomas C. Tuberculosis as an endemic and nosocomial infection among the elderly in nursing homes. *N Engl J Med.* 1985;312:1483–1487.

106. Comstock G, Livesay VT, Woolpert SF. Evaluation of BCG vaccination among Puerto Rican children. *Am J Pub Health.* 1974;64: 283–291.

107. IUAT. Efficacy of various durations of isoniazid preventive therapy for tuberculosis: five years of follow-up in the IUAT trial. *Bull WHO.* 1982;60:555–564.

108. Edwards L, Livesay VT, Acquaviva FA, Palmer CE. Height, weight, tuberculosis infection and tuberculous disease. *Arch Environ Health.* 1971;22:106–112.

109. Horwitz O. Epidemiologic basis of tuberculosis eradication. 10. Lung studies on the risk of tuberculosis in the general population of a low-prevalence area. *Bull WHO.* 1969;41:95–113.

110. Comstock G, Cauthen GM. Epidemiology of tuberculosis. In: Reichman L, Hershfield ES, eds. *Tuberculosis: A Comprehensive International Approach.* New York, NY: Marcel Dekker, Inc; 1993:23–48.

111. Horwitz O. Tuberculosis risk and marital status. *Am Rev Respir Dis.* 1971;104:22–31.

112. Lurie M. *Resistance to Tuberculosis: Experimental Studies in Native Acquired Defensive Mechanisms.* Cambridge, Mass: Harvard University Press; 1984.

113. O'Brien S. Ghetto legacy. *Curr Biol.* 1991;i:209–211.

114. Motulsky A. Metabolic polymorphisms and the role of infectious disease in human evolution. *Hum Biol.* 1960;32:28–62.

115. Stead W, Senner JW, Reddick WT, et al. Racial differences in susceptibility to infection by *Mycobacterium tuberculosis. N Engl J Med.* 1990;322:422–427.

116. Comstock G. Tuberculosis in twins: a re-analysis of the Prophit survey. *Am Rev Respir Dis.* 1978;117:621–624.

117. Kallmann F, Reisner D. Twin studies on the significance of genetic factors in tuberculosis. *Am Rev Tuberc.* 1942;47:549–574.

118. Simonds B. *Tuberculosis in Twins.* London, UK: Pitman Medical Publishing Company; 1963.

119. Overfield T, Klauber MR. Prevalence of tuberculosis in Eskimos having blood group B gene. *Hum Biol.* 1980;52:87–92.

120. Bellamy R, Ruwende C, Corrah T, McAdam KP, Whittle HC, Hill AV. Variations in the NRAMP1 gene and susceptibility to tuberculosis in West Africans. *N Engl J Med.* 1998;338:640–644.

121. Goldfeld A, Delgado JC, Thim S, et al. Association of an HLA-DQ allele with clinical tuberculosis. *JAMA.* 1998;279:226–228.

122. Casanova J-L, Blanche S, Emile J-F, et al. Idiopathic disseminated bacillus Calmette-Guerin infection: a French national retrospective study. *Pediatrics.* 1996;98:774–778.

123. Jouanguy E, Altare F, Lamhamedi S, et al. Interferon-γ-receptor deficiency in an infant with fatal bacille Calmette-Guerin infection. *N Engl J Med.* 1996;335:1956–1961.

124. Rwangabwoba J, Humphrey J, Coberly J, Moulton L, Desormeaux J, Halsey N. Vitamin A status and development of tuberculosis and or mortality. In: *The XI International Conference on AIDS.* Vancouver, Canada: International Conference on AIDS; 1996.

125. Sterling T, Pope DS, Bishai WR, Harrington S, Gershon RR, Chaisson RE. Transmission of *Mycobacterium tuberculosis* from a cadaver to an embalmer. *N Engl J Med.* 2000;342:246–248.

126. Geisseler J, Nelson KE, Crispen RG, Moses VK. Tuberculosis in physicians: a continuing problem. *Am Rev Respir Dis.* 1986;133:733–738.

127. McKenna M, Hutton M, Cauther G, Onorato IM. The association between occupation and tuberculosis: a population-based survey. *Am J Respir Crit Care Med.* 1996;154:587–593.

128. Barrett-Connor E. The epidemiology of tuberculosis in physicians. *JAMA.* 1979;241:33–38.

129. Gajalakshmi V, Peto R, Kanaka TS, Jha P. Smoking and mortality from tuberculosis and other diseases in India: retrospective study of 43000 adult male deaths and 35000 controls. *Lancet.* 2003;362:507–515.

130. Leung C, Li T, Lam TH, et al. Smoking and tuberculosis among the elderly in Hong Kong. *Am J Resp Crit Care Med.* 2004;170:1027–1033.

131. Abal A, Jayakrishnan B, Parwer S, ElShamy A, Abahussain E, Sharma PN. Effect of cigarette smoking on sputum smear conversion in adults with active pulmonary tuberculosis. *Respir Med.* 2005;99:415–420.

132. Boelaert J, Gomes MS, Gordeuk VR. Smoking, iron, and tuberculosis. *Lancet.* 2003;362:1243–1244.

133. Hopewell P, Chaisson RE. Tuberculosis and human immunodeficiency virus infection. In: Reichman L, Hershfield ES, eds. *Tuberculosis: A Comprehensive International Approach.* New York, NY: Marcel Dekker Inc; 2000.

134. Daley C, Small PM, Schecter GF, et al. An outbreak of tuberculosis with accelerated progression among persons infected with human immunodeficiency virus: an analysis using restriction-fragment-length polymorphisms. *N Engl J Med.* 1992;326:321–325.

135. Yinai H, Uthaivoravit W, Panich V, et al. Rapid increase in HIV-related tuberculosis, Chiang Rai, Thailand, 1990–1994. *AIDS.* 1996;10: 527–531.

136. Markowitz N, Hansen N, Hopewell PC, et al. Incidence of tuberculosis in the United States among HIV-infected patients. *Ann Intern Med.* 1997;126:123–132.

137. Antonucci G, Girardi E, Raviglione MC, Ippilito G. Risk factors for tuberculosis in HIV infected persons: a prospective cohort study. *JAMA.* 1995;274:143–148.

138. Selwyn P, Sckell BM, Alcabes P, et al. High risk of active tuberculosis among intravenous drug users with cutaneous anergy. *JAMA.* 1992;268:504–509.

139. Caiaffa W, Graham NHM, Vlahov D, et al. Instability of delayed-type hypersensitivity (DTH) skin test anergy in human immunodeficiency infection. *Arch Int Med.* 1996;155:2111–2117.

140. Theuer C, Hopewell PC, Elias D, et al. Human immunodeficiency virus infection in tuberculosis patients. *J Infect Dis.* 1990;162:8–12.

141. De Cock K, Soro B, Coulibay IM, Lucas SB. Tuberculosis and HIV infection in sub-Saharan Africa. *JAMA.* 1992;268:1581–1587.

142. ten Dam H. BCG vaccination: an old idea revisited. In: Rossman M, MacGregor RR, eds. *Tuberculosis.* New York, NY: McGraw-Hill; 1995:109–128.

143. Ayvazian L. History of tuberculosis. In: Reichman L, Hershfield ES, eds. *Tuberculosis: A Comprehensive International Approach.* New York, NY: Marcel Dekker Inc; 1993:1–22.

144. Fine P, Sterne JAC, Ponnighaus JM, Rees RJW. Delayed-type hypersensitivity, mycobacterial vaccines and protective immunity. *Lancet.* 1994;344:1245–1249.

145. Hagwood B. Doctor Albert Calmette 1863–1933: founder of antivenomous serotherapy and antituberculous BCG vaccination. *Toxicon.* 1999;37:1241–1258.

146. Smith P. Case-control studies of the efficacy of BCG against tuberculosis. In: *XXVIth IUAT World Conference, 1986.* Professional Post Graduate Services, International; 1987.

147. Shapiro C, Cook N, Evans D, et al. A case-control study of BCG and childhood tuberculosis in Cali, Colombia. *Int J Epidemiol.* 1985;14:441–446.

148. Sutrisna B, Utomo P, Komalarini S, Swatriani S. Penelitian efekitfitas vaksin BCG dan beberapa faktor lainnya pada anak yang mederita TBC berat di 3 Rumah sakit di Jakarta 1981–1982. *Medika.* 1983;9: 143–150.

149. Kenyon T, Mwasekaga MJ, Huebner R, Rumisha D, Binkin N, Maganu E. Low levels of drug resistance admidst rapidly increasing tuberculosis and human immunodeficiency virus co-epidemics in Botswana. *Int J Tuberc Lung Dis.* 1999;3:4–11.

150. IUATLD. *Tuberculosis Guide for Low Income Countries.* 3rd ed. Paris, France: International Union Against Tuberculosis and Lung Disease; 1994.

151. Ferebee S. Controlled chemoprophylaxis trials in tuberculosis: a general review. *Adv Tuberc Res.* 1970;17:28–106.

152. WHO/IUATLD. *Antituberculosis Drug Resistance in the World.* Geneva, Switzerland: WHO/IUATLD; 1997.

153. Kimerling M, Kluge H, Vezhnina N, et al. Inadequacy of the current WHO re-treatment regimen in a central Siberian prison: treatment failure and MDR-TB. *Int J Tuberc Lung Dis.* 1999;3:451–453.

154. Weis SE, Slocum PC, Blais FX, King B, Nunn M. The effect of directly observed therapy on the rates of drug resistance and relapse in tuberculosis. *N Engl J Med.* 1994;330:1179–1184.

CHAPTER NINETEEN

THE EPIDEMIOLOGY OF ACUTE RESPIRATORY INFECTIONS

Neil M.H. Graham, Kenrad E. Nelson, and Mark C. Steinhoff

Introduction

As recently as 1997, acute respiratory infections were termed a "forgotten pandemic."[1] These infections, which are composed of pneumonia, bronchitis, bronchiolitis, otitis media, sinusitis, pharyngitis, laryngitis, measles, and pertussis, continue to cause 19% of all deaths worldwide among children aged less than 5 years and 8.2% of all disability and premature mortality.[1] Children living in developing countries have especially high morbidity and mortality rates. Despite the pandemicity of acute lower respiratory infections, investigators of these illnesses receive only 0.15% of all health-related research and development dollars.[1] This translates to $0.51 per disability-adjusted life-year (DALY), compared with $13 for asthma and $10 for rheumatic diseases.[1]

Although slow in coming, substantial gains in the battle against acute respiratory infections have been made with the public health approach to prophylaxis and treatment. Major advances have occurred to facilitate our understanding of the epidemiology and etiology of these infections. Data about risk factors continue to accumulate, with most information coming from the developed world, where funding, logistics, and infrastructure are available to support large multidimensional epidemiologic studies. Promising areas of epidemiologic investigation have been pursued since the 1980s, such as nutritional risk factors, the effects of indoor and outdoor air pollution, and the development of new vaccines. In this chapter, the impact on public health, etiology, and risk factors for acute respiratory infections are reviewed, and the major methodologic problems and requirements for future research are delineated.

Impact on Public Health

Developing Countries

Over the past 25 years, published data have indicated huge differences in mortality rates from acute respiratory infections between developing and developed countries. A World Health Organization (WHO) study in 1990 revealed that, in the world as a whole, the number of deaths attributable to respiratory infections was 12 times greater in developing countries than in developed countries (Table 19-1).[2] A recent report from the World Health Organization has estimated that 19% of mortality in children aged less than 5 years is attributable to acute respiratory infections.[3] If developed countries can be defined as those with infant mortality rates of less than 25 per 1000, 98% of deaths from acute respiratory infections in infants and 99% of those in children aged 1 to 4 years can be expected to occur in less developed countries.[4] Conversely, countries with infant mortality of approximately 100 per 1000 can be expected to contribute 58% of the deaths in infants and 66% of those in children aged 1 to 4 years.[4] As these estimates are based on national mortality reporting systems of varying quality, underestimation of the true mortality rate is possible.

Pneumonia causes more deaths in children in the developing world (2.0 million, annually) than respiratory illness caused by malaria and measles (1.3 million).[1] The Pan American Health Organization reported pneumonia deaths in Peru as being 37 times higher in infants and 43 times higher in children aged 1 to 4 years than rates in North America.[5] Infant deaths from pneumonia and influenza in 1977 were five times higher in Costa Rica, and 30 times higher in Paraguay, than in the United States.[6] In infants in the Philippines, pneumonia death rates have been reported to be 24 times higher than in Australian infants and 73 times higher than in Australian children aged 1 to 4 years.[7]

In contrast to these mortality data, acute respiratory infection-related morbidity appears to differ little between developing and developed countries. Among developing countries, mean episodes of respiratory illness per year have been reported as 7.3 in children aged less than 3 years and 6.2 in children aged 3 to 5 years in India,[8] 7.9 in children aged less than 3 years and 6.6 in children aged 3 to 5 years in Ethiopia,[9] and 4.9 and 5.7 in urban settings in Costa Rica.[10]

TABLE 19-1   WHO Estimated Deaths from Respiratory Infections (excluding tuberculosis), 1990

	Respiratory Infections	All Causes of Death
World	4,314,400 (8.6%)	49,971,100
Developed countries	330,000 (3.0%)	10,883,100
Developing countries	3,984,400 (10.2%)	39,088,000

Source: C.J.L. Murray and A.D. Lopez, Global Comparative Assessments in the Health Sector, World Health Organization, 1994.

Similarly, in the developed world, data from the National Research Council studies of respiratory infection in young children in 12 countries suggest that the incidence in the first year of life ranges from five to nine episodes.[11] In the Seattle Virus Watch from 1965–1969, infants experienced four and one half mean episodes per year.[12] In Tecumseh, Michigan, infants experienced a mean of slightly more than six episodes of respiratory illness per year, and children aged 1 to 4 years experienced a mean of just more than five episodes per year.[13] It should be cautioned, however, that the studies from which these data were culled used widely differing methodologies and, thus, prevalence rates may not be directly comparable.

The incidence of chronic bronchitis (chronic obstructive pulmonary disease) is generally similar in developing and developed countries.[14] For example, Lai et al found 6.8% of an elderly group of Chinese living in Hong Kong to have chronic bronchitis,[15] and pharmaceutical research indicated a 6.9% incidence in Taiwan.[14] However, Pandey found a high incidence of chronic bronchitis (18%) in Nepal,[16] with women and men equally affected. Indonesia also appears to have an especially high incidence of chronic bronchitis, although available data do not differentiate chronic bronchitis from acute bronchitis or account for multiple episodes during the observation period.[14] An age profile in a sample of nearly 250,000 persons in Indonesia noted the incidence of chronic bronchitis was 15.7% in those aged 30 to 39 years, 19.3% for those aged 40 to 54 years, and approximately 6% for those aged 55 years or older.[14]

Developed Countries

In developed countries acute respiratory infections are the leading cause of morbidity, accounting for 20% of medical consultations, 30% of absences from work, and 75% of all antibiotic prescriptions.[1] Of all the acute respiratory infections, pneumonia has been the most thoroughly studied. In 1900, pneumonia was the second most likely cause of death in the United States after tuberculosis.[17] Mortality rates per 100,000 population between 1910 and the present are shown in Figure 19-1.[17] In 1918, pneumonia mortality skyrocketed from the great influenza pandemic, which that year killed more than 540,000 Americans. Since that time, the pneumonia-related mortality rate has fallen significantly because of better hygiene practices and the availability of effective treatment, including antipneumococcal serum, sulfa drugs, penicillin, and other effective antibiotics. The slight increase in pneumonia-related deaths since 1990 is primarily because of the increase in the elderly population, who have a high pneumonia risk.[17] Currently, in the United States mortality rates from community-acquired pneumonia range from 1% to 5% in outpatients and from 15% to 30% in inpatients, making it the sixth leading cause of death.[18-20] Community-acquired pneumonia incurs hospitalization in 20% of patients and 65 million days of restricted activity.[21]

Figure 19-2 pinpoints where in the United States deaths from pneumonia occurred between 1979 and 1992.[17] Although it was long theorized that a higher mortality rate from pneumonia occurred during winter and that cold temperatures promote pneumonia, these ideas are not consistent with the pattern of mortality shown in Figure 19-2.[17] Indeed, no definitive pattern with regard to climate is apparent: California had the highest pneumonia-related

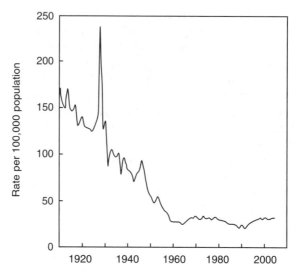

FIGURE 19-1   Rates in the graph are for the death registration area, which comprised 12 states in 1900 and 48 states by 1933. Alaska was added in 1959 and Hawaii in 1960. Not adjusted for changing age composition.
Source: Roger Doyle © 2000.

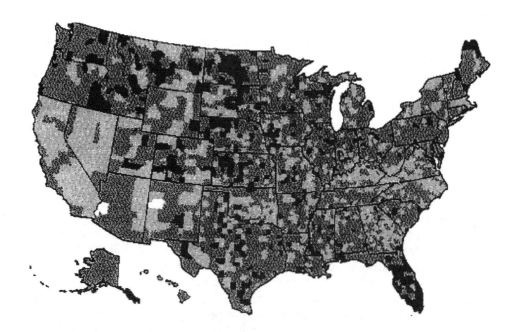

Age-adjusted rate per 100,000 people SS and over, by county, 1979–1992

■ UNDER 50   ▨ 50 TO 79.9   ▧ 80 OR MORE

FIGURE 19-2   Deaths from pneumonia in the United States.
Source: Roger Doyle © 2000.

mortality rates; Georgia and Massachusetts had high rates; and North Dakota had the third lowest rate. The fact that pneumonia-related deaths occurred least often in Florida is believed to be due to the "healthy retiree" effect, that is, the tendency of healthy older people to retire to places such as Florida, whereas less healthy people in the older age group remain at home.[17]

Hospital-acquired (nosocomial) pneumonia is the second most common nosocomial infection in the United States, but it is the type of nosocomial infection most frequently associated with a fatal outcome.[22] The annual incidence is 5 to 10 cases per 1000 hospital admissions, and up to 20 times this figure in patients on ventilators.[22] Mortality rates run as high as 33% to 50% in patients on ventilators.[23,24] The availability of penicillin and other antibiotics to treat pneumonia has greatly reduced the mortality and morbidity associated with this infection.

Age-specific incidence rates of minor episodes of respiratory illness (primarily upper respiratory tract infections) in the United States have varied little since 1933, as indicated by the results of studies that evaluated populations of varying compositions and used differing study methodologies and definitions of acute respiratory illness.[13,25-27] Over this period, however, pneumonia mortality rates have decreased in all age groups, except the elderly (Table 19-2). Indeed, since 1981, mortality rates have increased in pneumonia patients aged 55 years or older. It is unclear why this is occurring, although alterations in the types and pathogenicity of organisms causing pneumonia and changing host factors may be contributory factors.[28] Despite decreasing mortality rates for pneumonia and influenza in young children and infants, lower respiratory tract illness (croup, bronchitis, bronchiolitis, and pneumonia) remains an important cause of morbidity, annually affecting approximately 25% of children aged less than 1 year and 18% of children aged 1 to 4 years.[29-31] In 1989, Wright et al reported the cumulative incidence of first episodes of lower respiratory tract infection in infants to be 32.9% in children of families participating in a prepaid health plan.[32] This higher rate may have been seen because of differing diagnostic criteria compared with previous studies,[29-31] an active rather than a passive follow-up regimen, and increased physician attendance because of lack of a financial disincentive in a prepaid health plan. In older children and adults in the United Kingdom, acute respiratory infections accounted for almost one fourth of all primary care contacts, and one third of days taken off work were attributable to acute respiratory illness.[32] In a survey in Australia, 17% of patients aged 15 years or older and 43% of children aged less than 15 years consulted a doctor for respiratory symptoms during the 2 weeks presurvey.[33] A study in Adelaide, South Australia, showed that children younger than 5 years experienced a mean of seven episodes of respiratory illness per year, which prompted three doctor visits, 15 days of medication, and 52 days of respiratory symptoms annually.[34,35]

The incidence of chronic bronchitis is similar in the United States and Europe.[14] In 1994, Enright et al reported that 5.1% to 5.4% of the middle-aged to elderly population in the United States have chronic bronchitis, with a lower prevalence in nonsmokers.[36] In Europe, chronic bronchitis has been reported to affect 3.7% of people in Denmark,[37] 4.5% in Norway,[38] 6% and 6.4% in Barcelona and Valencia, Spain, respectively,[39,40] and 6.7% in Sweden.[41]

TABLE 19-2   Age-Specific Mortality Rates from Pneumonia and Influenza in the United States, 1968–1996

Age (years)

Year	<1	1–4	5–14	15–24	25–34	35–44	45–54	55–64	65–74	75–84	≥85
1968	234.9	9.9	1.8	2.8	4.4	9.3	19.9	41.9	106.0	330.7	1,167.8
1970	180.8	7.6	1.6	2.4	3.8	8.5	17.3	36.2	90.2	272.8	814.5
1971	147.2	6.9	1.3	2.2	3.3	7.0	13.4	29.3	77.0	253.8	855.9
1973	115.7	5.9	1.4	2.0	3.1	6.9	14.5	31.6	82.1	295.6	910.4
1975	71.5	4.1	1.0	1.7	2.5	5.3	11.1	27.0	70.2	264.4	777.1
1977	53.2	3.1	0.9	1.3	2.0	4.4	9.6	21.9	58.5	236.2	731.2
1979	33.0	2.0	0.6	0.8	1.5	3.2	7.1	16.4	47.8	184.2	694.9
1981	22.6	1.8	0.5	0.8	1.5	3.3	7.4	18.4	52.5	209.3	845.8
1983	21.0	1.7	0.4	0.7	1.4	2.8	6.7	16.8	51.1	205.8	859.9
1986	17.6	1.4	0.4	0.7	1.7	3.6	7.0	18.6	58.6	242.8	1,032.1
1996	—	1.1	0.4	0.6	2.4[†]	2.4[†]	10.6[‡]	10.6[‡]	221.4[§]	221.4[§]	221.4[§]

[†] Ages 25 to 44 years grouped together this year.
[‡] Ages 45 to 64 years grouped together this year.
[§] Ages ≥65 years grouped together this year.
Source: Reprinted from Monthly Vital Statistics Report, U.S. Public Health Service, National Center for Health Statistics, 1968–1988, and National Vital Statistics Report 1998, Vol. 47, No. 9.

In the United States in 1998, community-acquired pneumonia accounted for an estimated $3.6 billion for treating patients aged less than 65 years and $4.8 billion for treating patients aged 65 years or older.[42] In 1999, costs associated with acute exacerbations of chronic bronchitis were $419 million in patients aged less than 65 years and three times that much ($1.2 billion) for patients aged 65 years and older.[43]

Classification of Acute Respiratory Infections

Two basic systems are most commonly used to classify acute respiratory infections: the case-management classification system, and the "traditional" clinical classification system (Table 19-3).

Case-Management Classification

In an effort to reduce pneumonia-related mortality, the World Health Organization has developed a simple case-management approach to be followed by village health care workers. Before 1988, simplified case classifications, as used in India,[44] Papua New Guinea,[45] and other developing countries,[46] were applied successfully by health workers to determine when children should be given antibiotics or referred to secondary or tertiary level care. Adherence with these classifications resulted in reductions in both pneumonia-related mortality and in overall mortality. The simplified case definitions were based on respiratory rates recorded among children with symptoms of respiratory infections. The sensitivity and specificity of increased respiratory rate were determined using clinically confirmed or chest radiograph-confirmed pneumonia (or, "lower respiratory tract infection") as the putative gold standard. For example, using receiver operating characteristic (ROC) curves, Cherian et al showed that higher respiratory rates were more sensitive and specific for infants than for older children aged less than 5 years (Figure 19-3).[47]

In 1988, changes were made to improve the specificity of case-management guidelines.[46,48-50] Although the primary focus remained on pneumonia, classification and management of syndromes causing stridor and wheezing were directly addressed, and otitis media was classified separately (Table 19-3). Other major differences from the earlier classification were in the less-than-2-month-old age group, about whom the newer classification recognized that a respiratory rate greater than 50 breaths/minute and some chest indrawing could be considered normal[48]; with regard to cough, which is often absent in neonates with pneumonia, the newer classification specified that this sign is not sufficiently sensitive to be used as an indicator of severe disease. The newer case-management classification recommended that signs of general sepsis should be sought (i.e., fever, feeding problems, drowsiness, convulsions, abdominal distention, hypothermia) as well as more specific signs of pneumonia (respiratory rate greater than 60 breaths/minute, severe chest indrawing, respiratory grunt) when determining whether to prescribe antibiotics and to hospitalize.[48]

TABLE 19-3 Classification of Acute Respiratory Infection Clinical Syndromes

	Case-Management Classification (children aged 2 months to 4 years)			"Traditional" Classification
Stridor	**Wheezing**	**No wheezing**		
Mild	Mild	Mild		Upper respiratory tract syndromes
Hoarseness plus "barking" cough; no stridor when calm = mild croup	Improves with bronchodilator; respiratory rate <50/min = mild bronchiolitis or asthma	Cough; nasal obstruction; respiratory rate <50/min = URI,* cold		Common cold; URI* / Acute otitis media / Pharyngitis/tonsillitis / Acute sinusitis
Home care; no antibiotic	Oral salbutamol	No antibiotic; home care		Middle respiratory tract syndromes
	Moderate	Moderate		Croup Laryngotracheo-bronchitis / Epiglottitis / Laryngitis / Tracheitis
	Improves with bronchodilator; respiratory rate 50–70/min = mild bronchiolitis or asthma	Respiratory rate >50/min; no chest indrawing = pneumonia		
	Consider antibiotic; oral salbutamol; home care	Antibiotic; home care		
Severe	Severe	Severe		Lower respiratory tract syndromes
Stridor when calm; chest indrawing = severe croup or epiglottis	No improvement with bronchodilator; respiratory rate >70/min = severe bronchiolitis or asthma	Respiratory rate >50/min; chest indrawing = severe pneumonia		Bronchiolitis / Bronchitis / Pneumonia
Admit; antibiotic; manage airway	Admit; bronchodilators; consider oxygen and antibiotics	Admit; antibiotic		
	Very severe	Very severe		
	Cyanosis or inability to drink = very severe bronchiolitis or asthma	Cyanosis or inability to drink = very severe pneumonia		
	Admit; bronchodilators; oxygen and consider antibiotic	Antibiotic; admit; oxygen		

* URI, upper respiratory infection.

Source: N.M.H. Graham, The Epidemiology of Acute Respiratory Infection in Children and Adults: A Global Perspective, Epidemiologic Reviews, Vol. 12, pp. 149–178, © 1990, Oxford University Press.

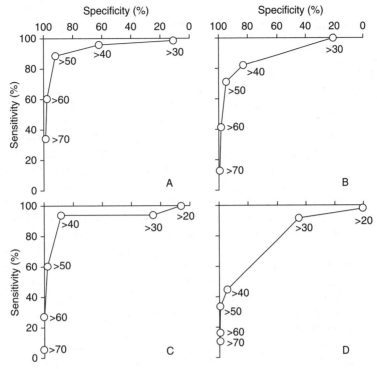

FIGURE 19-3 Receiver operating characteristic (ROC) curves for respiratory rates as indicators of lower respiratory tract infections in infants and children.
Source: T. Cherian et al., Evaluation of Simple Clinical Signs for the Diagnosis of Acute Lower Respiratory Tract Infection, *The Lancet*, Vol. 2, pp. 125–128, © by The Lancet Ltd., 1998, with permission from Elsevier.

Clinical Classification

Acute respiratory infections can be classified by the site of primary pathology (Table 19-3). This system is preferred by most physicians, and it is compatible with the International Classification of Diseases system. However, such classification can lead to some confusion because infections are not always limited to one part of the respiratory tract. Moreover, clinicians may disagree on whether an acute respiratory infection can be termed "upper," "middle," or "lower." Stridor-causing conditions often have been classified as upper respiratory tract infections, thus suggesting mild disease, which can be a misleading assumption. As stridor can cause severe, and possibly fatal, respiratory distress, consideration has been given to classifying stridor-causing conditions as acute lower respiratory infections.[51]

Pathogens Responsible for Acute Respiratory Infections

In a large percentage of patients with acute respiratory infections, the pathogens responsible for infection are not known. This problem is especially notable with regard to community-acquired pneumonia, for which the causative organism is unknown in approximately 98% of those treated as outpatients and 50% to 60% of those treated as hospital inpatients.[52,53]

Viruses

Upper respiratory viral infections in children and adults are caused by rhinoviruses (30% to 50%) or coronaviruses (5% to 20%), with the remainder (30% to 65%) due to influenza virus, parainfluenza virus, respiratory syncytial virus, adenoviruses, and certain enteroviruses.[54,55] These infections are generally mild, self-limiting, and do not involve respiratory distress.

In children, viral causes of the acute lower respiratory tract infections, pneumonia, bronchiolitis, and croup generally appear to be similar in both developed and developing countries,[56-65] the primary pathogens being respiratory syncytial virus; parainfluenza virus types 1, 2, and 3; influenza virus types A and B; adenoviruses; and enteroviruses. Respiratory syncytial virus is most commonly associated with bronchiolitis, and parainfluenza virus (especially type 1) is more often associated with croup.[66-69] In developing countries, measles contributes to croup and serious morbidity in other lower respiratory infections more than it does in the developed world.[70,71] Approximately 90% of cases of acute bronchitis are caused by viruses, including influenza virus, parainfluenza virus, and rhinovirus.[72]

In adults, viral causes of pneumonia are generally less important than nonviral causes. However, influenza has been associated with a significant proportion of cases in adults, perhaps causing as many as half of all virus-associated cases and approximately 8% to 10% of all pneumonias in general.[28,73] Respiratory syncytial virus and parainfluenza also have been identified in some adult cases of pneumonia, but these viruses are less commonly implicated than influenza.[74] In developed countries, influenza epidemics in elderly patients (older than 65 years of age) are associated with especially high mortality and hospitalization rates from acute respiratory infections; thus, influenza poses a major health risk to this age group.[75] More than 50% of excess hospitalizations and more than 80% of influenza-related deaths occur in persons aged 65 years and older, in whom mortality is 30 to 50 times greater than in younger adults.[76] In developing countries, viral causes of adult lower respiratory tract infections have not been widely studied. No indication is seen that viral pathogens are implicated to any greater degree in pneumonia cases in developing countries than they are in developed countries, although the mode of transmission in the poorer nations (unwashed hands, contaminated water) can differ from those in the developed world (day-care facilities, contaminated aerosols).[76]

Several viruses have been identified recently to be important causes of acute respiratory infection. The SARS coronavirus caused a major pandemic when it emerged in Southern China in 2002. This virus is a new human pathogen that crossed species to infect humans. The epidemiology of the SARS pandemic is covered in detail in the chapter on emerging infections.

In 2001, investigators in the Netherlands isolated a new virus from children and adults with acute respiratory tract infection.[77] This RNA virus is closely related to avian pneumovirus. In the last few years, metapneumovirus has been isolated from patients with acute respiratory infection in the United States, Australia, Canada, and the United Kingdom.[78-81] A study was published recently from Vanderbilt University in Nashville, Tennessee, in which nasal washes were collected prospectively from 463 infants and children who were seen for acute lower respiratory infection between 1976 and 2001.[313] A viral cause other than metapneumovirus was detected in 41% of these children. Of 248 specimens available for which no other pathogen was detected, 49 (20%) contained metapneumovirus[82]; 28% of illnesses occurred between December and April; and 2% of infected children were hospitalized. The seasonal distribution of metapneumoviruses and other viral pathogens in this study is shown in Figure 19-4.

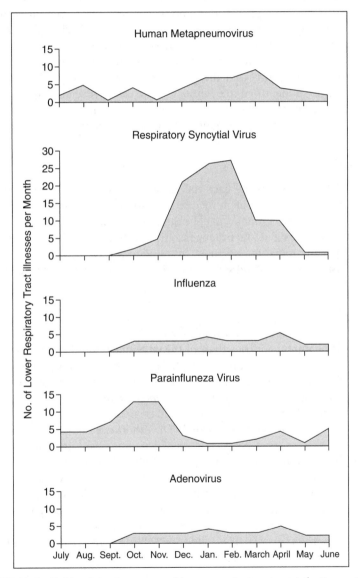

FIGURE 19-4 Epidemiologic pattern of lower respiratory tract infections with human metapneumovirus and other viruses.
Source: Williams et al. Human Metapneumovirus and Lower Respiratory Tract Disease in Otherwise Healthy Infants and Children. NEJM. Volume 350:443–450. Copyright 2004 by the Massachusetts Medical Society.

Sinnombre virus is another recently identified virus that is responsible for lower respiratory infections during epidemic or endemic transmission from its reservoir in rodents. The epidemiology of the Hantavirus pulmonary syndrome associated with sinnombre virus infections is discussed in the chapter on emerging infections.

Most epidemiologic studies have been hampered by the limited laboratory techniques available to isolate viral pathogens. Isolation of virus from 20% to 25% of specimens has been the maximal rate in several well-conducted studies.[31,67,83–85] Recent improvements in these techniques might be expected to result in higher isolation rates being more common. When combinations of viral culture and immunofluorescence techniques were used in one study of lower respiratory infections in infants to identify viral pathogens from throat and nasopharyngeal swabs, a 66% isolation rate was reported.[32]

The use of nucleic acid amplification methods to identify respiratory viruses has increased the proportion of illnesses in which a viral pathogen has been identified to over 50%.[80] The use of reverse transcriptase polymerase chain reaction has also identified human metapneumovirus (HMPV) and SARS coronavirus as important human pathogens.

Bacteria

Some studies of the bacterial causes of pneumonia have been marred by the methodologic problem of contamination of sputum specimens by nasopharyngeal and oropharyngeal organisms.[86] Therefore, sputum cultures may be of limited value. As bronchoscopic and transtracheal aspirates are also at risk of contamination,[87,88] most investigators rely on percutaneous needle lung aspirates and blood culture for accurate diagnosis of pneumonia.[89]

Developing Countries

Bacteria-caused lower respiratory infections are more common in children in developing countries than in the developed world, where viral infections are more often encountered.[29,31] Reliable data regarding pathogens responsible for pneumonia in adults in developing countries have come chiefly from hospital studies.[73] *Streptococcus pneumoniae* is by far the most important cause of pneumonia in adults: it is associated with up to 70% of cases in which a pathogen is isolated,[73,90] with *Haemophilis influenzae* and *Staphylococcus aureus* being relatively less important in adults than in children (together accounting for approximately 10% of cases). *Streptococcus pyogenes* and *Corynebacterium diphtheriae* most commonly cause pharyngitis and tonsillitis. Acute epiglottitis is caused chiefly by *H. influenzae* type B, and whooping cough by *Bordetella pertussis*.[55,91,92] In otitis media, *S. pneumoniae* and *H. influenzae* are the most commonly isolated bacteria,[93] but *Moraxella catarrhalis* has been isolated in 27% of patients in some series.[94] *S. pneumoniae* and *H. influenzae* are also important in acute sinusitis in children[95] and in adults.[96,97]

Berman and McIntosh[55] have reviewed studies of bacteria isolated from children in developing countries using lung aspiration techniques. The most frequently isolated pathogens were *H. influenzae*, *S. pneumoniae* (together accounting for 54% of isolates), and *S. aureus* (accounting for 17% of isolates). A subsequent study in Zimbabwe found a similar pattern of pathogens responsible for lower respiratory infections.[98]

Developed Countries

The key bacterial pathogens responsible for community-acquired pneumonia in the developed world appear to be the same as those in developing countries. A literature review of 15 published reports from North America showed the most common bacterial pathogens to be *S. pneumoniae* (20% to 60% of isolates) and *H. influenzae* (3% to 10%) (Table 19-4). A meta-analysis of 122 published studies between 1966 and 1995 (*N* = 7057) indicated that *S. pneumoniae* was responsible for 66% of deaths in community-acquired pneumonia cases.[99] A review of nosocomial pneumonia indicated that gram-negative bacteria account for 50% to 70% of cases (Table 19-5).[99] The most frequently isolated pathogen is *Pseudomonas aeruginosa*, followed by a diverse array of Enterobacteriaceae. These bacteria reach the lower airways by aspiration of gastric contents.

Approximately 50% to 75% of infective exacerbations of chronic bronchitis are bacterial in origin.[14] Studies conducted in the Northern Hemisphere have consistently shown *H. influenzae* to be the major pathogen and *M. catarrhalis* to be the second most common pathogen.[72]

TABLE 19-4   Pathogens Most Commonly Involved with Community-Acquired Pneumonia

Pathogen	%
Bacterial	
–Gram-negative bacilli	50–70
—*Pseudomonas aeruginosa**	
—*Enterobacteriaceae**	
–*Staphylococcus aureus**	15–30
–Anaerobic bacteria	10–30
–*Haemophilus influenzae*	10–20
–*Streptococcus pneumoniae*	10–20
–Legionella*	4
Viral	10–20
–Cytomegalovirus	
–Influenza virus*	
–Respiratory syncytial virus*	
Fungal	<1
–Aspergillus*	

*May cause nosocomial epidemics.
Source: J.G. Bartlett, Approach to the Patient with Pneumonia, In Infectious Diseases, 2nd Ed., pp. 553–564, © 1998, Lippincott Williams and Wilkins.

TABLE 19-5   Pathogens Most Commonly Involved in Nosocomial Pneumonia

Microbial Agents	Literature Review* (%)	The British Thoracic Society[+] (%)	Meta-analysis[+]	
			Cases (%)	Deaths (%)
Bacteria				
–*Streptococcus pneumoniae*	20–60	60–75	65	66
–*Haemophilus influenzae*	3–10	4–5	12	7
–*Staphylococcus aureus*	3–5	1–5	2	6
–Gram-negative bacilli	3–10	Rare	1	3
–Miscellaneous agents[§]	3–5	(Not included)	4	9
Atypical pathogens	10–20	—	12	6
–*Legionella* sp.	2–8	2–5	4	5
–*Mycoplasma pneumoniae*	1–6	5–18	7	1
–*Chlamydia pneumoniae*	4–6	(Not included)	1	<1
Viral	2–15	8–16	3	≤1
Aspiration pneumonia	6–10	(Not included)	—	—
No diagnosis	30–60	—	—	—

*Based on analysis of 15 published reports from North America.[98] Low and high values are deleted.
[+]Estimates are based on analysis of 453 adults in prospective study of community-acquired pneumonia in 25 British hospitals.[98]
[+]Meta-analysis of 122 published studies of community-acquired pneumonia in the English language literature 1966 to 1995; data are limited to 7057 patients who had an etiologic diagnosis.[98] Percentage of death column refers to percentage of all deaths attributed to the designated pathogen.
[§]Includes *Moraxella catarrhalis*, group A streptococcus, and *Neisseria meningitidis* (each 1% to 2%).
Source: J.G. Bartlett, Approach to the Patient with Pneumonia, In Infectious Diseases, 2nd Ed., pp. 553–564, © 1998, Lippincott Williams and Wilkins.

Other Pathogens

Mycoplasma pneumoniae, Chlamydia species, *Legionella* species, and *Pneumocystis carinii* are the nonviral respiratory pathogens most frequently responsible for pneumonia and acute bronchitis in both children and adults.[31,68,100,101] *M. pneumoniae* can also cause upper respiratory infections.[100,102] Of the *Chlamydia* species, *C. trachomatis* is implicated more in cases of pneumonia in young infants,[103] and *C. pneumoniae* (also called TWAR, based on the names of the first two isolates, TW-183 and AR-39) is responsible primarily for pneumonia cases among older children and adults.[103-105] Most of the cases of *P. carinii* pneumonia that have been reported since the early 1980s have been in patients with the acquired immune deficiency syndrome (AIDS). *P. carinii* pneumonia occurs as an opportunistic infection in patients with AIDS most frequently when their CD4+ lymphocyte counts fall below 200 cells/mm³. Approximately 60% to 80% of AIDS patients will develop *P. carinii* pneumonia at some stage during the course of their illness.[106,107] In developed countries, both children and adults with AIDS and other conditions associated with immunosuppression are at significant risk of *P. carinii* pneumonia. In countries in sub-Saharan Africa, AIDS-associated *P. carinii* pneumonia is less common, but the reasons for this are unclear.[108] Human immune deficiency virus (HIV)–infected patients have a greater incidence of community-acquired pneumonia caused by the intracellular bacterial pathogens *Salmonella* and *Legionella* than patients not infected with HIV.[109]

Risk Factors

The risk factors for community-acquired pneumonia and nosocomial pneumonia are summarized in Tables 19-7 and 19-8, respectively.[110] Specifics pertaining to key risk factors are provided below.

Demographic Factors

Age

The incidence of viral respiratory illness peaks in infancy and early childhood and steadily decreases with age because of changes in patterns of exposure and age-related acquisition of specific immunity to an increasing number of virus types encountered over time (Table 19-6).[12,25–27,111]

On examination of markers of more severe conditions (e.g., pneumonia and influenza mortality rates), a different pattern of age-related change is observed. Although infants are at greater risk from pneumonia than older children and young to middle-aged adults, mortality rates are highest in the elderly (Table 19-2). Elderly patients have reduced vital capacity and respiratory muscle strength, and impaired local and general immune defenses, all of which make them more susceptible than younger adults to severe acute lower respiratory infection. Pneumonia and influenza mortality rates, in particular, have increased in the elderly population over the past 15 years (Table 19-2). The most likely explanation for this is that many more at-risk persons (e.g., those with cardiovascular disease and chronic airways obstruction) are surviving into old age and suffering pneumonia as a terminal event. It is also possible that some of these deaths may have been attributable to changing virulence of respiratory pathogens and increased cumulative exposures to environmental factors, such as smoking and air pollution.

In developing countries, data on pneumonia-related mortality rates over the entire age range are sparse because many nations, especially those in Africa and Asia, do not report information to the World Health Organization.[112] However, Costa Rica and Cuba have contributed data, and both developing countries show an excess burden of mortality in infants and young children (Table 19-9).[6] Mortality rates in older children and young adults in Costa Rica are not much higher than those in the United States. As in the United States, mortality rates rise rapidly in the elderly in Costa Rica and Cuba, the rise being especially pronounced in Cuba.

Gender

The incidence of acute respiratory infections has been known to vary according to gender since the 1920s. In Baltimore, between 1928 and 1930, van

TABLE 19-6 Acute Respiratory Infection Morbidity Rates in Four US Cohort Studies

Investigators	Years	Population	Mean Incidence per Year by Age Group (years)											
			<1	1–2	3–4	5–9	10–14	15–19	20–24	25–29	30–39	40–49	50–59	≥60
van Volkenburgh and Frost[25]	1924	Public health service families		3.0		2.7	1.9	1.4		2.0*	1.8†	1.6‡	1.4§	
	1928–1929	Baltimore, MD, families		4.5		3.5	3.5	2.4	2.8		2.7	2.4	1.7	
	1929–1930	Baltimore, MD, families		4.5		3.8	2.8	2.3	2.7		2.6	2.3	2.1	
Gwaltney et al.[26]	1963–1966	Insurance company employees						2.5		2.1	2.2	1.7		
Fox et al.[27]	1965–1969	Seattle, WA, families	5.1	5.8	5.8	3.8	2.3							
Monto and Ullman[13]	1969–1971	Tecumseh, MI, families	6.1	5.7	4.7	3.5	2.7	2.4	2.8	2.7	2.3	1.7	1.6	1.3

* 25–34 years of age.
† 35–44 years of age.
‡ 45–54 years of age.
§ ≥55 years of age.
¶ ≥45 years of age.

Source: N.M.H. Graham, The Epidemiology of Acute Respiratory Infection in Children and Adults: A Global Perspective, Epidemiologic Reviews, Vol. 12, pp. 149–178, © 1990, Oxford University Press.

TABLE 19-7   Risk Factors of Community-Acquired Pneumonia

1. Old age
2. Smoking (>20 cigarettes a day)
3. Air pollution
4. Chronic diseases (e.g., diabetes, chronic hepatopathies, renal, cardiac, respiratory failure)
5. Malnutrition, precarious social and economic situations
6. Acute and chronic alcoholism
7. Chronic obstructive pulmonary disease
8. Primitive ciliary dyskinesia, bronchiectasis, cystic fibrosis
9. Congestive cardiomyopathies
10. Neuromuscular diseases
11. Dementia
12. Autoimmune diseases (LES, rheumatoid arthritis, and other collagen diseases)
13. Malignancy
14. Immunodeficiencies
15. Splenectomy
16. Immunosuppressive therapies
17. Drug addiction
18. Inadequate use of antibiotics

Source: Reprinted with permission from F. Ginesu and P. Pirina, Etiology and Risk Factors of Adult Pneumonia, *Journal of Chemotherapy*, Vol. 7, pp. 277–285, © 1995.

Volkenburgh and Frost reported higher rates of acute respiratory infections in boys aged younger than 9 years, and the reverse pattern above that age.[25] Similar findings were reported by Monto and Ullman, with higher rates of infection in boys aged less than 3 years, but lower rates in older age groups.[13] Gwaltney et al found that young women aged 16 to 24 years experienced more upper respiratory tract illness than did young men of similar age, even after adjusting for number of children and smoking status, with no differences being seen in patients aged more than 24 years.[26] A review of pneumonia cases between 1979 and 1992 showed men to be at greater risk of pneumonia than women; this was considered partly due to men being more susceptible because of increased exposure to two key pneumonia risk factors—alcoholism and nicotine.[17]

Fox et al found that mothers in Seattle families experienced more upper respiratory illness than did their husbands, but not more lower respiratory illness.[27] This could have been due to the mothers' more frequent exposure to young children. However, a subsequent study of viral chest infections in infants found no differences in incidence by sex.[32] Pneumonia-related mortality rates in older adults are higher in men than in women (Table 19-9), although this is not the case with mortality rates from upper respiratory tract infection. The reason for this greater susceptibility of older men is not certain, but it may be because of their generally higher rates of cardiovascular disease and chronic airway obstruction as compared to women.

TABLE 19-8   Risk Factors for Nosocomial Pneumonia

1. Advanced age (>65 years)
2. Chronic diseases (e.g., diabetes, cardiopathies, chronic obstructive pulmonary disease, chronic hepatopathies, chronic alcoholism, respiratory, cardiac, renal failure, obesity)
3. Malignancy
4. Prolonged immobilization (stroke, neuromuscular diseases)
5. Immunosuppressive therapies (cytotoxics, steroids)
6. Immunodeficiencies
7. Thoracic and abdominal surgery
8. Burns
9. Traumas (thorax and abdomen, multiple, rib fractures, pulmonary contusions, pneumothorax, hemothorax)
10. Treatment with antacids and/or H2 blockers
11. Antibiotic therapy and prophylaxis
12. Increase in number of hospitalized patients susceptible to infections
13. Increase in invasive techniques for diagnosis and therapy
14. Mechanical ventilation (MV):—Reintubation—MV duration (>3 d)—Positive end-expiratory pressure—Persistence of coma during MV—Severity of underlying disease—Gastric content aspiration—Oropharyngeal aspiration—Intensive care unit
15. Airway instrumentation
16. Previous intubations and endotracheal prostheses
17. Ultrasound nebulizers and humidifier systems
18. Increase in number of staff members caring for the patient
19. Visitors, relatives, friends, and so on
20. Moving the patient inside the hospital
21. Health staff not adequately educated to prevent nosocomial infections
22. Inadequate hospital structures and facilities
23. Organ transplantation
24. Periodontitis, dental caries, gingivitis

Source: Reprinted with permission from F. Ginesu and P. Pirina, Etiology and Risk Factors of Adult Pneumonia, *Journal of Chemotherapy*, Vol. 7, pp. 277–285, © 1995.

Outdoor Air Pollution

Outdoor air pollution has been known to affect the incidence of acute respiratory infections since the early 1930s. Episodes of acute, severe, particulate air pollution in the Meuse Valley, Belgium (1930), Donora, Pennsylvania (1948), New York City (1953 and 1962), and greater London, England (1948, 1952, and 1956), were associated with increases in all-cause mortality, primarily because of more deaths from pneumonia and cardiovascular disease.[113-120] An estimated 4000 excess deaths were reported in the disastrous London fog of 1952.[113] The elderly and very elderly in greater London were the groups most greatly affected.

TABLE 19-9 Pneumonia Mortality Rates (per 100,000 Population) by Age and Sex in the United States, Costa Rica, and Cuba, 1987

Country	Sex	Age (years)										
		<1	1–4	5–14	15–24	25–34	35–44	45–54	55–64	65–74	≥75
United States	Male	19.2	1.4	0.3	0.8	2.3	4.7	9.2	23.6	78.8	505.2
	Female	15.7	1.2	0.3	0.6	1.2	2.2	4.7	12.0	48.6	360.1
Costa Rica	Male	206.6	10.0		0.3		2.8	1.1	3.2	46.5	464.3
	Female	127.6	5.2	0.3		0.4	1.4	2.1	6.1	28.4	383.4
Cuba	Male	115.0	4.7	0.9	1.5	3.0	3.2	9.5	34.1	139.2	943.1
	Female	102.9	4.3	0.6	1.7	2.2	3.6	7.9	28.4	89.8	766.8

Source: World Health Statistics Annual, p. 105, © 1989, World Health Organization.

These studies prompted research to evaluate the effects of much lower levels of air pollution on the outcomes of acute respiratory illnesses. The components of air pollution most widely studied have been suspended respirable particulates, sulfur dioxide, nitrogen dioxide, and ozone. Although studies in the 1960s and 1970s provided somewhat contradictory results,[121] they were instrumental in changing the focus on outcomes from mortality to both mortality and morbidity. Indeed, morbidity was considered a more sensitive outcome measure than mortality in studies of relatively low levels of air pollution. In 1964, Toyama reported a correlation between bronchitis mortality and level of suspended particulates in all ages.[122] He also found that respiratory morbidity rates were higher for all age groups and ventilatory function poorer in children in air-polluted cities compared with relatively nonpolluted rural areas. Lunn et al studied respiratory illness patterns in children exposed to relatively high and low levels of particulate matter (smoke) and sulfur dioxide in Sheffield, United Kingdom.[123,124] These investigators found a relationship between exposure to high levels of particles and sulfur dioxide in air and repeated episodes of acute upper and lower respiratory tract illness, after adjusting for socioeconomic status. Conversely, Colley and Reid found a relationship between air pollution (urban/rural comparison) and acute lower, but not upper, respiratory illness in children.[125] This effect was most marked in the lower social classes. Cassel et al also found no relationship between air pollution and upper respiratory illness.[126] In infants in England and Wales who were examined and followed between 1958 and 1964, pneumonia and respiratory disease mortality were strongly associated with air pollution.[127] Lawther et al in 1970 related acute exacerbations of chronic bronchitis to daily variations in smoke and sulfur dioxide.[128]

Health effects in adults have been estimated to occur above $500 \mu g/m^3$ of sulfur dioxide and $250 \mu g/m^3$ of particular in adults, and $180 \mu g/m^3$ and $120 \mu g/m^3$, respectively, in children older than age 4 years.[121] A weaker but still significant relationship was also seen in children aged 1 to 4 years. In the Great Salt Lake Basin and the Rocky Mountains, high levels of sulfur dioxide and suspended sulfate were associated with excess reports of croup in children (age-, sex-, social class–adjusted rates) who resided in a high pollution area for more than 3 years.[129] Durham found that upper respiratory symptoms reported by Los Angeles college students presenting to campus health centers were significantly correlated with sulfur dioxide and nitrogen dioxide levels independent of the effects of age, weather, and smoking levels.[130] Levy et al found that high levels of sulfur dioxide and particulate matter, but not nitrogen dioxide, carbon monoxide, or pollen, predicted hospital admission for acute respiratory disease in children and adults, after adjusting for the effects of temperature.[131] In Chicago, acute upper and lower respiratory tract illness attack rates were reported to be higher in both adults and children, but in New York only lower respiratory tract illness attack rates were significantly higher in residents of high pollution areas.

Studies in the 1980s sought to examine the effects of air pollution at much lower levels than earlier studies and have tried to determine which components of air pollution were of primary importance. Studies designed to allow concurrent comparisons of similar demographic areas and adjustment for confounding factors (e.g., the Six Cities Study[132]) were instrumental in clarifying the role of outdoor air pollution in increasing susceptibility to acute respiratory illness. Ware et al found that between-city annual mean differences in particulate and suspended sulfate concentrations as low as $80\,\mu g/m^3$ doubled the risk of acute cough and substantially increased risk of bronchitis and other lower respiratory illness in children.[132] These investigators also found significant, but weaker, associations with sulfur dioxide. Mean monthly peaks of sulfur dioxide did not exceed a range of 80 to $200\,\mu g/m^3$. In a study by Pope, 24-hour fine-particulate levels as low as $50\,\mu g/m^3$ were associated with significantly increased hospitalization rates in children and adults for acute respiratory disease.[133] The associations were stronger for bronchitis and asthma than for pneumonia and pleurisy, and persisted when adjustments were made for meteorologic variables. Derriennic et al observed that sulfur dioxide levels, but not levels of particulates or nitrogen dioxide, predicted deaths from respiratory disease in adults aged more than 65 years.[134] Other studies have confirmed the importance of the association between particulates, sulfur dioxide, and respiratory symptoms in children.[135,136] The evidence is now supportive of the hypothesis that suspended particulates, suspended sulfates, and sulfur dioxide at levels currently being measured in ambient air significantly increase the risk of morbidity from acute respiratory illness in adults and children. Because most studies do not include virologic sampling, it is unclear whether morbidity is chiefly caused by bronchial reactivity and respiratory tract irritation or by infection. Studies supported by virologic culture and serology are needed to answer this question.

Ozone exposures below the US ambient air quality standard have been associated with acute changes in ventilatory function[137] and increased risk of cough and lower respiratory illness.[138] The importance of ambient levels of nitrogen dioxide as a risk factor for respiratory illness is less clear.[135,139]

Indoor Air Pollution

Indoor air pollution from passive smoke, nitrogen dioxide from gas cooking or heating, and smoke from biomass fuels have been investigated for their impact on acute respiratory infections. A 1999 review of studies published during the 1990s showed that the incidence of respiratory illnesses and middle ear infection was greater in children living in homes where either parent smoked, with odds ratios between 1.2 and 1.6.[140] The odds ratios were much higher in preschool than in school-aged children. For sudden infant death syndrome, the odds ratio for maternal smoking was about two. Exposure to maternal cigarette smoke approximately doubles the risk of lower respiratory tract infection in children aged less than 2 years.[141,142] Paternal smoking seems less contributory to infection rates, possibly because fathers are generally around their children less than mothers during their children's first 2 years of life.[143,144] Passive smoking is believed to increase respiratory infection rates in children by reducing mucociliary clearance.[140] Although negative studies have also been reported,[145-147] these either involved small numbers of patients,[147] or they did not report on smoking effects in children aged less than 2.[145,146]

In studies linking maternal smoking during pregnancy with respiratory infections in infants, prenatal smoking was found to be a stronger risk factor for bronchitis in infants than postnatal smoking.[148,149] As the number of women who change their smoking habit during or after pregnancy is few, it is difficult to identify sufficiently large comparison groups to fully settle this question.

Heating stoves and natural gas cooking increase exposure of household members to nitrogen dioxide.[150,151] However, studies designed to investigate a relationship between the low levels of nitrogen dioxide and enhancement of risk of acute respiratory illness have yielded equivocal results.[132,152-156] One study showed that children in Adelaide who lived in homes using gas heating were more likely to develop acute respiratory illness than those living in homes with electric heating, but the level of significance was marginal (odds ratio [OR] = 1.6; 95% confidence interval [CI] 1.0–2.6).[150] Based on current data, any effects attributable to nitrogen dioxide exposures are likely to be very small, if they exist at all.[158]

In developing countries, the negative public health impact of smoke from biomass fuels used for cooking is well established. Exposure to firewood or other biomass smoke during cooking can occur in up to 50% of the world's households.[159] Wood smoke, in particular, is thought to be responsible for almost 50% of all cases of obstructive airways disease.[14] In 1996, a multivariate analysis of a case-control study in Colombia found wood smoke to be more highly associated (OR, 3.43) with development of chronic bronchitis in women than either tobacco use or passive smoking (ORs, 2.22 and 2.05, respectively).[160] Children in many developing countries are exposed to respirable particles from these fuels at peak and daily indoor concentrations approximately 20 times greater than the levels present in developed countries where two packs of cigarettes are smoked per day[158] (a level at which the risk of many respiratory symptoms approximately doubles[142]). In a study in Nepal, Pandey et al found a relationship between hours per day spent near a stove and episodes of severe acute lower respiratory tract illness in children aged less than 2 years.[161] However, this study was flawed by the lack of adjustment made for confounding factors, such as parental smoking. In a small, poorly controlled study, Kossove found that Zulu infants presenting to a medical clinic with acute lower respiratory illness were more likely to be exposed to cooking smoke at home than children without respiratory illness.[162] Campbell et al reported that children carried on their mother's back during cooking periods were at a 2.8 times greater risk of an episode of "fast or difficult breathing" (predictive of acute lower respiratory infection) than children who were not carried in this way.[163,164] All of these studies had methodologic problems because they were conducted in high acute respiratory infection incidence areas where exposure to indoor smoke is universally high and exposure dose was not measured. Intervention studies in high incidence areas need to be conducted to evaluate respiratory infection rates in persons living in homes using wood fuel compared with those living in homes using smokeless fuel or fluted stoves.

In the developed world, one US study of children from homes with wood-burning stoves found children experienced more acute upper and lower respiratory tract illness than children from homes without such stoves.[165,166] Levels of the many gases, chemicals, and respirable particulates in wood smoke were not reported, which would have been desirable to assess the stove–illness connection in more detail. However, the greater incidence of respiratory illness was not explained by social class, smoking, or other indoor sources of air pollution. Another study in the United States, using a retrospective design, found no relationship between wood smoke exposure and respiratory illness in school-aged children.[166] By inference, this suggests that preschool children may be more at risk of acute respiratory infection in living environments heated by wood-burning stoves than are older children.[167]

Smoking

A relationship between smoking and acute respiratory infection was first established in several prospective studies conducted in the late 1950s.[168-174] These data indicated that smokers were at increased risk of dying from pneumonia and influenza, their overall pneumonia:influenza mortality ratio being 1.4 (range, 0.7 to 2.6). Four subsequent studies showed that smoking is associated with increased severity and incidence of influenza.[175-178] Kark et al reported that the attributable proportion of influenza ascribable to smoking was 31% for all influenza cases and 41% for severe influenza cases.[178] Tobacco smoking is undoubtedly the most common cause of chronic bronchitis.[14]

In the Tecumseh family-based study, Monto et al assessed the incidence of respiratory illness in smokers and nonsmokers.[179] In otherwise healthy index cases, both male and female smokers experienced more episodes of acute respiratory illness than nonsmokers. Studies in adolescents and young adults have also reported more respiratory symptoms in smokers than nonsmokers.[180-182] Reingold found that smoking significantly increased the incidence of pneumonia and pneumonia-related mortality, and that smoking is an important independent risk factor for Legionnaires' disease.[183] Lipsky et al found that smoking independently increased the risk of pneumococcal infections four-fold in their study of "high risk" adults.[184] Petitti and Friedman also found smokers to be at greater risk of pneumonia and influenza, but the risk was lower in those smoking low-tar cigarettes.[185] Conversely, Simberkoff et al found no relationship between pneumonia mortality and smoking in patients at high risk.[186] In a community-based study in which the prevalence of smoking was assessed among patients with pneumonia, Woodhead et al reported that 100 of 236 patients with pneumonia (42%) were current smokers, and that 175 of them (74%) had smoked "at some time."[187] However, a control group was not used in this study to see if smoking was associated with higher pneumonia rates.

In the American Cancer Society's 25-state study from 1959 to 1965, male smokers were at greater risk of dying from influenza and pneumonia (International Classification of Diseases, 7th revision, codes 480–481, 490–493) than male nonsmokers (relative risk [RR] = 1.82; 95% CI, 1.45–2.27).[188] This study did not show female smokers to be at increased risk. However, in the 50-city study in 1982–1986, risk of mortality from pneumonia and other respiratory disease (International Classification of Diseases, 9th revision, codes 010–012, 480–489, 493) was significantly increased in current female smokers (RR = 2.18; 95% CI, 1.60–2.97) as well as current male smokers (RR = 1.99; 95% CI, 1.52–2.61) aged 35 years and older.[188]

Crowding

Crowding favors the propagation of respiratory infections, as it does all contagious diseases. As early as 1927, a highly significant correlation was seen between the proportion of overcrowded houses in a borough (two or more persons per room) and pneumonia mortality in England and Wales.[189] The strongest correlation was in the age group 0 to 5 years, although an effect was also seen in the age groups 45 to 64 and 65 to 74 years. Pneumonia epidemics were observed in crowded living conditions in South African mining camps, during the construction of the Panama Canal, and in Civilian Conservation Corps barracks.[190] In 1945, Payling-Wright and Payling-Wright showed strong correlations between crowding (persons per room and number of children per family) and mortality from bronchopneumonia in children aged less than 2 years.[191] Another study demonstrated a significant correlation between crowding and death from bronchopneumonia in infants, although the investigators cautioned that the relationship was confounded by indices of air pollution, social class, and educational status.[127]

Family Size

Since the 1970s, studies have focused on family size as a measure of crowding. The number and age of siblings in families predict the rates of acute lower respiratory tract infection in infants,[147] incidence of bronchitis and pneumonia in infants,[192] and rates of acute respiratory illness in older children and adults.[193] In developing countries, given the extreme level of confounding between malnutrition and crowding as risk factors for acute respiratory infection, it is difficult to separate out the relative contribution of each.

Day-Care Centers

In developed countries, increased reliance on day-care centers for children has led to another type of crowding. Children attending group day-care centers are at increased risk of acute upper and lower respiratory tract infections.[147,194] In particular, day-care attendance greatly increases the risk of acute otitis media in children.[195-198]

Refugee Camps

During the 1990s, acute respiratory infections, along with measles and diarrheal disease, were the most frequent causes of death among refugees who escaped Somalia during the 1992–1993 famine[199] and among Bhutanese refugees emigrating into southeastern Nepal during 1991–1992 to escape ethnic persecution.[200]

Marfin et al examined the morbidity and mortality among 73,500 Bhutanese refugees who emigrated into southeastern Nepal (six refugee camps) between February 1991 and June 1992 to escape ethnic persecution in Bhutan.[200] Crude mortality rates up to 1.15 per 10,000 deaths per day were reported during the first 6 months of surveillance. The leading causes of death were measles, diarrhea, and acute respiratory infections.

Nutrition

As malnutrition is so closely correlated with poverty, crowding, poor housing, and poor education in developing countries, it has proved difficult to identify an independent effect of this factor on risk for respiratory infection.[201-203] Nevertheless, epidemiologic studies evaluating certain nutritional interventions (vitamin A and breastfeeding) have shown that malnutrition is at least contributory to respiratory health.

In a study in Costa Rica, James assessed the relationship of malnutrition (comparison of weight with standard measures) and respiratory illness in poor children under the age of 5 years.[10] His unadjusted analysis indicated that malnourished children experienced 2.7 times more bronchitis and 19 times more pneumonia, and they were far more likely to be hospitalized than well-nourished children. Children of low weight experienced no more upper respiratory illness than did children of normal weight, but their episodes lasted longer. Tupasi et al reported a 27-fold increased relative risk for pneumonia-related mortality in hospitalized children with third-degree malnutrition, with relative risks of 11.3 and 4.4 for second- and first-degree malnutrition, respectively.[203] However, their multivariate analyses indicated that malnutrition was not related to incidence of respiratory morbidity, possibly because of strong confounding from socioeconomic status. Berman et al found a significant relationship between malnutrition and pneumonia, but not between malnutrition and bronchitis or tracheobronchitis, in children attending health centers in Cali, Colombia.[70] Escobar et al observed that in children hospitalized with lower respiratory illness, mortality increased in relation to the level of malnutrition (weight for age).[57]

In a case-control study reported in 1996, Fonseca et al used a risk factor questionnaire to determine key factors contributing to childhood pneumonia among 650 children aged less than 2 years living in urban poor areas of Forteleza, Brazil.[204] Age-matched controls were recruited from the neighborhood where the children with pneumonia lived. Malnutrition was the most important risk factor, although low birth weight, non-breast-feeding, attendance at a day-care center, crowding, high parity, and incomplete vaccination status each posed a significant risk. Children who had suffered from previous episodes of wheezing or who had been hospitalized for pneumonia had a greater than three-fold increased risk of contracting the disease. Pneumonia risk in this study was not influenced by socioeconomic status or by environmental variables.

In the early 1980s, vitamin A deficiency in children was found to be a risk factor associated with both increased morbidity from respiratory infection and increased overall mortality.[205,206] In Thailand, children with deficient serum retinol were four times more likely to experience respiratory morbidity than children who were not deficient.[207] This study also found that supplementation with vitamin A offered some protection against respiratory illness; however, this varied by age and length of follow-up, probably because of small sample size. In well-nourished children in Adelaide, Australia, Pinnock et al conducted two placebo-controlled vitamin A intervention studies.[208,209] In the first study, respiratory morbidity in children with a history of frequent respiratory illness was reduced by 19% in those taking the supplement.[208] However, in the second study, vitamin A supplementation did not affect respiratory morbidity significantly in children aged 2 to 7 years who had an episode of bronchiolitis in the first year of life and who were followed for 12 months.[209] In view of the disparate findings between retinol-deficient and well-nourished children, the beneficial effects of vitamin A supplementation are likely to be limited to populations whose diets are significantly deficient.

In developing countries, breastfeeding has shown a protective effect against respiratory infections. In Brazil, for instance, breastfeeding reduced the incidence of upper respiratory morbidity, otitis media, and pneumonia in young infants in one study,[210] and respiratory infection mortality in children in another.[211] It is unclear whether the protective effect of breast milk was from its conferred anti-infective properties,[212] from improved hygiene, or from nutritional factors per se. Similarly, in Rwanda, mortality from acute lower respiratory infection in hospitalized children aged less than 2 years was lower in those who were breast-fed.[213] In developed countries, breastfeeding appears to be clearly protective against the risk of acute otitis media[212,213] but perhaps not against other types of respiratory morbidity. Many studies in which bivariate analyses were conducted have reported that breast-fed babies were at significantly lower risk of respiratory illness, but the relationship was not seen after adjustments were made for confounding factors.[214-218]

Certain other nutritional factors have been suggested as possibly influencing respiratory health, although the link is weak or inconclusive. Obesity was reported to be associated with increased incidence of respiratory illness in infants in one study,[219] but these findings were confounded by the fact that the normal weight comparison group was of higher socioeconomic status and had been breast-fed much longer. Although vitamin C supplementation has been suggested to prevent or to treat upper respiratory tract infections, the results of placebo-controlled trials have been too unimpressive to prompt a global recommendation for use of this vitamin.[220-222]

Lower Respiratory Tract Infection in Early Infancy

Several studies have reported a relationship between acute lower respiratory tract infection in the first 2 years of life and the development in adulthood of chronic cough,[181,223] reduced ventilatory function,[224-227] and increased bronchial reactivity.[224-227] In a case-control study in 1985,[157] young children who experienced high levels of respiratory illness morbidity were 11 times more likely to have experienced an episode of bronchitis, bronchiolitis, or pneumonia in the first year of life than children who had experienced low levels of morbidity (controls). The relationship remained strong (OR, 9.5; 95% CI, 5.5–16.6) even after adjustments were made for number of siblings, use of child care, sex, parental history of respiratory illness, breastfeeding, maternal stress levels, exposure to gas heating, parental occupational status, and low birth weight. In a 3-year study of pneumococcal vaccine in young children, the strongest predictor of acute respiratory morbidity (recorded in respiratory symptom diaries by the mothers) in any 6-month period was the level of morbidity the previous 6 months.[208,228] In England and Wales, Barker and Osmond found an increased incidence of mortality among people with chronic bronchitis who had a history of childhood respiratory infection.[229]

It is unclear whether lower respiratory infection in early life acts as a true risk factor by causing long-term damage to the lower respiratory tract or whether it acts as an early marker for genetically preprogrammed subsequent respiratory morbidity (chronic or acute). It will be difficult to determine which factor is more important until an effective intervention is available (e.g., a vaccine for respiratory syncytial virus). If previous respiratory morbidity predicts the level of subsequent morbidity from respiratory infections, implications also are seen for statistical analyses of these types of data. For autocorrelation of this type, a need is seen to control or adjust for repeated episodes of acute lower respiratory illness; alternatively, the first episode can be used as the outcome for analysis. In prospective studies, Kaplan-Meier curves and Cox regression analysis are then often used to estimate "survival time."[32] Where frequent outcomes occur, as with upper respiratory tract infections, use of the first episode as an outcome would result in loss of too much data. Autoregression techniques,[230] which have not been widely used in studies of acute respiratory infections, allow adjustment for autocorrelated variables in multivariate models.

Psychosocial Factors

The relationship between psychosocial factors and respiratory infections has been investigated in cross-sectional and retrospective studies,[230-236] in prospective epidemiologic studies,[237-239] and in experimental settings.[240-242] Upper respiratory infections or illnesses were the outcomes of interest in these studies, and no data regarding lower respiratory illness were presented. Two cross-sectional studies reported a relationship between respiratory infection and social isolation, life changes, illness behavior, maladaptive coping, and unresolved role crises.[233,234] However, these studies did not address the effect of psychosocial factors on respiratory infection rates. Another cross-sectional study indicated a relationship between anxiety and upper respiratory illness, but it was unclear how the outcome was measured.[230] In a longitudinal study that controlled for the effects of age, sex, race, family income, and family size in the analyses by Boyce et al, high life-event scores and strict family routines were associated with increased duration and severity of acute respiratory illness in children.[233] However, these investigators did not measure stress levels or rigidity of family routines until the end of the study. Other cross-sectional studies have found relationships between poor family functioning and doctor visits for acute respiratory infections in children,[236] type A personality and respiratory illness in college students,[234] and maternal stress and bronchitis in children.[235] None of these three studies controlled for confounding factors, nor did they address the temporal relationship between psychosocial factors and respiratory illness.

Several prospective studies have shown that psychosocial factors can increase susceptibility to upper respiratory tract infections.[238-243] Kasl et al evaluated the relationship between a combination of high motivation and poor academic performance with clinical infectious mononucleosis in US Military Academy cadets at West Point, New York.[238] Over a 4-year period, cadets who seroconverted to Epstein-Barr virus were monitored, and those with high motivation, a poor academic record, and an "overachieving" father were significantly more likely to have clinical infectious mononucleosis than a subclinical infection. Poor academic record and high motivation interacted in this study to increase the risk of clinical disease significantly. Disease severity was confirmed by ascertaining the heterophil antibody titers in the clinical and subclinical cases.

In a series of studies involving experimentally induced colds at the Common Cold Unit in the United Kingdom, introversion was associated with higher symptom and virus-shedding scores and certain life changes that resulted in decreased activity predicted virus shedding; cognitive dissonance was associated with increased symptoms.[240-242] Although patients who appear to be more introverted and those reporting higher stress or anxiety levels might be expected to report more symptoms, the finding that these factors were also associated with virus shedding in two of the studies substantiates objective validation of a psychosocial–illness relationship.

Graham et al[237] studied the relationship between stress and upper respiratory tract infection in a prospective study in Adelaide, Australia. In a blinded fashion, episodes of illness were divided into definite, uncertain, and doubtful, which were confirmed, where possible, by a study nurse, virologic culture, or both. To optimize the precision of stress measurement, a combination of three measures (major life events, minor life events, and psychological distress) was used in the initial analyses. Prestudy stress variables predicted nurse-confirmed episodes and symptom days in "definite" episodes even after adjusting for a range of confounding factors. Prestudy stress levels also predicted both episodes and symptom days of respiratory illness. Finally, in a longitudinal study of 16 families ($N = 100$), Meyer and Haggerty reported that stressful life events in families were four times more likely to precede an episode of streptococcal pharyngitis than to follow it.[239] High stress levels were also significantly associated with rises in antistreptolysin O titer in this study. Although no adjustments were made for confounding factors, the objective outcome measures and prospective design were strengths of this study.

Two mechanisms have been suggested to account for why stress and anxiety might predispose to respiratory infection.[4] First, because psychological stress and other psychological factors appear to suppress many components of immune function,[243] this may lead to increased susceptibility to respiratory infection. However, it is possible that the immune function fluctuations observed to be associated with psychological factors may not have high clinical relevance. Second, high stress levels or anxiety may lead to reduced adherence to normal hygiene measures (e.g., hand washing and use of tissues) usually used to reduce transmission of respiratory viruses.[244-246] This mechanism is questionable, however, because in experimental cold studies, transmission factors were controlled.[240-242]

Socioeconomic Status

In general, socioeconomic status, whether measured by rankings of occupational prestige,[125,181] level of income,[191] or educational status,[127] appears to be associated with increased susceptibility to acute lower, but not upper, respiratory tract infections. Gardner et al used a combined measure of family income, insurance status, and parental educational level to measure socioeconomic status, which they found to be related only to lower respiratory illness.[147] Measures of proportion of families with incomes below the poverty line and of occupational prestige have been linked with increased mortality from bronchitis and pneumonia in children,[191] as has educational status.[127] The differentials in pneumonia and influenza mortality observed between economically developing and developed countries (Table 19-9) reflect the association of low socioeconomic development with susceptibility to pneumonia, in particular. However, the relatively similar levels of upper respiratory illness reported in developing and developed countries lends support to findings in developed countries that low socioeconomic status does not increase the risk of these conditions.[8-13,25-27]

The results of a retrospective study by Schenker et al differ from those of the studies mentioned above.[247] These investigators found a relationship between low socioeconomic status (occupational status or educational level of parents) and severe chest illness in the first 2 years of life, as well as with chronic respiratory symptoms, but not with pneumonia or bronchitis. The disparity between the conclusions of this study and the others may be attributed to its presentation of differential symptom reporting rates by lower and high educational groups. This illustrates how differently alternate measures of socioeconomic status can behave in predicting respiratory illness; it may also indicate that lower social class could be a stronger risk factor for lower rather than upper respiratory illness. Tupasi et al confirmed that low socioeconomic status within developing countries also strongly predicts risk of acute respiratory infection.[203] However, these investigators did not differentiate between upper and lower tracts of respiratory infection, nor did they separate out the effects of factors such as crowding, malnutrition, and immunization status. This adjustment is very important in analyzing the results from epidemiologic studies investigating socioeconomic risk factors. Indeed, bivariate analyses performed in a study in Adelaide showed that children of parents of lower occupational status had increased susceptibility to respiratory illness.[248] However, after adjusting for factors such as sex, maternal smoking, number of siblings, parental history of respiratory illness, breastfeeding, use of child care, and maternal stress levels, the relationship between social class and increased risk of respiratory infection was no longer observed.

Meteorologic Factors

Epidemics of acute respiratory infections have correlated best with low temperature, humidity, precipitation, or all of those factors, which are associated with increased time spent indoors, either at home or at school.[249-251] Any situation in which crowding is present facilitates efficient viral transmission. It is not clear whether meteorologic factors alone cause increased host susceptibility or enhanced viral integrity, or whether crowding must be a concomitant. The effects of low temperature or "chilling" on host susceptibility has been well studied.[252-254] In studies conducted in the United States and the United Kingdom, volunteers experimentally infected with rhinoviruses and exposed to combinations of cold temperatures, wet clothes, and fatigue had no greater than normal susceptibility to infection.[252-254] Studies as early as the 1920s suggested a correlation between low temperatures and increases in mortality from pneumonia and bronchitis[191,255]; however, the results of these studies were confounded by increased time spent indoors (resulting in crowding) and higher levels of air pollution during winter. The latter factor may be an important contributor to respiratory illness. After all, in the Northern Hemisphere, peak levels of respirable particulate air pollution occur in midwinter, presumably because condensation, cloud cover, and precipitation prevent dispersal of particulates and gases; thus, trapped pathogens in the ambient air would be more likely. In a study by Pope,[133] low temperature was the meteorologic variable most closely correlated with hospitalization for respiratory disease and together with mean fine particulate levels explained 83% of the variance in total monthly hospital admissions for respiratory disease.

Humidity could also be a meteorologic factor contributing to respiratory morbidity. As rhinoviruses survive better at higher humidities, Gwaltney has postulated that rhinovirus-caused infections may be more easily transmitted in places where, or in seasons when, humidity is high.[256] As high humidity is often associated with the rainy season in temperate or warm climates, meteorologic studies investigating a humidity–respiratory infection correlation would need to factor the effect of crowding into analyses, as more of the study population would be expected to stay indoors to avoid the rain, thus confounding study results.

Care-Seeking Behavior

The care-seeking behavior of families and their expectations regarding appropriate treatment affect the morbidity and mortality associated with acute respiratory infections.[257] Factors influencing the choice of provider are the mother's perceptions of the cause of illness, distance from a provider, cost of care, availability and accessibility of a provider, and past experience with that provider. Some families demonstrate a "wait-and-see attitude" because of limited funds, distance from a health provider, not recognizing the severity of the illness, waiting for home remedies to work, or local custom prohibiting a mother to leave her home for any purpose.[258–260] In developing countries, patients can seek care from several different people (e.g., physicians, healers, shamans), making assessment of treatment difficult.

Human Immunodeficiency Virus Infection

Human immunodeficiency virus infection predisposes people to several different types of acute respiratory infections, the most common of which is *Pneumocystis carinii* pneumonia.[261] In 60% of newly diagnosed cases of AIDS, *P. carinii* pneumonia is the initial AIDS-defining illness, and an additional 20% of patients with AIDS will develop *P. carinii* pneumonia during the course of their illness.[106,107] Children with AIDS are also at risk from *P. carinii* but at a slightly lower rate than adults.[262–264] *P. carinii* pneumonia does not appear to be an important pulmonary complication of AIDS in Africa.[108] This lack of association in Africa may, in part, be because of the difficulty of diagnosing this condition when bronchoscopy is not readily available.[106] However, introduction of sputum induction techniques currently used in developed countries may prove useful in improving the diagnostic accuracy of studies in Africa.[265] This should lead to a more definitive picture of the incidence of *P. carinii* pneumonia in HIV-infected persons on that continent.

Adults and children infected with HIV are also at increased risk from bacterial pneumonia.[106,266] *Streptococccus pneumoniae* and *Haemophilus influenzae* are the most commonly isolated organisms in community-acquired, HIV-associated bacterial pneumonia. Risk of pneumonia appears to be increased in HIV-infected patients with and without AIDS.[267-271] The most common viral pulmonary infection found in both adults and children with AIDS is cytomegalovirus.[106,263,264] However, the pathogenicity of this virus in the lung is not always entirely clear, because it is sometimes isolated in the absence of histologic evidence of cytopathic change to lung parenchyma.[272] The causative agents of acute lower respiratory tract infections in HIV-infected patients in Africa have yet to be completely elucidated.

In general, gastrointestinal and dermatologic complications are more common in Africa than in the United States, where pulmonary complications most often manifest.[108] In one study, only 14% of HIV-infected Africans living in Europe had *P. carinii* pneumonia.[273] The most common pulmonary complication of HIV infection in Africa appears to be tuberculosis,[274,275] although few studies have used appropriate microbiologic techniques to establish accurate estimates of risk in comparison with other organisms. It seems likely that HIV-infected children and adults in Africa will be at greatly increased risk from pneumonia caused by pyogenic bacteria such as *S. pneumoniae, H. influenzae,* and *Staphylococcus aureus,* because these organisms are already important causes of pneumonia in that part of the world.

Whether HIV infection is associated with increased susceptibility to upper respiratory tract infections or respiratory viruses in general is not known. It is also not known whether these less serious conditions can predispose to secondary bacterial invasion and pneumonia in patients with AIDS. If immune system activation is important in the pathogenesis of AIDS, as has been postulated, another issue that needs to be explored is whether viral respiratory infections play a role in accelerating disease progression.

Low Birth Weight

Low birth weight may be an important risk factor for acute respiratory infections, as evidenced by the higher mortality rates of infants with low birth weight compared to normal-weight infants in developing countries in the first year of life.[6] Drillien reported that babies with low birth weight (<4 lb, 8 oz [<2000 g]) experienced higher rates of respiratory illness in the first 2 years of life.[276] This relationship persisted when this investigator stratified by a "maternal care" index, although what was meant by maternal care was not well defined. After stratification by quality of housing and maternal care, low birth weight did not predict respiratory illness. In a 7-year birth cohort study, Chan et al found that low birth weight (<2000 g) was associated with subsequent chronic cough, but not wheeze.[277] However, as acute respiratory symptoms were not reported in this study, the effect of low birth weight on respiratory infection rate could not be assessed.

Victora et al found that a birth weight of less than 2500 g was associated with increased mortality from respiratory infections, and this relationship persisted after adjustment for parental employment status, income, and education.[278] In a study in India, Datta et al observed that, during the first year of life, infants with low birth weights (<2500 g) had the same respiratory illness attack rate as normal-weight infants (4.65 versus 4.56 episodes), but a much higher case fatality rate (24.6 versus 3.2 per 100 episodes of moderate or severe respiratory illness).[279] These data suggest that low-birth-weight children may experience more severe respiratory infections; however, these infections are no more frequent than in normal-weight control populations. As low birth weight is associated with crowding, poverty, and poor nutritional status, these factors may cause too much confounding to allow any conclusions about the independent contribution of low birth weight on respiratory health.

Overprescribing of Antibiotics and Misuse of Medication

Shann et al have estimated that 75% of antibiotic prescriptions are written for acute respiratory infections.[1] Most of these prescriptions are probably unnecessary because the infections treated are predominantly viral in origin and, therefore, are unresponsive to drugs directed against bacterial pathogens. The annual costs incurred by inappropriate antibiotic prescribing is estimated at $8 billion worldwide.[1] Overprescribing of antibiotics poses a public health risk because it hastens the development of antibiotic resistance.

In developing countries, overprescribing of antibiotics by unqualified medical practitioners is especially common.[257] Self-medication with drugs that can mask the symptoms of respiratory infections, inappropriate courses of medication prescribed by health care providers, and premature discontinuation of therapy also contribute to increased morbidity in cases of acute respiratory infections.[258,280-282] In China, herbal remedies are still commonly used to treat these infections. Liu and Douglas identified 27 articles published primarily in Chinese language journals between 1985 and 1996 that described favorable effects of herbal remedies for acute respiratory infections.[283] These authors found limitations in the study design and data presentation of the clinical trials. They believed that definitive conclusions about efficacy could not be made in view of insufficient information on randomization and baseline comparisons, the use of outcome measures that were either complicated or of doubtful validity, the use of poorly defined terms to connote efficacy (e.g., "effect rate"), and inadequate or missing statistical analysis. Therefore, it is possible that millions of Chinese are currently receiving inadequate treatment of acute respiratory infections.

Increasing Resistance to Antibiotics

Clinical response to antibiotics, especially penicillins and oral cephalosporins, has been greatly affected by the rise of antibiotic resistance since the 1980s. Resistance rates of *H. influenzae* to penicillin and amoxicillin have been reported to be 30% to 40% in Singapore, Indonesia, Thailand, Taiwan, Hong Kong, and the Philippines, and 15% in Malaysia and Korea.[14] In Latin America, the prevalence of amoxicillin resistance to *H. influenzae* varies greatly among countries. It has been reported to be almost 50% in hospital isolates in Guatemala, 25% to 30% in the general population of Argentina and Venezuela, 10% in Colombia and Uruguay, and 2.5% in Ecuador.[14] Pneumococcal resistance is more than 70% among patients in hospitals in Manila, Philippines; 30% to 40% in Hong Kong, Korea, and Taiwan; and 10% to 20% in Singapore and Malaysia.[14] The prevalence of pneumococcal resistance is generally lower in Latin America than Southeast Asia, although it has reached 15% to 25% in some areas.[14]

Other Host Factors

Primarily uncontrolled studies have mentioned many other factors as possibly increasing the risk of pneumonia in adults. In high-risk outpatients, Simberkoff et al found that chronic pulmonary, cardiac, and renal disease predicted the incidence of pneumonia, but they did not observe an association with hepatic disease, alcoholism, or diabetes mellitus.[186] Lipsky et al noted that dementia, cerebrovascular disease, and institutionalization independently predicted pneumonia.[184] They also confirmed that increasing age, smoking, chronic obstructive lung disease, and congestive cardiac failure increased pneumonia risk, but that diabetes mellitus, malignancy, or heavy alcohol use did not.

Maternal antibodies to respiratory syncytial and influenza viruses in cord blood appear to be protective against subsequent infection in infants.[284,285] If maternal immunity can be passively transferred to infants, it would be expected that vaccination of pregnant women would be beneficial in protecting the infant against these viruses. A family history of asthma is associated with increased risk of bronchiolitis in infancy, and it appears to strongly interact with exposure factors such as presence of an older sibling in the house and passive smoking.[286] The contribution of genetic factors to the risk of respiratory infection in children appears to be supported by other studies reporting increased rates of wheeze-related respiratory infection in infants with higher virus-specific immunoglobulin E responses to respiratory syncytial viruses,[287] parainfluenza viruses,[288] and in those with small airway diameters.[289]

Efficient Methods of Data Collection to Evaluate Respiratory Epidemiology

No standardized questionnaires exist for collection of acute respiratory infection symptom data, although standardized instruments developed by the American Thoracic Society and the British Medical Research Council are available to measure chronic respiratory symptomatology.[290,291] As the focus of the latter questionnaires is set on symptoms of airway reactivity and allergy, they cannot be readily adapted for studies of acute respiratory infections. This situation has prompted many researchers to create and use either nonstandardized respiratory symptom diaries (Figure 19-5) or recall questionnaires. Respiratory diaries have three advantages over questionnaires: (1) they practically eliminate recall bias; (2) they are useful in studies in which specific symptom complexes are important; and (3) they are more likely to be accurate records of symptom duration. The main drawback of respiratory symptom diaries is that they require daily recording by the study participant, which could be viewed by participants as such a burden that they may stop making entries, as happens especially in multiyear studies.

Alternatively, research assistants can call or visit study participants on a weekly or biweekly basis to inquire via a questionnaire about symptom frequency and duration in the preceding period. Although this approach has all the problems associated with recall data, it has advantages of sustainability

CHILD'S NAME ID RESPIRATORY EVENTS IN EARLY CHILDHOOD

DECEMBER 1998	1	2	3	4	5	6	7	8	9	10	11	.12	13	14	15	16	17	18	19	20	21	22	23	24	25	26	27	28	29	30 31
Is he/she completely well? Y=Yes N = No																														
Do you think he/she has a cold? Y or N																														
Record each symptom he/she experiences each day. Mark with X.																														
Runny nose																														
Stopped-up nose																														
Hoarse throat																														
Wheezy/noisy breathing																														
Moist cough																														
Dry cough																														
Fever (feels hot)																														
Pulling at ears																														
Medication given (M)*																														
* Doctor visits (D)*																														
Hospital visits (V)/ Hospital stays (S)* (*more details on back)																														
OTHER ILLNESSES (give brief details)																														

FIGURE 19-5 Example of an acute respiratory illness symptom diary used in a 2-year cohort study of infants in Adelaide, Australia, 1988–1990.
Source: Direct and Indirect Effects of Routine Vaccination of Children with 7-Valent Pneumococcal Conjugate Vaccine on Incidence of Invasive Pneumococcal Disease—United States, 1998–2003. MMWR. September 16, 2005/54(36);893–897.

over long periods and the ability of the interviewer to define symptoms more clearly than would otherwise be possible using a diary approach. Questionnaires, which are easier to standardize than symptom diaries, have been shown to be associated with higher compliance rates over a 2-year period in patients with lower respiratory infections.[292,293]

Standardized questionnaires are especially needed in developing countries.[294] Often, the clinical and laboratory expertise and facilities are not available to confirm a diagnosis, and many difficulties exist regarding standardizing measures of exposure between studies. The National Research Council's project in 12 countries was a major attempt to standardize data collection and study protocols.[11] Although some variation in methods was inevitable, these data are probably the most comparable of any collected to date. Much effort has been given to developing criteria for identifying acute lower respiratory infections from simple clinical signs. Several studies have now shown that tachypnea and a history of fast breathing[45,294-295] are highly sensitive and specific predictors of lower respiratory tract infections in both community and hospital settings.[45,294-296] The sensitivity and specificity of tachypnea as a diagnostic criterion is improved when chest indrawing is considered.[296] Campbell et al reported that the best predictors of lobar pneumonia in infants were temperature above 38.5°C and a respiratory rate greater than 60 per minute.[297] Diagnoses more specific than "acute lower respiratory infection," such as severe pneumonia, may not be predictable based only on the presence of a respiratory rate of more than 50 per minute. Nevertheless, to conduct epidemiologic studies in developing countries, the high sensitivity and specificity of maternal history of fast breathing as a predictor of acute lower respiratory tract infection is still very valuable.

Prevention

The epidemiology of acute respiratory infections is well understood today primarily because of research that has been conducted during the past three decades. Clear associations between acute respiratory infections and chronic disease in adults, direct smoking, passive smoking, crowding, and breastfeeding have been well documented. The relatively higher incidence of acute respiratory infections in developing countries compared with the developed world results from a combination and interaction of factors associated with poverty and lower social status—large family size, crowded living conditions, less access to medical care, higher smoking rates, potential for nutritional deficit, lower breastfeeding rates, exposure to environmental pollutants (tobacco smoke, wood smoke, urban air pollution), and stressful living environments.

In developed countries, certain issues remain to be better defined, including the relationship between air pollution and acute respiratory infections, the relation between maternal antibody levels and passive immunity in infants, and the reasons for the increase in pneumonia mortality in older age groups. Standardization of acute symptom questionnaires and symptom diaries still needs to be done to facilitate more complete and thorough epidemiologic studies in both developing and developed countries.

Prevention of Respiratory Infections

The knowledge gained about the epidemiology and risk factors associated with acute respiratory infection has been accompanied by public health programs to prevent these serious infections.

Cigarette Smoking

In the United States many successful programs have been initiated to reduce the prevalence of cigarette smoking. These have involved health education programs targeted to individuals, laws regulating or prohibiting smoking in public places, increased taxes on cigarettes, and successful court cases to force tobacco companies to pay some of the health costs incurred from cigarette-related illnesses. These efforts have reduced the population prevalence of smoking to 21.6% in the United States—24.1% in men and 19.2% in women in 2003, which has decreased the effect of one important risk factor for morbidity and mortality from acute respiratory infection.[298]

Similar programs to prevent tobacco smoking in developing countries have not been either comprehensive or successful to date. For example, it has been estimated that 68% of the adult male population of China smokes cigarettes at present.[299] In the same survey, only 9.5% of those who had ever smoked cigarettes had quit, only 10% of current smokers said they intended to quit, and their knowledge of many of the adverse health effects of smoking was much lower than comparable populations in the United States.[300] In contrast, in the United States over half of those who had ever smoked had quit and most current smokers said they would like to quit.[298]

Vaccines

Pneumococcal Conjugate Vaccine

In 2000, a 7-valent pneumococcal (PCV-7) conjugate vaccine was licensed in the United States for routine use in children under 5 years of age.[301] The seven serotypes in the vaccine were selected to include 80–90% of pneumococcal serotypes causing invasive disease in US children. Surveillance data from 2001–2003 have indicated substantial declines in invasive pneumococcal disease in children and adults compared to prevaccine years.[302] The effectiveness of PCV-7 at the population level has been evaluated using population-based data from the Active Bacterial Core (ABC) of the Emerging Infections Program Network, a cooperative surveillance program conducted by several state health departments and the CDC.[303]

This surveillance includes active identification of invasive pneumococcal disease by staff who contact microbiology laboratories and secure *S. pneumoniae* isolates obtained from a normally sterile body site, from infected individuals in five states, and from several counties in California, representing a catchment area of about 16 million persons.[303]

This surveillance has shown the following:

- Routine immunization of young children with PCV-7 has resulted in significant declines in the incidence of invasive pneumococcal disease in the group targeted to receive the vaccine.

- The vaccine prevented more than twice as many cases of invasive pneumococcal disease in adults in 2003 through indirect effects on pneumococcal transmission (i.e., herd immunity) than through its direct effect of protecting vaccinated children.
- Increases in disease caused by pneumococcal serotypes not included in the vaccine (i.e., replacement disease) occurred; however, this increase was smaller than the declines in vaccine-serotype disease. See Figures 19-6, 19-7, 19-8, and Table 19-10.

The PCV-7 vaccine is expensive (estimated at $56.00 per dose in the United States) but has been estimated to be cost-effective in DALYs in developed industrialized countries.[304] The Global Alliance for Vaccines and Immunization (GAVI) has begun a new pneumococcal vaccine accelerated development and introduction program that aims to make the vaccine more widely available.

The results of a randomized, placebo-controlled, double-blind trial of an investigational 9-valent pneumococcal conjugate vaccine among children aged 6–51 weeks in the Gambia was reported recently.[305] This vaccine included the serotypes in the 7-valent vaccine licensed in the United States, plus serotypes 1 and 5, which are important causes of invasive pneumococcal disease among children in Africa. In this study 8218 children received vaccine and 8219 were given placebo. The efficacy of the vaccine against WHO-defined radiological pneumonia was 37% (95% CI, 27–45%). The

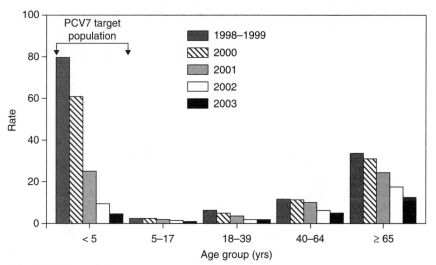

* Per 100,000 population.
† For each age group, the decrease in VT IPD rate for 2003 compared with the 1998–1999 baseline is statistically significant ($P < .05$).

FIGURE 19-6 Rate of vaccine-type (VT) invasive pneumococcal disease (IPD) before and after introduction of pneumococcal conjugate vaccine (PCV7), by age group and year—Active Bacterial Core surveillance, United States, 1998–2003. *Source:* Direct and Indirect Effects of Routine Vaccination of Children with 7-Valent Pneumococcal Conjugate Vaccine on Incidence of Invasive Pneumococcal Disease—United States, 1998–2003. MMWR. September 16, 2005/54(36);893–897.

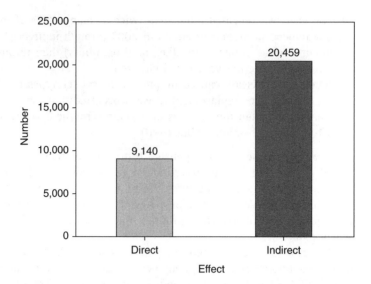

* Direct VT IPD cases prevented in 2003 = 1998 – 1999 average number of VT IPD cases in children aged < 5 years x 2003 PCV7 coverage with 3 doses (68.1%) x PCV7 effectiveness for VT IPD (93.9%).
† Indirect VT IPD cases prevented in 2003 = (1998 – 1999 average number of VT IPD cases across all age groups – 2003 number of VT IPD cases across all age groups) – 2003 direct VT IPD cases prevented. Calculation of indirect cases prevented does not account for replacement disease.

FIGURE 19-7 Estimated number of cases of vaccine-type (VT) invasive pneumococcal disease (IPD) prevented by direct and indirect effects of pneumococcal conjugate vaccine (PCV7)—Active Bacterial Core surveillance, United States, 2003.
Source: Whitney et al. Decline in Invasive Pneumococcal Disease After the Introduction of Protein–Polysaccharide Conjugate Vaccine. NEJM. Volume 348:1737–1746.

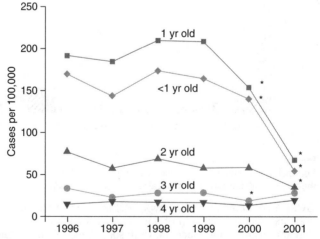

FIGURE 19-8 Rates of invasive pneumococcal disease among children under 5 years old, according to age and year.
Source: Williams et al. Human Metapneumovious and Lower Respiratory Tract Disease in Otherwise Healthy Infants and Children. NEJM. Volume 350:443–450.

TABLE 19-10 Changes in Projected Numbers of Invasive Pneumococcal Disease (IPD) Cases, by Age Group and Serotype Category—Active Bacterial Core Surveillance (ABCs), United States, 1998–1999, 2003

Age Group (yrs)	Serotype Category*	1998–1999 Average Projected No. of Cases[†]	2003 Projected No. of Cases[†]	Change in Annual Projected No. of Cases
<5				
	Vaccine	14,293	876	−13,417
	Nonvaccine	2,947	3,578	631
	Total	17,240	4,454	−12,786
5–17				
	Vaccine	1,195	569	−626
	Nonvaccine	880	824	−56
	Total	2,075	1,393	−682
18–39				
	Vaccine	5,023	1,610	−3,413
	Nonvaccine	3,419	3,407	−12
	Total	8,442	5,017	−3,425
40–64				
	Vaccine	8,945	4,167	−4,778
	Nonvaccine	7,545	10,237	2,692
	Total	16,490	14,404	−2,086
≥65				
	Vaccine	11,595	4,230	−7,365
	Nonvaccine	9,169	10,635	1,466
	Total	20,764	14,865	−5,899
All ages				
	Vaccine	41,051	11,452	−29,599
	Nonvaccine	23,960	28,681	4,721
	Total	65,011	40,133	−24,878

*Serotypes included in the 7-valent pneumococcal conjugate vaccine are defined as vaccine serotypes (4, 6B, 9V, 14, 18C, 19F, and 23F). All other serotypes are considered nonvaccine serotypes.
[†]Annual national projections of IPD cases were calculated by applying age- and race-specific disease rates for the aggregate ABCs surveillance area to the age and racial distribution of the US population on the basis of 2000 US Census data.
Source: Direct and Indirect Effects of Routine Vaccination of Children with 7-Valent Pneumococcal Conjugate Vaccine on Incidence of Invasive Pneumococcal Disease—United States, 1998–2003. MMWR. September 16, 2005/54(36);893–897.

efficacy of the vaccine against any invasive pneumococcal disease caused by vaccine serotypes was 72% (95% CI, 51–90%), and it was 50% (95% CI, 21–69%) against all serotypes and 16% (95% CI, 3–28%) against nonvaccine serotypes.

Another randomized, placebo-controlled trial of three doses of 9-valent pneumococcal conjugate vaccine among 39,836 children was done in Soweto, South Africa.[306] In this study vaccine efficacy was measured in children with and without HIV infection and in the setting of frequent antibiotic-resistant invasive pneumococcal infections. Among children who were HIV-negative the vaccine efficacy was 83% (95% CI, 39–97%) in preventing invasive pneumococcal disease from serotypes included in the vaccine; among HIV-positive children the efficacy was 65% (95% CI, 24–86%) against these serotypes. The episodes of radiographically confirmed pneumonia among HIV-negative children were reduced by 20% (95% CI, 2–35%). The incidence of invasive pneumococcal disease caused by penicillin-resistant strains was reduced by 67%, and the incidence of that disease caused by trimethoprim-sulfamethoxazole resistant-strains was reduced by 56%. These two studies among high-risk infants and children in Africa suggest that the routine use of a proposed pneumococcal vaccine with 11 of the most prevalent serotypes could be an important strategy to reduce the most important cause of childhood mortality in developing countries.

The diagnosis of pneumonia by health workers in the field and antibiotic treatment together with referral of those with severe infections for treatment, as described earlier in this chapter, are also important components of the public health strategy to reduce mortality from childhood pneumonia. However, the reports of invasive pneumococcal infections from organisms resistant to trimethoprim-sulfamethoxazole or penicillin might somewhat limit the effectiveness of antibiotic treatment.[307] Therefore, the use of an effective conjugated pneumococcal vaccine with appropriate spectrum of serotypes (i.e., a 9- or 11-valent vaccine) would be an important part of the strategy to reduce pneumonia mortality among children in developing countries.

Conjugated Haemophilus Influenzae Vaccines

Haemophilus influenzae is another organism that is an important cause of invasive respiratory infections among infants and children in developed industrialized countries. Prior to the availability of specific vaccines, *H. influenzae* type B (Hib) was estimated to cause meningitis in about 25/100,000 children less than 5 years of age per year and to be responsible for 50–100/100,000 cases of invasive disease in children of this age annually in the United States.[308] Among Native Americans and Australian aboriginals the rates of Hib meningitis prior to vaccine use were reported to be 152–254/100,000 per year in children under age 5.[309] After protein-conjugated Hib vaccines were found to have more than 90% efficacy in the prevention of *H. influenzae* meningitis and invasive disease with bacteremia, these vaccines were licensed and incorporated into routine childhood immunization schedules in the United States in 1980 and Europe during the 1990s. The implementation of conjugated Hib vaccines into routine vaccine schedules has led to an 80–90% decrease in the incidence of Hib-related diseases, especially meningitis.[308,310] Nevertheless, Hib vaccine has not been included in immunization schedules in many developing countries, especially in Asia. In part, this relates to their high cost compared to other vaccines. But also, some public health officials in developing countries, especially those in Asia, believe that invasive Hib disease is much less common in Asia than in the West,[311] as there is varying data on the burden of Hib pneumonia.

The results of a clinical trial was reported recently among children under age 2 on Lombok Island, Indonesia.[312] In this study 28,147 children were given DTP-PRP-T (i.e., conjugated Hib vaccine with DTP) and 26,926 were given DTP alone. This study found that there was no effect of the Hib vaccine in the prevention of radiologically confirmed pneumonia, but severe pneumonia, or clinical pneumonia was reduced by approximately 4%. However, the Hib vaccine group had 50% lower incidence of proven and likely bacterial hospitalized meningitis than children who received only the DTP vaccine. The incidence of all Hib vaccine-prevented pneumonia was $1561/10^5$ children under 2 years, about 1.5 cases of pneumonia averted for every 100 vaccinated children. With regard to radiological pneumonia, this study contrasts with a trial of a conjugated Hib vaccine in young children in the Gambia, which found the vaccine prevented 21% (95% CI, 5-35%) of episodes of radiologically defined pneumonia.[313] A study in Chile also showed no effect against radiological pneumonia, but "likely bacterial pneumonia" (defined by clinical and laboratory criteria) was reduced by 20% (95% CI, 1-36%).[301] The conjugated Hib and pneumococcal vaccines can be incorporated into routine immunization of children in developing countries in Africa, Asia, and elsewhere. The cost of the pneumococcal vaccine and the remaining uncertainty regarding the burden of Hib disease in Asia are challenges that will be confronted by GAVI and its developing country partners.

References

1. Bryce J, Boschi-Pinto C, Shibuyo K, Black RE, WHO Child Health Epidemiology Reference Group. WHO estimates of death in children. *Lancet.* 2005;365:1147-1150.
2. Murray CJL, Lopez AD. *Global Comparative Assessments in the Health Sector.* Geneva, Switzerland: World Health Organization; 1994.
3. Leowski J. Mortality from acute respiratory infections in children under 5 years of age: global estimates. *World Health Stat Q.* 1986;39: 138-144.
4. Graham NMH. The epidemiology of acute respiratory infection in children and adults: a global perspective. *Epidemiol Rev.* 1990;12: 149-178.
5. Pan American Health Organization. Acute respiratory infections in the Americas. *Epidemiol Bull.* 1980;1:1-4.
6. Pio A, Leowski J, ten Dam HG. The magnitude of the problem of acute respiratory infections. In: Douglas RM, Kerby-Eaton E, eds. *Acute Respiratory Infections: Proceedings of an International Workshop.* Adelaide, South Australia: University of Adelaide; 1985:3-16.
7. Douglas RM. *Acute Respiratory Infections.* (WHO/WPR/RC30/TP/1). Manila, Philippines: World Health Organization; 1979.
8. Kamath KR, Feldman RA, Sundar Rao PSS, et al. Infection and disease in a group of South Indian families. II. General morbidity patterns in families and family members. *Am J Epidemiol.* 1969;89: 375-383.
9. Freij L, Wall S. Exploring child health and its ecology. The Kirkos study in Addis Ababa. An evaluation of procedures in the measurement of

acute morbidity and a search for causal structure. *Acta Paediatr Scand Suppl.* 1977;267:1–18.

10. James JW, Longitudinal study of the morbidity of diarrheal and respiratory infections in malnourished children. *Am J Clin Nutr.* 1972;25:690–694.

11. Berman S. Epidemiology of acute respiratory infections in children of developing countries. *Rev Infect Dis.* 1991;13(suppl 6):S454-S462.

12. Fox JP, Cooney MK, Hall CE. The Seattle virus watch. V. Epidemiologic observations of rhinovirus infections, 1965–1969, in families with young children. *Am J Epidemiol.* 1975;101:122–143.

13. Monto AS, Ullman B. Acute respiratory illness in an American community. *JAMA.* 1974;227:164–169.

14. Ball P, Make B. Acute exacerbations of chronic bronchitis. An international comparison. *Chest.* 1998;113(suppl 3):199S-204S.

15. Lai CKW, Ho SC, Lau J, et al. Respiratory symptoms in elderly Chinese living in Hong Kong. *Eur Respir J.* 1995;8:2055–2061.

16. Pandey MR. Domestic smoke pollution and chronic bronchitis in a rural community of the hill region in Nepal. *Thorax.* 1984;39:337–339.

17. Doyle R. U.S. deaths from pneumonia. Available at: http://www.sciam .com/0297issue/0297scicit6.html. Accessed February 22, 2006.

18. Meeker DP, Longworth DL. Community-acquired pneumonia: an update. *Cleve Clin J Med.* 1996;63:16–30.

19. Fine MJ, Chowdhry T, Ketema A. Outpatient management of community-acquired pneumonia. *Hosp Pract (Off Ed).* 1998;3:123–133.

20. Marrie TJ. Community-acquired pneumonia: epidemiology, etiology, treatment. *Infect Dis Clin North Am.* 1998;13:723–740.

21. Farber MO. Managing community-acquired pneumonia. Factors to consider in outpatient care. *Postgrad Med.* 1999;105:106–114.

22. Mandell LA, Campbell GD Jr. Nosocomial pneumonia guidelines. An international perspective. *Chest.* 1998;113(suppl 3):188S-193S.

23. Fagon JY, Chastre J, Hance A, et al. Nosocomial pneumonia in ventilated patients: a cohort study evaluating attributable mortality and hospital stay. *Am J Med.* 1993;94:281–288.

24. American Thoracic Society. Hospital-acquired pneumonia in adults: diagnosis, assessment of severity, initial antimicrobial therapy, and preventative strategies. *Am J Respir Crit Care Med.* 1996;153: 1711–1725.

25. van Volkenburgh VA, Frost WH. Acute minor respiratory diseases prevailing in a group of families residing in Baltimore, Maryland, 1928–1930. Prevalence, distribution and clinical description of observed cases. *Am J Hygiene.* 1933;17:122–153.

26. Gwaltney JM Jr, Hendley JO, Simon C, et al. Rhinovirus infections in an industrial population. I. The occurrence of illness. *N Engl J Med.* 1966;275:1261–1268.

27. Fox JP, Hall CE, Cooney MK, et al. The Seattle virus watch. II. Objectives, study population and its observation, data processing and summary of illnesses. *Am J Epidemiol.* 1972;96:270–285.

28. Bates JH. Microbiologic etiology of pneumonia. *Chest.* 1989;95(suppl 5):194S-197S.

29. Glezen W, Denny FW. Epidemiology of acute lower respiratory disease in children. *N Engl J Med.* 1973;288:498–505.

30. Henderson FW, Clyde WA, Collier AM, et al. The etiologic and epidemiologic spectrum of bronchiolitis in pediatric practice. *J Pediatr.* 1979;95:183–190.

31. Denny FW, Clyde WA. Acute lower respiratory tract infections in non-hospitalized children. *J Pediatr.* 1986;108:635–646.
32. Wright AL, Taussig LM, Ray CC, et al. The Tucson children's respiratory study. II. Lower respiratory tract illness in the first year of life. *Am J Epidemiol.* 1989;129:1232–1246.
33. Cole P, Wilson R. Host-microbial interrelationships in respiratory infection. *Chest.* 1989;95(suppl):217S–221S.
34. Australian Bureau of Statistics. *Australian Health Survey.* Preliminary bulletin no. 1. Canberra, Australia: Australian Bureau of Statistics; 1977.
35. Douglas RM. ARI—the Cinderella of communicable diseases. In: Douglas RM, Kerby-Eaton E, eds. *Acute Respiratory Infections in Children.* Proceedings of an international workshop. Adelaide, South Australia: University of Adelaide; 1985:1–2.
36. Enright PL, Krumla RA, Higgins MW, et al. Prevalence and correlates of respiratory symptoms in the elderly. *Chest.* 1994;106:827–834.
37. Lange P, Groth S, Nyboe J, et al. Chronic obstructive lung disease in Copenhagen: cross-sectional epidemiological aspects. *J Intern Med.* 1989;226:25–32.
38. Bakke PS, Baste V, Hanoa R, et al. Prevalence of obstructive lung disease in a general population: relation to occupational title and exposure to some airborne agents. *Thorax.* 1991;46:863–870.
39. Alonso J, Anto JM. *Encuesta de salut de Barcelona. 1986* (government publication). Barcelona, Spain; 1989.
40. Brotons B, Perez JA, Sanchez-Toril F, et al. Prevalencia de la enfermedad obstructiva cronica y el asma: estudio transversal. *Arch Bronconeumol.* 1994;103:481–484.
41. Lundback B, Nystrom L, Rosenhall L, et al. Obstructive lung disease in northern Sweden: respiratory symptoms assessed by postal questionnaire. *Eur Respir J.* 1991;4:257–266.
42. Niederman MS, McCombs JS, Unger AN, Kumar A, Popovian R. The cost of treating community-acquired pneumonia. *Clin Ther.* 1998;20:820–837.
43. Niederman MS, McCombs JS, Unger AN, Kumar A, Popovian R. Treatment cost of acute exacerbations of chronic bronchitis. *Clin Ther.* 1999;21:576–591.
44. McCord C, Kielmann AA. A successful programme for medical auxiliaries treating childhood diarrhea and pneumonia. *Trop Doct.* 1978;8:220–225.
45. Shann FA, Hart K, Thomas D. Acute lower respiratory tract infections in children: possible criteria for selection of patients for antibiotic therapy and hospital admission. *Bull WHO.* 1984;62:749–753.
46. World Health Organization. *Case Management of Acute Respiratory Infections in Children: Intervention Studies.* (WHO/ARI/88.2). Geneva, Switzerland: World Health Organization; 1988.
47. Cherian T, John TJ, Simoes E, Steinhoff MC, John M. Evaluation of simple clinical signs for the diagnosis of acute lower respiratory tract infection. *Lancet.* 1988;2:125–128.
48. World Health Organization. *ARI Programme Report. 1988.* (WHO/ARI/89.3). Geneva, Switzerland: World Health Organization; 1989.
49. World Health Organization. Programme of acute respiratory infections. *Report of the Fourth Meeting of the Technical Advisory Group.* (WHO/ARI/89.4). Geneva, Switzerland: World Health Organization; 1989.

50. World Health Organization. *Case Management of Acute Respiratory Infections in Children in Developing Countries.* (WHO/RSD/85.151). Geneva, Switzerland: World Health Organization; 1985.

51. World Health Organization. *Proposal for the Classification of Acute Respiratory Infections and Tuberculosis for the Tenth Revision of the International Classification of Diseases.* (WHO/RSD/88.25). Geneva, Switzerland: World Health Organization; 1985.

52. Bartlett JG, Breiman RF, Mandell G, et al, for the Infectious Diseases Society of America. Community-acquired pneumonia in adults: guidelines for management. *Clin Infect Dis.* 1998;26:811–838.

53. Reimer LG, Caroll KC. Role of the microbiology laboratory in the diagnosis of lower respiratory tract infections. *Clin Infect Dis.* 1998;26:742–748.

54. Reed SE. The etiology and epidemiology of common colds and the possibilities of prevention. *Clin Otolaryngol.* 1981;6:379–387.

55. Berman S, McIntosh K. Selective primary healthcare: strategies for control of disease in the developing world. XXI. Acute respiratory infections. *Rev Infect Dis.* 1985;7:674–691.

56. Berman S, Duenas A, Bedoya A, et al. Acute lower respiratory tract illnesses in Cali, Colombia: a two-year ambulatory study. *Pediatrics.* 1983;71:210–218.

57. Escobar JA, Dover AS, Duenas A, et al. Etiology of respiratory tract infections in children in Cali, Colombia. *Pediatrics.* 1976;57:123–130.

58. Shann F, Gratten M, Germer S, et al. Aetiology of pneumonia in children in Goroka Hospital, Papua New Guinea. *Lancet.* 1984;2:537–541.

59. Sobeslavsky O, Sebikari SRK, Harland PSEG, et al. The viral etiology of acute respiratory infections in children in Uganda. *Bull WHO.* 1977;55:625–631.

60. Ogunbi O. Bacterial and viral etiology of bronchiolitis and bronchopneumonia in Lagos children. *J Trop Med Hyg.* 1970;73:138–140.

61. Monto AJ, Johnson KM. Respiratory infections in the American tropics. *Am J Trop Med Hyg.* 1968;17:867–874.

62. Chanock R, Chambon L, Chang W, et al. WHO respiratory disease survey in children: a serological study. *Bull WHO.* 1967;37:363–369.

63. Spence L, Barratt N. Respiratory syncytial virus associated with acute respiratory infections in Trinidadian patients. *Am J Epidemiol.* 1968;88:257–266.

64. Kloene W, Bang FB, Chakraborty SM, et al. A two-year respiratory virus survey in four villages in West Bengal, India. *Am J Epidemiol.* 1970;92:307–320.

65. Olson LC, Lexomboon U, Sithisarn P, et al. The etiology of respiratory tract infections in a tropical country. *Am J Epidemiol.* 1973;97:34–43.

66. Belshe RB, Van Voris LP, Mufson MA. Impact of viral respiratory diseases on infants and young children in a rural and urban area of southern West Virginia. *Am J Epidemiol.* 1983;117:467–474.

67. Foy HM, Cooney MK, Maletzky AJ, et al. Incidence and etiology of pneumonia, croup and bronchiolitis in preschool children belonging to a prepaid medical care group over a four-year period. *Am J Epidemiol.* 1973;97:80–92.

68. Mufson MA, Krause HE, Mocega HE, et al. Viruses, *Mycoplasma pneumoniae* and bacteria associated with lower respiratory tract disease among infants. *Am J Epidemiol.* 1970;91:192–202.
69. Murphy TF, Henderson FW, Clyde WA Jr, et al. Pneumonia: an eleven-year study in a pediatric practice. *Am J Epidemiol.* 1981;113:12–21.
70. Berman S, Duenas A, Bedoya A, et al. Acute lower respiratory tract illnesses in Cali, Colombia: a two-year ambulatory study. *Pediatrics.* 1983;71:210–218.
71. Wesley AG. Indications for intubation in laryngotracheobronchitis in black children. *S Afr Med J.* 1975;49:1126–1128.
72. Bariffi F, Sanduzzi A, Ponticiello A. Epidemiology of lower respiratory tract infections. *J Chemother.* 1995;7:263–276.
73. MacFarlane JT. Treatment of lower respiratory infections. *Lancet.* 1987;2:1446–1449.
74. Marrie TJ, Durant H, Yates L. Community-acquired pneumonia requiring hospitalization: 5 year prospective study. *Rev Infect Dis.* 1989;11:586–599.
75. Clezen WP. Serious morbidity and mortality associated with influenza epidemics. *Epidemiol Rev.* 1982;4:25–44.
76. Hayden FG. Respiratory viral infections. In: Federman DD, ed. *Scientific American Medicine.* New York: Scientific American, Inc; 1997:1–12.
77. van de Hoogen BG, de Jong JC, Groen J, et al. A newly discovered human pneumovirus isolated from young children with respiratory tract disease. *Nat Med.* 2001;7:719–724.
78. Peret TC, Bolvin G, Li Y, et al. Characterization of human metapneumoviruses isolated from patients in North America. *J Infect Dis.* 2002;185:1660–1663.
79. Nissen MD, Siebert DJ, Mackay IM, Sloots TP, Withers SJ. Evidence of human metapneumovirus in Australian children. *Med J Aust.* 2002;176:188.
80. Stockton J, Stephenson I, Fleming D, Zambon M. Human metapneumovirus as a cause of community-acquired respiratory illness. *Emerg Infect Dis.* 2002;8:897–901.
81. Esper F, Boucher D, Weibel C, Martinello RA, Kahn JS. Human metapneumovirus infestations associated with a newly emerging respiratory infection in children. *Pediatrics.* 2003;111:407–410.
82. Williams JV, Harris PA, Tollefson SJ, et al. Human metapneumovirus and lower respiratory tract disease in otherwise healthy infants and children. *N Engl J Med.* 2004;350:443–450.
83. Monto AS, Napier JA, Metzner HL. The Tecumseh study of respiratory illness. I. Plan of study and observations on syndromes of acute respiratory disease. *Am J Epidemiol.* 1971;94:269–279.
84. Monto AS, Cavallaro JJ. The Tecumseh study of respiratory illness. II. Patterns of occurrence of infection with respiratory pathogens. 1965–1969. *Am J Epidemiol.* 1971;94:280–289.
85. Maletzky AJ, Cooney MK, Luce R, et al. Epidemiology of viral and mycoplasma agents associated with childhood lower respiratory illness in a civilian population. *J Pediatr.* 1971;78:407–414.
86. Barrett-Connor E. The nonvalue of sputum culture in the diagnosis of pneumococcal pneumonia. *Am Rev Resp Dis.* 1971;103:845–848.
87. Davidson M, Tempest B, Palmer DL. Bacteriologic diagnosis of acute pneumonia: comparison of sputum, transtracheal aspirates and lung aspirates. *JAMA.* 1976;235:158–163.

88. Halperin SA, Suratt PM, Gwaltney JM Jr, et al. Bacterial cultures of the lower respiratory tract in normal volunteers with and without experimental rhinovirus infection using a plugged double catheter system. *Am Rev Respir Dis.* 1982;125:678–680.

89. Silverman M, Stratton D, Diallo A, et al. Diagnosis of acute bacterial pneumonia in Nigerian children. Value of needle aspirations of lung and counter current electrophoresis. *Arch Dis Child.* 1977;52:925–931.

90. Macfarlane JT, Finch RG, Ward MJ, et al. Hospital study of adult community acquired pneumonia. *Lancet.* 1982;2:255–258.

91. Molleni RA. Epiglottitis: incidence of extraepiglottic infection. Report of 72 cases and review of the literature. *Pediatrics.* 1976;58:526–531.

92. Miller DL, Alderslade R, Ross EM. Whooping cough and whooping cough vaccine: the risks and benefits debate. *Epidemiol Rev.* 1982;4:1–24.

93. Howie VM, Ploussard JH, Lester RL Jr. Otitis media: a clinical and bacteriological correlation. *Pediatrics.* 1970;45:29–35.

94. Engelhardt D, Cohen D, Strauss N, et al. Randomized study of myringotomy, amoxycillin/clavulanate or both for acute otitis media in infants. *Lancet.* 1989;2:141–143.

95. Wald ER, Milmoe GJ, Bowen A, et al. Acute maxillary sinusitis in children. *N Engl J Med.* 1981;304:749–754.

96. Evans FO, Sydnor JB, Moore WEC, et al. Sinusitis of the maxillary antrum. *N Engl J Med.* 1975;293:735–739.

97. Hamory BH, Sande MA, Snydor A, et al. Etiology and antimicrobial therapy of acute maxillary sinusitis. *J Infect Dis.* 1979;139:197–202.

98. Ikeogu MO. Acute pneumonia in Zimbabwe: bacterial isolates by lung aspirations. *Arch Dis Child.* 1988;63:1266–1267.

99. Bartlett JG. Approach to the patient with pneumonia. In: Gorbach SL, Bartlett JG, Blacklow NR, eds. *Infectious Diseases.* 2nd ed. Philadelphia, Pa: WB Saunders Co; 1998.

100. Grayston JT, Alexander E, Kenny G, et al. *Mycoplasma pneumoniae* infections. *JAMA.* 1965;19:369–374.

101. Jansson E, Wager O, Stenstrom R, et al. Studies on Eaton PPLO pneumonia. *Br Med J.* 1964;1:142–145.

102. Komaroff AL, Aronson MD, Pass TM, et al. Serologic evidence of chlamydia and mycoplasma pharyngitis in adults. *Science.* 1983;222:927–929.

103. Stagno S, Brasfield DM, Brown MB, et al. Infant pneumonitis associated with cytomegalovirus, chlamydia, pneumocystis and ureaplasma. *Pediatrics.* 1981;68:322–329.

104. Grayston JT, Kuo CC, Wang SP, et al. A new *Chlamydia psittaci* strain, TWAR, isolated from acute respiratory tract infections. *N Engl J Med.* 1986;315:161–168.

105. Marrie TJ, Grayston JT, Wang SP, et al. Pneumonia associated with TWAR strain of chlamydia. *Ann Intern Med.* 1987;106:507–511.

106. Murray JF, Felton CP, Garay SM, et al. Pulmonary complications of the acquired immunodeficiency syndrome. Report of a National Heart, Lung, and Blood Institute workshop. *N Engl J Med.* 1984;310:1682–1688.

107. Centers for Disease Control. Update: acquired immunodeficiency syndrome–United States. *MMWR.* 1985;34:245–248.

108. Quinn TC, Mann JM, Curran JW, et al. AIDS in Africa: an epidemiologic paradigm. *Science.* 1986;234:955–963.

109. Cunha BA. Community-acquired pneumonia in human immunodeficiency virus-infected patients. *Clin Infect Dis.* 1999;28:410–411.
110. Ginesu F, Pirina P. Etiology and risk factors of adult pneumonia. *J Chemother.* 1995;7:277–285.
111. Fox JP, Cooney MK, Hall CE, et al. Rhinoviruses in Seattle families, 1975–1979. *Am J Epidemiol.* 1985;122:830–846.
112. World Health Organization. *World Health Statistics Annual.* Geneva, Switzerland: World Health Organization; 1989.
113. Logan WPD. Mortality in the London fog incident, 1952. *Lancet.* 1953;1:336–338.
114. Firket J. The cause of the symptoms found in the Meuse Valley during the fog of December, 1930. *Bull Acad R Med Belg.* 1931;11:683–741.
115. Gore AT, Shaddick CW. Atmosphere pollution and mortality in the county of London. *Br J Prev Soc Med.* 1958;12:104–113.
116. Ciocco A, Thompson DJ. A follow-up of Donora ten years after: methodology and findings. *Am J Public Health.* 1961;51:155–164.
118. Greenberg L, Jacobs MB, Droletti BM, et al. Report of an air pollution incident in New York City, November, 1953. *Public Health Rep.* 1962;77:7–16.
119. Greenberg L, Erhardt C, Field F, et al. Intermittent air pollution episodes in New York City, 1962. *Public Health Rep.* 1963;78:1061–1064.
120. Daley C. Air pollution and causes of death. *Br J Prev Soc Med.* 1959;13:14–27.
121. Holland WW, Bennett AE, Cameron IR, et al. Health effects of particulate air pollution: reappraising the evidence. *Am J Epidemiol.* 1979;110:527–659.
122. Toyama T. Air pollution and its effects in Japan. *Arch Environ Health.* 1964;8:153–173.
123. Lunn JR, Knowelden J, Handyside AJ. Patterns of respiratory illness in Sheffield infant school children. *Br J Prev Soc Med.* 1967;21:7–16.
124. Lunn JE, Knowelden J, Roe JW. Patterns of respiratory illness in Sheffield infant school children. *Br J Prev Soc Med.* 1970;24:223–228.
125. Colley JRT, Reid DD. Urban and social origins of childhood bronchitis in England and Wales. *Br Med J.* 1970;2:213–217.
126. Cassel EJ, Lebowitz M, McCarroll JR. The relationship between air pollution, weather, and symptoms in an urban population. *Am Rev Respir Dis.* 1972;106:677–683.
127. Collins JJ, Kasap HS, Holland WW. Environmental factors in child mortality in England and Wales. *Am J Epidemiol.* 1971;93:10–22.
128. Lawther PJ, Waller RE, Henderson M. Air pollution and exacerbations of bronchitis. *Thorax.* 1970;25:525–539.
129. French JC, Lowrimore C, Nelson WC, et al. The effect of sulphur dioxide and suspended sulphates on acute respiratory disease. *Arch Environ Health.* 1973;27:129–133.
130. Durham WH. Air pollution and student health. *Arch Environ Health.* 1974;28:241–254.
131. Levy D, Gent M, Newhouse MT. Relationship between acute respiratory illness and air pollution levels in an industrial city. *Am Rev Respir Dis.* 1977;116:167–173.
132. Ware JH, Ferris BC, Dockery DW, et al. Effects of ambient sulphur oxides and suspended particles on respiratory health of preadolescent children. *Am Rev Respir Dis.* 1986;133:834–842.

133. Pope CA. Respiratory disease associated with community air pollution and a steel mill, Utah Valley. *Am J Public Health.* 1989;79:623–628.

134. Derriennic F, Richardson S, Mollie A, et al. Short-term effects of sulphur dioxide pollution on mortality in two French cities. *Int J Epidemiol.* 1989;18:186–187.

135. Dockery DW, Speizer FE, Stram DO, et al. Effects of inhalable particles on respiratory health of children. *Am Rev Respir Dis.* 1989;139:587–594.

136. Dales RE, Spitzer WO, Suissa S, et al. Respiratory health of a population living downwind from natural gas refineries. *Am Rev Respir Dis.* 1989;139:595–600.

137. Kinney PL, Ware JH, Spangler JD, et al. Short-term pulmonary function change in association with ozone levels. *Am Rev Respir Dis.* 1989;139:56–61.

138. Schwartz J, Dockery DW, Wypii D, et al. Acute effects of air pollution on respiratory symptom reporting in children [abstract]. *Am Rev Respir Dis.* 1989;139(suppl):A27.

139. Goings SAJ, Kulla TJ, Bascom R, et al. Effect of nitrogen dioxide exposure on susceptibility to influenza A virus infection in healthy adults. *Am Rev Respir Dis.* 1989;1075–1081.

140. Cook DG, Strachan DP. Summary of effects of parental smoking on the respiratory health of children and implications for research. *Thorax.* 1999;54:357–366.

141. Fergusson DM, Horwood LJ, Shannon FT. Parental smoking and respiratory illness in infancy. *Arch Dis Child.* 1980;55:358–361.

142. Ferris BG, Ware JH, Berkey CS, et al. Effects of passive smoking on health of children. *Environ Health Perspect.* 1985;62:289–295.

143. Colley JRT, Holland WW, Corkhill RT. Influence of passive smoking and parental phlegm on pneumonia and bronchitis in early childhood. *Lancet.* 1974;2:1031–1034.

144. Fergusson DM, Horwood LJ. Parental smoking and respiratory illness during early childhood: a six-year longitudinal study. *Pediatr Pulmonol.* 1985;1:99–106.

145. Lebowitz MD, Burrows B. Respiratory symptoms related to smoking habits of family adults. *Chest.* 1976;69:48–50.

146. Love GJ, Lan S, Shy CM, et al. The incidence and severity of acute respiratory illness in families exposed to different levels of air pollution, New York metropolitan area, 1971–2. *Arch Environ Health.* 1981;36:66–73.

147. Gardner G, Frank AL, Taber L. Effects of social and family factors on viral respiratory infection and illness in the first year of life. *J Epidemiol Community Health.* 1984;38:42–48.

148. Taylor B, Wadsworth J. Maternal smoking during pregnancy and lower respiratory tract illness early in life. *Arch Dis Child.* 1987;62:786–789.

149. Comstock GW, Meyer MB, Helsing KJ, et al. Respiratory effects of household exposures to tobacco smoke and gas cooking. *Am Rev Respir Dis.* 1981;124:143–148.

150. Melia RJW, Florey CduV, Darby SC, et al. Differences in NO2 levels in kitchens with gas or electric cookers. *Atmospheric Environ.* 1978;12:1379–1381.

151. Spangler JD, Duffy CP, Letz R, et al. Nitrogen-dioxide inside and outside 137 homes and implications for ambient air quality standards and health effects research. *Environ Sci Technol.* 1983;17:164–168.

152. Ware JH, Dockery DW, Spiro A, et al. Passive smoking, gas cooking and respiratory health of children living in six cities. *Am Rev Respir Dis.* 1984;129:366–374.

153. Melia RJ, Florey CduV, Altman DC, et al. Association between gas cooking and respiratory disease in children. *Br Med J.* 1977;2: 149–152.

154. Melia RJ, Florey C duV, Chinn S. The relation between respiratory illness in primary school children and the use of gas for cooking. I. Results from a national survey. *Int J Epidemiol.* 1979;8:333–338.

155. Keller MD, Lanese RR, Mitchell RI, et al. Respiratory illness in households using gas and electricity for cooking. I. Survey of incidence. *Environ Res.* 1979;19:495–503.

156. Keller MD, Lanese RR, Mitchell RI, et al. Respiratory illness in households using gas and electricity for cooking. II. Symptoms and objective findings. *Environ Res.* 1979;19:504–515.

157. Graham NMH. *Psychosocial Factors in the Epidemiology of Acute Respiratory Infection* [MD thesis]. Adelaide, South Australia: University of Adelaide; 1987.

158. Samet JM, Marbury MC, Spangler JD. Health effects and sources of indoor air pollution. Part 1. *Am Rev Respir Dis.* 1987;136: 1486–1508.

159. Smith KR, Aggarwal AL, Dave RM. Air pollution and rural biomass fuel in developing countries: a pilot study in India and implications for research and policy. *Atmospheric Environ.* 1983;17:2343–2362.

160. Dennis RJ, Maldonado D, Norman S, et al. Woodsmoke exposure and risk for obstructive airways disease among women. *Chest.* 1996;109:115–119.

161. Pandey MR, Boleij JSM, Smith KR, et al. Indoor air pollution in developing countries and acute respiratory infection in children. *Lancet.* 1989;1:427–429.

162. Kossove D. Smoke-filled rooms and lower respiratory disease in infants. *S Afr Med J.* 1982;61:622–624.

163. Campbell H, Armstrong JRM, Byass P. Indoor air pollution in developing countries and acute respiratory infection in children. *Lancet.* 1989;1:1012.

164. Campbell H, Byass P, Greenwood BM. Simple clinical signs for the diagnosis of acute respiratory infections. *Lancet.* 1988;2:742–743.

165. Honicky RE, Osborne JS, Akpom CA. Symptoms of respiratory illness in young children and the use of wood-burning stoves for indoor heating. *Pediatrics.* 1985;75:587–593.

166. Osborne JS III, Honicky RE. Chest illness in young children and indoor heating with wood [abstract]. *Am Rev Respir Dis.* 1989;139(suppl): A29.

167. Tuthill RW. Woodstoves, formaldehyde, and respiratory disease. *Am J Epidemiol.* 1984;120:952–955.

168. Doll R, Hill AB. Lung cancer and other causes of death in relation to smoking. *Br Med J.* 1956;2:1071–1081.

169. Hammond EC, Horn D. Smoking and death rates: report on forty-four months of follow-up on 187,783 men. I. Total mortality. *JAMA.* 1958;166:1159–1172.

170. Hammond EC, Horn D. Smoking and death rates: report on forty-four months of follow-up on 187,783 men. II. Death rates by cause. *JAMA.* 1958;166:1294–1308.

171. Dorn HF. The mortality of smokers and nonsmokers. *Am Stat Assoc Proc Soc Stat Sect.* 1958;1:34–71.

172. Dunn JE, Linden G, Breslow L. Lung cancer mortality experience of men in certain occupations in California. *Am J Public Health.* 1960;50:1475–1487.

173. Bes EWR, Josie GH, Walker CB. A Canadian study of mortality in relation to smoking habits, a preliminary report. *Can J Public Health.* 1961;52:99–106.

174. US Public Health Service. *Smoking and Health.* Report of the advisory committee to the Surgeon General of the Public Health Service. Atlanta, Ga: US Department of Health, Education and Welfare, Public Health Service, Centers for Disease Control; 1964 (PHS publication no. 1103).

175. Finklea JF, Sandifer SH, Smith DD. Cigarette smoking and epidemic influenza. *Am J Epidemiol.* 1969;90:390–399.

176. Mackenzie JS, Mackenzie IM, Holt PG. The effect of cigarette smoking on susceptibility to epidemic influenza and on serological responses to live attenuated and killed subunit influenza vaccines. *J Hyg (Camb).* 1976;77:409–417.

177. Kark JD, Lebuish M. Smoking and epidemic influenza-like illness in female military recruits: a brief survey. *Am J Public Health.* 1981;71:530–532.

178. Kark JD, Lebuish M, Rannon L. Cigarette smoking as a risk factor for epidemic a (h1n1) influenza in young men. *N Engl J Med.* 1982;307:1042–1046.

179. Monto AS, Higgins MW, Ross HW. The Tecumseh study of respiratory illness. VIII. Acute infection in chronic respiratory disease and comparison groups. *Am Rev Respir Dis.* 1975;111:27–36.

180. Holland WW, Elliott A. Cigarette smoking, respiratory symptoms and antismoking propaganda. *Lancet.* 1968;1:41–43.

181. Colley JRT, Douglas JWB, Reid DD. Respiratory disease in young adults: influence of early childhood lower respiratory tract illness, social class, air pollution and smoking. *Br Med J.* 1973;3:195–198.

182. Rush D. Respiratory symptoms in a group of American secondary school students: the overwhelming association with cigarette smoking. *Int J Epidemiol.* 1974;3:153–165.

183. Reingold AL. Role of *Legionellae* in acute infections of the lower respiratory tract. *Rev Infect Dis.* 1988;10:1018–1028.

184. Lipsky BA, Boyko EJ, Inui TS, et al. Risk factors for acquiring pneumococcal infections. *Arch Intern Med.* 1986;146:2179–2185.

185. Petitti DB, Friedman GD. Respiratory morbidity in smokers of low and high yield cigarettes. *Prev Med.* 1985;14:217–225.

186. Simberkoff MS, Cross AP, Al-Ibrabim M, et al. Efficacy of pneumococcal vaccine in high risk patients. Results of a Veterans Administration cooperative study. *N Engl J Med.* 1986;315:1318–1327.

187. Woodhead MA, MacFarlane JT, McCracken JS, et al. Prospective study of the aetiology and outcome of pneumonia in the community. *Lancet.* 1987;1:671–674.

188. US Department of Health and Human Services. *Reducing the Consequences of Smoking; 25 Years of Progress.* Atlanta, Ga: US Department of Health and Human Services, Public Health Service, Centers for Disease Control; 1989 (DHHS publication no. (CDC)89–8411).

189. Woods HM. The influence of external factors on the mortality from pneumonia in childhood and later adult life. *J Hyg (Camb)*. 1927;26:36–43.

190. Finland M. Pneumococcal infections. In: Evans AS, Feldman HA, eds. *Bacterial Infections in Humans. Epidemiology and Control*. New York, NY: Plenum; 1982.

191. Payling-Wright G, Payling-Wright H. Etiological factors in broncho-pneumonia amongst infants in London. *J Hyg (Camb)*. 1945; 44:15–30.

192. Leeder S, Corkhill R, Irwig LM, et al. Influence of family factors on the incidence of lower respiratory illness during the first year of life. *Br J Prev Soc Med*. 1976;30:203–212.

193. Monto AS, Ross HW. Acute respiratory illness in the community: effect of family composition, smoking and chronic symptoms. *Br J Prev Soc Med*. 1977;31:101–108.

194. Strangert K. Respiratory illness in preschool children with different forms of day care. *Pediatrics*. 1976;57:191–196.

195. Bell DM, Gleiber UW, Mercer AA, et al. Illness associated with child day care: a study of incidence and cost. *Am J Public Health*. 1989;79:479–484.

196. Strangert K. Otitis media in young children in different types of day-care. *Scand J Infect Dis*. 1977;9:113–123.

197. Vinther B, Pederson CB, Elbrond O. Otitis media in childhood. Sociomedical aspects with special reference to day care conditions. *Clin Otolaryngol*. 1984;9:3–8.

198. Silipa M, Karma P, Pukander J, et al. The Bayesian approach to the evaluation of risk factors in acute and recurrent otitis media. *Acta Otolaryngol*. 1988;106:94–101.

199. Moore PS, Marfin AA, Quenomoen LE, et al. Mortality rates in displaced and resident populations of central Somalia during the famine of 1992. *Lancet*. 1993;341:935–938.

200. Marfin AA, Moore J, Collins C, et al. Infectious disease surveillance during emergency relief to Bhutanese refugees in Nepal. *JAMA*. 1994;272:377–381.

201. Aaby P, Bukh J, Lisse IM, et al. Decline in measles mortality: nutrition, age at infection or exposure. *Br Med J*. 1988;296:1226–1228.

202. Aaby P. Malnutrition and overcrowding/intensive exposure in severe measles infection: review of community studies. *Rev Infect Dis*. 1988;10:478–491.

203. Tupasi TE, Velmonte MA, Sanvictores MEG, et al. Determinants of morbidity and mortality due to acute respiratory infections: implications for intervention. *J Infect Dis*. 1988;157:615–623.

204. Fonseca W, Kirkwood BR, Victora CG, Fuchs SR, Flores JA, Misago C. Risk factors for childhood pneumonia among the urban poor in Fortaleza, Brazil: a case-control study. *Bull WHO*. 1996;74:199–208.

205. Sommer A, Tarwotjo I, Hussaini G, et al. Increased mortality in mild vitamin A deficiency. *Lancet*. 1983;2:585–588.

206. Sommer A, Katz J, Tarwotjo I. Increased risk of respiratory disease and diarrhea in children with pre-existing mild vitamin A deficiency. *Am J Clin Nutr*. 1984;40:1090–1095.

207. Bloem MW, Wedel M, Egger RJ, et al. Mild vitamin A deficiency and risk of respiratory tract diseases and diarrhea in preschool and school children in northeastern Thailand. *Am J Epidemiol*. 1990;131: 332–339.

208. Pinnock CB, Douglas RM, Badcock NR. Vitamin A status in children who are prone to respiratory tract infections. *Aust Paediatr J.* 1986;22:95–99.

209. Pinnock CB, Douglas RM, Martin AJ, et al. Vitamin A status of children with a history of respiratory syncytial virus infection in infancy. *Aust Paediatr J.* 1988;24:286–289.

210. Forman MR, Gravbard BI, Hoffman HJ, et al. The Pima infant feeding study: breast feeding and respiratory infections in the first year of life. *Int J Epidemol.* 1984;13:447–453.

211. Victora C, Smith PG, Vaughan JP, et al. Evidence of protection by breast feeding against infant deaths from infectious diseases in Brazil. *Lancet.* 1987;2:319–322.

212. Saarinen UM. Prolonged breast feeding as a prophylaxis for recurrent otitis media. *Acta Paediatr Scand.* 1982;71:567–571.

213. Teele DW, Klein JO, Rosner B, et al. Epidemiology of otitis media during the first seven years of life in children in greater Boston: a prospective cohort study. *J Infect Dis.* 1989;160:83–94.

214. Pullan CR, Toms GL, Martin AJ, et al. Breast feeding and respiratory syncytial virus infection. *Br Med J.* 1980;281:1034–1036.

215. Watkins CJ, Leeder SR, Corkhill RT. The relationship between breast and bottle feeding and respiratory illness in the first year of life. *J Epidemiol Community Health.* 1979;33:180–182.

216. Taylor B, Wadsworth J, Golding J, et al. Breast-feeding, bronchitis, and admissions for lower respiratory illness and gastroenteritis during the first five years. *Lancet.* 1982;1:1227–1229.

217. Fergusson DM, Horwood LJ, Shannon FT, et al. Infant health and breast feeding during the first 16 weeks of life. *Austr Paediatr J.* 1978;14:254–258.

218. Fergusson DM, Horwood LJ, Shannon FT, et al. Breast feeding, gastrointestinal and lower respiratory illness in the first two years. *Austr Paediatr J.* 1981;17:191–195.

219. Tracey VV, De NC, Harper JR. Obesity and respiratory infection in infants and young children. *Br Med J.* 1971;1:16–18.

220. Wright AL, Holberg CJ, Martinex FD, et al. Breast feeding and lower respiratory tract illness in the first year of life. *Br Med J.* 1989;229:946–949.

221. Tyrell DAJ, Wallace-Craig J, Meade TW, et al. A trial of ascorbic acid in the treatment of the common cold. *Br J Prev Soc Med.* 1977;31:189–191.

222. Pitt HA, Costrini AM. Vitamin C prophylaxis in marine recruits. *JAMA.* 1979;241:908–911.

223. Strachan DP, Anderson HR, Bland JM, et al. Asthma as a link between chest illness in childhood and chronic cough and phlegm in young adults. *Br Med J.* 1988;296:890–893.

224. Weiss ST, Tager IB, Muñoz A, et al. The relationship of respiratory infections in early childhood to the occurrence of increased levels of bronchial responsiveness and atrophy. *Am Rev Respir Dis.* 1985;131:573–578.

225. Woolcock AJ, Leeder SR, Pear JK, et al. The influence of lower respiratory illness in infancy and childhood and subsequent cigarette smoking on lung function in Sydney school children. *Am Rev Respir Dis.* 1979;120:5–14.

226. Kattan M, Keens TG, Lapierre JG, et al. Pulmonary function abnormalities in symptom-free children after bronchiolitis. *Pediatrics.* 1977;59:883–888.

227. Mok JYQ, Simpson H. Outcome for acute bronchitis, bronchiolitis, and pneumonia in infancy. *Arch Dis Child.* 1984;59;306–309.

228. Douglas RM, Miles HB. Vaccination against *Streptococcus pneumoniae* in childhood: lack of a demonstrable benefit in young Australian children. *J Infect Dis.* 1984;149:861–869.

229. Barker DJP, Osmond C. Childhood respiratory infection and adult chronic bronchitis in England and Wales. *Br Med J.* 1986;293: 1271–1275.

230. Belfer ML, Shader RI, DiMascio A, et al. Stress and bronchitis. *Br Med J.* 1968;3:805–806.

231. Jacobs MA, Spilken AZ, Norman MM, et al. Life stress and respiratory illness. *Psychosom Med.* 1970;32:233–242.

232. Belfer ML, Shader RI, DiMascio A, et al. Stress and bronchitis. *Br Med J.* 1968;3:805–806.

233. Boyce WT, Jensen EW, Cassel JC, et al. Influence of life events and family routines on childhood respiratory tract illness. *Pediatrics.* 1977;60:609–615.

234. Stout CW, Bloom LJ. Type A behavior and upper respiratory infections. *J Human Stress.* 1981;8:4–7.

235. Hart H, Bax M, Jenkins S. Health and behavior in preschool children. *Child Care Health Dev.* 1984;10:1–16.

236. Foulke FG, Reeb KG, Graham AV, et al. Family function, respiratory illness and otitis media in urban black infants. *Fam Med.* 1988;20: 128–132.

237. Graham NMH, Douglas RM, Ryan P. Stress and acute respiratory infection. *Am J Epidemiol.* 1986;124:389–401.

238. Kasl SV, Evans AS, Niederman JC. Psychosocial risk factors in the development of infectious mononucleosis. *Psychosom Med.* 1979;41:445–466.

239. Meyer RJ, Haggerty RJ. Streptococcal infections in families: factors altering susceptibility. *Pediatrics.* 1962:29:539–549.

240. Totman R, Kiff J, Reed SE, et al. Predicting experimental colds in volunteers from different measures of life stress. *J Psychosom Res.* 1950;24:155–163.

241. Totman R, Reed SE, Craig JW. Cognitive dissonance, stress and virus-induced common colds. *J Psychosom Res.* 1977;21:51–61.

242. Broadbent DE, Broadhent MHP, Philpotts RJ, et al. Some further studies on the prediction of experimental colds in volunteers by psychological factors. *J Psychosom Res.* 1984;28:511–523.

243. Kiecolt-Glaser JK, Glaser R. Psychological influences on immunity. *Psychosomatics.* 1986;27:621–624.

244. Dick EC, Houssain SV, Mink KA, et al. Interruption of transmission of rhinovirus colds among human volunteers using virucidal paper handkerchiefs. *J Infect Dis.* 1986;153:352–356.

245. Gwaltney JM, Moskolski PB, Hendley JO. Hand-to-hand transmission of rhinovirus colds. *Ann Intern Med.* 1978;88:463–467.

246. Gwaltney JM Jr, Hendley JO. Transmission of experimental rhinovirus infection by contaminated surfaces. *Am J Epidemiol.* 1982;116: 828–833.

247. Schenker MB, Samet JM, Speizer FE. Risk factors for childhood respiratory disease. The effect of host factors and home environmental exposures. *Am Rev Respir Dis.* 1983;128:1038–1043.

248. Graham NMH, Woodward AJ, Ryan P, et al. Acute respiratory illness in Adelaide children. II. The relationship of maternal stress, social supports and family functioning. *Int J Epidemiol.* 1990;19:937–944.

249. Dingle JM, Badger GF, Jordan WS Jr. *Illness in the Home. A Study of 25,000 Illnesses in a Group of Cleveland Families.* Cleveland, Ohio: Western Reserve University; 1964.

250. Beem MO. Acute respiratory illness in nursery school children: a longitudinal study of the occurrence of illness and respiratory viruses. *Am J Epidemiol.* 1969;90:30–44.

251. Hendley JO, Gwaltney JM Jr, Jordan WS Jr. Rhinovirus infections in an industrial population. IV. Infections within families of employees during two fall peaks of respiratory illness. *Am J Epidemiol.* 1969;89:184–196.

252. Douglas RG Jr, Lindgram KM, Cough RB. Exposure to cold environment and rhinovirus cold. Failure to demonstrate an effect. *N Engl J Med.* 1968;279:742–747.

253. Christie AB. *Infectious Diseases: Epidemiology and Clinical Practice.* Edinburgh, Scotland: Churchill Livingstone; 1974.

254. Jackson GG, Muldoon RL, Johnson GC, et al. Contribution of volunteers to studies of the common cold. *Am Rev Respir Dis.* 1963;88(suppl):120–127.

255. Young M. The influence of weather conditions on the mortality from bronchitis and pneumonia in children. *J Hyg.* 1924;23:151–175.

256. Gwaltney JM. Epidemiology of the common cold. *Ann N Y Acad Sci.* 1980;353:54–60.

257. D'Souza RM. Care-seeking behavior. *Clin Infect Dis.* 1999;28:234.

258. D'Souza RM. *Household Determinants of Childhood Mortality: Illness Management in Karachi Slums.* Canberra, Australia: National Centre for Epidemiology and Population Health, the Australian National University; 1997:316.

259. Kundi MZM, Anjum M, Mull DS, Mull JD. Maternal perceptions of pneumonia and pneumonia signs in Pakistani children. *Soc Sci Med.* 1993;37:649–660.

260. Rahaman MM, Aziz KMS, Munshi MH, Patwari Y, Rahman M. A diarrhea clinic in rural Bangladesh: influence of distance, age and sex on attendance and diarrheal mortality. *Am J Public Health.* 1982;72:1124–1128.

261. Hughes WT. *Pneumocystis carinii* pneumonia. *N Engl J Med.* 1987;317:1021–1023.

262. Rubinstein A, Sicklick M, Gupta A, et al. Acquired immunodeficiency with reversed T4/T8 ratios in infants born to promiscuous and drug addicted mothers. *JAMA.* 1983;249:2350–2356.

263. Oleske J, Minnefar AB, Cooper B, et al. Immune deficiency syndrome in children. *JAMA.* 1983;249:2345–2349.

264. Scott GB, Buck BE, Leterman JG, et al. Acquired immunodeficiency syndrome in infants. *N Engl J Med.* 1984;310:76–81.

265. Leigh TR, Parsons P, Hume C, et al. Sputum induction for diagnosis of *Pneumocystis carinii* pneumonia. *Lancet.* 1989;2:205–206.

266. Bernstein LJ, Krieger BZ, Novick B, et al. Bacterial infection in the acquired immunodeficiency syndrome. *Pediatr Infect Dis J.* 1985;4:472–475.

267. Schlamm HT, Yancowitz SR. *Haemophilus influenzae* pneumonia in young adults with AIDS, ARC, or risk of AIDS. *Am J Med.* 1989;86:11–14.

268. Rolston KVI, Uribe-Botero G, Mansell PWA. Bacterial infections in adult patients with the acquired immune deficiency syndrome

(AIDS) and AIDS-related complex. *Am J Med.* 1987;83: 604–605.

269. Witt DJ, Craven DE, McCabe WR. Bacterial infections in adult patients with the acquired immune deficiency syndrome (AIDS) and AIDS-related complex. *Am J Med.* 1987;82:900–906.
270. White S, Tsou E, Waldhorn RE, et al. Life-threatening bacterial pneumonia in male homosexuals with laboratory features of the acquired immunodeficiency syndrome. *Chest.* 1985;87: 486–488.
271. Selwyn PA, Feingold AR, Martel D, et al. Increased risk of bacterial pneumonia in HIV-infected intravenous drug users without AIDS. *AIDS.* 1988;2:267–272.
272. Murray JF, Garay SM, Hopewell PC, et al. Pulmonary complications of the acquired immunodeficiency syndrome: an update. *Am Rev Respir Dis.* 1987;135:504–509.
273. Biggar RJ, Bouvet E, Ebbeen P, et al. Clinical features of AIDS in Europe. *Eur J Cancer Clin Oncol.* 1984;20:165–167.
274. Hira SK, Ngandu N, Wadhawan D, et al. Clinical and epidemiological features of HIV infection at a referral clinic in Zambia. *J Acquir Immune Defic Syndr.* 1990;3:87–91.
275. Piot P, Laga M, Ryder R, et al. The global epidemiology of HIV infection: continuity, heterogeneity, and change. *J Acquir Immune Defic Syndr.* 1990;3:403–412.
276. Drillien CM. A longitudinal study of the growth and development of prematurely and maturely born children. Part IV. Morbidity. *Arch Dis Child.* 1959;14:210–217.
277. Chan KN, Elliman A, Bryan E, et al. Respiratory symptoms in children of low birth weight. *Arch Dis Child.* 1989;64:1294–1304.
278. Victora CG, Smith PG, Barros FC, et al. Risk factors for deaths due to respiratory infections among Brazilian infants. *Int J Epidemiol.* 1989;18:918–925.
279. Datta N, Kumar V, Kumar L, et al. Application of a case management approach to the control of acute respiratory infections in low birth weight infants: a feasibility study. *Bull WHO.* 1987;65:77–82.
280. Caldwell JC, Reddy PH, Caldwell P. The social component of mortality decline: an investigation in South India employing alternative methodologies. *Population Studies.* 1983;37:185–205.
281. Abosede OA. Self-medication: an important aspect of primary health care. *Soc Sci Med.* 1984;19:699–703.
282. Colson AC. The differential use of medical resources in developing countries. *J Health Soc Behav.* 1971;12:226–237.
283. Liu C, Douglas RM. Chinese herbal medicine in the treatment of acute respiratory tract infections: review of randomized and controlled clinical trials. *Clin Infect Dis.* 1999;28:235–236.
284. Puck JM, Glezen WP, Frank AL, et al. Protection of infants from infection with influenza A virus by transplacentally acquired antibody. *J Infect Dis.* 1980;142:844–849.
285. Glezen WP, Paredes A, Allison JE, et al. Risk of respiratory syncytial virus infection for infants from low income families in relationship to age, sex, ethnic group and maternal antibody level. *J Pediatr.* 1981;98:708–715.
286. McConnochie KM, Roghmann KJ. Parental smoking, presence of older siblings and family history of asthma increase risk of bronchiolitis. *Am J Dis Child.* 1986;140:806–812.

287. Welliver RC, Wong DT, Sun M, et al. The development of respiratory syncytial virus specific IgE and the release of histamine in nasopharyngeal secretions after infection. *N Engl J Med.* 1981;305:841–846.

288. Welliver RC, Wong DT, Middleton E, et al. Role of parainfluenza virus specific IgE in pathogenesis of croup and wheezing subsequent to infection. *J Pediatr.* 1982;101:889–896.

289. Martinez FD, Morgan WJ, Wright AL, et al. Diminished lung function as a predisposing factor for wheezing respiratory illness in children. *N Engl J Med.* 1988; 319:1112–1117.

290. Speizer F, Comstock G. Recommended respiratory disease questionnaires for use with adults and children in epidemiological research. *Am Rev Respir Dis.* 1978;118:7–53.

291. Fletcher CM. Standardized questionnaire on respiratory symptoms. A statement prepared for and approved by the Medical Research Council's Committee on the Etiology for Chronic Bronchitis. *Br Med J.* 1960;2:1665.

292. Gold DR, Weiss ST, Tager IB, et al. Comparison of questionnaire and diary methods in acute childhood respiratory illness surveillance. *Am Rev Respir Dis.* 1989;139:847–849.

293. Miller DL. *Some Problems in the Classification of Acute Respiratory Infection in Young Children and Questionnaire Design.* (WHO/RSD/81.8). Geneva, Switzerland: World Health Organization; 1981.

294. Leventhal JM. Clinical predictors of pneumonia as a guide to ordering chest roentgenograms. *Clin Pediatr.* 1982;21:730–734.

295. Cherian T, John TJ, Simoes E, et al. Evaluation of simple clinical signs for the diagnosis of acute lower respiratory tract infection. *Lancet.* 1988;2:125–128.

296. Campbell H, Byass P, Greenwood BM. Simple clinical signs for the diagnosis of acute lower respiratory infections. *Lancet.* 1988;2:742–743.

297. Campbell H, Byass P, Lamont AC, et al. Assessment of clinical criteria for identification of severe acute lower respiratory tract infections in children. *Lancet.* 1989;1:297–299.

298. Centers for Disease Control and Prevention. Cigarette smoking among adults–United States, 2003. *MMWR.* 2005;54:509–512.

299. Yang G, Fan L, Tan J, et al. Smoking in China: findings of the 1996 National Prevalence Survey. *JAMA.* 1999;282:1247–1253.

300. Yang G, Ma J, Chen A, et al. Smoking cessation in China: findings from the 1996 National Prevalence Survey. *Tobacco Control.* 2001;10:170–174.

301. Centers for Disease Control and Prevention. Preventing pneumococcal disease among infants and young children: recommendations of the Advisory Committee on Immunization Practices (ACIP). *MMWR.* 2000;49(No RR-9).

302. Centers for Disease Control and Prevention. Direct and indirect effects of routine vaccination of children with 7-valent pneumococcal conjugate vaccine on incidence of invasive pneumococcal disease–United States, 1998-2003. *MMWR.* 2005;54:893–897.

303. Centers for Disease Control and Prevention. Behavioral Risk Factor Surveillance System (BRFSS). Available at: http://www.cdc.gov/brfss/index.htm. Accessed February 22, 2006.

304. Lieu TA, Ray GT, Black SB. Projected cost-effectiveness of pneumococcal conjugate vaccination of healthy infants and young children. *JAMA.* 2000;283:1460–1468.

305. Cutts FT, Zaman SMA, Enware G, et al. Efficacy of nine-valent pneumococcal conjugate vaccine against pneumonia and invasive pneumococcal disease in the Gambia: randomized, double-blind, placebo-controlled. *Lancet.* 2005;365:1139–1146.

306. Klugman KP, Madhi SA, Huebner RE, Kobberger R, Mbelle N, Pierce N. A trial of a 9-valent pneumococcal conjugate vaccine in children with and those without HIV infection. *N Engl J Med.* 2003;349:1341–1348.

307. Straus WL, Qazi SA, Kundi Z, Nomani NK, Shwartz B, the Pakistan Cotrimoxazole Study Group. Antimicrobial resistance and clinical effectiveness of cotrimoxazole versus amoxicillin for pneumonia among children in Pakistan: randomized controlled trial. *Lancet.* 1998;352:270–274.

308. Levine OS, Schwartz B, Pierce N, Kane M. Development, evaluation and implementation of *Haemophilus influenzae* type B vaccines for young children in developing countries: current status and priority actions. *Pediatr Infect Dis J.* 1998;17:S95–S113.

309. Heath PT. *Haemophilus influenzae* type b conjugate vaccines: a review of efficacy data. *Pediatr Infect Dis J.* 1998;17:S117–S122.

310. Peltola H, Kilpi T, Anttila M. Rapid disappearance of *Haemophilus influenzae* meningitis after routine childhood immunization with conjugate vaccines. *Lancet.* 1992;340:592–594.

311. Lee JW. *Haemophilus influenzae* in Asia. *Pediatr Infect Dis J.* 1998; 17:S92.

312. Gessner BD, Sutanto A, Linchn M, et al. Incidences of vaccine-preventable *haemophilus influenzae* type b pneumonia and meningitis in Indonesian children: hamlet-randomized vaccine-probe trial. *Lancet.* 2005;365:43–52.

313. Mulholland EK, Adegbola RA. The Gambian *Haemophilus influenzae* type 1 vaccine trial: what does it tell us about the burden of *Haemophilus influenzae* type b disease. *Pediatr Infect Dis J.* 1998;17: S123–S125.

314. Lagos R, Levine OS, Avendano A, Horwitz I, Levine MM. The introduction of routine *Haemophilus influenzae* type b conjugate vaccine in Chile: a framework for evaluating new vaccines in newly industrializing countries. *Pediatr Infect Dis J.* 1998;(suppl):S139–S148.

DIARRHEAL DISEASES

CHAPTER TWENTY

DIARRHEAL DISEASES

Robert E. Black and Claudio F. Lanata

Introduction

Diarrheal diseases are an important global problem, causing high rates of morbidity and mortality, particularly in developing countries.[1] Although mortality from infectious diarrheal diseases has been reduced to a low rate in economically developed countries, substantial morbidity and associated costs continue.[2-3] In addition, high rates of diarrhea in some settings, such as hospitals and day-care centers, and outbreaks of food-borne diarrhea have resulted in increased concern.[4-5]

Diarrheal diseases occur most frequently in the conditions of poor environmental sanitation and hygiene, inadequate water supplies, poverty, and limited education found especially in developing country settings. As these conditions improved over the last century in the now more economically developed countries, the burden of diarrheal diseases was greatly diminished.[6] Likewise, many developing countries are undergoing a similar economic, social, and epidemiologic transition with decreasing rates of diarrheal diseases. Unfortunately, nearly all countries in the world have populations still living in poor environmental conditions and poverty who will continue to have high rates of diarrhea and diarrheal mortality.

From the beginning of the 1980s, substantial global efforts were directed at reduction of diarrheal disease mortality.[7] It was recognized that dehydration as a result of diarrhea played a substantial part in the fatal illnesses and that this dehydration could be prevented or treated with oral fluid and electrolyte replacement, along with continued feeding. This low-tech approach made effective therapy more widely available through national diarrheal disease control programs in developing countries. Similar clinical approaches have also improved the management of diarrhea in the United States, resulting in improved therapy and a reduction in diarrhea-related mortality. With the consequent reduction in diarrheal deaths due to dehydration, attention has been directed at dysentery and persistent diarrhea, which are also major causes of diarrhea-related mortality. In addition, increased efforts are being directed at prevention of diarrhea through research on the etiology, epidemiology, and transmission patterns of diarrheal diseases.

General Epidemiology

Definitions

Diarrhea is a symptom complex characterized by stools of decreased consistency and increased number. Although it is possible to define diarrhea as the occurrence of these symptoms simply in comparison to that individual's prior bowel pattern, epidemiologic studies have usually used a more generalizable definition.[8] Most studies now define diarrhea as three or more liquid stools during a 24-hour period. At least 2 days free of diarrhea are usually required to define an episode as terminated. Dysentery is a diarrheal disease defined by the presence of blood in loose or liquid stools.

Although most diarrheal episodes resolve within a week, a small proportion continue for 2 weeks or more.[9] Studies in many countries show that the distribution of episode durations is continuous, but skewed toward the longer durations. Thus, any definition of "persistent" diarrhea is arbitrary, but nevertheless having a definition is useful for research and disease control purposes. The World Health Organization defines persistent diarrhea operationally as an episode that lasts for at least 14 days. This definition of persistent diarrhea identifies children that tend to have a very high prevalence of diarrhea from both acute and persistent episodes.[10-11] The term *persistent diarrhea*, as used by WHO, encompasses episodes that begin acutely and continue for longer than their expected duration and is not intended to include infrequent diarrheal disorders, such as hereditary syndromes, gluten-sensitive enteropathy, or other noninfectious conditions.

Sources of Data

Data to describe the epidemiology of diarrheal diseases come from three main sources: (1) prospective studies in households or health facilities, (2) passive or active surveillance systems, and (3) outbreak investigations. Surveys may also provide limited types of information.

Prospective studies in households in developing countries have generally used visits by health workers at an interval of no more than one week to collect data on symptoms and to obtain specimens of stool for etiologic testing. Such studies in more developed countries often use a combination of household visits and telephone contacts. Prospective studies in health facilities may be done in general outpatient clinics, hospital wards, or special populations, such as studies of nosocomial infections in newborn nurseries.

Passive surveillance is based on routine reports by health care workers of a specified disease to public health officials. Active surveillance is when cases are ascertained by the researcher querying health workers or laboratories about a specific disease. Passive surveillance can be done on a wide scale and is relatively inexpensive, but its value may be limited by reporting that is incomplete, biased, and delayed. Active surveillance of selected diseases might be appropriate if there is a need for more complete and timely information. In general, developing countries do not have useful passive or active surveillance as a routine system for diarrheal diseases. In the United States, surveillance systems exist for only a limited number of diarrheal diseases or pathogens that are reported through laboratory-based passive surveillance.

Investigation of outbreaks of diarrheal diseases can be very useful to rapidly develop information on the risk factors, transmission patterns, and control measures for enteric pathogens. Such investigations can lead to controls to contain that outbreak, as well as help develop measures to prevent future outbreaks.

In developing countries, surveys are commonly conducted to obtain information about health conditions and the use of health services. Although information on the presence of diarrhea in the respondent on the day of survey can be reported accurately, these data may be a biased indicator of the incidence of infectious diarrhea because the symptom of diarrhea is frequent, commonly mild, and may be impacted by seasonal variations. Surveys of patients or their families may provide information on recent more clear and memorable events such as hospitalization or death from diarrheal diseases or medical care received for current episodes.

Incidence

A summary of prospective, community-based studies in developing countries concluded that the median annual incidence of all diarrhea in children under 5 years of age was 3.5 episodes.[12] Diarrheal incidence has varied in the different settings in which it has been studied (Table 20-1). This variation could be due to methodologic differences, such as the definition of diarrhea, or surveillance techniques used in the study. In community-based studies the incidence has been highest in studies with a small number of children under surveillance and with more frequent home visiting, suggesting that the other studies may have found lower rates because of underreporting.[13] At the same time, it is likely that there are actual differences in the incidence of diarrhea in different populations due to different environmental and host risk factors, as

TABLE 20-1   Diarrhea Incidence and Duration in Children Aged <6 Years in Community-Based Studies in Developing Countries

Study	Age Group (months)	Episodes	Diarrheal Incidence (per 100 child-years)	Diarrheal Duration (days)		
				1–7	8–14	≥15
Bangladesh	0–59	941	557	66	21	14
Brazil	0–71	519	600	82	15	3
India	0–71	471	61	35	55	10
Brazil	0–60	2896	1140	76	13	11
Peru	0–35	5302	807	88	9	3
Bangladesh	0–59	2609	455	71	22	7
Bangladesh	0–71	1074	195	50	27	23

well as the relative frequency of various enteropathogens. Both methodologic and setting-specific differences may also affect the distribution of diarrheal episode durations. Studies that have the most intensive and frequent surveillance are most likely to identify mild and short-duration episodes that might not otherwise be reported with less intensive case finding.

In developing countries, the incidence of diarrhea varies greatly with age. Generally the first 2 years of life have the highest incidence followed by a decline with increasing age. Peak incidence is often at 6–17 months of age (Figure 20-1). The incidence in boys and girls is generally similar, or slightly higher in boys; however, in some countries boys may be taken to health facilities more often, giving the appearance of higher rates of diarrhea.

In the United States the Centers for Disease Control and Prevention (CDC) has estimated that there are 21–37 million episodes of diarrhea each year in children under 5 years of age; approximately 10% of these illnesses led to a visit to a physician.[14] It has also been estimated that food-borne disease, which is predominantly diarrheal disease, accounts for over 80 million illnesses each year in the United States.[15] A prospective community-based study found an annual incidence rate of diarrhea in persons of all ages of 0.63 episodes per person-year of observation.[16] The highest incidence was in infants who had a rate of 1.43 episodes per person-year. In developed countries the elderly are also at particular risk of diarrheal diseases. Adults in long-term care facilities have greater morbidity and mortality from diarrheal diseases either because of underlying conditions or increased risk of

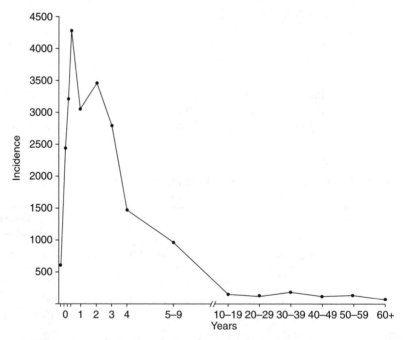

FIGURE 20-1   Annual age-specific incidence of diarrhea per 1000 person-years assessed by household surveillance.
Source: R.E. Black et al., Incidence and Severity of Rotavirus and *Escherichia coli* Diarrhea in Rural Bangladesh, *Lancet*, Vol. 1, p. 142, © by The Lancet Ltd., 1981, with permission from Elsevier.

nosocomial transmission. Children attending day-care centers have a higher incidence due to person-to-person transmission within these settings.

Another group of individuals from developed countries who are at increased risk of diarrhea are those who travel to developing countries.[17] Numerous studies have demonstrated that about half of such travelers will develop diarrhea during a trip of approximately 2 weeks.

Impact of Diarrhea

It is well appreciated that diarrheal diseases are important causes of death in developing countries. In 2005, WHO reported approximately 1.8 million diarrheal deaths in the developing world among children under 5 years of age each year.[1] This is substantially less than the estimate based on data from the 1980s (3.3 million child deaths)[13] or from the 1990s (2.5 million child deaths).[18] The diarrheal mortality rate is highest in the first year of life.

The case fatality rates in children in developing countries have been reported to range from 0.1% to 0.5% in settings as diverse as urban Central African Republic, rural Egypt, rural North India, and rural Indonesia. It has been estimated that overall the diarrheal case fatality rate in children under 5 years of age in developing countries is 0.2%. The case fatality rate is highest in the youngest children. In rural India, the case fatality rate for persistent diarrhea was reported to be 20 times higher than that for acute diarrhea.[19]

In more developed countries, the diarrheal mortality rate and the illness case fatality rate are very low.[2,14] Although the highest incidence of diarrheal disease is in children, it is likely that there are fewer than 100 deaths per year from diarrheal disease in the United States. Nearly all of the deaths in the United States are in adults, with two thirds of these being in the elderly.

In developing countries, the infectious diseases of childhood have an adverse effect on growth. Diarrheal diseases have the greatest effect of all the infectious diseases, possibly because of reduction in appetite, altered feeding practices, and decreased absorption of nutrients, along with the very high prevalence of diarrhea in young children in these settings.[20] The magnitude of the effect of diarrheal diseases on growth seems to be modified by a number of factors. Continued breast-feeding and continued feeding during diarrhea can prevent weight faltering. In addition, children who consume a good diet will not only better withstand the illness, but also have the potential to grow more rapidly after the illness to recover from any weight loss. Because most children in developed countries usually have appropriate treatment and are receiving an adequate diet, the growth effects of diarrhea, especially given the low prevalence of the illness, is probably very small. Infections in the first 6 months of life may result in greater long-term deficits in linear growth than later infections.[21]

Diarrheal diseases are an economic burden because of the costs of medical care, medications, and lost work. Because the illnesses can largely be managed by fluid and nutritional therapy, much of the medication use, such as antibiotics and so-called antidiarrheal drugs, are an unnecessary expense and are potentially hazardous. The micronutrient zinc, given orally, was recently recommended by the World Health Organization and UNICEF[22] as an inexpensive therapeutic adjunct to oral rehydration therapy for treatment of acute diarrhea.

Microbial Etiologies

Relative Importance of Enteropathogens

A large number of bacterial, viral, and parasitic agents have been associated with diarrhea in both developing and developed countries. Because the highest rates of diarrheal diseases and the most severe consequences are generally in young children, most studies have focused on this age group. Older children and adults may become ill from the same enteropathogens, but the relative frequencies of these organisms varies because of immunity acquired from prior infection or from differential exposure to the various pathogens.

Community-based studies are those in which household visits are made to identify cases of diarrhea and to collect fecal specimens for identification of enteropathogens. Because these studies ascertain cases without regard to severity or care seeking, they are the best measure of the overall incidence of diarrheal disease. Based on a review of 61 studies (published 1990–2002) with comprehensive microbiology from developing countries, enterotoxigenic *Escherichia coli* (ETEC) constituted the largest proportion of episodes with a median of 14.1% (Table 20-2). The next most commonly found organism has been *Giardia lamblia*. *Campylobacter* species, enteropathogenic *E. coli*, and rotavirus were identified in 7–8% of these diarrheal episodes. Other organisms were less frequent. The relative importance of these organisms was rather variable in the different studies.

Studies in health facilities, either outpatient clinics or hospital wards, represent a more selected group of patients who have sought care because of an illness of greater severity. A review of 98 studies done in health facilities in developing countries found that rotavirus was the most frequent enteropathogen with a median of 18% (Table 20-3). However, these studies demonstrated

TABLE 20-2   Percentage Identification of Selected Enteropathogens in Children with Diarrhea in Community-Based Studies in Developing Countries (61 studies)

Enteropathogen	Median (%)	Interquartile Range (%)
Campylobacter sp	7.6	3.9–13.4
Cryptosporidium parvum	5.7	3.8–8.5
Entameba histolytica	3.5	0.8–5.8
Enteropathogenic *Escherichia coli*	8.8	6.6–13.2
Enterotoxigenic *Escherichia coli*	14.1	6.7–22.6
Giardia lamblia	10.2	7.4–18.8
Rotavirus	8.0	4.2–15.3
Salmonella sp	0.9	0.2–3.1
Shigella sp	4.6	2.2–7.6

that bacterial pathogens predominated overall, accounting for about 40% of illnesses. Of these, the most common was *C. jejuni*. As illustrated in the range of percentage identification in Table 20-3, each of these bacterial pathogens can be very frequent in some settings. Among the parasites, *C. parvum* and *G. lamblia* were the most frequently identified. A review of 107 studies in hospitalized children found that rotavirus was the most common pathogen, followed by ETEC (Table 20-4). A number of recent studies in hospitalized children with diarrhea in East Asian countries have found that 40–60% had rotavirus identified.[23,24]

In general, community-based studies identified an enteropathogen in approximately half of the episodes, and the health facility-based studies identified an enteropathogen in about 75% of the episodes. The detection tests for many of the enteropathogens do not have optimal sensitivity, so these studies may have underestimated their incidence. In addition, there are other known enteropathogens that were not evaluated in most of these studies. Although it

TABLE 20-3   Percentage Identification of Selected Enteropathogens in Children with Diarrhea in Outpatient Clinic Studies in Developing Countries (98 studies)

Enteropathogen	Median (%)	Interquartile Range (%)
Campylobacter sp	12.6	4.0–16.7
Cryptosporidium parvum	2.5	0.8–4.0
Entameba histolytica	0.6	0.1–1.4
Enteropathogenic *Escherichia coli*	9.1	4.5–19.4
Enterotoxigenic *Escherichia coli*	8.7	5.2–15.3
Giardia lamblia	3.0	1.2–5.7
Rotavirus	18.0	13.3–30.7
Salmonella sp	3.2	1.3–6.7
Shigella sp	5.8	2.4–11.0

TABLE 20-4   Percentage Identification of Selected Enteropathogens in Children with Diarrhea in Hospital Studies in Developing Countries (107 studies)

Enteropathogen	Median (%)	Interquartile Range (%)
Campylobacter sp	4.5	2.3–9.9
Cryptosporidium parvum	3.4	1.3–7.9
Entameba histolytica	0.7	0.2–3.7
Enteropathogenic *Escherichia coli*	15.6	8.3–27.5
Enterotoxigenic *Escherichia coli*	9.5	6.4–16.1
Giardia lamblia	1.6	0.5–5.5
Rotavirus	25.4	17.0–37.7
Salmonella sp	4.4	2.9–8.4
Shigella sp	5.6	2.8–10.4

is likely that these enteropathogens may individually account for only a small proportion of the episodes, collectively they may cause many of the episodes not associated with one of the more common enteropathogens. Among the other enteropathogens are viral agents, such as adenovirus, astrovirus, and norovirus.[25,26] Noroviruses may be responsible for a substantial number of illnesses with diarrhea and/or vomiting. Other enteropathogens of unknown importance are *Bacteroides fragilis* and *Clostridium difficile*,[27] particularly among patients taking antibiotics.[28]

The identification of an enteropathogen from feces during diarrhea does not necessarily mean that that organism is causing the illness. In fact, studies that have performed comprehensive microbiology often find two or more enteropathogens simultaneously, and it is difficult to assign causality. These mixed infections could occur because the individual is exposed simultaneously or sequentially or an individual may have an asymptomatic infection with one enteropathogen at the time of exposure to another.

Asymptomatic enteric infections are common in developing country populations and less so in developed country settings. In community-based studies, routine assessment of enteropathogens allows for a comparison between times when the children have diarrhea and when they are healthy. Community-based studies often find a similar rate of identification of enteropathogens in children when they have diarrhea and when they do not. For example, in nine community-based studies in developing countries the median identification of *Campylobacter* species was 8% during diarrhea compared to 7% when they did not (Table 20-5). Some enteropathogens, such as rotavirus, may have a higher rate of identification during diarrhea episodes. In health facility–based studies, children who came to the same facility for a reason other than diarrhea may be used as controls. Often the relative prevalence of different enteropathogens is more distinct between diarrhea cases and controls in these studies.

The pathogenicity (i.e., the number of infections with diarrhea/the total number of infections) varies by enteropathogen and in some cases by age (Table 20-6). For example, the pathogenicity of rotavirus is lower in the first 6 months of life than in the second 6 months, presumably due to passive protection from maternally derived antibody in early infancy.[29] On the other hand, some pathogens, such as *Shigella* species, may have a higher pathogenicity early in childhood. This may be because the initial infection induces some immunity, which protects more against subsequent illness than against infection.

TABLE 20-5   Median Percentage Identification of *Campylobacter* sp and Rotavirus from Cases of Diarrhea and Controls without Diarrhea in Community-Based Studies in Developing Countries

Enteropathogen	Community-Based Studies			Health Facility–Based Studies		
	(N)	Diarrhea	Control	(N)	Diarrhea	Control
Campylobacter sp	9	8	7	29	7	2
Rotavirus	11	4	1	31	21	4

TABLE 20-6 Pathogenicity of Selected Enteropathogens by Age Group in Peruvian Infants in a Community-Based Study

Enteropathogen	Age 0–5 Months			Age 6–11 Months		
	Infections with Diarrhea (N)	Total Infections	Pathogenicity	Infections with Diarrhea (N)	Total Infections	Pathogenicity
Campylobacter sp	73	177	0.41	65	188	0.35
Enterotoxigenic *Escherichia coli*	42	119	0.35	40	103	0.39
Rotavirus	18	33	0.55	23	28	0.82
Shigella sp	14	17	0.82	16	34	0.47

The virulence (i.e., the number of severe illnesses/the total number of illnesses) may also vary by enteropathogen. This can be illustrated by the propensity of the organism to cause an illness that leads to dehydration. In community-based studies in Bangladesh,[30,31] children with rotavirus diarrhea or cholera are most likely to develop dehydration (Table 20-7). Those with ETEC had a modestly increased rate of dehydration compared with all other types of diarrhea.

In the United States the relative importance of the various enteropathogens differs from that in developing countries (Table 20-8). In studies done in health facilities, rotavirus is the most important enteropathogen associated with diarrhea, as it is in developing countries.[32] In general, the bacterial causes are less important in developed countries, although *Campylobacter* species and *Salmonella* species may be important in some settings. This pattern may be shifted closer to a developing country pattern in certain higher risk populations. For example, residents of Indian reservations in the United States have had higher rates of diarrhea than the general population, although good access to medical care has now reduced the diarrheal mortality to a very low level.[33,34] In such settings (Table 20-9), rotavirus is still the most important pathogen, but other organisms such as ETEC and *Campylobacter* species may play a more prominent role than they do in the general US population.

In the United States it is estimated that each year there are 5000 deaths, 325,000 hospitalizations, and 76 million illnesses caused by food-borne infections, counting both outbreaks and sporadic cases.[35] There are about 500 outbreaks of food-borne disease reported to the Centers for Disease Control and Prevention annually. In the 40% with a cause identified, a bacterial organism has been found in 75%. Traditionally *Salmonella, Staphylococcus,* and *Clostridium perfringens* have been considered the main responsible organisms, and they continue to be important. A number of other organisms, commonly spread by the food-borne route, notably *Campylobacter* and *E. coli* 0157:H7 have also caused substantial morbidity. However, a large number of bacterial parasitic and viral infections can be food-borne.[35] In an investigation of an outbreak of diarrhea possibly related to consumption of

TABLE 20-7   Percentage of Children <5 Years Experiencing Dehydration During Diarrheal Episodes by Enteropathogen in Two Community-Based Studies in Rural Bangladesh

Enteropathogen	Episodes (N)	Dehydration (N)	Dehydration (%)
Rotavirus	78	28	36
Vibrio cholerae	3	1	33
Enterotoxigenic *Escherichia coli*	322	17	5
Other	843	17	2
Total	1246	63	76

TABLE 20-8   Percentage Identification of Selected Enteropathogens in Children with Diarrhea and Controls Attending an Outpatient Clinic in the United States

Enteropathogen	Diarrhea Cases (*n* = 246)	Controls (*n* = 155)
Adenovirus (enteric)	4	0
Aeromonas sp	6	7
Campylobacter sp	<1	<1
C. parvum	<1	0
ETEC	0	0
G. lamblia	<1	0
Rotavirus	22	10
Salmonella sp	5	0
Shigella sp	0	—
Vibrios	<1	0

Source: Kotloff KL, Wasserman SS, Steciak JY, et al. Acute diarrhea in Baltimore children attending an outpatient clinic. *Pediatr Infect Dis J.* 1988;7:753–759.

TABLE 20-9   Percentage Identification of Selected Enteropathogens in Children with Diarrhea in Different Settings on a US Indian Reservation

Enteropathogen	Home	Outpatient Clinic (N = 535)	Hospital (N = 488)
Adenovirus	2	3	5
Aeromonas sp	1	1	2
Campylobacter sp	5	4	3
Enterotoxigenic *Escherichia coli*	5	5	14
Rotavirus	8	6	24
Salmonella sp	<1	1	1
Shigella sp	7	6	5
Vibrios	0	0	<1

Source: R.B. Sack et al., Journal of Diarrhoeal Disease Research, March 13 (1), pp. 12–17, © 1995, International Centre for Diarrhoeal Disease Research.

contaminated food, it is important to consider the different clinical presentations of these pathogens.[36] For example, *Staphylococcal* illness often has severe vomiting along with diarrhea, does not usually present with fever, and generally lasts about a day. *C. perfringens* usually has diarrhea without fever and also lasts less than a day. Salmonella often has diarrhea, vomiting, and fever that may last for several days. The incubation period of the causes of infectious food-borne diarrhea also differs. *Staphylococcus* has an incubation period of 2–7 hours, but *C. perfringens* has an incubation of 8–14 hours and *Salmonella* of 2–3 days.

Specific Enteropathogens

Bacterial Agents

Campylobacter jejuni or *Campylobacter coli* cause watery diarrhea and sometimes dysentery, especially in young children.[37] Immunity acquired from previous *Campylobacter* infections is the likely explanation for the low rate of illness in adults and the high prevalence of asymptomatic infection in developing countries. In the United States, *Campylobacter* species infection occurs in all age groups with peak incidence the first year of life and in young adults. The higher rate of disease in young adults has been linked to food-handling errors made by these individuals when cooking. There is often a summer seasonality with *Campylobacter* species infections.

Escherichia coli can produce diarrhea by a variety of mechanisms.[38] Although *E. coli* organisms are part of the normal flora of the intestine, this organism may also possess a variety of virulence properties. The diarrheagenic potential of *E. coli* was recognized decades ago with the so-called enteropathogenic *E. coli* (EPEC).[39] Previously these organisms were identified by their serotypes once they were implicated in a diarrhea outbreak. This nomenclature has now been superseded. Diarrheagenic *E. coli* are designated based on the demonstration of virulence properties or laboratory characteristics felt to be associated with virulence properties. Only some of the strains previously identified by serology as EPEC have been found to produce "attaching and effacing" lesions in the intestine and patterns of adherence in tissue culture assays.[38] EPEC strains are now identified by their adherence pattern in tissue cultures or by the presence of plasmids that confer that capacity. The pathogenic role of subgroups of these adherent *E. coli* in acute or persistent diarrhea has been well established; the role of others is still in question.[40-42] Persistent diarrhea in association with HIV infection is usually associated with the same enteropathogens as diarrhea in HIV-negative persons, but some additional organisms can be found.[43,44]

Other strains of enterotoxigenic *E. coli* produce a heat-labile toxin (LT) or heat-stable toxin (ST) or both, and a number of assays can now be used to evaluate these organisms for toxin production or the genetic capability to produce these toxins.[38] Although these assays are not optimally sensitive because they require testing of a small number of organisms in the feces, ETEC are still the most frequent cause of diarrheal illnesses in children in developing countries. It has been demonstrated further that many ETEC produce colonization factors that are important in pathogenesis, indicating that not all toxin-producing *E. coli* are necessarily pathogens.[38] This may be a partial explanation for the high frequency of asymptomatic infections with ETEC in developing countries, but it is also clear that acquired immunity may protect from illness, but not colonization.[45] An enteroinvasive type of *E. coli* has been described as resulting in dysentery and to have a pathogenesis similar to that found with *Shigella* species. These organisms may occasionally cause outbreaks but do not appear to be frequent causes of endemic diarrheal diseases.

In the early 1980s, *E. coli* O157:H7 was identified as an important cause of hemorrhagic colitis.[46] These organisms produce exotoxins, which resemble the Shiga toxin of *S. dysenteriae* type 1. These enterohemorrhagic *E. coli* (EHEC) have developed into a major public health problem in the United States and Canada, but appear to be very infrequent in developing countries. Large outbreaks of EHEC have occurred in which some cases developed hemolytic uremic syndrome or other serious complications, which can lead to death in approximately 2% of patients.[47] The primary reservoir for EHEC is cattle, and transmission to humans has been most commonly related to consumption of undercooked ground beef or unpasteurized milk. Outbreaks have also been traced to other foods and person-to-person transmission predominates in day-care centers and other types of institutions.

Salmonella species continue to be an important public health problem in developed countries, but their importance varies in developing countries. In the United States the highest attack rate for salmonellosis is in infants, but elderly and immunosuppressed individuals are also at higher risk.[48] *Salmonella* species have animal hosts, especially poultry. In fact, *S. enteritidis* can colonize the ovaries of egg-laying hens, which can result in infection of the egg before it is laid.[49] The rates of salmonellosis have increased in developed countries in the last decade, and nearly all of this is due to food-borne transmission. Salmonellosis often has a summer seasonality.

There are four serogroups of shigella. In developing countries *S. flexneri* is the most common followed by *S. sonnei*, *S. boydii*, and *S. dysenteriae*; however, outbreaks of *S. dysenteriae* type 1 (or Shiga's bacillus) have occurred in many countries.[50,51] The resulting illnesses are often severe, resulting in high case fatality, and these organisms may be resistant to most commonly used antibiotics. In the United States and most other developed countries *S. sonnei* is the most common serogroup with *S. flexneri* accounting for most of the remainder.[52] In endemic situations, shigellosis is primarily a disease of children, reflecting the likelihood of fecal-oral transmission in this age group. Food-borne and waterborne outbreaks occur occasionally, but the predominant route of transmission is from person to person. Shigellosis has a seasonality predominantly in the warm months, although in developing countries this may also be influenced by the availability of water and changes in the level of personal hygiene.

Cholera is a diarrheal illness caused by infection of the small intestine with *Vibrio cholerae*. It has been feared for centuries because cholera epidemics can result in high mortality and social disruption.[53] There have been a series of global pandemics of cholera. The seventh pandemic, which is still continuing, is generally thought to have begun in 1961. This pandemic, caused by the *V. cholerae* biotype El Tor, spread from Sulawesi throughout Asia, the Middle East, the Soviet Union, Africa, and into a few countries of Europe. North America had had no indigenous cases of cholera in this century until a single case was detected in Texas in 1973. It has subsequently been discovered that *V. cholerae* El Tor is endemic in the Gulf Coast area of Texas and Louisiana and cases have sporadically occurred in that area. Latin America had been spared from cholera epidemics since the end of the last century, but in 1991 cholera reappeared in Peru. It subsequently spread throughout much of South and Central America, with some cases being imported into the United States.[54]

All previous cholera pandemics had been due to *V. cholerae* serotype 01 until 1992 when cases of cholera associated with a *V. cholerae* strain that did not include agglutinate with 01 antisera were reported from India and Bangladesh. This strain, subsequently designated serotype 0139, caused epidemic disease throughout India and Bangladesh and cases in a number of other countries of Asia.[55] After the initial outbreaks due to this organism, the rates of disease have decreased, but the strain persists along with *V. cholerae* 01. These outbreaks demonstrate the potential for strains of *V. cholerae* other than serotype 01 to cause epidemic cholera and may represent the beginning of a new pandemic.

In endemic areas, cholera predominantly affects children 2–15 years of age, but may still cause a large proportion of severe watery diarrheal diseases in adults during the season of transmission.[53] Immunity develops after initial infection, although asymptomatic infections may still occur. In areas that have not had exposure to *V. cholerae* previously the entire population is susceptible, resulting in high outbreak attack rates in children and adults. *Vibrio cholerae* may have an environmental reservoir in marshes and rivers and is commonly spread by seafood, as well as directly by water.

A number of other vibrios may cause diarrhea, as well as bacteremia and other serious illness.[56] *V. parahemolyticus* can cause diarrhea, including outbreaks. These illnesses occur with low frequency in most countries, but in Japan *V. parahemolyticus* is a frequent cause of diarrhea and outbreaks.[57] There is recent evidence documenting that *V. parahemolyticus* serotype 03: K6 is spreading from Asia in a pandemic that has reached Africa and more recently South America.[58] In North America, as well as other countries, *V. vulnificus* and non-01 *V. cholerae* also cause diarrhea and systemic infection.[56,59]

Aeromonas hydrophila is often, and *Plesiomonas shigelloides* less frequently, found during diarrhea in developing countries.[60,61] These organisms appear to be much less frequent in developed country settings. At least for *A. hydrophila*, the higher rate of isolation of the organism during diarrhea compared with controls suggests a causative role.[62] However, the importance of these organisms and the mechanisms by which they may cause diarrhea are unknown.

Yersinia enterocolitica may cause diarrhea and other abdominal symptoms. It is a common cause of disease in Western Europe, and outbreaks have occurred in the United States, primarily from contaminated meat and milk.[63] This organism has been assayed for in a number of developing countries, but has been rarely found in cases of diarrhea.[64]

Clostridium difficile causes colitis associated with the use of a variety of antibiotics. Although this organism can be found in acute diarrhea, the causative relationship is unclear.[65]

A number of other bacterial enteropathogens are associated with diarrheal diseases. These organisms are primarily involved in food-borne disease outbreaks, but may also cause sporadic cases of diarrhea. *Bacillus cereus* has been associated with outbreaks related to consumption of cooked rice, and *Clostridium perfringens* is usually associated with outbreaks in which the spores of the organism germinate in anaerobic conditions after cooking of meat, resulting in the production of the toxin that causes diarrhea.[66] *Staphylococcus aureus* outbreaks of diarrhea are often caused by a food handler contaminating food. *S. aureus* produces a heat-stable enterotoxin that when ingested causes the illness.

Strains of *Bacteroides fragilis* that produce an enterotoxin have recently been associated with diarrheal diseases, both in the United States and in Bangladesh.[27,67] Because of limited availability of the diagnostic assay, the importance of this enteropathogen is unknown.

Viral Agents

Rotaviruses are the most important viral agent causing diarrheal diseases. Illness largely occurs in the first two years of life throughout the world.[68] Rotavirus diarrhea has a winter seasonality in most developed countries, but the seasonality in developing countries is less marked with disease occurring throughout the year. In addition to the role of rotavirus as an endemic enteropathogen, outbreaks have occurred in day-care centers and hospitals. The organism may be a cause of a small proportion of disease in adults, such as caregivers for small children and in travelers from developed countries to developing countries.

Enteric adenoviruses of serotypes 40 and 41 are the second most important cause of viral diarrhea.[69,70] These organisms appear to occur worldwide. Norovirus (previously referred to as Norwalk agent and related 27-nm caliciviruses, such as Hawaii and Snow Mountain agents) cause watery diarrhea and/or vomiting.[26,71] Several studies indicate that norovirus agent alone may account for 2–5% of childhood diarrheas in developing countries.[72] It may have a similar or greater importance in the United States.

Other viruses or viruslike particles have been proposed as causes of diarrhea, coronaviruses, astroviruses, as well as small round virus-like particles have been found during diarrhea.[25,73,74] Pestivirus has also been reported in association with diarrhea.[75] The causative role of these agents and their importance are unknown.

Parasitic Agents

Cryptosporidium parvum, a coccidian parasite, is likely the most important parasitic cause of diarrheal diseases.[76] It has a global distribution as an endemic disease, but may also occur in outbreaks, including large waterborne outbreaks from municipal water systems. Cryptosporidial cysts are very resistant to chlorine and must be removed from drinking water by filtration. Related organisms of the true coccidia, such as *Isospora belli*, may cause diarrhea but appear to be uncommon except possibly is association with AIDS.[77]

Diarrhea associated with microsporidia also occurs with AIDS, but the role of this organism in immunocompetent individuals is not described.[78]

Cyclospora cayetanensis, previously referred to as "cyanobacterium-like bodies" and by other names, is a newly described enteropathogen.[79] These coccidian parasites have been found in a number of developing countries and may be of comparable importance to *C. parvum*. In developed countries, these organisms have been known to cause diarrheal disease in AIDS patients and in travelers to developing countries.[79,80] Outbreaks have been reported from consumption of imported raspberries.

Giardia lamblia is a common protozoan with a very high carriage rate in many developing country populations, particularly in children.[81] However, it does not appear to be an important diarrheal pathogen in most developing countries.[82,83] In developed countries, *G. lamblia* may be a frequent parasitic cause of diarrhea.[84] Infections are passed from person to person and are common in day-care centers and other institutions. Water- or food-borne outbreaks have also occurred. Like *C. parvum*, *G. lamblia* is resistant to chlorine, particularly in cold water, and prevention of waterborne giardiasis depends on adequate water filtration to remove the parasitic cysts.

E. histolytica can cause amebiasis and may be associated with extraintestinal complications, such as liver abscess.[85,86] This parasite appears to be an infrequent cause of childhood diarrhea or dysentery in developing countries and is rare in developed countries. Other protozoan infections can be associated with diarrhea, including those due to *Balantidium coli* and *Chilomastix mesnili*. *Blastocystis hominis* is of uncertain pathogenicity.[87]

Most intestinal helminthic infections are not associated with diarrhea, but dysentery and even rectal prolapse has been associated with severe *Trichuris trichiura* infections and diarrhea with other intestinal parasites.[88]

Transmission Routes

General Factors

Diarrheal diseases result from exposure of a susceptible host to a pathogenic organism. Nearly all enteropathogens are transmitted by direct contact with human feces or indirectly through contact with feces through water, food, or eating utensils. Some enteropathogens have an animal or environmental reservoir, and contact with the pathogen from these sources may then result in infection. It is clear that populations of lower socioeconomic status or educational level may have a higher exposure to enteropathogens due to residence in poorer environmental conditions or less hygienic practices, particularly in child care.

Water

Waterborne transmission has been documented for most enteropathogens.[89] For some, such as *V. cholerae* and norovirus, this may be the predominant form of transmission, but even for these pathogens food-borne transmission also may be common. The use of contaminated sources of water for bathing, washing, swimming, cleaning, and cleaning feeding utensils have been implicated in transmission, as well as consumption of contaminated water.[90]

In developing country settings without access to tap water in the home, poor handling practices of water stored in the house, mainly by introduction of contaminated hands or utensils into water containers, have been linked to an increased risk for diarrheal diseases.[91] Studies have now documented that water quantity is in many situations more important than water quality for diarrheal diseases.[89] This is because water availability is important for hygienic behaviors that would prevent much of the transmission by person to person or through food.

Food

Breast-feeding, especially exclusively, protects against diarrheal diseases.[92,93] This is in part because breast-fed children are less exposed to enteropathogens that might be in food or water. Furthermore, breast milk may provide passive immunologic protection against some of the organisms. Especially in developing countries, the incidence of diarrheal diseases increases sharply with the introduction of weaning foods.[94] These foods are often heavily contaminated, and studies have demonstrated the relationship between consumption of more contaminated foods and illness related to organisms such as ETEC.[95] The level of bacterial contamination may vary by the type of food and by food-handling practices.[96] It is strongly influenced by the storage time between initial preparation and consumption because many of the bacterial enteropathogens can multiply in the food during storage at ambient temperature.[95] Food may be contaminated in the home or before it reaches the home. In developing countries, most foods must be assumed to be contaminated. This applies even to uncooked fruits and vegetables that might become contaminated from being irrigated with sewage or through improper handling. In the United States and other developed countries some foods, such as chicken, must also be assumed to be contaminated with *Salmonella* species and *Campylobacter* species.[66] In addition, the recent outbreaks of *E. coli* O157:H7 suggest that all ground beef must be considered potentially contaminated with this organism. Until further control of these infections in the reservoir and at the processing level are implemented, the primary control is proper cooking.

In developing countries, much of the food production is still done in small scale at the local level. In contrast, in developed countries there is an increasing trend toward large-scale production and distribution of food. These production and slaughtering techniques, such as of poultry, make contamination with enteropathogens much more widespread. In addition, developed countries are increasingly importing food from all over the world.[66] This means that consumers are at risk of exposure to contaminated fruits and vegetables, as well as other products.

Feeding Utensils

In developing countries, baby bottles, bottle nipples, cups, spoons, and food containers are frequently contaminated with fecal bacteria, as well as specific enteropathogens.[29,97] These utensils are difficult to keep clean in unhygienic environments. Although boiling or the use of sterilizing solution is effective in eliminating contamination, the use of these methods may be inconsistent. The risk of contamination of feeding utensils, as well as of water and food, makes breast-feeding that much more desirable in settings with poor environmental sanitation.

Animals

Animals may be the reservoir for a variety of enteropathogens.[47,98,99] Poultry is the primary source for *C. jejuni* and *Salmonella* species; the main animal reservoir for *E. coli* O157:H7 is cattle. *C. perfringens* is also commonly associated with animals and *Y. enterocolitica* commonly with pigs and cows. Shellfish may be a reservoir for *V. cholerae* and other vibrios.

Flies

A variety of enteropathogens have been isolated from flies, including bacteria, viruses, and parasites.[100] The organisms may be carried on the external surface of the fly or may be ingested in which case the survival of bacteria may be prolonged. Flies contaminate food or even water in a house when feeding. Evidence for flies as a means of transmission is inconclusive.[100,101] Intervention studies have shown that fly control at a military camp in Israel decreased diarrhea and particularly shigellosis.[102] These findings were confirmed in Pakistan.[103] More such studies are needed to evaluate the value of fly control as a major public health intervention in developing countries.

Hygiene

Personal hygiene practices are closely linked with person-to-person transmission of diarrhea.[104] Of hygiene practices, hand washing is probably the most widely studied. The increased risk of diarrhea with inadequate hand washing, in particular after defecation or cleaning a child, has been documented. Intervention studies have confirmed this by demonstrating a reduction in the incidence of diarrhea with proper hand washing.[105,106] Hand washing with soap is effective in eliminating fecal contamination, even viruses. In developing countries where soap may not be available, hand washing with mud, ash, or other agents that facilitate removal of contaminants from the hands has also been found to be effective, but rinsing with water alone less so.[107] Hand washing promoting programs seem effective in reducing diarrheal diseases as well as respiratory and skin diseases and require further evaluation for wide implementation.[108,109] Another important hygiene behavior is proper disposal of fecal material. In developing countries with poor sanitation, defecation in the yard or in open areas as well as nonhygienic methods of feces disposal are demonstrated risk factors for diarrhea.[110] Crawling infants who may come in contact with the feces on the ground are at particular risk.[111] The appropriate use of potty chairs in these settings has been proposed as a potential intervention.[112] There may also be transmission risk from unhygienic latrines or school toilets.

Host Risk Factors

Malnutrition

Malnutrition and diarrheal diseases are often found together in developing countries because they coexist in children living in poor socioeconomic and environmental conditions. In addition, malnutrition may be a direct risk factor for diarrheal diseases through compromised immunologic function and tissue regenerative capability. Malnourished children in developing countries have been found in some studies to have a risk of diarrhea increased by up to 70%.[113-115] Other studies have found no increase in diarrheal incidence in malnourished children.[116] Nearly all studies show that malnourished children have diarrheal episodes of longer duration and often greater severity.[116]

Micronutrient Deficiencies

In addition to general malnutrition, specific micronutrient deficiencies may result in either a higher incidence or greater severity of diarrhea. Vitamin A deficiency is associated with more severe diarrhea, and in populations deficient in vitamin A, supplementation reduces diarrheal mortality.[117,118] Zinc deficiency is also related to diarrhea. Zinc supplementation in populations presumed to be deficient reduces the incidence and duration of diarrheal episodes.[119,120] Other micronutrients may be related to diarrhea as well. As with malnutrition in general, these specific micronutrient deficiencies may result in immunologic compromise or reduced ability to repair damaged intestinal mucosa.

Gastric Acid

The acidic contents of the stomach are an important barrier to ingested enteropathogens, especially many of the bacterial agents. Hypochlorhydria may increase the likelihood that sufficient quantity of the pathogen would reach the small intestine and cause infection.[121] Thus, medical conditions that reduce gastric acid or medications that neutralize the acid may lead to a greater frequency or severity of diarrheal diseases. Furthermore, *Helicobacter pylori* infection in the stomach is common in children in developing countries.[122] Because this infection may result in hypochlorhydria, it may result in a greater risk of diarrhea.

Genetic Factors

There may be some genetic predisposition to diarrheal diseases, but current evidence is very limited. Persons of blood group O have a greater risk of developing cholera and have more severe illness than persons of other blood groups.[123] Few studies have been done to examine such a relationship between blood group and other enteropathogens, but limited data do not demonstrate a strong relationship for ETEC or vibrios other than *V. cholerae* 01.[124,125]

Immunity

Immunity plays an important role in susceptibility to enteropathogens. Maternal antibody is provided to the infant through breast milk and this protects against a variety of enteric infections. Transplacental antibody may also play a role in some. Immunity is actively acquired by the individual who has a diarrheal disease or in some cases even an asymptomatic infection.

There is also evidence that competence of the immune system can be compromised, such as by micronutrient deficiencies, reducing the resistance to enteric infection. Studies have shown that depressed cell-mediated immunity is associated with an increase in both acute and persistent diarrhea.[114,126] Immunocompetence in a child can be compromised by previous viral infections, such as measles or influenza, or by other infections, such as tuberculosis or typhoid fever. These infections, along with micronutrient deficiencies, could place individuals at a greater risk of diarrhea or of more severe illness through alteration in immune function or by other mechanisms.

Cholera was the first diarrheal disease for which a vaccine was available. A parenteral cholera vaccine provides approximately 50% protection lasting for less than 6 months. New killed or live *V. cholerae* vaccines may offer greater efficacy and duration of protection. An oral vaccine consisting of killed vibrios resulted in 52% efficacy for preventing cholera during a 3-year period in Bangladesh and also resulted in herd immunity.[127] This vaccine has been effective in mass vaccination against cholera as well,[128] although its public use has been limited to travelers and in the control of outbreaks in refugee populations.

An effective rhesus-based rotavirus vaccine introduced in the United States in 1998 was withdrawn from the market in 1999 due to rare side effects (intussusception). A new human-based rotavirus vaccine was introduced in 2005 into the market of Mexico and other Latin American countries after being proved to be effective and safe in large-scale trials. A bovine-based rotavirus vaccine will soon be introduced into the US market and evaluated in developing countries. Vaccines for many of the other important enteropathogens, such as ETEC and shigella, are also in development and under evaluation.

Antimicrobial Resistance

Among the bacterial enteropathogens, there has been a progressive increase in resistance to antibiotics.[129] For some of the enteropathogens for which there is an animal reservoir, this resistance may be the result of large-scale use of antimicrobial agents to prevent or treat infections in the animals. Also, the use of low-dose antibiotics in animal feed to enhance weight gain is suspected to increase the risk of the emergence of antibiotic resistance. Certainly extensive use of antibiotics for human infections also plays a part in the development of antimicrobial resistance. Especially problematic is the extensive use of antibiotics in developing countries without prescription or medical supervision. This has resulted in outbreaks caused by organisms such as *V. cholerae* and *Shigella dysenteriae* type 1 that are resistant to most commonly used antibiotics. Unfortunately, in developing countries alternative antibiotics are often unavailable or unaffordable.

Strategies for Control

Reduction of mortality from diarrheal diseases by appropriate treatment is the mainstay of diarrheal disease control programs.[7] Correction of dehydration by oral rehydration therapy, or intravenous therapy if necessary, and maintenance of nutrition by continued feeding during illness have played an important role in reducing diarrheal disease mortality throughout the world. Zinc supplements are now recommended in addition.[22] Antibiotic therapy of dysentery as presumed shigellosis and of cholera can reduce the illness severity and case fatality rate, and a few of the parasitic agents can also be specifically treated with antimicrobial agents.

For developing countries, reduction in the incidence of diarrheal diseases is a continuing challenge. Reviews of intervention research concluded that promotion of breast-feeding and improved weaning practices are a high priority for diarrheal prevention.[130] It was estimated that successful breast-feeding promotion programs could reduce diarrheal incidence early in infancy and childhood diarrheal mortality rates by up to 9%.[128] Improved weaning practices could have the added advantage of improving the nutritional content of the diet as well as decreasing microbial contamination.[131,132] Improved water supply, sanitation, and hygiene behaviors would also be expected to reduce diarrheal incidence. If both water supply and sanitation were improved in a typical developing country setting, it is estimated that diarrheal incidence and mortality could be reduced by about one quarter.[89] Hygiene education may further enhance the impact. In fact, hand washing education programs have been found to reduce diarrheal incidence by 14–48%.[104] It may be expected that programs combining water supply, sanitation, and hygiene education may reduce diarrheal morbidity by 25–50%. The recent demonstration that disinfection of water at the point of use can reduce diarrhea points to another feasible means of reducing diarrhea incidence.[133]

Measles causes transient immunosuppression, and measles immunization, which is currently being widely implemented in developing country programs, will likely result in a slight reduction in diarrheal incidence and a more substantial reduction in diarrheal mortality.[134] The use of cholera vaccines may have a role for control of this disease in selected populations.[135] The newly developed rotavirus vaccines could potentially have widespread applicability as rotavirus may be responsible for 5% of all diarrheal episodes and for about 25% of diarrheal deaths.[135] Because rotavirus diarrhea is also an important cause of morbidity and health care costs in developed countries, a vaccine would likely be a cost-effective preventive strategy in these settings as well.[3]

Routine zinc supplementation has been found to reduce diarrhea incidence, as well as pneumonia and other infectious diseases, and to reduce mortality.[120,136,137]

Although reduction in the incidence of diarrhea and its complications will follow from general economic development and improved environmental conditions, it is clear that particular interventions could speed progress in this regard. Efforts must continue to provide effective case management for diarrhea, but increased emphasis should be given to prevention of diarrheal morbidity. This is feasible, even in developing countries, through improved feeding practices and nutrition and an enhanced water supply, sanitation, and hygiene. Because numerous enteropathogens cause diarrhea, especially in the developing countries, and because vaccines protect only against specific organisms, these more general control measures are essential.

References

1. Bryce J, Boschi-Pinto C, Shibuya K, Black RE, and the WHO Child Health Epidemiology Reference Group. "WHO estimates of the causes of death in children." *Lancet.* 2005;365:1147–1152.
2. Kilgore PE, Holman RC, Matthew MS, et al. Trends of diarrheal disease-associated mortality in US children, 1968 through 1991. *JAMA.* 1995;274:1143–1148.
3. Smith JC, Haddix AC, Teutsch SM, Glass RI. Cost-effectiveness analysis of a rotavirus immunization program for the United States. *Pediatrics.* 1995;96:609–615.
4. Holmes SJ, Morrow AL, Pickering LK. Child-care practices: effects of social change on the epidemiology of infectious diseases and antibiotic resistance. *Epidemiol Reviews.* 1996;18:10–28.
5. Voetsch AC, Van Gilder TJ, Angulo FJ, et al for the Emerging Infections Program FoodNet Working Group. FoodNet estimate of the burden of illness caused by nontyphoidal *Salmonella* infections in the United States. *Clin Infect Dis.* 2004;38:S127–S134.
6. Newsholme A. *Fifty Years in Public Health.* London, UK: George Allen and Unwin; 1939:321–360.
7. Claeson M, Merson MH. Global progress in the control of diarrheal diseases. *Pediatr Infect Dis J.* 1990;9:345.
8. Baqui AH, Black RE, Yunus MD, Hoque ARA, Chowdhury HR, Sack RB. Methodological issues in diarrhoeal diseases epidemiology: definition of diarrhoeal episodes. *Int J Epidemiol.* 1991;20: 1057–1063.
9. Black RE. Persistent diarrhea in children of developing countries. *Pediatr Inf Dis J.* 1993;12:751–761.
10. McAuliffe JF, Shields DS, de Souza MA, Sakell J, Schorling J, Guerrant RL. Prolonged and recurring diarrhea in the northeast of Brazil: examination of cases from a community-based study. *J Pediatr Gastroenterol Nutr.* 1986;5:902–906.
11. Baqui AH, Black RE, Sack RB, Yunus MD, Siddique AK, Chowdhury HR. Epidemiological and clinical characteristics of acute and persistent diarrhea in rural Bangladeshi children. *Acta Paediatr.* 1992;381(suppl):15–21.
12. Diarrhea (WHO web site); http://www.who.int/child-adolescent-health/New_Publications/CHILD_HEALTH/EPI/Improving_Diarrhoea_Estimates.pdf.
13. Bern C, Martines J, de Zoysa I, Glass RI. The magnitude of the global problem of diarrheal disease: a ten-year update. *Bull WHO.* 1992;70:705–714.
14 Glass RI, Lew JF, Gangarosa RE, et al. Estimates of morbidity and mortality rates for diarrheal disease in American children. *J Pediatr.* 1991;118:27–33.
15. Archer DL, Kvenberg JE. Incidence and cost of food-borne diarrheal disease in the United States. *J Food Protect.* 1985;48:887–894.
16. Monto AS, Koopman JS. The Tecumseh Study: XI. Occurrence of acute enteric illness in the community. *Am J Epidemiol.* 1980;112: 323–333.

17. Black RE. Epidemiology of travelers, diarrhea and relative importance of various pathogens. *Rev Infect Dis.* 1990;12(suppl):S73–S79.

18. Kosek M, Bern C, Guerrant RL. The global burden of diarrhoeal disease, as estimated from studies published between 1992 and 2000. *Bull WHO.* 2003;81:197–204.

19. Bhan MK, Arora NH, Ghai KR, Khoshoo V, Bhandari N. Major factors in diarrhoea-related mortality among rural children. *Indian J Med Res.* 1986;83:9–12.

20. Black RE. Would control of childhood infectious diseases reduce malnutrition? *Acta Paediatr Scand Suppl.* 1991;374:133–140.

21. Checkley W, Epstein LD, Gilman RH, Cabrera L, Black RE. Effects of acute diarrhea on linear growth in Peruvian children. *Am J Epidemiol.* 2003;157:166–175.

22. WHO/UNICEF Geneva, Switzerland Joint Statement. Clinical management of acute diarrhoea. World Health Organization and United Nations Children's Fund; 2004.

23. Fang ZY, Wang B, Kilgore PE, et al. Sentinel hospital surveillance for rotavirus diarrhea in the People's Republic of China, August 2001–July 2003. *J Infect Dis.* 2005;192:S94–S99.

24. Man NV, Luan LT, Trach DD, et al for the Vietnam rotavirus surveillance network. *J Infect Dis.* 2005;192:S127–S132.

25. Unicomb LE, Banu NN, Azim T, et al. Astrovirus infection in association with acute persistent and nosocomial diarrhea in Bangladesh. *Pediatr Infect Dis J.* 1998;17:611–614.

26. Parashar UD, Li JF, Cama R, et al. Human caliciviruses as a cause of severe gastroenteritis in Peruvian children. *J Infect Dis.* 2004;190:1088–1092.

27. San Joaquin VH, Griffis JC, Lee C, Sears CL. Association of *Bacteroides fragilis* with childhood diarrhea. *Scand J Infect Dis.* 1995;27:211–215.

28. Thomas C, Stevenson M, Williamson DJ, Riley R. *Clostridium difficile*-associated diarrhea: epidemiological data from Western Australia associated with a modified antibiotic policy. *Clin Infect Dis.* 2002;365:1457–1462.

29. Black RE, Lopez de Romana G, Brown KH, Bravo N, Bazalar OG, Kanashiro HE. Incidence and etiology of infantile diarrhea and major routes of transmission in Huascar, Peru. *Am J Epidemiol.* 1989;129:785–799.

30. Black RE, Merson MH, Huq I, Alm ARMA, Yunus MD. Incidence and severity of rotavirus and *Escherichia coli* diarrhoea in rural Bangladesh. *Lancet.* 1981;1:141–143.

31. Black RE, Brown KH, Becker S, Abdul Alim ARM, Huq I. Longitudinal studies of infectious diseases and physical growth of children in rural Bangladesh. II. Incidence of diarrhea and association with known pathogens. *Am J Epidemiol.* 1982;115:315–324.

32. Kotloff KL, Wasserman SS, Steciak JY, et al. Acute diarrhea in Baltimore children attending an outpatient clinic. *Pediatr Infect Dis J.* 1988;7:753–759.

33. Sack RB, Santosham M, Reid R, et al. Diarrhoeal diseases in the White Mountain Apaches: clinical studies. *J Diarrhoeal Dis Res.* 1995;13: 12–17.

34. Santosham M, Sack RB, Reid R, et al. Diarrheal diseases in the White Mountain Apaches: epidemiologic studies. *J Diarrhoeal Dis Res.* 1995;13:18–28.

35. Mead PS, Slutsker L, Dietz V, et al. Food-related illness and death in the United States. *Emerg Infect Dis.* 1999;5:607–625.

36. Horwitz MA. Specific diagnosis of food-borne diseases. *Gastroenterology.* 1977;73:375–381.

37. Nachamkin I, Blaser MJ, Tompkins LS, eds. *Campylobacter jejuni; Current Status and Future Trends.* Washington, DC: American Society for Microbiology; 1992.

38. Levine MM. *Escherichia coli* that cause diarrhea: enterotoxigenic, enteropathogenic, enteroinvasive, enterohemorrhagic, and enteroadherent. *J Infect Dis.* 1987;155:377–388.

39. Robins-Browne RM. Traditional enteropathogenic *Escherichia coli* of infantile diarrhea. *Rev Infect Dis.* 1987;9:28–53.

40. Clausen CR, Christie DL. Chronic diarrhea in infants caused by adherent enteropathogenic *Escherichia coli. J Pediatr.* 1982;100: 358–361.

41. Korzeniowski OM, Dantas W, Trabulsi LR, Guerrant RL. A controlled study of endemic sporadic diarrhoea among adult residents of southern Brazil. *Trans R Soc Trop Med Hyg.* 1984;84:363–369.

42. Lanata CF, Black RE, Gilman RH, Lazo F, Del Aquila R. Epidemiologic, clinical, and laboratory characteristics of acute vs. persistent diarrhea in periurban Lima, Peru. *J Ped Gastroenterol Nutr.* 1991;12:82–88.

43. Carcamo C, Hooten T, Wener MH, et al. Etiologies and manifestations of persistent diarrhea in adults with HIV-1 infections: a case-control study in Lima, Peru. *J Infect Dis.* 2005;191:11–19.

44. Bern C, Kawai V, Vargas D, Rabke-Verani J, et al. The epidemiology of intestinal microsporidiosis in patients with HIV/AIDS in Lima, Peru. *J Infect Dis.* 2005;191:1658–1664.

45. Black RE, Merson MH, Rowe B, et al. Enterotoxigenic *Escherichia coli* diarrhoea: acquired immunity and transmission in an endemic area. *Bull WHO.* 1981;59:263–268.

46. Riley LW, Remis RS, Helgerson SD, et al. Hemorrhagic colitis associated with a rare *Escherichia coli* serotype. *N Engl J Med.* 1983; 308:681.

47. Griffin PM, Tauxe RV. The epidemiology of infections caused by *Escherichia coli* 0157:H7, other enterohemorrhogic *E. coli,* and the associated hemolytic uremic syndrome. *Epidemiol Rev.* 1991;13: 60–98.

48. Chalker RB, Blaser MJ. A review of human salmonellosis: III. Magnitude of salmonella infections in the United States. *Rev Infect Dis.* 1987;7:111–124.

49. Gast RK, Beard CW. Production of *Salmonella enteritidis* contaminated eggs by experimentally infected hens. *Avian Dis.* 1990;34:438–446.

50. Khan MD, Roy NC, Islam R, Huq I, Stoll B. Fourteen years of shigellosis in Dhaka: an epidemiological analysis. *Int J Epidemiol.* 1985;14: 607–613.

51. Ebright JR, Moore EC, Sanborn WR, Schaeberg D, Kyle J, Ishida K. Epidemic shiga bacillus dysentery in Central Africa. *Am J Trop Med Hyg.* 1984;33:1192–1197.

52. Lee LA, Shapiro CN, Hargrett-Bean N, et al. Hyperendemic shigellosis in the United States: a review of surveillance data for 1967–1988. *J Infect Dis.* 1991;164:894–900.

53. Glass RI, Black RE. The epidemiology of cholera. In: Barua D, Greenough WB III, eds. *Cholera.* New York, NY: Plenum Medical Book Company; 1992:129–154.

54. Ries AA, Vugia DJ, Beingolea L, et al. Cholera in Piura, Peru: a modern urban epidemic. *J Infect Dis.* 1992;166:1429–1433.

55. Cholera Working Group, International Centre for Diarrhoeal Diseases Research, Bangladesh. Large epidemic of cholera-like disease in Bangladesh caused by *Vibrio cholerae* 0139 synonym Bengal. *Lancet.* 1993;342:387–390.

56. Black PA, Weaver RE, Hollis DG. Diseases of humans (other than cholera) caused by *vibrios. Ann Rev Microbiol.* 1980;34:341.

57. Fukami T, Saku K. Clinical epidemiology of infectious enteritis of outpatients at Tokyo Metropolitan Bokuto General Hospital. In: Saito M, Nakaya R, Matsubara Y, eds. *Infectious Enteritis in Japan.* Tokyo, Japan: Saikon Publishing; 1986:211–220.

58. Matsumoto C, Okuda J, Ishibashi M, et al. Pandemic spread of O3: K6 clone of *Vibrio parahaemolyticus* and emergence of related strains evidenced by arbitrarily primed PCR and *toxRS* sequence analysis. *J Clin Microbiol.* 2000;38:578–585.

59. Levine WC, Griffin PM, and the Gulf Coast Working Group. Vibrio infections on the Gulf Coast: results of first year of regional surveillance. *J Infect Dis.* 1993;167:479–483.

60. Holmberg SD, Farmer JJ III. *Aeromonas hydrophila* and *Plesiomonas shigelloides* as causes of intestinal infections. *Rev Infect Dis.* 1984;6:633–639.

61. Rennels MB, Levine MM. Classical bacterial diarrhea: perspectives and update—salmonella, shigella, *Escherichia coli,* aeromonas, and plesiomonas. *Pediatr Infect Dis.* 1986;5(suppl 1):S91–S100.

62. Gracey M, Burke V, Robinson J. Aeromonas-associated gastroentertis. *Lancet.* 1982;2:1304–1306.

63. Black RE, Jackson RJ, Tsai IF, et al. Epidemic *Yersinia enterocolitica* infection due to contaminated chocolate milk. *N Engl J Med.* 1978;298:76–79.

64. Samadi AR, Wachsmuth K, Huq MI, Mahbub M, Agbonlahor DE. An attempt to detect *Yersinia entero colitica. Trop Geograph Med.* 1982;34:151–154.

65. Torres JF, Cedillo R, Sanchez J, Dillman C, Giono S, Munoz O. Prevalence of *Clostridium difficile* and its cytotoxin in infants in Mexico. *J Clin Microbiol.* 1984;20:274–275.

66. Bean NH, Griffin PM. Foodborne disease outbreaks in the United States, 1973–1987: pathogens, vehicles and trends. *J Food Protect.* 1990;53:804–817.

67. Sack RB, Myers LL, Almeido-Hill J, et al. Enterotoxigenic *Bacteroides fragilis:* epidemiologic studies of its role as a human diarrhoeal pathogen. *J Diarrhoeal Dis Res.* 1992;10:4–9.

68. Anderson EV, Weber SG. Rotavirus infection in adults. *Lancet.* 2004;4:91–99.

69. Gary GW Jr, Hierholzer JC, Black RE. Characteristics of noncultivable adenoviruses associated with diarrhea in infants: a new subgroup of human adenoviruses. *J Clin Microbiol.* 1979;10:96–103.

70. Uhnoo I, Wadell G, Svensson L, Johansson ME. Importance of enteric adenoviruses 40 and 41 in acute gastroenteritis in infants and young children. *J Clin Microbiol.* 1984;20:365–372.

71. Greenberg HB, Valdesuso J, Kapikian AZ, et al. Prevalence of antibody to the Norwalk virus in various countries. *Infect Immun.* 1979;26:270–273.

72. Black RE, Greenberg HB, Kapikian AZ, Brown KH, Becker S. Acquisition of serum antibody to Norwalk virus and rotavirus and relation to diarrhea in a longitudinal study of young children in rural Bangladesh. *J Infect Dis.* 1982;145:483–489.

73. Tiemessen CT, Wegerhoff FO, Erasmus MJ, Kidd AH. Infection by enteric adenoviruses, rotaviruses, and other agents in a rural African environment. *J Med Viral.* 1989;28:176–182.

74. Kurtz JB, Lee TW, Pickering D. Astrovirus associated gastroenteritis in a children's ward. *J Clin Path.* 1977;30:948–952.

75. Yolken R, Dubovi E, Leister F, et al. Infantile gastroenteritis associated with excretion of pestivirus antigens. *Lancet.* 1989;1:517–520.

76. Leav BA, Mackay M, Ward HD. *Cryptosporidium* species: new insights and old challenges. *Clin Infect Dis.* 2003;36:903–908.

77. Guerrant RL, Bobak DA. Bacterial and protozoal gastroenteritis. *N Engl J Med.* 1991;325:327–340.

78. Shadduck JA. Human microsporidiosis and AIDS. *Rev Infect Dis.* 1989;11:203–207.

79. Ortega YR, Sterling CR, Gilman RH, Cama VA, Diaz F. *Cyclospora* species: a new protozoan pathogen of humans. *N Engl J Med.* 1993;328:1308–1312.

80. Elder GH, Hunter PR, Codd GA. Hazardous freshwater cyanobacteria (blue-green algae). *Lancet.* 1993;341:1519–1520.

81. Stevens DP. Selective primary health care: strategies for control of disease in the developing world. XIX. Giardiasis. *Rev Infect Dis.* 1985;7:530–535.

82. Gilman RH, Marquis GS, Miranda E, Vestegui M, Martinez H. Rapid reinfection of *Giardia lamblia* after treatment in hyperendemic third world community. *Lancet.* 1988;1:343–345.

83. Sullivan PS, DuPont HL, Arafat RR, et al. Illness and reservoirs associated with *Giardia lamblia* infection in rural Egypt: the case against treatment in developing world environments of high endemicity. *Am J Epidemiol.* 1988;127:1272–1281.

84. Flanagan PA. Giardia—diagnosis, clinical course and epidemiology: a review. *Epidemiol Infect.* 1992;109:1–22.

85. Wanke C, Butler I, Islam M. Epidemiologic and clinical features of invasive amebiasis in Bangladesh: a case control comparison with other diarrheal diseases and postmortem findings. *Am J Trop Med Hyg.* 1988;38:335–341.

86. Nanda R, Bavaja U, Anand BS. *Entamoeba histolytica* cyst passers: clinical features and outcome in untreated subjects. *Lancet.* 1984;2:301–303.

87. Casemore DP. Foodborne protozoal infection. *Lancet.* 1990;336: 1427–1443.

88. Genta RM. Diarrhea in helminthic infections. *Clin Infect Dis.* 1993;16(suppl 2):S122–S129.

89. Esrey SA, Feachem RG, Hughes LM. Interventions for the control of diarrhoeal diseases among young children: improving water supplies and excreta disposal facilities. *Bull WHO.* 1985;63:757–772.

90. Hughes LM, Boyce LM, Levine RJ, et al. Epidemiology of El Tor cholera in rural Bangladesh: importance of surface water in transmission. *Bull WHO.* 1982;60:395–404.

91. Swerdlow DL, Mintz ED, Rodriguez M, et al. Waterborne transmission of epidemic cholera in Trujillo, Peru: lessons for a continent at risk. *Lancet.* 1992;340:28–33.

92. Arifeen S, Black RE, Antelman G, Baqui A, Caulfield L, Becker S. Exclusive breastfeeding reduces acute respiratory infection and diarrhea deaths among infants in Dhaka slums. *Pediatrics*. 2001; 108:1–8.

93. Bhandari N, Bahl R, Mazumdar S, Martines J, Black RE, Bhan MK, and the other members of the Infant Feeding Study Group. Effect of community-based promotion of exclusive breastfeeding on diarrhoeal illness and growth: a cluster randomized controlled trial. *Lancet*. 2003;361:1418–1423.

94. Barrell RAE, Rowland MGM. Infant foods as a potential source of diarrhoeal illness in rural West Africa. *Trans R Soc Trop Med Hyg*. 1979;73:85–90.

95. Black RE, Brown KH, Becker S, Abdul Alim ARM, Merson MH. Contamination of weaning foods and transmission of enterotoxigenic *Escherichia coli* diarrhoea in children in rural Bangladesh. *Trans R Soc Trop Med Hyg*. 1982;76:259–264.

96. Lanata CF. Studies of food hygiene and diarrhoeal disease. *Int J Environ Health Res*. 1003;13:S175–S183.

97. Cherian A, Lawande RV. Recovery of potential pathogens from feeding bottle contents and teats in Zaria, Nigeria. *Trans R Soc Trop Med Hyg*. 1985;79:840–842.

98. Rodrigue DC, Tauxe RV, Rower B. International increase in *Salmonella enteritidis*: a new pandemic? *Epidemiol Infect*. 1990;105:21–27.

99. Blaser MJ, LaForce FM, Wilson NA, Wang WL. Reservoirs for human campylobacteriosis. *J Infect Dis*. 1980;141:665–669.

100. Esrey SA. *Interventions for the Control of Diarrhoeal Diseases among Young Children: Fly Control*. Geneva, Switzerland: World Health Organization; 1991. WHO/CDD/91.37.

101. Nichols GI. Fly transmission of *Campylobacter. Emerg Infect Dis*. 2005;11:361–364.

102. Cohen D, Green M, Block C, et al. Reduction of transmission of shigellosis by control of houseflies (*Musca domestica*). *Lancet*. 1991;337:993–997.

103. Chavasse CD, Shier RP, Murphy OA, Huttly SR, Cousens SN, Akhtar T. Impact of fly control on childhood diarrhoea in Pakistan: community-randomised trial. *Lancet*. 1999;353:22–25.

104. Feachem RG. Interventions for the control of diarrhoeal diseases among young children: promotion of personal and domestic hygiene. *Bull WHO*. 1984;62:467–476.

105. Black RE, Dykes AC, Anderson KE, et al. Handwashing to prevent diarrhea in day-care centers. *Am J Epidemiol*. 1981;113:445–451.

106. Khan MD. Interruption of shigellosis by handwashing. *Trans R Soc Trop Med Hyg*. 1982;76:164–168.

107. Hoque BA, Briend A. A comparison of local handwashing agents in Bangladesh. *J Trop Med Hyg*. 1991;94:61–64.

108. Luby SP, Agboatwalla M, Painter J, Altaf A, Billhimer WL, Hoekstra RM. Effect of intensive handwashing promotion on childhood diarrhea in high-risk communities in Pakistan. A randomized controlled trial. *JAMA*. 2004;291:2547–2554.

109. Luby SP, Agboatwalla M, Painter J, Altaf A, Billhimer WL, Hoekstra RM. Effect of handwashing on child health. A randomized controlled trial. *Lancet*. 2005;366:225–233.

110. Huttly SRA, Lanata CF, Yeager BAC, Fukumoto M, Del Aguila R, Kendall C. Feces, flies, and fetor: findings from a Peruvian shantytown. *Pan Am Public Health*. 1998;4(2):75–79.

111. Zeitlin MF, Guldan G, Klein RE, Ahmad N, Ahmad K. Sanitary Conditions of Crawling Infants in Rural Bangladesh. Report to the USAID Asia Bureau and to the HHS Office of International Health, Bangladesh.

112. Yeager BAC, Huttly SRA, Diaz J, Bartolini R, Marin M, Lanata CF. An intervention for the promotion of hygienic feces disposal behaviors in a shanty town of Lima, Peru. *Health Education Research.* 2002;17:761–773.

113. Sepulveda J, Willett W, Munoz A. Malnutrition and diarrhea. A longitudinal study among urban Mexican children. *Am J Epidemiol.* 1988;127:365–376.

114. Baqui AH, Black RE, Sack RB, Chowdhury HR, Yunus M, Siddique AK. Malnutrition, cell-mediated immune deficiency and diarrhea: a community-based longitudinal study in rural Bangladeshi children. *Am J Epidemiol.* 1993;137:355–365.

115. Checkley W, Gilman RH, Black RE, et al. Effects of nutritional status on diarrhea in Peruvian children. *J Pediatr.* 2002;140: 210–218.

116. Black RE, Brown KH, Becker S. Malnutrition is a determining factor in diarrheal duration, but not incidence, among young children in a longitudinal study in rural Bangladesh. *Am J Clin Nutr.* 1984; 37:87–94.

117. Sommer A, Katz J, Tarwotjo L. Increased risk of respiratory disease and diarrhea in children with preexisting mild vitamin A deficiency. *Am J Clin Nutr.* 1984;40:1090–1095.

118. Sommer A, Dijunaedi E, Loeden AA, et al. Impact of vitamin A supplementation on childhood mortality. *Lancet.* 1986;1169–1173.

119. Sazawal S, Black RE, Bhan MK, et al. Efficacy of zinc supplementation in reducing the incidence and prevalence of acute diarrhea–a community-based, double blind, controlled trial. *Am J Clin Nutr.* 1997;66:413–418.

120. Bhutta ZA, Black RE, Brown KH, et al. Prevention of diarrhea and pneumonia by zinc supplementation in children in developing countries: pooled analysis of randomized controlled trials. *J Pediatr.* 1999;135:689–697.

121. Schiraldi O, Benvestito V, Di Bari C, et al. Gastric abnormalities in cholera: epidemiological and clinical considerations. *Bull WHO.* 1974;51:349–352.

122. Sullivan PB, Thomas JE, Wight DGD, et al. *Helicobacter pylori* in Gambian children with chronic diarrhoea and malnutrition. *Arch Dis Child.* 1990;65:189–191.

123. Glass RI, Holmgren J, Haley CE, et al. Predisposition for cholera of individuals with O blood group. Possible evolutionary significance. *Am J Epidemiol.* 1985;121:791–796.

124. Black RE, Levine MM, Clements ML, Hughes T, O'Donnell S. Association between O blood group and occurrence and severity of diarrhoea due to *Escherichia coli. Trans R Soc Trop Med Hyg.* 1987;81:120–123.

125. van Loon FPL, Clemens JD, Sack DA, et al. ABO blood groups and the risk of diarrhea due to enterotoxigenic *Escherichia coli. J Infect Dis.* 1991;163:1243–1246.

126. Black RE, Lanata CF, Lazo F. Delayed cutaneous hypersensitivity: epidemiologic factors affecting and usefulness in predicting diarrheal incidence in young Peruvian children. *Pediatr Infect Dis J.* 1989;8: 210–215.

127. Ali M, Emch M, von Seidlein L, et al. Herd immunity conferred by killed oral cholera vaccines in Bangladesh: a reanalysis. *Lancet.* 2005;10:1–6.

128. Lucas MES, Deen JL, von Seidlein L, et al. Effectiveness of mass oral cholera vaccination in Beira, Mozambique. *N Engl J Med.* 2005;352:757–767.

129. Lederberg J, Shope RE, Oaks SC Jr, eds. *Emerging Infections: Microbial Threats to Health in the United States.* National Academies Press; 1992:105.

130. Feachem RG, Koblinsky MA. Interventions for the control of diarrhoeal disease among young children: promotion of breast-feeding. *Bull WHO.* 1984;62:271–291.

131. World Health Organization. Research on improving infant feeding practices to prevent diarrhoea or reduce its severity: memorandum from a JHU/WHO meeting. *Bull WHO.* 1989;67:27–33.

132. Ashworth A, Feachem RG. Interventions for the control of diarrhoeal diseases among young children: weaning education. *Bull WHO.* 1985;63:1115–1117.

133. Mintz ED, Reiff FM, Tauxe RV. Safe water treatment and storage in the home. *JAMA.* 1995;273:948–953.

134. Feachem RG, Koblinsky MA. Interventions for the control of diarrhoeal diseases among young children: measles immunization. *Bull WHO.* 1983;61:641–652.

135. de Zoysa I, Feachem RG. Interventions for the control of diarrhoeal diseases among young children: rotavirus and cholera immunization. *Bull WHO.* 1985;63:569–583.

136. Sazawal S, Black RE, Menon VP, et al. Zinc supplementation in infants born small for gestational age reduces mortality: a prospective, randomized, controlled trial. *Pediatrics.* 2001;108:1280–1286.

137. Fischer Walker C, Black RE. Zinc and the risk for infectious disease. *Annu Rev Nutr.* 2004;24:255–275.

PART IV

BLOOD AND BODY FLUID AS A RESERVOIR OF INFECTIOUS DISEASES

HUMAN IMMUNODEFICIENCY VIRUS INFECTIONS AND THE ACQUIRED IMMUNE DEFICIENCY SYNDROME

Kenrad E. Nelson, Rohit Chitale, and David D. Celentano

Introduction

The AIDS epidemic was first recognized in the United States in 1980–1981 among men who have sex with men (MSM). The disease was recognized originally as clusters of *Pneumocystis carinii* pneumonia (PCP) and Kaposi's sarcoma (KS) (or both) occurring in MSM in Los Angeles, New York, and a few other cities, many of whom had reported sexual contact with another case (Figure 21-1).[1-4] Subsequently, similar patterns of disease occurred among injection drug users, persons with hemophilia, and some transfusion recipients.[5,6] The unusual increase in PCP among these populations led to a rapid growth in requests for the controlled antiparasitic drug, pentamidine, from the Centers for Disease Control and the early recognition that a new health problem was emerging.

Several research groups investigated the causes of the immunosuppression underlying the occurrence of these opportunistic infections. In 1984, Robert Gallo and colleagues at the National Cancer Institute of the NIH and Luc Montagnier and coworkers at the Pasteur Institute reported the discovery of the cause of AIDS, a novel human retrovirus, the human immunodeficiency virus (HIV).[7,8]

In retrospect, the disease likely had been present in Central and Eastern Africa much earlier, manifested by increases in cryptococcal meningitis and disseminated tuberculosis. Serological evidence of HIV infection was found in stored serum samples from subjects from Zaire that had been collected in 1959.[9] The probable origin of HIV-1 was from *Pan troglodytes* (chimpanzees) in West and Central Africa, which was transmitted to humans during hunting for "bush meat."[10] Another human immunodeficiency virus, HIV-2, was discovered subsequently in African Green monkeys in the wild in West Africa.[11] Humans can be infected either by HIV-1 or HIV-2, and both can cause immunodeficiency and AIDS, although the virulence of HIV-2 is considerably less than HIV-1.[12-13]

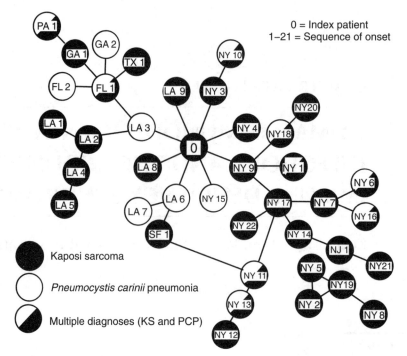

0 = Index patient
1–21 = Sequence of onset

Kaposi sarcoma

Pneumocystis carinii pneumonia

Multiple diagnoses (KS and PCP)

Cities: LA, Los Angeles; NY, New York City; SF, San Francisco.
States: FL, Florida; GA, Georgia; NJ, New Jersey; PA, Pennsylvania;
          TX, Texas.

FIGURE 21-1   Sexual contacts among homosexual men with AIDS. Each
circle represents an AIDS patient. Lines connecting the circles represent sexual
exposures. Indicated city or state is place of residence of a patient at the time of
diagnosis. "0" indicates Patient 0 (described in text).
Source: D. Auerbach et al., *American Journal of Medicine,* Cluster of Cases of the
Acquired Immune Deficiency Syndrome, Patients Linked by Sexual Contact, Vol.
76, pp. 487–492, Copyright 1984. Excerpta Medica Inc.

The AIDS Pandemic

Since AIDS was originally identified in the early 1980s, the disease has spread
to nearly every country in the world. AIDS has become a global pandemic of
extraordinary importance. The disease is most frequent in sub-Saharan Africa,
where the population prevalence among adults is estimated to be over 7%.[14]
The prevalence among adults worldwide is estimated by WHO to be 1.1%.[14]
AIDS decreases the life expectancy of its victims by 20 or more years, and it
has become the main cause of death in many sub-Saharan African countries.
Because of its relentless increase, involving primarily adolescents and young
adults during their prime of life, the AIDS epidemic has had a catastrophic
effect on many societies and economies.

The HIV Virus

The HIV virus is a retrovirus, signifying that the double-stranded RNA undergoes reverse transcription to form double-stranded DNA in the cytoplasm of

an infected cell (Figure 21-2). The viral genome consists of three structural genes, termed *env*, *pol*, and *gag*. The genome codes for several regulatory proteins, including Tat, Rev, Vif, Vpu, Vpr, and Nef. The p16/p14 Tat proteins activate viral transcription. The p14 Rev protein is responsible for the transport and stability of viral RNA. The p27/p25 Nef proteins are active in the down regulation of CD4 cells.

The HIV virus attaches to the CD4 cell through high-affinity interactions between the viral envelope protein, Gp120, and a specific region of the CD4 molecule (Figure 21-3). The CD4 molecule is present in abundance on both immature T lymphocytes and mature CD4+ helper T lymphocytes. It is also present in lower concentrations on monocytes, macrophages, and antigen-presenting dendritic cells. In addition, coreceptors termed *CCR5* and *CXCR4* are involved in binding and entry of HIV into the cell. Cells of the monocyte/macrophage origin generally only express CCR5; however, many lymphocyte populations express both receptors. The transmitted viruses are usually macrophage or lymphocytotropic and utilize the CCR5 coreceptors. However, occasionally CXCR4 strains are more commonly transmitted.

Some viruses are able to cause lymphocytes to fuse together causing the formation of syncytia. The syncytia-forming viruses (CXCR-4 or C-4 strains) infect lymphocytes and are commonly associated with more rapid progression of disease, whereas the CCR5 strains are transmitted and usually predominate early in infection.

After the virus enters the cell, the viral RNA is converted to DNA using the viral enzyme reverse transcriptase. The double-stranded DNA molecules then enter the nucleus and are integrated into the host cell chromosomal DNA. In quiescent cells the transcription and integration may be incomplete and viral DNA may remain in the cytoplasm. The unintegrated DNA is short lived; however, integrated DNA can persist for long periods in resting T lymphocytes.[15]

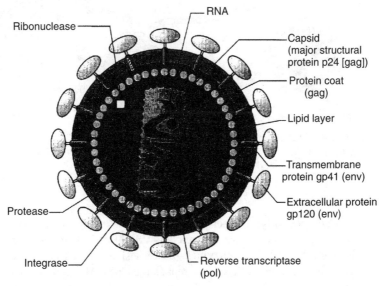

FIGURE 21-2 Antigenic structure of HIV.
Source: HIV/AIDS Learning system, Section 2.3, *The Prime Deceiver: HIV*, Figures 14 and 15 © GlaxoSmithKline, Inc.

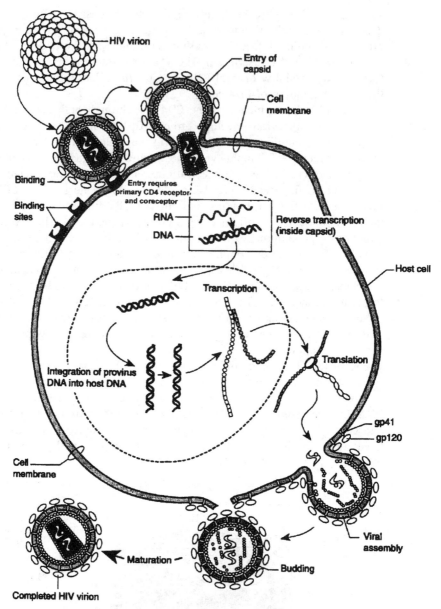

FIGURE 21-3 Schematic drawing of the HIV life cycle.
Source: HIV/AIDS Learning system, Section 2.3, *The Prime Deceiver: HIV*, Figures 14 and 15 © GlaxoSmithKline, Inc.

Subsequently, transcription of the HIV genome occurs to form RNA transcripts, which leave the nucleus. Modification of the viral polyproteins by cellular and viral enzymes (proteases) are essential for viral assembly. The virus is then spliced and repackaged near the cell surface and released from the host cell.

HIV has a high replication rate, with approximately 10 billion viral particles produced each day.[16,17] The generation time of HIV averages 2.6

days, with the half-life of the virus lasting about 6 hours and the half-life of an infected cell lasting 1.3 days. Using these data, it has been calculated that 140 generations of HIV are produced each year in an infected patient. A second, much slower, plateau phase has been described, which involves latently infected CD4+ T lymphocytes and macrophages. The viral genome is archived in the genome of these resting lymphocytes so that HIV is not eradicable even with several years, or even decades, of highly active anti-retroviral therapy.[15] The presence of this reservoir has essentially eliminated the possibility of a permanent cure of HIV infection with currently available therapy even with aggressive therapy early after infection.

There are several major targets of anti-HIV chemotherapy designed to interfere with viral replication. Several drugs have been developed to inhibit the reverse transcriptase (RT) enzyme. The RT enzyme is responsible for copying the viral genetic material into DNA. However, this enzyme has a high error rate—about one mutation per virus replication event. This means that mutants are constantly being generated that have the potential for drug resistance. Another target, for which drugs have been developed, is the protease enzymes that are important for viral assembly. Resistance also can develop to the protease inhibitors (PIs). The third drug target is the attachment of the virus to the CD4 cell receptor. One drug has been licensed that inhibits attachment and entry. Other drugs are being developed to inhibit viral DNA integration (integrase inhibitors) and to inhibit attachment to coreceptors; however, these drugs have not yet been licensed for therapy.

HIV Natural History

After HIV infection either by sexual contact or parenterally, the virus is present in the blood and the viral RNA can be detected within 7–10 days. About 7–21 days later HIV antibodies appear in the blood. Early in the infection, the viral load is usually very high.[18] Subsequently an immune response occurs, which includes the appearance of antibodies and a cellular response with CD8+ cytotoxic T lymphocytes directed against the virus. At this point, the level of viremia declines and a viral "set point" is established in 3–4 months (Figure 21-4). The level of the viral set point can vary considerably and is predictive of the rate at which the disease will progress. The AIDS mortality among untreated persons with very high viral load at the set point, that is, greater than 100,000 copies/mL, is quite rapid and averages about 4.5 years, whereas persons with lower viral loads at the set point survive more than 10 years after their infection.[19] After the set point is reached, a gradual decline in the level of CD4+ T lymphocytes occurs with an elevated level of CD8+ T lymphocytes, so that the total number of CD3+ T cells is relatively stable for several years. Nevertheless, the CD4/CD8 lymphocyte ratio is significantly decreased (i.e., less than 1.0) compared to the uninfected state. About 18–24 months prior to the development of clinical AIDS, the level of total CD3+ cells decreases more rapidly, meaning there is loss of T-cell homeostasis.[20] The loss of T-cell homeostasis signifies an inability to keep up with the virus-induced destruction of the immune system. This is often accompanied by a "switch" in the coreceptor utilization of the dominant HIV, from a CCR5, or non-syncitium-inducing cell type, to a CXCR-4

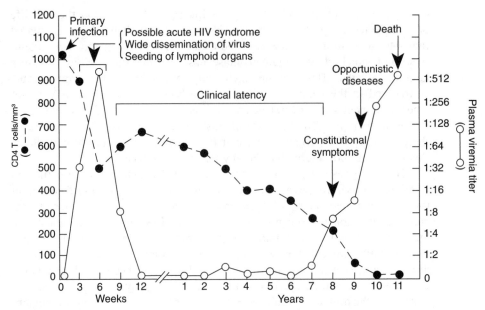

FIGURE 21-4 Typical course of HIV infection in persons who receive no treatment. Following primary infection, a chain of events occurs over the next decade of the person's life—widespread dissemination of HIV in peripheral blood accompanied by an abrupt fall in CD4+ lymphocytes; a clinical latency period lasting about 5 years; further declines in CD4 cells marked by constitutional symptoms, opportunistic diseases, and death. *Source:* Pantaleo et al. Mechanisms of Disease: The Immuno-pathogenesis of Human Immunodeficiency Virus Infection, *New England Journal of Medicine,* Vol. 328, pp. 327–335. Copyright © 1993, Massachusetts Medical Society.

(syncitium-inducing or duotropic) type. Occasionally, CXCR-4 viruses are transmitted initially and predominate even early in the infection; in such cases the progression to clinical AIDS is more rapid.[21]

During the acute stage, 2–4 weeks after infection when HIV levels in the blood are maximal, an "acute HIV infection syndrome" commonly occurs, which has been reported in about 50% or more of patients in some closely observed cohorts in developed countries.[22-24] The symptoms resemble infectious mononucleosis and include fever (95%), adenopathy (75%), pharyngitis (70%), rash (70%), and other systemic symptoms, including meningitis, Guillain-Barré syndrome, peripheral neuropathy, and Bell's palsy.[22-24] Generally, HIV serology is negative during this acute seroconversion syndrome, but patients have demonstrable viremia but seroconversion occurs within a few weeks after symptoms resolve spontaneously.

A meta-analysis of the time from HIV-1 seroconversion to AIDS and death (before the widespread use of highly active antiretroviral therapy [HAART]) among 13,030 HIV-1 seroconverters enrolled in 38 studies in Europe, North America, and Australia has been published—the CASCADE study.[25] These data are the most comprehensive evaluation of the time to AIDS and death among persons in developed countries in the pre-HAART era. The CASCADE investigators found that the median time to AIDS was about 9.5–11.0 years, and the median survival was 10.5–11.8 years after infection in patients not receiving effective therapy (Figure 21-5). There were

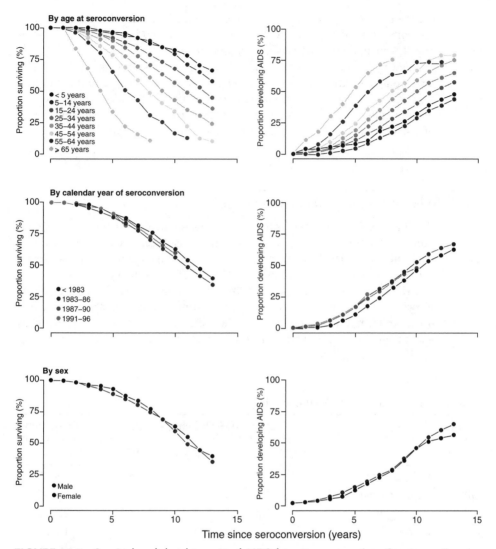

FIGURE 21-5 Survival and development of AIDS from seroconversion. Curves continue until fewer than 10 individuals remain at risk. Data shown in upper graphs are adjusted for study. Data shown in middle graphs are based on individuals aged 15–54 years at seroconversion, adjusted for age at seroconversion to age 25–29 years and for study. Data shown in lower graphs are based on individuals exposed through injecting drug use and sex between men and women, aged 15–54 years at seroconversion, adjusted for age at seroconversion to age 25–29 years, and for exposure category and study.
Source: CASCADE study. Time from HIV seroconversion to AIDS and death before widespread use of highly-active antiretroviral therapy: a collaborative re-analysis. Lancet 2000;355:1131–1137, with permission from Elsevier.

no significant differences in progression by exposure category, gender, or year of infection between 1983 and 1996. However, the age of the person at the time of infection substantially affected the progression rate. Persons who were older when they were infected progressed more rapidly. Among persons aged 15–24 years at the time of infection, the median survival was 12.5 years (95% CI, 12.0–12.9), and the median time to AIDS was 12.0 years

(95% CI, 10.7–11.7 years). In contrast, among persons 45–54 years old at seroconversion, the median AIDS-free interval was 7.7 years (95% CI, 7.1–8.6) and the median survival was 11.0 years (10.7–11.7).

Fewer data are available on the rate of progression among persons in developing countries. However, a recent study in Thailand found that progression was more rapid among young adults compared to HIV-infected persons of comparable age in developed industrialized countries, with median survival of 7.4–8.4 years after seroconversion among infected Thais.[26]

AIDS-Related Opportunistic Infections

The diagnostic hallmark of AIDS is the development of opportunistic infections (OIs) secondary to the immunocompromise caused by HIV infection. A large number of OIs have been identified in immunosuppressed HIV-infected persons and have been classified as "AIDS-defining illnesses."

The CDC lists 28 conditions as "AIDS-defining illnesses." However, *Pneumocystis carinii* pneumonia, the HIV wasting syndrome, Kaposi sarcoma, oropharyngeal and esophageal candidiasis, extrapulmonary cryptococcus, and tuberculosis account for most initial AIDS-defining OIs in patients in the United States (Table 21-1).

TABLE 21-1   Frequency of AIDS-Defining Diagnosis

	Initial AIDS-Defining Diagnosis[a]			Frequency Among All Patients (%)[b]
	1990 (%)	1995 (%)	1997 (%)	
Pneumocystis carinii pneumonia	49	28	42	75–85
HIV wasting syndrome[c]	17	14	11	70–90
Candida esophagitis	13	11	15	20–30
Kaposi's sarcoma	11	6	11	15–25
HIV-associated dementia	6	4	4	40–70
Disseminated CMV	6	6	4	80–90
Toxoplasmosis encephalitis	5	3	3	5–15
Disseminated *M. avium* infection	4	4	5	30–40
Lymphoma	3	2	4	3–5
Chronic mucocutaneous herpes simplex[c]	3	4	1	10–25
Cryptococcal meningitis	3	4	—	8–12
Cryptosporidiosis	2	2	2	5–10
Tuberculosis	—	5[c]	5	4–20

[a] Frequency according to CDC criteria for AIDS 1987–1992 as reported for newly diagnosed cases in 1990 and for 1995.
[b] Estimated lifetime frequency among all patients with AIDS without prophylaxis.
[c] Added in the revised case definition of 1993.
Source: Data from the Centers for Disease Control and Prevention.

The frequency of the initial AIDS-defining diagnosis among cases reported to the CDC in 1990, 1995, and 1997, using the pre-1993 clinical definition is shown in Table 21-1.

AIDS-related OIs in developing countries often have a different distribution at the onset of AIDS than has been reported among patients in the United States and other industrialized countries. In Thailand, for example, the distribution of the top 10 AIDS-defining illnesses among 101,945 cases of symptomatic AIDS that were reported between 1994 and 1998 is shown in Table 21-2.[27]

Thailand is similar to many other developing countries in Asia and Africa in that tuberculosis is the most frequent AIDS-defining illness, followed closely by the wasting syndrome and several systemic fungal infections, namely candidiasis, cryptococcosis, and penicilliosis. Also, PCP, which has been classified as a fungous infection caused by *Pneumocystis javonecki*, is common in Thailand. The frequent occurrence of PCP differs from the clinical reports of AIDS in Africa, where PCP among adults has been reported to be rare, although it appears to occur commonly in pediatric AIDS cases.[28] Infection with *Penicillium marneffei* is limited to AIDS patients in Southeast Asia, where the organism is endemic and is geographically localized to this area.[29] Kaposi's sarcoma is relatively rare among AIDS patients in Asia but is quite common among such patients in Africa and the Caribbean.[27,30]

Disseminated histoplasmosis is a common AIDS-defining illness among patients in the histoplasmosis belt in the US Midwest.[31] Leishmaniasis is a common AIDS-related OI in Spain and other areas where this organism is endemic.[32]

TABLE 21-2   AIDS-Defining Illnesses Among Patients >10 Years of Age in Thailand, 1994–1998

Illness	Number	%
Tuberculosis	29,437	28.9
Wasting syndrome	28,729	28.2
Pneumocystic carinii pneumonia	20,145	19.8
Disseminated cryptococcosis	18,821	18.5
Esophageal candidiasis	5,989	5.9
Pneumonia, bacterial	3,691	3.6
Penicillium marneffei	3,054	3.0
Cerebral toxoplasmosis	3,133	3.1
HIV encephalopathy	1,987	1.9
Cryptosporidiosis	895	0.9

Source: Chariyalertsak S et al, Clinical presentation and risk behaviors of patients with acquired immunodeficiency syndrome in Thailand, 1994–1998: regional variation and temporal trends. Clin Infect Dis 2001;32:955–962. Copyright University of Chicago Press.

Timing of AIDS-Related Opportunistic Infections

The time of occurrence of AIDS-related opportunistic infections during the natural history of HIV infection varies with each OI (Figure 21-6). Typically, oropharyngeal and esophageal candidiasis, oral hairy leukoplakia, and tuberculosis occur relatively early in an HIV infection when the CD4+ count may be between 200–300 cells/μL. Disseminated cytomegalovirus infections (CMV), toxoplasmosis, and *Mycobacterium avium* infections usually do not occur until the CD4+ cell count is below 50–100 cell/μL. This knowledge of the natural history of HIV has been used to develop antibiotic protocols to prevent frequently occurring OIs in patients with HIV. In some cases, antibiotic prophylaxis of an opportunistic infection has been shown to delay the progression of HIV/AIDS and to prolong survival of HIV-positive patients. Prolonged survival has been shown for prophylaxis of PCP, tuberculosis, and *M. avium* infections.[33] It is equally likely, but no clear data have been reported, that prevention of fungal infections may also prolong survival of antiretroviral naive patients.

A CDC task force has reviewed the published literature and the available scientific evidence and published recommendations for the use of prophylactic regimens for the prevention of specific AIDS-related OIs.[33] It is clear that HAART has substantially reduced the risk of OIs. The use of effective antiretroviral therapy with HAART clearly is the most effective way to prevent OIs. However, OI prophylaxis is still important among patients who cannot take or who fail to respond to HAART. In developing countries where HAART regimens are being introduced but are not yet widely available, effective OI prophylaxis should be provided to patients in need to allow them to survive long enough to eventually receive effective HAART when treatment availability expands.

The conditions shown in Table 21-3 were felt by the CDC task force to be "strongly recommended" as the standard of care for AIDS patients or "generally recommended."

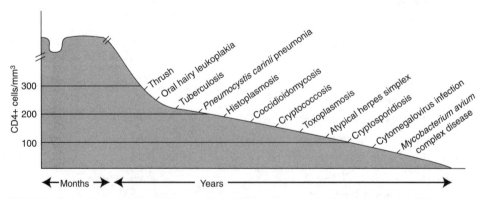

FIGURE 21-6 Occurrence of opportunistic illnesses that typically occur as the CD4+ lymphocyte count in peripheral blood progressively decreases over time in an untreated HIV-infected patient.
Source: Schooley, R., *Acquired Immune Deficiency Syndrome, Infectious Disease,* Scientific American Medicine, Vol. 2. Dale DC, Federman DD, Eds. Copyright 1998 WebMD, New York, NY.

TABLE 21-3   Diseases for Which CDC Task Force Recommends Prophylaxis in HIV-Infected Patients to Prevent AIDS-Related OIs and Progression

Disease	Prophylaxis	Level
Tuberculosis (latent), i.e., PPD+	INH and pyramethamine	Strong
Pneumocystis carinii pneumonia	TMP-SMX	Strong
Toxoplasmosis (*T. gondii* antibody-positive pts)	Toxoplasma-IgG antibody pos TMP-SMX	Strong
M. avium complex	(<100 CD4+) clarithromycin or azithromycin	Strong
Strep. pneumonia	Pneumovax	General
Influenza	Influenza vaccine	General
Hepatitis B virus	HBV vaccine	General
Hepatitis A virus	HAV vaccine	General (esp. for HCV carriers)

Note: Consult CDC. *MMWR.* 2002;51:RR-6 for details of recommendations.
Source: Data from the Centers for Disease Control and Prevention.

In patients who develop a sustained CDC+ count above 200 cells/mm³, it is felt to be safe to discontinue prophylaxis for PCP. Because of the different distribution of AIDS OIs in many developing countries, decisions for when to use prophylaxis and which agents to use may differ. For example, in Thailand and many other developing countries in Asia and Africa, where fungal infections are much more common than in the United States and Europe, prophylaxis with an antifungal drug such as itraconizole has been evaluated and recommended.[34]

Host Factors in Susceptibility or Resistance to HIV Infection and Disease Progression

After infection with HIV the host mounts an immune response consisting of both cellular and humoral immunity. This response usually results in some control of viral replication with a substantial decrease in the viral load. The decrease in viral load coincides with the appearance of HIV-specific CD8+ cytotoxic T lymphocytes and replication of the CD4+ T-cell population. The CD8+ and/or CD4+ cytotoxic T cells kill HIV-infected cells, which present viral peptides associated with HLA molecules. Memory CD4+ T lymphocytes persist and respond to active HIV replication. However, the HIV virus eventually destroys the CD4+ T-cell population sufficiently that T-cell homeostasis fails, and the patient progresses to clinical AIDS and succumbs to the infection.[20]

Mucosal IgA and IgG antibodies and CD8+ T cells may inhibit HIV at the mucosal surface and prevent or clear HIV infection after exposure. Also, CD8+ and CD4+ T cells may clear infection after the virus has penetrated the mucosal barrier early in infection. Clearance of virus may occur prior to the appearance of neutralizing antibodies; however, exposed persons may harbor T lymphocytes that respond specifically to HIV peptides by proliferation and cytokine secretion.[35-36] The ability of this acquired immunity after HIV exposure in some frequently exposed persons and nonprogression of the infection for prolonged periods in other infected persons have given rise to some optimism that the disease could be controlled with a vaccine or antiviral drugs.

In addition to the acquired immune response, several genetic host factors have been discovered that influence resistance or susceptibility to infection. Among these host factors is a common genetic mutation, a 32 base pair deletion, that was discovered in the chemokine receptor, CXCR-5, the coreceptor for entry of most transmitted viruses into host cells. Persons who are homozygous for this mutation are resistant to infection with CXCR-5 utilizing viruses.[37] Persons who are heterozygous for the deletion have lower viral loads and slower progression to AIDS.[38] More recently, additional host genetic factors have been identified that affect the resistance or susceptibility to HIV-1 infection or the rate of progression to AIDS after infection. These include a mutation in the CCR5 promoter, a CCR2–641 mutation, and a mutation in the stromal-derived factor (SDF13′A/3′A).[39,40] The number of segmental duplications of two CC chemokine genes, CCL3L1 and CCL4L1, on chromosome 17q were recently shown to be associated with the susceptibility to HIV infection and the rate of progression after infection in several human populations.[41]

Persons who are homozygous at one, two, or three HLA class 1 loci or have a polymorphism for interleukin 10 (IL-10+/5′A or 5′A/5′A) have more rapid progression after they are infected.[42] However, homozygosity of class 1 HLA alleles has not been shown to increase the risk of HIV infection. In contrast, HLA class 1 allele sharing between an infected person and an exposed seronegative recipient, either a sexual contact or mother-infant pair, has been shown to increase the risk of transmission.[43,44] Also, one study has found discordance of an HLA class II allele, HLA-DRB3, to be protective for the sexual transmission of HIV-1 among a sample of couples.[45]

Specific HLA alleles have also been shown to influence the genetic susceptibility to HIV-1 infection. The alleles HLA-B*27 and B*57 have been consistently associated with a favorable prognosis after infection, mostly by influencing early viral equilibration,[42] although they do not protect against HIV infection. In contrast, HLA-B*35 and HLA-B*53 have been associated with an unfavorable prognosis and higher viral load in infected individuals.[42] No other single HLA-B allele has been thus far shown to have a significant influence on the disease progression, nor have any associations between HLA-A or HLA-C alleles and natural history been demonstrated convincingly. However, research in the genetic influences on HIV susceptibility and natural history is being pursued by several research groups at present.

The combined effect of several of these genetic host factors on the natural history of HIV infection has been studied among 525 homosexual men in the MACS cohort who seroconverted between 1984 and 1996, prior to the advent of HAART.[46] On the basis of a regression tree analysis using a Cox proportional hazard model for times to AIDS, it was estimated that 30% of the men enrolled in MACS had one or more genetic resistance factors. The participants with the genetic resistance determinants had slower progression early after their infection, although the effect was limited to the first four years after infection. Clearly, additional evaluation of host resistance factors influencing HIV infection and progression will be important. However, such studies require large cohorts of carefully followed subjects in various populations in whom genetic diversity can be evaluated. Some of the host factors currently believed to be related to susceptibility or resistance to HIV-1 infection and progression are listed in Table 21-4.

Recent research has discovered several cellular factors that suppress HIV-1 replication. It has been known for some time that several human and primate cell lines were naturally resistant to infection with HIV-1. One mechanism of this natural resistance has been identified to be due to a protein called tripartite motif (TRIM) 5-alpha, which has ubiquiton ligase activity. When the TRIM 5-alpha gene from monkey cells that were resistant to HIV-1 infection were transferred into and expressed by normally susceptible human cells resistance to HIV-1 infection was induced.[47] This finding could eventually be important for the development of new therapeutic approaches to control HIV-1 infection.

Another cellular mechanism to defend against infection with HIV-1 and other retroviruses has been described recently. This resistance is mediated by a cytidine deaminase termed APOBEC3G (an acronym for Apolipoprotein B mRNA catalytic polypeptide).[48] The activity of APOBEC3G in deaminating HIV-1 DNA is neutralized by the vif (viral infectivity factor) gene of HIV-1 viruses. The successful replication of HIV-1 in cells is determined by a balance between cellular APOBEC3-6 and viral. Recently, vif Importantly mutations in APOBEC3G have been discovered.[49] One such mutation, H186 RR, has been associated with a more rapid decline in T lymphocytes and progression to AIDS. This codon-changing variant gene was found to be common among

TABLE 21-4   Association Between Human Genetic Markers and Polymorphisms and Susceptibility to HIV-1 Infection and Progression

Genetic Marker	Effect on Risk
CCR5	
Homozygous 32 base pair deletion	Absolute protection from CCR5 viruses
Heterozygous 32 base pair deletion	Slower progression
Promoter P1/-P1	Slower progression
CCR2-641	Slower progression
Increased CCL3L1 segmented duplication	Increased resistance
HLA Class 1 homozygous	Rapid progression
HLA-DR B3+ homozygous (couples)	Increased transmission
HLA concordance (in couples)	Increased transmission
HLA-B*57, HLA-B*27	Slower progression
HLA-B*35, HLA-B*53	More rapid progression
HLA-A2/6802 and HLA-A0205/6802	Decreased transmission
TRIM 5a	Slower progression associated with some SNPs due to an uncoating block
APOBEC3G (RR Genotype)	More rapid disease progression
NK (natural killer) KIR alleles (e.g., 3DS1 and 3D1 in pts. with BW4 genotype)	Slower progression

African Americans ($f = 37\%$) but rare in European Americans ($f = 5\%$) with HIV-1 infection.[50]

HIV Genotypes

HIV-1 has been classified into three groups, based on genetic relatedness, namely, groups M, N, and O. The latter two groups are geographically limited to countries in West Africa. Group M strains of HIV-1 have been divided into 11 genetic subtypes, designated A–K. Particular subtypes are found more commonly in certain areas of the world. In the Americas and Europe, subtype B strains have predominated, whereas in Africa various subtypes have been more common in different countries. In India, subtype C has predominated, and in Thailand and other countries in Southeast Asia, subtype E (now called CRF01_AE) has predominated.

In the last 10 years the frequency and importance of viral recombination has been recognized. Recombinants are becoming more common over time, and genetic subtypes are showing significant dynamism between and across countries, risk groups, and regions. Data from Africa, Asia, and South America have shown that a significant percentage of circulating strains represent mosaics of two or more subtypes. Coinfection by different subtypes is apparently not uncommon. Packaging of RNA from different subtypes into the same viral particle, coupled with the strand-switching activity of reverse transcriptase, generates recombinant HIV in coinfected individuals. Since full-length viral sequencing became more efficient in the past 5 years, it has become clear that subtypes and recombinants are equally important in the pandemic. Recombinant viruses are now identified as *circulating recombinant forms* (CRFs), if the same recombinants are commonly found, or Unique Recombinant Forms (URFs) if found in only a few individuals. The distribution of HIV-1 genotypes in 3 East African countries (Uganda, Tanzania, and Kenya) included 35–45% URFs, emphasizing the frequency of coinfections or super infections with different HIV-1 geneotypes in these populations.[51] Subtype E has been classified as a recombinant subtype when the first full-genome sequences were done and is now designated CRF01_AE; several other strains have been recognized as recombinants based on full-length or partial sequences.[51] It is now possible to amplify virtually the full-length 9.0 kilobase genome as a single amplicon, permitting the refined classification of HIV genotypes and recombinant forms.

A recent classification of the subtypes and their geographic distribution is shown in Table 21-5 and Figure 21-7. In some areas the CRF strains have become the most commonly transmitted viral subtype, such as CRF01_AE in Southeast Asia. Worldwide, the most frequent subtype among HIV-infected individuals is subtype C, which predominates among infected individuals in Southern Africa and India.

The relevance of subtype infection to such biological variables as infectivity, rate of progression after infection, and response to therapy is currently being evaluated. One study reported higher replication rates of subtype E (CRF01_AE) and C viruses than subtype B viruses in Langerhans cell cultures.[52] However, other investigators were unable to replicate these results.[53] A cross-sectional study of heterosexual couples in Thailand found a higher

TABLE 21-5 Full Genome Sequences of HIV-1 and Their Geographic Origins

	Category*	Number	Geographic Origins
Subtypes	A	14	Uganda, Tanzania, Kenya, Somalia
	B	17	USA, Europe, China, Africa
	C	21	Eastern and Southern Africa, India, Brazil, USA
	D	17	Uganda, DRC, Kenya
	F and F2	6	DRC, Kenya, Congo, Cameroon
	G	4	Nigeria, Kenya, Congo, DRC
	H	3	Belgium, CAR
	I	2	DRC, Sweden
	K	2	Cameroon
Circulating, recombinant forms	CRF01_AE CM240	9	Thailand, China, CAR, USA
	CRF02_AG IbNG	11	Djibouti, Ivory Coast, Cameroon, USA
	CRF03_A8 Kal153	1	Russia
	CRF04_cpx CY032	3	Cyprus, Greece
	CRF05_FD V11310	2	DRC
	CRF06_cpx BFP90	2	Burkina Faso, Mali
	CRF07_BC c34	2	China
	CRF08_BC GX-6F	3	China
	CRF09_cpx p2911	4	Senegal, USA
Unique recombinant forms	AC recombinant	10	Tanzania, Zambia, Rwanda, Ethiopia, India, Uganda
	AD recombinant	10	Uganda, Kenya
	BE recombinant	2	Thailand, USA
	Other recombinant	11	Various
Other	Unclassified	5	Cameroon, DRC, Gabon

*The designations F and F2 represent sub-subtypes, CRF are numbered in the order discovered, "cpx." A complex recombinant combining three or more subtypes. The structures of CRF are given by reference to a prototype strain, as indicated. The names CRF07_BC, CRF08_BC, and CRF09_cpx are provisional. "Unique," recombinant forms so far identified only in a single individual and without current evidence of epidemic spread. Unclassified strains fail to cluster with known subtypes in all genome regions examined. "USA" includes US Military seroconverters, many of whom may have been infected while on deployment overseas. DRC, Democratic Republic of Congo, formerly Zaire; CAR, Central African Republic.
Source: McCutchan, FE. Understanding the diversity of HIV-1. AIDS. 14(suppl 3): S31-S44.

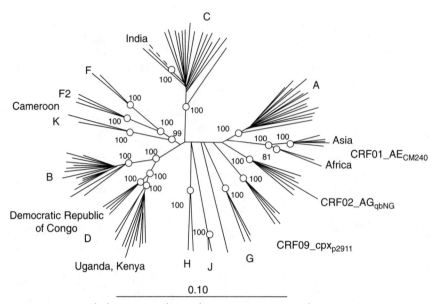

FIGURE 21-7   Phylogenetic relationships among HIV-1 subtypes.
Source: McCutchan FE. Understanding the diversity of HIV-1. AIDS. 14(suppl 3): S31–S44. Copyright American Medical Association.

risk of sexual transmission of subtype E (CRF01_AE) than subtype B virus.[54] Also, subtype E strains have become more frequent among injection drug users (IDUs) in Bangkok, as the Thai epidemic has evolved, possibly suggesting greater infectivity.[55] In the early stages of HIV-1 infection the plasma viral load of subtype E–infected patients has been found to exceed that of those with subtype B infections, but the viral load equalizes 18 months after infection.[56]

However, there is also evidence against significant differences in infectivity of various genotypes. For example, there are many persons infected with subtypes other than B in Europe, but there is no evidence of more efficient spread of non-B subtypes by sexual transmission. Studies of maternal-infant transmission of HIV-1 in different regions of the world suggest similar rates of vertical transmission of the various subtypes in the absence of preventive interventions.

The relationship between HIV subtypes and clinical progression has been investigated in several populations with diverse strains. For example, in over 2000 hospitalized patients in Thailand, the level of immune suppression, spectrum of opportunistic infections, and mortality were similar with subtype B- and CRF01_AE-infected patients.[57] However, a study of survival after infection with subtype CRF01_AE strains among Thai military conscripts found significantly shorter median survival (7.8–8.4 years) than has been reported among cohorts of persons from Western countries infected with subtype B strains.[26] Whether the decreased survival was due to viral, host, or environmental factors is not clear. In Kenya, where subtypes A, C, and D cocirculate, the plasma RNA levels were highest and the CD4 counts were lowest in persons infected with subtype C viruses.[58] In Uganda, subtype D infection has been reported to be associated with more rapid progression than subtype A.[59] However, a study in Sweden showed no differences in the rate of CD4 cell decline or clinical progression among persons infected with subtypes A, B, C, or D.[60] In a prospective study in Senegal, persons infected with subtypes C, D, or G were eight times more likely to develop AIDS during follow-up than those infected with subtype A.[61] It is difficult to determine whether the apparent variation in progression among persons infected with different subtypes is due to genetic differences in the viruses, host characteristics, or other factors.

Studies of the genetic diversity of HIV strains have been very useful in tracing epidemiologic patterns of HIV-1 transmission in populations. Among IDUs in Russia, several subtypes of HIV-1 have been recovered, including subtype A, subtype B, and a recombinant A/B strain, isolated from patients in Kaliningrad, a Russian enclave on the Baltic Sea.[62] Shortly thereafter, the same strain appeared in patients in distant areas of Russia, apparently having been spread by contaminated heroin. In Southeast Asia genetic sequencing of HIV-1 viruses has been used to identify four overland heroin-trafficking routes (Figure 21-8).[63] CRF01_AE strains from Northern Vietnam and in Guangxi province in neighboring Southern China are linked. A B/C recombinant strain has been found among IDUs that was introduced into Guangxi from a different route from Yunnan province in Southern China north of Laos and Thailand. A distinct B/C recombinant strain has been identified by full-genome sequencing that originated in Myanmar and spread through Yunnan to the North and West and reached its highest concentration in Xinjiang Province in Northern China.[63] The use of genetic sequencing of HIV-1 isolates to map the transmission routes, especially those associated with the distribution of illicit drugs, appears to have yielded important epidemiologic data.

Impact of Coinfections on HIV

It is now widely accepted that the progression to AIDS among HIV-1-infected individuals is highly correlated with HIV-1 viral load and the CD4 cell count.[19,64] It is also likely that differential immune activation is the primary driver of the variability in progression to AIDS in persons infected with HIV-1.[65-67] Over the last several years, evidence has accumulated in support of the theory that coinfections, through chronic immune activation and its consequent effect on host immunity and HIV progression, may account for the enhanced HIV infection rate, accelerated progression of disease, and reduced survival seen in sub-Saharan Africa.[71]

Sexually Transmitted Diseases (STDs)

The HIV epidemic in sub-Saharan Africa has developed in a population with a preexisting burden of infectious diseases, and these concurrent infections appear to have important interactions with HIV. Sexually transmitted diseases (STDs) are known to have a direct effect on HIV-1 transmission, especially those with genital ulceration, such as *Treponema pallidum*, HSV-2, and *Haemophilus ducreyi*.[68-73] Both ulcerative and nonulcerative STDs also

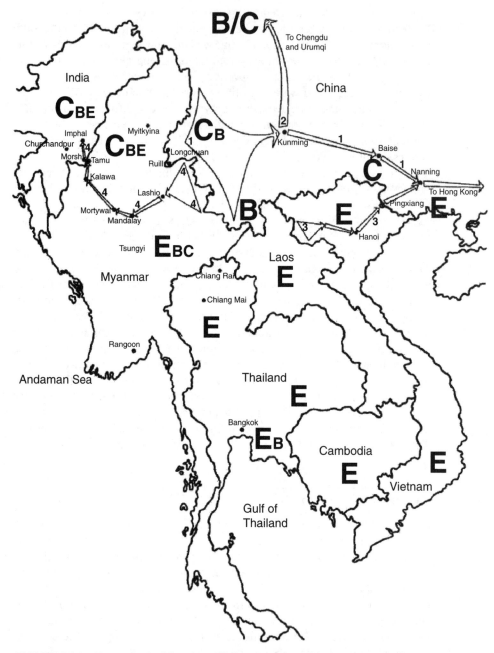

FIGURE 21-8 Four principal heroin trafficking routes and known HIV-1 subtypes (B, C, E, B/C recombinant) in south and Southeast Asia, 1999.
Source: Beyrer, C. et al. Overland heroin trafficking routes and HIV-1 spread in south and south-east Asia. AIDS. 2000 Jan 7;14(1):75–83.

have been associated with an increased viral load in the genital tract.[71,74] Nonulcerative STDs have also been shown to increase HIV-1 transmission, possibly via increased CD4+ cell recruitment and activation at the genital tract.[75-76] In vitro studies have shown that *T. pallidum* can induce HIV gene expression in monocytes through a nuclear factor NF-κ B pathway.[77] Studies have found a substantial increased concentration of HIV in the genital tract of persons infected with *N. gonorrhea* or other STDs, which decreased after successful treatment of the STD.[78,79] The increased HIV viral load in the genital tract of HIV-positive persons during frequent STDs has been postulated to explain, in part, the rapid dissemination of HIV in sub-Saharan Africa and Asia.[77,78,80–82]

Tuberculosis

Worldwide, tuberculosis is the most common major opportunistic infection among HIV-infected individuals. Since the inception of the HIV epidemic, there has been a resurgence of tuberculosis.[83] Though HIV infection puts an individual at increased risk for tuberculosis infection or reactivation, the converse also seems to hold true—the host response to tuberculosis infection sets in motion a cascade that increases the risk of HIV acquisition and disease progression. The usual host response to tuberculosis infection is that of cellular activation following a Th1 cytokine response.[84] In individuals infected with HIV and tuberculosis, tumor necrosis factor (TNF)-α is upregulated and present at much higher levels than among HIV-1-negative individuals; certain Th2 pathway cytokines (e.g., IL-6) are also decreased in coinfected individuals. These elevated levels of TNF-α are associated with enhanced HIV replication, in part due to the activation of the NF-κ B.[85]

Helminths

It has been hypothesized that parasitic infections, specifically helminths, (schistosomiasis, ascaris, book worm, and taenia) may be responsible, in part, for the increased susceptibility and spread of HIV in the developing world.[65-67] Specifically, the immune activation caused by helminthic infections is thought to increase the susceptibility to and progression of HIV in coinfected persons. The evidence supporting this hypothesis comes in part from studies of Ethiopian Jews who have emigrated to Israel, as well as residents of the Western Cape region of South Africa. The majority of Ethiopian immigrants were infected with helminths, and their immunological profiles were dominated by activation of a Th2 response.[65-67] There is some evidence that Th2 clones are more permissive for HIV-1 infection, and a Th2 predominance or a Th2 immune activation may impede the development of antiviral immunity.[85] This immune activation is also marked by increased expression of HIV coreceptors and decreased secretion of β–chemokines in vitro.[67] Further, studies in some populations have found that antihelminthic treatment has been associated with decreased HIV plasma viral load. However, the reduction in HIV viral load after antihelminth therapy has not been observed in all African populations.[86] The dominant cytokine response in *M. tuberculosis* infection is Th1, and 90% of individuals newly infected with *M. tuberculosis* do not develop active TB, in part, due to the Th1 immune response. However, when there is a Th1/Th2 shift, the predominant Th2 response may predispose such individuals to an increased risk of both HIV and active *M. tuberculosis* when they are exposed.[66]

Malaria

Together, malaria and HIV cause more than 4 million deaths per year, with more than 90% of these in sub-Saharan Africa. These highly disease-burdened regions overlap geographically, further prompting speculation about the possibility of a direct interaction between HIV and malaria. Early studies failed to find a significant direct impact of malaria on the prevalence or progression of HIV.[87] However, children with severe anemia due to malaria are at risk of transfusion-transmitted HIV. With the creation of the WHO Roll Back Malaria partnership in 1998, as well as increased funding for both of these diseases from the Global Fund for HIV, Tuberculosis, and Malaria, increased attention has been paid to these three significant diseases of poverty in developing countries in the tropics. The possibility of interactions between HIV and malaria has major public health implications, and the growing body of evidence lending support to this possibility justifies the need to better understand these interactions (Table 21-6). Recent studies

TABLE 21-6   Overview of the Interactions Between HIV and Malaria

OVERVIEW OF THE INTERACTIONS BETWEEN HIV AND MALARIA

Type of Interaction	Pregnant Women	Children	Adult Men and Non-Pregnant Women
The effect of HIV on malaria			
— Increased risk of infection with malaria	+	?	+
— Increased malaria parasite density	+	?	+
— Decreased response to standard antimalarial treatment	+	?	+
The effect of malaria on HIV			
— Increased HIV viral load	+	?	+
— Increased risk of HIV transmission	?[1]	+[2]	?
Effects of dual infection			
— Increased risk of illness	+	+	+
— Increased risk of anemia	+	+	+
— Increased risk of low birth weight	+	−	−

Notes:
+ Evidence for interaction available
? Lack of direct evidence of data
− Interaction is not applicalbe
[1] Through mother-to-child transmission
[2] Through unscreened blood transfusions to cleat anaemia
Source: Reprinted from *Malaria and HIV/AIDS: Interactions and Implications*, June 2004, © Roll Back Malaria/WHO.

have demonstrated an increased HIV-1 viral load in persons with malaria, which decreased with successful treatment of malaria.[88] Studies of pregnant women have found an increased rate of mother-to-child transmission (MTCT) of HIV-1 associated with placental malaria.[89] A study in Uganda of patients with partial immunity to malaria found that HIV-1-infected persons more frequently developed clinical malaria and had higher parasite levels than those who were HIV negative.[90]

Hepatitis C Virus

Because of shared routes of transmission, hepatitis C virus (HCV) infection is common in HIV-positive individuals and is considered an opportunistic infection of HIV.[91-93] In the United States, 15–30% of HIV-infected persons are also infected with HCV; however, the prevalence of HIV-HCV coinfection varies markedly by the route of acquisition of HIV infection (risk category). For example, among HIV-positive patients seen at the Johns Hopkins HIV Clinic (n = 1955), HCV coinfection prevalence rates were as follows: 85.1% of those reporting injection drug use, 14.3% of those reporting heterosexual contact, and 9.8% of those reporting male homosexual contact.[91]

HCV infection in patients with HIV infection has been associated with higher HCV RNA viral load and accelerated progression of HCV-related liver disease.[92-94] One study reported that HCV RNA levels were higher in persons with hemophilia who became infected with HIV than in those who did not, and that liver failure occurred exclusively in those coinfected with HIV and HCV.[94] In a study of liver disease and hepatocellular carcinoma among 4865 men exposed to HCV-contaminated blood products, at all ages the risk for liver-related death after HCV exposure was 1.4% and 6.5% for HIV- and HIV+ individuals, respectively.[95] Data from most studies confirm the detrimental impact of HIV infection on hepatitis C infection. As survival of HIV-infected persons has been extended due to HAART and the prophylaxis of traditional OIs, it is likely that hepatitis C morbidity and mortality will increase.[96]

The issue of whether HCV infection also adversely affects progression of HIV disease remains controversial.[93] In a prospective study of 416 HIV seroconverters in Italy, those with and without HIV infection progressed to AIDS at similar rates.[97] Among the 1955 men seen at the Johns Hopkins HIV Clinic, there was no difference in progression to AIDS or death associated with HCV infection after adjusting for HAART and HIV suppression.[91] Conversely, one study of 3111 persons receiving HAART reported that HCV-infected persons had a modestly increased risk for progression to a new AIDS-defining event or death, even among the subgroup with continuous suppression of HIV replication.[98] This same study found that CD4 increases were smaller after effective anti-HIV therapy in persons with HCV infection than in those without. However, a review of the literature, including two subsequent studies evaluating the immunologic response to potent antiretroviral therapy, failed to confirm these observations.[99,100,101] Given the significant clinical impact of HIV-HCV coinfection, it seems prudent that the coinfected patient be recognized to have a distinct and separate clinical condition from

HIV or HCV monoinfection, with appropriate modifications made in screening, diagnosis, management, and therapy.[101]

GB Virus-C

GB virus-C (GBV-C) is a flavivirus that is closely related to hepatitis C virus. Although GBV-C was first detected by nucleic acid amplification in patients with non-A, non-B hepatitis, the virus does not replicate in hepatocytes and is not a hepatitis virus. In fact, GBV has not been associated consistently with any human disease, although infections are quite common among injection drug users and homosexual men. GBV-C replicates in CD4+ T cells.[102] Patients coinfected with GBV-C and HIV were found to have lower mortality rates, higher baseline CD4+ T cell counts, a slower rate of decline in the number of CD4+ T cells, and in some studies, lower plasma HIV RNA levels than HIV-positive people who did not have GBV-C viremia.[103-109] However, other studies have not shown an effect of coinfection with GBV-C on the progression of HIV-1 infection.[110-112]

Most of these studies were done among cohorts of prevalent HIV-1-infected persons, in whom the duration of HIV-1 infection was not precisely known but was estimated by modeling.[103-109] However, a recent study of the effect of coinfection on survival and progression among subjects in the MACS cohort found that 5 to 6 years after HIV seroconversion men without GBV-C viremia were 2.78 times more likely to die than men with persistent GBV-C infection.[113] Men in the MACS cohort who cleared their GBV-C viremia also had more rapid progression and poorer survival than either those with persistent infection or HIV-positive men who never experienced a GBV-C coinfection.[113] A report from the Amsterdam cohort of homosexual men found no association between GBV-C persistent viremia and survival or progression to AIDS; instead, men who lost their GBV-C viremia were three times more likely to progress than men who never had GBV-C virus infection in their cohort.[112] These authors postulated that loss of GBV-C viremia was a marker for loss of sufficient CD4+ T cells to support continued GBV-C replication.

In vitro experiments have found that GBV-C-infected CD4+ T cells are more resistant to infection with HIV-1.[114] Also the expression of a gene for the chemokines RANTES, MIP 1-a, MIP-1-b, and SDF-1 and secretion of the chemokines into the culture supernates were higher in GBV-C-infected cells. Surface expression of CCR5 was also significantly lower in GBV-C-infected cells.[114]

Further research on the effect of coinfections of HIV-1-positive persons with GBV-C and other infectious agents could provide important insight into the pathogenesis of HIV-1.

Other Agents

Several other coinfections have been reported to be associated with transient decreases in HIV-1 viral load, including measles,[115-126] dengue fever,[117] and scrub typhus.[118] The mechanism of the suppression of HIV replication during these acute infections is believed to be associated with immune activation and elevated cytokine and/or chemokine levels from the coinfection. However, these acute infections are associated with only transient reductions in the viral load.

Antiretroviral Therapy

A detailed description of antiretroviral therapy is beyond the scope of this text. However, since antiretroviral therapy is often discussed not only in the context of treating the individual patient but as a public health strategy to affect the epidemic, some treatment issues are worthy of mention, especially as they influence the epidemiology of HIV infection.

Several advances in our knowledge of HIV/AIDS in the past decade, especially in recent years, have changed the predominant ideas about treatment. The use of drug therapy to model the dynamics of HIV replication demonstrated that about 10 billion virions were produced daily throughout the disease.[16,17] After it became possible to quantitate HIV viral RNA in the plasma, it was shown that the levels of virus in the plasma during the set point were predictive of the subsequent rate of HIV progression and could be combined with the CD4+ count to more accurately predict the time of onset of AIDS and death in HIV-infected patients.[18,19] In fact, the combination of the viral RNA (i.e., viral load) with the CD4+ count more accurately predict the time to AIDS than the CD4+ count alone.[19] The CD4 count indicates the degree of immunosuppression, and a higher viral load correlates with more rapid progression.

With the development and licensure of protease inhibitors it became possible to dramatically reduce the levels of virus in the blood in most patients to below the threshold of detectability with the licensed viral load assays (i.e., <50 copies/μL). This led to the hypothesis that with aggressive therapy for several years the infection might be "cured" with the combined effect of the drugs and the host's immune system. The catchphrase for HAART during this period became "Hit hard, hit HIV early."[119] Subsequently, the latent viral reservoir in long-lived resting lymphocytes and macrophages was described, leading to a change in thinking about appropriate antiretroviral therapy.[15] Modeling the time to the natural elimination of this reservoir of latent virus suggested that the reservoir of these cells or their daughter cells would persist for 60 years or more.[15] Adding to this discovery of the latent reservoir was the recognition that patients who were treated for several years with repeatedly undetectable viral load commonly returned to their pretreatment viral load within a few weeks after withdrawal of treatment. This observation led to the rejection of the hypothesis that HIV infection could be cured with currently available drugs. The strategy shifted to delaying treatment until required because of symptoms or immune suppression. More recently many experts have recommended starting treatment earlier, prior to significant immunocompromise.

The guidelines of when to begin antiretroviral therapy have changed frequently. Deciding when to start treating a patient is based, in part, on considerations of whether a patient is ready to be treated and agrees to adhere to the regimen that is prescribed, since adherence below 80% is associated with the frequent emergence of resistant viruses.

The most important questions regarding antiretroviral therapy in an HIV-infected treatment-naive patient are when to start treatment, what drugs to start with, when to change, and what to change to. In 1995, physicians with specific expertise in HIV-related basic science and clinical research were invited by the International AIDS Society-USA to serve on a volunteer panel to evaluate the scientific evidence on therapy and to make broad recommendations. This panel, augmented since 1999 by international experts, meets periodically to evaluate the evidence and update their recommendations. The reader should refer to their reports, which are usually published in the *Journal of the American Medical Association*, for their detailed recommendations. The recently published recommendation for when to start and what to start with are presented in Table 21-7.

Therapy should include three drugs to maximize efficacy and limit the emergence of resistant viruses.

The panel does not recommend a single drug combination as optimal for all patients. However, several combinations of antiretroviral drugs are mentioned, namely:

- 2 NRTIs + 1 NNRTI
- 2 NRTIs + 1 PI
- 3 NRTIs (e.g., Abacavir, Zidovudine, and Lamivudine)

The reader is referred to the panel's published recommendations for more detail.

Complications of therapy include a variety of conditions, especially lactic acidosis, lipodystrophy, visceral fat accumulation, insulin resistance, and diabetes, especially with thymidine analogs, such as d4T (stavudine), AZT

TABLE 21-7   Recommendations for Initiating Therapy in Treatment-Naive Individuals

Disease Type	Recommendation
Symptomatic HIV disease	Treatment recommended
Asymptomatic HIV disease, ≤200 CD4 cells/µL	Treatment recommended
Asymptomatic HIV disease, >200 CD4 cells/µL	Treatment decision should be individualized; recommendations are based on: • CD4 cell count and rate of decline[†] • HIV RNA level in the plasma[‡] • Patient interest in and potential to adhere to therapy • Individual risks or toxicity and drug-drug pharmacokinetic interaction

[†]Some clinicians and guidelines use a CD4 count threshold of 350 cells/µL to initiate therapy and/or a high rate of CD4 cell count decline >100 cells/µL per annum.
[‡]A high HIV RNA level is above 50,000–100,000 copies/mL. The frequency of CD4 cell measurements before therapy is initiated may be guided by the plasma HIV RNA level.
Source: Yeni PG. Antiretroviral Treatment for Adult HIV Infection in 2002: Updated Recommendations of the International AIDS Society-USA Panel. JAMA 2002;288:222–235, American Medical Association. All rights reserved.

(zidovudine), and protease inhibitors. Also, peripheral neuropathy, hepatitis, rash (including Stevens-Johnson syndrome), and renal toxicity have been reported as complications of therapy with antiretroviral drugs. The reader should consult references describing HIV/AIDS therapy for more details (see below).

It is important to consider the fact that HAART therapy has delayed the progression and mortality from HIV/AIDS, but the treatment has increased the risks of several other diseases, especially cardiovascular and hepatic diseases. Although the benefits of treatment clearly outweigh the risks of complications, the risks of these chronic complications have increased in the era of HAART treatment.

Therapeutic Regimens to Treat HIV

As therapy of HIV has been integrated into the prevention of infection, the topic will be reviewed briefly. However, a detailed discussion of antiretroviral therapy is beyond the scope of this text. Several excellent references are available for the interested reader, including *The Johns Hopkins Hospital 2005-2006 Edition, Medical Management of HIV infection*, by John G. Bartlett, M.D. and Joel E. Gallant, M.D., M.P.H. (hopkins-aids.edu/mmhiv/order.html.)

There have been several sequential changes in the use of antiretroviral therapy since zidovudine (AZT), the first antiretroviral drug, was licensed in 1987. When patients were receiving antiretroviral therapy prior to 1992, they were usually given only monotherapy. Between 1992 and 1996, many HIV-infected patients were given two agents simultaneously, the era of so-called dual therapy. After protease inhibitors were licensed in 1996, patients were usually treated with combinations of several drugs. These treatment regimens were often referred to as *highly active anti-retroviral therapy* (HAART). HAART is usually defined as including the following combinations of ARVs:

- Use of two or more NRTIs (nucleoside reverse transcriptase inhibitors) plus one PI (protease inhibitor)
- One NRTI, one NNRTI (nonnucleoside reverse transcriptase inhibitor), and one PI
- Ritonavir and Saquinavir or one NRTI
- An Abacavir-containing regimen with three NRTIs

The number of drugs approved for use in the United States and the date of their approval are shown in Table 21-8.

More antiviral drugs are approved for the treatment of HIV/AIDS than for any other viral infection in humans. However, the fairly large number of drugs available for the treatment of HIV infections in the United States, in part, reflects the fact that none are capable of eradicating the virus or producing a permanent cure, and many have significant toxicity, are expensive, or difficult to take. The development of viral resistance to many drugs is quite common, especially when adherence is not excellent (i.e., over 80%). In addition, adverse drug reactions are quite common, so that drug regimens must be changed frequently. Nevertheless, antiretroviral therapy has had a profound effect on the natural history of HIV in countries where HAART is

TABLE 21-8 Antiretroviral Drugs Approved by the FDA

Trade Name	Generic Name	Class	License Date
Retrovir	Zidovudine (AZT)	NRTI	March 1987
Videx	Didanosine (ddl)	NRTI	October 1991
Hivid	Zalcitabine (ddC)	NRTI	June 1992
Zerit	Stavudine (d4T)	NRTI	June 1994
Epivir	Lamivudine (3TC)	NRTI	November 1995
Ziagen	Abacavir (ABC)	NRTI	February 1999
Viread	Tenofovir (TDF)	NRTI	October 2001
Truvada	Tenofovir/Emtricitabine	NRTI	July 2004
Emtriva	Emtricitabine	NRTI	July 2003
Aptivus	Tipranavir (TPV)	NRTI	June 2005
Viramune	Nevirapine	NNRTI	June 1996
Rescriptor	Delavirdine (DLV)	NNRTI	April 1997
Sustiva	Efavirenz	NNRTI	September 1998
Crixivan	Indinavir	PI	March 1996
Norvir	Ritonavir	PI	March 1996
Invirase	Saquinavir (hard gel)	PI	December 1995
Fortovase	Saquinavir (soft gel)	PI	November 1997
Viracept	Nelfinavir	PI	March 1997
Agenerase	Amprenavir	PI	April 1997
Kaletra	Lopinavir/Ritonavir	PI	September 2000
Reyataz	Atazanavir	PI	July 2004
Lexiva	Fosamprenavir	PI	September 2004
Fuzean (T20	Enfuvirtide	EI	April 2003
Combivir	Zidovudine and lamivudine	2 NRTIs	September 1997
Trizivir	Zidovudine, lamivudine, and abacavir	3 NRTIs	November 2000
Atripla	Efavarenz/Emtricitabine/Tonofovir	1 NNRTI + 2 NRTIs	July 2006

Abbreviations: NRTI, nucleoside reverse transcriptase inhibitor; NNRTI, nonnucleoside reverse transcriptase inhibitor; NTRTI, nucleotide reverse transcriptase inhibitor; PI, protease inhibitor; EI, entry inhibitor. *Source:* United States Food and Drug Administration.

available. The success of antiretroviral therapy in decreasing AIDS mortality in industrialized countries has fueled the development of strategies by WHO to provide effective treatment for resource-limited countries. Recently several effective anti-retroviral drugs have been combined in a single tablet to more effectively treat HIV infection with HAART with a simplified regimen and improve adherence to therapy. The most recent of these drugs, Atripla, was licensed by the US. FDA in July, 2006. It combines 3 drugs into a single tablet, which effectively treats HIV as a single daily dose.

Clinical trials that measured the effect of therapy on the two key determinants of HIV progression (CD4+ cell count and HIV viral load) found progressively more effective suppression of viral load and elevation of the CD4+ cell count in persons receiving combination therapy or HAART. Often 80% or more of patients receiving HAART in a clinical trial had reductions of HIV viral load to less than 400 copies/mL, or 50 copies/mL with more sensitive assays. Some patients followed in clinical practice have not had as good results as those reported in clinical trials. Nevertheless, most patients have good clinical, virological, and immunological responses to HAART.

There has been a marked improvement in the natural history of HIV infections when responses are measured at the population level. An evaluation of the proportion of men in the Multicenter AIDS Cohort Study (MACS) who were receiving various forms of therapy between 1986 and 1999 and their progression to AIDS documented the benefits of various regimens in a cohort of HIV-infected men. A comparison of the progression of infection among HIV-positive MACS participants, after adjusting for the duration of infection at baseline, found the relative hazard of progression to AIDS during the era of no treatment to be 1.52 (95% CI, 0.93–2.49) compared with men in the monotherapy era.[120] The hazard of progression in the era of combination therapy was 1.03 (95% CI, 0.77–1.38), and during the era of HAART it has been 0.31 (95% CI, 0.21–0.45).[35]

Mortality from AIDS in the general population in the United States declined dramatically with the availability of HAART after 1996. A CDC-sponsored HIV outpatient study (HOPS) reported the use of HAART therapy and mortality among 1000 patients with AIDS and CD4+ cell counts less than 100 cells/mm³.[96] In these patients, about 80% were using PIs by 1997, and the mortality declined from 29.4 deaths/100 person-years in 1995 to 8.8 deaths/100 person-years in 1997 (Figure 21-9). In addition to decreased mortality, the incidence of AIDS-defining opportunistic infections have been reduced dramatically in the HAART era (Figure 21-10).

Modes of Transmission and Risk Factors

HIV infection is transmitted by sexual intercourse, injection drug use or other parenteral exposures, transfusion of blood or blood products, organ transplantation, and by occupational exposure to HIV-contaminated blood or body fluids.

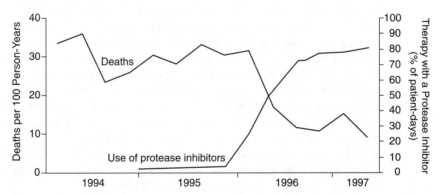

FIGURE 21-9 Mortality and frequency of use of combination antiretroviral therapy including a protease inhibitor among HIV-infected patients with fewer than 100 CD4+ cells per cubic millimeter, according to calendar quarter, from January 1994 through June 1997. *Source:* Palella FJ et al. Declining morbidity and mortality among patients with advanced human immunodeficiency virus infection. HIV Outpatient Study Investigators. N Engl J Med. 1998 Mar 26;338(13):853–860. Copyright 1998 by the Massachusetts Medical Society.

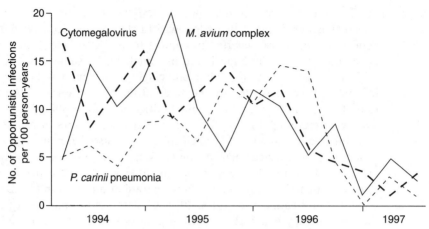

FIGURE 21-10   Rates of cytomegalovirus infection, *Pneumocystis carinii* pneumonia, and *Mycobacterium avium* complex disease among HIV-infected patients with fewer than 100 CD4+ cells per cubic millimeter, according to calendar quarter, from January 1994 through June 1997.
Source: Palella FJ et al. Declining morbidity and mortality among patients with advanced human immunodeficiency virus infection. HIV Outpatient Study Investigators. N Engl J Med. 1998 Mar 26;338(13):853–860. Copyright 1998 by the Massachusetts Medical Society.

Sexual Transmission

Transmission of HIV through sexual intercourse is estimated to account for 75–80% of the global HIV infections that have occurred to date.[76] Unprotected receptive anal intercourse is the most effective means of sexual transmission. The risk varies according to various factors but probably is on the order of 0.5–1.0% per contact.[76] Both males and females are equally vulnerable to infection by anal intercourse. The transmission from infected males to females by vaginal intercourse has been estimated to occur at an average rate of about 0.3% per contact, and transmission from an infected female to a male at a somewhat lower rate.[76,121] However, a study in Uganda found similar rates of transmission from men to women and vice versa.[80,122] Traumatic sex, such as from fisting among MSM or rough heterosexual sex, is associated with an increased rate of transmission. Sociocultural situations that increase the likelihood of traumatic sex, such as rape, use of vaginal tightening agents, or sex while under the influence of cocaine or alcohol, increase the risk of HIV transmission. The presence of a sexually transmitted infection in either partner increases the risk of transmission by about five-fold.[78] The increased risk is greatest with a genital ulcer disease, such as syphilis, herpes, or chancroid. However, nonulcerative STDs also increases the risk of transmission in part because of the activated inflammatory cells in the genital tract, many of which may be quite susceptible to HIV infection.[75]

Another important factor in the risk of HIV-1 transmission is the viral load in the infected partner. Studies in Uganda and Thailand have estimated a 2.5-fold increased risk of transmission for each log increment in the viral load.[80,81] No transmission occurred in these populations when the viral load was below 1500 copies/μL, despite unprotected sex.

Because of the high viral load occurring in primary infection prior to an immune response, the risk of transmission is high at this time.[78,122] It has been postulated that early in an epidemic, the risk per sexual contact may be higher than it is in a more mature epidemic because a higher proportion of infected persons has recent infections with high viral loads.[78] High viral load also occurs late in the natural history, after the onset of AIDS. However, at this time patients are frequently quite ill, so unprotected sex, when it occurs, is less frequent. In addition, most persons are well aware of their HIV infection after the onset of AIDS and may be more likely to use barrier precautions during sex.

Cervical ectopy (replacement of the multilayered squamous cells at the cervical os with single-layered columnar epithelium) increases the risk of HIV transmission.[76] The higher prevalence of cervical ectopy in adolescent girls after menarche may partially explain the higher HIV seroprevalence among 15–24-year-old females than in older women in sub-Saharan African countries.[123] The method of contraception also affects the risk of transmission. The regular use of condoms is highly protective. No infections occurred among subjects in the European discordant couples study when condoms were reported to have been used regularly.[124] However, among couples who used condoms intermittently during intercourse, the incidence of HIV did not differ from nonusers of condoms. The "100% condom" public health program in Thailand demonstrated the effectiveness of condom promotion as a public health approach to controlling an HIV/AIDS epidemic.[125,126]

Hormonal contraceptives (in the absence of condom use) have been shown in some studies to increase the risk of HIV transmission,[127] whereas other studies have failed to confirm this association.[128,129] Women using hormonal contraceptives may have more frequent intercourse or use barrier methods less often, which may confound this association. However, it is biologically plausible that some hormonal contraceptives could increase the risk of HIV transmission by increasing cervical ectopy. The specific hormonal composition of the contraceptive used may also influence the risk and explain some of the discrepant results reported by various researchers. Contraceptives containing progesterone, which have a greater effect on the cervical epithelium, may be associated with a greater risk.[130] Unprotected sex during pregnancy and menstruation has been shown to increase the risk of transmission in some studies.[121,131]

Vaginal microbicides containing nonoxynol 9 increase the risk of HIV transmission, especially if they are used frequently, such as by sex workers having many partners each day.[132] The development of safer effective microbicides is an important public health priority. An effective microbicide could be an important method of prevention, since it could be controlled by a female in situations where condom use might be difficult to negotiate.

Several studies have found a protective effect for male circumcision both for transmission and acquisition of HIV.[80,133,134] The foreskin contains abundant Langerhans/dendritic cells, which are highly susceptible to HIV infection. However, populations in which most men are circumcised are culturally different with regard to their usual sexual practices from those where most men are uncircumcised. The control of possible confounders in the available data has been difficult. For this reason, two controlled clinical trials are in progress in East Africa to determine whether circumcision of adult men decreases the risk of HIV infection. One controlled trial of circumcision was completed recently in South Africa among 3274 uncircumcised HIV-seronegative men, aged 18–24 years who were randomly allocated to circumsized or not and followed afterwards. After a mean follow-up of 18 months the relative risk of HIV infection was 0.40 (95% CI, 0.24–0.68) in the circumcised men.[134] Circumcision of adult men will be a difficult intervention be to implement in many cultures, so a clear demonstration of the benefit with additional controlled trials is needed.

An important factor influencing the risk of HIV transmission and the rate at which an epidemic emerges in a country is the pattern of sexual partnerships. The numbers of different sexual partners and the frequency of sexual contact are important risk variables for HIV transmission. But even more important is whether sexual partnerships are concurrent or sequential. The spread of HIV is much more likely in a population in which partnerships are commonly concurrent.[135-137] In many cultures, most HIV-infected women's sole risk factor is marriage, and their infection was due to their husbands' concurrent extramarital sexual relationships. One study in several countries found that reported, or suspected, concurrent sexual partnerships were significantly more common among married couples in sub-Saharan Africa than in couples in developing countries elsewhere (Figure 21-11).[137]

In all regions of sub-Saharan Africa, the predominant method of transmission of HIV-1 is believed by most experts to be heterosexual. However, there is considerable heterogeneity in the prevalence of HIV infection in different regions of the continent. In particular, the rates of infection in populations in Western Africa are considerably lower than those in Eastern and Southern Africa.[138] To explore some of the determinants of these regional differences, an ecological study was done in four cities in sub-Saharan Africa.[133,139] This study enrolled 900–1000 persons in Catonou, Benin, and in Yaoundé, Cameroon, where the adult population HIV prevalence was about 4%, compared to Kisumu, Kenya, and Ndola, Zambia, where the prevalence was 25–30%. The participants were questioned about their sexual practices, condom use, STD history, and other potential factors that might explain the differences in HIV-1 prevalence in their country. Although sexual behavior variables were strongly correlated with HIV-1 prevalence at the individual level, there were only moderate differences in the frequency of these factors at the population level that could explain the variation in country-level HIV-1 prevalence. A stronger ecological association was seen with HSV-2 infection and male circumcision rates and adult HIV-1 prevalence than with sexual behavior variables. The prevalence of HSV-2 was higher and circumcision rates were lower in areas with higher HIV-1 prevalence, possibly explaining some of the differences seen.[133] Although many of the important factors that affect HIV-1 transmission have been identified, their combined interaction at the population level can be complex.

Injection Drug Use

Injection drug use is the second most important risk behavior associated with HIV infection worldwide. It accounts for an estimated 15–25% of HIV infections globally. However, in some areas of the world, especially Eastern

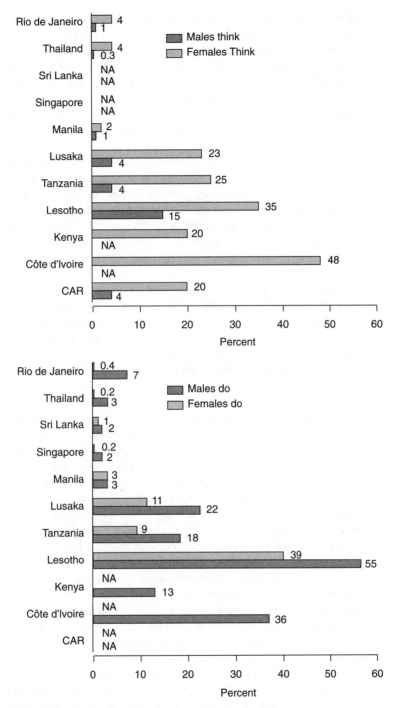

FIGURE 21-11 Frequency of concurrent and suspected concurrent sexual relationships.
Source: Halperin DT. Concurrent sexual partnerships help to explain Africa's high HIV prevalence: implications for prevention. Lancet. 2004 Jul 3–9;364(9428):4–6, with permission from Elsevier.

Europe, the Russian Federation, Southern China, East Asia, and the Middle East, IDUs account for the great majority of HIV-infected persons.[14]

The predominant risk behavior associated with HIV transmission among injection drug users is sharing of contaminated injection equipment.[140-144] Most IDUs initiate the injection of illicit drugs with another experienced drug user, who is often older. At the time of initiation of drug injection and early after starting to inject, drugs and injection equipment are commonly shared. Therefore, IDUs are at especially high risk of HIV infections early in their injection careers.

Social situations that increase the likelihood that injection equipment will be shared, such as injection in "shooting galleries" (defined as places such as abandoned buildings, private homes, or other areas where drugs and equipment can be purchased or rented for injection), put a drug user at especially high risk of acquiring HIV.[140] Injection of drugs in shooting galleries is necessitated by paraphernalia laws that define carrying syringes as a crime and thus discourages IDUs from having their own injecting equipment on their person.

Some drug injection practices, such as "booting," the practice of drawing a small amount of blood into the syringe prior to injection, can increase the risk of HIV transmission to those who share equipment. Also, the "cooker," or equipment used to dissolve the drugs, can become contaminated, when the dissolved drugs are drawn into several syringes. Both "back loading," where the syringe is used to mix and measure out aliquots of drugs, and "front loading," where the needle is replaced between syringes, can lead to transmission of HIV from one user to another.[145]

In addition to the specific injection practices, the risk of infection increases with a larger number of needle-sharing partners. Also, injection of cocaine compared to heroin is associated with a higher risk of infection among drug users in the northeastern United States. These users commonly inject both heroin and cocaine (commonly referred to as "speedballing").[146] Cocaine has a shorter half-life than heroin and is often injected more frequently, sometimes in binges, with a larger number of needle-sharing partners.[146] Cocaine injection, which is a stimulant, is commonly associated with concomitant high-risk sexual practices. Crack cocaine use has been linked to outbreaks of syphilis and other STDs.[147]

Treatment of drug abuse with methadone or bupernorphine replacement has been shown to decrease the risk of HIV infection.[148] However, there is insufficient access to methadone or other drug treatment programs in the United States to accommodate the numbers of persons injecting drugs. Furthermore, methadone treatment is most effective for persons using opiates alone rather than those also injecting cocaine or other illicit drugs. Also, many drug users do not feel "ready" to enroll in a treatment program. Therefore, a public health strategy of "harm reduction" has been developed to decrease the risk of HIV, other infections, and other adverse consequences of using contaminated injection equipment.[149] These programs offer clean syringes in exchange for used injection equipment to out-of-treatment injection drug users. Such programs have generated political controversy in the United States and many developing countries by persons who believe they condone, tolerate, or support illegal injection drug behavior.[150-151] Therefore, no syringe exchange harm reduction programs have been funded by the federal government in the United States. Nevertheless, many syringe exchange programs are operating in the United States with funding by foundations, NGOs, or local governments.[152] Evaluation of these programs has indicated that they commonly attract the heaviest drug users who are not in drug treatment.[153-156] These programs allow medical and public health contact with a seriously addicted population, who can sometimes be referred for needed medical care as well as reduce their high-risk behavior for HIV transmission.[153,156] An evaluation of the evidence of their effectiveness by a committee of the Institute of Medicine concluded that harm reduction programs were effective in reducing transmission of HIV.[157-158]

The epidemic of HIV among drug users in the United States is geographically diverse. In most large cities in the northeastern United States the HIV prevalence is higher than in western or midwestern cities. The HIV prevalence among IDUs in several northeastern cities such as Hartford, New York, Newark, Philadelphia, Baltimore, and Washington, DC, ranges from 25–40%, whereas in western cities such as Denver, Phoenix, San Diego, Los Angeles, and Portland, only 2.7–12.0% of IDUs are HIV positive.[159] These discrepant seroprevalence rates among IDUs have persisted from the mid-1980s to the present, whereas the prevalence of HIV among MSM does not differ widely in large cities in the United States.[159]

One study of sexual and drug use variables among 1528 East Coast IDUs compared to 1149 West Coast IDUs found a nearly 10-fold higher prevalence in HIV (21.5%) among East Coast IDUs compared to West Coast IDUs (2.3%). However, the differences in reported sexual or injection behaviors were insufficient to explain the difference in HIV infection rates.[160]

Another study raised the novel hypothesis that differences in the types of heroin available in West Coast and East Coast cities could explain much of the difference in HIV infection rates.[161] Heroin on the West Coast commonly is grown and processed in Mexico and is called "black tar heroin." It is quite viscous and requires fairly extensive heating to dissolve the drug prior to injection. It also is likely to clot in the syringe, so extensive rinsing is necessary after it is injected. Furthermore, it is likely to sclerose veins, so IDUs commonly transition rapidly from intravenous injection to subcutaneous or intramuscular injection and sharing or reuse of syringes is less feasible. All of these behavioral characteristics of the injection routine differ from drug users on the East Coast, where the heroin originates in South Asia and South America and consists primarily of a white or light brown powder. This heroin is more easily dissolved and may not require heating or subsequent extensive rinsing of syringes after an injection.[161] Reuse and sharing of syringes is facilitated by the heroin available to drug users in eastern cities in the United States (Figure 21-12).

The epidemic of HIV related to injection drug use is strongly affected by the sociocultural environment.[162] Several researchers have demonstrated that being in prison constitutes a high risk for exposure to HIV through injection drug use.[162-163] Other high-risk urban environments in inner-city populations facilitate the transmission of HIV directly or are indirectly related to drug use. Therefore, preventive interventions directed only at individual behavior are likely to be less successful than structural interventions directed at changing the social environment in preventing drug use–related HIV epidemics.[162]

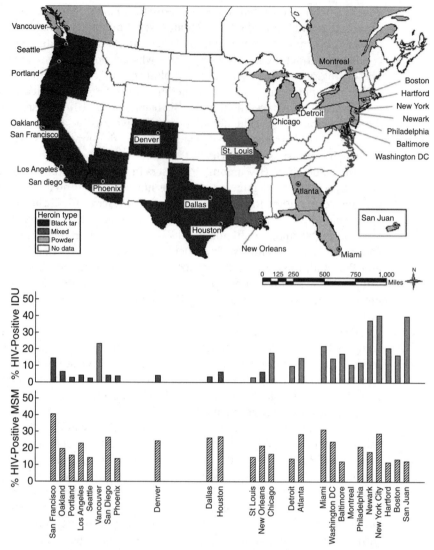

FIGURE 21-12 Geographical variation of HIV among IDUs in the United States. *Source:* Ciccarone P. Explaining the Geographical Variation of HIV Among Injection Drug Users in the United States. Substance Use and Misuse. 38, 14:2049–2063. Produced by permission of Taylor and Francis Group, LLP.

Perinatal Transmission

The risk of perinatal transmission from an HIV-infected woman to her infant was first recognized in 1982. About 90% of HIV/AIDS cases in children are perinatally acquired; the remainder occurs in children with hemophilia or those who have received a contaminated blood transfusion. In the absence of a preventive intervention, about 20–25% of HIV-infected women who deliver vaginally in the United States or Europe and 25–40% in sub-Saharan Africa transmit the infection to their infants.[164–168] Approximately 20% of HIV transmission from a mother to her infant occurs in utero, about 60–65%

during delivery, and about 12–15% from breast-feeding. Most breast-feeding transmission occurs in developing countries where breast-feeding is common, formula is too expensive, or no clean water supply is available to facilitate formula feeding. Transmission in utero is operationally defined as detection of HIV by culture or nucleic acid amplification in the infant within the first 48 hours after birth.[169] Peripartum infection is defined as children who were not breast-fed and who have negative HIV culture and/or nucleic acid amplification (PCR) tests in the first few days of life followed by a positive test on days 7 to 90. Transmission by breast-feeding can occur at any time. The risk appears to be greatest during the early weeks after birth but continues throughout the duration of breast-feeding.[170-173] In developing countries, where the absence of breast-feeding is associated with very high infant mortality, exclusive breast-feeding has been shown to be associated with a lower risk of HIV transmission than when other foods are given to the infant who is being breast-fed.[173] Elective cesarean section performed prior to rupture of the membranes appears to reduce the risk of HIV transmission. A meta-analysis that included data from 8533 mother-infant pairs from 15 international cohorts of non-breast-feeding women showed that, after adjustment for receipt of antiretroviral therapy, maternal disease stage, and infant birth weight, elective cesarean section decreased HIV transmission by approximately 50% (adjusted odds ratio, 0.43; 95% CI, 0.33–0.56).[168] When elective cesarean section was combined with zidovudine during the antepartum, intrapartum, and neonatal periods, HIV transmission was reduced by about 87%, compared with vaginal delivery and nonuse of zidovudine therapy (adjusted OR = 0.13; 95% CI, 0.09–0.19).[168] With effective therapy of the mother with HAART regimens that have resulted in very low viral loads at the time of delivery (<400 copies/μL), cesarean section probably has no added benefit. Perinatal transmission rates with effective HAART therapy of the mother are approximately 1.2%.[174-175]

Risk factors that increase the risk of mother-to-infant transmission include internal fetal monitoring, prolonged labor and delivery, chorioamnionitis, high viral load in the mother, primary HIV infection during pregnancy, and advanced HIV disease in the mother. Several studies have shown that women with low serum vitamin A levels were more likely to transmit HIV to their infant during delivery. However, controlled trials of vitamin A supplementation during pregnancy failed to decrease the transmission rate.[176,177] Thus, vitamin A deficiency is now regarded as a marker of increased risk rather than a cofactor for perinatal transmission of HIV. Irrigation of the birth canal with chlorhexidine in order to lower the HIV viral load in the birth canal prior to delivery did not reduce HIV transmission to the infant.[178-179] However, the rates of bacterial neonatal sepsis were significantly reduced by vaginal cleansing.[180] Treatment of chorioamnionitis during pregnancy also did not decrease the rates of maternal-to-child transmission of HIV.

A landmark study that was published in 1994, the ACTG-076 trial, found that zidovudine given to pregnant women after the first trimester, during delivery, and to the infant for the first 6 weeks of life decreased the mother-to-child transmission by 67%, from 25% in those receiving placebo to 8% in those given AZT.[181] There was only a modest decrease in the viral load in the mother from baseline (median decrease of 0.28 log copies/μL).[182] This landmark study found that most infections were transmitted during the last trimester or during labor and delivery into this non-breast-feeding population and that reductions in the viral load explained only a part of the protective efficacy.[182] This complex and expensive regimen, though effective, was not suitable for implementation in developing countries, where most mother-to-child infections were occurring. Therefore, a study was done in Thailand with a modified AZT regimen. In this study, AZT was started in pregnant women at the 36th week of pregnancy and given during delivery but not to the infant. This simpler regimen had a 50% efficacy and reduced transmission from 18.9% to 9.4% at a fraction of the cost of the ACTG-076 regimen.[183] The Thai infants in this study were fed formula after delivery.

Another important study was done of a simpler regimen in Uganda (HIVNET 012). In this study a single dose of nevirapine was given during labor and another dose to the infant during the first week of life.[184] Despite breast-feeding, the maternal-infant transmission was reduced from 25.1% to 13.1% (47% efficacy) at 14–16 weeks and persisted until 18 months, at which time the infants who had received nevirapine had a 15.2% infection rate compared to 25.8% in the controls (41% efficacy).[185] This greatly simplified regimen was well tolerated. However resistance mutations to nevirapine (especially $K^{103}N$) were demonstrated at 6 weeks postpartum in about 20% of women who had received a single dose of the drug,[186] although the mutant virus became less frequent in untreated women after several months.[187] This raised the concern that widespread use of nevirapine might eventually increase the risk of the transmission of resistant viruses or that subsequent therapy of women with those resistance mutations with other nonnucleoside RT inhibitors might fail.[188] Despite these concerns, a review of the risks and benefits of single-dose nevirapine for the prevention of mother-to-child transmission by a WHO committee concluded that the benefits outweigh the risk in resource-limited settings.[189]

The positive results of these prevention trials have raised hopes that mother-to-child transmission (MTCT) of HIV could be prevented or reduced dramatically at the population level. Several additional trials were done of ARV treatment of pregnant women in developing countries aimed at improving the efficacy, simplifying the regimen, or reducing the cost or toxicity.

The PETRA trial was done in five sites in South Africa, Tanzania, and Uganda.[190] It was designed to find a regimen with improved efficacy in a breast-feeding population. This study compared ZDV/3TC given in three different regimens. In one regimen the drugs were given starting at 36 weeks, during labor and delivery, and for 1 week postpartum; in another regimen the drugs were given only intrapartum and postpartum; in the third regimen, the drugs were only given intrapartum. There was no effect on HIV transmission in the intrapartum-only arm. However, the other two regimens were 41–63% effective at 6 weeks and 19–33% effective after 18 months in preventing HIV infection in these breast-feeding populations.[190] An identical regimen to the short-course ZDV trial in Bangkok in which the drug was started at 36 weeks and given during labor but not to infants in a breast-feeding population in the Ivory Coast found a 38% efficacy at 6 months and a 30% efficacy at 15 months in preventing HIV transmission.[191]

A study in Thailand compared four regimens of zidovudine (ZDV) prophylaxis.[192] In this study one group received ZDV starting at 28 weeks of gestation, similar to ACTG-076 (long regimen) plus 6 weeks of treatment for the infant (long regimen); another group received ZDV from 36 weeks of gestation (short regimen) with 3 days of treatment for the infant (short regimen); a third group received the long maternal and short infant regimen; and a fourth group received the short maternal and long infant regimen. The transmission rates were 6.5% for the long-long regimen, 4.7% for the long-short regimen, and 8.6% for the short-long regimen. The short-short regimen was stopped by the DSMB during the study because of lower efficacy. The rate of in utero transmission was significantly higher with the two regimens with shorter maternal treatment (5.1%) than the two with longer maternal treatment (1.6%). No placebo group was included in this "equivalency" study.

Because of the remarkable efficacy of nevirapine in preventing maternal-to-infant transmission in Uganda, another study was done among pregnant women in Thailand who received ZDV starting at 28 weeks. In this study, 1844 Thai women were randomized also to receive a single dose of nevirapine along with a single dose of nevaripine given to their infant (Group 1), one dose of nevirapine to the mother with placebo to the infant (Group 2), or placebo to the mother and infant (Group 3). The HIV transmission rate in Group 1 was 1.1% (95% CI, 0.3–2.2%), in Group 2 it was 2.8% (95% CI, 1.5–4.1%), and in the placebo-only group it was 6.3% (95% CI, 3.8–8.95).[193] Of interest, among women with CD4 counts below 250 cells/µL who were treated with nevirapine-containing regimes after delivery, 49% had HIV-1 RNA levels less than 50 copies/µL after 6 months compared to 68% of those women who were not given intrapartum nevirapine ($P = .03$).[193] Resistance mutations to nevirapine were detected in 32% of women who had received intrapartum nevirapine.[193] Women who had received nevirapine for prevention of vertical transmission were less likely to respond to a nevirapine-based regimen with HIV-1 RNA levels less than 50 copies/µL at 6 months postpartum than women who had not received nevirapine.[194]

Evaluation of mother-to-child transmission rates among HIV-positive pregnant women in the United States who were enrolled in the Women and Infants Transmission Study (WITS) between 1990 and 2000 found dramatic reductions in transmission over time when women were treated with more effective therapy to suppress viral replication. Among 396 women who were untreated, the transmission rate was 20.0%; for 710 women receiving ZDV monotherapy, the transmission rate was 10.4%; and for those receiving dual therapy the transmission rate was 3.8%; and for those receiving HAART, it was 1.2%.[195] Transmission also varied according to the maternal HIV-RNA level at delivery; it was 1% for less than 400 copies/µL, 5.3% for 400–3499, 9.3% for 3500–9999, 14.7% for 10,000–29,999, and 23.4% for greater than 30,000 copies.[195] In an analysis of transmission rates among women enrolled in seven European and United States prospective studies who had HIV RNA virus loads less than 1000 copies/µL at or near delivery, vertical transmission occurred to 44 (3.7%) of 1202 infants. For mothers receiving antiretroviral therapy during pregnancy or at the time of delivery, 1% (8 of 834) infants became infected, whereas among women not on therapy 9% (36 of 368) of their infants became infected.[196] Therefore, antiviral therapy plays an important role in reducing the risk of transmission even in women with relatively low viral loads. Infected women with low HIV viral loads when they are evaluated may have periodic increases in viral replication leading to transmission to their infant.

Current Guidelines for Prevention of MTCT of HIV in the United States

A US Public Health Service task force has reviewed the evidence relating to the prevention of vertical transmission of HIV and developed guidelines for the United States (Table 21-9).[197] These guidelines aim to maximally reduce the rates of transmission according to existing evidence. They are not feasible in resource-poor countries where the majority of vertical transmission of HIV continues to occur. Because of the lower rates of transmission in women with low viral loads, infected women should be treated with a HAART regimen that includes ZDV. If the viral load is above 1000 copies/μL, elective cesarean section should be done prior to the onset of labor. In women who have not received antepartum or intrapartum antiviral therapy, the committee recommended prophylactic therapy of the infant.

TABLE 21-9 Summary of US Public Health Service Task Force Guidelines for Prevention of Mother-to-Child HIV Transmission in the United States

---

- Maternal antenatal plasma HIV RNA >1000 copies/mL
  — Highly active antiretroviral therapy (ideally containing ZDV after the first trimester), plus ZDV given intravenously intrapartum and for 6 weeks to the infant
  — Elective cesarean delivery if plasma HIV RNA remains >1000 copies/mL near delivery
- Maternal plasma HIV RNA <1000 copies
  — ZDV given antepartum after the first trimester, intravenously intrapartum, and for 6 weeks to the infant

Or

  — Highly active antiretroviral therapy (ideally containing ZDV after the first trimester), plus ZDV given intravenously intrapartum and for 6 weeks to the infant
- No antiretroviral therapy before labor:
  — Several effective regimens are available to choose from for women who have had no prior therapy:
    - ZDV given intravenously during labor, followed by 6 weeks of ZDV for the infant

  Or

    - Nevirapine, given as a single dose at onset of labor to the woman, followed by a single dose of nevirapine for the newborn at age 48 hours

  Or

    - The intrapartum/postpartum ZDV regimen (above) plus the single-dose nevirapine regimen (above)
- No antiretroviral therapy before or during labor:
  — ZDV given for 6 weeks to the infant, started as soon as possible after delivery (preferably within 6–12 hours of birth)

Or

  — Some clinicians may choose to use ZDV in combination with additional antiretroviral drugs, but appropriate dosing regimens for neonates are incompletely defined, and the additional efficacy of this approach in reducing transmission is not known.

Note: To access the most recent guidelines, see http://AIDSInfo.nih.gov.
Source: MMWR Rec Rep 2002;51:1–4.

A critically important component of the successful prevention of mother-to-child transmission of HIV in the United States is the identification of HIV-infected pregnant women. It is currently recommended that all pregnant women be tested for HIV regardless of their perceived risk. The most effective strategy to obtain informed consent for testing is the "opt out" strategy in which women are told they will be tested unless they decline, rather than an "opt in" strategy where they are counseled and asked if they wish to be tested. The former strategy has resulted in testing of about 85% of pregnant women.[198]

Developing Countries

Despite the availability of several effective regimens to prevent mother-to-child transmission of HIV, an estimated 640,000–700,000 new HIV infections occurred in children under 15 years of age in 2004, and 510,000 children died from AIDS that year. Nearly all of these new HIV infections in children occurred in developing countries, especially in sub-Saharan Africa.[14] The dramatic increase in HIV infections among young women 15–24 years old in sub-Saharan African countries has escalated the problem of infant and childhood infections. About 90% of HIV infections in children were caused by maternal-to-infant transmission. Overall in sub-Saharan Africa the ratio of female:male HIV infection is about 1.3:1.0.[14] In several countries in Southern Africa, the HIV prevalence among 15–24-year-old females is 30% or higher. Therefore, it is especially urgent to implement programs to detect and treat HIV-infected pregnant women in order to prevent transmission to their infants.

There are several obstacles to implementing an effective public health program to prevent MTCT of HIV. Among these are that most deliveries in sub-Saharan Africa are at home, especially in rural areas. Many women do not receive prenatal care. The availability of screening for HIV is far from universal, and many women are fearful of being screened because of the stigma of being identified as HIV positive. Nevertheless, prevention of MTCT of HIV is a major component of the WHO "3 by 5 program." Access to HIV testing continues to expand. The availability of reliable rapid tests has been important in identifying HIV-positive women, especially when their first contact with health care is when they are in labor.

The WHO Expert Panel on Prevention of MTCT has made the following recommendations:

- Women who need ARV treatment for their own health should receive it in accordance with WHO guidelines on ARV treatment.
- HIV-infected pregnant women who do not have indications for ARV treatment, or do not have access to treatment, should be offered ARV prophylaxis to prevent MTCT using one of several regimens known to be safe and effective:
  - ZDV from 28 weeks of pregnancy plus single-dose NVP during labor and single-dose NVP and 1-week ZDV for the infant. This regimen is highly efficacious, as is initiating ZDV later in pregnancy.
  - Alternative regimens based on ZDV alone, short-course ZDV+ 3TC, or single-dose NVP alone are also recommended.

- In resource-constrained settings, elective cesarean delivery is seldom available and/or safe and refraining from breast-feeding is often not acceptable, feasible, or safe. Therefore, efforts to reduce MTCT in most resource-constrained settings have focused on ARV prophylaxis around the time of delivery, which can reduce HIV transmission almost two-fold in a breast-feeding population.

At the United Nations General Assembly Special Session on HIV/AIDS in June 2001, governments from 189 countries committed themselves to a comprehensive program of international and national action to fight the HIV/AIDS pandemic by adopting the Declaration of Commitment on HIV/AIDS. The declaration established specific goals, including reducing the proportion of infants infected with HIV by 20% by 2005 and by 50% by 2010.

A successful program to prevent MTCT of HIV has been implemented in Thailand. The nationwide program was implemented in 2000 after a successful pilot study in seven provinces. Between October 2000 and September 2001 data were reported from 822 public health hospitals in all regions in Thailand. Among 573,655 women giving birth during that period, 96.7% received prenatal care, and of those, 93.3% were tested for HIV prior to delivery. Among 6646 HIV-seropositive women, 70.1% received prophylactic antiretroviral therapy prior to delivery, 88.7% of the neonates of these seropositive women received prophylactic antiretroviral therapy, and 83.2% received infant formula.[199] These encouraging results suggest that rapid implementation of a public health program to prevent maternal-to-infant transmission in a developing country is feasible.

Transmission by Blood Transfusion, Blood Products, and Organ Transplantation

The transfusion of HIV-contaminated blood is the most effective way to transmit the virus. Over 90% of seronegative recipients are infected by transfusion of a single contaminated unit of blood.[200] The risk of transmission of HIV through the transfusion of blood or blood products was recognized very early in the AIDS epidemic. After the risk was recognized, and prior to the identification of the HIV virus, blood banks established procedures to exclude any man who had sex with another man since 1978 and other potential donors at high risk of infections from heterosexual or drug-use exposures. These donor exclusion criteria have remained in place to the present, despite the implementation of serological and nucleic acid testing (NAT) of all donations. Exclusion of potential donors at high risk and screening of all units with sensitive antibody and nucleic acid tests have resulted in a very low risk of HIV transmission by blood transmission in the United States and other industrialized countries at present. Lackritz et al estimated the risk of transmission of an HIV-infected unit of blood as 1 in 450,000–660,000 donations among 41 million blood donations in 19 American Red Cross centers in 1992–1993.[201]

The risk of transfusion-related transmission has been further reduced with the development of more sensitive ELISA assays and the implementation of NAT to identify infected donors (those in the window period) prior to seroconversion. The risk of an HIV-infected unit being accepted for transfusion was estimated to be only 1:2,135,000 units in 2001 after the implementation of a fairly extensive behavioral interview to screen donors, followed by EIA and NAT screening.[202] In the first 3 years after NAT screening of all blood donations was introduced in 1999, the Red Cross Blood Collection Centers in the United States identified 12 NAT-positive, antibody-negative units among 37,164,054 units screened, or 1 in 3.1 million donations.[203] A cost-effectiveness analysis found that NAT screening for HIV and hepatitis C virus (HCV) costs $4.7–11.2 million per quality-adjusted life-year (QALY) saved.[204] Despite this high cost, it is the current philosophy of FDA and other regulatory authorities that transfusion should be as close as possible to "100% safe" for the recipient, even though it is not possible to achieve perfect safety. Another advantage of the introduction of nucleic acid testing is that the testing can be multiplexed fairly easily by introducing additional primers to detect nucleic acids of other infectious agents. This was done recently during the West Nile virus (WNV) epidemic, after it was recognized that the incidence of WNV infectious donors was fairly high in some areas during the height of the transmission season.[205-206] Over 1000 WNV viremic donors have been identified in 2003 and 2004.[206]

Before HIV screening became available, 75–90% of recipients of factor VIII concentrate and 30% of all factor IX recipients had been infected.[207] The risk of HIV transmission from transplantation of a whole organ of an HIV-infected donor is nearly 100%.[208-210] Fresh-frozen, unprocessed bone from a donor who is HIV positive is highly likely to transmit an HIV infection if marrow elements and adherent tissue are not removed. Relatively avascular solid tissue poses a lower risk for HIV transmission, especially if it has been processed by techniques that might inactivate HIV.[210]

Despite the safety of the blood supply in industrialized countries, blood transfusion in many developing countries still carries a significant risk of HIV transmission. In some resource-poor countries, antibody screening of blood donors is not universal because of an inconsistent supply of testing reagents. Furthermore, donors are commonly paid or are replacement donors for individual patients. First-time donors, who are at higher risk of HIV than repeat donors, are more common in most developing countries. Paid and first-time donors have been found to be at higher risk of HIV, hepatitis B, and hepatitis C virus infections in most populations. Importantly, the HIV risk in many developing countries is not concentrated in populations of MSM and IDUs, but rather in the general heterosexual population. This complicates the development of a strategy to select a low-risk donor population. Outbreaks of HIV infection have been reported among plasmapheresis donors in China, Mexico, and other developing countries.[211-212]

Transmission in the Health Care Setting

HIV infection is a risk for health care workers and laboratory personnel who handle sharp instruments or may be exposed to body fluids from HIV-infected patients. Needlestick accidents pose a far greater risk than does intact skin or mucous membrane exposure to HIV-contaminated blood or body fluids. A 0.4% HIV seroconversion rate has been reported in health care workers who had percutaneous injuries with HIV-contaminated surgical instruments.[213-214] Most of these injuries have occurred in emergency situations involving resuscitation attempts and during surgery. The risk of HIV infection is greatest when the health care worker has been exposed to a quantity of blood from patients with advanced HIV disease and very high viral load. Exposure of mucosal and nonintact skin to HIV-contaminated body fluids accounts for a lower infection risk (less than 0.1%) than does penetrating exposures.[214-215] One large prospective study evaluating 2712 intact cutaneous exposures detected no infections,[216] although there have been reports of HIV transmission in cases where there was cutaneous exposure to HIV-contaminated fluids or blood splashes.[217]

An HIV-infected dentist was reported to be responsible for HIV spread to six of his patients.[218] Genetic sequencing of the viruses from the infected patients and the dentist indicated the viruses were from a common source.[219] The only reasonable explanation was transmission from the dentist to his patient.[218] In some developing countries, inadequate infection control practices regarding contaminated syringes and needles have resulted in HIV transmission to patients. The relative importance of parenteral versus sexual exposures in the transmission of HIV in developing countries has recently been debated.[220-221] Nevertheless, the adoption of universal precautions is strongly advocated to reduce occupational exposures among health care workers.

Environmental and Casual Contact Transmission

Environmental transmission of HIV is not believed to occur. Although studies of HIV survival in the environment revealed that HIV could be recovered by tissue culture 1–3 days after drying,[222] the clinical relevance of this finding is dubious because the virus concentration in this report was several thousand-fold higher than in blood in persons with HIV infection. However, environmental contamination could pose a risk for persons working in a research laboratory where concentrated virus preparations exist; at least one transmission has occurred in this setting.[223] Environmental spread of HIV is also unlikely, as inactivation of HIV is quite rapid. CDC studies have demonstrated that drying causes HIV concentrations to decrease 90–95% within several hours.[224] There have been no reports of HIV infection due to contact with an environmental surface because HIV is unable to reproduce, spread, or maintain infectivity outside its living host. There is no evidence to support the transmission of HIV by insects,[224-227] despite the common belief in many populations that this poses a risk.

Household transmission of HIV in the absence of sexual or percutaneous exposure is rare. HIV has not been shown to be transmitted through the sharing of household items, such as towels, plates, sheets, glasses, toilet, or bath or shower facilities that have been soiled by feces, saliva, urine, or tears from an infected patient. Studies in the United States and Europe of nonsexual, non-needle-sharing household contacts of persons with HIV infection have indicated no evidence of infection among family members.[228-230] HIV transmission has been reported in households where needles were shared for medical injections at home and where there was mucocutaneous exposure to blood or other body substances during home health care.[231-233] In one unusual case reported to the CDC involving HIV transmission between two brothers with hemophilia, the putative spread of infection was due to sharing the same shaving razor.[234]

Postexposure Prophylaxis (PEP) and Preexposure Prophylaxis (PREP)

Occupational Exposure

As of June 2003, CDC had received voluntary reports of 57 US health care workers with documented seroconversion temporally associated with an occupational exposure to an HIV-infected patient. An additional 138 seroconversions in health care workers are considered possibly due to occupational exposures.[235]

In a retrospective case-control study of occupational exposure, several factors were associated with an increased risk of HIV transmission.[236] Risk was increased if the exposure was to a larger quantity of blood, by a device visibly contaminated with blood, by a hollow-bore device as compared to a solid needle, by a procedure that involved a needle being placed directly in a vein or artery, or by a deep injury. The risk was also increased for exposure to blood from source persons with terminal illness.

Some evidence exists that host defenses possibly influence the risk for HIV infection. Studies of HIV-exposed but uninfected health care workers and sex workers demonstrated that several persons had an HIV-specific cytotoxic T-lymphocyte (CTL) response or mucosal IgA HIV-specific antibodies.[237–238]

Studies in animals suggest that postexposure prophylaxis (PEP) might have some prophylactic efficacy.[214] Although a randomized clinical trial comparing PEP versus no treatment in humans will not be conducted for ethical and logistical reasons, observational data comparing infection rates after known exposures among health care workers who received prophylaxis and those who did not after a known exposure indicate that PEP with ZDV was associated with an 81% (95% CI, 43–94%) decrease in transmission.[214]

The efficacy of prevention of maternal-to-child transmission by treatment of either mother or infant suggests that prophylaxis after exposure might be capable of preventing transmission under some circumstances. Nevertheless, failures of PEP to prevent HIV transmission have been reported in at least 21 cases, despite the prompt initiation of antiretroviral therapy.[235] Currently, CDC recommends a two-drug regimen be provided within 1–2 hours (if possible) for a less-severe exposure (e.g., solid needle, asymptomatic source case) for 28 days. The two drugs selected could be AZT/3TC (Combivir), 3TC and Stavudine, or Didanosine and D4T.[214] For more severe exposures or if the source patient has a known resistant virus, lopinavir, invirase, atazanavir, or tenofovir can be added to the 28-day regimen. Minor to moderate adverse reactions are commonly experienced by patients receiving these PEP regimens. However, serious side effects are unusual.

Nonoccupational Exposures

The suggestion that postexposure prophylaxis (PEP) with antiviral drugs may be capable of preventing infection among health care workers or infants born to HIV-positive women led to the consideration of the use of PEP for other exposures to HIV, especially sexual or parenteral (e.g., IDU) exposures.

After reviewing the available evidence, a CDC committee recommended that HAART PEP be given as soon as possible (48–72 hours) after sexual exposure, injection drug use exposure, or other parenteral exposure to a person who has been exposed to a source known to be HIV positive. The therapy should be continued for 28 days.[239] No specific recommendations were made concerning exposure to a source whose HIV status was unknown. In the past several years, a substantial number of MSMs have taken PEP following a possible exposure to HIV. There has been no clear evidence to date that the availability of PEP after a high-risk exposure has disinhibited the use of condoms or promoted other high-risk sexual behavior. However, this remains an issue of public health concern.

Recently studies have been initiated in several developing countries to evaluate the efficacy of tenofovir, a drug with a long half-life, to prevent HIV in persons who have frequent exposures, such as IDUs and sex workers. These studies of preexposure prophylaxis (PREP) could provide another method for prevention of HIV in highly exposed populations.

Rapid HIV Tests

HIV testing is a critical point of entry for providing information regarding HIV transmission, prevention, counseling, and referral. Unfortunately, almost one third of patients who have tested positive for HIV at CDC-funded public testing sites did not return for their results,[240] and many high-risk patients often do not get tested because of various factors, including the number of visits required to be tested and obtain their result. The need for accurate, noninvasive, and inexpensive rapid testing for HIV remains acute. Rapid tests for HIV have important applications in several testing situations, including in social venues such as bars; in acute care settings such as emergency rooms; and for military use in the field.[241] Rapid tests are believed to be an essential component of the WHO "3 by 5" scale-up access program to antiretroviral therapy in Africa. To address these needs, rapid tests have been in development for more than a decade. At present, over 60 HIV rapid tests have been developed and are available worldwide; four of these are US FDA approved.[242]

The first FDA HIV rapid test, Oraquick Advance, received FDA approval in November 2002. This test can be performed using whole blood, oral fluid, or plasma; it can detect HIV-1 and HIV-2; and results are available in 20 minutes. Using whole blood, the sensitivity and specificity of this test is 99.6% and 100%, respectively; using oral fluid, 99.3% and 99.8%, respectively; and using plasma, 99.6% and 99.9%, respectively. A second test is Uni-Gold Recombigen, which can be performed using whole blood or serum/plasma. This test detects HIV-1 only and results can be obtained in 10 minutes. The sensitivity and specificity to detect established HIV infection are similar to the Oraquick test. A third test is the Multispot test, which can be performed using serum or plasma, can detect either HIV-1 or HIV-2, and results are available in 15 minutes. Using serum or plasma, the sensitivity and specificity are 100% and 99.9%, respectively. The fourth test is the Reveal G2 test, which can be performed using serum or plasma, can test for HIV-1 only, and results are available in 5 minutes. Using serum, the sensitivity and specificity are 99.8% and 99.1%, respectively; and using plasma, 99.8% and 98.6%, respectively. The high sensitivity of these tests indicates that most patients with established HIV infection will be correctly diagnosed. However, a rare false positive may occur; therefore, it is important to repeat or confirm the test. Persons who test positive should have their screening test results confirmed, be interviewed, counseled, and referred for medical evaluation and care.

Global Prevalence of HIV

UNAIDS has estimated that 40.3 million persons were living with HIV infection in 2005 (Table 21-10). Of these, 38.0 million were adults and 17.5 million were women. A total of 2.3 million children under age 15 years were HIV infected.[14] In 2005 there were an estimated 4.9 million newly infected persons and 3.1 million deaths.[14]

The regional HIV/AIDS statistics for 2003 and 2005 are shown in Table 21-11A, and the projected expenditures on prevention and care and support are lested in Table 21-11B. Between 2002 and 2004 there was a 7% increase in the number of HIV-infected persons worldwide, rising from 36.6 million to 40.0 million.

The AIDS epidemic is affecting females in increasing numbers. Globally, just under half of HIV-infected persons are females. In Africa, 57% of persons aged 15–48 years are women; however, among HIV-positive persons 15–24 years of age, 76% are females, reflecting sexual partnering of younger women with older males.[14] The proportion of HIV-infected persons who are female is increasing worldwide (Figure 21-13). Understanding and dealing with gender inequality regarding prevention and care, which often limits women's choices, are critical to prevent new HIV infections.

Southern Africa

Southern Africa has experienced the greatest burden of HIV/AIDS in the world. Data from antenatal clinics in the Republic of South Africa (the country with the most infections in the world) indicate that HIV prevalence

TABLE 21-10   Global Summary of the AIDS Epidemic, December 2005

Number of people living with HIV in 2005	**Total**	**40.3 million (36.7–45.3 million)**
	Adults	38.0 million (34.5–42.6 million)
	Women	17.5 million (16.2–19.3 million)
	Children under 15 years	2.3 million (2.1–2.8 million)
People newly infected with HIV in 2005	**Total**	**4.9 million (4.3–6.6 million)**
	Adults	4.2 million (3.6–5.8 million)
	Children under 15 years	700,000 (630,000–820,000)
AIDS deaths in 2005	**Total**	**3.1 million (2.8–3.6 million)**
	Adults	2.6 million (2.3–2.9 million)
	Children under 15 years	570,000 (510,000–670,000)

Note: The ranges around the estimates in this table define the boundaries within which the actual numbers lie, based on the best available information.
Source: Reproduced by kind permission of UNAIDS. www.unaids.org.

TABLE 21-11　Regional HIV and AIDS Statistics and Features, 2003 and 2005

	Adults and Children Living with HIV	Adults and Children Newly Infected with HIV	Adult Prevalence (%)*	Adult and Child Deaths Due to AIDS
Sub-Saharan Africa				
2005	25.8 million (23.8–28.9 million)	3.2 million (2.8–3.9 million)	7.2 (6.6–8.0)	2.4 million (2.1–2.7 million)
2003	24.9 million (23.0–27.9 million)	3.0 million (2.7–3.7 million)	7.3 (6.7–8.1)	2.1 million (1.9–2.4 million)
North Africa and Middle East				
2005	510,000 (230,000–1.4 million)	67,000 (35,000–200,000)	0.2 (0.1–0.7)	58,000 (25,000–145,000)
2003	500,000 (200,000–1.4 million)	62,000 (31,000–200,000)	0.2 (0.1–0.7)	55,000 (22,000–140,000)
South and Southeast Asia				
2005	7.4 million (4.5–11.0 million)	990,000 (480,000–2.4 million)	0.7 (0.4–1.0)	480,000 (290,000–740,000)
2003	6.5 million (4.0–9.7 million)	840,000 (410,000–2.0 million)	0.6 (0.4–0.9)	390,000 (240,000–590,000)
East Asia				
2005	870,000 (440,000–1.4 million)	140,000 (42,000–390,000)	0.1 (0.05–0.2)	41,000 (20,000–68,000)
2003	690,000 (350,000–1.1 million)	100,000 (33,000–300,000)	0.1 (0.04–0.1)	22,000 (11,000–37,000)

continued

TABLE 21-11 continued

	Adults and Children Living with HIV	Adults and Children Newly Infected with HIV	Adult Prevalence (%)*	Adult and Child Deaths Due to AIDS
Oceania				
2005	74,000	8,200	0.5	3,600
	(45,000–120,000)	(2,400–25,000)	(0.2–0.7)	(1,700–8,200)
2003	63,000	8,900	0.4	2,000
	(38,000–99,000)	(2,600–2,700)	(0.2–0.6)	(910–4,900)
Latin America				
2005	1.8 million	200,000	0.6	68,000
	(1.4–2.4 million)	(130,000–380,000)	(0.5–0.8)	(52,000–86,000)
2003	1.6 million	170,000	0.6	59,000
	(1.2–2.1 million)	(120,000–310,000)	(0.4–0.8)	(46,000–77,000)
Caribbean				
2005	300,000	30,000	1.6	24,000
	(200,000–510,000)	(17,000–71,000)	(1.1–2.7)	(16,000–40,000)
2003	300,000	29,000	1.6	24,000
	(200,000–510,000)	(17,000–68,000)	(1.1–2.7)	(16,000–40,000)
Eastern Europe and Central Asia				
2005	1.6 million	270,000	0.9	62,000
	(990,000–2.3 million)	(140,000–610,000)	(0.6–1.3)	(39,000–91,000)
2003	1.2 million	270,000	0.7	38,000
	(740,000–1.8 million)	(120,000–630,000)	(0.4–1.0)	(24,000–52,000)

continued

TABLE 21-11   continued

	Adults and Children Living with HIV	Adults and Children Newly Infected with HIV	Adult Prevalence (%)*	Adult and Child Deaths Due to AIDS
Western and Central Europe				
2005	720,000	22,000	0.3	12,000
	(570,000–890,000)	(15,000–39,000)	(0.2–0.4)	<15,000
2003	700,000	20,000	0.3	12,000
	(550,000–870,000)	(13,000–37,000)	(0.2–0.4)	<15,000
North America				
2005	1.2 million	43,000	0.7	18,000
	(650,000–1.0 million)	(15,000–120,000)	(0.4–1.1)	(9,000–30,000)
2003	1.1 million	43,000	0.7	18,000
	(570,000–1.0 million)	(15,000–120,000)	(0.3–1.1)	(9,000–30,000)
TOTAL				
2005	40.3 million	4.9 million	1.1	3.1 million
	(36.7–45.3 million)	(4.3–6.6 million)	(1.0–1.3)	(2.8–3.6 million)
2003	37.5 million	4.6 million	1.1	2.8 million
	(34.0–41.9 million)	(4.0–6.0 million)	(1.0–1.2)	(2.5–3.1 million)

Source: Reproduced by kind permission of UNAIDS. www.unaids.org.

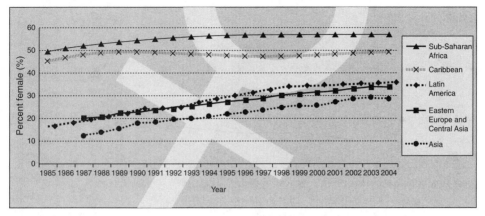

FIGURE 21-13 Percentage of adults (15–49) living with HIV who are female, 1985–2004. *Source:* Reproduced by kind permission of UNAIDS. www.unaids.org.

has increased steadily from under 5% in 1991–1993 to 25% or higher in 2003 (Figure 21-14).

Very high HIV prevalence, in excess of 30%, has been reported in Botswana, Lesotho, Namibia, and Swaziland.[14,138] In South Africa the HIV prevalence has increased dramatically in the past 10 years, especially in females; one study reported an increase in HIV prevalence from 4.8% among 15–19-year-old girls to 16.5% in 20–24-year-olds. Among young women 15–24 years of age the prevalence was 24.5%; among similar aged men it was 7.6%.[14]

East Africa

The epidemic in East Africa is older than the Southern African epidemic. Some countries in this region, especially Uganda, have shown evidence of a decline in HIV prevalence since the mid-1990s (Figure 21-15).[243] The estimated national prevalence in Uganda fell from 13% in the early 1990s to 4.1% by the end of 2003.[14,243] The decreased HIV prevalence in Uganda has been especially marked in adolescents and young adults. A 60% reduction in casual sex, a delay in onset of sex, and an increase in the use of condoms have been important in reducing HIV in Uganda. Some other countries in the region have shown more modest decreases in HIV prevalence as well. Comparisons of HIV prevalence among antenatal clinic attendees in East Africa have shown an overall decline from 12.9% in 1997–1998 to 8.5% in 2002. Modest declines in the HIV prevalence among antenatal patients have also been reported in Kenya, Tanzania, Ethiopia, and Burundi. However, there is no evidence of an overall decline in HIV prevalence in any other East African country. Despite these decreases in HIV prevalence in several areas of East Africa, HIV/AIDS continues to be the major health problem faced by all countries in the region.

West Africa

The epidemic in West Africa has been more focal and less intense overall than in East, Central, and Southern Africa. The median HIV prevalence

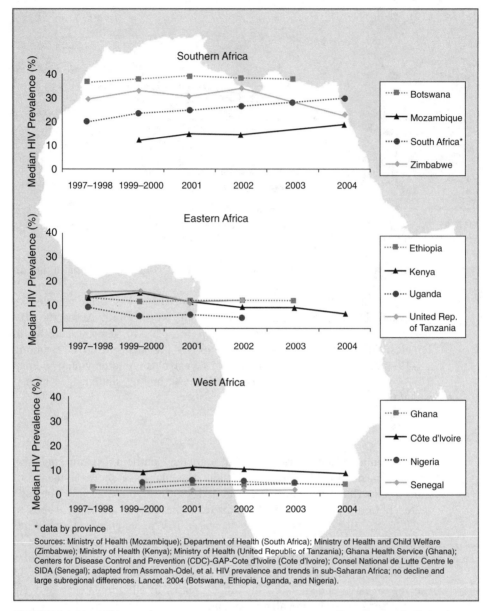

FIGURE 21-14 HIV prevalence among pregnant women attending antenatal clinics in sub-Saharan Africa, 1997/98–2004.
Source: Reproduced by kind permission of UNAIDS. www.unaids.org.

among women in 112 antenatal clinics in West Africa has remained steady at 3–4% between 1997 and 2002.[14,138] HIV prevalence is lowest in the Sahel countries and highest in Burkina Faso, Côte d'Ivoire, and Nigeria. The HIV epidemic in Nigeria is expanding rapidly. Nigeria's 2003 HIV sentinel survey estimated the national HIV prevalence to be 5%, with a prevalence over 7% in the North Central areas. Nigeria is estimated to have the third largest number of HIV-infected persons of any country in the world, behind South Africa, and India.

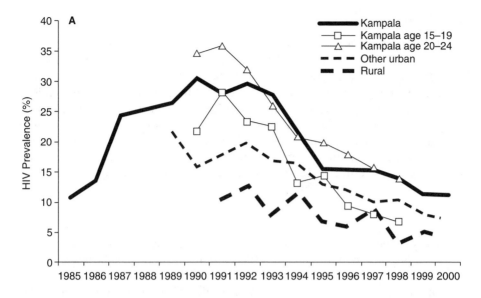

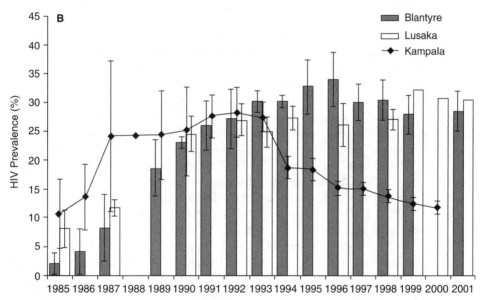

FIGURE 21-15   (A) HIV prevalence rates (%) in pregnant women surveyed at antenatal sentinel surveillance sites in Uganda in urban Kampala, other urban sentinel sites, and rural sites from 1985 to 2001. (B) A comparison of HIV prevalence rates (%) in pregnant women surveyed at antenatal sentinel surveillance sites between 1985 and 2001 in urban Kampala, Uganda; Lusaka, Zambia; and Blantyre, Malawi. Error bars represent 95% CI around the sample mean.
Source: Stoneburner et al. Population-Level HIV Declines and Behavioral Risk Avoidance in Uganda. *Science*, Vol. 304, Issue 5671, 714–718. Copyright 2004 AAAS.

Côte d'Ivoire has had the highest reported HIV prevalence in the region since the beginning of the epidemic, although the estimated prevalence of HIV among adults in Abidjan in 2002 decreased to an estimated 6.4% from 13% in 1999.[14]

The Caribbean

The Caribbean is the second-most affected region in the world. Among persons 15–44 years of age, AIDS is now the leading cause of death. The adult HIV prevalence has been estimated to be 2–3%, and about 440,000 adults and children are living with HIV infection.[14] In five countries in the region, (the Bahamas, Belize, Guyana, Haiti, Trinidad and Tobago), the national prevalence exceeds 2%.[14] The epidemic in the Caribbean is occurring largely through heterosexual intercourse, although sex between men, which is stigmatized, is a significant contributor. Cuba is notable for having a very low HIV prevalence in a region characterized by a high HIV burden.[14]

Asia

While national HIV rates in many Asian countries are much lower than those in most of sub-Saharan Africa, the population of Asia is very large and heterogeneous. Large numbers of persons are infected with HIV, and many are at high risk of becoming infected. Asia comprises both well-established, generalized epidemics (i.e., general population HIV prevalence ≥1%) and recent concentrated epidemics (i.e., HIV prevalence ≥5% in risk groups), each having unique epidemiologic features and HIV prevention and control needs. Long-term generalized epidemics are found in Thailand, Cambodia, and Myanmar. Others, such as selected areas in India and China, have localized but significant epidemics in specific populations, particularly migrants, sex workers, and drug users. Some countries have only recently experienced expanding epidemics. These countries include Indonesia, Nepal, Vietnam, Malaysia, and several provinces in China. Other Asian countries continue to have low rates of HIV, even among persons at high risk of HIV, including Bangladesh, East Timor, Laos, Pakistan, and the Philippines. Overall, UNAIDS has estimated that there are 8.2 million adults and children living with HIV in Asia as of December 2005 compared to 7.2 million in 2002. About 1.2 million persons were newly infected in 2005; the adult population prevalence in Asia has been estimated to be about 0.4%.[14]

In China, HIV has spread to all 31 provinces, autonomous regions, and principalities. In some areas, such as Henan, Anhui, and Shandong, HIV has spread extensively among rural adults who sold their plasma repeatedly to supplement their incomes and acquired HIV through contaminated plasmapheresis coupled with reinfusion of red blood cells to prevent anemia from frequent donation.[211,212] In Southern and Western China the prevalence of HIV is high among injection drug users and commercial sex workers.[14]

In India, the HIV epidemic is more diverse. It is estimated that in 2003 about 5.1 million persons were living with HIV, second only to South Africa in the number of persons with HIV/AIDS.[14] A severe epidemic of HIV among injection drug users has been under way for several years in the state of Manipur in northeastern India. However, HIV prevalence is high among IDUs elsewhere, notably Chennai where 64% of IDUs have been reported to be HIV positive in one study.[14] The HIV epidemic is more severe in southern India than in the very populous northern states at present and is fueled primarily by heterosexual transmission. The course of the HIV/AIDS epidemic in India, China, and Indonesia will be a major determinant of the size of the future global pandemic because of the very large populations potentially at risk of infection in these areas.

The HIV/AIDS epidemic emerged rapidly among injection drug users in Thailand in early 1988. This was followed soon thereafter by increasing HIV prevalence among sex workers and their clients seen at STD clinics, especially in the upper northern provinces. In 1991 the Thai government instituted an aggressive and successful prevention program to prevent the heterosexual transmission of HIV during commercial or casual sex.[125,126] The program has often been called the 100% Condom Program, since it emphasized the use of condoms during commercial sex to prevent HIV infection. However, the promotion of condoms was only one feature of the AIDS prevention effort in Thailand. The campaign also included a strong and integrated political and financial commitment to prevention of HIV at all levels of Thai society, directed by Prime Minister Anand Panyarachun in cooperation with governmental organizations and ministries and nongovernmental organizations. Extensive health education messages aimed at the public about the risks of HIV and methods of protection, including condoms, were distributed through widely available media. Laws were enacted to prevent discrimination and AIDS was destigmatized to some extent.

A nationwide semiannual HIV seroprevalence sentinel surveillance system included anonymous surveys of HIV prevalence in several populations at risk (i.e., "direct" or brothel-based female sex workers and "indirect" female sex workers, STD patients, injection drug users, blood donors, and pregnant women) was begun in June 1989 and expanded nationally in 1991. These prevalence data allowed monitoring of the temporal trends and spread of HIV infection in the various risk groups throughout the country and helped to evaluate the needs and progress of the control program. The sentinel surveillance data showed decreasing HIV prevalence among all of these populations, except for injection drug users, during the mid and late 1990s (Figure 21-16).

The effective HIV prevention program in Thailand was partially replicated in neighboring Cambodia and has been associated with reduced HIV prevalence among high-risk groups. In addition to public health programs to prevent HIV by reducing the frequency of high-risk sex, programs to prevent transmission through injection drug use and expanded voluntary counseling and testing and treatment programs are needed in Asia to more effectively control the epidemic. In 2004 fewer than 6% of the estimated 170,000 persons who needed antiretroviral treatment in Asia were being treated. However, several countries are now expanding treatment access with the help of the Global Fund. Thailand is likely to reach its target of providing antiretroviral treatment for 50,000 persons by the end of 2005.

Eastern Europe and Central Asia

The number of persons infected with HIV in Eastern Europe has increased dramatically in the past few years, reaching an estimated 1.4 million by the end of 2004.[14] Several countries in Eastern Europe, including the Ukraine, the Russian Federation, Estonia, and Latvia, have severe HIV epidemics. An estimated 210,000 people in the region were newly infected with HIV in the past year, while 60,000 died of AIDS. The epidemic in the Ukraine is the most

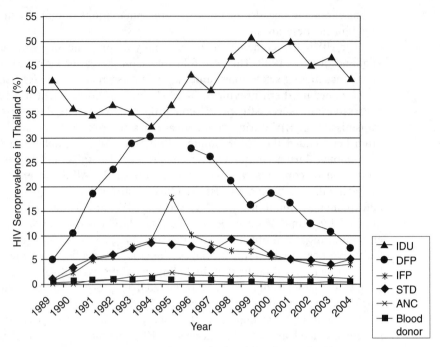

FIGURE 21-16 HIV seroprevalence, Thailand 1989–2004.
Source: Produced from Thai Ministry of Health data.

severe and illustrates an epidemic fueled by widespread injection of illicit drugs. About 80% of HIV-infected injecting drug users are young adults (i.e., under age 30). Injection equipment is very commonly reused by drug users in the Ukraine. In some areas drug users are females who frequently engage in commercial sex to gain finances to support their drug use. All of the elements are in place for an explosive epidemic.

The epidemic in the Russian Federation accounts for about 70% of the persons infected with HIV in the region. An estimated 800,000 people were living with HIV in Russia at the end of 2003; 80% of them were 15–29 years of age and more than a third were women.[14] In Russia, aggressive (and previously mandatory) testing was conducted under the Soviet system. Tens of millions of persons have been tested in the past 15 years or so. In addition, HIV infections are reportable and included in the official statistics. Recent data show a decline in new infections to 39,699 in 2003 compared to 52,349 reported in 2002 and 88,577 cases in 2001.[14,244] It is not clear why the numbers of reported new infections are decreasing. However, it is possible that previous widespread testing among injection drug users, who have constituted 80% of the reported cases, has identified many of the HIV-positive IDUs. The reported decline in HIV prevalence probably does not mean that the incidence of new infections has declined but more likely reflects widespread serological screening of high-risk groups. The epidemic is concentrated in 10 oblasts, mostly in western areas, in the Russian Federation. Although most reported HIV infections have been among injection drug users, there is evidence of an increased infection rate among sex workers and their partners, especially in St. Petersburg.[14,245] It has been estimated that there are 1.5–3.0 million drug users in Russia. Methadone replacement therapy for opiate users is illegal in Russia, as is buprenorphine, and harm reduction programs are not widespread. The number of female sex workers has expanded significantly in the past decade after the break-up of the former Soviet Union. The proportion of prisoners with a history of drug use has increased, which has fueled epidemics of HIV and tuberculosis in the prison system. The future of the HIV epidemic in Russia and Eastern Europe will be influenced substantially by the movement of HIV infections from drug users to sex workers and their clients and the numbers of new drug users.

Latin America

More than 1.7 million people are living with HIV infection in Latin America. In 2004 about 95,000 people died of AIDS, and 240,000 people were newly infected.[14] Among persons aged 15–24 years, an estimated 0.5% of women and 0.8% of men were HIV-infected at the end of 2004.

Two countries in the region, Guatemala and Honduras, have HIV prevalence rates over 1% of the general population, meaning they are having a generalized epidemic. However, several other countries have substantial focal epidemics.

Brazil accounts for more than one third of the people with HIV infections in Latin America. The HIV epidemic in Brazil has spread to all regions of the country. Originally, the main risk behavior for HIV infection was rectal sex among males. However, more recently injection drug use, especially in southern Brazil,[246] and heterosexual transmission have become important in the epidemic. Infection is significantly associated with lower socioeconomic status among drug users and those who have acquired HIV through sexual contact.[247] Bisexuality is significantly more common among men who have sex with men in Latin America than in North America or Europe. Also rectal intercourse is more common among heterosexual couples in Latin America, thereby increasing the risk of male-to-female transmission of HIV.[248]

The national AIDS program in Brazil is unique among developing countries in that it was the first to integrate HIV/AIDS prevention with care and treatment of persons with HIV/AIDS.[249] Although it is now generally recognized that prevention and treatment are both essential components of an effective AIDS control program, access to treatment was very limited until antiretroviral medication prices were dramatically reduced due to worldwide demand and price reduction. Because of the cost and complexity of HIV treatment, most developing countries focused their early efforts entirely on prevention. However, in Brazil the overthrow of a military dictatorship in the late 1980s fostered a democracy movement, which included access to health care as a basic human right. This included the development of needle exchange programs for IDUs in Santos and Salvador and antiretroviral treatment, beginning with access to AZT, in Santos in 1989.[250] Early in the epidemic MSM and IDUs were primarily infected. However, the epidemic later evolved to primarily affect heterosexuals in the late 1990s.[250]

When effective combination antiretroviral therapy was developed and licensed in the United States in 1996, the Brazilian government included free AIDS treatment in the national health care system. Although this required substantial initial cost, the results have been impressive: mortality rates from AIDS declined by 50% and inpatient hospitalization days were reduced 70% over the past 7 years.[250] The number of HIV-infected persons in the country is now about 600,000; whereas it was estimated 10 years ago that the figure would increase to 1,200,000 by 2005.[14] Of the estimated 600,000 HIV-infected persons, 200,000 are aware of their infection and 135,000 were receiving highly active antiretroviral therapy in 2003.[14,249] The cost of implementing the program by 2001 was estimated to be about US$232 million, which has resulted in a total savings of US$1.1 billion due to reduced hospitalization costs.[250]

A critical feature of the success of the AIDS program in Brazil was the local manufacture of several important antiretroviral drugs. In addition, Brazil imported several generic antiretroviral drugs and negotiated reduced prices of name-brand drugs with pharmaceutical manufacturers. Therefore, the drug treatment costs were reduced to an average of US$180–250 per year, compared with US$5000 or more in the United States. The patent violations by the Brazilian program were challenged initially by the United States through the World Trade Organization, after pressure from the pharmaceutical manufacturers. However, these challenges were withdrawn in June 2001. These events have paved the way for the acceptance of the importance of access to affordable antiretroviral treatment as a critical component of the global AIDS prevention effort.

Spread of HIV has been common in Latin America among men who have sex with men, especially in Costa Rica, Venezuela, Panama, and Nicaragua. Commonly men who have a history of male sex in Latin America are bisexual, placing their regular female partners at risk.[14] Most countries in Latin America have focused their official HIV/AIDS prevention efforts on populations of female commercial sex workers, so there is often a mismatch between prevention spending priorities and the main epidemiological features of the epidemic.[14]

Oceania

An estimated 35,000 persons in Oceania are HIV infected. Although 1700 persons are believed to have died of AIDS, an estimated 5000 persons were newly infected with HIV in 2004.[14] Among young people 15–24 years of age an estimated 0.2% of women and 0.2% of men were infected with HIV by the end of 2004.[14]

The annual number of new HIV diagnoses in Australia has gradually increased from 650 in 1998 to about 800 in 2002. Transmission of HIV in Australia and New Zealand continues to be mainly through sexual intercourse between men, which accounted for more than 85% of new HIV diagnoses between 1997 and 2002. Remarkably, injection drug use was responsible for only about 4% and heterosexual intercourse for 8.5% of newly required HIV infections in that period. Australia is perhaps the best example of prevention of spread of HIV among injection drug users through a well-organized and functional harm reduction program to prevent HIV among injection drug users.

Papua New Guinea has the highest prevalence of HIV infection in the Pacific. An estimated 0.6% of adults, roughly 16,000 people in an adult population of about 2.6 million, were living with HIV at the end of 2003.[14] The annual number of new HIV infections has been increasing annually since the mid-1990s. In 2003, 1.4% of pregnant women at antenatal clinics in the capital city of Port Moresby tested HIV positive. The main risk factor for transmission in New Guinea is commercial and casual heterosexual sex. Also in New Guinea there is a high incidence of rape, sexual aggression, and other forms of violence against women. In one study as many as 70% of women had experienced domestic violence.[14,251]

Middle East and North Africa

It has been estimated that about 540,000 persons in this region were infected with HIV at the end of 2004.[14] An estimated 92,000 adults and children were newly infected in 2004, and the adult HIV prevalence was 0.3%. There were some 28,000 deaths among adults and children due to AIDS in 2004. All routes of transmission occur among recognized cases. In most countries, the epidemics are still at a very early stage. However, surveillance is not adequate in most countries in this region.

The most severely affected country in the region is Sudan, which has been wracked by a civil war and humanitarian crises. Recent estimates are that 2% of the adult population was living with HIV at the end of 2003; approximately 400,000 persons were infected, and they accounted for about 80% of all HIV infections in the entire region.[14]

Injection drug use has accounted for the majority of the persons known to be HIV infected in several countries in North Africa and the Middle East. This appears to be the case in Libya, Algeria, Egypt, Iran, Bahrain, Kuwait, and Oman.[14]

Western and Central Europe

Because of the general availability of effective antiretroviral therapy in the countries of Western Europe, the incidence of AIDS has become less representative of the underlying trends of HIV transmission. Therefore, the reporting of new HIV diagnoses was begun in Europe in 1999. Reports include a new standardized format of individual anonymous data of new HIV diagnoses and AIDS cases, which are reported at 6-month intervals. Although HIV reporting is widely implemented, coverage is incomplete. Reporting has started only recently in Portugal, the Netherlands, and France; reporting is not done in all regions of Italy and Spain; and there are no reports from Austria.[14,252] Furthermore, reported new HIV diagnoses are not equivalent to HIV incidence because of the long latency between incident infections and symptoms or screening for HIV in many cases. Also, the widespread availability of effective antiretroviral therapy has resulted in more widespread screening of persons at risk than previously.

UNAIDS and WHO have estimated that 520,000–680,000 people were living with HIV in Western Europe at the end of 2003. Many have been infected for several years, and about 20% have AIDS. By the end of June 2003 a cumulative total of 259,000 persons had been diagnosed with AIDS, of whom 152,000 had died and 107,000 were alive (Figure 21-17). Despite substantial reductions in HIV-related morbidity and mortality in the countries of Western and Central Europe, HIV continues to be a major public health problem in the region.

In the 12 Western European countries, newly diagnosed HIV infections attributable to heterosexual contact increased 122% between 1997 and 2002. Also, there was an increase in HIV among MSM by 22% between 2001 and 2002.[14,252]

Migrants from countries with generalized HIV epidemics, especially from sub-Saharan Africa, account for a large and increasing proportion of infections in Western Europe. In the 12 countries with available data, two thirds of all heterosexually acquired HIV infections during 1997–2002 occurred in people who had immigrated to Europe from countries in Africa with generalized HIV epidemics. Western Europe is the destination of many migrants from sub-Saharan Africa, where the HIV epidemic is most severe and the HIV genotypes most diverse. However, there was a 34% increase of heterosexu-

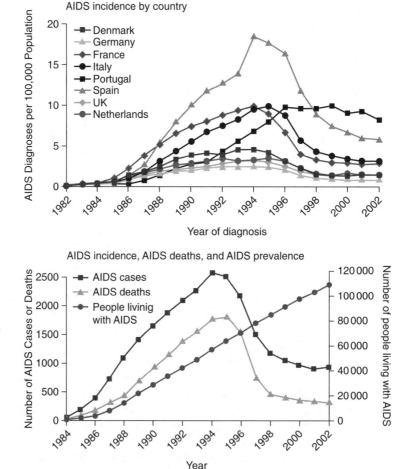

FIGURE 21-17 Trends in AIDS incidence, AIDS deaths, and AIDS prevalence in Western Europe.
Source: Hamers FF et al. The changing face of the HIV epidemic in western Europe: what are the implications for public health policies? Lancet. 2004 Jul 3–9;364(9428):83–94, with permission from Elsevier.

ally transmitted HIV between 1997 and 2002 among persons who were not migrants.[14]

Between 1997 and 2002 the number of new HIV diagnoses decreased gradually by 16% among injection drug users. Along with these changes in transmission patterns, the proportion of women among persons newly diagnosed with HIV infection increased from 25% in 1997 to 38% in 2002.

Available data indicate that although HIV/AIDS is widely distributed throughout Europe, the epidemic is most severe in the countries of southern Europe.[14] There are several challenges for the future control of the epidemic in Western Europe. Among them are the evidence of increased risky sexual behavior among MSM based on the belief that HIV can be prevented with postexposure prophylaxis or that AIDS is now easily treatable. Since the late 1990s increases in the rates of syphilis and gonorrhea have been reported among homosexual and bisexual men in Europe and other industrialized countries. These increases in STDs among MSM are very troubling and suggest that the HIV epidemic in Europe is not under control despite the declining AIDS mortality. Many of the STD cases occurred among older MSM, suggesting that the fear of AIDS morbidity and mortality has declined with the advent of successful HIV therapy.

The detection and control of HIV among migrants is a continuing challenge, since these populations often are affected by substantial barriers to HIV prevention and care. Providing effective HIV prevention and treatment to migrant populations will be an important goal to prevent the future spread of HIV in Europe.

North America

United States

In the United States, AIDS surveillance data are reported to the states, which are responsible for reporting their data to the CDC for compilation in a national database. Patient and physician names and personal identifiers may be reported to the state and local health departments but these data are not included in the CDC database. Some 35 states collect data on patients who are HIV positive who do not have AIDS, meaning HIV prevalence and incidence. According to CDC guidelines, AIDS is defined by the occurrence of an opportunistic infection (OI) in an HIV-positive, immunocompromised patient or a person with a CD4 count of 200 or less who is HIV positive but is free of an OI.

By 2003 the surveillance data indicated that 902,223 cases of AIDS had occurred and 505,801 (56%) persons had died of AIDS in the United States.[253] The number of AIDS cases increased substantially with a change in the AIDS case definition in 1993 to include HIV-positive persons with a CD4 count less than 200 cells/μL as an AIDS case in 1993. The definition was changed to be more inclusive of the total HIV-related immunosuppressed population because of concerns that a proportion of AIDS cases and deaths were missed because an AIDS-related OI did not occur or was not diagnosed prior to death.

After the initial increase in reported cases following the new case definition in 1993, the number of reported AIDS cases leveled off. A more significant decrease in the incidence of AIDS and AIDS mortality occurred after the licensure and widespread use of protease inhibitors and combination HAART to treat HIV and AIDS in 1996 (Figure 21-18). However, the estimated prevalence of HIV infections in the US population has continued to increase because there has not been a concomitant decline in HIV incidence. The CDC has estimated that about 40,000 new HIV infections occur annually in the United States. Reliable estimation of HIV incidence is more difficult than AIDS surveillance, as it depends on routine serological testing of persons at risk and reporting of results to CDC. Of epidemiologic importance is the shift in the distribution of risk groups, with more heterosexuals, more women, and more African Americans and other minority populations becoming infected in the most recent years (Figure 21-19).

HIV Prevalence and Incidence

The CDC has estimated that in December 2003 there were 1,039,000 to 1,185,000 persons in the United States who were living with HIV/AIDS, with about 27% unaware of their HIV infection.[253] In 2003, the estimated number of deaths of persons with AIDS was 18,017, including 17,934 adults and adolescents and 83 children under age 13.

HIV/AIDS by Experience Category

The majority of people with HIV infection are MSM. Among newly diagnosed HIV infections in 2003, CDC has estimated that about 63% were among MSM; of these, 50% were among African Americans, 32% were among whites, and 16% were among Hispanics.[253]

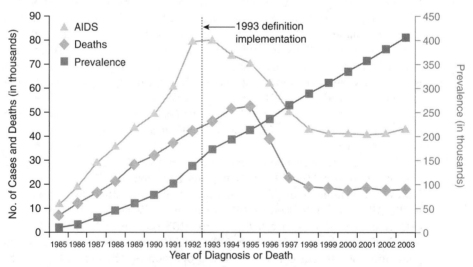

Note: Data adjusted for reporting delays.

FIGURE 21-18 Estimated number of AIDS cases, deaths, and persons living with AIDS, 1985–2003, United States.
Source: Centers for Disease Control and Prevention.

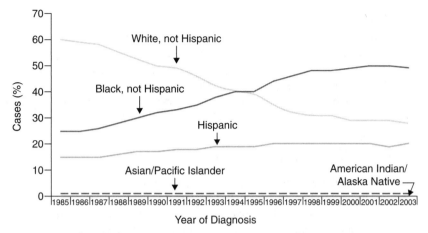

Year of Diagnosis

Note: Data adjusted for reporting delays.

FIGURE 21-19 Proportion of AIDS cases among adults and adolescents, by race/ethnicity and year of diagnosis, 1985–2003—United States.
Source: Centers for Disease Control and Prevention.

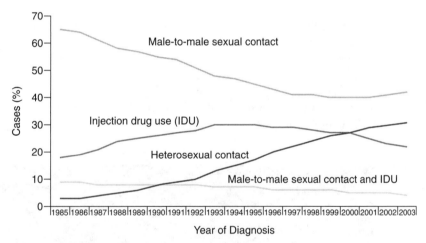

Year of Diagnosis

Note: Data adjusted for reporting delays and estimated proportional redistribution of cases in persons initially reported without an identified risk factor.

FIGURE 21-20 Proportion of AIDS cases among adults and adolescents by transmission category and year of diagnosis, 1985–2003—United States.
Source: Centers for Disease Control and Prevention.

There has been an increase in reported AIDS cases due to heterosexual contact each year between 1999 and 2002. Over the same time period, AIDS cases decreased among IDUs, MSM who were also injection drug users, and among children. In 2002, MSM accounted for 44% of all new HIV/AIDS cases, and persons exposed through heterosexual contact accounted for 35%; together these two groups accounted for 79% of all new HIV/AIDS reports (Figure 21-20).

HIV/AIDS by Age Group

In 2002 persons aged 35–44 years represented 41% of all new cases of AIDS reported to the CDC. The AIDS incidence decreased 61% among children and 24% in persons 25–34 years of age. There has been a dramatic reduction in the estimated number of children less than 13 years of age with AIDS, from 952 in 1992 to 92 in 2002. This decrease primarily reflects the efficacy and wide use of antiretroviral therapy to prevent mother-to-child transmission.

HIV/AIDS by Race/Ethnicity and Sex

The AIDS incidence declined among whites and Hispanics but increased among African Americans, Asians/Pacific Islanders, and American Indians/Alaskan Natives. In 2002 the rates of AIDS diagnoses ranged from 58.7/100,000 in the black population to 4.0/100,000 among Asians/Pacific Islanders. Increasingly, the HIV/AIDS epidemic in the United States is becoming concentrated among minority populations, homosexual men (both white and black), and heterosexual women, 72% of whom were African American.

HIV/AIDS by Geographic Area

The rates of HIV and AIDS for 2002 for the various states and territories in the United States are depicted in Figure 21-21 for only the 30 states that have had name-based reporting. The highest AIDS case rate of 1685.8/100,000 was from the District of Columbia; however, the district is not a state, so these rates cannot be compared to those from the states. New York had the highest rate of AIDS among the states at 400.8/100,000 persons.

In 2003 the highest rate of AIDS occurred in urban areas (population of metropolitan statistical area [MSA] over 500,000), next in smaller urban areas

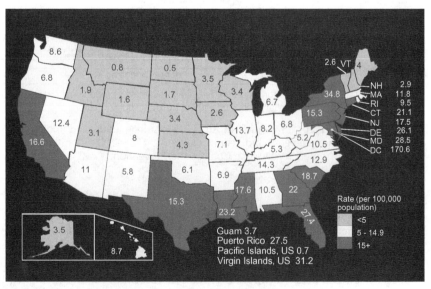

FIGURE 21-21   AIDS rates, reported in 2003, United States.
Source: Centers for Disease Control and Prevention.

Population	2003		Cumulative through 2003
	Number	Rate/100,000	
MSA of >500,000	35,757	23.5	732,141
MSA of 50,000–500,000	4,288	10.9	75,521
Nonmetropolitan	3,317	7.1	52,375

Note: Data based on residence at time of AIDS diagnosis.

FIGURE 21-22 Reported AIDS cases among adults and adolescents by population of area of residence, 2003, and cumulative 50 states and D.C. *Source:* Centers for Disease Control and Prevention.

(MSA 50,000–500,000), and least in rural areas (under 50,000) (Figure 21-22). However, the AIDS rates among rural residents was substantially greater in the South than in other areas of the country.

AIDS Mortality

About 70% of all deaths due to HIV infection and AIDS occur among persons 25–44 years of age in the United States. HIV disease was the leading cause of death among 25–44-year-old persons in 1994 and 1995, after increasing steadily since 1987 (Figure 21-18). In 1995 HIV disease caused 20% of all deaths in this age group. Starting in 1996 the rank of HIV disease among deaths in these young adults fell to fifth place from 1997–2000 and to sixth place in 2001 and 2002. In 2002, HIV disease caused about 7500 deaths, or 6% of all deaths in this age group. However, among non-Hispanic African-American men, deaths from HIV infection were nearly equal to homicide, unintentional injury, and heart disease in 2002 and accounted for 2600 deaths, or 15% of all deaths in this age group.

Mexico

The first AIDS cases in Mexico were reported in 1983. Since then approximately 50,000 cases of AIDS have been reported nationwide, and it has been estimated that over 150,000 persons are HIV infected.[254] The epidemic is less intense than in the United States: about 0.2% of the general adult population is infected, compared to about 0.6% of the general adult population of the United States. Overall, about 40% of reported cases are in homosexual or bisexual men, 7% in transfusion recipients, 20% in heterosexuals, 0.2% in IDUs, and 1% in paid plasma donors. Mexico experienced a significant epidemic of HIV infections in paid plasmapheresis donors in the early and mid-1980s, when donors were infected during donation by contaminated blood collection equipment.[254,255] Over 400 cases of AIDS among paid donors and over 2500 cases have been reported among transfusion recipients in Mexico.[254] Many of these transfusion-acquired cases were among women who required blood transfusions for bleeding during delivery. The epidemic related to plasma donation and blood transfusions was eventually controlled by closing commercial plasmapheresis centers, outlawing paid donors, and establishing licensed state blood transfusion centers with adequate infection control procedures.

Another contribution to the HIV/AIDS epidemic in Mexico is migrant workers, who account for 12.7% of the reported AIDS cases in Mexico.[256] Behavioral studies have found that migrant workers report greater frequencies of high-risk sexual and drug-using behaviors during their migration to the United States for seasonal employment.[256]

Canada

A total of 56,523 positive HIV tests were reported to the Centers for Infectious Diseases Prevention and Control in Canada between November 1985 and June 30, 2004.[257] The highest proportion of reports involved persons 15–29 years of age; MSM represent the highest proportion of risk categories. Injecting drug use was the second exposure category until 1998, peaking at 33% in 1996 and 1997 and decreasing to 18% in 2003 and 2004. Starting in 1999 the heterosexual category became the second largest exposure category, increasing from 7.5% prior to 1995 and reaching 30% of all reported HIV-positives by 2001.

A total of 19,466 AIDS cases were reported up to June 30, 2004. The proportion of females among reported AIDS cases increased from 6.1% during the period 1979–1994 to 25.2% by 2004.

Estimating HIV Incidence

Estimating the incidence of HIV-1 infection is important in order to evaluate the current status of transmission dynamics, to identify high-risk populations, and to determine needs and evaluate prevention programs. Incidence estimates are critical for calculating sample sizes needed for clinical trials of vaccines or other preventive interventions.

The traditional method of measuring the incidence of HIV-1 infection involves repeated testing of cohorts of persons at risk routinely during extended periods of follow-up. These could be cohorts of persons enrolled in a study or those who undergo routine repeated screening, such as for blood donation, pregnancy, or other indications. These selected populations may not provide reliable data for other groups in the population who are at higher risk (e.g., STD clinic patients, sex workers). Cohort members are repeatedly counseled to prevent infection, and those at higher risk may be more likely to be lost to follow-up, leading to an underestimate of the incidence. Prospective studies are expensive, and the data may not be generalizable to key subgroups in the population. Blood donors are screened for behavioral risks and selected by blood banks so they are at significantly lower risk of infection, while younger pregnant women are sexually active and therefore may be at greater HIV risk. UNAIDS uses seroprevalence rates of pregnant women (adjusting for sexual activity, mortality, and fertility) to estimate the seroprevalence in the general population in developing countries.[258,259]

Various models have been described to estimate the incidence and total numbers of persons who are HIV-infected in a population. The "back calculation model" was first described in the 1980s.[260] This model relied on accurate reporting of AIDS cases and an assumption that trends in new AIDS cases reflected existing and past trends in HIV infection. The incidence of AIDS together with the incubation period from HIV infection to AIDS allowed the size of the HIV-positive population to be estimated. However, these models are not useful if AIDS case reporting is incomplete. As the availability of effective antiretroviral therapy has changed the natural history, prolonged the incubation period, and decreased the mortality from AIDS, these models are no longer applicable in populations with access to HAART. Various statistical models have been developed to estimate incidence from cross-sectional, age-specific, prevalence surveys. The simplest of these models assumes that HIV incidence rates in the population are stable over time and that the prevalence increases linearly with age, so that the slope of the regression line provides a crude estimate of HIV incidence.[261] More complex models adjust for mortality, cohort effects, or other factors.

Other methods to estimate the incidence of HIV-1 utilize virological or serological markers; for example, p24 antigen prevalence among HIV-negative persons in the population can be used to estimate incidence. A study in India reported a 19.6% 1-year incidence based on the p24 antigen-positive/antibody-negative prevalence compared to a 11.7% annual incidence based upon the seroconversion rate among prospectively followed STD patients.[262] In this study the duration of the p24 antigen-positive window prior to EIA seroconversion was estimated as 22.5 days, and the p24 antigen-positive/EIA-negative prevalence was used to calculate the incidence that was then compared with the seroconversion rate in prospective follow-up. Other investigators have utilized HIV RNA prevalence among seronegative subjects (the seronegative window period) to estimate the incidence of infection.[263]

The most common method for estimating HIV incidence at present relies on a sensitive/less-sensitive serological testing strategy. In this algorithm, sera that are reactive with a sensitive EIA are retested using an EIA in which the sera have been diluted 1:20,000 instead of 1:400, and the incubation period is shortened from 60–120 minutes to 30 minutes to make the assay less sensitive.[264] The original sensitive/less-sensitive testing strategy (also called "detuned" or standard algorithm for recent HIV-1 seroconversion [STARHS] assay) used a modified commercial HIV-1 antibody assay (Abbott 3A11) and calculated an incubation period of 129 days for the seroconversion from the more sensitive standard assay to the detuned, less-sensitive assay among persons with HIV subtype B infections.[264] Subsequently, the assay was modified to use the licensed Vironostika EIA assay after the Abbott 3A11 assay was no longer available.[265] However, when sera were studied from persons in Thailand who were infected with subtype E infections, the window period was found to be much longer and variable, that is, 270–350 days.[266-267] Because the window period varies with different viral subtypes, the test is less useful in international settings.

Recently an IgG capture enzyme immunoassay (BED-EIA) has been developed, which indirectly measures an increasing proportion of HIV IgG in the serum.[268-269] This assay captures both HIV and non-HIV IgG in the same proportion present in the serum and includes a multi-subtype-derived branched synthetic peptide (BED) from the gp41 immunodominant region of HIV-1. This assay has been shown to detect recent infections with various

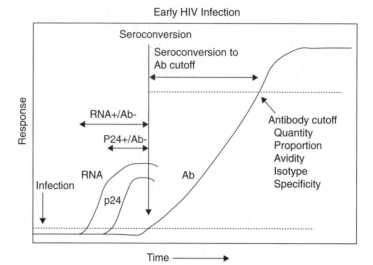

Early HIV Infection

FIGURE 21-23 A schematic diagram showing various parameters that define early HIV-1 infection.
Source: Parekh BS et al. Application of laboratory methods for estimation of HIV-1 incidence. Ind J Med Res. April 2005, pp. 501–518. Copyright 2005 IJMR.

subtypes of HIV, including subtypes B and E in Thailand; A, D, and C, in Africa; and B in the United States and Europe with a similar duration of the seroconversion window of about 160 days.[269] Because of the loss of antibody-producing cells with advanced HIV infection, these sensitive/less-sensitive antibody assays can become positive among some patients with advanced AIDS. However, these persons can be identified by their very low CD4 counts or AIDS symptoms. To calculate incidence, the seroprevalence and the proportion of prevalent infections that are recent, as defined by the sensitive/less-sensitive EIA, must be available. The effect of measurement of RNA and p24 on decreasing the duration of the seronegative window period is shown in Figure 21-23.

Other investigators have reported on the evolution of antibody patterns during infection and have used these patterns to estimate recent infections. Antibodies to gag (p24 and p17) and env (gp120 and gp47) usually appear earlier than those to polymerase gene products (p31, p51, and p66). Antibody affinity and avidity also vary during the course of infection and can be used to differentiate recent from more chronic infections.[270]

It has been reported recently that anti-p24 IgG3 antibodies are elicited only early in HIV-1 infection.[271] The IgG3 antibodies to p24 disappeared by about 4 months after infection and were present only 34 to 120 days after infection (total duration 86 days) among sera from 17 seroconversion panels. If these data can be generalized to persons infected with different subtypes, this assay could become a very useful epidemiological tool.

Social and Cultural Factors

Urbanization has been associated with a higher prevalence of STDs in many parts of the world because bringing people closer together increases the likelihood of sexual encounters, which may occur because single people migrate from rural to urban areas or that cities provide greater anonymity. In the United States, HIV/AIDS has been observed more frequently in urban than in rural areas. Sexual mixing patterns can define how rapidly HIV-1 spreads in a population. In cities with a high male/female ratio, such as Nairobi, Bombay, and Harare, the rate of casual and commercial sex has increased. This has led to high HIV-1 prevalence rates in sex workers and their clients and ultimately to an increased incidence of HIV infection in the general population of these cities. Sexual practices certainly vary between countries and regions of the world. For example, unprotected receptive anal intercourse is unusual in sub-Saharan Africa, whereas it plays a significant role in the spread of HIV in the United States, Latin America, and some Caribbean countries.[272-273] Bisexuality appears to be more common in Latin American than in many other Western countries.[274] In most developing countries, expression of a homosexual lifestyle is repressed; therefore, MSM in these countries may be more hesitant in surveys to admit to anal intercourse. Cultural conceptions of sexual identity vary considerably and must be considered when reviewing the local epidemiology of HIV prevalence and incidence.

Significant rural-to-urban migration is occurring throughout the developing world. The use of migrant labor (which may be seasonal or for weeks at a time) exposes the worker to long absences, increasing the possibility of family breakdown and seeking of other sexual partners.[275] Higher HIV incidence is seen among women who are poor and who have few options to make money other than commercial sex. Poverty predisposes to commercial sex, homelessness in adults, the presence of street children, poor education, and migration, all of which may enhance the possibility of spreading HIV infection.

UNAIDS and the World Health Organization (WHO) conducted an international study in 1998 to evaluate the effect of literacy on HIV incidence.[276] In 161 countries for which literacy and HIV data were available, there was a strong correlation between higher rates of literacy and lower rates of HIV infection. Better-educated people have greater access to information about HIV, how it is spread, and how it can be avoided. However, in sub-Saharan Africa, the opposite literacy-HIV incidence pattern also has been observed.[276] In this region, the rapid social changes that have accompanied development and increased educational opportunities have prompted behaviors that increase the risk of HIV infection. Higher-paying jobs among the educated in this region have apparently served to support high-risk behaviors, which may include increased alcohol consumption, supporting a younger female partner, or visiting sex workers. Education has provided access to income and has emancipated many women of sub-Saharan Africa, resulting in their greater social mobility and increased likelihood of being involved in more sexual relationships, albeit not usually concurrently.

Condoms

Discussions of condom use are largely focused on male latex condoms. Other male condoms used consist of plastic or lambskin, but latex condoms are the most effective against HIV and are also the most studied.[277] It is now well known that water-based lubricants are the only recommended lubricant or additive to be used with condoms. Petroleum-based lubricants render latex condoms less effective against HIV transmission, and nonoxynol-9 has been implicated in increasing the risk of HIV transmission (see Microbicides section later in this chapter).

Latex condoms have been shown in in vitro permeability tests to block the passage of HIV.[278] However, studies of effectiveness, as opposed to laboratory or efficacy studies, are the most useful in determining the real-life (or use-effectiveness) potential of condoms to prevent HIV transmission. A large European prospective study of serodiscordant subjects who were stable partners showed the following rates of transmission according to reported condom use: none (0%) of the HIV-negative partners became infected among couples who consistently and correctly used condoms, despite a cumulative 15,000 episodes of intercourse when the negative partner was at putative risk; among couples using condoms inconsistently, the rate of seroconversion was 4.8/100 person-years (95% CI, 2.5–8.4).[279] The risk of transmission increased with advanced stages of HIV infection in the positive partner ($P < .04$), and withdrawal to avoid ejaculation in the vagina had a protective effect in uninfected women ($P < .02$).

Because randomized controlled trials of condom use for the prevention of HIV transmission are not considered ethical, the best data on condom effectiveness come from observational studies comparing subjects who were "always users" as compared to "never users" of condoms. A recent meta-analysis of studies conducted with subjects who either always (100%) or never (0%) use condoms provides the most convincing evidence of their effectiveness.[280] Studies used in this meta-analysis of "always users" yielded a homogenous HIV infection incidence of 1.14 (95% CI, 0.56–2.04) per 100 person-years. References of "never users" were more heterogeneous, but yielded an incidence rate of 5.75 (95% CI, 3.16–9.66). The preventable fraction (proportionate reduction) of HIV infection with consistent condom use was about 80%.

Most experts suggest that condoms may reduce HIV infection risk by as much as 90%.[280] Model-based estimates concur, indicating that condoms decrease the per-contact probability of male-to-female transmission of HIV by about 95%.[281-282] Even occasional condom use, based on some statistical models, has been shown to be of significant value, with a roughly linear relationship between the proportion of sexual contacts in which a condom is used and the resultant reduction in the risk of infection. For example, using a condom half the time will result in about half the potential reduction obtained through consistent condom use. Such results suggest that harm reduction strategies need to be reconsidered to include the message that some condom use can be protective, for those who are unable to use condoms 100% of the time.[283] Most risk reduction counseling protocols currently recommend using condoms for all sexual acts, and do not take into consideration the protection provided by at least some condom use.

Female condoms can also be used for the prevention of HIV transmission. They can be inserted several hours before intercourse, and can be reused after proper care (disinfecting after use is commonly done for reuse if the package insert does not state that the device is single use).[284] A paucity of data exists on the effectiveness of female condoms against HIV transmission, and most studies have measured non-HIV STD prevention. Based on STD and pregnancy prevention studies, it is estimated that the female condom is 94–97% effective in HIV risk reduction when used correctly and consistently.[284] Finally, the female condom provides a method for a female-controlled prevention method, which is an urgent need given the increasing feminization of the global HIV/AIDS epidemic.

An expert committee of the World Health Organization reviewed the evidence in the role of condoms the control of HIV and other sexually transmitted diseases. They concluded, "Condom use is a critical element in a comprehensive, effective and sustainable approach to HIV prevention and treatment."[285]

Microbicides

Because more than 90% of global HIV transmission occurs via heterosexual sex, there remains an urgent need to expand interventions that can curtail the sexual transmission of HIV between males and females.[286] Due to power inequities between men and women in many cultures throughout the world, women at risk have little or no ability to negotiate the use of a male condom with their partner.[287] Though there has been a large focus on mitigating the risk of women, specifically adolescent women, another key risk group includes those participating in recipient anal sex (both men and women), primarily because of the delicate nature of the epithelial lining of the rectum and the consequent potential for HIV infection. To address these risks, efforts have been directed toward the development of intravaginal, intrarectal, and topical penile microbicides.[288]

Long before the HIV epidemic the first microbicidal product to be clinically evaluated in the 1970s contained nonoxynol-9 (N-9), a nonionic surfactant as the active ingredient.[286-289] Nonoxynol-9, in addition to being a condom lubricant and a spermicide, has been shown to be effective against a number of organisms, including herpes simplex virus (HSV), *Neisseria gonorrhea*, *Treponema pallidum*, *Trichonomonas vaginalis*, *Chlamydia trachomatis*, and other pathogens. Several trials of N-9 in women have been conducted over the last decade, with varying results; recent clinical studies, most notably the COL-1492 randomized trial, have shown significant negative results.[287] Trial results indicated that N-9 gel actually increased the risk of HIV infection in women using the gel more than 3–4 times per day, as compared to placebo.[132] Increased susceptibility to HIV infection was associated with a higher incidence of lesions with epithelial disruption, indicating that N-9 may have an adverse effect on the integrity of the mucosa.[132,289] As a consequence, N-9 is no longer considered to be a safe microbicide.

Over the last five years, increasing attention has been focused on the development of microbicides, many with novel mechanisms of action.[290-292] Currently 60 candidate agents have been shown to have in vitro activity against HIV, and 23 of them have advanced to clinical testing. Microbicides are now categorized according to their mode of action, including (1) anionic polymers, which are all viral entry inhibitors; (2) detergents; (3) vaginal fortifiers; and (4) viral replication inhibitors. Anionic polymers are thought to work by shielding the positive sites of the V3 loop of gp120, thus blocking the binding of HIV to CD4+ cells. These polymers are being evaluated as potential vaginal topical microbicides for prevention of the sexual transmission of HIV. Detergents belong to a category of surfactants, which includes N-9. Because of the epithelial disruption and inflammation seen in previous trials of N-9, detergent agents are not suitable for use intrarectally or intravaginally. However, their use in other forms, such as penile wipes, is currently being evaluated. Vaginal fortifiers work by increasing the number of hydrogen peroxide–producing lactobacilli in the vagina. The hypothesis that could explain their possible efficacy is that lactobacilli in the vagina secrete hydrogen peroxide that reduces the prevalence of bacterial vaginosis, a known risk factor for HIV. Viral replication inhibitors include both nucleoside reverse transcriptase (NRTI) and nonnucleoside reverse transcriptase (NNRTI) inhibitors, which function in the same manner as when they are used for HIV treatment. Finally, other agents under development include inhibitors of viral binding, fusion, entry, replication, and chemokines. Plant antiviral proteins and monoclonal antibodies are also being considered as potential microbicides.[293,294]

Microbicide development faces many challenges, and hence designing a safe, efficacious anti-HIV microbicide remains an elusive target. Microbicidal development has long been impeded by lack of funding from large pharmaceutical manufacturers, and has been left primarily to the government, privately funded organizations, and smaller biotechnology firms.[295-296] Fortunately, there is a commitment to funding the development of a microbicide by some major funding sources, including the Bill and Melinda Gates Foundation, the HIV Vaccine Trials Network (HVTN), the CDC Microbicide Working Group, and the Global Campaign for Microbicides. Other issues that have curtailed the development of microbicides include the lack of consensus on the important outcomes in clinical trials, a lack of agreement on the choice of comparison compounds or placebos for clinical trials (e.g., lower dose of the same agent, condoms only, or placebo), the lack of US FDA approval criteria, and the selection of study subjects for trials—specifically, the need for a balance between the protection of the rights of study subjects for appropriate counseling and condom promotion and validity and efficiency in testing potential candidate microbicides. Though these represent some key challenges, successful microbicide development will require an approach that combines the evaluation of microbicides coupled with harm reduction strategies in order to protect the participants from HIV. Web sites containing information about harm reduction and microbicides developed by WHO include a site related to IDUs (http://www.who.int/hiv/topics/harm/reduction/en/) and a site on microbicides (http://www.who.int/hiv/topics/microbicides/microbicides/en/).

Voluntary Counseling and Testing (VCT)

HIV voluntary counseling and testing (VCT) is an important component of most national AIDS prevention and control programs in developed and developing countries. VCT provides persons knowledge of their HIV infection status, risk assessment, and promotes risk reduction. It also serves as the gateway to HIV care for those who are infected. If effective, it may reduce the risk of further transmission of the virus by promoting safer sex and injection practices. Therefore, the availability of easily accessible, reliable, and user friendly VCT services are critical for successful AIDS prevention. One of the major obstacles to implementing a comprehensive HIV control program in many countries in sub-Saharan Africa has been the unavailability of reliable VCT services to many populations, particularly those in rural areas.[297] In the United States, the CDC has recently begun a major effort to promote HIV testing for persons at high risk in order to control the epidemic.[298] It has been estimated that almost 30% of HIV-infected persons in the United States are unaware of their infection. In some inner-city populations, the proportion of infected persons who are unaware of their infection is considerably higher.[299] In developing countries in sub-Saharan Africa, the vast majority of infected persons are unaware of their infection.

A fundamental research question remains: what is the effect of HIV counseling and testing on high-risk sexual behavior and, subsequently, on HIV incidence? Many studies have been done in diverse populations in order to evaluate the effect of VCT on behavior. A meta-analysis of 27 published studies, which included 19,597 participants, concluded that VCT was effective in increasing condom use, reducing the frequency of unprotected sex, and reducing the numbers of partners among persons who tested HIV positive. However, the effect of VCT on HIV-negative persons was not significantly different from untested controls (Figure 21-24).[300] A study of 5758 heterosexual, HIV-negative STD clinic patients enrolled from five STD clinics in the United States who were assigned to specific counseling (enhanced or brief) or to receive general didactic messages only in conjunction with counseling, found that 30% fewer participants in the counseling arms had STDs within 12 months than those who only received didactic information.[301] This large study suggested that even brief directed counseling of an STD clinic population had some effect in reducing high-risk behavior.

A large international trial was done to assess the efficacy of VCT among 3120 individuals and 586 couples enrolled in Kenya, Tanzania, and Trinidad. This study found a significantly greater reduction in those reporting unprotected intercourse with nonprimary partners among those randomized to receive counseling as well as testing (35–39%) compared with those only receiving health information (17–13%).[302] Behavior change was greatest among HIV positives and HIV-discordant couples. This study was not adequately powered to evaluate the effect of VCT on HIV transmission.

Because HAART has been shown to dramatically reduce the viral load in HIV-1-infected persons and transmission is directly related to viral load, an important question is whether, or to what extent, expanding widespread testing and provision of therapy would decrease the epidemic. It seems intuitive that treatment could, in some instances, reduce the risks of transmission. However, if a high proportion of transmission occurs in the early stages of infection, antiretroviral therapy would not affect transmission in these couples with current indications for initiating therapy.[78] A recent analysis of the stage of infection at the time that HIV transmission occurred among couples in the Rakai Uganda study indicates that half of all transmission occurred in the first few months after infection.[122] Also, if HIV-positives receiving treatment were less likely to practice safe sex, believing that the risk of transmission was low, the protective effect of treatment could be nullified. The effect of antiretroviral therapy of HIV positives on the course of the epidemic remains unknown, but future research on this question is critical.

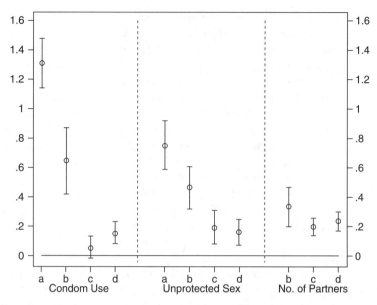

Note: a, HIV-serodiscordant couples; b, HIV-positive participants; c, HIV-negative participants; d, untested participants.

FIGURE 21-24   Weighted mean effect size (with 95% confidence interval) for HIV counseling and testing from 27 published studies, by type of risk behavior and participants' HIV serostatus group.
Source: Weinhardt LS et al. Effects of HIV counseling and testing on sexual risk behavior: A meta-analytic review of published research 1985–1997. Am J Public Health 1999;89:1397–1405.

Recently the US Preventive Services Task Force reviewed the evidence on HIV screening and concluded that there were clear benefits from HIV screening, especially among high-risk populations, but that data are insufficient to estimate the effects of screening on transmission rates.[240]

Preventing HIV Infection Through Behavior Intervention

In this chapter, we have presented the evidence for the effectiveness of prevention for selected topics, including the use of antiretroviral treatment incorporated with HIV prevention, the utility of HIV voluntary counseling and testing, the efficacy of condoms to prevent HIV acquisition and transmission, microbicides to protect women and men from sexual transmission of HIV, and the utility of antiretroviral treatment of pregnant HIV-infected women to prevent perinatal transmission. In this section, we review summary data on the effectiveness of behavioral interventions to prevent HIV infection. It is beyond the scope of this review to cover all aspects of prevention trials (such as educational strategies and communication approaches), and where feasible, references are made to published meta-analyses. In addition, the reader is directed to the CDC's HIV/AIDS Prevention Research Synthesis Project, which updates HIV prevention interventions with evidence of effectiveness.[303]

Individual Behavior Change for HIV Risk Reduction

Counseling strategies, using individual or small groups focusing on skills-building for condom use and communication strategies to improve condom negotiation, combined with STD recognition and care seeking have been shown to be effective in risk reduction for both men and women as well as in decreasing recurrent STDs.[301,304] Voluntary counseling and testing focused on individuals and primary and nonprimary partners has been shown to reduce risk in several developing country settings in a cost-effective program that is sustainable.[302,305] Recently, a multisite two-group randomized controlled trial tested the efficacy of an intervention consisting of 10 one-on-one counseling sessions among 4295 men who have sex with men in the United States. After adjustment for baseline covariates, the EXPLORE study intervention effect was estimated to produce a 5.7% reduced rate of HIV-1 acquisition, which held for 12–18 months, achieved primarily through a 20% reduction in the rate of unprotected receptive anal intercourse with HIV-infected partners or partners with unknown serostatus.[306] An early intervention among STD patients in Los Angeles randomized clients to one of three single session interventions: condom skills, social influence, and access to condoms. Although there was no impact on recurrent STDs, among men assigned to the condom skills group, rates of incident STI were half that of men in the control group.[307] A four-session counseling intervention among 393 STD patients in San Francisco found little influence of intensive counseling on recurrent STD rates or in self-reported unprotected sex at five months postintervention.[308] Recent summaries of the intervention literature focused on STI and HIV conclude that individual counseling strategies are effective, but depend largely upon the knowledge base of the counselor and the amount of time that is spent with clients.[309,310] Counseling approaches are more effective for HIV-infected individuals than those who are HIV-negative but of high risk, and for older than younger persons. Manhart and Holmes identified a total of 28 individual-level trials in a meta-analysis of the published literature that evaluated efficacy of trials to prevent STI and HIV, and virtually all addressed issues of acquisition of infection, including 4 on behavior change, 2 on antimicrobial prophylaxis, 7 addressed STI vaccines or passive immunization, and 10 assessed microbicides.[309]

Group Counseling Behavioral Interventions

Group interventions have been widely evaluated for their efficacy in promoting risk reduction and reducing acquisition of infection. An early report evaluated an intense, three small-group intervention with sessions lasting 3–4 hours with African-American and Hispanic women focused on susceptibility, skills development, and commitment to change, as compared to a control condition that received standard STD counseling.[311] Rates of reinfection with chlamydia and gonorrhea were significantly lower in the intervention group compared to the control over the 12 months of follow-up. Another RCT to reduce sexual risk behaviors, STD, and pregnancy among 522 sexually experienced African-American girls recruited from four community health agencies compared four 4-hour group sessions.[312] The intervention group focused on ethnic and gender pride, HIV knowledge, communication, condom-use skills, and health relationships, while the control group emphasized nutrition and exercise. There were trends in reductions of STDs over time, including a reduction in chlamydia infection. A large, multisite randomized controlled trial among adults in the USA, recruited from STD clinics and primary care settings, including large proportions of minorities, evaluated a seven session small group risk-reduction intervention on self-reported behavior and STD endpoints over a 12-month follow-up.[313] There were significant increases in condom use and significant decreases in self-reported STD symptoms, including incident gonorrhea among men. However, there were no differences in incident gonorrhea and *Chlamydia* documented using the ligase chain reaction.

Overall, intensive interventions appear promising if targeted toward specific population segments. Few biological endpoints appear to be affected by these interventions, and the cost-effectiveness of most programs has not been rigorously evaluated. The logistics of conducting these studies and the translation of research findings from specialized clinics into sustainable programs have been continuing issues confronting prevention researchers.

Community-Level Behavioral Interventions

Community-level interventions that were conducted over the past decade in the United States have established their effectiveness when rigorously conducted. Kelly has developed one type of community-level program that is based on the "popular opinion leader" approach, in which ethnographic methods are used to identify and recruit popular and influential members of a target group, and then systematically train them to become peer leaders, educating their friends and reinforcing risk-reduction messages.[314] This intervention is based on the diffusion of innovations theory and is predicated on the statement that behavior change can be initiated and diffused to others once a sufficient number of visible opinion leaders enact the behavior.[315] A series of interventions has shown that high-risk sexual behavior can be reduced (in the range of 30%) in MSM.[316,317] This approach has been replicated,[318] and it has been shown to work similarly with inner-city women,[319] male sex workers,[320] and young gay men.[321] Although some studies have failed to demonstrate effective behavior change based on this approach,[322,323] they generally suffer from severe methodological flaws or have misinterpreted the steps involved in conducting this type of community-level research.[313]

Other community-oriented prevention programs have found teacher training and peer education, workplace programs, and condom social marketing to be particularly successful.[324] These programs are also identified to be effective by the Institute of Medicine and the NIH Consensus Development Conference.[325,326] One example of a workplace intervention was a community randomized controlled trial conducted in the Royal Thai Army.[327] In this study, military camps and companies were randomized based on military mission to either an intense, peer-led HIV education intervention that continued for a 2-year period, or to a control condition, which offered HIV counseling and testing. At discharge, the cumulative STD infection rate in the intervention arm was 85% lower than that of the control condition (P < .001). Some community-based interventions using information, education, and communication (IEC) approaches, which are less intensive, have not proved to be beneficial for all population segments, although some positive results have been reported.[328]

Structural-Level Behavioral Interventions

Changes in national policy that directly affect HIV risk behavior are considered to be the most effective approaches for HIV prevention. For example, decriminalizing the possession of injecting equipment allows injection drug users to carry their own injection equipment and thereby avoid being forced to use others' needles when using drugs.[151,157] A widely regarded structural intervention has been alluded to earlier in this chapter, the "100 Percent Condom Campaign" in Thailand, which required the use of condoms in brothel-based sex work.[125,126] This policy led to nearly universal condom use in these settings and resulted in a dramatic decline in STD rates in female sex workers and their clients. An independent evaluation of the impact of this campaign on young men demonstrated a major decline in incident STDs after this policy was enacted.[126,329,330]

The other commonly cited successful structural intervention is the ABC program in Uganda (abstain and delay sexual initiation; be safer by being faithful or reducing number of sexual partners; and use condoms correctly and consistently). The campaign, which began in the late 1980s, with the full support of the president (again, signaling political will to confront an epidemic that was all but ignored by Uganda's neighbors), was considered effective; however, the essential components of the ABC program could not be precisely quantified.[331] As a result, during the past decade HIV prevalence in adults decreased from 15% to 5%, with partner reduction viewed by some to be of critical importance,[332] although there is some debate as to the veracity of the data used to make claims of program success.[333]

Behavioral Interventions Focused on Specific Risk Behaviors

Several behavioral interventions have targeted specific risk groups or high risk groups.

Drug Use

Injection drug use is a major factor in the HIV epidemic in the United States and in many parts of the developed and the developing world. Access to drug abuse treatment is one of the principal HIV prevention strategies that exists, yet all too often treatment services are lacking. Studies have clearly shown that drug abuse treatment is effective in reducing illicit drug use,[151,326,334] and methadone replacement therapy has been the most rigorously evaluated treatment modality.[148,335] Needle exchange programs have shown reductions in the frequency with which participants share injection equipment, they do not lead to increased drug use frequency, and do not encourage initiation of injection in community residents.[336,337] A recent meta-analysis of the effect of HIV preventive interventions on sexual risks of drug users in the United States concluded that in 33 rigorous studies that multiple-session, intensive interventions lead to sexual risk reductions among drug users.[338] Prospective follow-up of a large cohort of injection drug users in Baltimore (The ALIVE Study) has documented substantial reductions in HIV incidence between 1990 and 1998 accompanied by decreases in reported high-risk injection behavior.[339]

MSM

Men who have sex with men comprise a large proportion of new cases of HIV infection in many Western countries, and an increasing number internationally. The remarkable reduction in behavioral risk taking seen early in the HIV epidemic was replaced by an upsurge in STDs in the late 1990s.[340-341] A meta-analyses on nine behavioral interventions conducted and reported through June 1998 showed a 26% reduction in the proportion of men practicing unprotected anal intercourse.[342] A more recent review of 33 studies completed by July 2003 reported that interventions were associated with a 23% overall reduction in unprotected anal intercourse, a 15% reduction in number of sexual partners, and a 61% increase in the use of condoms during anal intercourse.[343] Successful interventions included behavioral skills training, used multiple channels to provide information, and were delivered in multiple sessions over at least a 3-week period.

HIV Prevention Needs for HIV-Infected Persons

The continued transmission of HIV is attributed to HIV-infected persons who are unaware of their infection status and to HIV-infected persons who know their HIV status. The CDC estimates that approximately 25% of the 900,000 persons living with HIV in the United States are not aware of their HIV status.[344,345] Interventions are essential to promote HIV testing to reduce behavioral risks (through pre- and posttest counseling), and to link HIV-infected persons to appropriate medical care and, where warranted, to pharmacotherapy. A recent meta-analysis compared high-risk sexual behaviors of male and female HIV-positive persons who were aware of their HIV status with persons who were infected but unaware of their status.[346] The results were that prevalence of high-risk sexual behavior was substantially reduced (45-75%) when HIV-infected people were aware of their serostatus, and the results were the same for both men and women. Thus, efforts to expand voluntary counseling and testing (VCT) must address issues of accessibility and acceptability.[298]

In 2000, Auerbach and Coates called for a greater focus on HIV prevention among infected individuals, as improvement in HIV/AIDS treatment was anticipated as well as expanded international availability of HAART medications.[346] A meeting organized by the National Institute of Mental Health (NIMH) and the CDC in 2003 outlined the state-of-the-science of behavioral interventions for HIV-infected persons in order to prioritize research needs. In a special issue of *JAIDS*, papers from that conference address interventions that demonstrate efficacy, including overviews of two large randomized trials and patient reports of risk reduction counseling in HIV primary care settings.[347] Future research priorities included maintenance of behavior change, where the longest follow-up period has been limited to 12 months, and a new focus on effectiveness studies, addressing issues of diffusion, translation, and operational research. Integration of effective interventions into health service settings remains a significant challenge.

Future HIV Prevention Needs—What Should Be Our Priorities?

The Committee on HIV Prevention Strategies at the Institute of Medicine noted in its landmark 2001 report that "the nation does not have a comprehensive, effective, and efficient strategy for preventing the spread of the human immunodeficiency virus."[325] They point out a lack of federal leadership in this effort, as well as the growing sense of complacency in government and the public, as well as in some segments of the HIV-infected population and high-risk persons. The integration of HIV prevention at the primary (to prevent HIV acquisition) and secondary (to prevent HIV transmission) levels with HIV voluntary counseling and testing and HIV treatment is essential, although the critical personnel needed to implement each approach may not always be skilled at carrying out effective prevention activities. The complexity of this approach at a national level was presented in detail by Wasserheit et al, who carefully reviewed the multiple components of HIV prevention programs at multiple levels, using a clearly articulated conceptual framework.[348] A review of this work suggests why there are so few documented evaluations of comprehensive prevention programs. When extrapolated from a single nation to the global level, the task becomes even more daunting and requires multisectoral responses that are exceptionally difficult to coordinate. Setting priorities in resource-constrained contexts, balancing care and prevention, is the true challenge of this decade.

Auerbach and Coates suggest three overarching challenges in HIV prevention: scientific challenges, political and cultural challenges, and ethical considerations.[346] The major scientific challenges for the coming decade include methodological issues. Because HIV risk behaviors cannot be directly measured, there is considerable measurement error, which is a function of bias, memory, embarrassment, and perhaps concerns about stigma and discrimination. Coming to consensus on what to measure and how to measure it would propel the field forward. Many prevention programs have been evaluated in limited groups and have not been taken to scale or replicated in other settings. Research translation to the field setting has not been commonly reported, and reports on sustainability of pilot prevention projects that have been integrated into existing public structures are needed.

Political will seems to be as important for HIV prevention as the evidence base from scientifically valid studies.[349] This is particularly true for prevention science, where we must overcome obstacles related to decision makers providing limited resources for prevention versus care, for complacency or distrust of specific risk populations (injection drug users, commercial sex workers [CSW], gay men), and for legal structures that prohibit prevention programs shown to be effective (e.g., needle exchange bans).

Finally, ethical considerations dictate that prevention must incorporate the local community concerns within prevention programs. Demonstration programs that fail to integrate community concerns are certainly on the road to failure. Community advisory boards provide one linkage between the research and program proponents and the community. The ethical concerns in HIV prevention have been widely discussed, although by no means should we consider this resolved; rather, it is an ongoing issue that will undoubtedly be influenced by future social, political, and economic events.

The Search for an HIV/AIDS Vaccine

Soon after the virus was identified it was predicted by the Secretary of the Department of Health and Human Services that it would be possible to develop an effective HIV vaccine within 2 years. However, 20 years after the discovery of HIV the development of an effective vaccine is currently not imminent. Two phase III efficacy trials of an envelope-derived gp120 vaccine have been completed among injection drug users in Thailand and persons at high risk of sexual transmission in the United States.[350-352] This vaccine failed to prevent, delay, or modify HIV infection in both of these trials.[351-354]

These discouraging trial results were accompanied by laboratory evidence indicating that the levels of neutralizing antibodies stimulated by existing vaccines are only low to moderate and that neutralization of primary isolates from infected patients, compared to laboratory-derived viruses, was very poor.[351] Studies of the time course of the decrease in HIV viral RNA after primary infection suggested that the decrease in viral RNA to a set point level correlated better with the appearance of cellular immune responses (i.e., CD8 CTL activity and CD4 responses) than antibodies.[355] Also studies of "long-term nonprogressors" found that many such persons had cellular immune responses involving CD4+ and CD8+ recognition of multiple HIV epitopes; these CTL responses were more often robust in nonprogressors than in persons with progressing infection.[356-358] Many persons who have been exposed repeatedly to HIV but remained uninfected had cytotoxic T-cell recognition of various HIV peptide epitopes, although they remained negative for HIV antibodies and viral RNA.[359] These data suggest that cellular immunity involving CD8+ cytotoxic lymphocytes and CD4+ memory lymphocytes directed at critical HIV proteins might be capable of either preventing an HIV infection or converting an HIV infection from one that progressed to immune deficiency to one that was chronic but stable.

Because of these considerations, the HIV vaccine development effort has shifted to producing vaccines capable of stimulating a cytotoxic T-lymphocyte (CTL) response to HIV proteins, along with a CD4-T-lymphocyte memory response. However, one expert believes that technological advances might possibly lead to a more effective vaccine that could produce "sterilizing immunity" based on high levels of neutralizing antibodies.[360] In mid-2005, there was only one large phase III efficacy trial of a preventive HIV vaccine under way in Thailand among 16,000 volunteers testing the efficacy of a combination of two separate vaccines. This vaccine trial involves immunizing with *ALVA6 vCP1521,* which is a poxvirus-vectored vaccine containing the genes of subtype E env and gag/pol genes of subtype B (designed to stimulate a CTL response), followed by AIDS/VAX, a vaccine containing subtype B and E gp120 envelope proteins, designed to stimulate neutralizing antibodies to the HIV envelope.[361]

In addition to this phase III trial, 15 new phase I and II trials of AIDS vaccine candidates in seven different countries began in 2004 and were designed to evaluate safety and immunogenicity of vaccine candidates.[361] For further information on ongoing HIV vaccine trials, the interested reader should consult the *International AIDS Vaccine Initiative* newsletter at www .iavireport.org and/or the National Institutes of Health Web site at www .niaid.nih.gov.

Addressing the AIDS Pandemic

As described earlier in this chapter, the HIV/AIDS pandemic represents an unprecedented crisis treating human health. Virtually every country in the world has been affected to some extent by the AIDS epidemic. However, many countries in sub-Saharan Africa have been devastated, with life expectancy of their populations declining by 20 years or more and substantial proportions of young adults dead or seriously ill from the disease.[14] The AIDS epidemic has destabilized societies as it has spread.

In recognition of the societal impact of the AIDS pandemic, a United Nations General Assembly Special Session (UNGASS) on HIV/AIDS was held on June 25–27, 2001, the first special session of the UN General Assembly devoted to coping with the effects of a single disease. At this session, governments from 189 countries committed themselves to a comprehensive program of international and national action to fight the HIV/AIDS pandemic by adopting the Declaration of Commitment on HIV/AIDS. The declaration also included a pledge on the part of the United Nations General Assembly that it would devote itself at least one full day annually to reviewing the progress achieved in realizing the goals of the commitment. To facilitate this review, the joint United Nations Programme on HIV/AIDS (UNAIDS) and its partners have developed a set of core indicators for monitoring the progress of the various international and national organizations in meeting the goals. These core indicators can be found at www.unaids.org.

Numerous serious barriers exist to implement the commitment to reverse the effects of the AIDS pandemic in resource-limited countries in sub-Saharan Africa and other regions of the world. Effective antiretroviral drug combinations are very expensive, associated with some toxicity, difficult to take, and require a high degree of adherence to be effective. Even more important, the absence of an adequate public health and medical infrastructure for diagnosing and treating HIV infections, monitoring the response, and the stigmatization of persons who are HIV infected in many developing countries are serious barriers to the development of an effective global AIDS control program.

Despite these obstacles, the United Nations followed the UNGASS meeting with the establishment of a Global Fund to Control HIV, Tuberculosis, and Malaria, the three major lethal epidemic infectious diseases affecting less-developed countries. Contributions were solicited from developed industrialized countries to support the global fund. Developing countries could develop a disease control plan directed at one or more of these diseases and submit a request for funding to the United Nations Global Fund. By the end of 2003 the global fund had approved 227 grants totaling US$2.1 billion to 124 countries and had already disbursed US$232 million; about 60% of these grants were for AIDS prevention.

In 2001, scientists at UNAIDS, WHO, and other organizations calculated that, under optimal conditions, 3 million people living in developing countries with HIV infection could be provided with antiretroviral therapy and access to medical services by the end of 2005. Despite these estimates, treatment enrollment among persons in developing countries continued to lag. In 2003, only an estimated 400,000 (7%) of the 5,900,000 believed to need antiretroviral therapy in developing countries were receiving treatment.[362-363] On September 22, 2003, the "Treat 3 Million Persons by 2005" ("3 by 5") initiative was announced by Dr. Lee Jung-Wok, Director General of WHO.[362] This important initiative helped energize the urgent effort to deal with the AIDS crisis in sub-Saharan Africa and other developing, resource-limited countries with major AIDS epidemics. The challenge was put forward to meet a specific goal—treat 3 million persons within 2 years.

Implementation of the 3 by 5 Program

When the "3 by 5" program was announced by the WHO in 2003, major hurdles existed to its implementation, including the expense and difficulties of using HAART, inadequate public health and medical infrastructure, widespread stigmatization of AIDS, and uncertain and uneven political commitment. Although most developed market economy countries supported the 3 by 5 program philosophically, their level of financial support for the program was uncertain.

To begin implementation of the 3 by 5 program WHO developed a series of guidelines at a meeting in Lusaka, Zambia, in November 2003 as follows[362]:

1. Strengthen and expand prevention, care, treatment support, and other services provided directly by communities.
2. Promote and protect the human rights of people living with HIV/AIDS and everyone affected by HIV, especially poor and vulnerable populations, including sex workers, injection drug users, men who have sex with men, displaced persons, and migrant workers. This must be done in an environment in which people living with HIV/AIDS are encouraged and supported to volunteer, learn, and disclose their HIV status.
3. Assure quality of care by involving communities in monitoring and evaluating antiretroviral services.
4. HIV testing and counseling should be available in health facilities at all levels.
5. Simple rapid finger-prick tests should be the test of choice to scale up testing and counseling services.
6. Strengthen existing HIV prevention services while antiretroviral therapy is being introduced.
7. Ensure that people living with HIV/AIDS receive key HIV prevention services and commodities.

WHO recommended initial therapy with a simplified first-line drug combination of stavudine, lamivudine, and nevirapine in a fixed-dose combination.

This multidrug tablet has been produced, along with various second-line combinations, by several private and government pharmaceutical firms in India, Thailand, China, and Brazil at a cost of about $300–500 per patient per year.

As of June 2005, about 1 million persons in resource-limited countries were receiving combination antiretroviral therapy.[363] UNAIDS/WHO recommends that therapy should be started in persons with WHO stage III or IV (symptomatic) HIV disease or in those with a CD4+ cell count less than 200 cells/μL. When CD4+ cell counting is unavailable, a total lymphocyte count less than 1200 was recommended to be used as a surrogate.

PEPFAR Program

A major boost to the global effort to control the AIDS pandemic came in January 2003 when President Bush announced in his State of the Union Message the intention of the United States to initiate the President's Emergency Plan for AIDS Relief (PEPFAR), with funding of $15 billion over the next 5 years. The initial funds were provided by the US Congress in 2003. The Emergency Plan reached 155,000 people with antiretroviral treatment in the first 8 months of its operation.[364] In addition, 1.2 million women were provided services to prevent mother-to-child transmission of HIV, and more than 1.7 million persons received some health care through the PEPFAR program.

The PEPFAR program is targeted to 15 countries in Africa, the Caribbean, and Vietnam. It provides both treatment and preventive services and supports the care of children orphaned by AIDS.[364] In contrast to the UN Global Fund and the 3 by 5 program, the antiretroviral drugs used in the PEPFAR program have to be licensed by the US FDA. In response to this requirement, the FDA created a mechanism for the rapid review and licensure of antiretroviral drug combinations allowing the use of cheaper, simpler-to-use, generic drug combinations in countries included in PEPFAR programs.

The prevention activities in PEPFAR were modeled after the ABC program that successfully reduced the HIV incidence in Uganda. This program includes a focus on abstinence (A), being faithful (B), and current and consistent use of condoms (C), as appropriate. Prevention activities for sex workers have been hampered in the PEPFAR program by the requirement to "not support prostitution," which has been interpreted differently in various settings. Also, among injection drug using populations, the program focused on efforts to reduce drug use and needle sharing and substitution or replacement therapy. However, full harm reduction programs, including needle/syringe exchange, were not supported initially under PEPFAR. Recently, this restriction has been somewhat relaxed. Specific targets were set for the PEPFAR program, including the provision of antiretroviral therapy for 200,000 HIV-infected persons by June 2005 and 2 million persons by 2008. However, the political and philosophical restrictions on developing effective prevention programs with marginalized populations, such as sex workers and IDUs, have compromised the effectiveness of these programs.

In addition to the United Nation program and PEPFAR, a number of bilateral collaborations between developed and developing countries in sub-Saharan Africa have been established. The United States, through USAID and the Centers for Disease Control and Prevention, has established the Global AIDS Program (GAP). This program has provided technical consultation and resources to many countries in Africa, Asia, and the Caribbean for the prevention and control of the HIV/AIDS epidemic.

The Bill and Melinda Gates Foundation, in collaboration with CDC, the Harvard AIDS Institute, and the Merck Research Foundation, has developed an HIV/AIDS prevention and treatment program in Botswana, the country with the highest proportion of adults who are HIV positive. To improve the capacity of sub-Saharan African countries to begin to deal with the AIDS pandemic, there is a critical need to greatly improve their medical and public health capability. To begin this effort a group of academic infectious disease specialists affiliated with the Infectious Diseases Society of America, with seed funding from Pfizer Pharmaceutical, have established a training program for clinicians at the Mulago Hospital of Makrere University in Kampala, Uganda, to train health care workers in Africa in the care of patients with HIV/AIDS.[365]

Estimating the Cost of the WHO/UNAIDS Prevention and Treatment Program for Developing, Resource-Limited Countries

Estimating HIV Incidence and Prevalence

The first step in estimating the costs of an HIV/AIDS prevention and treatment program involves estimating the prevalence and incidence of HIV. Next, a set of assumptions about the survival time after HIV infection, the sex ratio, and prevalence curves is used to derive estimates of HIV incidence and AIDS mortality for adults and children. The HIV prevalence data come from the national AIDS program along with ad hoc selective, sentinel surveillance and other data such as prevalence among pregnant women and blood donors, which tend to be readily available in most developing countries.[366]

AIDS epidemics are classified by UNAIDS as:

1. *Generalized* when the HIV prevalence among the general population (i.e., pregnant women) is above 1%
2. *Concentrated* when the prevalence in pregnant women is below 1%, but the prevalence is above 5% in populations at higher risk (e.g., IDUs, CSWs, MSM, or STD patients)
3. *Nascent* in countries with some HIV infections but with prevalence below 5% in high-risk populations

Although most countries have some information about HIV prevalence, a major determinant of the quality of estimates of the number of HIV positive persons is the availability of reliable data.

Estimating the Costs of Prevention and Treatment

Following the UNGASS statement of commitment to launch a program to deal with the global AIDS pandemic, an estimate was made of the costs to institute a program of prevention and HIV/AIDS care in low- and middle-income countries (those with per capita incomes less than $10,000/year).[367] Estimates were made of the finances needed for both preventive interventions and HIV/AIDS care and support. Overall, it was estimated that by 2005 US$9.2 billion would be needed to support an expanded response to HIV/AIDS in 135 low- and middle-income countries. Of this total, US$4.8 billion would be needed for prevention interventions and US$4.4 billion for care and support of HIV-positive persons. Half of the total resources are needed for countries in sub-Saharan Africa (Table 21-12). The majority of the resources in Africa are needed for care and support. This proportion is much lower for Asia (32%) and other regions (Figure 21-25).

An estimate of the need for health care (excluding prevention needs) from 2001 to 2007 for low- and middle-income countries was recently published.[368] This estimate indicated that the need will increase from US$4.4 billion to at least US$7.5 billion by 2007, as the epidemic continues to grow and the numbers of HIV-positive persons needing care and services continue to accumulate (Figure 21-26).

These sobering estimates emphasize the magnitude of the need. Also, they indicate that the efforts to date, while an important beginning, have not nearly been sufficient to stem the rising tide of this pandemic. It is clear that a broad and sustained effort will be needed by governments worldwide if the AIDS pandemic is to be contained. However, it has been

TABLE 21-12   Projected Annual Expenditures by 2005 (in US$ millions)

PROJECTED ANNUAL EXPENDITURES BY 2005		
Region	**Prevention**	**Care and Support**
Sub-Saharan Africa	1560	3070
South and Southeast Asia	1440	670
East Asia, Pacific	810	80
Latin America, Caribbean	590	550
Eastern Europe, Central Asia	250	20
North Africa, Middle East	160	50
Total	**4810**	**4440**

Source: Schwartländer, B. AIDS. Resource needs for HIV/AIDS. Science. 2001 Jun 29;292(5526):2434–2436. Copyright 2001 AAAS.

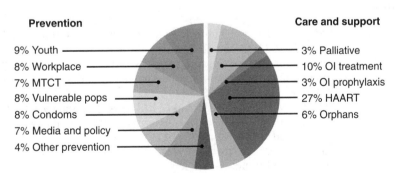

FIGURE 21-25   Distribution of estimated resource need for prevention, care, and support for 2005 (total US$9.2 billion) by type of intervention.
Source: Schwartländer, B. AIDS. Resource needs for HIV/AIDS. Science. 2001 Jun 29;292(5526):2434–2436. Copyright 2001 AAAS.

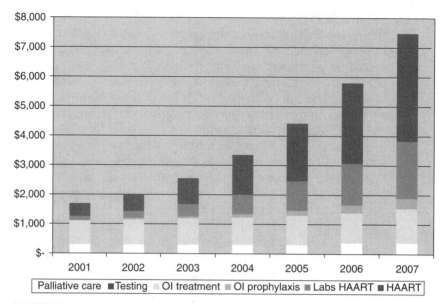

FIGURE 21-26 Estimated needs for HIV/AIDS-related health care by type of care, 2001–2007.
Source: Bertozzi SM et al. Estimating resource needs for HIV/AIDS health care services in low-income and middle-income countries. Health Policy. 2004 Aug;69(2):189–200.

estimated that if the successful control efforts already accomplished in a few resource-limited countries (Thailand, Uganda, Senegal, and Brazil) were applied globally, over 26 million AIDS deaths could be averted. Furthermore a cost-benefit analysis has found that preventive interventions, such as condom promotion and treatment of STDs and tuberculosis are highly cost-effective in the African setting, and that antiretroviral therapy is feasible in terms of disability-adjusted life-years saved (DALYs). Clearly, a broader, more effective global AIDS control program will be worth the effort.

References

1. Centers for Disease Control. Pneumocystic pneumonia: Los Angeles. *MMWR*. 1981;30:250–252.
2. Centers for Disease Control. Kaposi's sarcoma and pneumocystic pneumonia among homosexual men. New York City and California. *MMWR*. 1981;30:305–308.
3. Gottlieb M, Schroff R, Schanker HM, et al. Pneumocystic pneumonia and mucosal candidiasis in previously healthy homosexual men. *N Engl J Med*. 1981;305:1425–1431.
4. Auerbach DM, Darrow WM, Jaffe HW, Curran JW. Cluster of cases of the acquired immune deficiency syndrome: patients linked by sexual contact. *Am J Med*. 1984;76:487–492.
5. Selik RM, Haverkos HH, Curran JW. Acquired immune deficiency syndrome (AIDS) trends in the United States, 1978–1982. *Am J Med*. 1984;76:493–500.

6. Chamberland MO, Lastrok G, Haverkos HH, et al. Acquired immunodeficiency in the United States: an analysis of cases outside high-incidence groups. *Ann Inter Med.* 1984;101:617–623.

7. Gallo RL, Salahuddin SZ, Popovic M, et al. Frequent detection and isolation of cytopathic retroviruses (HTLV-III) from patients with AIDS and at risk for AIDS. *Science.* 1984;224:497–500.

8. Klatzmawn D, Barre-Sinousi F, Nugeyre MT, et al. Selective tropism of lymphadenopathy associated virus (LAV) for helper-inducer T lymphocytes. *Science.* 1984;225:59–63.

9. Nahmias AJ, Weiss J, Yao X, et al. Evidence for human infection with an HTLVII/LAV-like virus in Central Africa, 1959. *Lancet.* 1986; 1:1297.

10. Gau F, Bailes E, Robertsen DL, et al. Origin of HIV-1 in the chimpanzee, *Pan troglodytes. Nature.* 1999;397:436–437.

11. Hirsch VM, Olnsted RA, Murphey-Corb M, Purcell RH, Johnson PR. An African primate lentivirus (SIVson) closely related to HIV-2. *Nature.* 1989;339:389–392.

12. Marlink R, Kanki P, Thior I, et al. Reduced rate of disease development after HIV-2 infection as compared to HIV-1. *Science* 1994;265: 1587–1590.

13. DeKock KM, Adjorlolo G, Ekpini E, et al. Epidemiology and transmission of HIV-2: why there is no HIV-2 pandemic. *JAMA.* 1993;270:2083–2086.

14. UNAIDS/WHO. AIDS epidemic update, December, 2005. UNAIDS/WHO; Genevor, Switzerland.

15. Siliciano JD, Kajdas J, Finzi D, et al. Long-term latent reservoir for HIV-1 in resting CD4+ T cells. *Nat Med.* 2003;9:727–728.

16. Perelson AS, Neumann AU, Markowitz M, Leonard JM, Ho DD. HIV-1 dynamics in vivo: virion clearance rate, infected cell life span and viral generation time. *Science.* 1996;271:1582–1586.

17. Perelson AS, Essunger P, Lao YZ, et al. Decay characteristics of HIV-1 compartments during combination therapy. *Nature.* 1997;387: 188–191.

18. Lyles R, Munoz A, Yamashita TE, et al. Natural history of human immunodeficiency virus type-1 viremia after seroconversion and proximal to AIDS in a large cohort of homosexual men, in the Multicenter AIDS Cohort Study. *J Infect Dis.* 2000;18:872–880.

19. Mellors JW, Munoz A, Giorgi JV, et al. Plasma viral load and CD4+ lymphocytes as prognostic markers of HIV-1 infection. *Ann Intern Med.* 1997;126:946–954.

20. Margolick JB, Munoz A, Donnenberg AD, et al. Failure of T-cell homeostasis preceding AIDS in HIV-1 infection. The Multicenter AIDS Cohort Study. *Nat Med.* 1995;1:674–680.

21. Tersmette M, Lange JME, De Goede REY, et al. Differences in risk for AIDS and AIDS mortality associated with biological properties of HIV variants. *Lancet.* 1989;1:983–985.

22. Kassatto S, Rosenberg ER. Primary HIV type 1 infection. *Clin Infect Dis.* 2004;38:1447–1453.

23. Schacker T, Collier AC, Hughes J, Shea T, Corey C. Clinical and epidemiologic features of primary HIV infection. *Ann Intern Med.* 1996;125:257–264.

24. Niu MT, Stein DS, Schnittman SM. Primary HIV type-1 infection: review of pathogenesis and early treatment interventions in humans and animal retrovirus infections. *J Infect Dis.* 1994;168:1490–1501.

25. CASCADE study. Time from HIV seroconversion to AIDS and death before widespread use of highly-active antiretroviral therapy: a collaborative re-analysis. *Lancet.* 2000;355:1131–1137.
26. Rangsin R, Chio J, Khamboonruang C, et al.The natural history of HIV-1 infection in young Thai men after seroconversion. *JAIDS.* 2004;36:622–629.
27. Chariyalerksak S, Sirisanthana T, Saengwonloey O, Nelson KE. Clinical presentation and risk behaviors of AIDS patients in Thailand, 1994–1998: regional variation and temporal trends. *Clin Infect Dis.* 2001;32:955–962.
28. Allen S, Batongwanayo J, Kerlikowski K, et al. Two year incidence of tuberculosis in cohorts of HIV-infected and uninfected Rwandan women. *Am Rev Respir Dis.* 1992;146:1439–1444.
29. Supparatpinyo K, Uthammachai C, Baosong V, Nelson KE, Sirisanthana T. Disseminated *Penicillium marneffei*: an emerging HIV-associated opportunistic infection in SE Asia. *Lancet.* 1994;344:110–113.
30. Ablashi D, Chatlynne L, Cooper H, et al. Seroprevalence of human herpes virus 8 in countries of Southeast Asia, compared to the USA, Carribean and Africa. *Br J Cancer.* 1999;81:893–897.
31. Wheat CJ, Connolly-Stringfield PA, Baker RL. Disseminated histoplasmosis in the acquired immunodeficiency syndrome: clinical findings diagnosis and treatment and review of the literature. *Medicine.* 1990;60:361–375.
32. Alvar J, Canavete C, Gutierrez-Sohr E, et al. Leishmania and human immunodeficiency virus, co-infection: the first 10 years. *Clin Microbiol Rev.* 1997;10:298–319.
33. Centers for Disease Control. Recommendations for the prophylaxis of opportunistic infection in patients with HIV infection. *MMWR.* 2002;51:RR-6.
34. Chariyalerksak S, Supparatpinyo K, Sirisanthana T, Nelson KE. A controlled trial of itraconazole as primary prophylaxis for systemic fungus infections in patients with HIV infection in Thailand. *Clin Infect Dis.* 2002;34:227–234.
35. Rowland-Jones SL, Doug T, Fowke KR, et al. Cytotoxic T cell responses to multiple conserved HIV epitopes in HIV-resistant prostitutes in Nairobi. *J Clin Invest.* 1998;102:1758–1765.
36. Promedej N, Costello C, Wernett MM, et al. Broad human immunodeficiency virus-specific T cell responses to conserved HIV proteins in HIV-seronegative women highly exposed to a single HIV-infected partner. *J Infect Dis.* 2003;187:1053–1063.
37. Dean M, Carrington M, Winkler C, et al. Genetic restriction of HIV-1 infection and progression to AIDS by a deletion allele of the CKR5 structural gene. *Science.* 1996;273:1856–1862.
38. Huang Y, Paxton WA, Wolinsky SM, et al. The role of a mutant CCR5 allele in HIV-1 transmission and disease progression. *Nature Med.* 1996;2:1240–1243.
39. Smith MW, Dean M, Carrington M, et al. Contrasting genetic influence of CCR2 and CCR5 variants in HIV-2 infection and disease progression. *Science.* 1997;277:959–965.
40. Winkler C, Medi W, Smith MW, et al. Genetic restriction of AIDS pathogenesis by an SDF-1 chemokine gene variant. *Science.* 1998;279:389–393.
41. Gonzalex E, Kulkarni H, Boivar H, et al. The influence of CCL3L1 gene-containing segmental duplications on HIV-1/AIDS susceptibility. *Science.* 2005;307:1434–1440.

42. Kaslow RA, Dorak T, Tang J. Influence of host genetic variation on susceptibility to HIV type 1 infection. *J Infect Dis.* 2005;191 (suppl 1):S68-S77.

43. MacDonald KS, Embree J, Njenga S, et al. Mother-child class 1 HLA concordance increases perinatal human immunodeficiency type-1 transmission. *J Infect Dis.* 2000;182:123-132.

44. Dorak MT, Tang J, Penman-Aguilar A, et al. Transmission of HIV-1 and HLA-B allele sharing within serodiscordant heterosexual Zambian couples. *Lancet.* 2004;363:2132-2139.

45. Hader SL, Hodge TW, Buchacz KA, et al. Discordance at human leukocyte antigen-DR-B3 and protection from human immunodeficiency virus type 1 transmission. *J Infect Dis.* 2002;185: 1729-1735.

46. Silverberg MJ, Smith MW, Chimiel JS, et al. Fraction of cases of acquired immunodeficiency syndrome prevented by interactions of identified restriction gene variants. *Am J Epidemiol.* 2004;159: 239-241.

47. Stremlau M, Owens CM, Perron MJ, Klessling M, Autissler P, Sodroski J. The cytoplasmic body component TRIM 5a restricts HIV-1 infection in old world monkeys. *Nature.* 2004;427:848-857.

48. Sheehy AM, Gaddis NC, Choi JD, Malim MH. Isolation of a human gene that inhibits HIV-1 infection and is suppressed by the viral Vif protein. *Nature.* 2002;418:646-650.

49. Harris RS, Liddament MT. Retroviral restriction by APOBEC proteins. *Nature Reviews/Immunology* 2004; 4:868-876.

50. An P, Blieber G, Duggal P, et al. APOBEC3G genetic variants and their influence on the progression to AIDS. *J Virol.* 2004;78: 11070-11076.

51. McCutchan FE. Understanding the genetic diversity of HIV-1. *AIDS.* 2000;14(suppl 3):S31-S44.

52. Soto-Ramirez LE, Renjifo B, McLane MC, et al. HIV-1 Langerhan's cell tropism associated with heterosexual transmission of HIV. *Science.* 1996;271:1291-1293.

53. Pope M, Frankel SS, Masgola JR, et al. Human immunodeficiency virus type 1 strains of subtypes B and E replicate in cutaneous dendritic cell T cell mixtures without displaying subtype-specific tropism. *J Virol.* 1997;71:8001-8007.

54. Kunanasont C, Foy HM, Kreiss JK, et al. HIV-1 subtypes and male to female transmission in Thailand. *Lancet.* 1995;345:1078-1083.

55. Limpakarnjanarat K, Ungchusak K, Mastro TD, et al. The epidemiological evaluation of HIV-1 subtypes B and E and heterosexuals and injection drug users in Thailand, 1992-1997. *AIDS.* 1998;12:1108-1109.

56. Hu DJ, Vanichseni S, Mastro TD, et al. Viral load differences in early infection with two HIV-1 subtypes. *AIDS.* 2001;15:683-691.

57. Amornkul PN, Tansuphaswadikul S, Limpakarnjanarat K, et al. Clinical disease associated with HIV-1 subtype B and E infection among 2104 patients in Thailand. *AIDS.* 1999;13:1963-1969.

58. Neilson JR, John GL, Carr JK, et al. Subtypes of human immunodeficiency virus type 1 and disease stage among women in Nairobi, Kenya. *J Virol.* 1999;73:4393-4403.

59. Kaleebu PFN, Mahe C, Yirrell D, et al. The role of HIV-envelope subtypes A and D on disease progression in a large cohort of HIV-1 positive individuals in Uganda. 13th International Conference on AIDS, Durban, S. Africa, July 2000 (abstract A 3079).

60. Aleus A, Lidman K, Bjorkmon A, Gieseke J, Albert J. Similar rate of disease progression among individuals infected with HIV-1 genetic subtypes A–D. *AIDS*. 1999;13:901–907.
61. Kanki PJ, Hamel DJ, Sankale JL, et al. Human immunodeficiency virus type 1 subtypes differ in disease progression. *J Infect Dis*. 1999;179: 68–73.
62. Bobkov A, Kazenna E, Selimova L, et al. A sudden epidemic of HIV type 1 among injecting drug users in the former Soviet Union: identification of subtype A, subtype B and novel gag A/env B recombinants AIDS. *Res Hum Retroviruses*. 1998;14:669–676.
63. Beyrer C, Razak HH, Lisam K, Chen J, Lui W, Yu XF. Overland heroin trafficking routes and HIV-1 spreading in south and south-east Asia. *AIDS*. 2000;14:75–83.
64. Graziosi C, Soudeyns H, Rizzardi GP, Bart P-A, Chapuis A, Pantaleo G. Immunopathogenesis of HIV infection. *AIDS Res Hum Retroviruses*. 1998;14:S135–S142.
65. Bentwich Z, Maartens G, Torten D, Altaf AL, Lal RB. Concurrent infections and HIV pathogenesis. *AIDS*. 2000;14:2071–2081.
66. Lawn SD. AIDS in Africa: the impact of coinfections on the pathogenesis of HIV-1 infection. *J Infection*. 2004;48:1–12.
67. Bentwich Z, Kalinkovich A, Weisman Z, Borkow G, Beyers N, Beyers AD. Can eradication of helminthic infections change the face of AIDS and tuberculosis? *Immunol Today*. 1999;20:485–487.
68. Wasserheit JN. Epidemiological synergy: interrelationships between human immunodeficiency virus infection and other sexually transmitted diseases. *Sex Trans Dis*. 1992;19:61–77.
69. Rompalo AM, Shepherd M, Lawlor JP, et al. Definitions of genital ulcer disease and variation in risk for prevalent human immunodeficiency virus infection. *Sex Trans Dis*. 1997;24:426–442.
70. Nelson KE, Celentano DD, Eiumtrakul S, et al. The association of herpes simplex-type 2, *Haemophilus ducreyi* and syphilis infections with genital ulcer disease and HIV infection among young men in northern Thailand. *JAIDS*. 1997;16:293–300.
71. Dyer JR, Eron JJ, Hoffman IF, et al. Association of CD4 cell depletion and elevated blood and seminal plasma human immunodeficiency virus type 1 (HIV-1) RNA concentrations with genital ulcer disease in HIV-1 infected men in Malawi. *J Infect Dis*. 1998;177:224–227.
72. Reynolds SJ, Risbud AP, Shepherd ME, et al. Recent herpes simplex virus type 2 infection and the risk of human immunodeficiency virus type 1 acquisition in India. *J Infect Dis*. 2003;187:1513–1521.
73. Serwadda D, Gray RH, Sewankambo N, et al. Human immunodeficiency virus acquisition associated with genital ulcer disease and herpes simplex virus type 2 infection: a nested case-control study in Raki, Uganda. *J Infect Dis*. 2003;188:1492–1497.
74. Nelson KE, Suriyanon V, Rongruangthankit K, et al. High rate of transmission of subtype E human immunodeficiency virus type 1 among heterosexual couples in northern Thailand: role of sexually transmitted diseases and immune compromise. *J Infect Dis*. 1999;180:337–343.
75. Laga M, Manoka A, Kivuvu M, et al. Non-ulcerative sexually transmitted diseases as risk factors for HIV-1 transmission in women: results from a cohort study. *AIDS*. 1993;7:95–102.
76. Royce RA, Sena A, Cates W, Cohen MS. Sexual transmission of HIV. *N Engl J Med*. 1997;336:1072–1078.

77. Theus SA, Harrich DA, Gaynor R, Radolf JD, Norgard MV. *Treponema pallidum*, lipoproteins, and synthetic lipoprotein analogues induce human immunodeficiency virus type 1 gene expression in monocytes via NF-κ B activation. *J Infect Dis.* 1998;177:941–950. Available at: http://www.who.int/hiv/pub/prev_care/en/WHO%20Malaria%20and%20AIDS.pdf. Accessed July 3, 2005.

78. Pilcher CD, Tien HC, Eron JL, et al. Brief but efficient: acute HIV infection and the sexual transmission of HIV. *J Infect Dis.* 2004;189:1785–1792.

79. Cohen MS, Hoffman IF, Royce RA, et al. Reduction of concentration of HIV-1 in semen after treatment of urethritis: implications for prevention of sexual transmission of HIV-1. *Lancet.* 1997;349: 1868–1873.

80. Quinn TC, Wawer MJ, Sewankambo N, et al. Viral load and heterosexual transmission of human immunodeficiency virus type 1. *N Engl J Med.* 2000;342:921–929.

81. Tovanabutra S, Robison V, Wongtrakul J, Kawichai S, Duerr A, Nelson KE. Male viral load and heterosexual transmission of HIV-1 subtype E in northern Thailand. *JAIDS.* 2002;29:275–287.

82. Gray RH, Wawer MI, Bookmeyer R, et al, for the Rakai Project Study Group. Probability of HIV-1 transmission per coital act in monogamous, heterosexual HIV-1 discordant couples in Rakai, Uganda. *Lancet.* 2001;357:1149–1153.

83. Dolin PF, Raviglione MC, Kochi A. Global tuberculosis incidence and mortality during 1990–2000. *Bull WHO.* 2004;72:213–220.

84. Schluger NW, Rom WN. The host immune response to tuberculosis. *Am J Respir Crit Care Med.* 1998;157:679–691.

85. Lawn SD, Shattock RJ, Achenmpong JW, et al. Sustained plasma TNF-a and HIV-1 load despite resolution of other parameters of immunoactivation during treatment of tuberculosis in Africans. *AIDS.* 1999;13:2231–2237.

86. Modjarrad K, Zulu I, Redden DJ, et al. Treatment of intestinal helminthes does not reduce plasma concentrations of HIV-1 RNA in coinfected Zambian adults. *J Infect Dis.* 2005;192:1277–1283.

87. Greenburg AL, Ryder RW, Medi M, et al. *Plasmodium falciparum* malaria and perinatally acquired human immunodeficiency virus type 1 infection in Kinshasa, Zaire. *N Engl J Med.* 1991;325:105–109.

88. Kublin JG, Patnaik P, Jere CS, et al. Effect of *Plasmodium falciparum* malaria on concentration of HIV-1 RNA in the blood of adults in rural Malawi: a prospective cohort study. *Lancet.* 2005;365:233–240.

89. Xiao L, Owen SM, Rudolph DL, Lal RB, Lal AA. *Plasmodium falciparum* antigen-induced human immunodeficiency virus type 1 replication is mediated through induction of tumor necrosis factor-alpha. *J Infect Dis.* 1998;177:437–445.

90. French N, Nakiyingi J, Lugada E, Watera L, Whitworth Jag, Gilks CF. Increasing rates of malarial fever with deteriorating immune status in HIV-1 infected Ugandan adults. *AIDS.* 2001;15:899–906.

91. Sulkowski MS, Thomas DL. Hepatitis C in the HIV-infected person. *Ann Intern Med.* 2003;138:197–207.

92. Monga HK, Rodriguez-Barradas MC, Breaux K, et al. Hepatitis C virus infection-related morbidity and mortality among patients with human immunodeficiency virus infection. *Clin Infect Dis.* 2001;33:240–247.

93. Rockstroh JK, Spengler U. HIV and hepatitis C virus co-infection. *Lancet Infect Dis.* 2004;4:437–444.

94. Eyster Fried MW, Di Bisceglie AM, Goedert JJ, et al. Increasing hepatitis C virus RNA levels in hemophiliacs: relationship to human immunodeficiency virus infection and liver disease. Multicenter Hemophilia Cohort Study. *Blood.* 1994;84:1020–1023.

95. Darby SC, Ewart DW, Giangrande PL, et al. Mortality from liver disease in haemophilic men and boys in UK given blood products contaminated with hepatitis C. UK Haemophilia Centre Directors' Organisation. *Lancet.* 1997;350:1425–1431.

96. Palella FJ Jr, Delaney KM, Moorman AC, et al. Declining morbidity and mortality among patients with advanced human immunodeficiency virus infection. HIV Outpatient Study Investigators. *N Engl J Med.* 1998;338:853–860.

97. Dorrucci M, Pezzotti P, Phillips AN, Lepri AC, Rezza G. Coinfection of hepatitis C virus with human immunodeficiency virus and progression to AIDS. Italian Seroconversion Study. *J Infect Dis.* 1995;172: 1503–1508.

98. Greub G, Ledergerber B, Battegay M, et al. Clinical progression, survival, and immune recovery during antiretroviral therapy in patients with HIV-1 and hepatitis C coinfection: the Swiss HIV Cohort Study. *Lancet.* 2000;356:1800–1805.

99. Sulkowski MS, Moore RD, Mehta SH, Chaisson RE, Thomas DL. Hepatitis C and progression of HIV disease. *JAMA.* 2002;288:199–206.

100. Chung RT, Evans SR, Yang Y, Theodore D, et al. Immune recovery is associated with persistent rise in hepatitis C virus RNA, infrequent liver test flares, and is not impaired by hepatitis C virus in co-infected subjects. *AIDS.* 2002;16:1915–1923.

101. Gonzalez SA, Talal AH. Hepatitis C virus in human immunodeficiency virus-infected individuals: an emerging comorbidity with significant implications. *Sem Liver Dis.* 2003;23:149–166.

102. Xiang J, Wunschmann S, Schmidt WN, Shao J, Stapleton JT. Full-length GB virus C (hepatitis G virus) RNA transcripts are infectious in primary CD4-positive T cells. *J Virol.* 2000;74:9125–9133.

103. Heringlake S, Ockenga J, Tillmann HI, et al. GB virus C/ hepatitis G virus infection: a favorable prognostic factor in human immunodeficiency virus-infected patients? *J Infect Dis.* 1998;177:1723–1726.

104. Toyoda H, Fukuda Y, Hayakawa T, Takamatsu J, Saito H. Effect of GB virus C/hepatitis G virus coinfection on the course of HIV infection in hemophilia patients in Japan. *J Acquir Immune Defic Syndr Hum Retrovirol.* 1998;17:209–213.

105. Lefrère JJ, Roudot-Thoraval F, Morand-Joubert L, et al. Carriage of GB virus C/hepatitis G virus RNA is associated with a slower immunologic, virologic, and clinical progression of human immunodeficiency virus disease in coinfected persons. *J Infect Dis.* 1999;179:783–789.

106. Yeo AET, Matsumoto A, Hisada M, Shih JW, Alter HJ, Goedert JJ. Effect of hepatitis G virus infection on progression of HIV infection in patients with hemophilia: Multicenter Hemophilia Cohort Study. *Ann Intern Med.* 1000;132:959–963.

107. Xiang J, Wunschmann S, Diekema DJ, et al. Effect of coinfection with GB virus C on survival among patients with HIV infection. *N Engl J Med.* 2001;345:707–714.

108. Tillman HL, Heiken H, Knapik-Botor A, et al. Infection with GB virus C and reduced mortality among HIV-infected patients. *N Engl J Med.* 2001;345:715–724.

109. Sabin CA, Devereux H, Kinson Z, et al. Effect of coinfection with hepatitis G virus on HIV disease progression in hemophilic men. *J Acquir Immun Defic Syndr Human Retrovirol.* 1998;19:546–548.

110. Birk M, Lindback S, Lidman C. No influence of GB virus C replication on the prognosis in a cohort of HIV-1 infected patients. *AIDS.* 2002;16:2482–2485.

111. Brust D, Jagannatha S, Herpin B, et al. Hepatitis G virus (HGV) infection does not prolong survival of patients with early-stage HIV disease: importance of baseline HIV viral load as a predictor of mortality. In: Abstracts of the 14th International AIDS Conference, Barcelona, Spain, July 7–12, 2002.

112. Van der Bij AK, Kloosterboen N, Prins M, et al. GB virus C coinfection and HIV-1 disease progression: the Amsterdam Cohort Study. *J Infect Dis.* 2005;181:678–685.

113. Williams CF, Kliazman D, Yamashita TE, et al. Persistent GB virus C infection and survival in HIV-infected men. *N Engl J Med.* 2004;350:980–990.

114. Xiang J, George SL, Wunshchmann S, Chang Q, Klinzman D, Stapleton JT. Inhibitors of HIV-1 replication by GB virus C infection through increases in RANTES, MIP-1a, MIP-1b and SDF-1. *Lancet.* 2004;363:2040–2046.

115. Moss WJ, Ryan JT, Monze M, et al. Suppression of human immunodeficiency virus replication during acute measles. *J Infect Dis.* 2002;185:1035–1042.

116. Grivel JC, Garcia M, Moss WJ, Margolis LB. Inhibition of HIV-1 replication in human lymphoid tissues ex vivo by measles virus. *J Infect Dis.* 2005;192:71–78.

117. Watt G, Kanti-Pong P, Jongsakul K. Decrease in human immunology virus type 1 load during acute dengue fever. *Clin Infect Dis.* 2003;36:1067–1069.

118. Watt G, Kant-Pong P, de Souza M, et al. HIV-1 suppression during acute scrub-typhus infection. *Lancet.* 2000;356:475–479.

119. Ho DD. Time to hit HIV, early and hard. *N Engl J Med.* 1995;333:450–451.

120. Tarwater P, Mellors J, Gore ME, et al. Methods to assess population effectiveness of therapies in human immunodeficiency virus incident and prevalent cohorts. *Am J Epidemiol.* 2001;154:675–681.

121. European Study Group on Heterosexual Transmission of HIV. Comparison of female to male and male to female transmission of HIV in 563 stable couples. *BMJ.* 1992;304:809–813.

122. Wawer MJ, Gray RH, Serwadda NK, et al. Rates of HIV-1 transmission per coital act, by stage of HIV-1 infection, Rakai, Uganda. *J Infect Dis.* 2005;191:1403–1409.

123. Laga M, Schwartlander B, Risani E, Sow PS, Carael M. To stem HIV in Africa, prevent transmission to young women. *AIDS.* 2001;15:931–934.

124. de Vincenzi I. A longitudinal study of human immunodeficiency virus transmission by heterosexual partners. *N Engl J Med.* 1994;331:341–346.

125. Rojanapithayakurn W, Hanenberg R. The 100% condom program in Thailand. *AIDS.* 1996;10:1–7.

126. Nelson KE, Celentano DD, Eiumtrakul S, et al. Changes in sex and behavior and a decline in HIV infection among young men in Thailand. *N Engl J Med.* 1996;335:297–303.

127. Nagachinta T, Duerr A, Suriyanon V, et al. Risk factors for HIV-1 transmission from seropositive male blood donors to their regular female partners in northern Thailand. *AIDS.* 1997;11:1763–1772.

128. Nicolosi A, Correa Leite ML, Musico M, Arici L, Garazzeni G, Lazzaria A. The efficiency of male-female and female to male sexual transmission of HIV: a study of 730 stable couples. *Epidemiology.* 1994;5:570–575.

129. Mati SK, Hunter DJ, Maggwn BN, Tukei PM. Contraceptive use and the risk of HIV infection in Nairobi, Kenya. *Int J Gynacecol Obstet.* 1995;48:61–67.

130. Marx PA, Spira AL, Gettie A, et al. Progesterone implants enhance HIV vaginal transmission and early virus load. *Nat Med.* 1996;2:1084–1089.

131. Henin Y, Mendelbrot I, Henrion R, Pradinavd R, Couland JP, Montagnier L. Virus excretion in the cervicovaginal secretions of pregnant and nonpregnant HIV-infected women. *JAIDS.* 1993;6:72–75.

132. Roddy R, Zekeng L, Ryan KA, Tamoufe U, Weir SS, Wong EL. A controlled trial of nonoxynol 9 film to reduce male-to-female transmission of sexually transmitted diseases. *N Engl J Med.* 1998;339:504–510.

133. Auvert B, Buve A, Lagarde E, et al. Male circumcision and HIV infection in four cities in sub-Saharan Africa. *AIDS.* 2001;15(suppl 4):S31–S40.

134. Auvert B, Jaljaard D, Lagarda E, Sobngwin-Tambekou J, Sitta Z, Purea A. Randomized controlled intervention trial of male circumcision for reduction of HIV infection risk: the ANR5 1205 trial. *PLoS Medicine.* 2005;2:0001–0010. Available at: http://www.plosmedicine.org. Accessed July 2006.

135. Anderson R, May R, Boily M, Garnet G, Rowley J. The spread of HIV-1 in Africa: sexual contact patterns and the predicted demographic impact of AIDS. *Nature.* 1991;352:581–589.

136. Morris M, Kretzschmar M. Concurrent partnerships and the spread of HIV. *AIDS.* 1997;11:681–683.

137. Halperin DT, Epstein H. Concurrent sexual partnerships help to explain Africa's high HIV prevalence implications for prevention. *Lancet.* 2004;364:4–6.

138. Asamoah-Odei E, Garcia-Callga JM, Boerma T. HIV prevalence and trends in sub-Saharan Africa: no decline and large subregional differences. *Lancet.* 2004;364:35–40.

139. Buve A, Carael M, Hayes RJ, et al. The multicenter study to determine the differential spread of HIV in four cities in Africa: summary and conclusions. *AIDS.* 2001;(suppl 4):S127–S131.

140. Vlahov D, Munoz A, Anthony JC, Cohen S, Celentano DD, Nelson KE. Association of drug-injection patterns with antibody to HIV type-1 among injection drug users in Baltimore. *Am J Epidemiol.* 1990;132:847–856.

141. Sassi H, Salmas S, Conti S, et al. Risk behaviors for HIV-1 infection in Italian drug users: report from a multi-center study. *JAIDS.* 1989;2:486–496.

142. Marror M, Des Jarlais DC, Cohen H, et al. Risk factors for infection with HIV among intravenous drug users in New York City. *AIDS.* 1987;1:39–44.

143. Battjes RJ, Rickens RW, Haverkos HW, Sloboda Z. HIV risk factors among injecting drug users in five U.S. cities. *AIDS.* 1994;8; 681–687.

144. Schoenbaun EE, Harter D, Selwyn PA, et al. Risk factors for human immunodeficiency virus infection in intravenous drug users. *N Engl J Med.* 1989;321:874–879.

145. Jose B, Friedman SR, Neaigus A, et al. Syringe-mediated drug-sharing (backloading): a new risk factor for HIV among injecting drug users. *AIDS.* 1993;7:1653–1660.

146. Anthony JC, Vlahov D, Nelson KE, Cohen S, et al. New evidence on intravenous cocaine use and the risk of infection with HIV. *Am J Epidemiol.* 1991;134:1179–1184.

147. Chirgwin K, DeHovitz JA, Dillion S, et al. HIV infection, genital ulcer disease and crack cocaine use among patients attending a clinic for sexually transmitted diseases. *Am J Public Health.* 1991;81: 1576–1579.

148. Metzger DS, Woody GE, McClellan AT, et al. Human immunodeficiency virus seroconversion among intravenous drug users in- and out-of-treatment: an 18 month prospective follow-up. *JAIDS.* 1993;6: 1049–1056.

149. van Ameijden EJC, van den Hock JAR, Hangtrecht HJA, Coutinho RA. The harm reduction approach and risk factors for human immunodeficiency virus seroconversion in injecting drug users, Amsterdam. *Am J Epidemiol.* 1992;136:236–243.

150. Ball AL, Rana S, Dehne K. HIV prevention among injecting drug users: responses in developing and transitional countries. *Public Health Rep.* 1998;113(suppl 1):170–181.

151. Lurie P, Drucker E. An opportunity lost: HIV infections associated with lack of a national needle-exchange program in the USA. *Lancet.* 1997;349:604–608.

152. Centers for Disease Control. Update: Syringe Exchange Programs—United States, 2002. *MMWR.* 2005;54:673–676.

153. Strathdee SA, Celentano DD, Shah N, et al. Needle exchange attendance and health care utilization promote entry into detoxification. *J Urban Health.* 1999;98:448–453.

154. Han JA, Vranizam KM, Moss AR. Who uses needle exchange? A study of injection drug users in San Francisco, 1989–1990. *JAIDS.* 1997;15:157–164.

155. Archibald CP, Ofner M, Strathdee SA, et al. Factors associated with frequent needle exchange program attendance in injection drug users in Vancouver, Canada. *JAIDS.* 1998;17:160–166.

156. Vlahov D, Unge B, Brookmeyer R, et al. Reductions in high-risk drug use behaviors among participants in the Baltimore needle exchange program. *JAIDS.* 1997;16:400–406.

157. Normand J, Vlahov D, Moses LE. Preventing HIV transmission: the role of sterile needles and bleach. Washington, DC: National Academies Press; 1995.

158. Lurie P, Reingold A, Bower B, et al. The public health impact of needle exchange programs in the United States and abroad. Vol. 1. Atlanta, Ga: Centers for Disease Control and Prevention; 1996.

159. Holmberg SD. The estimated prevalence and incidence of HIV in 96 large U.S. metropolitan areas. *Am J Public Health.* 1996;86: 642–654.

160. Garfein RS, Monterroso ER, Tong TC, et al. Comparison of HIV injection risk behaviors among injection drug users from East and West Coast US cities. *J Urban Health.* 2004;81:260–267.

161. Ciccarone D, Bourgois P. Explaining the geographic variation for HIV among injection drug users in the United States. *Substance Use and Abuse.* 2003;14:2049–2063.

162. Rhodes T, Singer M, Bourgois P, Friedman SR, Strathdee SA. The social structural production of HIV risk among injecting drug users. *Soc Sci Med.* 2005;61:1026–1044.

163. Beyrer C, Jittiwutikarn J, Teokol W, et al. Drug use, increasing incarceration rates and prison-associated HIV risks in Thailand. *AIDS Behavior.* 2003;7:153–161.

164. Blanche S, Rouzioux C, Guihard Moscato ML, et al. A prospective study of infants born to women seropositive for human immunodeficiency virus type 1. *N Engl J Med.* 1989;320:1643–1648.

165. European Collaborative Study. Mother-to-child transmission of HIV infection. *Lancet.* 1988;2:1039–1043.

166. European Collaborative Study. Risk factors for mother-to-child transmission of HIV-1. *Lancet.* 1992;339:1007–1012.

167. Hutton C, Parks WP, Lai SH, et al. A hospital-based prospective study of perinatal infection with human immunodeficiency virus type. *J Pediatr.* 1991;118:347–353.

168. The International Perinatal HIV Group. The mode of delivery and the risk of vertical transmission of human immunodeficiency virus type-1: a meta-analysis of 15 prospective cohort studies. *N Engl J Med.* 1999;340:977–987.

169. Bryson YJ, Luzuriaga K, Sullivan JL, Wara DW. Proposed definitions for utero versus intrapartum transmission of HIV-1. *N Engl J Med.* 1992;326:1246–1247.

170. Van de Perre P, Simonon A, Msellati P, et al. Postnatal transmission of human immunodeficiency virus type-1 from mother to infant. *N Engl J Med.* 1991;325:593–598.

171. Wiktor SZ, Ekpini E, Nduati RW. Prevention of mother-to-child transmission of HIV-1 in Africa. *AIDS.* 1997;11(suppl B):S79–S87.

172. Nduati R, John G, Mobori-Ngacha D, et al. Effect of breastfeeding and formula feeding on transmission of HIV-1: a randomized trial. *JAMA.* 2000;283:1167–1174.

173. Coutsoudis A, Pillay K, Kuhn L, et al. Method of feeding and transmissions of HIV-1 from mothers to children by 15 months of age: prospective cohort study from Durban, South Africa. *AIDS.* 2001;15:379–387.

174. Cooper ER, Charurat M, Mofenson L, et al. Combination antiretroviral strategies for treatment of pregnant HIV-1 infected women and prevention of prenatal HIV-1 transmission. *J Acquir Immune Defic Syndr.* 2002;484–494.

175. Centers for Disease Control and Prevention. Successful implementation of perinatal HIV guidelines: a multistate surveillance evaluation. *MMWR Recomm Rep.* 2001;50:17–28.

176. Fawzi WW, Msamanga G, Hunter D, et al. Randomized trial of vitamin supplements in relation to vertical transmissionof HIV-1 in Tanzania. *J Acquir Immune Defic Syndr.* 2000;23:246–254.

177. Coutsoudis A, Pillay K, Spooner E, et al. Randomized trial testing the effect of vitamin A supplementation on pregnancy outcomes and early mother to child HIV-1 transmisson in Durban, South Africa. *AIDS.* 1999;13:1517–1524.

178. Biggar RJ, Miotti PG, Taha TE, et al. Perinatal intervention trial in Africa: effects of a birth canal cleansing intervention to prevent HIV transmission. *Lancet.* 1996;347:1647–1650.

179. Gallard P, Mwanyumba F, Verhofstede C, et al. Vaginal lavage with chlorhexidine during labor to reduce mother-to-child HIV transmission: clinical trial in Mombasa, Kenya. *AIDS*. 2001;15: 389–396.

180. Taha TE, Biggar RJ, Broadhead RL, et al. Effect of cleansing the birth canal with antiseptic solution on maternal and newborn morbidity and mortality in Malawi: clinical trial. *BMJ*. 1997;315:216–220.

181. Connor EM, Sperling RS, Gelber R, et al. Reduction of maternal-infant transmission of human immunodeficiency virus type-1 with zidovudine treatment. *N Engl J Med*. 1994;331:1173–1180.

182. Sperling RS, Shapiro DE, Coombs RW, et al. Maternal viral load, zidovudine treatment, and the risk of transmission of human immunodeficiency virus type-1 from mother to infant. *N Engl J Med*. 1996;335:1621.

183. Shaffer N, Chuachoowong PA, Mock C, et al. Short-course zidovudine for perinatal HIV-1 transmission in Bangkok, Thailand: a randomized controlled trial. *Lancet*. 1999;353:773–780.

184. Guay L, Musoke P, Fleming T, et al. Intrapartum and neonatal single-dose nevirapine compared with zidovudine for prevention of mother-child transmission of HIV-1 in Kampala, Uganda: HIVNET 012 randomized trial. *Lancet*. 1999;354:795–802.

185. Jackson JB, Musoke P, Fleming T, et al. Intrapartum and neonatal nevirapine compared with zidovudine for prevention of mother-to-child transmission of HIV-1 in Kampala, Uganda: 18 month follow-up of the HIVNET 012 randomized trial. *Lancet*. 2003;362:859–868.

186. Jackson JB, Backer-Pergola G, Guay LA, et al. Identification of the K103N resistance mutation in Ugandan women receiving nevirapine to prevent vertical HIV-1 transmission. *AIDS*. 2000;14:F111–F115.

187. Eschleman SH, Mracna M, Guay L, et al. Selection and fading of resistance mutations in women and infants receiving nevirapine to prevent HIV-1 vertical transmission (HIVNET 012). *AIDS*. 2001;15:1951–1957.

188. Nolan M, Fowler MG, Mofenson LM. Antiretroviral prophylaxis of perinatal HIV-1 transmission and the potential impact of antiretroviral resistance. *J Acquir Immune Defic Syndr*. 2002;30:216–229.

189. WHO. *Antiretroviral Drugs and the Prevention of Mother-to-Child Transmission of HIV Infection in Resource-Limits Settings*. Report of a Technical Consultation. Geneva, Switzerland; February 5–6, 2004.

190. The Petra Study Team. Efficacy of three short-course regimens of zidovudine and lamivudine in preventing early and late transmission of HIV-1 from mother to child in Tanzania, South Africa, and Uganda (Petra study): a randomized, double-blind, placebo-controlled trial. *Lancet*. 2002;359:1178–1186.

191. Wiktor S, Ekpini E, Karon J, et al. Short course oral zidovudine for prevention of mother-to-child transmission of HIV-1 in Abidjan, Cote D'Ivoire: a randomized trial. *Lancet*. 1999;353:781–785.

192. Lallemant M, Jourdain G, Le Coeur S, et al. A trial of shortened zidovudine regimens to prevent mother-to-child transmission of human immunodeficiency virus type-1. *N Engl J Med*. 2000;343:982–991.

193. Lallemant M, Jourdain G, LeCoeur S, et al. Single-dose perinatal nevirapine plus standard zidovudine to prevent mother-to-child transmission of HIV-1 in Thailand. *N Engl J Med*. 2004;351:217–228.

194. Jourdain G, Houng G, LeCour S, et al. Intrapartum exposure to nevirapine and subsequent maternal responses to nevirapine-based anti-retroviral therapy. *N Engl J Med*. 2004;351:229–240.

195. Mofenson LM. Advances in the prevention of vertical transmission of human immunodeficiency virus. *Sem Pediatr Infect Dis.* 2003;14: 295–308.

196. Loannidis JPA, Abrams EJ, Ammann A, et al. Perinatal transmission of human immunodeficiency virus type 1 by pregnant women with RNA virus loads <1000 copies/mL. *J Infect Dis.* 2001;183:539–545.

197. Centers for Disease Control and Prevention. U.S. Public Health Service Task Force recommendations for use of antiretroviral drugs in pregnant HIV-1 infected women for maternal health and interventions to reduce perinatal HIV-1 transmission in the United States. *MMWR Recomm Rep.* 2002;51:1–4.

198. Centers for Disease Control and Prevention. HIV testing among pregnant women—United States and Canada, 1998–2001. *MMWR Recomm Rep.* 2002;51:1013–1016.

199. Amornwichet P, Teeraratkul A, Simonds RJ, et al. Preventing mother-to-child HIV transmission: the first year of Thailand's national program. *JAMA.* 2002;288:245–248.

200. Busch MP, Operskalski EA, Mosley JW, et al. Factors influencing human immunodeficiency virus type 1 transmission by blood transfusion. *J Infect Dis.* 1996;174:26–33.

201. Lackritz EM, Satten GA, Aberle-Grasse J, et al. Estimated risk of transmission of the human immunodeficiency virus by screened blood in the United States. *N Engl J Med.* 1995;333:1721–1725.

202. Dodd RY, Notari EP, Stramer SL. Current prevalence and incidence of infectious disease markers and estimated window-period risk in the American Red Cross blood donor population. *Transfusion.* 2002;42:973–979.

203. Stramer SL, Glynn SA, Kleinman SH, et al. Detection of HIV-1 and HCV infections among antibody-negative blood donors by nucleic acid-amplification testing. *N Engl J Med.* 2004;351:760–768.

204. Jackson JB, Busch MP, Stramer SL, Aubuchon JP. The cost-effectiveness of NAT for HIV, NCV and HBV in whole blood donations. *Transfusion.* 2003;43(6):721–729.

205. Pealer LN, Marfin AA, Petersen LR, et al. Transmission of West Nile virus through blood transfusion in the United States in 2002. *N Engl J Med.* 2003;349:1236–1245.

206. Busch MP, Laglio HS, Robertson EE, et al. Screening the blood supply for West Nile virus RNA by nucleic acid amplification testing. *N Engl J Med.* 2005;353:460–467.

207. Caussy D, Goedert J. The epidemiology of human immunodeficiency virus and acquired immunodeficiency syndrome. *Sem Oncol.* 1990;17:244–250.

208. Simonds RJ, Holmberg SD, Hurwitz RL, et al. Transmission of human immunodeficiency virus type 1 from a seronegative organ and tissue donor. *N Engl J Med.* 1992;326:726–732.

209. Centers for Disease Control and Prevention. Guidelines for preventing transmission of human immunodeficiency virus through transplantation of human tissues and organs. *MMWR.* 1994;43: RR-8.

210. Ratijan Ga, Strengers PEW, Persijn HM. Prevention of transmission of HIV by organ and tissue transplantation. *Transpl Int.* 1993;6: 165–172.

211. Shan H, Wang J-X, Reu F-R. Blood banking in China. *Lancet.* 2002;360:1770–1775.

212. Volkow P, Del Rio L. Paid donation and plasma trade: unrecognized forces that drive the AIDS epidemic in developing countries. *Int J STD AIDS*. 2005;16:5–8.
213. Tokars JI, Marcus R, Culver DH, et al. Surveillance of HIV infection and zidovudine use among health care workers after occupational exposure. *Ann Intern Med*. 1993;48:913–919.
214. Centers for Disease Control. Public Health Service guidelines for the management of occupational exposures to HBV, HCV and HIV and recommendations for post exposure prophylaxis. *MMWR*. 2001;50: RR-11.
215. Ippolito G, Puro V, DeCarli G. The risk of occupational human immunodeficiency virus infection in health care workers: the Italian Study Group on occupational risk of HIV infection. *Arch Intern Med*. 1993;153:1451–1458.
216. Henderson DK, Fahey BJ, Willy M, et al. Risk for occupational transmission of human immunodeficiency virus type 1 (HIV-1) associated with clinical exposures: a prospective evaluation. *Ann Intern Med*. 1990;113:740–746.
217. Ippolito G, Puro V, Petrosillo N, et al. Simultaneous infection with HIV and hepatitis C virus following occupational conjunctive blood exposure. *Scand J Infect Dis*. 1993;25:270–271.
218. Ciesielski C, Marianos D, Ou CY, et al. Transmission of human immunodeficiency virus in a dental practice. *Ann Intern Med*. 1992;116:798–805.
219. Ou C-Y, Ciesielski C, Myers G, et al. Molecular epidemiology of HIV transmission in a dental practice. *Science*. 1992;256:1165–1171.
220. Gisselguist D, Rothenberg RB, Potterat J, et al. HIV infections in sub-Saharan Africa not explained by sexual or vertical transmission. *Int J STD AIDS*. 202;13:657–666.
221. Kiwanaka N, Gray RH, Serwadda D, et al. The incidence of HIV-1 associated with injecting and transfusions in a prospective cohort, Rakai, Uganda. *AIDS*. 2004;18:341–344.
222. Reinik L, Verea K, Salahoddin SZ, Tondreau S, Markham PD. Stability and inactivation of HTLV-III/LAV under clinical and laboratory environments. *JAMA*. 1986;255:1887–1891.
223. Beaumont T, van Nuenen A, Broersen S, et al. Reversal of human immunodeficiency virus type 1 IIIB to a neutralization-resistant phenotype in an accidentally infected laboratory worker with a progressive clinical course. *J Virol*. 2001;75:2246–2252.
224. Centers for Disease Control. Recommendation for prevention of HIV transmission in healthcare settings. *MMWR*. 1987;36:28.
225. Webb PA, Happ CM, Maupin G, et al. Potential for insect transmission of HIV: experimental exposure of *Limex hemipterus* and *Toxobychites amboinensis* to human immunodeficiency virus. *J Infect Dis*. 1989;160:970–977.
226. Srinivasan A, York D, Bohen C. Lack of HIV replication in arthropod cells. *Lancet*. 1987;1:1094–1095.
227. Jupp PG, Lyons SF. Experimental assessment of bedbugs and mosquitoes as vectors of human immunodeficiency virus. *AIDS*. 1987;1:171–174.
228. Friedland GH, Saltzman BR, Rogers MF, et al. Lack of transmission of HTLV-III/LAV infection to household contacts of patients with AIDS or AIDS-related complex with oral candidiasis. *N Engl J Med*. 1986;314:344–349.

229. Friedland GH, Kahl P, Saltzman B, et al. Additional evidence for lack of transmission of HIV infection by close interpersonal casual contact.

230. Rogers ME, White C, Sanders T, et al. Lack of transmission of human immunodeficiency virus from infected children to their household contacts. *Pediatrics*. 1990;84:210–214.

231. Wahn V, Kramer H, Voit T, et al. Horizontal transmission of HIV infection between two siblings. *Lancet*. 1986;2:694.

232. Koenig RE, Gautier T, Levy JA. Unusual intrafamilial transmission of human immunodeficiency virus. *Lancet*. 1986;2:627.

233. Fitzgibbon JE, Gaur S, Frenkel CD, et al. Transmission from one child to another of human immunodeficiency virus type 1 with a zidovudine-resistance mutation. *N Engl J Med*. 1993;329: 1835–1841.

234. Centers for Disease Control and Prevention. HIV transmission between two adolescent brothers with hemophilia. *MMWR*. 1993;42:948–951.

235. Gerberding JC. Occupational exposure to HIV in health care settings. *N Engl J Med*. 2003;348:826–833.

236. Cardo DM, Culuer DH, Ciesielski LA, et al. A case-control study of HIV seroconversion in health care workers after percutaneous exposure. *N Engl J Med*. 1997;337:1485–1490.

237. Clerici M, Levin JM, Kessler HA, et al. HIV-specific T-helper activity in seronegative health care workers exposed to contaminated blood. *JAMA*. 1994;221:42–46.

238. Broliden K, Hinkula J, Devito C, et al. Functional HIV-1 specific IgA antibodies in HIV-1 exposed, persistently IgG seronegative female sex workers. *Immunol Letter*. 2001;79:29–36.

239. Centers for Disease Control and Prevention. Antiretroviral postexposure prophylaxis after injection-drug use or other nonoccupational exposure to HIV in the United States. *MMWR*. 2005;54(RR-02):1–20.

240. Chon R, Hoffman LH, Fu R, Smits AK, Korthuis PT. Screening for HIV: a review of the evidence for the U.S. Preventive Services Task Force. *Ann Intern Med*. 2005;143:85–93.

241. Branson BM. Point-of-Care Rapid Tests for HIV Antibodies. *J Lab Med*. 2003;27:288–295.

242. CDC Quick Facts: Rapid Testing. HHS approves wider access to rapid HIV test. AMFAR Web site. February 4, 2003. Available at: http://www.amfar.org. Accessed July 25, 2005.

243. Stoneburner RL, Low-Beer D. Population-level HIV declines and behavioral risk avoidance in Uganda. *Science*. 2004;304:714–718.

244. Rhodes T. HIV transmission and HIV prevention associated with injecting drug use in the Russian Federation. *Inter J Drug Policy*. 2004;15:1–16.

245. Smolskaya T, et al. Sentinel sero-epidemiological and behavioral surveillance among female sex workers, St. Petersburg, Russian Federation, 2003 [abstract]. XV International AIDS Conference. Bangkok, Thailand; July 11–17, 2004. Abstract ThOrC1371.

246. Caiaffai WJ. The dynamics of the human immunodeficiency virus epidemics in the south of Brazil: increasing role of injection drug users. *Clin Infect Dis*. 2003;37(suppl 5):5376–5381.

247. Granato N, Morell MGG, Areco K, Peres CA. Association factors for HIV infection in commercial sex workers in Sao Paolo, Brazil [abstract]. XV International AIDS Conference, Bangkok, Thailand; July 11–16, 2004. WePcC6202.

248. Guimaraes MD, Munoz A, Boschi-Pinto C, Castilho CA. HIV infection among female partners of seropositive men in Brazil. *Am J Epidemiol.* 1995;142:538–547.
249. Galvao J. Brazil and access to HIV/AIDS drugs: a question of human rights and public health. *Am J Public Health.* 2005;95:1110–1016.
250. Mesquita F, Doneda D, Gaudolfi D, et al. Brazilian response to the AIDS epidemic among injection drug users. *CID.* 2003;37 (suppl 5):5382–5385.
251. Brouwer C, Harris BM, Tanaka S. *Gender Analysis in Papua, New Guinea, 1998.* Washington, DC: World Bank; 1998.
252. Hamers FF, Downs AM. The changing face of the HIV epidemic in Western Europe: what are the implications for public health policies? *Lancet.* 2000;364:83–94.
253. Centers for Disease Control and Prevention. *HIV/AIDS Surveillance Report, 2003.* Vol. 15. Atlanta, Ga: CDC; 2004:1–46.
254. Del Rio C, Sepulvida J. AIDS in Mexico: lessons learned and implications for developing countries. *AIDS.* 2002;16:1445–1457.
255. Volkow P, Velasco SR, Mueller N, et al. Transfusion-associated HIV infection in Mexico related to paid blood donors; HIV epidemic. *Int J STDs AIDS.* 2004;15:337–342.
256. Magis-Rodriguez C, Gayet C, Negroni M, et al. Migration and AIDS in Mexico: an overview based on recent evidence. *JAIDS.* 2004;37: S215–S226.
257. Public Health Agency of Canada. *HIV and AIDS in Canada.* Surveillance Report to June 30, 2004. Surveillance and Risk Assessment Division, Center for Infectious Diseases Prevention and Control, Public Health Agency of Canada; 2004.
258. Schwartlander B, Stanecki K, Brown T, et al. Country-specific estimates and models of HIV and AIDS: methods and limitations. *AIDS.* 1999;13:2445–2458.
259. Walker N, Stanecki K, Brown T, et al. Methods and procedures for estimating HIV/AIDS and its impact: the UNAIDS/WHO estimates for the end of 2001. *AIDS.* 2003;17:2215–2225.
260. Brookmeyer R, Gail MH. AIDS epidemiology: a quantative approach. New York, NY: Oxford University Press; 1992.
261. Williams B, Gouws E, Wilkinson D, Karim SA. Estimating HIV incidence rates from age prevalence data in epidemic situations. *Statis Med.* 2001;20:2003–2016.
262. Brookmeyer R, Quinn T, Shepherd M, et al. AIDS epidemic in India: a new method for estimating current human immunodeficiency virus (HIV) incidence rates. *Am J Epidemiol.* 1995;142:209–213.
263. Busch M, Satten GA, Henrard DR, et al. Time course of detection of viral and serological makers for HIV infection. *Transfusion.* 1995;35:91–97.
264. Janssen RS, Satten GA, Stramer SL, et al. New testing strategy to detect early infection for use in incidence estimates and for clinical and prevention purposes. *JAMA.* 1998;280:42–48.
265. Rawal BD, Degola A, Lebedeoa L, et al. Development of a new less-sensitive enzyme immunoassay for detection of early HIV-a infection. *JAIDS.* 2003;33:349–355.
266. Young CL, Hu DJ, Byers R, et al. Evaluation of a sensitive/less sensitive testing algorithim using the biomerieux vironostika-LS assay for recent HIV-1 subtype B1 or E infection in Thailand. *AIDS Res Hum Retroviruses.* 2003;19:481–486.

267. Parekh BS, Hu DJ, Vanichseni S, et al. Evaluation of a sensitive/less sensitive testing algorithim using the 3 A11-LS assay for detecting recent HIV seroconversion among individuals with HIV-1 subtype B or E infection in Thailand. *AIDS Res Hum Retrovirus*. 2001;17:453–458.

268. Dobbs T, Kennedy S, Pau C-P, McDoug S, Parekh BS. Performance characteristics of the immunoglobulin G-Capture BED-enzyme immunoassay, an assay to detect recent human immunodeficiency virus type 1 seroconversion. *J Clin Micro*. 2004;42:2623–2628.

269. Parekh BS, McDoug JS. Application of laboratory method's for estimation of HIV-1 incidence. *Indian J Med Res*. 2005;121:510–518.

270. Thomas HI, Wilson S, O'Toole CM, et al. Differential maturation of avidity of IgG antibodies to gp41, p24 and p14 following infection with HIV-1. *Clin Exper Immun*. 1996;103:185–191.

271. Wilson KM, Johnson EM, Croom HA, et al. Incidence immunoassay for distinguishing recent from established HIV-1 infection in therapy naïve populations. *AIDS*. 2004;18:2253–2259.

272. Baily MC, Anderson RM. Sexual contact patterns between men and women and the spread of HIV-1 in urban centers in Africa. *IMA J Math Appl Med Biol*. 1991;8:221–247.

273. Quinn TL, Mann JM, Curran JW, et al. AIDS in Africa: an epidemiological paradigm. *Science*. 1986;16:516–519.

274. Parker RG, Tawil O. Bisexual behavior and HIV transmission in Latin America. In: Tielman R, Caballo M, Hendriks A, eds. Bisexuality and HIV/AIDS. New York, NY: Prometheus Press; 1991.

275. Hunt CW. Migrant labor and sexually transmitted disease and AIDS in Africa. *J Health Soc Behav*. 1989;30:353–373.

276. UNAIDS/WHO. *Report on the Global HIV/AIDS Epidemic*. Geneva, Switzerland: WHO; 1998.

277. Auerbach J, Byram EP, Kandathil SM. The effectiveness of condoms in preventing HIV transmission. AMFAR Web site. Issue Brief 1. 2005. Available at: http://www.amfar.org. Accessed July 25, 2005.

278. Moss AR, Osmond D, Bacchetti P, et al. Risk factors for AIDS and HIV seropositivity in homosexual men. *Am J Epidemiol*. 1987;125:1035–1047.

279. De Vincenzi I, European Study Group on Heterosexual Transmission of HIV. A Longitudinal study of human immunodeficiency virus transmission by heterosexual partners. *N Engl J Med*. 1994;331:341–346.

280. Weller S, Davis K. Condom effectiveness in reducing heterosexual HIV transmission. *Cochrane Database Syst Rev*. 2004;2:CD003255.

281. Hearst N, Chen S. Condom promotion for AIDS prevention in the developing world: is it working? *Stud Fam Plann*. 2004;35:39–47.

282. Pinkerton SD, Abramson PR. Effectiveness of condoms in preventing HIV transmission. *Soc Sci Med*. 1997;44:1303–1312.

283. Pinkerton SD, Abramson PR. Occasional condom use and HIV risk reduction. *J Acquir Immune Defic Syndr Hum Retrovirol*. 1996;13:456–460.

284. Trussel J, Sturgen K, Strickler J, Dominick R. Comparative contraceptive efficacy of the female condom and other barrier methods. *Family Planning Perspectives*. 1994;26.

285. Holmes KK, Levine R, Weaver M. Effectiveness of condoms in preventing sexually transmitted infections. *Bull WHO*. 2004;82:454–461.

286. Stephenson J. Microbicides: ideas flourish, money to follow? *JAMA*. 2000;283:1811–1812.

287. Van Damme L. Clinical microbicide research: an overview. *Trop Med and Intl Health*. 2004;9:1290–1296.

288. D'Cruz OJ, Uckun FM. Clinical development of microbicides for the prevention of HIV infection. *Current Pharm Design*. 2004;10: 315–336.

289. Hillier SL, Moench T, Shattock R, Black R, Reichelderfer P, Veronese F. In vitro and in vivo: the story of nonoxynol 9. *J Aquir Immune Defic Syndr Hum Retrovirol*. 2005;39:1–8.

290. Alliance for Microbicide Development Web site. Available at: http://www.microbicide.org/. Accessed July 5, 2005.

291. CDC Microbicide Working Group. Available at: http://www.cdc.gov/hiv/PUBS/microbicides/members.htm. Accessed July 5, 2005.

292. D'Cruz OJ, Venkatachalam TK, Uckun FM. Novel thiourea compounds as dual-function microbicides. *Biol Reprod*. 2000;63:196–205.

293. Kawamura T, Gulden FO, Sugaya M, et al. R5 HIV productively infects Langerhans cells, and infection levels are regulated by compound CCR5 polymorphisms. *Proc Natl Acad Sci USA*. 2003;100:8401–8406.

294. O'Hara BM, Olson WC. HIV entry inhibitors in clinical development. *Curr Opin Pharmacol*. 2002;2:523–528.

295. Expanding microbicide research. AMFAR Web site. Available at: http://www.amfar.org/cgi-bin/iowa/td/feature/print.html?record=123. Accessed.

296. Agreeing to Disagree. AMFAR Web site. Available at: http://www.amfar.org/cgi-bin/iowa/td/feature/print.html?record=106.

297. Glick P. Scaling up HIV voluntary counseling and testing in Africa. *Evaluation Review*. 2005;29:331–357.

298. Johnson RS, Holtgrave DR, Valdiserri RO, Shepherd M, Gayle HD, DeKock KM. The serostatus approach to fighting the HIV epidemic: prevention strategies for infected individuals. *Am J Public Health*. 2001;91:1019–1024.

299. Hilton C, Sabundayo BP, Langan SJ, Quinn TC, Margolick JB, Nelson KE. Screening for HIV infection in high risk communities by urine antibody testing. *JAIDS*. 2002;31:416–421.

300. Weinhardt LS, Carey MP, Johnson BT, Bickham NL. Effects of HIV counseling and testing on sexual risk behavior: a meta-analytic review of published research 1985–1997. *Am J Public Health*. 1999;89: 1397–1405.

301. Kamb ML, Fishbein M, Douglas JM. Efficacy of risk-reduction counseling to prevent human immunodeficiency virus and sexually transmitted virus. *JAMA*. 1998;280:1161–1168.

302. The Voluntary HIV-1 Counseling and Testing Efficacy Study Group. Efficacy of voluntary HIV-1 counseling and testing in individuals and couples in Kenya, Tanzania and Trindidad: a randomized trial. *Lancet*. 2000;356:103–112.

303. Centers for Disease Control and Prevention. *Compendium of HIV Prevention Interventions with Evidence of Effectiveness (Revised)*. Atlanta, Ga: Centers for Disease Control and Prevention; 2001.

304. The National Institute of Mental Health (NIMH) Multisite HIV Prevention Trial Group. The NIMH Multisite HIV Prevention Trial: reducing HIV sexual risk behavior. *Science*. 1998:280:1889–1894.

305. Sweat M, Sangiwa G, Furlonge C, et al. Cost-effectiveness of voluntary HIV-1 counseling and testing in reducing sexual transmission of HIV-1 in Kenya and Tanzania. *Lancet*. 2000;356:113–121.

306. The EXPLORE Study Team. Effects of a behavioural intervention to reduce acquisition of HIV infection among men who have sex with men: the EXPLORE randomized controlled study. *Lancet.* 2004;364: 41–50.

307. Cohen DA, Dent C, MacKinnon D, et al. Condoms for men, not women. Results of brief promotion programs. *Sex Transm Dis.* 1992;19: 245–251.

308. Boyer CB, Barrett DC, Peterman TA, et al. Sexually transmited disease (STD) and HIV risk in heterosexual adults attending a public STD clinic: evaluation of a randomized controlled behavioral risk-reduction intervention trial. *AIDS.* 1997;11:359–367.

309. Manhart L, Holmes KK. Randomized controlled trials of individual level, population-level, and multi-level interventions for preventing sexually transmitted infections: what has worked? *J Infect Dis.* 2004;190(suppl):S1–S17.

310. Golden MR, Manhart LE. Innovative approaches to the prevention and control of bacterial sexually transmitted infections. *Infect Dis Clin N Am.* 2005;19:513–540.

311. Shain RN, Piper JM, Newton ER, et al. A randomized, controlled trial of a behavioral intervention to prevent sexually transmitted disease among minority women. *New Eng J Med.* 1999;340:93–100.

312. DiClemente RJ, Wingood GM, Harrington KF, et al. Efficacy of an HIV prevention intervention for African American adolescent girls; a randomized controlled trial. *JAMA.* 2004;292(2):171–179.

313. The National Institute of Mental Health (NIMH) HIV Prevention Trial Group. The NIMH Multisite HIV Prevention Trial: reducing HIV sexual risk behavior. *Science.* 1998;280:1889–1894.

314. Kelly JA. Popular opinion leaders and HIV prevention peer education: resolving discrepant findings, and implications for the development of effective community programs. *AIDS Care.* 2004;16:139–150.

315. Rogers EM. *Diffusion of Innovations.* 2nd ed. New York, NY: Free Press; 1983.

316. Kelly JA, St. Lawrence JS, Diaz YE, et al. HIV risk behavior reduction following intervention with key opinion leaders of a population: an experimental analysis. *Am J Public Health.* 1991;81:168–171.

317. Kelly JA. *Changing HIV Risk Behavior: Practical Strategies.* New York, NY: Guilford; 1995.

318. Kelly JA, Murphy DA, Sikkema KJ, et al. Randomized, controlled, community-level HIV prevention intervention for sexual risk behaviour among homosexual men in U.S. cities. *Lancet.* 1997;350: 1500–1505.

319. Sikkema KJ, Kelly JA, Winett RA, et al. Outcomes of a randomized community-level HIV prevention intervention for women living in 18 low-income housing developments. *Am J Public Health.* 2000;90: 57–63.

320. Miller RL, Klotz D, Eckholdt HM. HIV prevention with male prostitutes and patrons of hustler bars: replication of an HIV prevention intervention. *Am J Comm Psychol.* 1998;26:97–131.

321. Kegeles SM, Hays RB, Coates TJ. The MPowerment Project: a community-level HIV prevention intervention for young gay men. *Am J Public Health.* 1996;86:1129–1136.

322. Elford J, Bolding G, Sherr L. Peer education has no significant impact on HIV risk behaviours among gay men in London. *AIDS.* 2001;15:535–537.

323. Flowers P, Hart GJ, Williamson LM, Frankis JS, Der GJ. Does bar-based, peer-led health promotion have a community-level effect amongst gay men in Scotland? *Int J STD AIDS.* 2002;13:102–108.
324. Valdiserri RO, Ogden LL, McCray E. Accomplishments in HIV prevention science: implications for stemming the epidemic. *Nat Med.* 2003;9:881–886.
325. Institute of Medicine. *No Time to Lose: Getting More from HIV Prevention.* Washington, DC: National Academies Press; 2001.
326. National Institutes of Health. Interventions to prevent HIV risk behaviors. NIH Consensus Statement (11–13 February 1997);15:1–41.
327. Celentano DD, Bond KC, Lyles C, et al. Preventive intervention to reduce sexually transmitted infections: a field trial in the Royal Thai Army. *Arch Intern Med.* 2000;160:535–540.
328. Quigley MA, Kamali A, Kinsman J, et al. The impact of attending a behavioural intervention on HIV incidence in Masaka, Uganda. *AIDS.* 2004;18:2055–2063.
329. Hanenberg RS, Rojanapithayakorn W, Kunasol P, Sokal DC. Impact of Thailand's HIV-control programme as indicated by the decline of sexually transmitted diseases. *Lancet.* 1994;344:243–245.
330. Celentano DD, Nelson KE, Lyles CM, et al. Decreasing incidence of HIV and sexually transmitted diseases in young Thai men: evidence for success of the HIV/AIDS control and prevention program. *AIDS.* 1998;12:F29–F36.
331. Singh S, Darroch JE, Bankole A. *A, B and C in Uganda: The Roles of Abstinence, Monogamy and Condom Use in HIV Decline.* Occasional Report No. 9. New York, NY: Alan Guttmacher Institute; December 2003. Available at: http://www.synergyaids.com/documents/UgandaABC.pdf. Accessed October 25, 2005.
332. Shelton JD, Halperin DT, Nantulya V, Potts M, Gayle HD, Holmes KK. Partner reduction is crucial for balanced "ABC" approach to HIV prevention. *BMJ.* 2004;328:891–894.
333. Parkhurst JO. The Ugandan success story? Evidence and claims of HIV-1 prevention. *Lancet.* 2002;360:78–80.
334. General Accounting Office. *Drug Abuse Treatment: Efforts Underway to Determine Effectiveness of State Programs.* Washington, DC: GAO; 2000.
335. Metzger DS, Navaline H, Woody GE. Drug-abuse treatment as AIDS prevention. *Public Health Rep.* 1998;113(suppl 1):S97–S106.
336. Hurley S, Jolley D, Kaldor J. Effectiveness of needle-exchange programmes for prevention of HIV infection. *Lancet.* 1997;349: 1797–1800.
337. Vlahov D, Junge B. The role of needle exchange programs in HIV prevention. *Public Health Rep.* 1988;113(suppl 1):S75–S80.
338. Semaan S, Des Jarlais DC, Sogolow E, et al. A meta-analysis of the effect of HIV prevention interventions on the sex behaviors of drug users in the United States. *JAIDS.* 2002;30(suppl 1):S73–S93.
339. Nelson KE, Galai N, Safaeia M, Strathdee SA, Celentano DD, Vlahov D. Temporal trends in the incidence of human immunodeficiency virus infection and risk behavior among injection drug users in Baltimore, Maryland 1988–1998. *Am J Epidemiol.* 2002;156: 641–653.
340. Stall RD, Hays RB, Waldo CR, et al. The Gay 90's: a review of research in the 1990s on sexual behavior and risk among men who have sex with men. *AIDS.* 2000;14(suppl):S101–S114.

341. Fox KK, del Rio C, Holmes KK, et al. Gonorrhea in the HIV era: a reversal in trends among men who have sex with men. *Am J Public Health.* 2001;91:959–964.

342. Johnson WD, Hedges LV, Ramirez G, et al. HIV prevention research for men who have sex with men: a systematic review and meta-analysis. *JAIDS.* 2002;30(suppl):S118–S129.

343. Herbst JH, Sherba RT, Crepaz N, et al. A meta-analytic review of HIV behavioral interventions for reducing sexual risk behavior of men who have sex with men. *JAIDS.* 2005;39:228–241.

344. Centers for Disease Control and Prevention. Advancing HIV prevention: new strategies for a changing epidemic–United States, 2003. *MMWR.* 2003;52:329–332.

345. Marks G, Crepaz N, Senterfitt JW, Janssen RS. Meta-analysis of high-risk sexual behavior in persons aware and unaware they are infected with HIV in the United States; implications for HIV prevention programs. *JAIDS.* 2005;39:446–453.

346. Auerbach JD, Coates TJ. HIV prevention research: accomplishments and challenges for the third decade of AIDS. *Am J Public Health.* 2000;90:1029–1032.

347. Gordon CM, Stall R, Cheever LW. Preventive interventions with persons living with HIV/AIDS; challenges, progress and research priorities. *JAIDS.* 2004;27(suppl 2):S53–S57.

348. Brindis CD, Loo VS, Adler NE, Bolan Ga, Wasserheit JN. Service integration and teen friendliness in practice: a program assessment of sexual and reproductive health services for adolescents. *J Adolesc Health.* 2005;37:155–162.

349. del Rio C. AIDS: the second wave. *Arch Med Res.* 2005;36:682–688.

350. Vanichseni S, Tappero JW, Pitsutiithum P, et al. Recruitment screening and characteristics of injection drug users participating in the AIDS VAX B/E HIV vaccine trial, Bangkok, Thailand. *AIDS.* 2004;18: 311–316.

351. Francis DR, Heyward W, Poporic V, et al. Candidate HIV/AIDS vaccines: lessons learned from the world's first phase III efficacy trials. *AIDS.* 2003;17:147–156.

352. The rgp120 HIV Vaccine Study Group. Placebo-controlled phase 3 trial of a recombinant glycoprotein 120 vaccine to prevent HIV-1 infection. *J Infect Dis.* 2005;191:654–665.

353. Gilbert PB, Peterson ML, Fullmann D, et al. Correlation between immunologic responses to a recombinant glycoprotein 120 vaccine and incidence of HIV-1 infection in a phase 3 HIV-1 preventive vaccine trial. *J Infect Dis.* 2005;191:656–677.

354. Graham BS, Mascola JR. Lessons from failure–preparing for future HIV-1 vaccine efficacy trials. *J Infect Dis.* 2005;191:647–649.

355. Koup RA, Safrit JT, Lao Y, et al. Temporal association of cellular immune responses with the initial control of viremia in primary human immunodeficiency virus type 1 syndrome. *J Virol.* 1999;23:6715–6720.

356. Patke DS, Langan JJ, Carroth LM, et al. Association of gag-specific T lymphocyte responses during the early phase of human immunodeficiency virus type 1 infection and lower virus set-point. *J Infect Dis.* 2002;186:1177–1180.

357. Lubaki NM, Shepherd ME, Brookmeyer RS, et al. HIV-1-specific cytolytic T-lymphocyte activity correlates with lower viral load, higher CD4 count and CD8+ CD38-DR-phenotype: comparison of statistical methods for measurement. *JAIDS.* 1999;22:19–30.

358. Rinaldo CR Jr, Bettz LA, Huang XL, Gupta P, Fan Z, Torpey DJ III. Anti-HIV type 1 cytotoxic T lymphocyte suppressive activity and disease progression in the first 8 years of HIV-type 1 infection of homosexual men. *AIDS Res Hum Retroviruses.* 1995;11:481–489.
359. Lo Caputo S, Trabattoni D, Vichi F, et al. Mucosal and systemic HIV-1 specific immunity in HIV-1 exposed but uninfected heterosexual men. *AIDS.* 2003;17:531–539.
360. Gallo RC. The end or the beginning of the drive to an HIV-preventive vaccine: a view from over 20 years. *Lancet.* 2005;366:1894–1898.
361. International AIDS Vaccine Initiative. *IRVI Bulletin, 2004: Year in Review.* Available at: http://www.IAVI.org. Accessed 2005.
362. World Health Organization. *Scaling Up Antiretroviral Therapy in Resource-Limited Settings; Treatment Guidelines for a Public Health Approach.* Geneva, Switzerland: WHO; 2003:1–58.
363. World Health Organization/UNAID. *Progress on Global Access to HIV Antiretroviral Therapy: An Update on "3 by 5."* Geneva, Switzerland: WHO/UNAIDS; 2005.
364. Centers for Disease Control and Prevention. Report to Congress on the President's Emergency Program for AIDS Relief (PEPFAR). Available at: http://www.cdc.gov. Accessed 2005.
365. Scheld JM. *Emerging infectious diseases.* Volume (6) 2005.
366. Walker N, Garcia-Calleja JM, Heaton L, et al. Epidemiological analysis of the quality of HIV sero-surveillance in the world: how well do we track the epidemic? *AIDS.* 2001;15:1545–1554.
367. Schwartlander B, Stover J, Walter N, et al. Resource needs for HIV/AIDS. *Science.* 2001;292:2434–2436.
368. Bertuzzi S, Guitiervez J-P, Opuni M, Walker N, Schwartlander B. Estimating resource needs for HIV/AIDS health care services in low-income and middle-income countries. *Health Policy.* 2004;69:189–200.

VIRAL HEPATITIS

Kenrad E. Nelson and David L. Thomas

Introduction

Hepatitis is inflammation of the liver, which may be caused by viral or other infections, toxins, and a number of other conditions. This chapter considers the epidemiology of the five diverse viruses that share the name *hepatitis* as they all cause hepatitis as their primary clinical syndrome. These include hepatitis A virus (HAV) and hepatitis E virus (HEV), which are transmitted by fecal-oral exposures from an infected to a susceptible individual, and hepatitis B virus (HBV), hepatitis C virus (HCV), and hepatitis delta virus (HDV), which are transmitted by blood or through sexual or perinatal contact.

Other viruses, such as cytomegalovirus (CMV), Epstein-Barr virus (EBV), yellow fever virus, Lassa fever virus, Ebola virus, and other agents may also infect the liver and cause hepatitis (Exhibit 22-1). However, their clinical manifestations usually reflect infection of other tissues, so they are not considered to be hepatitis viruses.

As early as the 1600s, epidemics of jaundice and other manifestations of liver disease were associated with military campaigns and were especially problematic during World War II.[1] Hepatitis following use of glycerinated human lymph to prevent smallpox was described in 1885.[2] Outbreaks of jaundice related to the administration of pooled human serum to prevent mumps[3] or to prepare a yellow fever vaccine[4] suggested that a transmissible agent was present in human blood. Blood transmission of hepatitis was also suggested by the frequent recognition of hepatitis in syphilis patients treated in clinics where injection equipment was not sterilized between patients.[5] Conversely, hepatitis was uncommon in patients attending clinics with good infection control practices.[5]

Exhibit 22-1   Conditions That Cause Hepatitis in Humans

Hepatitis viruses
  Hepatitis A virus
  Hepatitis B virus
  Hepatitis C virus
  Hepatitis D virus
  Hepatitis E virus

Other viruses
  Epstein-Barr virus
  Human immunodeficiency virus
  Lassa fever virus
  Yellow fever virus
  Adenovirus
  Herpes simplex virus
  Human herpes-6 virus
  Ebola virus

Nonviral infectious agents
  Pneumococcal pneumonia
  Leptospirosis
  Syphilis
  Coxiella burnetti
  Toxoplasmosis

Noninfections
  Alcohol
  Medications
    Dilantin
    Isoniazid
    Ritonavir
    Chlorpromazine
    Rifampin, etc.
  Anesthesia (halothane)

Along with the appreciation that human blood could transmit hepatitis came the recognition that many cases of hepatitis, including epidemics of the disease, did not follow blood exposure. The suspicion that there were at least two different epidemiologic types of hepatitis virus was confirmed by studies of Krugman et al at the Willowbrook State School in New York.[6] These studies showed that viruses he labeled MS-2 strains were exclusively transmitted parenterally; whereas other MS-1 strains could be transmitted orally. Furthermore, heat-inactivated convalescent sera obtained after MS-2 infection could prevent MS-2 infection. These studies laid the basis for the classification of hepatitis into serum hepatitis (MS-2 viruses) and infectious hepatitis (MS-1 viruses). In the 1950s and 1960s, there were numerous attempts to isolate the viruses or infect experimental animals with the agents responsible for hepatitis. In 1965 the "Australia antigen" was isolated from the blood of Australian aboriginals by Blumberg and associates.[7] This antigen was subsequently found to be the hepatitis B surface antigen (HBsAg).[8]

Within a decade of this discovery, the HBV virus and its major antigens had been fully characterized, and serologic tools became available for epidemiologic studies. After the introduction of the routine screening of blood donors for HBsAg in 1973, the incidence of posttransfusion hepatitis decreased by about 50%. Yet posttransfusion hepatitis that was not due to hepatitis B continued to occur indicating that another parenterally transmitted hepatitis virus existed.[9] HCV was discovered in 1989 and was shown to be the cause of most parenterally transmitted non-A, non-B (PT-NANB) hepatitis worldwide.[10-12] The hepatitis delta virus (HDV) was discovered by Rizzetto in 1977 and was initially described as a new antigen detectable in patients with HBV-associated chronic liver disease.[13] Studies in chimpanzees subsequently established that HDV was a unique RNA virus that was transmissible but dependent on the presence of active HBV infection to cause infection in humans.[14]

Viral particles of HAV were identified in stool samples of patients with infectious hepatitis in 1973.[15] Over the next several years, the immunologic and virologic aspects of HAV and its natural history were more clearly defined. In 1979, HAV was first grown in tissue culture[16]; subsequently, vaccines were developed from cell culture-derived virus and shown to be effective.[17,18]

However, large epidemics of waterborne hepatitis, most notably a very large epidemic that occurred in New Delhi, India, in 1955, were found not to be due to HAV.[18] Researchers found that convalescent sera from persons who were infected during this large epidemic did not have HAV antibodies.[19] The agent of these outbreaks was called enterically transmitted non-A, non-B hepatitis (ET-NANB).[20] Viruslike particles were identified in the feces of patients by immune electron microscopy in the early 1980s and named hepatitis E virus (HEV). Subsequently, an animal model of hepatitis E was developed in cynomolgus monkeys.[20,21]

Biologic Basis for Transmission

These five viruses differ markedly in their genetic composition and biology (Table 22-1). The viral characteristics can explain differences in transmission routes. HBV, HCV, and HDV are not transmitted through fecal-oral exposure as their lipid envelopes are unstable in the biliary excretory tract, rendering them noninfectious in stool. HAV and HEV do not have envelopes, are infectious in stool, and are relatively stable under environmental conditions. In contrast, the capability of hepatitis viruses to be spread by blood relates to the total time and viral levels in serum. All hepatitis viruses can cause infection if they are percutaneously inoculated. However, HAV and HEV exist in blood for very brief intervals and, thus, only rarely contaminate percutaneous transmission vehicles, such as blood products or needles. In contrast, HBV, HCV, and HDV may be detected in the blood of asymptomatic carriers for decades.

Clinical Syndrome

All hepatitis viruses may cause the same general syndrome (Exhibit 22-2). After exposure, there is an incubation period lasting from 2 to 10 weeks for

TABLE 22-1   Characteristics of Hepatitis Viruses

Virus	Nucleic Acid	Routes of Transmission	Mortality	Risk of Chronic Illlness
HAV	Unenveloped single-stranded RNA	Fecal-oral	Low	None
HBV	Enveloped double-stranded DNA	Parenteral (sex, perinatal)	Moderate–high	High
HCV	Enveloped single-stranded RNA	Parenteral (sex, perinatal)	Moderate–high	High
HDV	Enveloped single-stranded RNA	Parenteral (sex)	High	High
HEV	Unenveloped single-stranded RNA	Fecal-oral	Low–moderate	None

Exhibit 22–2   Clinical Course of Viral Hepatitis

Incubation	Time from exposure to first symptoms ranges from 2–4 weeks for HAV to 6–12 weeks for HBV.
Prodrome	A flulike illness can precede jaundice.
Icterus	Jaundice (dark urine and yellow discoloration of sclera) occurs variably in adults, most with HAV and least with HCV infection.
Convalescence	Period of resolution of jaundice.
Recovery or persistence	In the months after HCV, HBV, and HDV infections, it becomes evident whether an infection will persist or resolve; HAV and HEV infections always resolve and never become chronic.

HAV and HEV, from 4 to 10 weeks for HCV, and from 6 to 20 weeks for HBV. This may be followed by a flulike prodromal illness with fever, chills, anorexia, vomiting, and fatigue. A few patients with HBV infection develop an urticarial rash, arthralgia, arthritis, or glomerulonephritis during the acute illness, which are cause by immune complexes. As the systemic symptoms improve, jaundice may occur, followed by a period of convalescence. The hallmark of hepatitis is an elevation in the blood of levels of enzymes contained in the liver, specifically alanine aminotransferase (ALT) and aspartate aminotransferase (AST). The blood bilirubin may also rise, with levels greater than 3.0 mg/dL producing jaundice. Rarely, patients will develop acute fulminant hepatic necrosis and liver failure. This is less frequent with HCV than with the other hepatitis viruses.

Hepatitis A Virus

Virology

The hepatitis A virus (HAV) is a small (27 nm) nonenveloped RNA virus belonging to the family Picornaviridae. The virus, which has icosohedral symmetry and contains about 2500 nucleotides, is composed of at least four major structural polypeptides, VP1 to VP4. The genomic organization and replication of HAV are similar to that of polio virus and other picornaviruses. However, HAV has little nucleotide or amino acid homology with other enteroviruses, and there is less evidence that HAV replicates in intestinal tissues. HAV was originally classified in the genus *Enterovirus*, but it is now classified in a separate genus, designated *Hepatovirus*.

HAV is quite stable in the environment after it is shed in the feces, retaining infectivity for at least 2 to 4 weeks at room temperatures. The virus is resistant to nonionic detergents, chloroform, or ether, and it retains infectivity at pH 1.0 at 38°C for 90 minutes. It is only partially inactivated at 60°C for 1 hour. Temperatures of 85° to 95°C for 1 minute are required to inactivate HAV in shellfish. It is also relatively resistant to free chlorine, especially when the virus is associated with organic matter. These features explain the occurrence of HAV outbreaks from consumption of shellfish and other foods or beverages and outbreaks associated with swimming pools.

HAV exists as a single serotype, and HAV infection—whether symptomatic or not—confers lifelong immunity in people infected with strains from any location worldwide. Only man and several nonhuman primates (e.g., marmosets, tamarins, owl monkeys, and chimpanzees) are known to be naturally infected with HAV.

In 1979, HAV was cultured in fetal rhesus monkey kidney cells after the virus had been passaged multiple times in marmosets.[16] Since then, HAV has been cultivated directly from clinical or environmental samples, but adaptation periods of 4 to 10 weeks have been required for detection of significant amounts of HAV antigen in infected cells. Generally, HAV isolates do not produce cytopathology in tissue cultures, although cytopathic variants have been isolated that produce plaques in cell culture.

The isolation of the virus has allowed comparative virologic studies to be done and diagnostic reagents to be developed to confirm current or past infection and immunity.

Clinical Features and Diagnosis

In the individual, the clinical features of acute HAV infection are not sufficiently distinctive to allow differentiation from other types of acute viral hepatitis. However, prodromal symptoms, including anorexia, nausea, abdominal discomfort, diarrhea, and fever may be more prominent than in patients infected with HBV or HCV, and they often begin abruptly. Rarely, arthritis, urticarial rash, arteritis, or aplastic anemia has been reported in patients with acute HAV infection. HAV infection can cause 2.0% to 27% of cases of acute fulminant hepatitis in developed countries.[22,23] Unlike HBV and HCV infections, there is no evidence that HAV causes chronic hepatitis. However, about 10% to 15% of patients with acute HAV have a relapse of their illness within a few weeks of their recovery. These relapses include excretion of virus in the stool, indicating that patients are infectious during a clinical relapse.[24]

An important clinical feature of HAV infection is the inverse correlation of symptoms with the age of the patient. Most infants and children under age 6 have mild, often nonspecific symptoms or, more commonly, their acute infection is completely asymptomatic. Among children under age 3, only about 5% develop jaundice. The rate of icteric disease is about 10% in children 4 to 6 years of age. In contrast, most adolescents and adults develop jaundice, and 75% develop characteristic prodromal symptoms. The public health importance of HAV infections in developed countries is related to the high rates of morbidity, which can persist for a few weeks. As noted above, some patients will have a recurrence of symptoms that prolongs morbidity.

The specific diagnosis of HAV infection is confirmed by testing a serum specimen for IgM antibodies to HAV. The antibody assay is highly sensitive and specific. Antibodies of the IgM class usually develop by the time the patient is symptomatic and persist for 3 to 6 months. Total Ig or IgG antibodies in the absence of IgM antibodies usually signify previous infection. Most patients, even those who are not icteric, will have elevated serum ALT and AST levels during the acute infection. Although HAV is present in the stool in the presymptomatic and preicteric phases of the illness, viral cultures are not generally done because of the difficulty in isolation of this virus in tissue culture.[25]

Transmission Routes

The principal means of HAV transmission is by ingestion of infectious feces. Infection can occur by direct person-to-person transfer of virus on hands or fomites, or by consumption of contaminated food or water. As noted earlier, blood-borne transmission is uncommon as HAV is only present in the blood from the middle of the incubation period until early in the clinical illness. Infectivity titers in the stool are very high, up to 10^8 infectious units per gram of feces in the late incubation period and first week of the illness.[26] Virus can also be present in saliva at titers of 10^{2-3} or lower per ml.[27] Household or sexual contact with a person with hepatitis is the most common exposure reported by patients with HAV infections reported to the Centers for Disease Control and Prevention (CDC), accounting for about 22% of cases (Figure 22-1).[28] To be counted as a secondary case, the most recent exposure to a case of hepatitis should have been 2 to 6 weeks before onset of illness. Transmission among homosexual men has been well documented; whether this occurs through sexual contact or simply by nonsexual intimate contact is not clear.[29,30]

Transmission of HAV by blood occurs infrequently.[31,32] However, a large outbreak of parenterally transmitted HAV was reported in 1994 among European hemophiliacs infected by contaminated clotting factor concentrates.[33] The clotting factor concentrate was purified from a large pool of plasma donors who did not have neutralizing antibodies so that HAV in the preparation was not inactivated.[34] Injection drug users are believed to be at increased risk of infection, but the route of transmission could be parenteral or fecal-oral transmission from poor hygienic practices.[29,35,36] Common-source outbreaks have occurred from contamination of food and water supplies.[37,38] Food-borne

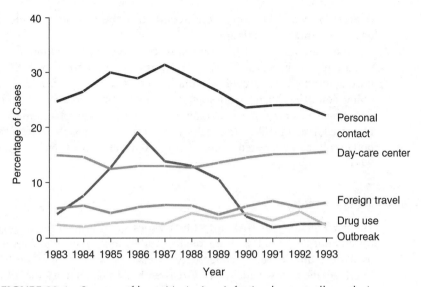

FIGURE 22-1   Sources of hepatitis A virus infection by mutually exclusive groups, United States, 1983–1993.
Source: Reprinted from Viral Hepatitis Surveillance Program, Centers for Disease Control and Prevention.

outbreaks usually result from contamination of food by an infected food handler who is asymptomatic or is in the incubation period. Uncooked foods, such as salads, fruit, lettuce, sandwiches, glazed or iced pastries, and some dairy products are particularly susceptible.[39,40] Some food-borne outbreaks have involved consumption of shellfish harvested from sewage-contaminated waters that have been eaten with little or no cooking.[41,42] Bivalve mollusks, such as clams, oysters, and mussels, are at particular high risk of transmission of HAV because they filter large volumes of water and concentrate infectious HAV and other viruses in their digestive system.[43] In addition, outbreaks of HAV have been reported from consumption of foods contaminated at the time of harvest or processing that were subsequently served raw, such as lettuce, onions, strawberries, and raspberries.[39,40] Nevertheless, hepatitis traced to contaminated food or water accounts for only about 8% of HAV cases reported to the CDC.[44,45]

Transmission in the day-care setting has been studied, especially in Maricopa County (Phoenix), Arizona. Studies in this area in the late 1970s identified a two-fold increase in HAV cases; most of the increase could be traced to direct or indirect contact with an infected child or employee in a day-care center.[46-48]

In centers enrolling children in diapers, hepatitis A outbreaks may be common. In this setting, HAV may be spread not only among children but also to adult contacts in the center, at home, or in the community. Infected infants and young children are rarely jaundiced, but they may transmit HAV to adult contacts, who are more likely to become symptomatic. Adult contacts of 1- to 2-year-old children are at highest risk of infection. In centers not enrolling children in diapers, outbreaks are much less common.[46] In addition to the absence of symptoms in infected children, prolonged viral secretion in infants has been linked to transmission in day-care centers and hospitals.

Over 15% of all HAV infections reported to the CDC have been related to day-care center transmission.

International travel to developing countries with contaminated food or water supplies may also result in HAV infection. The risk of HAV infection during international travel is highest among long-term residents of developing countries, such as missionaries, Peace Corps volunteers, and military and peacekeeping force personnel.[49-51] Although short-term tourists are at increased risk of HAV, the risk is not great as most travelers can avoid potentially contaminated water and foods during short travel periods (Figure 22-1).

Worldwide Epidemiology

The epidemiology of HAV infections varies greatly in different populations throughout the world. Seroprevalence studies in various countries have been used to define levels of endemicity to classify areas into those with high, intermediate, or low endemicity. Areas with high endemicity for HAV include countries in Africa, Asia, Central and South America, and the Middle East (Figure 22-2). In these areas, the prevalence of HAV antibody reaches 90% among adults, and most children become infected by age 10. However, persons of upper socioeconomic class may not become infected until they reach adolescence or adulthood.

In more developed countries in Europe and Asia, the endemicity of HAV is intermediate, and the prevalence of HAV antibody varies widely. In countries such as Italy, Greece, Thailand, Taiwan, and Korea, the prevalence of HAV antibody in adults reaches 80% or higher, but in children under age 10,

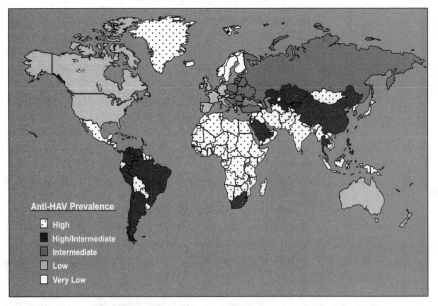

FIGURE 22-2 Geographic distribution of HAV infection.
Source: Viral Hepatitis Surveillance Program, Centers for Disease Control and Prevention.

antibody prevalence is only 20% to 30%, and the major increase in antibody occurs in persons between the ages of 10 and 20 years (Figure 22-3).[52-55] These data indicate a cohort effect in which older adults belong to cohorts that were infected in childhood. Paradoxically, this delay in the occurrence of infection actually increases morbidity, because early childhood infection is usually asymptomatic.[51]

In Europe and the United States, HAV antibody prevalence in adults varies from 30% to 50% but is less than 10% in children under age 10. However, low socioeconomic status is associated with high rates of infection.[56]

In some northern European countries and in Japan, HAV infection has become quite unusual. The antibody prevalence is well below 10% in children and adolescents. However, adults over age 40 have antibody prevalence of 30% to 60%, indicating a cohort effect when HAV infections were more common.

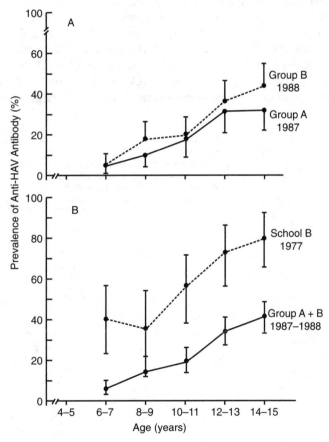

FIGURE 22-3   Age-specific hepatitis A (HAV) antibody prevalence (with 95% confidence intervals) among schoolchildren in Bangkok: A, rates measured in 1987 (group A) and 1988; B, combined antibody prevalence rates for groups A and B contrasted to those in the group B school in 1977.
Source: B.L. Innis, R. Snitbhan, and C.H. Hoke et al., The Declining Transmission of Hepatitis A in Thailand, *Journal of Infectious Diseases*, Vol. 163, pp. 989–995, Copyright 1991, University of Chicago Press.

In countries with high endemicity of HAV infection, most acute hepatitis in children under age 15 is due to HAV; however, HAV is rarely the cause of hepatitis in adults. In areas of intermediate endemicity, studies have shown that a relatively high proportion (50% to 60%) of adult cases of hepatitis are due to HAV. In low endemicity areas in Western Europe and the United Sates, the majority of acute hepatitis cases in children is caused by HAV, but in adults, the proportion varies from 10% to 50%.[56]

Despite the fact that the United States is considered to be a country where the endemicity of HAV is low, there is considerable geographic variation among HAV incidence rates within the country. In the United States, counties having more than 10% of the population classified as American Indian have HAV incidence rates 3.5 times higher than other counties.[56,57] Similarly, counties with 15% or more of the population classified as Hispanic have average rates 2.1 times higher than other counties. The incidence rate by age is highest in persons under age 40.

In the United States and many other countries with low or intermediate endemicity, HAV incidence is cyclical, with 7- to 10-year peaks in the number of reported cases (Figure 22-4). Recent peak years occurred in 1971 (59,000 cases; 29/100,000), 1989 (36,000 cases; 14/100,000), and 1995 (31,582 cases; 12/100,000) (Figure 22-4).[44,58-60] The cyclical pattern of HAV is even more apparent in surveillance data from Shanghai, China (Figure 22-5). These data show a substantial epidemic of HAV in 1989, over 300,000 cases, due to consumption of contaminated raw clams.[42] This large food-borne epidemic

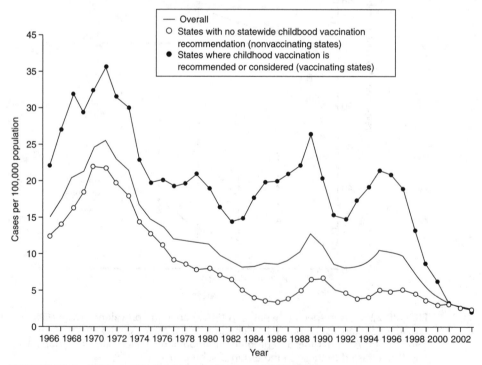

FIGURE 22-4   US hepatitis A incidence by year, 1966–2003.
Source: Wasley A et al. Incidence of Hepatitis A in the United States in the Era of Vaccination. JAMA. Vol. 294 No. 2. 194–201.

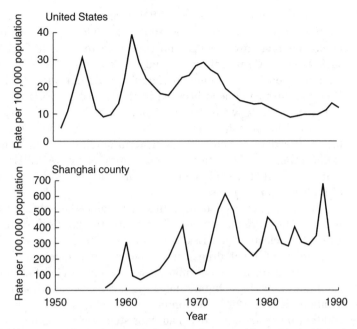

FIGURE 22-5 Incidence patterns of reported cases of hepatitis A, United States and Shanghai County, People's Republic of China.
Source: A.S. Evans and R.A. Kaslow, *Viral Infections of Humans,* p. 269, © 1997, Plenum Publishing Corporation.

illustrates the potential for explosive epidemics of HAV in a country where the endemicity has been reduced in recent years by improvements in the hygiene. Low transmission results in the accumulation of a large susceptible population in which a large outbreak can occur.

Prevention

Improved environmental sanitation to prevent fecal contamination of food and water has been the most important means of preventing infection.[52-55] Prior to development of a vaccine, passive immunization with pooled human immunoglobulin (IG) was used as post- or preexposure prophylaxis against hepatitis A. IG is highly effective in preventing symptomatic HAV infections if given before or within 2 weeks after exposure to the virus.[61,62] If given prior to exposure, IG is nearly 100% effective in preventing symptomatic infection. However, depending on the dose, this protection may last for 1 to 6 months. If given after exposure, IG is only 75% to 85% effective[63]; HAV infection may occur, but symptoms are rare, and fecal shedding of the virus is limited. The decreased symptoms in patients who receive IG after infection may be due to control of the spread of HAV within the liver until a protective immune response is mounted. The use of IG as postexposure prophylaxis is also called passive-active immunization.[37]

For postexposure prophylaxis of adult household contacts of acute cases, the usual recommended dose of IG is 0.02 mL/kg, or about 1.5 to 2.0 mL given intramuscularly. IG is often not recommended or is ineffective in common-source food-borne or waterborne outbreaks when exposure is identified too late for infection to be prevented.[64,65] Prior to the licensure of effective HAV vaccines, repeated preexposure prophylaxis with IG was recommended at 6-month intervals for persons who continued to be at high risk of exposure, such as Peace Corps volunteers and medical missionaries.[63] However, active immunization is now a much preferable preventive strategy. Two inactivated HAV vaccines have been licensed in the United States. These vaccines were tested in 1- to 16-year-olds in Thailand[18] and in 2- to 16-year-olds living in a Hassidic Jewish community in New York state.[17] Both vaccines are highly effective. Although the long-term durability of the immune response is uncertain, the high efficacy in preventing acute HAV raises the possibility that HAV morbidity could be reduced dramatically with selective vaccination of high-risk populations.

After the licensure of hepatitis A vaccine the Advisory Committee on Immunization Practices of the Centers for Disease Control recommended in 1996 that selected high-risk populations, such as men who have sex with men, users of illicit drugs, and travelers to endemic countries, be given vaccine.[66] Also routine vaccination was recommended for children living in communities with the highest hepatitis A incidence, such as Native American communities. In 1999, the committee recommended routine vaccination of children living in states that had consistently elevated hepatitis A rates and a distinctive pattern of hepatitis A epidemiology (Figure 22-6).[67] These recommendations included 11 states with reported rates of hepatitis A infection over 20/100,000 and an additional 6 states with rates of 10/100,000 or more. An evaluation of the results of these recommendations showed a dramatic decline in the incidence of HAV, so that by 2002 the rates in the states with

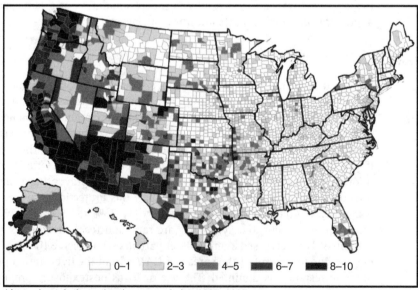

□ 0–1   ▦ 2–3   ▨ 4–5   ▩ 6–7   ▪ 8–10

*Approximately the national average during 1987–1997.
Source: National Notifiable Diseases Surveillance System.

FIGURE 22-6 Number of years that reported incidence of hepatitis A exceeded 10 cases per 100,000,* by county—1987–1997.
Source: MMWR. October 1, 1999 / Vol. 48 / No. RR-12.

previously high incidence was the same as that in the other states (Figure 22-4).[1] However, the incidence of HAV has declined overall in the United States since the licensure and use of the hepatitis A vaccine. Research on the development of a live attenuated HAV vaccine is continuing in the hope that a less expensive, easier-to-administer vaccine can be developed to control HAV globally. An immunization program was started in Israel in 1999 in which toddlers aged 18–24 months were given two doses of HAV vaccine. This resulted in a 95% reduction in reported hepatitis A infections, from 50.4 per 100,000 in 1993–1998 to 2.4 per 100,000, suggesting a profound effect of herd immunity by vaccination of toddlers.

Hepatitis B Virus

Virology

Hepatitis B virus is a partially double-stranded DNA virus that is a member of the family Hepadnaviridae. This family includes several other animal viruses, including woodchuck hepatitis virus, duck hepatitis virus, and ground squirrel hepatitis virus. The HBV genome has about 3200 nucleotides and replicates through an RNA intermediate that is transcribed by a gene product with reverse transcriptase activity. The proteins encoded by the HBV genome are the envelope, the nucleocapsid, the X protein, and a DNA polymerase. The envelope proteins encoded by the HBV genome include pre-S, pre-S2, and the HBsAg, which is a glycosylated lipoprotein that contains the major site for binding of neutralizing antibody. HBsAg can circulate as a part of the complete virion (i.e., the Dane particle) or independently of viral particles. Four subtypes of HBsAg have been identified, which are designated adw, ayw, adr, and ayr. The "a" epitope, which is common to all HBsAg subtypes, is the binding epitope for neutralizing antibodies.

Therefore, antibodies to HBsAg are protective for all subtypes.[68] However, occurrence of the other subtype determinants varies geographically, such that HBsAg subtyping has been used in epidemiologic studies to establish patterns of transmission.[69] The subtypes do not appear to differ in infectivity or virulence. Nonlethal mutations can also occur in the S gene, sufficiently altering expression of this protein to permit viral escape from neutralizing antibodies.

HBV encodes nucleocapsid proteins, which include HBeAg and HBV core antigen (HBcoreAg). HBeAg is a marker for current active viral replication. However, mutations can occur that truncate expression of "e" antigen without substantially altering virion production. The resultant viral phenotype results in clinical infection with HBV DNA and HBsAg but no detectable HBeAg in the blood. Some individuals infected with these HBeAg-negative mutant viruses have developed fulminant hepatitis.[70,71] The HBcoreAg is the major nucleocapsid protein and is not detected in the serum but is present in the liver. The cellular immune response to HBcoreAg in the liver is believed by some investigators to be responsible for hepatic necrosis associated with chronic liver disease in HBV carriers.[72–75] Persons infected with HBV form antibodies to HBcoreAg that are persistent, making them useful in the diagnosis of current or previous infection. Humans are the only natural host for HBV infection. The chimpanzee is the primary experimental model for infection, but the disease has also been studied in gibbons, marmosets, and other primates.[76] HBV can retain infectivity for at least 1 month at room temperature and much longer when frozen. Heating to 90°C for 1 hour renders HBV noninfectious.

Clinical Features and Diagnosis

The clinical features of HBV infection are similar to those of other hepatitis viruses and range from asymptomatic infection to jaundice following a flulike prodromal illness. However, persons with acute HBV infection are more likely to develop a serum sickness–like illness (arthritis, arthralgia, urticarial rash), and chronic infection is associated with glomerulonephritis or vasculitis resembling periarteritis nodosa.[77]

As with HAV infection, a direct relationship exists between the age of the patient and the likelihood that an acute HBV infection will be symptomatic. Infections in infants and children rarely cause jaundice, and they usually remain completely asymptomatic; whereas 10% to 20% of children over age 6 and 40% to 50% of adults develop jaundice with acute HBV infection.[78]

The probability that chronic infection will develop is inversely related to the rates of jaundice during acute infection. In infants born to a mother who is an HBeAg-positive carrier, the risk of infection with chronic carriage (defined as carriage for over 1 year) is about 80%.[79] The risk of chronic infection decreases with increasing age.[80] By age 6, chronic infection occurs in 5% to 10% of individuals. The risk of chronic infection in adolescents and adults is 1% to 5%. Persons who are immunosuppressed, such as patients on dialysis, oncology or transplant patients, or persons with HIV infection or AIDS, have high rates of chronic carriage of HBV after acute infection.

Most persons with persistent HBV infection do not develop chronic liver disease, and a spectrum of histologic disease has been described.[81-83] Some patients have normal liver biopsies; chronic persistent hepatitis is diagnosed in patients with low-grade focal inflammation, and chronic active hepatitis is characterized by diffuse active inflammation with bridging necrosis between hepatic lobules. Cirrhosis is characterized by scarring, diffuse necrosis, and regeneration and disruption of hepatic lobular architecture.

The probability of clinically significant chronic liver disease is higher in persons infected as infants or children than when infection occurs during adult life.[84] Prospective studies in Taiwan have estimated that 25% of persons infected as infants or children who become chronic HBV carriers develop primary hepatocellular carcinoma (PHC) during their lifetime.[84-88]

Hepatitis B Virus and Primary Liver Cancer

In the last 30 years, considerable evidence has been published describing chronic HBV infection as a cause of PHC in humans The evidence includes ecologic data that indicate geographic areas where the HBV carrier rates are highest (Figure 22-7), as well as the areas where PHC is most common. More persuasive are several prospective cohort studies of infection with HBV and the subsequent development of PHC. In the largest and most comprehensive of these studies, Beasley et al studied 22,707 male civil servants between the

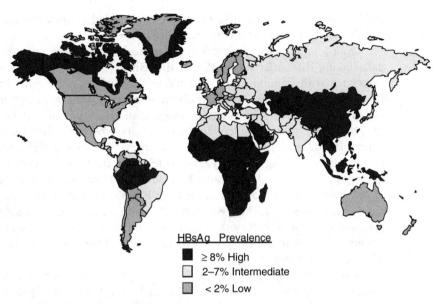

HBsAg Prevalence
- ≥ 8% High
- 2–7% Intermediate
- < 2% Low

FIGURE 22-7   Geographic distribution of chronic HBV infection.
Source: Division of Viral Hepatitis, Centers for Disease Control and Prevention.

ages of 40 and 59 in Taiwan between March 15, 1976 and June 3, 1978.[86] These men were all healthy and free of liver cancer at baseline. By December 1985, 151 of these men experienced incident PHC in a cumulative 186,000 person-years of follow-up, an average of 8.2 per 100 person-years. Overall, 141 of the men who developed PHC were HBsAg carriers at baseline; the rate of PHC in the HBsAg carriers was 505 per 100 person-years of follow-up. Among non-HBsAg carriers, the rate of PHC was only 5.3 per 100 person-years. The relative risk of PHC for HBsAg carriers was 104 times higher than for noncarriers at baseline.

Additional prospective studies of the risk of PHC in areas where this neoplasm is common have shown similar strong associations with chronic HBV infection.[85] The risk is especially high in China, and prospective studies suggest that 40% of Chinese males with chronic HBV infection will die from PHC.[86] The World Health Organization has estimated that 80% of all PHC cases in the world occur in persons with chronic HBV infection.[85]

Although the precise molecular mechanism of carcinogenesis is not known, HBV DNA is often clonally integrated into the cellular DNA of carcinoma cells, indicating that these tumors have arisen by a clonal expansion in a cell with HBV integration.[87-89] The oncogenic potential of HBV is supported by data from studies of carcinogenesis of other animal hepadnaviruses. Chronic hepatitis and liver cancer have been documented in woodchucks in the United States and in ducks in China that are infected with other hepadnaviruses closely related to HBV. The association of PHC with persistent hepadnavirus infections in woodchucks and the Beachey ground squirrel is even stronger than the association between HBV and PHC in humans. In fact, the risk of liver cancer in animals who have carried these hepadnaviruses for 3 years or more approaches 100%.[90-94] Oncogenesis may also be the result of

HBV-induced increased cell turnover. Other chronic liver diseases are linked to PHC, and this may be a common mechanism.

From a public health perspective, the most encouraging and persuasive data linking HBV infection to PHC is the reduction in the incidence of PHC associated with immunization for HBV in Taiwan.[95] A nationwide hepatitis B vaccination program of all newborn infants of HBsAg-carrier mothers began in July 1984. The program was expanded to include all newborns in 1987, then to include children and adults who were HBV-uninfected between 1987 and 1990. The rates of primary liver cancer reported to the tumor registry among 6- to 9-year-olds fell from 0.52 per 100,000 (82 cases among 15,739,570 children) born between July 1978 and June 1984, prior to the immunization program, to 0.13 per 100,000 (3 cases among 2,281,106 children) in those born between July 1984 and June 1986. This significant decrease was not seen for other neoplasms and strongly suggests that HBV immunization of newborns prevented subsequent liver cancer in this cohort of immunized children.

A study in Shanghai, China, found a synergistic interaction between chronic HBV infection and aflatoxin biomarkers in the urine of patients with PHC.[96] The relative risk for PHC was 7.3 in those with HBsAg alone and 3.4 in subjects with aflatoxin biomarkers only, but it was 59.4 in subjects who were aflatoxin positive in addition to having chronic HBV infection.

Diagnosis

The diagnosis of HBV infection is usually confirmed using serologic tests. The glycoprotein coat of HBV contains HBsAg, which is produced in excess and can circulate independent of the virus. Detection of HBsAg has evolved from first-generation immunodiffusion methods to third-generation methods, including reverse passive hemagglutination (RPHA) and more sensitive methods that utilize radioimmunoassay (RAI) or enzyme immunoassay (EIA).

The presence of HBsAg indicates active HBV infection, but testing for IgM antibody to hepatitis B core (anti-HBc) is needed to determine whether the HBV infection is acute or chronic. Detection of HBsAg is possible in acute infections during the incubation period prior to the increase in liver enzymes or the appearance of jaundice and for several weeks thereafter (Figure 22-8). In persons who develop chronic HBV infection, HBsAg persists in the serum, and symptoms during acute infection are uncommon (Figure 22-9).

Antibody to HBsAg (anti-HBs) appears with recovery from acute infection and after immunization with HBV vaccine, which is prepared from purified HBsAg. Anti-HBs titers have been measured to document the levels of protective antibodies after immunization, and anti-HBs of 10 IU/mL or more are felt to be protective. Commonly, anti-HBs levels may not rise for several months after acute HBV infection, and initially they complex with HBsAg and may be undetectable.

Hepatitis B core antigen (HBcAg) is part of the viral nucleocapsid. No serologic test for HBcAg is available because this antigen doesn't circulate but is localized within hepatic cells. However, antibodies to HBcAg (anti-HBc) are commonly used to diagnose current or past HBV infection. Anti-HBc develops soon after HBV infection and persists for the lifetime of an individual.[97,98] Therefore, it is a good marker of past HBV infection. IgM

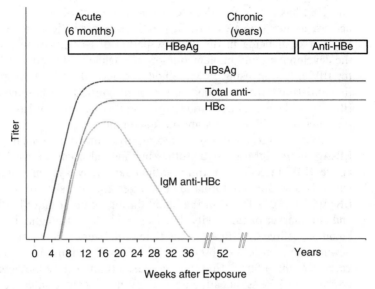

FIGURE 22-8 Progression to chronic hepatitis B infection.
Source: Division of Viral Hepatitis, Centers for Disease Control and Prevention.

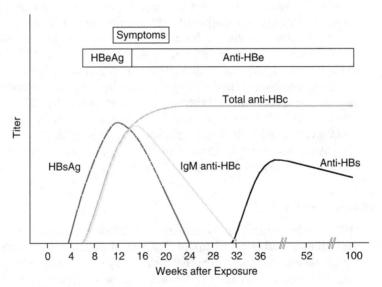

FIGURE 22-9 Acute hepatitis B infection with recovery.
Source: Division of Viral Hepatitis, Centers for Disease Control and Prevention.

anti-HBc persists for the first 3 to 6 months after an acute HBV infection and is a good marker of acute infection. Antibodies to HBcAg (anti-HBcAg) can be useful in measuring infection after HBV vaccine, because the vaccine will produce only anti-HBs. Anti-HBc testing has also been used to screen blood donors since 1987, because these antibodies were found to be a useful surrogate marker for hepatitis C virus infection (HCV) prior to the licensure of specific antibody tests for HCV in 1990.[99,100] Screening of blood donors for anti-HBc has continued, despite the development of sensitive tests for HCV because donors who are anti-HBc positive also are believed to be at somewhat higher risk of being in the window period of HIV infection. However, with the development and implementation of nucleic acid testing of blood donors for HIV infection using PCR methods, some authorities have recommended that anti-HBc testing of blood donors be discontinued. But screening for anti-HBcore has been retained largely because it is a marker of HBV infection and false-negative HBsAg tests are not uncommon.

Although the diagnosis of recent HBV infection is made by detecting HBsAg and/or IgM anti-HBc, other methods also can be used to document active HBV infection. A third antigen–antibody system involves HBeAg, which is a soluble conformational antigen that consists of a portion of the HBcAg. HBeAg is found in the blood during acute or chronic HBV infection and is a marker of infectivity. For example, 90% of pregnant women whose blood is positive for HBeAg at the time of delivery will transmit HBV to their newborn infants in the absence of the administration of immunoglobulin or vaccine to the infant.[79] However, because infants whose mothers are HBsAg-positive but HBeAg negative at delivery may become infected, decisions to use HBV vaccine for prevention of transmission are not based on the HBeAg status of the mother. On the other hand, the potential infectivity of health care personnel and subsequent work restrictions are judged largely by HBeAg results. The enzyme HBV DNA polymerase can also be measured in the serum and, like HBeAg, is a marker of active replication of HBV.

In addition to the serologic methods described above, HBV DNA can be detected in serum by nucleic acid hybridization or PCR amplification. Although these diagnostic methods are primarily available in research laboratories, monitoring HBV DNA levels can be a useful method of following patients receiving antiviral therapy and for screening for HBsAg mutants (see above). HBV DNA can be detected in tissue by in situ hybridization or PCR amplification. HBV does not replicate reliably to high titers in cell cultures. The dynamics of the appearance of HBV antigens and antibody responses to infection are depicted in Figures 22-8 and 22-9.

Transmission Routes

HBV can be transmitted by percutaneous blood exposure, sexual intercourse, and from a mother to her infant. The risk of parenteral transmission of HBV in developed countries has been greatly reduced in recent years by the screening of blood donors for HBsAg and the use of sterile disposable injection equipment. However, parenteral transmission still occurs in some situations. Persons who inject illicit drugs commonly share injection equipment and have a very high prevalence and incidence of HBV infection.[101,102] Persons receiving pooled blood products also have high rates of HBV infection because very large pools may include a rare donor who was in the seronegative window period or had a false-negative test for HBsAg at the time of donation.

In many developing countries, where the HBsAg carrier rate is very high (i.e., 10% or higher) in the general population and disposable injection equipment is not available, HBV transmission by medical injections continues to be common. Also, parenteral exposures, such as acupuncture, tattoos, and body piercing, are risks for HBV transmission.

Because of the very high concentration of virus in some persons with acute or chronic HBV infection, up to 10^{10} virions/mL, exposures to minute amounts of blood that occur from activities such as sharing of toothbrushes, razors, wash cloths, or towels and the presence of eczematous skin lesions that exude serum can result in transmission in the household setting.[103-105] HBV transmission has also been demonstrated to occur in children or teachers in a classroom.[106] Other populations who are at high risk of HBV infection include clients of institutions for the developmentally disabled and prisoners.

HBV is also transmitted by sexual intercourse. Numerous studies in various populations have shown that the prevalence of HBV increases with the number of sex partners.[107-109] Populations with large numbers of partners, such as commercial sex workers and both homosexuals and heterosexuals with multiple partners, have very high prevalence of HBV infection.[107-109] In households, the sexual partners of an HBsAg carrier are at much greater risk of HBV infection than are others in the household.[103,107,108] Virologic studies have shown that HBV is present in semen and other secretions, although at levels 100- to 1000-fold lower than in the blood.

In many parts of the world, HBV infection is commonly acquired during the perinatal period or in early childhood. Infants born to a mother who is an HBsAg carrier and is HBeAg positive have a 90% risk of acquiring an HBV infection if they are not given hepatitis B immunoglobulin or HBV vaccine.[79] Infants of women who are HBsAg positive but HBeAg negative have a lower (but still elevated) risk.

Worldwide Epidemiology

The prevalence of HBV infection varies greatly worldwide. In some areas of the world, HBV infections are highly endemic, and 8% or more of the total population are chronic carriers of HBsAg. These areas constitute 45% of the global population and include China and Southeast Asian countries, sub-Saharan Africa, and several areas in the Arctic, including Alaska, Northern Canada, and Greenland (Figure 22-7). In most of these areas, primary liver cancer is also very common and is often the most frequent cancer in adult males. Nearly all HBV infections occur during the perinatal period or in early childhood in these areas. Because acute HBV infections in infancy and early childhood result in a high rate of chronic carriage, the high endemicity is perpetuated from one generation to the next.

In developed countries of North America, Western Europe, Australia, and some areas of South America, the rates of HBV infection are much lower. Less than 2% of the population are chronic carriers, and the overall infection rate, measured by the prevalence of anti-HBc antibodies, is 5% to 20% (Figure 22-7). In these areas, which constitute 12% of the global population, the frequency of perinatal or early childhood infection is low; however, they may account for a disproportionately high number of chronic HBV infections. Also, immigrants from highly endemic areas may contribute substantially to the subset of HBV infections that are transmitted during the perinatal and early childhood period.[107,108] In these areas, most infections occur among high-risk adult populations, including injection drug users; homosexual men; persons with multiple sex partners; patients with multiple exposures to pooled blood products, such as hemophiliacs; and health care workers.[107]

The remaining parts of the world, which constitute about 43% of the global population, have an intermediate rate of HBV infection (Figure 22-7). The prevalence of HBsAg positivity ranges from 2% to 8%, and serologic evidence of past infection is found in 20% to 60% of the population. In these areas, there are mixed patterns of infant, early childhood, and adult transmission.

The CDC has estimated the risk factors for acute hepatitis B virus infection by detailed epidemiologic assessment of the behaviors associated with infection in the sentinel counties study of viral hepatitis in several representative US counties. The CDC estimate of the proportion of persons with acute HBV infections associated with known risk factors in 1992–1993 was as follows: heterosexual contact, 41%; injection drug use, 15%; homosexual activity, 9%; household contact, 2%; health care employment, 1%; others, 1%; and unknown, 31% (Figure 22-10). It is likely that the relative contribution of injection drug use to HBV infections may be much higher in large inner-city populations in the United States.

The number of chronic carriers of HBV in the United States has probably increased in recent years. It is estimated that at least 5% of the US population has been infected with HBV, based on testing the sera obtained in the national health and nutrition survey in 1978–1980, which is a probability sample of the US population.[109,110] However, African Americans were found to have a four-fold greater risk of infection than whites in this study. Also, persons who have immigrated from China or Southeast Asia have much higher rates of HBV infections than do other residents of the United States.[107] Other countries also have subpopulations with higher rates of HBV infections. Eskimo populations in Canada and the United States have high rates of HBV, and immigrants to Israel from Africa have high rates.[111,112] The endemicity of

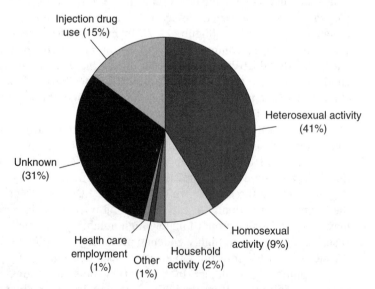

FIGURE 22-10   Risk factors for acute hepatitis B, United States, 1992–1993. *Source:* CDC Sentinel Counties Study of Viral Hepatitis. Reprinted from Sentinel Counties Study of Viral Hepatitis, Centers for Disease Control and Prevention.

HBV is high in residents of the Amazon basin in South America, but lower in other areas of South America.[113]

The increased rates of chronic HBV infection in the United States in recent years is related to a number of factors. Among them are an increase in the sizes of the populations of injection drug users, an increase in the population with multiple sex partners, increased immigration from Southeast Asia, and the influence of the AIDS epidemic with its increased rates of chronic carriage of HBV in persons who are immunosuppressed.[107] Also, there has been some transmission in the health care setting. Outbreaks of hepatitis B were common among hemodialysis patients during the 1960s and 1970s, related to percutaneous exposures to blood. Health care workers have been infected from needlesticks from contaminated needles used in infected patients for blood drawing or suturing and dental procedures.[114] Laboratory workers or phlebotomists who have frequent contact with blood are at relatively high risk of infection. Rarely, infected health care workers have transmitted HBV to their patients.[115-117] However, transmission in the hospital setting has become much less common with the implementation of HBV vaccination of staff and patients, institution of "universal precautions" for infection control, and testing and isolation of HBsAg carriers in some settings, such as dialysis. Despite the recent decrease in the risk of HBV transmission in the health care setting in the United States, the risk of nosocomial transmission in developing countries where HBV is highly endemic remains significant.

The risk of transfusion-transmitted HBV infections in the United States has declined substantially in the last few decades. Screening of blood donors for HBsAg was instituted in 1973. More effective screening of blood donors for drug use or sexual risk behavior and exclusion of male homosexual donors was implemented to reduce the risk of HIV transmission in the early 1980s.

A recent study of the incidence of hepatocellular carcinoma in the United States has estimated that the disease has increased by 46% between 1976–1980 and 1991–1995.[118] This increased incidence of liver cancer probably reflects the combined effects of an increased rate of chronic HBV and HCV infections, combined with the effects of alcohol use among carriers of these viruses.

Prevention

Studies of strategies to prevent HBV infection began in the 1970s. Krugman et al[119] showed that heat-inactivated whole virus preparations from HBV carriers could prevent infection. Also, it was shown that immunoglobulin containing high titers of antibodies to surface antigen was effective in preventing infection after acute exposure.

The initial vaccines were prepared from the plasma of persons chronically infected with HBV. The plasma was treated to inactivate adventitious viruses with chemical-physical inactivation steps, and HBsAg was purified. These plasma-derived vaccines were found to be highly effective and safe.[120,121] The overall preventive efficacy was 92%; however, nearly 100% of subjects who developed anti-HBs above 10 MIU/mL were protected, especially from developing chronic HBV infection.[120]

The donors for the original HBV human-derived vaccine later developed HIV disease and it was highly likely that the pooled plasma used for the first vaccine was contaminated with HIV. Fortunately, the vaccine preparation method inactivated both HBV and HIV, and no cases of HIV from the human-derived HBV vaccine were ever reported. Subsequently, hepatitis B vaccines were produced using recombinant DNA technology to express HBsAg in yeast or mammalian cells.[121] These new subunit vaccines were found to be comparable to plasma-derived vaccines in preventing acute and chronic infections and were highly purified and free of other viral components and, as they were not derived from pooled human sera, they could not accidentally expose recipients to other human-derived contaminates.[122-124] This was the first successful use of molecular genetic methods to produce a human vaccine.

Preexposure vaccination requires three or more doses to induce a protective immune response. HBV vaccines provide good long-term protection—at least 10 years—among persons who respond to the initial vaccine series (Table 22-2). In persons whose level of antibody declines, exposure to HBV rarely results in clinically apparent acute or chronic infection. However, some individuals develop anti-HBc, and a few develop HBsAg. Although it is currently not known whether HBV vaccine provides a lifelong immunity to infections, available data suggest that persons who respond well to vaccine are protected for at least 10 years.[125]

HBV vaccines are poorly immunogenic if given subcutaneously rather than by the intramuscular route.[126,127] Also, when HBV vaccines are frozen, their immunogenicity declines. Therefore, it is important that HBV vaccine be administered in the deltoid area in adults to ensure that the vaccine is given intramuscularly. Even with proper handling and administration, some persons respond poorly to HBV vaccines, based on genetic factors. One study found that persons who were homozygous for a certain major histocompatibility haplotype (HLA-B8, SCO1, DR 3) responded poorly to HBV vaccines.[128] Although most persons responded to vaccine, up to 50% of vaccine responders have anti-HBs titers less than 10 MIU/mL several years later. These true responders are protected against disease but years later are difficult to distinguish from nonresponders. Thus, when checking vaccine response, it is necessary to measure anti-HBs titers about 2 months after the third vaccine dose.

Strategies for the use of HBV vaccines to prevent HBV infections must consider the epidemiology of the infection and populations in whom the

TABLE 22-2   Combined Effects (Relative Risks) of HBsAg Positivity and Presence of Urinary Aflatoxin on Risk of Hepatocellular Carcinoma in Shanghai, China

HBsAg	Negative	Urinary Aflatoxin Positive
Negative	1.0	3.4 (1.1, 10.0)
Positive	7.3 (2.2, 24.4)	59.4 (16.6, 212.0)

Source: Qian G-S et al Cancer, Epidemiol, Biomarkers Prev 1994;3:3–10.

risk of infection is greatest. In many developing countries, especially in Asia where the endemicity of HBV is high and perinatal infection accounts for a large proportion of HBV infections, vaccine should be given soon after birth. Where the rate of HBeAg positivity among pregnant women is low and perinatal transmission is less of a risk, the first dose of HBV vaccine can be given to newborns, or the vaccine series can be started with the series of diphtheria-tetanus-pertussis vaccine (see Chapter 11).

The World Health Organization has recommended that HBV vaccines be included with the vaccines given in the Expanded Programme of Immunization (EPI) for countries having high or moderate endemicity of hepatitis B virus infection.[129] Unfortunately, many countries in sub-Saharan Africa have not yet included HBV vaccine in their EPI programs because of economic constraints and lack of appreciation of the sequelae of chronic HBV infections in their countries.

Initially, in the United States, HBV vaccine was used selectively in high-risk adults and children. However, this strategy did not substantially affect the incidence of HBV infection because it proved to be very difficult to identify and immunize persons who were at risk. Recently, the strategy has been changed to include HBV vaccine in the regular childhood immunization schedule, in addition to targeted immunization of persons at higher risk, such as illicit drug users, persons with multiple sex partners, and health care workers. An economic analysis of the routine use of HBV vaccine for the immunization of infants found this strategy to be cost-effective in the United States over a wide range of assumptions.[130] There is some evidence that the incidence of HBV has declined in the United States in the past few years. The decline may not be due entirely to a change in vaccination policy but also to a wider implementation of methods to prevent the sexual and parenteral transmission of other infectious diseases.

It is particularly important to periodically screen persons who are chronic HBV carriers for PHC. A tumor marker, alpha fetoprotein (AFP), has been found to be elevated in persons with liver cancer. Neither the sensitivity nor specificity of the test is ideal for early detection of PHC. Nonetheless, a program of periodic AFP screening of chronic HBsAg carriers, followed by ultrasound evaluation of those with elevated levels and resection of hepatic tumors, has lowered the mortality from hepatitis B–associated liver cancer.[131] More recent studies have found that precore mutations in the X gene of HBV may precede the occurrence of PHC by several years.[132,133] Further research to confirm this finding is needed.

Treatment

Infection can be suppressed or eradicated in some chronic carriers. Currently, there are five approved therapies for chronic hepatitis B in the United States: interferon alfa-2b, lamivudine, adefovir, entecavir, and pegylated interferon alfa-2a.[128–131,134–138] Generally these drugs were approved based upon the results of treatment of HBV carriers for one year. Treatment responses were judged based upon loss of serum HBV DNA, HBeAg seroconversion, loss of HBsAg, (which occurs very rarely), normalization of alanine aminotransferase levels, and/or histologic improvement.[138] Treatment of HBV often suppresses but does not eradicate infection. The goal of treatment is to suppress active

TABLE 22-3 Long-Term Protection from Hepatitis B Virus Infection Among Cohorts of Children and Adults Known to Have Responded to Hepatitis B Vaccination

	Study Group No.*	Follow-up (yr)	Anti-HBs Loss† (%) Anti-HBc (+)	HBV Infections	HBsAg (+)
Postexposure immunoprophylaxis: infants of HBeAg-positive mothers					
Passive-active					
Taiwan	199	5	3	0	0
Taiwan	654	5	9	46	4
United States	315	4–11	12	30	0
Active					
China	55	5	17	6	1
Routine preexposure immunization of infants/children					
Senegal	100	6	22	8	4
Alaska	600	10	17	4	0
Venezuela	280	6	29	6	0
Preexposure immunization of adults					
Homosexual men	634	9	54	48	4
Homosexual men	127	11	61	26	0
Alaskan Eskimos	272	10	38	6	0

*Number of cases; some studies used person-years of follow-up.
†Less than 10 MIU/mL of anti-HBs.
Source: A.S. Evans and R.A. Kaslow, Viral Infections of Humans, p. 385, © 1997, Plenum Publishing Corporation.

infection to prevent or delay the progression of liver damage. The permanent eradication of HBV infection is not likely because of the integration of HBV DNA into the host genome and the presence of an intracellular conversion pathway that replenishes the pool of transcripts and templates (i.e., covalently closed circular HBV DNA) in the hepatocytes.[139] Because of treatment toxicity, cost, and the development of resistance to the drugs, therapy is generally targeted to patients with elevated alanine aminotransferase levels or histologic evidence of moderate or severe inflammation or fibrosis. The goal of treatment is to prevent cirrhosis, hepatic failure, or hepatocellular carcinoma.

The first nucleoside analogue antiviral drug to be evaluated for the treatment of chronic HBV infection was lamivudine. In three large-scale placebo-controlled trials, lamivudine treatment was associated with histological improvement in 52–60% of patients, HBeAg seroconversion in 16%, suppression of HBV DNA in 48–65%, and normalization of ALT in 41–72% of patients.[138,140] However, prolonged treatment with lamivudine results in the emergence of resistant HBV viruses because of mutations of the tyrosine-methionine-aspartate-aspartate (YMDD) motif at the catalytic domain of the viral reverse transcriptase/DNA polymerase gene.[141] The incidence of mutants increases from 15–32% in the first year to about 70% by the fifth year of treatment.[143,144] However, these YMDD mutant viruses appear to be less fit and pathogenic than wild strains, so the drug still retains some efficacy.[140,145-147] Lamivudine, unlike interferon alpha, is safe and effective in patients with decompensated liver disease. Many such patients will show improved liver function and prolonged survival.[138,140]

Adefovir dipivoxil is the second nucleotide analogue to be approved for the treatment of chronic hepatitis B virus infection in the United States and Europe.[138,148,149] Controlled trials of 10 mg of adefovir given daily for 48 weeks to patients who were HBeAg positive or HBeAg negative with elevated ALT levels at baseline showed significant improvement of fibrosis and necroinflammatory scores in their biopsies (Figure 22-11). In addition, the treated patients had reduction in HBV DNA, lowered ALT levels, and cleared HBeAg more frequently than the patients who received placebo.

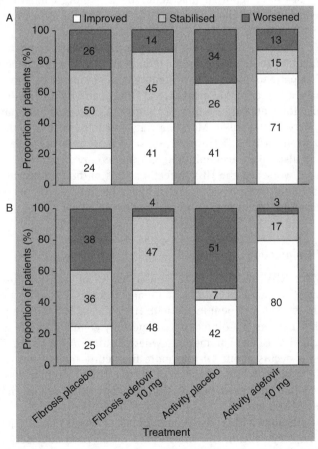

FIGURE 22-11   Effect of 10 mg adefovir on fibrosis stage and necroinflammatory activity grade in patients with chronic hepatitis B. (A) antigen HBe positive: 168 patients with baseline biopsy given adefovir, 161 given placebo. (B) antigen HBe negative: 121 patients with baseline biopsy given adefovir, 57 given placebo. There was a significant difference (P < .001) both for fibrosis and necroinflammatory (activity) scores.
Source: Reprinted from *The Lancet*, 2003 Dec 20; 362(9401): 2089–94, Lai CL et al., Viral Hepatitis B, Copyright (2003), with permission from Elsevier.

Hepatitis B Genotypes

There are eight major genotypes of HBV (A to H). The genotypes have different geographic distributions. Genotype A is pandemic, B and C are found in Asia, D in Southern Europe and the United States, E in Africa, F in the United States, G in the United States and France, and H in Central and South America.[139] There is somewhat conflicting data on the association of HBV genotypes with differing natural history. Most information on the association of the HBV genotype with the natural history has come from studies in Asia, where genotype B and C predominate.[139] As most chronic HBV infections in Asia arise from perinatal infections, the duration of infection is somewhat easier to assess. Most studies in Asia have found that compared to genotype C, genotype B infections are associated with spontaneous HBeAg seroconversion at a younger age, less active liver disease, a slower rate of progression to cirrhosis, and better responses to interferon treatment.[150-155] Some studies have reported that genotype C is more common than B in patients with hepatocellular carcinoma in Asia, but the data are conflicting on this association.[150,154]

There is considerably less data on the natural history of chronic HBV infection in genotypes other than B and C. However, studies have suggested that patients infected with genotype A compared to those with genotype D have a higher rate of clearance of HBeAg and HBV DNA and a more favorable histologic appearance on liver biopsy. A cluster of fulminant hepatitis among American Indians in Montana was associated with infection with a genotype D strain of HBV.[156] However, most of these patients with fulminant hepatitis had also taken acetaminophen, a potentially hepatotoxic drug, which could have worsened the HBV infection. This outbreak illustrates the difficulty in assessing the role of viral genotypes because of the possible effect of other hepatotoxins in many infected patients.

HBV-HIV Coinfection

Since HBV and HIV have similar modes of transmission, coinfection with these two viruses is very common. Whereas 40 million persons worldwide are estimated to be infected with HIV, almost 400 million persons are chronic HBV carriers.[157] Coinfection is especially common in sub-Saharan Africa and Asia, but is also common elsewhere. In the United States chronic HBV infections occurs about 10-fold more frequently in HIV-positive persons than in those who are HIV negative.[157] Active HBV infection was associated with a two-fold increased rate of HIV seroconversion among homosexual men in the MACS study.[158]

Persons with anti-HB core are at increased risk of reactivation of HBsAg after they develop HIV infection.[157] Coinfection adversely affects the chronic viral illnesses associated with infection with either virus. The liver-related mortality among participants in the Multicenter AIDS Cohort Study was 17 times greater in men who were HIV positive than in those who were only HBsAg carriers.[159] Also, HBV infection can increase the toxicity of antiretroviral medications. Several studies have reported that the incidence of grade 3-4 hepatotoxicity among HBV-HIV coinfected persons was 9-10 times more frequent than in those with only HIV infection.[157]

The treatment of either HBV or HIV in persons who are coinfected is further complicated by the fact that some drugs are effective against both viruses, so that single drug therapy for HBV may lead to resistance mutations in HIV. Drugs with these characteristics include lamivudine and tenofovir. Also, there are concerns that the use of adefovir as monotherapy for HBV could induce resistance to tenofovir.[148-150] Therefore, the US FDA currently recommends the use of entecavir, which has no anti-HIV activity, or interferon monotherapy for HBV carriers who are HIV positive.[160] Alternatively, lamivudine or tenofovir can be used in a multidrug regimen for the therapy of both HBV and HIV. Clearly, more data are needed on the short-term and long-term efficacy of various treatment regimens for coinfected individuals. The recommendations of an expert panel that examined the complex issues in the care of patients with HIV-HBV coinfections was published recently.[160]

Orthotopic liver transplantation has also been used for the treatment of chronic carriers; however, the transplanted liver is almost always reinfected, and this is not an option for most persons worldwide.

Delta Hepatitis

Virology

Hepatitis delta virus (HDV) was discovered by Rizzetto and colleagues in Italy in 1977.[13] The virus was originally described as a new antigen in patients with chronic HBV infection. The virus could be transmitted to chimpanzees only if they were infected with HBV.[14] It was then recognized that HDV virus relies on HBV for essential viral components and cannot cause infection in those who are not also infected with HBV. HDV infections can be established in other species, such as woodchucks, ducks, and ground squirrels, that are chronically infected with their respective hepadnaviruses. However, natural HDV infections have not been identified in these animals.

The HDV is a 35- to 38-nm enveloped particle that contains a small circular single-stranded RNA; the internal protein is the delta antigen, and the outer coat is the HBsAg. The virus appears to be related to some disease-causing viruses of plants. Only one serotype of HDV is known to occur. However, three genotypes have been described, based on nucleic acid homology of isolates from different locations: one from North America, Europe, and Asia; one from Japan; and one from tropical South America.

Clinical Features and Diagnosis

The clinical features of acute and chronic HDV infection are similar to those with other forms of hepatitis. However, persons who are coinfected with HBV and HDV from the same source may have more severe acute hepatitis than persons who have only HBV infection.[142] Anicteric hepatitis occurs in only 20% to 30% of adult patients with HBV and HDV coinfections, but it occurs in over 50% of adults who are infected with HBV alone.[143] Also, some persons who are coinfected with HDV and HBV may have a biphasic illness.[143] Fulminant hepatitis may occur in some persons who are coinfected with these two viruses and appears to be much more common than in persons infected with only HBV.

Superinfection occurs in persons chronically infected with HBV who are exposed to HDV. Jaundice and further elevation in the liver enzymes may occur very soon after HDV superinfection in a person who is a chronic HBsAg carrier. However, serologic evidence of HDV infection may not occur for 2 to 6 weeks (Figure 22-12). Jaundice precedes serologic evidence of infection, due to the fact that liver cells are already infected with HBV. Such patients generally develop chronic infection and are at high risk of severe chronic liver disease.[144] Some data suggest that patients who are coinfected with HDV have a higher risk of developing primary liver cancer than do those with HBV infection alone; however, the risk of liver cancer in such patients has not been clearly defined.

HDV infection can be diagnosed serologically. Enzyme immunoassay tests are available for testing for HDV antigen and antibodies in serum. Persons who are coinfected will be positive for anti-HBcore and a marker of delta infection. Although delta antigen is detectable in liver tissue, it is not always observed in blood. Likewise, anti-HDV can be undetectable in some instances of acute self-limited infection. Antibodies to HDV appear soon after acute HDV infection, so coinfected patients may also be HDV antibody positive.

HDV superinfection of HBsA carriers will be HDV antigen or antibody positive and IgM anti-HBc negative. HDV antigen is usually cleared, but HDV antibody can persist for years. Also, patients infected with HDV will have HDV RNA in their serum.

Transmission Routes

HDV transmission can occur either by parenteral exposure to blood from HDV-infected persons or by sexual contact with a carrier. Outbreaks of HDV have been reported among injection drug users in Los Angeles and Worcester,

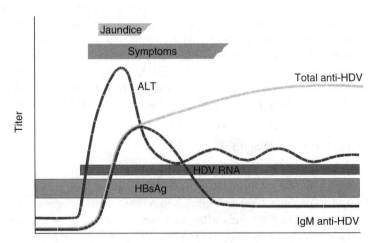

FIGURE 22-12   HBV-HDV superinfection.
Source: Division of Viral Hepatitis, Centers for Disease Control and Prevention.

Massachusetts.[161] Indirect exposure to infected blood may account for most of the cases in epidemic areas of South America.[162] Sexual transmission is much less efficient, and HDV infections are uncommon in homosexual men who are HBsAg carriers.

Worldwide Epidemiology

Infections with HDV have been reported throughout the world, but generally correspond to areas where HBV is highly endemic, with some exceptions (Figure 22-13). The regions with the highest prevalence of HDV are in northern Colombia, Venezuela, the Amazon basin of Brazil, Romania, Italy, and parts of Africa. The prevalence of HDV is low in the United States and Western Europe but is higher among some populations of injection drug users in these areas. The prevalence of HDV is very low in China and Southeast Asia, despite the high level of HBV endemicity in this region.

Prevention

Methods for the control and prevention of HDV infection are the same as those used to prevent hepatitis B virus infection. Successful immunization with HBV vaccine of persons at risk for HBV would also prevent HDV. In addition, the risk of HDV superinfection should be a major incentive for injection drug users who are HBsAg carriers to avoid further high-risk exposures. All HBsAg carriers should be counseled to avoid parenteral or sexual exposure to possible HBV-HDV carriers.

Hepatitis C Virus

Virology

HCV is a spherical, enveloped, RNA virus approximately 50 nm in diameter that contains a positive-sense, single-stranded genome approximately 9.7 kb

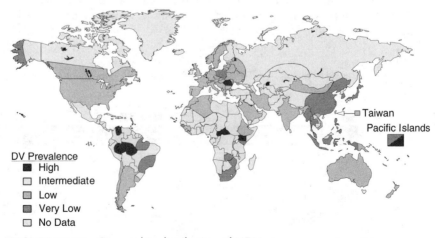

FIGURE 22-13   Geographic distribution of HDV.
Source: Division of Viral Hepatitis, Centers for Disease Control and Prevention.

in length.[163,164] HCV is a member of the family Flaviviridae, classified within its own *Hepacivirus* genus. The RNA contains a single large (approximately 3000[165]) open reading frame (ORF) flanked by highly conserved 5′ and 3′ untranslated regions.[165] The approximate 9.0 kb ORF encodes a polyprotein that is cotranslationally processed into at least 10 proteins. These include, from the amino terminus, structural proteins (the viral nucleocapsid or "core" protein, the envelope proteins E1 and E2, and a short, possibly transmembrane protein, p7 or NS2A), and six nonstructural proteins that are involved in replication of the viral RNA (Figure 22-14).

The liver is presumed to be the primary source of virus present in blood, because HCV-specific antigens and both negative- and positive-strand HCV RNA have been identified within hepatocytes.[163,166,167] Some data suggest that the virus may also replicate within peripheral mononuclear cells of lymphoid or perhaps bone marrow origin.[168,169] However, when assays are done with strand-specific rTth, Lanford et al showed that extra hepatic replication is insufficient to explain HCV RNA detected in blood.[170] Mathematical models of viral kinetics suggest a half-life of approximately 2.5 hours for virions in the bloodstream and that up to 10^{12} virions are produced each day in a chronically infected human.[171] This rate exceeds comparable estimates of the production of HIV by more than an order of magnitude. The high level of virion turnover, coupled with the absence of proofreading by the NS5B RNA polymerase, results in relatively rapid accumulation of mutations within the viral genome. Multiple HCV variants can be recovered from the plasma and liver of an infected individual at any time. Thus, like many RNA viruses, HCV exists in each infected person as a quasispecies, or "swarm" of closely related but distinct genetic sequences.[172,173] For example, in the blood of a recently infected individual, up to 85% of cDNA clones recovered from viral RNAs may represent unique genetic variants.[174]

HCV infections are often persistent (see below), indicating that the virus has evolved mechanisms to escape immune surveillance. Because of limitations in experimental models and the infrequent recognition of natural acute infection, these mechanisms are poorly understood. It has been proposed that the quasispecies nature of the infection is responsible for persistence, and individuals with a more complex infection were more likely to have persistent infection in one study.[175] However, because single clone

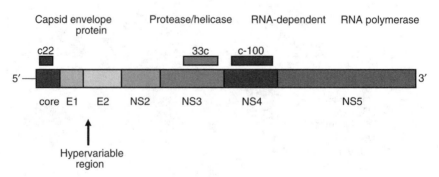

FIGURE 22-14 Hepatitis C virus.
Source: Division of Viral Hepatitis, Centers for Disease Control and Prevention.

infections of chimpanzees can persist, viral complexity is clearly not necessary and could be a result of persistence, rather than the cause.[176] One paradox is that HCV persistence occurs despite a broad humoral and cellular immune response. It has been suggested that HCV sequence variation may contribute to viral persistence. Mutations may alter the amino acid sequences of critical epitopes, leading to the escape of a new quasispecies variant from a previously suppressive immune response, either cellular or humoral.[177-179] Viral escape from a cytotoxic lymphocyte clone has been reported in a persistently infected chimpanzee and was shown to correlate with a single NS3 amino acid substitution.[179]

HCV transmission requires that infectious virions contact susceptible cells that sustain replication. It is difficult to ascertain which body fluids contain infectious hepatitis C virions. Using sensitive techniques, HCV RNA can be detected in blood (including serum and plasma), saliva, tears, seminal fluid, ascitic fluid, and cerebrospinal fluid.[180-184] HCV RNA-containing blood is infectious when administered intravenously, for example, by transfusion or experimental inoculation of chimpanzees. In addition, one chimpanzee was infected by intravenous inoculation of saliva.[185] However, there is very little information regarding the potential infectivity of other body fluids, both because the experiments have not been performed and because accidental percutaneous exposures to nonblood body fluids are rare.

The second requirement for transmission is contact of infectious virions with a susceptible cell. HCV replication occurs in the hepatocyte and possibly elsewhere. There are some data to suggest that HCV interacts with CD81 molecules.[186] However, their role as an HCV receptor is not established, and very little is known about cellular susceptibility to HCV infection. For example, seminal fluid may contain HCV RNA, but sexual transmission is uncommon. Whether this discrepancy is due to a paucity of infectious virions in seminal fluid or insufficient numbers of susceptible cells in the genital mucosa is unknown.

HCV diversity can be exploited for epidemiologic research. The nucleotide sequence corresponding to the HCV envelope and some nonstructural proteins is highly variable, and at least six distinct HCV genotypes have been described.[187,188] The genetic heterogeneity of HCV strains is sufficiently high that detection of the same or nearly identical nucleotide sequences in two individuals is strong evidence for a common source of infection. These comparisons have been used to demonstrate HCV transmission between sexual partners, within families, among patients, and from health care workers to patients.[189-192] HCV genotype/subtype classification also may be used epidemiologically but is less specific than nucleotide sequence analysis.

Clinical Features and Diagnosis

Acute HCV infection is usually unnoticed. Fewer than one fifth of persons will have jaundice or sufficient symptoms to seek medical care. When symptoms do occur, they are indistinguishable from those caused by other hepatitis viruses. After the acute infection, 85% of persons will have persistent viremia, and more than half will have elevated levels of liver enzymes[193-196] HCV infection may persist over 10 to 50 years without symptoms or with symptoms, such as malaise, that are too general to be attributed to HCV infection.

From 2% to 25% of individuals with persistent HCV infection will develop life-threatening cirrhosis and/or liver cancer.[196-199] Cirrhosis can cause liver failure, which manifests as esophageal varices, ascites, hypoprothrombinemia, and hepatic encephalopathy. HCV infection is also associated with vasculitis, essential mixed cryoglobulinemia,[200,201] membranoproliferative glomerulo-nephritis,[201,202] and sporadic porphyria cutanea.[203,204] Approximately 10,000 persons die of HCV infection each year in the United States.[205]

The laboratory diagnosis of HCV infection is based principally on detection by enzyme immunoassay of antibodies to recombinant HCV peptides.[206-208] The sensitivity of the latest, third-generation, HCV antibody assay is estimated to be 97%, and it can detect HCV antibody within 6 to 8 weeks of exposure.[209,210] These assays are measures of HCV infection, not immunity. Assays for IgM HCV antibodies are not clinically useful. The US FDA has licensed the recombinant immunoblot assay (RIBA) (Ortho Diagnostic Systems, Raritan, New Jersey) as a supplemental test to the enzyme immunoassay.[211,212] The RIBA generally identifies the specific antigens to which antibodies are reacting in the EIA and may be positive (≥2 antigens), indeterminate (1 antigen), or negative. EIA- and RIBA-positive sera often contain HCV RNA, as indicated by direct detection and by look-back studies of donations that caused infection after transfusion.[211,213,214] EIA-positive, RIBA-indeterminate sera may also contain HCV RNA, especially if the reactivity was to core or NS3 antigens (the c22-3 and c33-c bands). The RIBA assay is useful to confirm the specificity of a positive EIA test, especially if it is weakly positive. In populations at low risk of HCV infection, such as healthy blood donors, many weakly positive EIA tests are not HCV specific.[212]

HCV RNA can be detected in plasma and serum by reverse transcription polymerase chain reaction (PCR) and by branched DNA (bDNA) assays.[190-195] Detection of HCV RNA indicates ongoing infection, whereas clearance of serum HCV RNA, either spontaneously or following treatment, correlates with ALT normalization and improvement in liver histology.[196] Thus, HCV infection is usually diagnosed by detection of HCV antibody by enzyme immunoassay, followed by either detection of HCV RNA or supplemental (RIBA) antibody testing.

Some studies have shown poor interlaboratory agreement on HCV RNA detection assays. In one study, only 16% of 31 laboratories accurately identified all samples in a standardized panel.[215]

Transmission Routes

Transfusion of Blood Products

Transfusion of HCV RNA-containing blood or organs almost always results in transmission.[214,223-226] Prior to screening blood donations for HCV antibodies and surrogate markers, approximately 17% of HCV infections in the United States were caused by transfusion.[227] After routine screening, the risk of transfusion transmission of HCV has been reduced substantially.[228,229] In 1987, routine screening of blood donors for elevations in the liver enzyme, alanine aminotransferase (ALT), and antibodies to HBcAg were instituted primarily to decrease the risk of transmitting hepatitis C virus. It is estimated that these surrogate markers for HCV infection reduced the risk of transfusion transmission of HCV by about 50%.[100] In May 1990, the first-generation two-antigen serologic test for HCV was licensed and used to screen all blood donors in the United States. The use of this specific HCV screening test further reduced the risk of the transmission of HCV by blood products. The probable rate of transmission of viral infections by transfusion was estimated by calculating the number of donors who were in the seronegative window period at the time of donation in 1991–1993 by modeling data from seroconverters among repeat donors at five large Red Cross blood banks. This study estimated that about 1 in 63,000 donors who were HBV infected and 1 in 103,000 who were HCV infected were in the seronegative window period at the time of their donation.[230] Transfusion transmission may still occur from donors with recent infection who have not yet developed antibodies and possibly from others who lose or never develop HCV antibodies.[231] However, this risk is estimated to be less than 1 in 100,000.[230] Accordingly, blood transfusion now causes less than 4% of HCV infections in the United States.[227]

Since 1999 all blood donors in the United States have been screened for HIV-1 and HCV RNA in a minipool format (i.e., pools of 16 or 24 samples) with the use of one of two nucleic acid-amplification tests.[232] Both assays are highly specific and sensitive, with 50% detection limits of 14 copies of HCV per milliliter. Among 39,721,404 donors screened between March 1999 and April 1, 2002, 170 (4.3 per million) were HCV RNA positive and 105 (2.9 per million) of these persons donated blood that was otherwise "transfusable" (i.e., had no other infectious markers).[232] The rate of transfusion-transmitted HCV is extremely low currently in the United States and Europe where RNA amplification is used for donor screening, and the prevalence of HCV infections in the donor population is low. However, in many developing countries, where screening is not done or utilizes only EIA, transfusion-transmitted HCV infections are much more common. The prevalence of HCV infection in the general population of many developing countries is higher than in the United States and western Europe due to illicit drug use and more frequent exposures to potentially contaminated injections.

HCV also has been transmitted by intravenous administration of contaminated blood products, including immunoglobulin (IG) and clotting factors, as illustrated in several large outbreaks.[233-236] Current IG viral inactivation procedures and recombinant clotting factor use has decreased the risk of further transmission by these products.

HCV can also be transmitted by percutaneous needlesticks, as occur among illicit injection drug users and inadvertently in the practice of medicine. From a single needlestick exposure, the risk of HCV transmission to a susceptible person is approximately 3%, intermediate between HBV (30%) and HIV (0.3%). Because of multiple needle-stick exposures, 50% to 95% of persons acknowledging drug use have HCV infection.[237-242] Injection drug users acquire HCV infection by sharing contaminated needles and drug use equipment, sometimes among groups of persons, such as in "shooting galleries." New initiates into drug use are at highest risk for HCV infection.[243] HCV infection that occurs in the context of drug use but without acknowledged injection use may be due to other blood exposures (such as sharing straws for intranasal ingestion of cocaine).[244] However, unacknowledged injection drug use is difficult to exclude, and the extent to which HCV transmission can occur through intranasal cocaine use remains unclear.

HCV transmission occurs in 3% to 8% of health care workers who experience needlestick exposures to HCV-infected patients.[245-247] Whereas hollow-bore needlestick exposures account for most transmission from patients to health care workers, HCV infection has also been reported from blood splashed on the conjunctiva and a solid bore needlestick.[248] Nonetheless, the prevalence of HCV infection among dental and medical health care workers is similar to the general population, demonstrating that chronic infection is uncommon after such exposures.[249-256]

Other forms of blood-borne nosocomial transmission also occur. Patient-to-patient HCV transmission has been documented. In one example, two patients acquired HCV infection 8 to 10 weeks after a colonoscopic procedure, which was performed with the same colonoscope as had been used hours earlier on an HCV-infected patient.[189] HCV isolates from all three patients had high nucleotide identity in a variable HCV genomic segment, essentially proving a common source of infection. Nosocomial HCV transmission also has been suggested by identification of clusters of untransfused patients with similar HCV nucleotide sequences. In one Swedish hematology ward, five clusters of identical or closely related viruses were found. All patients in each cluster had overlapping hospitalizations but not common sources of blood.[191] Similarly, there is evidence of patient-to-patient HCV transmission in several dialysis centers.[256-259]

Nosocomial transmission of HCV is rare in developed countries, where recent receipt or provision of health care is not commonly acknowledged by patients with new HCV infections.[260] However, in developed countries, traditional and nontraditional medical practices are probably the leading source of HCV transmission. Breaks in infection control practices have been detected in some instances of nosocomial HCV transmission and are impossible to exclude in others. Strict adherence to these guidelines must be rigorously maintained, especially when mucosal barriers frequently are broken, such as in dialysis units.

HCV has also been transmitted from health care providers to patients, although this is rare. In one instance, HCV infection was detected in six patients after cardiac surgery.[190] Blood donors for these patients were HCV negative. Five of six patients had a genetically similar, unusual HCV strain that later also was found in the surgeon. No infection control breaches were identified. However, percutaneous injuries occurred occasionally when the surgeon tied wires to close the sternum.

HCV can be transmitted by other unusual percutaneous exposures. Tattooing has been associated with HCV infection.[261,262] A human bite and acupuncture and scarification rituals have also been associated with HCV infection (see below).[263]

HCV is probably infrequently transmitted by sexual intercourse. Biologic plausibility exists for sexual transmission, as evidenced by detection of HCV RNA in semen and saliva.[180-183] However, as mentioned above, we do not know whether these fluids contain infectious virions in sufficient quantity to transmit infection or whether the mucosal barrier is protective. Evidence for sexual transmission is indirect. High rates of HCV infection have been found in persons with multiple sexual partners and commercial sex workers,[191,264-268] and acute HCV infection has been reported in instances where sexual, but not other exposures, are recognized.[269,270] In studies of families of HCV-infected patients, sexual partners are generally the only contacts at increased infection risk, a risk that increases with the duration of the relationship.[271-274] High nucleotide identity is often found in the HCV strains of the sexual partners.[191,272,274-276] Sexual transmission could explain these findings. However, it is virtually impossible to exclude other common exposures, such as sharing razors, other subtle percutaneous exposures, or unacknowledged drug use. The importance of the "indirect" nature of the evidence is underscored by other evidence suggesting that sexual transmission is rare. Studies of long-term sexual partners of HCV-infected hemophiliacs and transfusion recipients generally show little or no HCV transmission, even if there had been frequent unprotected sexual intercourse.[277-280] HCV prevalence rates among homosexual men also are generally lower than for other infections, such as HIV, HBV, and syphilis, for which sexual transmission is well established.[281-284] Although the risk of transmission attributable to intercourse per se may never be precisely defined, individuals with HCV-positive sexual partners and especially those with multiple partners generally are at increased risk of infection. Individuals in long-term monogamous relationships should be informed of the low documented risk of transmission and may elect not to use barrier precautions.

Perinatal Transmission

HCV infection occurs in 2% to 8% of infants born to HCV-infected mothers.[285-291] Because of passive transfer of maternal HCV antibody, infant HCV infection must be diagnosed through detection in infant serum of HCV RNA or HCV antibody after 18 months of age. HIV coinfection has been associated with more frequent transmission of HCV from mother to infant in some studies.[288,292] Higher maternal HCV viral load also has been associated with transmission of HCV from mother to infant.[287,293-296] The effect of maternal HIV on perinatal HCV transmission may be through increasing the HCV viral load.[297-300] HCV RNA has been detected in breast milk,[287,301,302] but the risk of transmission does not appear to be substantially increased in breast-feeding infants.[303]

Two large prospective studies of the perinatal transmission of HCV have been reported recently. The rates of perinatal transmission in these studies varied from 4.7% in 190 infants born to infected mothers in the US study to 6.2% in 1479 infants in a collaborator European study.[304,305] Both studies found an increased rate of transmission among women who were coinfected with HIV, had prolonged labor (i.e., over 6 hours), or had internal fetal monitoring. Of interest, in both studies the proportion of HCV transmission to female infants was about twice that of male infants. This curious finding is unexplained but could be due to greater intrauterine mortality of male infants.[306] However, the authors of the European study do not believe this is the explanation.[304]

Factors Affecting HCV Natural History

Although the viral genotype and level of viral RNA are not useful as predictors of the rate of progression of HCV to severe liver disease, several host characteristics are important. The progression of fibrosis in liver biopsies was

evaluated among 2235 HCV-infected patients in France.[307] In this study the
stage of fibrosis was graded using a 5-point scale, the METAVIR scale, with
0 being normal ranging to 4 being cirrhosis. The factors associated with more
rapid progression were age of infection older than 40 years, daily alcohol
consumption of 50 grams or more, and male sex (Figures 22-15, 22-16, 22-
17). These risk factors for more rapid progression after infection have been
confirmed in other populations.[308,309]

In addition, patients with HIV infection and severe immunosuppression
(i.e., CD4 T-cell counts <200 cells/μL) progress more rapidly than HIV-
uninfected subjects, after adjusting for age, sex, and alcohol consumption.[300,307,309-312] Also, patients with a high body mass index and diabetes
mellitus appear to progress more rapidly.[159]

Antiviral treatment of HCV infection has improved since 1991 when
interferon was first licensed as a therapeutic agent. Currently, with 12 months
treatment with pegylated interferon plus ribavirin sustained virological
response (i.e., cure) can be achieved in about 54% of patients infected with
genotype 1a or 1b strains.

Worldwide Epidemiology

It is estimated that there are more than 170 million persons infected with
HCV worldwide.[313] Through August 1997, 130 countries had reported HCV
prevalence rates to the World Health Organization or in the literature in at
least one population. HCV infection was found in all but three countries, and
it is difficult to imagine that infection would not be found there with further
investigation. In developed nations, general population HCV prevalence rates

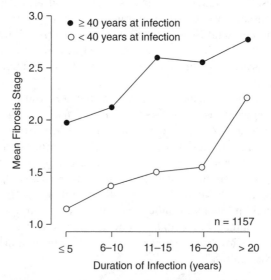

FIGURE 22-15   Fibrosis score by age of infection and estimated duration of
infection.
Source: Reprinted from *The Lancet*, 1997 Mar 22; 349(9055): 825–32, Poynard T
et al., *Natural history of liver fibrosis progression in patients with chronic hepatitis
C*, The OBSVIRC, METAVIR, CLINIVIR, and DOSVIRC groups, Copyright (1997),
with permission from Elsevier.

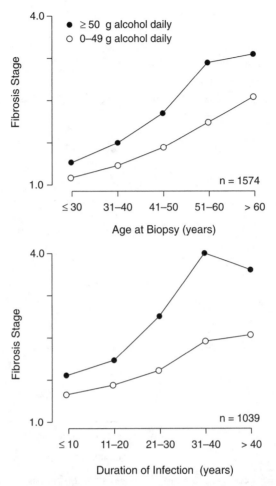

FIGURE 22-16 Association between stage of fibrosis and age at biopsy or duration of infection by alcohol consumption.
Source: Reprinted from *The Lancet,* 1997 Mar 22; 349(9055): 825–32, Poynard T et al., *Natural history of liver fibrosis progression in patients with chronic hepatitis C,* The OBSVIRC, METAVIR, CLINIVIR, and DOSVIRC groups, Copyright (1997), with permission from Elsevier.

are generally less than 3%; whereas among volunteer blood donors, they are less than 1%.

There are several highly endemic regions. In most of these countries, HCV infection is prevalent among persons over 40 years of age but uncommon in those less than 20 years of age.[314–317] This cohort effect suggests a time-restricted exposure that, in many instances, appears to have been receipt of a medical procedure. In Egypt, HCV prevalence rates from 10% to 30% have been reported.[318–323] A national campaign to treat schistosomiasis infections was responsible for a major epidemic of HCV infections. Up until the 1970s, parenteral antischistosomiasis therapies were administered to entire villages, and injection equipment was frequently not sterilized between injections. Similarly, in several areas in Italy and Japan, a high HCV prevalence among older persons was linked to receipt of medical or traditional injections.[314,315,317,324,325] In the isolated Arahiro region of Japan, 45% of individuals

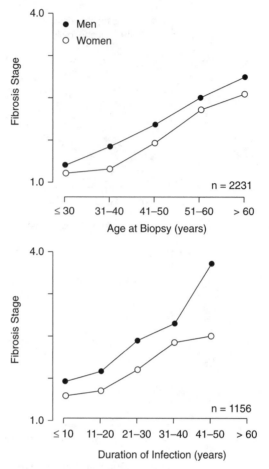

FIGURE 22-17   Association between stage of fibrosis and age at biopsy or
duration of infection by sex.
Source: Reprinted from *The Lancet,* 1997 Mar 22; 349(9055): 825–32, Poynard T
et al., *Natural history of liver fibrosis progression in patients with chronic hepatitis
C,* The OBSVIRC, METAVIR, CLINIVIR, and DOSVIRC groups, Copyright (1997),
with permission from Elsevier.

over 41 years of age had HCV infection, whereas in another area the same-
age prevalence was 2%.[326] Folk remedies, such as acupuncture and cutting of
skin with nonsterilized knives, were identified as likely transmission modes.
Percutaneous folk practices have occurred for thousands of years and probably account for the worldwide distribution of HCV.

High rates of HCV infection also have been reported in urban areas of
developed countries. In Baltimore, Maryland, HCV infection was found in
18% of patients attending an inner-city emergency department and 15%
attending a nearby clinic for sexually transmitted diseases.[265,327] Injection
drug use, not medical procedures, was chiefly responsible for transmission
in this setting.

The epidemiology of HCV infection has been carefully studied in several
developed nations, including the United States and France. In the United
States, the yearly incidence of HCV infection has declined since the 1980s.[205,328]
At least two thirds of community-acquired HCV infections are related to
injection drug use. Injection drug use in the 6 months prior to infection is

acknowledged by approximately 38% of subjects.[260,329] However, noninjection drug use and other indicators of injection use are acknowledged by another 44%. Sexual or household exposure to HCV is detected in approximately 10% of individuals with acute HCV infection; whereas transfusions, occupational exposures, and other factors are infrequently (<4%) identified.

The epidemiology and overall burden of HCV infection in the United States has been further characterized using the Third National Health and Nutrition Examination (NHANES) data.[330] A total of 23,527 persons, who were representative of the general population of the United States, were tested for HCV infection. Antibodies to HCV were detected in 1.8%, which translates to almost 4 million Americans. Active infection (HCV RNA) was detected in 74% of those who were HCV antibody (RNA) postive, suggesting that 2.7 million persons in the United States had ongoing infection. Illegal drug use and high-risk sexual exposures were associated with HCV infection, as were low socioeconomic indices, low levels of education, and poverty. This large-scale representative sampling improved our understanding of the burden and distribution of infection. However, it also points to the difficulty of ascertaining risk, because some of the factors identified, such as marijuana use and low education, represent unmeasured exposures (residual confounding). Furthermore, because a history of the injection of illicit drugs was not included in the NHANES interview, it is difficult to estimate the contribution of current or remote drug injection to the HCV prevalence in this sample. Because the NHANES survey only included persons with a stable residence, and excluded the homeless and imprisoned population, the measured prevalence of HCV underestimated the true rate.[331] A survey of HCV prevalence was repeated in the 1999–2002 NHANES population.[397] The HCV prevalence was 1.6% and the peak prevalence of HCV was in persons 40–49 years of age. Significant risk factors for HCV include: 1) any history of injection drug use, 2) a blood transfusion prior to 1992 and 3) an elevated ALT level. Taken together these 3 risk factors identified 85.1% of HCV infected persons.

HCV Genotypes

Various methods have been utilized to determine the genotype of a viral strain. The most commonly used tests detect subtype-specific point mutations in PCR-amplified cDNA. These include the line probe assay (LIPA), which is based on reverse dot-blot hybridization (Innogenetics, Zwijnaarde, Belgium), restriction fragment-length polymorphism assays, and PCR using subtype-specific primers.[219-222] Phylogenetic analysis of cDNA sequence is the gold standard for evaluating HCV genotypes.

Based on sequence analysis, six genotypes of HCV have been defined, numbered 1–6. Knowledge of the genotype or serotype (i.e., genotype-specific antibodies) is helpful for prediction of a response to antiviral therapy and the choice and duration of therapy. Viral clearance rates after treatment with the combination of pegylated interferon and ribavirin are about 70–80% for genotypes 2 and 3 but only about 48% for genotypes 1, 4, 5, and 6 (Figure 22-18).[388,332] The severity of the disease, measured by the fibrosis stage, is not related to the genotype. However, genotype 3 is associated with higher rates of hepatic steatosis and higher ALT levels.[333]

The genotypes are distributed geographically. Genotypes 1 and 2 account for about 90% of infections in the United States and are the most common in

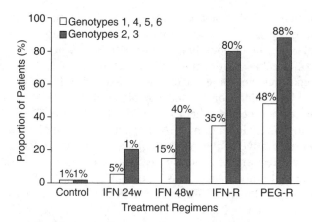

Note: IFN, interferon; w, weeks, R, ribavirin; PEG, pegylated interferon.

FIGURE 22-18   Progress in treatment of chronic hepatitis C. Data are proportions of patients with undetectable HCV RNA at the end of follow-up, according to genotype. IFN = interferon; w = weeks; R = ribavirin; PEG = pegylated interferon. *Source:* Reprinted from *The Lancet*, 2003; 362(9401): 2095–2100, Poynard T et al., *Viral Hepatitis C*, Copyright (2003), with permission from Elsevier.

Europe. Genotype 4 accounts for nearly all of the HCV infections in Egypt.[308] In Asia, genotypes 1, 3, and 6 each account for about one third of HCV infections.[232] Genotype 5 is geographically limited to Madagascar, South Africa, and France.[308] Viral recombination has been reported among injecting drug users in St. Petersburg, Russia, but appears to be very uncommon with HCV, in contrast to HIV infection.[332]

HCV-Related Hepatocellular Carcinoma

Despite the reduced incidence of HCV infections in the last several years, the burden of chronic disease from previous infections is increasing in the United States. The incidence of mortality from hepatocellular carcinoma has increased by 41% in the interval from 1991 to 1995 compared to 1976–1980.[118] Also, hospitalizations for liver cancer have increased by 46% in Veterans Administration hospitals between 1983 and 1997. Analysis of hospitalizations for primary liver cancer among veterans found a three-fold increase in the age-adjusted rates associated with hepatitis C virus infection in the 1990s; whereas the rates for liver cancer associated with hepatitis B virus infection and alcoholic cirrhosis have remained relatively stable.[334] Modeling the national HCV seroprevalence data from the NHANES study suggested that the numbers of persons with chronic HCV infection for 30 or more years, who are at risk for liver cancer or cirrhosis, will continue to increase for another decade (Figures 22-19 and 22-20).[335]

Prevention

HCV prevention is chiefly accomplished through efforts to prevent exposure. There are no vaccines available to prevent HCV infection. Exploratory vaccine development efforts are ongoing, but the complexity of the infection and poor

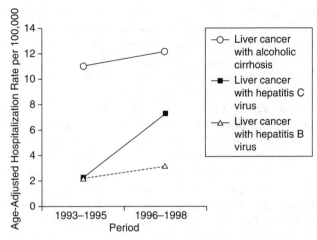

FIGURE 22-19 Temporal trends in age-adjusted proportional hospitalization rates for primary liver cancer broken down by the presence of risk factors for hepatocellular carcinoma. The rates are displayed for 2 periods: 1993 to 1995 and 1996 to 1998.
Source: El-Serag HB et al. Risk Factors for the Rising Rates of Primary Liver Cancer in the United States. Arch Intern Med. 2000;160:3227–3230.

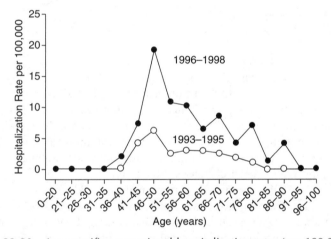

FIGURE 22-20 Age-specific proportional hospitalization rates (per 100,000) for primary liver cancer associated with hepatitis C virus infection from 1993 to 1995 and from 1996 to 1998.
Source: El-Serag HB et al. Risk Factors for the Rising Rates of Primary Liver Cancer in the United States. Arch Intern Med. 2000;160:3227–3230.

understanding of the immune response complicate this work. Postexposure administration of immunoglobulin to prevent HCV infection is not currently recommended because there is little evidence that it was effective in the past and even more reason to doubt the effectiveness of the newer products that do not contain HCV antibody.[205]

The incidence of HCV infection has declined in the United States. One reason is the practice of screening blood donations for HCV antibody and surrogate markers. In some but not all studies, use of needle exchange programs has also been associated with reductions in HCV incidence.[336,337]

However, HCV incidence has declined in areas where there are no needle exchange programs. Because most HCV infections in developed nations are due to illicit injection drug use, expanded efforts to treat drug dependence are urgently needed. In developing nations, it is urgent to begin programs to alter attitudes regarding blood exposures and to improve the safety of necessary percutaneous practices.

Research to develop a preventive HCV vaccine is under way. The facts that 20–30% of infected persons clear the virus spontaneously and that sequelae develop very slowly suggest that acquired immunity might be somewhat efficacious. Also, the HCV genome, unlike HIV, is not integrated into the human genome. Nevertheless, experiments showing that it was possible to reinfect chimpanzees with the same HCV strain that the animal had recently cleared and the frequent reinfection of injection drug users suggests that immunity after natural infection often may be weak or incompletely protective against reinfection.[338,339]

Nevertheless, a study of HIV-negative injection drug users who had cleared their HCV infection found them to be 12 times less likely to develop new HCV infection and to have two logs lower HCV RNA levels among those who were reinfected.[340] These data suggest that a preventive HCV vaccine may be feasible.

Hepatitis E Virus

Virology

Hepatitis E virus (HEV) is a single-stranded, positive sense RNA virus that is approximately 32 nm in diameter.[341-343] The virus is relatively sensitive to inactivation, being inactivated by Cesium Chloride, freeze-thawing, and pelleting. Like HAV, HEV lacks an envelope, making it stable in bile and, thus, transmissible by ingestion of fecally contaminated water. HEV is resistant to the pH extremes of the gastrointestinal tract, although it is assumed that water chlorination decreases infectivity.

The HEV genome is approximately 7.2 kb and consists of three open reading frames (ORFs). Recombinant antigens synthesized from the second and third ORFs are used in diagnostic assays. HEV isolates may have as little as 75% homology, and four major serotypes have been identified. Isolates collected in the Western Hemisphere are especially heterogeneous but phylogenetically cluster with a highly related virus from swine.[344] HEV shares certain morphologic and biophysical properties with caliciviruses, yet its genomic organization is notably different from others in this family.[345] Hepatitis E virus shows highest, but limited, amino acid similarity in its replicative enzymes with Rubella virus and alphaviruses of the Family Togaviridae and with plant Furovirus. However, recently, HEV has been classified as a Hepevirus in the Family Hepeviridae.

Although HEV does not proliferate well in cell culture, animal models have been developed. Most experiments have been conducted in nonhuman primate species using the cynomolgus macaque, *Macaca fascicularis*.[346] Laboratory infections of chimpanzees, tamarins, owl monkeys, rhesus monkeys, and even rats have also been reported.[347,348] Especially interesting is natural recovery of an HEV-like agent from swine.[343]

Clinical Features and Diagnosis

Clinically, HEV is impossible to distinguish from other hepatitis virus infections. As with HAV infection, the disease is self-limited, and most patients recover completely without complications or sequelae. No chronic or carrier state has been demonstrated after hepatitis E infection. The typical incubation period ranges from 15 to 60 days (mean 40 days) from the time of exposure.[349] The liver is probably the main site of HEV replication in infected humans. HEV infection is rarely fatal in the general population. However, fulminant hepatic failure can occur, especially in pregnant women.[350-352] During a 1993–1994 Pakistan HEV outbreak, attack rates of fulminant icteric hepatitis increased by trimester of pregnancy.[351]

As with all hepatitis virus infections, viremia can be detected before the onset of symptoms or liver enzyme elevations. HEV RNA is detectable in blood for 14 to 28 days in most patients with clinical disease, although it may be prolonged.[349,353] HEV has been detected in stool up to 9 days prior to the icteric phase of disease and typically lasts 7 to 14 days thereafter.[349,354]

The serologic course of HEV infection has been determined using nonhuman primate models, human volunteer studies, and outbreak investigations. Both IgG and IgM antibody responses occur soon after HEV infection, with peak antibody titers occurring 2 to 4 weeks after inoculation or infection.[349,355] The HEV IgM titers decline rapidly within 3 months after infection. Published data on the persistence of anti-HEV IgG are somewhat conflicting. A study of Egyptian children noted the disappearance of anti-HEV IgG within 6 to 12 months after infection,[356] and in Indonesia, 28% of persons involved in an HEV outbreak lost anti-HEV over 2 years of follow-up.[357] On the other hand, in some persons, IgG anti-HEV persists for 15 years or more.[355,358,359] Discrepancies in these results may relate to the laboratory tests, as demonstrated by Mast and colleagues who found that synthetic peptide-based EIAs were less sensitive for the detection of remote infections when compared with recombinant antigen assays.[358]

HEV diagnosis can be complicated by what may be serologic cross-reactivity with another unrecognized condition or infection. In one study, approximately 20% of blood donors from Maryland, New York, and California had IgG anti-HEV, although only a small number of human HEV infections have ever been demonstrated to originate in the United States.[360] Given the lack of familiarity of most laboratories with HEV testing, a practical approach is to collect sera, store it at −20°C in a cryovial, and contact a local reference laboratory for assistance. In the United States, practitioners with patients having unexplained acute jaundice and negative tests for HAV, HBV, and HCV should contact the hepatitis branch of the CDC at (404) 639-3048 for assistance.

Transmission Routes

The possible routes of HEV transmission are the same as with HAV. However, HEV infection appears to be more frequently linked to ingestion of contaminated water. In many Asian countries, epidemics of HEV infection have occurred during periods of monsoon rains.[361] Because there is a brief period of viremia, blood-borne transmission is also possible with HEV.[362] Similarly, mother-to-infant transmission has been reported.[363]

Direct comparisons of the efficiency of person-to-person transmission of HEV and HAV are difficult, because in most areas of the world where HEV infections occur, the majority of persons have already been infected with HAV by 10 years of age. However, person-to-person HEV transmission seems to be less efficient than HAV, as indicated by the lower secondary attack rates.[364] The propensity to cause large-scale outbreaks is associated more with HEV than HAV but may be an artifact of the more extensive population-wide immunity from HAV in areas where large outbreaks have been reported.[325] Fecal contamination of water supplies from a variety of causes is a frequent finding in evaluations of HEV outbreaks and probably explains the tendency for outbreaks to occur following the rainy season.

The reservoir for HEV infections is an area of renewed interest. Humans are the only proven reservoir for HEV. However, a highly related virus has been found in swine.[344,365] This HEV-like swine virus can cause infection of nonhuman primates and humans, and HEV can infect swine.[365] Moreover, antibody that cross-reacts with HEV antigens (and in some cases, neutralizes HEV) has been detected in swine, rats, and other animals.[366] These findings may explain the serologic evidence of HEV infection found in nonendemic areas. However, more research is needed to determine how extensive this family of viruses is and to what extent these viruses infect humans.[367] Of interest are recent reports of transmission of HEV to humans from contaminated uncooked deer meat and after consumption of uncooked wild boar liver in Japan.[368,369]

Worldwide Epidemiology

HEV infections are rare in developed countries. Only a few cases of HEV infection in humans have been documented to have been acquired in the United States; others have been imported by travelers. However several cases of hepatitis due to HEV have been reported among nontravelers in the UK, other European countries, and the United States.[370-372] As mentioned above, a far greater proportion of those living in developed nations may have serologic reactivity to HEV. However, this seroreactivity has not been associated with a history of jaundice or, for that matter, traditional markers of blood-borne or sexually transmitted infectious disease.[360]

Similar to HAV, HEV is endemic in many developing countries in Asia, Africa, and the Middle East (Figure 22-21). However, interesting epidemiologic differences have been observed between those two enterically transmitted viruses.[374] A striking increase in the age-specific HEV clinical attack rate and seroprevalence is seen, beginning in the third decade of life.[373,375] In contrast, HAV infection is almost universal in developing nations by the age of 10 years. This difference could be explained by less frequent transmission of HEV and, thus, postponement of infection for years, when it is clinically apparent (similar to what has happened with HAV infections in countries undergoing economic transition). The difference could also be explained if HEV infection of children did not result in durable immunity.

Development of serologic tests for HEV infection has not completely resolved this issue. Although HEV infection has been demonstrated in children,[356] in many studies the seroprevalence usually is low until the third decade of life.[375-378] However, some populations have substantially higher seroprevalence rates of HEV infection in children.[379] Thus, the conventional

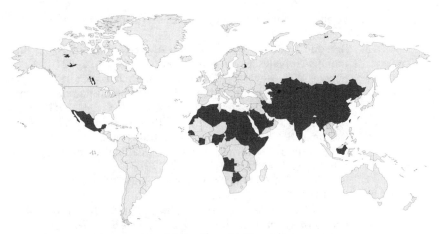

FIGURE 22-21   Geographic distribution of HEV.
Source: Division of Viral Hepatitis, Centers for Disease Control and Prevention.

wisdom that HEV infection is less common in children may relate to differences in the tools used to measure infection. No matter what the explanation, HEV remains unique among enteric viruses in having a peak in clinical attack rate beginning in the third decade of life.

Prevention

Because HEV infection rarely occurs in developed countries, the most important control measures involve improvements in hygiene, especially in the development of an uncontaminated water supply in countries where infections are endemic.

There is emerging data that indicate HEV infection can be prevented by vaccination and immunoglobulin administration.[380-384] A recent trial in Nepal of an experimental HEV subunit vaccine developed from an ORF-3 protein found this experimental vaccine to be 96% efficacious compared to placebo.[398]

Other Viruses

For 5% to 20% of persons with acute hepatitis syndromes, no etiology is found (non-A to E hepatitis). Other viruses, such as GB virus C (or the hepatitis G virus), TTV virus, and SEN-V virus, have been discovered among patients with clinical hepatitis.[385-387] However, most of these recently described viruses (e.g., GB-C, TTV) do not usually cause hepatitis and the viruses do not replicate in hepatic cells. Nevertheless, other viral agents, which are as yet undiscovered, likely are responsible for some cases of hepatitis.

References

1. Zuckerman AJ. The history of viral hepatitis from antiquity to the present. In: Deinhardt F, Deinhardt J, eds. *Viral Hepatitis Laboratory and Clinical Science.* New York, NY: Marcel Dekker; 1983:3–32.

2. Lürman A. Eine icterus epidemic. *Berl Klin Worchenschr.* 1885;22: 20–23.

3. Beeson PB, Chainey G, McFarlan AM. Hepatitis following injection of mumps convalescent plasma. *Lancet.* 1944;1:814–821.

4. Sawyer WA, Meyer KF, Eaton WD, et al. Jaundice in army personnel in the western region of the United States and its relation to vaccination against yellow fever. *Am J Hyg.* 1944;39:334.

5. MacCallum FO. Jaundice in syphilitics. *Br J Vener Dis.* 1943;19:63.

6. Krugman S, Giles JP, Hammond J. Infectious hepatitis: evidence for two distinctive, clinical, epidemiological and immunological types of infections. *JAMA.* 1967;200:365–373.

7. Blumberg BS, Alter HJ, Visnich S. A "new" antigen in leukemia sera. *JAMA.* 1965;191:541–546.

8. Prince AM. An antigen detected in the blood during the incubation period of serum hepatitis. *Proc Natl Acad Sci USA.* 1968;60: 814–821.

9. Feinstone SM, Kapikian AZ, Purcell RH, Alter AJ, Holland PV. Transfusion-associated hepatitis not due to viral hepatitis type A or B. *N Engl J Med.* 1975;292:767–770.

10. Alter HJ, Purcell RH, Shih JW, et al. Detection of antibody to hepatitis C in prospectively followed transfusion recipients with acute and chronic non-A, non-B hepatitis. *N Engl J Med.* 1989;321: 1494–1500.

11. Choo QL, Koo G, Weiner AJ, Overby LR, Bradley DW, Houghton M. Isolation of a cDNA clone derived from a blood borne non-A, non-B viral hepatitis genome. *Science.* 1989;244:351–362.

12. Kuo G, Choo QL, Alter HJ, et al. An assay for circulating antibodies to a major etiologic virus of human non-A, non-B hepatitis. *Science.* 1989;244:362–364.

13. Rizzetto M, Canese MC, Arico S, et al. Immunofluorescence detection of a new antigen-antibody system associated to the hepatitis B virus in the liver and in the serum of HBsAg carriers. *Gut.* 1977;18: 997–1003.

14. Rizzetto M, Canese MC, Gerin JC, et al. Transmission of the hepatitis virus associated delta antigen to chimpanzees. *J Infect Dis.* 1980;141:590–601.

15. Feinstone SM, Kapikian AZ, Purcell RH. Hepatitis A: detection by immune electron microscopy of a virus-like antigen association with acute illness. *Science.* 1973;182:1026–1028.

16. Provost PJ, Hilleman MR. Propagation of human hepatitis A virus in cell culture in vitro. *Proc Soc Exp Biol Med.* 1979;160:213.

17. Werzberger A, Mensch B, Kuter B, et al. A controlled trial of formalin-inactivated hepatitis A vaccine in healthy children. *N Engl J Med.* 1992;327:453–457.

18. Innis BL, Snitbban R, Kunasol P, et al. Protection against hepatitis A by an inactivated vaccine. *JAMA.* 1994;271:1328–1334.

19. Wong DL, Purcell RH, Sreentvasan MA, Prasad SR, Parri KM. Epidemic and endemic hepatitis in India: evidence for non A/non B hepatitis virus etiology. *Lancet.* 1980;2:876–878.

20. Bradley DW, Krawczynski K, Cook EH, et al. Enterically transmitted non-A, non-b hepatitis: serial passage of disease in cynomolgus monkeys and tamarins, and discovery of disease associated with 27 to 34 nm virus-like particles. *Proc Natl Acad Sci USA.* 1987;84: 6277–6281.

21. Kane MA, Bradley DW, Shrestha SM, et al. Epidemic non-A, non-B hepatitis in Nepal: recovery of a possible etiologic agent and transmission to marmosets. *JAMA*. 1984;252:3140-3145.
22. Acute Hepatic Failure Study Group. Etiology and prognosis in fulminant hepatitis. *Gastroenterology*. 1979;77:A33.
23. Mathieson CR, Skinholj P, Nielsen JO, Purcell RH, Wong DC, Ranek C. Hepatitis A, B and non-A, non-B in fulminant hepatitis. *Gut*. 1980;21:72-77.
24. Sjogren MH, Tanno H, Fay O, et al. Hepatitis A virus in stool during clinical relapse. *Ann Intern Med*. 1987;106:221.
25. Andre FE, D'Hondt E, Delem A, Safary A. Clinical assessment of the safety and efficacy of an inactivated hepatitis A vaccine. Rationale and summary of findings. *Vaccine*. 1992;10(suppl 1): S160-S163.
26. Conlepis AG, Locarnini SA, Lehmann NC, Gust D. Detection of hepatitis A virus in the feces of patients with naturally acquired infections. *J Infect Dis*. 1980;141:151.
27. Cohen JL, Feinstone S, Purcell RH. Hepatitis A virus infection in a chimpanzee: duration of viremia and detection of virus in saliva and throat swabs. *J Infect Dis*. 1989;180:887.
28. Shapiro CN, Coleman PJ, McQuillan GM, Alter MJ, Margolis HS. Epidemiology of hepatitis A: seroepidemiology and risk groups in the USA. *Vaccine*. 1992;10:S59-S62.
29. Villano SA, Nelson KE, Vlahov D, et al. Hepatitis-A among homosexual men and injection drug users: more evidence for vaccination. *Clin Infect Dis*. 1997;25:726-728.
30. Corey L, Holmes HK. Sexual transmission of hepatitis A in homosexual men. *N Engl J Med*. 1980;302:345-438.
31. Noble RC, Kane MA, Reeves SA, Roeckel I. Post transfusion hepatitis A in a neonatal intensive care unit. *JAMA*. 1984;252:2711-2715.
32. Rosenblum LS, Villarino ME, Nainan OV, et al. Hepatitis A outbreak in a neonatal intensive care unit: risk factors for transmission and evidence of prolonged viral excretion among preterm infants. *J Infect Dis*. 1991;164:476-482.
33. Mannucci PM, Gdorin S, Gringeri A, et al. Transmission of hepatitis A to patients with hemophilia by factor VIII concentrates treated with organic solvent and detergent to inactivate viruses. *Am Intern Med*. 1994;120:1-10.
34. Lemon SM, Murphy PC, Smith A, et al. Removal/neutralization of hepatitis A virus during manufacture of high purity, solvent/detergent factor VIII concentrate. *J Med Virol*. 1994;43:44-48.
35. Widell A, Hansson BG, Moestrup T, Nordenfelt E. Increased occurrence of hepatitis A with cyclic outbreaks among drug addicts in a Swedish community. *Infection*. 1983;11:198-204.
36. Centers for Disease Control. Hepatitis A among drug users. *MMWR*. 1988;37:297.
37. Lemon SM. Type A viral hepatitis. New developments in an old disease. *N Engl J Med*. 1985;313:1059-1067.
38. Bergeisen GH, Hinds MW, Skaggs JW. A waterborne outbreak of hepatitis A in Meade County, Kentucky. *Am J Public Health*. 1985;75:161-168.
39. Niu MT, Polish LB, Robertson BH, et al. A multi-state outbreak of hepatitis A associated with frozen strawberries. *J Infect Dis*. 1992;166:518-529.

40. Rosenblum LS, Mirkin IR, Allen DT, Safford S, Hadler SC. A multi-focal outbreak of hepatitis A traced to commercially distributed lettuce. *Am J Public Health.* 1990;80:1075–1079.

41. Desenclos JA, Klontz KC, Wilder MH, Nainan OV, Margolis HS, Gunn RA. A multi-state outbreak of hepatitis A caused by the consumption of raw oysters. *Am J Public Health.* 1991;81:1268–1272.

42. Halliday ML, Kang L, Lao Y, et al. An epidemic of hepatitis A attributable to the ingestion of raw clams in Shanghai, China. *J Infect Dis.* 1991;164:852–859.

43. Enriquez R, Frosner GG, Hochstein-Montzel V, Riedemann S, Reinhardt G. Accumulation and persistence of hepatitis A virus in mussels. *J Med Virol.* 1992;37:174–179.

44. Centers for Disease Control. *Hepatitis Surveillance Report.* 1994;55: 1–35.

45. Shapiro CM, Shaw FE, Mendel EI, Hadler SC. Epidemiology of hepatitis in the United States. In: Hollinger FB, Lemon SM, Margolis HS, eds. *Viral Hepatitis and Liver Disease.* Baltimore, Md: Williams & Wilkins; 1991:214–220.

46. Hadler SC, McFarland L. Hepatitis in day care centers. Epidemiology and prevention. *Rev Infect Dis.* 1985;8:548–557.

47. Hadler SC, Webster HM, Erben JJ, et al. Hepatitis A in daycare centers. A community-wide assessment. *N Engl J Med.* 1980;302:1222–1230.

48. Gingrich GA, Hadler SC, Elder HA, Asleko. Serologic investigation of an outbreak of hepatitis A in a rural daycare center. *Am J Public Health.* 1983;83:1190–1198.

49. Lange WR, France JD. High incidence of viral hepatitis among American missionaries in Africa. *Am J Trop Med Hyg.* 1990;43: 527–533.

50. Steffen R. Risk of hepatitis A in travelers. *Vaccine.* 1992;30: 569–572.

51. Bancroft WH, Lemon SM. Hepatitis A from the military perspective. In: Gerety RJ, ed. *Hepatitis A.* New York, NY: Academic Press; 1984:81–100.

52. Innis BL, Snithban R, Hoke CH, Muniudhorn W, Laorakpongse T. The declining transmission of hepatitis A in Thailand. *J Infect Dis.* 1991;163:989–995.

53. Hsu HY, Chang MH, Chen DS, Lee CY, Sung JL. Changing seroepidemiology of hepatitis A virus infection in Taiwan. *J Med Virol.* 17:297–301.

54. Kremastinis J, Kalapothaki V, Trichopoulos D. The changing epidemiologic pattern of hepatitis A infection in urban Greece. *Am J Epidemiol.* 1984;120:203–206.

55. Stroffolini T, Decrescenzo L, Giammacco A, et al. Changing patterns of hepatitis virus infection in children in Palermo, Italy. *Eur J Epidemiol.* 1990;6:84–87.

56. Shapiro CN, Coleman PJ, McQuillan GM, Alter HJ, Margolis HS. Epidemiology of hepatitis A: seroepidemiology and risk groups in the USA. *Vaccine.* 1992;10:S59–S62.

57. Shaw FGJ, Shapiro CN, Welty TK, Dill W, Reddington J, Hadler SC. Hepatitis transmission among the Sioux Indians of South Dakota. *Am J Public Health.* 1990;80:1091–1094.

58. Centers for Disease Control. *Hepatitis Surveillance Report.* 1996;56: 15–27.

59. Wasley A, Samandari T, Bell BP. Incidence of hepatitis A in the United States in the era of vaccination. *JAMA*. 2005;294:194–201.

60. Centers for Disease Control and Prevention. Prevention of hepatitis A through active or passive immunization: recommendations of the Advisory Committee on Immunization. Practices (ACID). *MMWR*. 1999;48(RR-12):1–37.

61. Krugman S, Ward R, Giles JP, Jacobs AM. Infectious hepatitis, study on effect of gammaglobulin and on the incidence of apparent infection. *JAMA*. 1960;174:823–883.

62. Winokur PC, Stapleton JT. Immunoglobulin prophylaxis for hepatitis A. *Clin Infect Dis*. 1992;14:580–586.

63. Advisory Committee on Immunization Practices CDC. Recommendations for protection against viral hepatitis. *MMWR*. 1985;34:315–316.

64. Carl M, Francis DP, Maynard JE. Food-borne hepatitis: recommendations for control. *J Infect Dis*. 1983;148(6):1133–1135.

65. Centers for Disease Control. Protection against viral hepatitis: recommendation of the immunization practices advisory committee. *MMWR*. 1990;39:5–27.

66. Szmuness W, Stevens CE, Harley EJ, et al. Hepatitis B vaccine in medical staff on hemodialysis units: efficacy and subtype cross-protection. *N Engl J Med*. 1982;307:1481–1486.

67. Coursaget-Pauty AM, Plancoa A, Soulier JP. Distribution of HBsAg subtypes in the world. *Vox Sang*. 1983;44:197–211.

68. Brown JC, Carman WF, Thomas HC. The clinical significance of molecular variation within the hepatitis B virus genome. *Hepatology*. 1992;15:144–148.

69. Hawkins AE, Gilson RJC, Beath SV, et al. Novel application of a point mutation assay: evidence for transmission of hepatitis B viruses with precore mutations and their detection in infants with fulminant hepatitis B. *J Med Virol*. 1994;44:13–21.

70. Fingerote RJ, Bain VG. Fulminant hepatic failure. *Am J Gastroenterol*. 1993;88:1000–1010.

71. Terazawa S, Kojsma M, Yamanaka T, et al. Hepatitis B virus mutants with pre-core region defects in two babies with fulminant hepatitis and their mothers positive for antibodies to hepatitis B e antigen. *Pediatr Res*. 1991;29:5–9.

72. Penna A, Chisani FV, Bertolotti A, et al. Cytotoxic T lymphocytes recognize an HLA-DZ-restricted epitope within the hepatitis B virus nucleocapsid antigen. *J Exp Med*. 1991;174:1568–1570.

73. Ando K, Moriyama T, Guidotti LG, et al. Mechanism of class I restricted immunopathology. A transgenic mouse model of fulminant hepatitis. *J Exp Med*. 1993;178:1541–1554.

74. Yoakum GH, Korba BE, Lechner JR, et al. High-frequency transfusion and cytopathology of hepatitis B virus core antigen gene in human cells. *Science*. 1983;22:385–389.

75. Pignattelli M, Waters J, Brown D, et al. HLA class I antigens on hepatocyte membrane during recovery from acute hepatitis B virus infection and during interferon therapy in chronic hepatitis B virus infection. *Hepatology*. 1986;6:349–355.

76. Deinhardt F. Hepatitis in primates. In: Lauffer M, ed. *Advances in Virus Research*. Vol. 20. New York, NY: Academic Press; 1976:113–157.

77. Deinstag JL. Immunogenesis of the extra hepatic manifestation of hepatitis B virus infection. *Springer Semin Immunopathol.* 1981;3: 461–475.

78. McMahon BJ, Alward WLM, Ball DB, et al. Acute hepatitis B virus infection: relation of age to the clinic expression of disease and subsequent development of the carrier state. *J Infect Dis.* 1985;157:599–603.

79. Stevens CE, Neurath RA, Bensley RP, Szmuness W. HBeAg and anti-HBe detection by radioimmunoassay: correlation of vertical transmission of hepatitis B virus in Taiwan. *J Med Virol.* 1979;3: 237–241.

80. Ganem D. Persistent infection of human with hepatitis B virus, mechanisms and consequences. *Rev Infect Dis.* 1982;4:1026–1047.

81. Hoofnagle JH, Shafritz DA, Popper H. Chronic type B hepatitis and the "healthy" HBsAg carrier state. *Hepatology.* 1987;7:758–763.

82. McMahon BJ, Alberts SR, Wainwright RB, Bulkow L, Lanier AP. Hepatitis B related sequelae. Prospective study in 1400 hepatitis B surface antigen positive Alaska Native carriers. *Arch Intern Med.* 1990;150:1051–1054.

83. Beasley RP, Hwang LY, Stevens CE, et al. Efficacy of hepatitis B immunoglobulin for prevention of perinatal transmission of the hepatitis B virus: final report of a randomized double-blind, placebo-controlled trial. *Hepatology.* 1983;3:135–141.

84. Hsieh CC, Tzonoa A, Zaritsanos K, Kalaman E, Lan SJ, Trichopulos D. Age at first establishment of chronic hepatitis B virus infection and hepatocellular carcinoma risk. A birth order study. *Am J Epidemiol.* 1992;136:1115–1121.

85. Beasley RP. Hepatitis B virus. The major etiology of hepatocellular carcinoma. *Cancer.* 1988;61:1942–1956.

86. Beasley RP, Hwong LY, Lin CC, Chicu CS. Hepatocellular carcinoma and hepatitis B virus. A prospective study of 22,207 men in Taiwan. *Lancet.* 1981;2:1129–1133.

87. Aoki N, Robinson WS. Hepatitis B virus in cirrhosis and hepatocellular carcinoma nodules. *Mol Biol Med.* 1989;6:398–408.

88. Shih C, Burke K, Chou MJ, et al. Tight clustering of human hepatitis B virus integration sites in hepatomas near a triple-stranded region. *J Virol.* 1987;61:3491–3498.

89. Safritz DA, Shoural D, Sherman H, Hadziyannis S, Kew M. Integration of hepatitis B virus DNA into the genome of liver cells in chronic liver disease and hepatocellular carcinoma. *N Engl J Med.* 1981;305: 1067–1075.

90. Gerin JL. Experimental WHV infection of woodchucks: an animal model of hepadnavirus-induced liver cancer. *Gastroenterol Jpn.* 1990;25(suppl):38–42.

91. Korba BE, Weks FU, Baldwin B, et al. Hepatocellular carcinoma in woodchuck hepatitis virus-infected woodchucks: presence of viral DNA in tumor tissue from known carriers and animals serologically recovered from acute infections. *Hepatology.* 1989;9:465–470.

92. Marion PL, Van Davelano MJ, Knight SS, et al. Hepatocellular carcinoma in ground squirrels persistently infected with ground squirrel hepatitis virus. *Proc Natl Acad Sci USA.* 1983;33:4543–4546.

93. Popper HJ, Roth L, Purcell RH, Tennant BC, Gerin JH. Hepatocarcinogenicity of the woodchuck hepatitis virus. *Proc Natl Acad Sci USA.* 1987;84:855–870.

94. Popper HJ, Shih JW, Gerin JH, et al. Woodchuck hepatitis and hepatocellular carcinoma: correlation of histologic with virologic observations. *Hepatology.* 1981;1:91–98.

95. Chang M-H, Chen C-J, Lai M-S, et al. Universal hepatitis B vaccination in Taiwan and the incidence of hepatocellular carcinoma in children. *N Engl J Med.* 1997;336:1855–1859.

96. Qian G-S, Ross RK, Yu MC, et al. A follow-up study of urinary markers of Aflatoxin exposure and liver cancer, risk in Shanghai, People's Republic of China. *Cancer, Epidemiol, Biomarkers Prev.* 1994;3:3–10.

97. Hoofnagle JH, Di Bisceglie AM. Serologic diagnosis of acute and chronic hepatitis. *Semin Liver Dis.* 1991;11:73–83.

98. Seeff LB, Beebe BW, Hoofnagle JH, et al. A serologic follow-up of the 1942 epidemic of post-vaccination hepatitis in the United States Army. *N Engl J Med.* 1987;316:965–970.

99. Koziol DE, Holland PV, Allong DW, et al. Antibody to hepatitis B core antigen as a paradoxical marker for non-A, non-B hepatitis agents in donated blood. *Annals Intern Med.* 1986;104:488–495.

100. Donahue JG, Munoz A, Ness PM, et al. The declining risk of post-transfusion hepatitis C virus infection. *N Engl J Med.* 1992;327: 369–373.

101. Levine OS, Vlahov D, Nelson KE. Epidemiology of hepatitis B virus infections among injecting drug users: seroprevalence, risk factors and viral interactions. *Epidemiol Rev.* 1994;16:418–436.

102. Garfein R, Vlahov D, Galai N, Doherty MC, Nelson KE. Prevalence of hepatitis C virus, hepatitis B virus, human immunodeficiency virus and human T-lymphotrophic virus infections in short term injection drug users. *Am J Public Health.* 1996;86:655–661.

103. Bernier RH, Sampliner R, Gerety R, Tabor E, Hamilton F, Nathanson N. Hepatitis B infection in households of chronic carriers of hepatitis B surface antigen: factors associated with prevalence of infection. *Am J Epidemiol.* 1982;116:199–211.

104. Franks AL, Berg CJ, Kane MA, et al. Hepatitis B infection among children born in the United States to Southeast Asian refugees. *N Engl J Med.* 1089;321:1301–1305.

105. Hurie MB, Mart EE, Davis JP. Horizontal transmission of hepatitis B virus infection to United States-born children of Hmong refugees. *Pediatrics.* 1992;89:269–274.

106. Williams I, Smith MG, Sinha D, et al. Hepatitis B virus transmission in an elementary school setting. *JAMA.* 1997;278:2167–2169.

107. Margolis AS, Alter MJ, Hadler SC. Hepatitis B: evolving epidemiology and implications for control. *Semin Liver Dis.* 1991;11:84–92.

108. Alter MJ, Hadler SC, Judson FN, et al. The changing epidemiology of hepatitis B in the United States: need for alternative vaccination strategies. *JAMA.* 1990;263:1218–1222.

109. McQuillan GM, Coleman PJ, Kruszon-Maran D, Moyer LA, Lambert SB, Margolis HS. Prevalence of hepatitis B virus infection in the United States: the National Health and Nutrition Examination Surveys, 1976 through 1994. *Am J Public Health.* 1999;89:14–18.

110. McQuillan GM, Townsend TR, Fields HA, et al. The seroepidemiology of hepatitis B virus in the United States 1976–89. *Am J Med.* 1989;87:5–10.

111. Bogomolski-Yaholow V, Granot E, Linder N, et al. Prevalence of HBsAg carriers in native and immigrant pregnant female populations

in Israel and passive/active vaccination against HBV of newborns at risk. *J Med Virol.* 1991;34:217–222.

112. McMahon BJ, Schoenberg S, Bulkow L, et al. Seroprevalence of hepatitis B viral markers in 52,000 Alaskan Natives. *Am J Epidemiol.* 1993;138:544–549.

113. Fay OH, Hadler SC, Maynard JE, Pinherro F. Hepatitis in the Americas. *Bull Pan Am Health Org.* 1985;19:401–408.

114. Feldman RE, Schiff ER. Hepatitis in dental professionals. *JAMA.* 1975;232:1228–1230.

115. Mosley JW, Edwards VM, Casey G, Redeker AG, White E. Hepatitis B virus infection in dentists. *N Engl J Med.* 1975;293:729–734.

116. Carl M, Blakey DL, Francis DP, Maynard JE. Interruption of hepatitis B transmission by modification of gynecologists' surgical technique. *Lancet.* 1982;1:731–733.

117. Shaw FE Jr, Barrett CI, Hamm R, et al. Lethal outbreak of hepatitis B in a clinical practice. *JAMA.* 1986;255:3260–3264.

118. El-Serag HB, Mason AC. Rising incidence of hepatocellular carcinoma in the United States. *N Engl J Med.* 1999;340:745–750.

119. Krugman S, Giles JP, Hammond J. Hepatitis virus effect of heat on the infectivity and antigenicity of MS-1 and MS-2 strain. *J Infect Dis.* 1970;122:423–436.

120. Szmuness W, Stevens CE, Harley EJ, et al. Hepatitis B vaccine: demonstration of efficacy in a controlled clinical trial in a high-risk population in the United States. *N Engl J Med.* 1980;303:833–841.

121. Francis DP, Hadler SC, Thompson SE, et al. Prevention of hepatitis B with vaccine. Report from the Centers for Disease Control multi-center efficacy trial among homosexual men. *Ann Intern Med.* 1982;97:362–366.

122. Yu ZY, Liu CB, Francis DP, et al. Prevention of perinatal acquisition of hepatitis B virus carriage using vaccine: preliminary report of a randomized double-blind placebo-controlled and comparative trial. *Pediatrics.* 1985;76:713–718.

123. Pooduotawan Y, Sanpayat S, Pongpuniert W. Protective efficacy of a recombinant DNA hepatitis B vaccine in neonates of HBe antigen-positive mothers. *JAMA.* 1989;261:3278–3281.

124. Stevens CE, Taylor PR, Tong MJ, et al. Yeast-recombinant hepatitis B vaccine. Efficacy with hepatitis B immunoglobulin in prevention of perinatal hepatitis B virus transmission. *JAMA.* 1987;257:2612–2616.

125. Centers for Disease Control and Prevention. Update: recommendations to prevent hepatitis B virus transmission—United States. *MMWR.* 1995;44:574–575.

126. Ukena T, Esber H, Bessette R, et al. Site of injection and response to hepatitis B vaccine. *N Engl J Med.* 1985;313:579–580.

127. Centers for Disease Control. Suboptimal responses to hepatitis B vaccine given by injection in the buttock. *MMWR.* 1985;34:105–108.

128. Alper CA, Kruskall MS, Marcus-Bagley D, et al. Genetic prediction of non response to hepatitis B vaccine. *N Engl J Med.* 1989;321:708–712.

129. World Health Organization. Progression and control of viral hepatitis: memorandum from WHO meeting. *Bull WHO.* 1988;66:443–455.

130. Margolis HS, Coleman PJ, Brown RG, Mart EE, Sheingold SH, Arevelo JA. Prevention of hepatitis B virus transmission by immunization: an economic analysis of current recommendation. *JAMA.* 1995;274:1201–1208.

131. McMahon BJ, Lanier A, Wainwright RB, Kilkenny JJ. Hepatocellular carcinoma in Alaska Eskimos: epidemiology, clinical features and early detection. *Prog Liver Dis.* 1990;9:643–655.

132. Kuang S-Y, Lekawanvijut S, Maneekarn N, et al. Hepatitis B 1762T/1764A mutations, hepatitis C infection and codon 249 p53 mutations in hepatocellular carcinoma in Thailand. *Cancer, Epidemiol, Biomarkers Prev.* 2005;14:380–384.

133. Kuang SY, Jackson PE, Wang JB, et al. Specific mutations of hepatitis B virus in plasma predict liver cancer development. *Proc Natl Acad Sci USA.* 2004;101:3575–3580.

134. Korenman J, Baker R, Waggoner J, Everhart JE, Di Bisceglie AM, Hoofnagle JH. Long-term remission in chronic hepatitis B after alfa-interferon therapy. *Ann Intern Med.* 1991;114:629–634.

135. Perrillo RP, Schiff ER, Davis GL. A randomized controlled trial of interferon alfa-2b alone and after prednisone withdrawal for the treatment of chronic hepatitis B. *N Engl J Med.* 1990;323: 295–301.

136. Lai CL, Chien R-N, Leung NWY. A one-year trial of Lamivudine for chronic hepatitis B. *N Engl J Med.* 1998;339:61–68.

137. Dienstag JL, Schiff ER, Wright TL, et al. Lamivudine initial treatment for chronic hepatitis B in the United States. *N Engl J Med.* 1999;341:1256–1263.

138. Lok AS-F. The maze of treatments for hepatitis B. *N Engl J Med.* 2005;352:274–276.

139. Lee SM. Hepatitis B virus infection. *N Engl J Med.* 1997;337: 1733–1745.

140. Liaw Y-F, Sung JJY, Chow WC, et al. Lamivudine for patients with chronic hepatitis B and advanced liver disease. *N Engl J Med.* 2004;351:1521–1531.

141. Lai C-L, Dienstag J, Schiff E, et al. Prevalence and clinical correlates of YMDD variants during lumivudine therapy for patients with chronic hepatitis B. *Clin Infect Dis.* 2003;36:687–696.

142. Fields HA, Hadler SC. Delta hepatitis: a review. *J Clin Immunol.* 1986;9:128–142.

143. Arico S, Aragona M, Rizzetto M, et al. Clinical significance of antibody to the hepatitis delta virus in symptomless HBsAg carriers. *Lancet.* 1985;2:356–357.

144. Caredda F, Antinoni S, Re T, Pastechia C, Moroni M. Course and prognosis of acute HDV hepatitis. *Prog Clin Biol Res.* 1987;234: 267–276.

145. Perrillo RP, Lai C-L, Liaw Y-F, et al. Predictors of HBeAg loss after lamivudine treatment for chronic hepatitis B. *Hepatology.* 2002;36:186–194.

146. Fung SK, Wong F, Hussain M, Lok ASF. Sustained response after a 2 year course of lamivudine treatment of hepatitis Be antigen-negative chronic hepatitis B. *J Viral Hepatitis.* 2004;11:432–438.

147. Fung SK, Lok ASF. Management of hepatitis B patients with antiviral resistance. *Antivir Ther.* 2004;9:1013–1026.

148. Perrilo R, Schiff E, Yoshida E, et al. Adefovir dipivoxil for the treatment of lamivudine-resistant hepatitis B mutants. *Hepatology.* 2000;32:129–134.

149. Hadziyannis SJ, Tassopoulos MC, Heathcote EJ, et al. Adefovir dipivoxil for the treatment of hepatitis Be antigen-negative chronic hepatitis B. *N Engl J Med.* 2003;348:800–807.

150. Yuen M-F, Sablon E, Yuan H-J, et al. Significance of hepatitis B genotype in acute exacerbation, HBeAg seroconversion, cirrhosis-related complications and hepatocellular carcinoma. *Hepatology.* 2003;37:562–567.

151. Wai CT, Chu C-J, Hussain M, Lok ASF. HBV genotype B is associated with better response to interferon therapy in HBeAg(+) chronic hepatitis than genotype C. *Hepatology.* 2002;36:1425–1430.

152. Kao J-H, Wa N-H, Chen P-J, Lai M-Y, Chen D-S. Hepatitis B genotypes and the response to interferon therapy. *J Hepatol.* 2000;33:998–1002.

153. Chu C-J, Hussain M, Lok ASF. Hepatitis B virus genotype B is associated with earlier HBeAg seroconversion compared with hepatitis B virus genotype C. *Gastroenterology.* 2002;122:1756–1762.

154. Anzola M. Hepatocellular carcinoma: a role of hepatitis B and hepatitis C viruses proteins in hepatocarcinogenesis. *J Virol Hep.* 2004;11:383–393.

155. Sanchez-Tapias JM, Costa J, Mas A, Bruguera M, Rodes J. Influence of hepatitis B virus genotype on the long-term outcome of chronic hepatitis B in western patients. *Gastroenterology.* 2002;123:1848–1856.

156. Garfein RS, Bower WA, Loney CM, et al. Factors associated with fulminant liver failure during an outbreak among injecting drug users with acute hepatitis B. *Hepatology.* 2004;40:865–873.

157. Thio CL. Hepatitis B in the human immunodeficiency virus infected patient: epidemiology, natural history and treatment. *Sem Liver Dis.* 2003;3:125–136.

158. Twu SJ, Detels R, Nelson KE, et al. Relationship of hepatitis B virus infection to human immunodeficiency virus type 1 infection. *J Infect Dis.* 1993;167:299–304.

159. Thio CL, Seaburg EC, Skolasky R, et al. HIV-1, hepatitis B virus and risk of liver-related mortality in the Multicenter AIDS Cohort Study (MACS). *Lancet.* 2002;360:1921–1926.

160. Soriano V, Puoti M, Bonacini M, et al. Care of patients with chronic hepatitis B and HIV coinfection: recommendations from an HIV-HBV international panel. *AIDS.* 2005;19:221–240.

161. Lettau L, McCarthy JG, Smith MH, et al. An outbreak of severe hepatitis due to delta and hepatitis B virus in injection drug users and their contacts. *N Engl J Med.* 1987;317:1256–1261.

162. Hadler SC, De Monson M, Ponzotto A, et al. Delta virus infection and severe hepatitis: an epidemic in the Yupca Indians of Venezuela. *Ann Intern Med.* 1984;100:339–344.

163. Shimizu YK, Feinstone SM, Kohara M, Purcell RH, Yoshikura H. Hepatitis C virus: detection of intracellular virus particles by electron microscopy. *Hepatology.* 1996;23:205–209.

164. Kaito M, Watanabe S, Tsukiyama-Kohara K, et al. Hepatitis C virus particle detected by immunoelectron microscopic study. *J Gen Virol.* 1994;75:1755–1760.

165. Choo QL, Richman KH, Han JH, et al. Genetic organization and diversity of the hepatitis C virus. *Proc Natl Acad Sci USA.* 1991;88:2451–2455.

166. Negro F, Pacchioni D, Shimizu Y, et al. Detection of intrahepatic replication of hepatitis C virus RNA by in situ hybridization and comparison with histopathology. *Proc Natl Acad Sci USA.* 1992;89:2247–2251.

167. Krawczynski K, Beach MJ, Bradley DW, et al. Hepatitis C antigens in hepatocytes. Immuno-morphologic detection and identification. *Gastroenterology.* 1992;103:622–629.

168. Lerat H, Berby F, Trabaud MA, et al. Specific detection of hepatitis C virus minus strand RNA in hematopoietic cells. *J Clin Invest.* 1996;97:845–851.

169. Shimizu YK, Igarashi H, Kanematu T, et al. Sequence analysis of the hepatitis C virus genome recovered from serum, liver, and peripheral blood mononuclear cells of infected chimpanzees. *J Virol.* 1997;71:5769–5773.

170. Lanford RE, Chavez D, Von Chisari F, Sureau C. Lack of detection of negative-strand hepatitis C virus RNA in peripheral blood mononuclear cells and other extrahepatic tissues by the highly strand-specific rTth reverse transcriptase PCR. *J Virol.* 1995;69: 8079–8083.

171. Neumann AU, Lam NP, Dahari H, et al. Hepatitis C viral dynamics in vivo and the antiviral efficacy of interferon-alpha therapy. *Science.* 1998;282:103–107.

172. Martell M, Esteban JI, Quer J, et al. Hepatitis C virus (HCV) circulates as a population of different but closely related genomes: quasispecies nature of HCV genome distribution. *J Virol.* 1992;66:3225–3229.

173. Kato N, Ootsuyama Y, Tanaka T, et al. Marked sequence diversity in the putative envelope proteins of hepatitis C viruses. *Virus Res.* 1992;22:107–123.

174. Wang Y, Ray SC, Laeyendecker O, Ticehurst JR, Thomas DL. Assessment of hepatitis C virus sequence complexity by the electrophoretic mobility of both single- and double-stranded DNA. *J Clin Micro.* 1998;36:2982–2989.

175. Ray SC, Wang YM, Laeyendecker O, Ticehurst J, Villano SA, Thomas DL. Acute hepatitis C virus structural gene sequences as predictors of persistent viremia: hypervariable region 1 as decoy. *J Virol.* 1998;73:2938–2946.

176. Major ME, Mihalik K, Fernandez J, et al. Long-term follow-up of chimpanzees inoculated with the first infectious clone for hepatitis C virus. *J Virol.* 1999;73:3317–3325.

177. Weiner AJ, Geysen HM, Christopherson C, et al. Evidence for immune selection of hepatitis C virus (HCV) putative envelope glycoprotein variants: potential role in chronic HCV infections. *Proc Natl Acad Sci USA.* 1992;89:3468–3472.

178. Shimizu YK, Hijikata M, Iwamoto A, Alter HJ, Purcell RH, Yoshikura H. Neutralizing antibodies against hepatitis C virus and the emergence of neutralization escape mutant viruses. *J Virol.* 1994;68:1494–1500.

179. Weiner A, Erickson AL, Kansopon J, et al. Persistent hepatitis C virus infection in a chimpanzee is associated with emergence of a cytotoxic T lymphocyte escape variant. *Proc Natl Acad Sci USA.* 1995;92: 2755–2759.

180. Liou TC, Chang TT, Young KC, Lin XZ, Lin CY, Wu HL. Detection of HCV RNA in saliva, urine, seminal fluid, and ascites. *J Med Virol.* 1992;37:197–202.

181. Chen M, Yun Z-B, Sällberg M, et al. Detection of hepatitis C virus RNA in the cell fraction of saliva before and after oral surgery. *J Med Virol.* 1995;45:223–226.

182. Wang JT, Wang TH, Sheu JC, Lin JT, Chen DS. Hepatitis C virus RNA in saliva of patients with posttransfusion hepatitis and low efficiency of transmission among spouses. *J Med Virol.* 1992;36:28–31.

183. Fiore RJ, Potenza D, Monno L, et al. Detection of HCV RNA in serum and seminal fluid from HIV-1 co-infected intravenous drug addicts. *J Med Virol.* 1995;46:364–367.

184. Mendel I, Muraine M, Riachi G, et al. Detection and genotyping of the hepatitis C RNA in tear fluid from patients with chronic hepatitis C. *J Med Virol.* 1997;51:231–233.

185. Abe K, Inchauspe G. Transmission of hepatitis C by saliva. *Lancet.* 1991;337:248.

186. Pileri P, Uematsu Y, Campagnoli S, et al. Binding of hepatitis C virus to CD81. *Science.* 1998;282:938–941.

187. Bukh J, Miller RH, Purcell RH. Genetic heterogeneity of hepatitis C virus: quasispecies and genotypes. *Semin Liver Dis.* 1995;15:41–63.

188. Simmonds P, Holmes EC, Cha T-A, et al. Classification of hepatitis C virus into six major genotypes and a series of subtypes by phylogenetic analysis of the NS-5 region. *J Gen Virol.* 1993;74:2391–2399.

189. Bronowicki JP, Venard V, Botté C, et al. Patient-to-patient transmission of hepatitis C virus during colonoscopy. *N Engl J Med.* 1997;337:237–240.

190. Esteban JI, Gómez J, Martell M, et al. Transmission of hepatitis C virus by a cardiac surgeon. *N Engl J Med.* 1996;334:555–560.

191. Thomas DL, Zenilman JZ, Alter HJ, Shih JW, Galai N, Quinn TC. Sexual transmission of hepatitis C virus among patients attending Baltimore sexually transmitted diseases clinics—an analysis of 309 sexual partnerships. *J Infect Dis.* 1995;171:768–775.

192. Allander T, Gruber A, Naghavi M, et al. Frequent patient-to-patient transmission of hepatitis C virus in a haematology ward. *Lancet.* 1995;345:603–607.

193. Villano SA, Vlahov D, Nelson KE, Cohn S, Thomas DL. Persistence of viremia and the importance of long-term follow-up after acute hepatitis C infection. *Hepatology.* 1999;29:908–914.

194. Inglesby TV, Rai R, Astemborski J, et al. A prospective, community-based evaluation of liver enzymes in individuals with hepatitis C after drug use. *Hepatology.* 1999;29:590–596.

195. Farci P, Alter HJ, Wong D, et al. A long-term study of hepatitis C virus replication in non-A, non-B hepatitis. *N Engl J Med.* 1991;325:98–104.

196. Alter MJ, Margolis HS, Krawczynski K, et al. The natural history of community acquired hepatitis C in the United States. *N Engl J Med.* 1992;327:1899–1905.

197. Tong MJ, El-Farra NS, Reikes AR, Co RL. Clinical outcomes after transfusion-associated hepatitis C. *N Engl J Med.* 1995;332:1463–1466.

198. Kiyosawa K, Sodeyama T, Tanaka E, et al. Interrelationship of blood transfusion, non-A, non-B hepatitis and hepatocellular carcinoma: analysis by detection of antibody to hepatitis C virus. *Hepatology.* 1990;12:671–675.

199. Kenny-Walsh E. Clinical outcomes after hepatitis C infection from contaminated anti-D immune globulin. Irish Hepatology Research Group. *N Engl J Med.* 1999;340:1228–1233.

200. Agnello V, Chung RT, Kaplan LM. A role for hepatitis C virus infection in Type II cryoglobulinemia. *N Engl J Med.* 1992;327:1490–1495.

201. Misiani R, Bellavita P, Fenili D, et al. Hepatitis C virus infection in patients with essential mixed cryoglobulinemia. *Ann Intern Med.* 1992;117:573–577.

202. Johnson RJ, Gretch DR, Yamabe H, et al. Membranoproliferative glomerulonephritis associated with hepatitis C virus infection [see comments]. *N Engl J Med.* 1993;328:465–470.

203. Fargion S, Piperno A, Cappellini MD, et al. Hepatitis C virus and porphyria cutanea tarda: evidence of a strong association. *Hepatology.* 1992;16:1322–1326.

204. DeCastro M, Sanchez J, Herrera JF, et al. Hepatitis C virus antibodies and liver disease in patients with porphyria cutanea tarda. *Hepatology.* 1993;17:551–557.

205. Centers for Disease Control and Prevention. Recommendations for prevention and control of hepatitis C virus infection and HCV-related chronic disease. *MMWR.* 1998;47(RR-19):1–39.

206. McHutchinson JG, Person JL, Govindarajan S, et al. Improved detection of hepatitis C virus antibodies in high-risk populations. *Hepatology.* 1992;15:19–25.

207. Nakatsuji Y, Matsumoto A, Tanaka E, Ogata H, Kiyosawa K. Detection of chronic hepatitis C virus infection by four diagnostic systems: first-generation and second-generation enzyme-linked immunosorbent assay, second-generation recombinant immunoblot assay and nested polymerase chain reaction analysis. *Hepatology.* 1992;16:300–305.

208. Chien DY, Choo QL, Tabrizi A, et al. Diagnosis of hepatitis C virus (HCV) infection using an immunodominant chimeric polyprotein to capture circulating antibodies: reevaluation of the role of HCV in liver disease. *Proc Natl Acad Sci USA.* 1992;89:10011–10015.

209. Couroucé A-M, Le Marrec N, Girault A, Ducamp S, Simon N. Anti-hepatitis C virus (anti-HCV) seroconversion in patients undergoing hemodialysis: comparison of second- and third-generation anti-HCV assays. *Transfusion.* 1994;34:790–795.

210. Vallari DS, Jett BW, Alter HJ, Mimms LT, Holzman R, Shih JW. Serological markers of posttransfusion hepatitis C viral infection. *J Clin Micro.* 1992;30:552–556.

211. van der Poel CL, Cuypers HTM, Reesink HW, et al. Confirmation of hepatitis C virus infection by new four-antigen recombinant immunoblot assay. *Lancet.* 1991;337:317–319.

212. Buffet C, Charnaux N, Laurent-Puig P, et al. Enhanced detection of antibodies to hepatitis C virus by use of a third-generation recombinant immunoblot assay. *J Med Virol.* 1994;43:259–261.

213. McGuinness PH, Bishop GA, Lien A, Wiley B, Parsons C, McCaughan GW. Detection of serum hepatitis C virus RNA in HCV antibody-seropositive volunteer blood donors. *Hepatology.* 1993;18:485–490.

214. Vrielink H, van der Poel CL, Reesink HW, et al. Look-back study of infectivity of anti-HCV ELISA-positive blood components. *Lancet.* 1995;345:95–96.

215. Zaaijer HL, Cuypers HTM, Reesink HW, Winkel IN, Gerken G, Lelie PN. Reliability of polymerase chain reaction for detection of hepatitis C virus. *Lancet.* 1993;341:722–724.

216. Bresters D, Cuypers HT, Reesink HW, et al. Comparison of quantitative cDNA-PCR with the branched DNA hybridization assay

for monitoring plasma hepatitis C virus RNA levels in haemophilia patients participating in a controlled interferon trial. *J Med Virol.* 1994;43:262–268.

217. Gretch DR, Dela Rosa C, Carithers RL Jr, Willson RA, Williams B, Corey L. Assessment of hepatitis C viremia using molecular amplification technologies: correlations and clinical implications. *Ann Intern Med.* 1995;123:321–329.

218. Miskovsky EP, Carella AV, Gutekunst K, Sun C, Quinn TC, Thomas DL. Clinical characterization of a competitive PCR assay for quantitative testing of hepatitis C virus. *J Clin Microbiol.* 1996;34:1975–1979.

219. Stuyver L, Rossau R, Wyseur A, et al. Typing of hepatitis C virus isolates and characterization of new subtypes using a line probe assay. *J Gen Virol.* 1993;74:1093–1102.

220. Stuyver L, Wyseur A, Van Arnhem W, Hernandez F, Maertens G. Second-generation line probe assay for hepatitis C virus genotyping. *J Clin Microbiol.* 1996;34:2259–2266.

221. Thiers V, Jaffredo F, Tuveri R, Chodan N, Bréchot C. Development of a simple restriction fragment length polymorphism (RFLP)-based assay for HCV genotyping and comparative analysis with genotyping and serotyping tests. *J Virol Methods.* 1997;65:9–17.

222. Widell A, Shev S, Mansson S, et al. Genotyping of hepatitis C virus isolates by a modified polymerase chain reaction assay using type specific primers: epidemiological applications. *J Med Virol.* 1994;44:272–279.

223. Esteban JI, Lopez-Talavera JC, Genesca J, et al. High rate of infectivity and liver disease in blood donors with antibodies to hepatitis C virus. *Ann Intern Med.* 1991;115:443–449.

224. Pereira BJG, Milford EL, Kirkman RL, et al. Prevalence of hepatitis C virus RNA in organ donors positive for hepatitis C antibody and in the recipients of their organs. *N Engl J Med.* 1992; 327:910–915.

225. Terrault NA, Wright TL. Hepatitis C virus in the setting of transplantation. *Semin Liver Dis.* 1995;15:92–100.

226. Pereira BJG, Milford EL, Kirkman RL, Levey AS. Transmission of hepatitis C virus by organ transplantation. *N Engl J Med.* 1991;325:454–460.

227. Centers for Disease Control and Prevention. Public Health Service interagency guidelines for screening blood, plasma, organs, tissue and semen for evidence of hepatitis B and C. *MMWR.* 1991;40:1–23.

228. Donahue JG, Munoz A, Ness PM, et al. The declining risk of post-transfusion hepatitis C virus infection. *N Engl J Med.* 1992;327: 369–373.

229. Blajchman MA, Bull SB, Feinman SV. Post-transfusion hepatitis: impact of non-A, non-B hepatitis surrogate tests. *Lancet.* 1995;345: 21–25.

230. Schreiber GB, Busch MP, Kleinman SH, Korelitz JJ. The risk of transfusion-transmitted viral infections. *N Engl J Med.* 1996;334: 1685–90.

231. Widell A, Elmud H, Persson MH, Jonsson M. Transmission of hepatitis C via both erythrocyte and platelet transfusions from a single donor in serological window-phase of hepatitis C. *Vox Sang.* 1996;71: 55–57.

232. Stramer SL, Glynn SA, Kleinman SH, et al. Detection of HIV-1 and HCV infection among antibody-negative blood donors by nucleic acid-amplification testing. *N Engl J Med.* 2004;351:760–768.

233. Yap PL, McOmish F, Webster ADB, et al. Hepatitis C virus transmission by intravenous immunoglobulin. *J Hepatol*. 1994;21:455–460.

234. Bjoro K, Froland SS, Yun Z, Samdal HH, Haaland T. Hepatitis C infection in patients with primary hypogammaglobulinemia after treatment with contaminated immune globulin. *N Engl J Med*. 1994;331:1607–1611.

235. Power JP, Lawlor E, Davidson F, Hepatitis C. Viraemia in recipients of Irish intravenous anti-D immunoglobulin. *Lancet*. 1994;344:1166–1167.

236. Bresee JS, Mast EE, Coleman FJ, et al. Hepatitis C virus infection associated with administration of intravenous immune globulin–a cohort study. *JAMA*. 1996;276:1563–1567.

237. Thomas DL, Vlahov D, Solomon L, et al. Correlates of hepatitis C virus infections among injection drug users in Baltimore. *Medicine*. 1995;74:212–220.

238. Bolumar F, Hernandez-Aguado I, Ferrer L, Ruiz I, Aviñó M, Rebagliato M. Prevalence of antibodies to hepatitis C in a population of intravenous drug users in Valencia, Spain, 1990-1992. *Int J Epidemiol*. 1996;25:204–209.

239. Girardi E, Zaccarelli M, Tossini G, Puro V, Narciso P, Visco G. Hepatitis C virus infection in intravenous drug users: prevalence and risk factors. *Scand J Infect Dis*. 1990;22:751–752.

240. Bell J, Batey RG, Farrell GC, Crewe EB, Cunningham AL, Byth K. Hepatitis C virus in intravenous drug users. *Med J Aust*. 1990;153:274–276.

241. Van Ameijden EJ, van den Hoek JA, Mientjes GH, Coutinho RA. A longitudinal study on the incidence and transmission patterns of HIV, HBV and HCV infection among drug users in Amsterdam. *Eur J Epidemiol*. 1993;9:255–262.

242. Patti AM, Santi AL, Pompa MG, et al. Viral hepatitis and drugs: a continuing problem. *Int J Epidemiol*. 1993;22:135–139.

243. Garfein RS, Doherty MC, Brown D, et al. Hepatitis C virus infection among short-term injection drug users. *JAIDS*. 1998;18:S11–S19.

244. Conry-Cantilena C, Vanraden MT, Gibble J, et al. Routes of infection, viremia, and liver disease in blood donors found to have hepatitis C virus infection. *N Engl J Med*. 1996;334:1691–1696.

245. Kiyosawa K, Sodeyama T, Tanaka E, et al. Hepatitis C in hospital employees with needlestick injuries [see comments]. *Ann Intern Med*. 1991;115:367–369.

246. Ridzon R, Gallagher K, Ciesielski C, et al. Simultaneous transmission of human immunodeficiency virus and hepatitis C virus from a needle-stick injury. *N Engl J Med*. 1997;336:919–922.

247. Mitsui T, Iwano K, Masuko K, et al. Hepatitis C virus infection in medical personnel after needlestick accident. *Hepatology*. 1992;16:1109–1114.

248. Sartori M, La Terra G, Aglietta M, Manzin A, Navino C, Verzetti G. Transmission of hepatitis C via blood splash into conjunctiva. *Scand J Infect Dis*. 1993;25:270–271.

249. Thomas DL, Gruninger SE, Siew C, Joy ED, Quinn TC. Occupational risk of hepatitis C infections among general dentists and oral surgeons in North America. *Am J Med*. 1996;100:41–45.

250. Thomas DL, Factor S, Kelen G, Washington AS, Taylor E, Quinn TQ. Hepatitis B and C in health care workers at the Johns Hopkins Hospital. *Arch Intern Med*. 1993;153:1705–1712.

251. Gerberding JL. Incidence and prevalence of human immunodeficiency virus, hepatitis B virus, hepatitis C virus, and cytomegalovirus among health care personnel at risk for blood exposure: final report from a longitudinal study. *J Infect Dis.* 1994;170:1410–1417.

252. Kuo MY, Hahn LJ, Hong CY, Kao JH, Chen DS. Low prevalence of hepatitis C virus infection among dentists in Taiwan. *J Med Virol.* 1993;40:10–13.

253. Campello C, Majori S, Poli A, Pacini P, Nicolardi L, Pini F. Prevalence of HCV antibodies in health-care workers from northern Italy. *Infection.* 1992;20:224–226.

254. Polish LB, Tong MJ, Co RL, Coleman PJ, Alter MJ. Risk factors for hepatitis C virus infection among health care personnel in a community hospital. *Am J Infect Control.* 1993;21:196–200.

255. Puro V, Petrosillo N, Ippolito G, et al. Occupational hepatitis C virus infection in Italian health care workers. *Am J Public Health.* 1995;85:1272–1275.

256. Schvarcz R, Johansson B, Nyström B, Sönnerborg A. Nosocomial transmission of hepatitis C virus. *Infection.* 1997;25:74–77.

257. Munro J, Biggs JD, McCruden EAB. Detection of a cluster of hepatitis C infections in a renal transplant unit by analysis of sequence variation of the NS5a gene. *J Infect Dis.* 1996;174:177–180.

258. Stuyver L, Claeys H, Wyseur A, et al. Hepatitis C virus in a hemodialysis unit: molecular evidence for nosocomial transmission. *Kidney Int.* 1996;49:889–895.

259. Sampietro M, Badalamenti S, Salvadori S, et al. High prevalence of a rare hepatitis C virus in patients treated in the same hemodialysis unit: evidence for nosocomial transmission of HCV. *Kidney Int.* 1995;47:911–917.

260. Alter MJ. Epidemiology of hepatitis C. *Hepatology.* 1997;26:62S–65S.

261. Ko YC, Ho MS, Chiang TA, Chang SJ, Chang PY. Tattooing as a risk of hepatitis C virus infection. *J Med Virol.* 1992;38:288–291.

262. Sun DX, Zhang FG, Geng YQ, Xi DS. Hepatitis C transmission by cosmetic tattooing in women. *Lancet.* 1996;347:541.

263. Dusheiko GM, Smith M, Scheuer PJ. Hepatitis C virus transmission by human bite. *Lancet.* 1990;336:503–504.

264. van Doornum GJJ, Hooykaas C, Cuypers MT, van Der Lind MMD, Coutinho RS. Prevalence of hepatitis C virus infections among heterosexuals with multiple partners. *J Med Virol.* 1991;35:22–27.

265. Thomas DL, Cannon RO, Shapiro C, Hook EWI, Alter MJ, Quinn TC. *J Infect Dis.* 1994;169:990–995.

266. Petersen EE, Clemens R, Bock HL, Friese K, Hess G. Hepatitis B and C in heterosexual patients with various sexually transmitted diseases. *Infection.* 1992;20:128–131.

267. Nakashima K, Kashiwagi S, Hayashi J, et al. Sexual transmission of hepatitis C virus among female prostitutes and patients with sexually transmitted diseases in Fukuoka, Kyushu, Japan. *Am J Epidemiol.* 1992;136:1132–1137.

268. Utsumi T, Hashimoto E, Okumura Y, et al. Heterosexual activity as a risk factor for the transmission of hepatitis C virus. *J Med Virol.* 1995;46:122–125.

269. Capelli C, Prati D, Bosoni P, et al. Sexual transmission of hepatitis C virus to a repeat blood donor. *Transfusion.* 1997;37:436–440.

270. Healey CJ, Smith DB, Walker JL, et al. Acute hepatitis C infection after sexual exposure. *Gut.* 1995;36:148–150.

271. Akahane Y, Kojima M, Sugai Y, et al. Hepatitis C virus infection in spouses of patients with type C chronic liver disease [see comments]. *Ann Intern Med.* 1994;120:748–752.

272. Kao JH, Chen PJ, Yang PM, et al. Intrafamilial transmission of hepatitis C virus: the important role of infections between spouses. *J Infect Dis.* 1992;166:900–903.

273. Kao JH, Hwang YT, Chen PJ, et al. Transmission of hepatitis C virus between spouses: the important role of exposure duration. *Am J Gastroenterol.* 1996;91:2087–2090.

274. Chayama K, Kobayashi M, Tsubota A, et al. Molecular analysis of intraspousal transmission of hepatitis C virus. *J Hepatol.* 1995;22: 431–439.

275. Piazza M, Sagliocca L, Tosone GM, et al. Sexual transmission of the hepatitis C virus and efficacy of prophylaxis with intramuscular immune serum globulin—a randomized controlled trial. *Arch Intern Med.* 1997;157:1537–1544.

276. Thaikruea L, Nelson KE, Thongsawat S, Maneekarn N, Netski D, Thomas DL. Risk factors for hepatitis C virus infection among blood donors in Northern Thailand. *Transfusion.* 2004;44:1433–1440.

277. Bresters D, Mauser-Bunschoten ED, Reesink HW, et al. Sexual transmission of hepatitis C. *Lancet.* 1993;342:210–211.

278. Everhart JE, Di Bisceglie AM, Murray LM, et al. Risk for non-A, non-B (Type C) hepatitis through sexual or household contact with chronic carriers. *Ann Intern Med.* 1990;112:544–555.

279. Brettler DB, Mannucci PM, Gringeri A, et al. The low risk of hepatitis C virus transmission among sexual partners of hepatitis C infected hemophilic males: an international, multicenter study. *Blood.* 1992;80:540–543.

280. Gordon SC, Patel AH, Kulesza GW, Barnes RE, Silverman AL. Lack of evidence for the heterosexual transmission of hepatitis C. *Am J Gastroenterol.* 1992;87:1849–1851.

281. Melbye M, Biggar RJ, Wantzin P, Krogsgaard K, Ebbesen P, Becker NG. Sexual transmission of hepatitis C virus: cohort study (1981–1989) among European homosexual men. *Br Med J.* 1990;301: 210–212.

282. Osmond DH, Charlebois E, Sheppard HW, et al. Comparison of risk factors for hepatitis C and hepatitis B virus infection in homosexual men. *J Infect Dis.* 1993;167:66–71.

283. Bodsworth NJ, Cunningham P, Kaldor J, Donovan B. Hepatitis C virus infection in a large cohort of homosexually active men: independent associations with HIV-1 infection and injecting drug use but not sexual behaviour. *Genitourin Med.* 1996;72:118–122.

284. Donahue JG, Nelson KE, Munoz A, et al. Antibody to hepatitis C virus among cardiac surgery patients, homosexual men, and intravenous drug users in Baltimore, Maryland. *Am J Epidemiol.* 1991;134: 1206–1211.

285. Roudot Thoraval F, Pawlotsky JM, Thiers V, et al. Lack of mother-to-infant transmission of hepatitis C virus in human immunodeficiency virus-seronegative women: a prospective study with hepatitis C virus RNA testing. *Hepatology.* 1993;17:772–777.

286. Reinus JF, Leikin EL, Alter HJ, et al. Failure to detect vertical transmission of hepatitis C virus. *Ann Intern Med.* 1992;117:881–886.

287. Ohto H, Terazawa S, Nobuhiko S, et al. Transmission of hepatitis C virus from mothers to infants. *N Engl J Med.* 1994;330:744–750.

288. Zanetti AR, Tanzi E, Paccagnini S, et al. Mother-to-infant transmission of hepatitis C virus. *Lancet.* 1995;345:289–291.

289. Lam JPH, McOmish F, Burns SM, Yap PL, Mok JYQ, Simmonds P. Infrequent vertical transmission of hepatitis C virus. *J Infect Dis.* 1993;167:572–576.

290. Novati R, Thiers V, Monforte AD, et al. Mother-to-child transmission of hepatitis C virus detected by nested polymerase chain reaction. *J Infect Dis.* 1992;165:720–723.

291. Wejstal R, Widell A, Mansson A-S, Hermodsson S, Norkrans G. Mother-to-infant transmission of hepatitis C virus. *Ann Intern Med.* 1992;117:887–890.

292. Weintrub PS, Veereman Wauters G, Cowan MJ, Thaler MM. Hepatitis C virus infection in infants whose mothers took street drugs intravenously. *J Pediatr.* 1991;119:869.

293. Thomas DL, Villano SA, Reister K, et al. Perinatal transmission of hepatitis C virus from human immunodeficiency virus type 1-infected individuals. *J Infect Dis.* 1998;177:1480–1488.

294. Matsubara T, Sumazaki R, Takita H. Mother-to-infant transmission of hepatitis C virus: a prospective study. *Eur J Pediatr.* 1995;154: 973–978.

295. Lin H-H, Kao J-H, Hsu H-Y, et al. Possible role of high-titer maternal viremia in perinatal transmission of hepatitis C virus. *J Infect Dis.* 1994;169:638–641.

296. Moriya T, Sasaki F, Mizui M, et al. Transmission of hepatitis C virus from mothers to infants: its frequency and risk factors revisited. *Biomed Pharmacother.* 1995;49:59–64.

297. Telfer PT, Brown D, Devereux H, Lee CA, Dusheiko GM. HCV RNA levels and HIV infection: evidence for a viral interaction in haemophilic patients. *Br J Haematol.* 1994;88:397–399.

298. Sherman KE, O'Brien J, Gutierrez G, et al. Quantitative evaluation of hepatitis C virus RNA in patients with concurrent human immunodeficiency virus infections. *J Clin Microbiol.* 1993;31: 2679–2682.

299. Eyster ME, Fried MW, Di Bisceglie AM, Goedert JJ. Increasing hepatitis C virus RNA levels in hemophiliacs: relationship to human immunodeficiency virus infection and liver disease. *Blood.* 1994;84:1020–1023.

300. Thomas DL, Shih JW, Alter HJ, et al. Effect of human immunodeficiency virus on hepatitis C virus infection among injecting drug users. *J Infect Dis.* 1996;174:690–695.

301. Ogasawara S, Kage M, Kosai K, Shimamatsu K, Kojiro M. Hepatitis C virus RNA in saliva and breast-milk of hepatitis C carrier mothers. *Lancet.* 1993;341:561.

302. Ohto H, Okamoto H, Mishiro S. Vertical transmission of hepatitis C virus. Reply. *N Engl J Med.* 1994;331:400.

303. Lin H-H, Kao J-H, Hsu H-Y, et al. Absence of infection in breast-fed infants born to hepatitis C virus-infected mothers. *J Pediatr.* 1995;126:589–591.

304. Hepatitis C Virus Network. A significant sex—but not elective cesarean section—effect on mother-to child transmission of hepatitis C virus infection. *J Infect Dis.* 2005;192:1872–1879.

305. Mast EE, Huvang L-Y, Seto DSY, et al. Risk factors for perinatal transmission of hepatitis C virus (HCV) and the natural history of HCV acquired in infancy. *J Infect Dis.* 2005;192:1880–1889.

306. Beasley RP. Nature usually favors females. *J Infect Dis* 2005;192:1865–1866.

307. Poynard T, Bedossa P, Opolon P, et al. Natural history of liver fibrosis progression in patients with chronic hepatitis C. *Lancet.* 1997;349: 825–832.

308. Poynard T, Yuen MF, Ratzine V, Lai CL. Viral hepatitis C. *Lancet.* 2003;362:2095–3000.

309. Thomas DL, Astembroski J, Rai R, et al. The natural history of hepatitis C virus infection: host, viral and environmental factors. *JAMA.* 2000;284:450–456.

310. Sulkowski MS. Hepatitis C virus infection as an opportunistic disease in persons infected with the human immunodeficiency virus. *Clin Infect Dis.* 2000;30:S77–S84.

311. Eyster ME, Diamondstone LS, Lien JM, Ehrmann WC, Quan S, Goedert JJ. Natural history of hepatitis C virus infections in multitransfused hemophiliacs: effect of coinfection with human immunodeficiency virus. The Multicenter Hemophilia Cohort Study. *JAIDS.* 1993;6: 602–610.

312. Benhamon Y, Bocket M, DiMartino V, et al. Liver fibrosis progression in HIV and HCV coinfected patients. The Multivirc Group. *Hepatology.* 1999;30:1054–1058.

313. World Health Organization. Hepatitis C: global prevalence. *Weekly Epidemiological Record.* 1997:341–348.

314. Osella AR, Misciagna G, Leone A, Di Leo A, Fiore G. Epidemiology of hepatitis C virus infection in an area of southern Italy. *J Hepatol.* 1997;27:30–35.

315. Chiaramonte M, Stroffolini T, Lorenzoni U, et al. Risk factors in community-acquired chronic hepatitis C virus infection: a case-control study in Italy. *J Hepatol.* 1996;24: 129–134.

316. Nakashima K, Ikematsu H, Hayashi J, Kishihara Y, Mitsutake A, Kashiwagi S. Intrafamilial transmission of hepatitis C virus among the population of an endemic area of Japan. *JAMA.* 1995;274:1459–1461.

317. Guadagnino V, Stroffolini T, Rapicetta M, et al. Prevalence, risk factors, and genotype distribution of hepatitis C virus infection in the general population: a community-based survey in southern Italy. *Hepatology.* 1997;26:1006–1011.

318. Arthur RR, Hassan NF, Abdallah MY, et al. Hepatitis C antibody prevalence in blood donors in different governorates in Egypt. *Trans R Soc Trop Med Hyg.* 1997;91:271–274.

319. Abdel-Wahab MF, Zakaria S, Kamel M, et al. High seroprevalence of hepatitis C infection among risk groups in Egypt. *Am J Trop Med Hyg.* 1994;51:563–567.

320. Kamel MA, Ghaffar YA, Wasef MA, Wright M, Clark LC, Miller FD. High HCV prevalence in Egyptian blood donors [letter; comment] [see comments]. *Lancet.* 1992;340:427.

321. Darwish MA, Raouf TA, Rushdy P, Constantine NT, Rao MR, Edelman R. Risk factors associated with a high seroprevalence of hepatitis C virus infection in Egyptian blood donors. *Am J Trop Med Hyg.* 1993;49:440–447.

322. Hibbs RG, Corwin AL, Hassan NF, et al. The epidemiology of antibody to hepatitis C in Egypt [letter]. [Review]. *J Infect Dis.* 1993;168: 789–790.

323. El-Sayed NM, Gomatos PJ, Rodier GR, et al. Seroprevalence survey of Egyptian tourism workers for hepatitis B virus, hepatitis C virus, human immunodeficiency virus, and *Treponema pallidum* infections: association of hepatitis C virus infections with specific regions of Egypt. *Am J Trop Med Hyg.* 1996;55:179–184.

324. Prati D, Capelli C, Silvani C, et al. The incidence and risk factors of community-acquired hepatitis C in a cohort of Italian blood donors. *Hepatology.* 1997;25:702–704.

325. Noguchi S, Sata M, Suzuki H, Mizokami M, Tanikawa K. Routes of transmission of hepatitis C virus in an endemic rural area of Japan— molecular epidemiologic study of hepatitis C virus infection. *Scand J Infect Dis.* 1997;29:23–28.

326. Kiyosawa K, Tanaka E, Sodeyama T, et al. Transmission of hepatitis C in an isolated area in Japan: community-acquired infection. *Gastroenterology.* 1994;106:1596–1602.

327. Kelen GD, Green GB, Purcell RH, et al. Hepatitis B and hepatitis C in emergency department patients [see comments]. *N Engl J Med.* 1992;326:1399–1404.

328. Alter MJ. Epidemiology of hepatitis C in the West. *Semin Liver Dis.* 1995;15:5–14.

329. Alter MJ, Hadler SC, Judson FN, et al. Risk factors for acute non-A, non-B hepatitis in the United States and association with hepatitis C virus infection. *JAMA.* 1990;264:2231–2235.

330. Alter MJ, Kruszon-Moran D, Nainan OV, et al. The prevalence of hepatitis C virus infection in the United States, 1988 through 1994. *N Engl J Med.* 1999;341:556–562.

331. Letter to NEJM Regarding NHANES Study of HEV.

332. Kalinina O, Norder H, Mukomolor S, Magnias LO. A natural intergenotypic recombinant of hepatitis C virus identified in St. Petersburg. *J Virol.* 2002;76:4034–4043.

333. Fried MW, Shiffman MI, Reddy RK, et al. Pegyalted interferon alpha-2a (Pegasys) in combination with ribavirin: efficacy and safety results from a phase III, randomized, actively controlled, multicenter trial [abstract]. *Gastronenterology.* 2001;120(suppl 1):288.

334. El-Serag HB, Mason AC. Risk factors for the rising rates of primary liver cancer in the United States. *Arch Intern Med.* 2000;160:3222–3230.

335. Armstrong GL, Alter MJ, McQuillan GM, Margolis HS. The past incidence of hepatitis C virus infection: implication for the future burden of chronic liver disease in the United States. *Hepatology.* 2000;31:772–782.

336. Hagan H, Jarlais DCD, Friedman SR, Purchase D, Alter MJ. Reduced risk of hepatitis B and hepatitis C among injection drug users in the Tacoma syringe exchange program. *Am J Public Health.* 1995;85:1531–1537.

337. Hagan H, McGough JP, Thiede H, Weiss NS, Hopkins S, Alexander ER. Syringe exchange and risk of infection with hepatitis B and C viruses. *Am J Epidemiol.* 1999;149:203–213.

338. Farci P, Alter HT, Govindarajan S, et al. Lack of protective immunity against reinfection with hepatitis C virus. *Science.* 1992;258:135–140.

339. Prince AM, Brotmar B, Lee D-H, et al. Protection against chronic hepatitis C virus infection after rechallenge with homologous, but no heterologous, genotypes in a chimpanzee model. *J Infect Dis.* 2005;192:1701–1709.

340. Mehta SH, Cox A, Hoover PR, et al. Protection against persistence of hepatitis C. *Lancet.* 2002;359:1478–1483.

341. Reyes GR, Purdy MA, Kim JP, et al. Isolation of a cDNA from the virus responsible for enterically transmitted non-A, non-B hepatitis. *Eur J Biochem.* 1990;247:1335–1339.

342. Ticehurst J. Identification and characterization of hepatitis E virus. In: Hollinger FB, ed. *Viral Hepatitis and Liver Disease.* Baltimore, Md: Williams & Wilkins; 1991:501–513.

343. Bradley DW. Hepatitis E virus: a brief review of the biology, molecular virology, and immunology of a novel virus. *J Hepatol.* 1995;22(suppl 1):140–145.

344. Meng XJ, Purcell RH, Halbur PG, et al. A novel virus in swine is closely related to the human hepatitis E virus. *Proc Natl Acad Sci USA.* 1997;94:9860–9865.

345. Scharschmidt BF. Hepatitis E: a virus in waiting. *Lancet.* 1995;346:519–520.

346. Longer CF, Denny SL, Caudill JD, et al. Experimental hepatitis E: pathogenesis in cynomolgus macaques (*Macaca fascicularis*). *J Infect Dis.* 1993;168:602–609.

347. Maneerat Y, Clayson ET, Myint KS, Young GD, Innis BL. Experimental infection of the laboratory rat with the hepatitis E virus. *J Med Virol.* 1996;48:121–128.

348. Bradley DW, Krawczynski K, Cook EH, et al. Enterically transmitted non-A, non-B hepatitis: serial passage of disease in cynomolgus macaques and tamarins and recovery of disease-associated 27 to 34 nm virus-like particles. *Proc Natl Acad Sci USA.* 1987;84: 6277–6281.

349. Chauhan A, Jamell S, Dilawari JB, Chawla YK, Kaur U, Ganguly NK. Hepatitis E transmission to a volunteer. *Lancet.* 1993;341:149–150.

350. Nanda SK, Yalcinkaya K, Panigrahi AK, Acharya SK, Jameel S, Panda SK. Etiological role of hepatitis E virus in sporadic fulminant hepatitis. *J Med Virol.* 1994;42:133–137.

351. Rab MA, Bile MK, Mubarik MM, et al. Water-borne hepatitis E virus epidemic in Islamabad, Pakistan: a common source outbreak traced to the malfunction of a modern water treatment plant. *Am J Trop Med Hyg.* 1997;57:151–157.

352. Acharya SK, Dasarathy S, Kumer TL, et al. Fulminant hepatitis in a tropical population: clinical course, cause, and early predictors of outcome [see comments]. *Hepatology.* 1996;23:1448–1455.

353. Nanda SK, Ansari IH, Acharya SK, Jameel S, Panda SK. Protracted viremia during acute sporadic hepatitis E virus infection. *Gastroenterology.* 1995;108:225–230.

354. Ticehurst J, Popkin TJ, Bryan JP, et al. Association of hepatitis E virus with an outbreak of hepatitis in Pakistan: serologic responses and pattern of virus excretion. *J Med Virol.* 1992;36:84–92.

355. Bryan JP, Tsarev SA, Iqbal M, et al. Epidemic hepatitis E in Pakistan: patterns of serologic response and evidence that antibody to hepatitis E virus protects against disease. *J Infect Dis.* 1994;170:517–521.

356. Goldsmith R, Yarbough PO, Reyes GR, et al. Enzyme-linked immunosorbent assay for diagnosis of acute sporadic hepatitis E in Egyptian children. *Lancet.* 1992;339:328–333.

357. Corwin A, Jarot K, Lubis I, et al. Two years' investigation of epidemic hepatitis E virus transmission in West Kalimantan (Borneo), Indonesia. *Trans R Soc Trop Med Hyg.* 1995;89:262–265.

358. Mast EE, Alter MJ, Holland PV, Purcell RH. Evaluation of assays for antibody to hepatitis E virus by a serum panel. Hepatitis E Virus Antibody Serum Panel Evaluation Group. *Hepatology.* 1998;27: 857–861.

359. Khuroo MS, Kamili S, Dar MY, Moecklii R, Jameel S. Hepatitis E and long-term antibody status [letter]. *Lancet.* 1993;341:1355.

360. Thomas DL, Yarbough PO, Vlahov D, et al. Seroreactivity to hepatitis E virus in areas where the disease is not endemic. *J Clin Microbiol.* 1997;35:1244–1247.

361. Labrique AB, Thomas DL, Stoszck SK, Nelson KE. Hepatitis E: new emerging infectious disease. *Epidemiol Rev.* 1999;21:162–178.

362. Wang CH, Flehmig B, Moeckli R. Transmission of hepatitis E virus by transfusion? [letter]. *Lancet.* 1993;341:825–826.

363. Khuroo MS, Kamili S, Jameel S. Vertical transmission of hepatitis E virus. *Lancet.* 1995;345:1025–1026.

364. Aggarwal R, Naik SR. Hepatitis E: intrafamilial transmission versus waterborne spread. *J Hepatol.* 1994;21:718–723.

365. Meng XJ, Halbur PG, Shapiro MS, et al. Genetic and experimental evidence for cross-species infection by swine hepatitis E virus. *J Virol.* 1998;72:9714–9721.

366. Kabrane-Lazizi Y, Fine JB, Elm J, et al. Evidence for widespread infection of wild rats with hepatitis E virus in the United States. *Am J Trop Med Hyg.* 1999;61:331–335.

367. Kwo PY, Schlauder GG, Carpenter HA, et al. Acute hepatitis E by a new isolate acquired in the United States. *Mayo Clin Proc.* 1997;72: 1133–1136.

368. Tei S, Kitajima N, Takahashi K, Mishiro S. Zoonatic transmission of hepatitis E virus from deer to human beings. *Lancet.* 2003;362: 371–373.

369. Matsuda H, Okada K, Takahashi K, Misbiro S. Severe hepatitis E virus infection after ingestion of uncooked liver from a wild boar. *J Infect Dis.* 2003;188:944.

370. Hepatitis E in the South West of France in individuals who have never visited an endemic area. *J Med Virol.* 2004;74:419–424.

371. Ijaz S, Arnold E, Banks M, et al. Non-travel-associated hepatitis E in England and Wales: demographic, clinical and molecular epidemiologic characteristics. *J Infect Dis.* 2005;1992;1166–1172.

372. Clemente-Casares P, Pina S, Buti M, et al. Hepatitis E virus epidemiology in industrialized countries. *Emerg Infect Dis.* 2003;9:448–454.

373. Wong DC, Purcell RH, Sreennivasan MA, Prasad SR, Parvi KM. Epidemic and endemic hepatitis in India: evidence for non-A, non-B hepatitis virus etiology. *Lancet.* 1980;2:876–878.

374. Khuroo MS. Study of an epidemic of non-A, non-B hepatitis: possibility of another human hepatitis virus distinct from post-transfusion non-A, non-B type. *Am J Med.* 1980;68:818–824.

375. Thomas DL, Mahley RW, Badur S, Palaoglu KE, Quinn TQ. Epidemiology of hepatitis E virus infection in Turkey. *Lancet.* 1993;341:1561–1562.

376. Clayson ET, Shrestha MP, Vaughn DW, et al. Rates of hepatitis E virus infection and disease among adolescents and adults in Kathmandu, Nepal. *J Infect Dis.* 1997;176:763–766.

377. Arankalle VA, Tsarev SA, Chadha MS, et al. Age-specific prevalence of antibodies to hepatitis A and E viruses in Pune, India, 1982 and 1992. *J Infect Dis.* 1995;171:447–445.

378. Lee SD, Wang YJ, Lu RH, Chan CY, Lo KJ, Moeckli R. Seroprevalence of antibody to hepatitis E virus among Chinese subjects in Taiwan. *Hepatology.* 1994;19:866–870.

379. Aggarwal R, Shahi H, Naik S, Yachha SK, Naik SR. Evidence in favour of high infection rate with hepatitis E virus among young children in India [letter]. *J Hepatol.* 1997;26:1425–1426.

380. Meng J, Pillot J, Dai X, Fields HA, Khudyakov YE. Neutralization of different geographic strains of the hepatitis E virus with anti-hepatitis E virus-positive serum samples obtained from different sources. *Virology.* 1998;249:316–324.

381. Bryan JP, Tsarev SA, Iqbal M, et al. Epidemic hepatitis E in Pakistan: patterns of serologic response and evidence that antibody to hepatitis E virus protects against disease. *J Infect Dis.* 1994;170:517–521.

382. Arankalle VA, Chadha MS, Chobe LP, Nair R, Banerjee K. Cross-challenge studies in rhesus monkeys employing different Indian isolates of hepatitis E virus. *J Med Virol.* 1995;46:358–363.

383. Tsarev SA, Tsareva TS, Emerson SU, et al. Successful passive and active immunization of cynomolgus monkeys against hepatitis E. *Proc Natl Acad Sci USA.* 1994;91:10198–10202.

384. Tsarev SA, Emerson SU, Tsareva TS, et al. Variation in course of hepatitis E in experimentally infected cynomolgus monkeys. *J Infect Dis.* 1993;167:1302–1306.

385. Simons JN, Leary TP, Dawson GJ, et al. Isolation of novel virus-like sequences associated with human hepatitis. *Nature Med.* 1995;1: 564–569.

386. Alter HJ, Nakatsuji Y, Melpolder JC, et al. The incidence and disease implications of transfusion associated hepatitis G virus infection. *N Engl J Med.* 1997;336:747–754.

387. Linnen J, Wages J Jr, Zhang-Keck ZY, et al. Molecular cloning and disease association of hepatitis G virus: a transfusion-transmissible agent. *Eur J Biochem.* 1996;271:505–508.

388. Manns MP, McHutchinson JG, Gordon SC, et al. Peginterferon alfa-2b plus ribavirin compared with interferon alfa-2b plus ribavirin for initial treatment of chronic hepatitis C: a randomized trial. *Lancet.* 2001;358:958–965.

SEXUALLY TRANSMITTED DISEASES

Jonathan M. Zenilman

Introduction

In the United States, 12 to 15 million new cases of sexually transmitted diseases (STDs) occur annually, primarily affecting adolescents and young adults.[1,2] This chapter will review the epidemiology of STDs, assessment of personal risk factors, and the community factors that contribute to STD morbidity. A number of specific diseases will be reviewed in detail focusing on the most common organisms, including *Neisseria gonorrhoeae*, *Chlamydia trachomatis*, *Treponema pallidum* (syphilis), *Hemophilus ducreyi* (chancroid), *Trichomonas vaginalis*, bacterial vaginosis, and chronic viral infections including herpes simplex and human papillomavirus (see Table 23-1 for a complete list of STDs). Understanding the pathophysiology and epidemiology of STDs is a critical first step in developing rational diagnostic, treatment, and control strategies. Diagnostic approaches have been revolutionized by such techniques as nucleic acid amplification testing. Treatment has become more complex, especially in bacterial infections, because of the emergence of antimicrobial resistance. STDs have been conclusively linked to increased risk of HIV transmission and acquisition. Traditional disease control program approaches have included clinic-based screening and partner notification. These have been supplemented by newer approaches to community-based STD control, which include use of computerized disease surveillance systems, geographic mapping, and use of noninvasive new diagnostic techniques and population-based screening in the nonclinical setting.

Transmission Mode: The Definition of a Sexually Transmitted Disease

Sexually transmitted diseases are transmitted through sexual intercourse. Sexual intercourse is defined as sexual contact including vaginal intercourse, oral intercourse (either receptive oral intercourse, i.e., fellatio or

TABLE 23-1   Sexually Transmitted Diseases

Bacterial Infection

Gonorrhea (*Neisseria gonorrhoeae*)

Syphilis (*Treponema pallidum*)

Chlamydia (*Chlamydia trachomatis*)

Chancroid (*Hemophilus ducreyi*)

Granuloma inguinbale (*Campylobacter granulomatis*)

Lymphogranuloma venereum (*Chlamydia trachomatis LGV serovars*)

Bacterial vaginosis (ecological disturbance of the vaginal flora)

Viral

Genital herpes (herpes simplex type 1 and type 2)

Human herpesvirus 8 (Kaposi sarcoma)
  Human papillomavirus infection
  Condylomata acuminate (genital warts)
  Cervical/anal dysplasia and epithelial cancers

Hepatitis B infection

Human immunodeficiency virus

Human T-cell lymphotropic virus type 1 (HTLV-1)

Cytomegalovirus

Parasitic

Trichomonas

Scabies

Pediculosis

---

cunnilingus), or rectal intercourse. Sexually transmitted diseases can be transmitted between heterosexual or homosexual partners. Different types of sexual activity may result in increased risks. Receptive rectal intercourse and vaginal intercourse carry the highest risks of STD transmission.[3]

STDs are unique in the infectious disease world as they are completely dependent on behavioral factors for transmission. Abstinent individuals will not contract an STD. Acquisition of STDs is also dependent on the probability that one will come into contact with an STD-infected partner, susceptibility of the host, and efficiency of transmission of the organism through sexual intercourse. Therefore, the epidemiological risk of the sexual *partner* is a key determinant.

STD incidence is highest in adolescents and young adults. For gonorrhea and chlamydia infections, where the largest bodies of data are available, over 95% of incident infections occur between the ages of 15 and 39.[4] Highest rates of incidence are seen in adolescent women (age 15–19) and in men who are between the ages of 20 and 24. These findings correlate very closely with sexual behavior patterns. For example, sexual partner turnover is highest in the adolescent and young adult age groups.

Not only is the absolute number of sexual partners important, but the *type* of sexual partner also contributes to potential infection risk. The constellation of an individual's sexual partners, and their partners' partners, constitute a sexual network.[5-7] Individuals with partners who are more likely to be infected with STDs (for example, those involved in commercial sex work or drug use) are much more likely to contract an STD than individuals who do not have high-risk sexual partners—even though the index patient may perceive him- or herself to be at low risk. Similarly, persons with serial partners (but only having one sexual partner at a time) are less likely to spread STDs than persons who have multiple concurrent sex partners.

STDs need to be evaluated within the context of overall morbidity attributable to unprotected sexual behavior.[2] Risky sexual behavior patterns also result in morbidity such as unintended pregnancy, low-birth-weight infants, the cost of pregnancy terminations, sexually transmitted diseases, direct costs attributable to STD care, and the long-term STD costs including complications of STDs such as pelvic inflammatory disease and ectopic pregnancy, HIV, and STD-facilitated HIV transmission. Table 23-2 shows common perinatal complications caused by STDs.

Developing effective prevention control strategies requires understanding patterns of sexual behavior. The particular events that are important include the following:

- The age of sexual debut: Individuals with younger age at first coitus are at higher risk for STDs.[8,9]
- Number of partners including delineation between serial partners (serial monogamy) or number of concurrent partners and development of a dense sexual network. Individuals with multiple concurrent partners are much more likely to spread STDs than individuals with serial partners.[10]
- Qualitative features of sex partners that impart greater risk, for example, commercial sex workers, anonymous sex partners, contacts in the context of gay bathhouses or drug use environments.
- Use of barrier protection methods including condom use patterns.
- Other comorbidities, especially drug use, socioeconomic status, and commercial sex.[11]

TABLE 23-2 Perinatal Complications of STDs

Gonorrhea, Chlamydia	Ophthalmia Neonata
	Pneumonia
	Low birth weight
Syphilis	Congenital syphilis
Trichomonas	
Bacterial vaginosis	Premature rupture of membranes
	Premature delivery
Herpes simplex	Congenital herpes syndrome
Human papillomavirus	Laryngeal papillomatosis
Hepatitis B	Perinatal transmission
HIV	

- Travel is particularly important for some populations.[12] In parts of the world such as Western Europe where STD rates are low, travelers to highly endemic areas account for over half of the new bacterial STD infections.

Assessing sexual behavior is critical to the development of behavior and disease control interventions. Major challenges in designing and implementing intervention strategies include using appropriate assessment tools, defining an individual's or population baseline status, and implementing the intervention.[13-15] A number of large cross-sectional national surveys have been very useful in assessing behavior and trends. In the United States, these have included the National Health and Nutritional Examination Survey (NHANES), the Behavioral Risk Factor Surveillance System, and the Youth Risk Behavioral Surveillance Survey (YRBSS). Each is subject to its own set of biases. For example, the YRBSS is conducted biannually at public high schools. The biases include that it does not represent either nonpublic high school students or persons who have dropped out of school. Nevertheless, the trends in these data strongly suggest that the overall age of sexual debut has stabilized at 15.5–16. Condom use has substantially increased, especially among inner-city African-American youth.[16]

Socioeconomic status has been linked to increased incidence of STDs in a number of different settings, including rural and urban areas in the United States and developing countries.[17] Areas where there has been a decrease in available health services, and especially preventive health services, have also been associated with increased incidence of STDs. Furthermore, STD incidence increases have also been linked to the imposition of fees for public health clinical services.[18] In Eastern Europe, where there has been tremendous social disruption, disintegration of the health system, and loosening of travel restrictions, these factors have coalesced to drive development of a very large STD epidemic.[19]

Urbanization in developing countries has been strongly associated with increased STD rates.[20] Urbanization and population migration are associated with changes in the social–sexual network. Because of economic development in the urban areas, males are attracted to the cities for job opportunities. In the absence of the regular female partners, commercial sex industries have developed. From an epidemiological standpoint, an accurate indicator of these types of risk is a high male/female ratio. These high ratios in turn have provided social networks for the easy spread of sexually transmitted diseases. In turn, when the males return home for holidays, spread of STDs to their spouses or other regular sexual partners has become a problem. The ramifications of these patterns were particularly demonstrated in many parts of the world where monogamous women were at risk for STD and HIV infection through the behaviors of their spouses.[21]

In the United States, drug use is particularly associated with STD incidence, especially syphilis.[22] In part, this is not related to direct pharmacologic activities of the drugs themselves, but rather the behaviors associated with drug use and the marketing of drugs, including prostitution.

In the United States when STDs are examined by race or ethnicity, very wide discrepancies are demonstrated between racial ethnic groups.[23] Race and ethnicity in the United States often correlate with other more fundamental determinants of health status such as socioeconomic status, access to good quality medical care, and efforts to receive good quality medical care. Reporting biases may also be at play, although these differences occur even when these biases are controlled.

Syphilis presents a scenario that demonstrates the interaction of disease and the social setting. Between 1999 and 2003, overall syphilis rates in the United States increased 20%, while the proportion in minority groups decreased from 74.7% in 1999 to 39.2%. The increase is related to substantial increases in sexually transmitted infections and in high-risk sexual behavior observed in gay men since the late 1990s. In some studies, up to 40–50% of homosexual men with incident syphilis are HIV positive. Furthermore, the syphilis increase has changed the male/female ratio of this disease from nearly 1:1 in 1991 to greater than 3:1 in 2004, reflecting the shift to a predominantly homosexual population.[24–29]

There are a number of hypotheses of why this trend developed. Hypotheses that have been proposed include the following:

- The availability of highly active antiretroviral therapy that essentially removed the stigma and threat of HIV/AIDS as an immediate death sentence. This has been hypothesized as being associated with seeing HIV as a manageable disease, as opposed to a fatal disease.
- "Prevention fatigue" among homosexual men after 20 years of reinforcing prevention messages in the gay community.
- Some have proposed that the increase in high-risk activity is an intergenerational rebellion effect, with younger gay men rebelling against the peer norms established by the older generation that came of age in the 1970s and 1980s.

Nevertheless, these trends are particularly troubling because of the implication and impact this would have on HIV transmission. In terms of illicit drug use, one of the most troubling trends has been the increasing availability of methamphetamine, especially in the western and midwestern states.[30–32] A stimulant, methamphetamine has been associated with hypersexual activity, as well as increased risk taking. There is also evidence that methamphetamine can adversely affect mucous membranes, making them more susceptible to trauma and bleeding, and therefore it could potentially increase susceptibility to sexually transmitted diseases.

Sexual Context Affects Interventions

Epidemiological risk assessment of STDs and other infectious diseases most frequently evaluate *individual-based risk.* A challenge in using STDs as intervention measures is that risk is also determined by environmental and contextual factors that are beyond the immediate sexual encounter situation, in particular, qualitative aspects not of the individual him- or herself but of the sexual partners. For example, the risk profile of a partner may dictate an individual's STD risk, independent of his or her own sexual behavior. The best examples of these are the high rates of STDs and HIV among monogamous women in sub-Saharan Africa and Asia, who had one lifetime sexual partner, yet have high disease rates because of the risk profile of their husband.[21]

Behavioral Models

When developing STD/HIV interventions, behavioral models are necessary for their design and evaluation.[33-35] Behavioral models are deterministic constructs of sexual behavior. These constructs are usually delineated in sequential steps, with each step being either an environmental factor, a behavioral attitude (e.g., positive or negative attitude for condom use), subject area knowledge, or a previous behavior. For STD research, risky behavior is a necessary precursor step to disease acquisition. These elements are assembled in a logical framework, with the end result being a risky behavior or a prevention behavior.

Behavior models provide a deterministic basis and underlying rationale for intervention. They also provide a process for evaluation mode as the predecessor key behavioral determinants can also be measured. Defined as a multiple-step process, the behavioral models allow for logical points for intervention. For example, if a model posits that the key determinant of a behavior is presence or absence of a specific attitude, then an intervention approach would be to change the underlying attitude. Evaluation methods would determine whether the intervention affected the attitude, usually defined by assessments before and after the interventions. The evaluation framework can also determine the validity of the underlying behavioral model. For example, if the model just cited was valid, then changes in attitudes should result in changed behaviors. Behavioral models also facilitate multiple-step intervention approaches (synergy). In this approach, interventions occur at multiple points of attack; simultaneously affecting knowledge, attitudes, and other factors should have an additive or even synergistic effect. Conceptually, a biomedical model analogue would be cancer chemotherapy in which multiple molecular targets are attached. Behaviors do not occur in a social vacuum. Structural and environmental factors related to STD control and prevention can affect an individual's ability to implement prevention behaviors, with the peer group often being most important. When developing an intervention, a common error is to focus on individual-level changes while being ignorant of whether the social or societal structure provides a supportive environment for STD/HIV behavior change.

Temporal sequence is also important to model development and interventions. The stages of change theory is a construct that was used in a number of interventions, including the widely reported project RESPECT.[36,37] This model has been particularly attractive in intervention development because it divides a behavior into five steps or stages that are on a continuum. *Precontemplation* is before an individual is even beginning to think of changing or adopting safer sexual behaviors. *Contemplation* is where an individual is considering a behavior change, but is not ready to act on it. *Preparation* ("ready for change") is where an individual is actively considering changing behavior and is taking steps in order to actualize that behavior change. *Action* is the process of changing behavior and moving toward a preventive behavior mode. *Maintenance* is the process of maintaining behavior change once it has occurred. This usually involves efforts such as continual education or encouragement.

Although the model describes sexual behavior change in a positive direction, regression is also possible, again following a behavioral biomedical model similar to remission and relapse that one may see with other chronic diseases. The advantage of this type of model construct is that it offers intervention designers an opportunity to rationally design interventions that can be adapted to an individual based on understanding that person's particular "stage" along the five-step continuum. From a population basis, this type of model offers the potential for attacking a risk behavior at multiple key decision points.

Project RESPECT was a large intervention study evaluated in five STD clinics in the United States. It compared four sessions of intensive post-HIV counseling, one session of post-HIV testing intervention that emphasized counseling skills and technical skills building, and a control group that was an educational intervention.[38] Outcomes evaluated included self-reported behavioral outcomes and incidence of sexually transmitted infections. Project RESPECT provides two major important lessons. First, skill building with a positive health outcome can be implemented in a high-risk setting. There were significant reductions in both self-reported behavior and biological outcomes among the two intervention groups. The second lesson is the importance of translation. RESPECT was developed and implemented as a research protocol. Almost 10 years after the results were first presented, this intervention has not been widely implemented because of funding constraints.

Another example of a successful intervention program based on skills building was developed by Celentano and Thai collaborators to prevent HIV/STDs in the Royal Thai Army in the early 1990s.[39] At that time, HIV seroincidence in draftees was greater than 4% per year, and STD rates were high. The intervention approach included an individual-based component, but also structural changes. The individual-based components included skills building, increasing knowledge, condom skills training, and improved risk perception. This program was developed simultaneously with the 100% condom program in Thailand,[40,41] which monitored brothels to ensure that condoms were used with all sex acts. The developers also recognized that the group dynamic in the Royal Thai Army field units was a critical part of high-risk sexual behavior with commercial sex workers. For example, soldiers in Royal Thai Army units based in rural areas were paid on a monthly basis. After payday there was a group dynamic that involved binge drinking and en-masse visits to commercial sex workers. By staggering paydays across the four weeks of the month, providing interventions in the field units—building on the cohesion and group dynamic that is integral to army units and the implementation of "buddy" systems to monitor condom use and safer sex practices among peers—the incidence of bacterial STDs and HIV dropped by 79%. A key feature is that *safer sex became the peer and recognized norm.*

Another important and often overlooked covariate is assessment of risk in the context of mental illness. Since the early 1980s, with the increased appreciation of sexual behavior as an important key determinant, intervention strategies have focused on reducing risky sexual behavior as the key to reducing STD risk. However, STD risk behavior is, in turn, impacted by other factors. In particular, what are the key determinates for high-risk behavior? Mental illness may actually be an important covariate, and STD risk behavior may actually be a result of either affective or Axis II disorders that are inadequately treated.[42-44] Under this more holistic scenario, STD control becomes integrated into other aspects of the health care system, especially mental health care, an area in which services are woefully inadequate in many parts of the world.

This latter concept brings also new conceptions of intervention. Traditional STD/HIV prevention interventions are based on preventing a long-term outcome. For example, patients or subjects are encouraged to use condoms or to forgo risky sexual activity because of their interest in preventing an outcome that will result in illness years hence. However, patients who have Axis II disorders or who have major affective disorders may respond more effectively to interventions that are based on present aspects of their behavior (for example, increased sensation seeking as part of an STD/HIV prevention intervention) as opposed to a long-term approach based on preventing an outcome (such as HIV or PID) in the future, which may be very abstract for many patients.

Gonorrhea

In 2003, 335,104 cases of gonorrhea were reported to the Centers for Disease Control and Prevention by local and state health departments,[4] representing a nationwide population-based rate of 116/100,000, which has been stable since 1997. An additional 1-2 cases are thought to occur for every reported case. The highest rates are seen in adolescent women (age 15-19) and young adult men (20-24) representing, in part, sexual behavior patterns. One of the problems with the CDC reported data is that they are based on a passive case-based reporting system. Population-based studies have demonstrated that the epidemiology of *incident* symptomatic disease, which passive reporting represents, is different from *prevalent* asymptomatic infection. For example, in a survey conducted in Baltimore in 1997-1998, a population-based sample of individuals age 18-35 was interviewed in their household, and urine samples were assayed by nucleic acid amplification tests for chlamydia and gonorrhea. Gonorrhea estimates using the population were over three times those reported by health departments.[46,47]

Although gonorrhea incidence has decreased by nearly 70% since the peak of the gonorrhea epidemic in the mid-1970s, the infection has become increasingly prevalent in inner-city areas affected by other social problems, especially drug use and pregnancy. In these areas, incidence rates among adolescents often exceed 15% per year.

Gonorrhea is a bacterial exudative infection caused by *Neisseria gonorrhoeae*, a fastidious gram-negative coccus.[48] In men, urethritis is the most common syndrome.[45] Discharge or dysuria usually appears within one week of exposure, although as many as 5-10% of patients never have signs or symptoms. Asymptomatic disease can exist in men up to several weeks after infection.[49] Nevertheless, the organism is potentially transmissible to sexual partners.

Symptomatic anorectal gonococcal disease occurs in persons with a history of receptive rectal intercourse.[50] Approximately 50% have symptoms of rectal pain, discharge, constipation, and tenesmus. Anorectal disease can also occur in women with endocervical gonorrhea and who have not necessarily had receptive rectal intercourse. In these cases infection is presumed to have occurred via tracking of secretion across the perineum. Indeed, up to

30% of such women often have coexistent rectal infection, but it is usually asymptomatic.

Because rectal gonorrhea in men implies a history of unprotected rectal intercourse, surveillance of rectal gonorrhea has been useful as a surrogate marker for HIV risk in gay men. For example, early in the AIDS epidemic, the rate of rectal gonorrhea declined.[51] In contrast, starting in 1997 troubling trends were reported of an increase of gonorrhea in homosexual men, which correlated with observed increases in HIV-risk behavior among homosexual adolescents.[52] These have continued and correlate with the increased syphilis rates as described above.

In women, gonorrhea typically causes cervical disease (cervicitis). Women with untreated gonococcal cervicitis develop upper tract infection and/or pelvic inflammatory disease (PID).[53-55] Semantically, PID represents infection of the soft tissues of upper genital tract structures and includes endometritis, salpingitis, oophoritis, and pelvic peritonitis. Fatalities from PID are rare. However, severe PID may lead to tubo-ovarian abscess and the necessity at times for hysterectomy. The chronic complications are more common. Women with previous history of PID are more likely to have tubal-factor infertility and are at higher risk for ectopic pregnancy.[56-59] The overall direct economic impact of PID alone was estimated to be $4.2 billion in 1990.[40]

Estimates of PID incidence vary and are made difficult by the lack of prospective studies, as well as difficulty in clinical diagnosis. The total burden of PID cases is estimated to be 500,000.

Gonococcal pharyngitis occurs in men or women after oral sexual exposure.[61] The disease is clinically indistinguishable from any other bacterial pharyngitis and is asymptomatic in as many as 60% of cases. Natural history studies have demonstrated that gonococcal pharyngitis is a self-limited syndrome, and uninfected patients become culture-negative after 4-6 weeks. However, transmission through oral sexual exposure can occur even while asymptomatic.

Disseminated gonococcal infection (DGI), or gonococcal septicemia, occurs in approximately 0.1-0.5% of total gonococcal cases.[62] DGI is more commonly seen in women, in particular during pregnancy, and is also more common in persons with deficiencies of the terminal complement components.[63]

Perinatal Disease

Perinatal infection is relatively rare in the United States, but it is still often found in the developing world.[64,65] Perinatal gonococcal disease is transmitted by direct exposure to an infant passing through the birth canal of an infected cervix. Gonococcal ophthalmia is a severe public health problem in the developing world and is effectively prevented by inexpensive prophylaxis. The incidence of gonococcal ophthalmia is estimated to be 42% of infants exposed to an infected cervical canal. These infants develop a purulent conjunctivitis that can then rapidly progress to keratitis and subsequent corneal blindness. Because of the severe sequelae of this, public health authorities instituted postnatal prophylaxis with ophthalmic silver nitrate as early as 1910, effectively preventing corneal infection in 95% of exposed infants.

Prevention of perinatal infection is the rationale for aggressive screening programs in pregnant women. Ophthalmia is also occasionally seen in adults, usually as a result of self-inoculation.

The traditional diagnostic approach is culture; culture involves many operational considerations, such as logistical requirements and environmental requirements. Nucleic acid amplification techniques (NAAT), such as polymerase chain reaction and standard displacement, are now widely used and are estimated to represent 75% of gonorrhea tests performed.[66,67] NAAT are more sensitive in certain situations and can be used on nongenital samples, such as urine. The use of urine as a diagnostic technique has facilitated expansion of gonorrhea screening efforts, especially in populations where clinical service provision is difficult and/or inadequate.

Treatment for mucosal gonorrhea infections is based on providing single-dose regimens, preferably oral, that are effective against most or all of the known resistant determinants.[68-70] Current regimens include either a quinolone (see below for discussion of resistance) or a third-generation cephalosporin. All patients treated for gonorrhea should also be treated for chlamydia, with either azithromycin 1 gram (single dose) or doxycycline 100 mg twice daily for 1 week. The chlamydia recommendation is based on the high rate of gonorrhea-chlamydia coinfection,[71,72] which may be as high as 30–40%. In most settings, it is more cost-effective to presumptively treat for chlamydia than to pursue a testing strategy.

N. gonorrhoeae has tremendous capacity to develop antimicrobial resistance.[73] For 30 years after World War II, penicillin was the antimicrobial therapy of choice. In 1976, the first case of plasmid-medicated penicillinase-producing *Neisseria gonorrhoeae* (PPNG) was reported.[74] PPNG rapidly developed into a major public health problem and made the penicillin class of antibiotics obsolete by the mid-1980s. Chromosomally mediated resistance to penicillin (CMRNG) was described in the early 1980s,[75] high-level plasmid-mediated tetracycline resistance (TRNG) developed in 1986,[76] and quinolone antibiotic resistance (QRNG) appeared in the late 1990s.[77,78] Development of standardized effective gonococcal treatment strategies has required accurate surveillance, which has occurred since the mid-1980s with the implementation of the national gonorrhea surveillance network.[79,80] This multisite surveillance system has provided standardized mechanisms for determining antimicrobial resistance. Baseline behavioral and treatment data are also collected. As a by-product of that system, recently, the CDC's Gonococcal Isolate Surveillance Project (GISP) described increased incidence of anorectal infection in the GISP cohort,[81] suggesting that risky practices were beginning to develop within the homosexual community served by the GISP program. This presents a very troubling public health issue.

Quinolone Resistance

Quinolone resistance has rapidly emerged as a major public health problem in gonorrhea treatment. Quinolone resistance is mediated by mutations in the gyrase and topoisomerase genes in the gonococcal genome, which render high-level resistance to the quinolone class of drugs. This has had major implications. For example, in parts of Southeast Asia, over 50% of gonococcal isolates are QRNG.[82,83] From 2002 to 2004, this development rapidly spread to the western United States and Hawaii. More recently, QRNG has been associated with up to 10–15% of isolates nationwide in homosexual men.[81] Therefore, in homosexual men, quinolones are no longer recommended as first-line therapy. There are two major implications for this. First, QRNGs are a very attractive, oral, single-dose treatment option that has essentially been eliminated as a therapeutic approach. Treatments that are available include third-generation cephalosporins, such as ceftriaxone and cefexime. Cefexime is an oral option, but it is not be widely available in the oral formulation. Therefore, in most venues, intramuscular therapy is the only option. Furthermore, because cephalosporins cross-react with penicillin class drugs (in the case of allergy), these drugs may not be utilized in patients with reported penicillin allergy, especially in outpatient clinical settings such as STD clinics, where there is no tertiary hospital services available. This is especially problematic because alternative therapeutic options such as spectinomycin are not recommended nor are they effective in the treatment of rectal and pharyngeal infections.[61,84] Furthermore, there are no new drugs that are currently in the pipeline that are effective against gonorrhea.

With the intersection of high-risk behaviors, poverty, and poor public health services, the importance of health care access is critical for an effective control strategy. Furthermore, many patients with gonorrhea have recurrent disease.[71,72,85] Recurrence is usually not the result of treatment failures, because with the implementation of adequate, single-dose effective regimens, treatment failures are rare. Recurrence often occurs through reexposure, and, with the exception of exposure to a similar serotype to gonorrhea (an extremely rare event), there is little evidence of effective development of protective immunity, which has major implications for the development of vaccines.

Chlamydia

Chlamydia trachomatis infection is the most common STD in the United States, with approximately four million cases estimated annually.[86,87] The syndromes for chlamydia are similar to those seen in gonorrhea; however, they tend to be less aggressive in the acute context but cause significant numbers of complications. In men, the most common syndrome is chlamydia urethritis, which in the United States accounts for approximately 40% of all cases of nongonococcal urethritis.[88–91] Urethritis in men typically presents as a mucoid discharge, associated often with dysuria. Asymptomatic infection occurs in over 30% of cases.[92] The time from infection to development of symptoms is longer than that for gonorrhea, usually about 7–14 days.

In women, cervical infection is the most commonly reported syndrome.[93,94] Over half of women with cervical infection are asymptomatic.[95] When symptoms occur they may manifest as vaginal discharge or poorly differentiated abdominal or lower abdominal pain.[96,97] At clinical examination, there are often no clinical signs present. When they are present, they include mucopurulent cervical discharge, cervical friability, and cervical edema. Although cervical ectopy has been traditionally associated with chlamydia, studies by our group have demonstrated that cervical ectopy, when strictly defined clinically, is actually not more significantly found in chlamydia than in other adolescent women.[98]

Left untreated, approximately 30% of women with chlamydial infection will develop pelvic inflammatory disease.[99] The PID of chlamydia is associated with lower rates of clinical symptoms than the PID seen in gonorrhea. However, this subacute PID is associated with higher rates of subsequent infertility,[72] because chlamydia induces an inflammatory reaction characterized by fibrosis. Rectal chlamydia infection occurs predominantly in homosexual men who have had receptive rectal intercourse.[100-102] As with other infection in gay men, rectal chlamydia has been increasing. Lymphogranuloma venereum (LGV) is a chlamydia syndrome causing inflammatory and ulcerative disease and is caused by the L1, L2, L3 serovars.[103,104] From 2003 to 2005, LGV outbreaks causing severe rectal inflammation were reported from the Netherlands and a number of US cities.[105] As with the other homosexual male outbreaks, there was a high proportion of HIV infections.

The epidemiology of chlamydia is interesting because there are a number of artifacts in the reporting scheme. Reported chlamydia infections are more common in women than in men, and rates have increased substantially since 1984 (Figure 23-1). Both of these trends are artifacts. The rate differential between women and men is due to different ascertainment practices.[106,107] Women are typically diagnosed with an etiologic diagnosis of chlamydia on the basis of a chlamydia screening test performed at physical examination. Clinical practice guidelines strongly recommend routine chlamydia screening for sexually active women below the age of 25. This has also been recently incorporated into quality assurance guidelines for managed care organizations (HEDIS).[108] In contrast, men are often treated for chlamydia infection on the basis of presentation of a syndrome of urethritis or as a contact to a woman with chlamydia and a definitive etiologic diagnosis is not made. Therefore these cases are not going to meet surveillance definitions for chlamydia and are not be reported.

The trend of increasing incidence of infection, with the most recent number of figures indicating 800,000 cases reported to CDC in 2003, results from increased screening activity. Figure 23-1 demonstrates chlamydia incidence in the United States since 1980. However, the trends are biased. Screening tests were not available prior to 1985. Furthermore, increased federal support for screening and implementation of reporting laws are both thought to contribute to an ascertainment bias, which appeals as an artificial increased incidence. Similarly, because women are routinely screened (and men are not) the ascertainment bias favors increased disease reporting in women. A true estimate of chlamydia prevalence is therefore not known, which presents major problems in evaluating trends.[109]

Advances in chlamydia screening technology since the early 1980s have resulted in easy, assessable chlamydia screening being available. Before 1984, chlamydia testing was available only by tissue culture, which is expensive and cumbersome. Currently, DNA and other nucleic acid amplification technologies can be performed both on anogenital specimens and on urine.[110-112] The development of new, noninvasive urine-based, nucleic acid-based technologies will result in substantial expansion of screening activities because of the reduced need to perform clinical exams. Many test formats have combined the gonorrhea and chlamydia assay into one test.

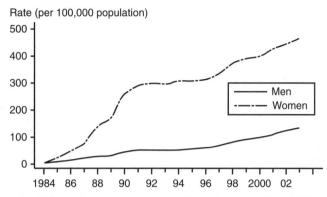

FIGURE 23-1 Chlamydia rates by gender—United states, 1984–2003.
Source: Division of STD Prevention, Centers for Disease Control and Prevention.

The rates of chlamydia are highest in adolescent women and drop off steeply past that age. For example, the reported rate for women between the ages of 15–19 is 2687/100,000 but drops off to 344/100,000 for women ages 30–34. There is strong suggestion that this steep drop-off in incidence may not be related only to behavior but also may be related to the development of partial immunity to clinical infection through periodic repeated exposures.

Chlamydia screening programs have been demonstrated to be effective.[113,114] Implementation of chlamydia screening results in an initial increase in chlamydia prevalence among women tested, followed by a nearly 50% decrease over four subsequent years. These data demonstrate that a screening intervention alone can affect chlamydia prevalence by removing infected individuals from the prevalent pool of the population.

A more important demonstration of this was published in 1997.[115] In this study from the group Health Cooperative of Puget Sound, individuals in a managed care organization, which had longitudinal tracking ability of all of its clients, demonstrated that periodic chlamydia screening resulted in a 44% reduction in pelvic inflammatory disease among the managed care population members.

Population-Based Surveys for Chlamydia and Gonorrhea Diagnostic Testing

The availability of nucleic acid amplification tests (NAATs) has revolutionized gonorrhea and chlamydia diagnostics. NAATs are highly sensitive and are able to detect as few as 10 organisms per specimen. NAATs have been applied in a large number of field settings including emergency departments, job centers, middle and high schools, and military training sites. The largest studies were done in military recruits being inducted at two large bases in the eastern United States that processed inductees from all 50 states. In a sample of more than 12,000 persons, the overall prevalence of chlamydial infection in the United States was estimated to be 4.2%.[116] Regional differences were evident with the South having the highest prevalence (5.4%). The prevalence was higher among women (4.7%) than men (3.7%).

Combining the new NAAT technology with population-based surveys provides new insights into the burden of these STDs in the general population.

A survey in Baltimore provided estimates that were representative of adults living in the city between the ages of 18 and 35 years.[117] The National Survey of Adolescent Males (NSAM), which was conducted in 1988 and 1995, provided a representative sample of adolescent and young men in the United States. NSAM provided a similar estimate of chlamydial infection. Based on a survey that was conducted in 1995 among approximately 500 men ages 18 and 19 and 1000 men ages 22 to 26 years, the prevalence of chlamydial infection was 3.1% and 4.5%. In the Baltimore study, the prevalence of chlamydial infection overall was 3.0% in adults who were aged 18 to 35 years. The prevalence ranged from 8% in 19- and 20-year-olds to 0.5% in 33- to 35-year-olds.

Pelvic Inflammatory Disease

The major complication of untreated or undertreated gonorrhea and chlamydia is pelvic inflammatory disease (PID).[118,119] PID actually represents a constellation of syndromes ranging from endometritis, oophoritis, and pelvic peritonitis. PID is a poorly defined syndrome, in part because it affects multiple organs and is soft tissue infection with no clear defined diagnostic criteria.

The microbiology of upper tract genital infection is complex.[120,121] Organisms that are isolated from the upper tract, for example, at laparoscopy or surgery, include *Neisseria gonorrhoeae*; *Chlamydia trachomatis*; organisms associated with vaginal flora, such as *Streptococcus* (group B), *Gardnerella*, *E. coli*, and *Veilonella*, and intra-abdominal colonic organisms such as *Bacteroides* and other anaerobes. The pathophysiological progression of PID is hypothesized to be a sexually transmitted lower tract (cervical) infection causing breakdown of the normal defense mechanisms, followed by ascent of bacteria into the uterus, fallopian tubes, and periovarian areas and causing consequent inflammation (Figure 23-2).[122-124]

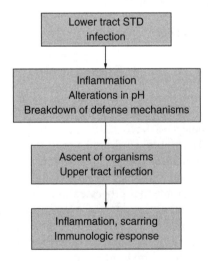

Note: STD, sexually transmitted disease.

FIGURE 23-2   Pelvic Inflammatory disease pathogenesis model.

Although sepsis can occur, mortality is rare in women with PID, probably because it is often a localized infection in an otherwise healthy age group. The tissue inflammation caused by PID often results in tubal scarring, which is the cause of the major sequelae of infertility and increased risk of ectopic pregnancy. The consequences of PID were eloquently shown by Westrom in a large cohort of Swedish women.[125-129] He diagnosed all cases of PID by laparoscopy (the "gold standard" diagnostic procedure) and followed them for over 25 years—from adolescence through the child-bearing years. He found that 10% of women with one PID episode had tubal infertility, 25% of those who had two episodes had tubal infertility, and over 60% of women with three episodes had tubal infertility. The relative risk of ectopic pregnancy was greater than 10 compared to women without one episode of PID. Because these complications occur long after the initial process, the epidemics of infertility and ectopic pregnancy track the initial epidemic of gonorrhea or chlamydial infection by a substantial latency period.

In the United States, an estimated 500,000–1,000,000 cases occur annually.[130-134] Ascertainment of disease burden is difficult because the PID syndrome is not a reportable disease. Changes in the health care system have emphasized outpatient management of STDs. Therefore, although hospital discharges for PID since 1990 have dropped sharply, these data are unreliable because of the confounding caused by changing practice patterns.

PID is associated with such risk factors as adolescence, increased number of sexual partners, a previous episode of PID, use of an intrauterine device, and douching.[135-141] Clinical criteria that have been traditionally used for diagnosis include two of three major criteria: lower abdominal pain, adnexal tenderness, or fever.[137] Some have also added the presence of a lower tract infection (gonococcal or chlamydial cervicitis). Careful studies of clinical criteria that have used laparoscopy as the standard found that the sensitivity and specificity of clinical criteria is 60–70% in expert hands.[142] Up to one quarter of PID cases may manifest no symptoms, especially disease associated with chlamydia.[54] Therefore, many practitioners currently will treat women with mild cervical motion tenderness with treatment regimens effective against PID under the assumption that the benefit of preventing pelvic inflammatory disease or curing early pelvic inflammatory disease outweighs the costs in terms of increased cost of treatment and potential side effects.[143]

Treatment strategies for PID are based on the underlying microbiology, including antimicrobial coverage for *N. gonorrhoeae*, *C. trachomatis*, streptococci, gram-negative rods, and anaerobes.[144,145] Treatment regimens are therefore complex and beyond the scope of this chapter.[70] Despite the efforts of developing effective antimicrobial regimens, treatment efficacy has been difficult to assess. Most clinical treatment studies use clinical criteria for determination of efficacy, despite the limitations of clinical diagnosis. Therefore, these studies are subject to both type I and type II statistical error. Furthermore, although the morbidity of PID is long term, few treatment studies have correlated effective antimicrobial therapy with better long-term outcomes in terms of reduced incidence of infertility and ectopic pregnancy.

Treatment of acute PID is secondary prevention. The consensus for primary prevention is that reducing gonococcal and chlamydial infections is the most effective approach. Screening interventions for chlamydia have demonstrated PID reductions of >60%.[146]

Syphilis

Syphilis is a bacterial sexually transmitted disease caused by *Treponema pallidum*.[147] Traditionally syphilis has been divided into three clinical stages: primary, secondary, and late (including tertiary and late benign syphilis). Latent syphilis is a serological diagnosis where symptoms are not apparent and which is differentiated into early (infection duration less than 1 year) or late (infection duration greater than 1 year).

Epidemiology

Transmission of syphilis is relatively inefficient. Studies have demonstrated that the transmission efficiency of syphilis between an infected and uninfected partner is only about 20%. After the initial exposure, there is a latency period of three weeks prior to the development of the initial symptoms. During this latency period (or in epidemiologic terms *critical period*), a newly infected individual is not infectious to his or her sexual partners. However, this status changes rapidly after development of the initial genital ulcerative lesion, or chancre. The chancre is a primary syphilis ulceration that occurs at the site of mucosal inoculation.

Syphilis occurs in settings where there is high turnover of sex partners. Commercial sex workers and other transient individuals with multiple sex partners are at increased risk. In the developed countries, syphilis has been associated with a variety of social and behavioral factors, including bathhouses frequented by homosexual men, prostitution related to drug abuse, and poor access to health care.[148-150] In the developing world, more important issues are prostitution, transience, and poor access to health care.

Syphilis rates in the United States reached a plateau in the late 1960s and continued to drop until 1975. Syphilis epidemiology often reflects broader societal social trends (see Figure 23-3). During 1975–1980, rates increased nearly 50%, but nearly all of the increase was due to increased incidence among homosexual men, which coincided with the "gay revolution" at that time. During 1980–1985, rates declined 40% in response to the HIV epidemic. Rates again increased nearly 100% between 1985 and 1991 (Figure 23-3).[151] This epidemic was due to increased rates among heterosexuals, especially racial and ethnic minorities, and corresponded to the use of crack cocaine, which was introduced in 1985 to the United States. Aggressive control programs, especially a large national syphilis elimination effort in African-American communities which included extensive medical ethnography and grassroots efforts, led to a sustained decrease in this community since 1991.[70,152-154] Recently, as described earlier, syphilis epidemiology more closely resembles the epidemic of the late 1970s, with increased incidence in homosexual men.

Clinical Course

Initial infection with *Treponema pallidum* occurs through sexual contact at a mucosal membrane. The incubation period ranges between 10 and 30 days. Typically, 3 weeks after the initial exposure, a chancre develops at the site of contact. The chancre is a painless lesion with an indurated border and has associated painless lymphadenopathy.

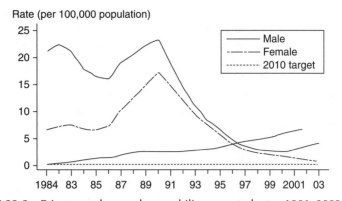

FIGURE 23-3   Primary and secondary syphilis—reported rates 1981–2003, by sex.
Source: Division of STD Prevention, Centers for Disease Control and Prevention.

Syphilis is a systemic disease. Even in primary syphilis, systemic dissemination may occur. Ten percent to 15% of patients in some studies with early primary syphilis will have cerebrospinal fluid (CSF) abnormalities.[155] Left untreated, the chancre spontaneously heals within 2–3 weeks. Four to eight weeks later, the secondary syphilis syndrome develops. Secondary syphilis is a systemic vasculitis caused by high levels of *T. pallidum* in the blood and associated immunologic responses. The most characteristic findings are dermatological including the classic palmar plantar rash, but patterns include papular, maculopapular, papulosquamous, and psoriasiform lesions. Patchy alopecia may develop especially on the scalp. On the mucosal surfaces their may be mucus patches. Condyloma lata, which are large fleshy wartlike lesions, may develop on the genitalia. Condyloma lata and mucus patches are highly infectious. Left untreated, the secondary syphilis syndrome spontaneously resolves usually within 1–2 months of onset.

Late complications of syphilis such as neurosyphilis, cardiovascular syphilis, and gummatous syphilis do not develop until 10–20 years after the resolution of early syphilis. In HIV patients, case reports have suggested that late complications may occur earlier.[156–158]

Early latent syphilis is a serologic diagnosis in which a four-fold increase in titer (i.e., two dilutions, see below) occurs within one year with previous documentation of the earlier serology. Late latent syphilis is a serologic diagnosis of syphilis occurring more than 1 year after baseline diagnosis. The differentiation between early latent and late latent syphilis has both treatment and public health implications.

Diagnosis of Syphilis

Diagnosis of syphilis is complex because the organism cannot be cultured, and serological tests have been largely unchanged for half a century. In primary cases, the organism can be visualized by darkfield microscopic examination, but realistically this procedure is not available in most settings. Serological diagnosis of syphilis is a two-step procedure.[159] Initially, a nontreponemal screening test is performed. The most widely used tests are the venereal disease research laboratory (VDRL) and the rapid plasma reagin

(RPR). Results for these tests are reported as titers (i.e., the dilutions required to achieve a negative reaction using standard reagents). Patients with a positive nontreponemal test should have a confirmatory test such as the fluorescent treponemal antibody-absorbed (FTA-ABS) or microhemagglutination (MHATP or HATS) tests. Up to 20% of patients with positive nontreponemal tests have negative confirmatory tests. These are termed *benign false positives* (BFP). Most frequently, these are seen in patients with past series of intravenous drug abuse, pregnancy, systemic disorders such as lupus, and other infectious processes such as Lyme disease. BFPs with titers greater than 1:16 are extremely unusual.

In primary syphilis, the sensitivity of serologic testing is 85%. The false-negative cases occur because seroconversion may occasionally take longer to develop than the genital ulcer. In secondary syphilis, sensitivity of serological diagnosis is close to 100%. Titers in secondary syphilis may be extremely high. Latent syphilis represents cases where the serological tests are positive, but there are no corresponding clinical symptoms.

Syphilis in HIV-Infected Patients

All stages of syphilis are seen more commonly in HIV-infected patients. Studies in STD clinics have demonstrated that HIV prevalence in patients with syphilis is up to three times higher than the number of nonsyphilis patients in these settings.[160,161] However, the serologic manifestations and serologic response to treatment are largely not affected by HIV status. Because of initial reports of treatment failure, many experts believed that all patients with syphilis, and especially patients with coexistent HIV infection, should be aggressively treated. Prospective studies presented by CDC investigators have demonstrated that in the majority of cases this is not necessary.[162-165]

Congenital Syphilis

In women who have untreated primary or secondary syphilis, the vertical transmission rate is estimated to be 75–95%.[163,166-168] Late congenital syphilis is rarely seen in the antibiotic era. Signs and symptoms of congenital syphilis may mimic those of adults (and may be similar to that of acute secondary syphilis). Transmission occurs transplacentally. Screening and treatment for congenital syphilis during pregnancy effectively prevents this disorder. Congenital syphilis is completely preventable through screening, diagnosis, and treatment during the prenatal period. Therefore, congenital syphilis is considered a sentinel public health event and warrants an investigation. These cases occur almost exclusively in situations where there was inadequate prenatal care or where there are deviations from medical practice.

Treatment

Treatment of primary, secondary, and early latent syphilis is recommended with benzathine penicillin.[70] In patients who are allergic to penicillin, doxycycline may be used. Pregnant women with syphilis should be treated only with penicillin-based regimens. There are an increased number of case reports of syphilis being resistant to macrolides,[169] so these are not recommended.

Intervention approaches to syphilis control have long capitalized on the unique clinical aspects of the disease. These include the following:

1. After treatment, an individual is noninfectious to sexual partners. With the advent of penicillin therapy this has became a major tool in developing intervention strategies.
2. The long latency period from time of infection to time of infectiousness offers an opportunity for reducing secondary spread contacts. This has been the basis of syphilis control programs based on partner notification and screening programs.
3. The availability of a cheap diagnostic screening test (the syphilis serological test) allows widespread screening opportunities.
4. Because treatment during pregnancy prevents vertical transmission, prenatal screening and treatment programs have been established.

Role of the Syphilis Registry

All state and many local health departments in the United States maintain a syphilis "reactor registry." Positive serological tests are reportable by law (by the laboratory); therefore, reporting is reasonably complete. Reactor registries compile test results and histories of treatment and can be useful in determining whether an individual patient had a previous serology and whether a positive test represents early latent, late latent, or previously treated disease. These are also useful epidemiological databases to conduct operational and clinical research.

Partner Notification

Syphilis presents the prototype disease for the use of partner notification and presumptive treatment of partners.[170] Although the empirical evidence strongly suggests that this has been an effective approach in syphilis control, no randomized trials to date have been performed to demonstrate this. Furthermore, partner notification is complicated in situations where large numbers of anonymous sex partners are the secondary spread contacts. This has been especially an issue in evaluation of disease intervention approaches in the homosexual bathhouses and in crack cocaine–associated epidemics.[26,171-173] In these situations, many public health intervention strategies have revolved around aggressive screening and presumptive treatment of partners.

Another intriguing aspect of syphilis is the relationship of immunology to infectiousness. The infectiousness of syphilis to sexual partners is largely concentrated in the primary and secondary stages. Individuals who are in late stages of syphilis (late latent, tertiary) are *infected* but not *infectious* and cannot be reinfected themselves during that time.[174] Theoretically, therefore, it is possible to "saturate" a community to the point where there are so many latent infections that the pool of susceptibles decreases and "burns out" the outbreak. Paradoxically, in this situation, treating infected persons would revert many individuals back to a susceptible state.

Chancroid

Chancroid is a genital ulcer disease caused by *Hemophilus ducreyi* and is predominantly seen in the developing world.[175-181] In the United States less than 1000 cases are seen annually and are usually associated with prostitution and drug use.[178] Chancroid was critically important in fomenting the spread of HIV in sub-Saharan Africa and South Asia. This genital ulcer disease is highly associated with increasing HIV transmission and acquisition risk.[182]

Chancroid is the most common genital ulcer disease in developing parts of the world, especially sub-Saharan Africa.[183-186] In addition, HIV has been successfully cultivated from the base chancroidal ulcers. Vertical transmission does not appear to occur with *Hemophilus ducreyi*. In the United States, outbreaks of chancroid have been generally associated with heterosexual, drug-using activity. No homosexually related epidemics have been reported in the United States. In addition, other risk factors that appear to play a role in the epidemiology of chancroid include alcohol use, intravenous drug use, and contact with commercial sex workers. Chancroid should also be considered in travelers to endemic areas presenting with a genital ulcer.

The incubation of chancroid is 4–7 days. The ulcer develops initially as a tender papule with erythema. Over the next 1–2 days pustular erosion develops leading to ulceration. The ulcer typically is undermined, and in contrast to syphilis it is often painful and is not indurated, and has a purulent exudate. Painful large adenopathy is seen in up to 50% of patients. These can develop into large purulent nodes that can spontaneously develop sinus tracts and rupture (buboes). Chancroid does not disseminate or cause systemic disease.

The classic identifying features of chancroidal ulcers are short incubation period; painful, tender ulcerations with undermined, beefy appearance; purulent exudate; and rapid resolution with appropriate antimicrobial treatment.

Diagnosis of chancroid is difficult because the organism grows only on special medium at 33°C. Culture media are not widely available outside of infectious disease reference centers. Newer diagnostic tests using DNA amplification techniques of ulcer exudates have been developed but are not yet widely available.[177]

In the United States, chancroid should be considered as a potential etiology of genital ulcer in the following groups:

1. Patients with genital ulcers in an area where chancroid is known to be endemic. Outbreaks over the past 20 years have occurred in New York City; Philadelphia, Pennsylvania; South Florida; Southern California; and Mississippi.
2. Patients with genital ulcer disease who have recent travel or exposure to an individual with travel to developing countries.
3. If there is any doubt about the diagnosis, presumptive treatment may be an option, as it is extremely effective.

Treatment

Chancroid is effectively treated with azithromycin.[200] There is widespread resistance to penicillin and Single-dose Ceftriaxone or trimethoprim sulfamethoxazole.

Epidemiological approaches in chancroid control are based on detection of disease and aggressive treatment. No studies have been performed to demonstrate effectiveness of partner notification. In addition, the issues of diagnosis are a major problem. Therefore, surveillance of cases of genital ulcer disease that do not respond to traditional therapies is useful for detecting the emergence of chancroid within a defined population. Subsequent to identification, aggressive partner notification and even presumptive treatment approaches have been successful in reducing outbreaks in the United States.[200]

Chancroid can be differentiated from syphilis and from herpes in that the genital ulcers do not respond to penicillin or to antiviral drugs, the genital ulcers do not spontaneously resolve, and the ulcer does respond very rapidly to ceftriaxone and the other recommended antichancroid therapies. In the United States, chancroid should be considered as a sentinel event causing an epidemiologic investigation including evaluation of travel patterns of potential partners.

Genital Herpes Infection

Genital herpes is typically due to herpes simplex type (HSV-2) 21 and is widely prevalent in the adult United States population.[188] Because of the difficulty in differentiating recurrences versus new infection, accurate incidence data are difficult to enumerate. Seroprevalence studies using type-specific research-grade assays have demonstrated that approximately 1 in 6 married sexually active Americans, or 40 million people, are infected with the herpes simplex virus,[189] most of whom are asymptomatic (Figure 23-4). Seropositivity has been associated with increased numbers of sexual partners, minority

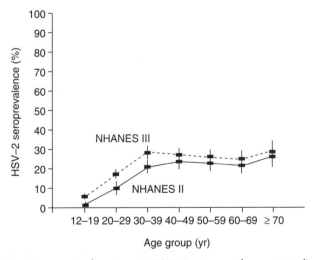

FIGURE 23-4   Herpes simplex virus 2 (HSV-2) seroprevalence according to age in NHANES II (1976 to 1980) and NHANES III (1988 to 1994). Bars indicate 95% confidence intervals (CIs).
Source: Fleming et al. Herpes Simplex Virus Type 2 in the United States, 1976 to 1994, *New England Journal of Medicine*, Vol. 337, pp. 1105–1111, Copyright © 1997, Massachusetts Medical Society.

race, and socioeconomic status. Interestingly, even when adjusting for reporting artifacts in socioeconomic differences, African Americans still have substantially higher rates of HSV-2 seropositivity than other ethnic groups.[190]

One of the most intriguing aspects of herpes epidemiology has been the shift in primary genital disease from HSV-2 to HSV-1.[191] HSV-1 usually causes orofacial herpes (cold sores). Although HSV-2 still causes the bulk of prevalent infection, this is because recurrences due to HSV-2 are much more common. In contrast, studies from a variety of places in the United States and Western Europe have demonstrated that HSV-1 can cause just as many primary outbreaks as HSV-2. There are two potential hypotheses to explain this epidemiological trend. One hypothesis posits that increased HSV-1 genital infection results from increased oral sexual behavior that has become much more prevalent in many areas in the past 10–15 years. An alternative hypothesis is based on immunologic susceptibility. For example, individuals from previous generations would have typically become infected with HSV-1 as a young child and therefore would become immune to genital HSV-1. In contrast, many college students are susceptible to HSV-1 because of the lack of prior exposure.

Genital herpes is almost exclusively sexually transmitted.[192,193] Approximately 90% of genital herpes is caused by herpes simplex type 2 (HSV-2); 10% is caused by HSV-1. The reversed ratio is seen in cases of orofacial herpes. Orofacial herpes due to herpes simplex type 1 is transmitted as an upper respiratory tract infection, usually in early childhood. HSV-1 and HSV-2 cause similar clinical syndromes at the respective mucosal sites.

Acute infection with herpes simplex occurs after inoculation of virus to the mucosal site. Primary infection is often asymptomatic. When symptomatic cases occur, a mucosal or epidermal ulcer develops. Simultaneously, viral particles enter the sensory nerve roots supplying the area and travel cephalad along the nerve axons to the dorsal root ganglia (DRG) where latency develops. For genital herpes, latency develops in the lumbosacral dorsal root ganglia, and for orofacial herpes the trigeminal ganglia. When recurrences develop, viral particles begin replication in the DRG and travel centripetally to the periphery, exit at the mucosa or skin surface, and cause a repeat genital ulceration. Because of prior priming of the humoral and cellular immune systems, outbreaks are typically shorter.

Clinical Features

Genital herpes can occur at any mucosal exposed site (genitalia, rectum, and mouth). In primary disease, the ulceration develops 5–10 days after exposure; there may also be associated systemic signs,[194] such as fever, myalgias, headache, and occasionally meningeal irritation. Recurrent herpes can develop at any time after the primary infection. In many settings, patients report a prodrome, which may consist of low-grade fever, pruritis, tingling at the site of recurrence. Patients often report that they are able to feel the recurrence developing with nonspecific signs and symptoms, which is most likely related to irritation of the peripheral nerve roots.

Because many patients have asymptomatic primary infection, differentiation of a clinical first episode into primary disease or recurrence (in patients who have had an asymptomatic primary episode) is often not possible. In the research setting, *primary* infections are defined as an initial clinical episode with no serological evidence of prior infection. Most patients, however, presenting with their initial episode, actually have serological evidence of prior infection.[195,196] This is termed *first clinical episode of recurrent disease*. This is often a very confusing point to clinicians and can be diagnosed by using type-specific serological tests. In some studies, over 90% of persons with recurrent herpes diagnosed serologically cannot identify a primary outbreak occurrence in the past.

Symptomatic recurrences are less symptomatic and heal faster than the primary episode.[197] Recurrences often occur most frequently within the first year after primary infection and frequency decreases thereafter. The factors involved in inducing recurrent episodes are not well characterized. Physical and physiological stresses have been classically cited as important cofactors, but there are few well-controlled studies that have been able to clearly elucidate these relationships. Methodologically, these investigations are difficult; therefore, most of the associations are based on anecdotal reports.

Asymptomatic shedding plays a major role in transmission of HSV. Asymptomatic shedding occurs between clinical outbreaks, especially in the first few years after diagnosis.[195,196,198] Initial culture studies of women with a recent diagnosis of primary herpes found that asymptomatic shedding occurred approximately 1% of the time. The asymptomatic culture-diagnosed shedding definitely represents a potential infectious inoculum (about 10^4 viral particles). Further recent work with PCR (polymerase chain reaction) demonstrated that shedding detectable by PCR occurred almost on a daily basis.[199] From a transmission and public health standpoint, the implications of the PCR data are not yet fully understood. Asymptomatic shedding rates are increased in persons with HIV or other immunodeficiencies.[200,201] Individuals who are asymptomatic shedders are the majority of primary HSV source contacts (or in other words, the patient for whom people with acute primary genital herpes got their disease from). Although asymptomatic shedding occurs only infrequently, the large numbers of infected individuals increases the attributable fraction of incident disease due to asymptomatic shedding.

Diagnosis of Genital Herpes

Culture or other direct viral-specific tests from a lesion specimen establish the virological diagnosis of herpes. The highest yield of samples is that from the base of a wet genital ulcer or an aspirate of a vesicular eruption prior to breakdown.

Serological testing using recombinant type-specific antigens are useful in ascertaining the presence of an IgG response to HSV-2.[202] This response is typically detectable 4–6 weeks after exposure. Persons who have positive cultures but who are seronegative are defined as *primary HSV infection*. In contrast, persons with a first clinical outbreak, but who are HSV-2 seropositive have *recurrent* infection. Serology can also be useful in defining whether an individual will benefit from suppressive therapy to reduce transmission (see below).

Herpes Simplex in Pregnancy

The major concern is preventing transmission to the neonate.[203,204] Recurrent herpes during pregnancy is not a severe clinical problem unless lesions are present in the birth canal at time of delivery, which is an indication for a cesarean section. Another approach advocated by some obstetricians and perinatologists is routine cultures of the birth canal at parturition. If herpes simplex is diagnosed (which usually occurs by culture within 1–2 days), the infant may be started on prophylactic antiviral therapy.

The major risk in pregnant women is development of primary herpes during the last trimester of pregnancy.[205] In those cases, up to one third of infants will be born with the neonatal herpes syndrome that may be fatal or lead to disability. Fetal infection is presumed to occur transplacentally. Primary infection during pregnancy can occur *only* if the pregnant woman is previously uninfected and has an infected male partner. This is the type of setting where serologic diagnoses of previously unrecognized HSV are useful.

Treatment

In acute primary or recurrent genital herpes, treatment with nucleoside analogs results in more rapid healing of symptoms and more rapid resolution of viral shedding and of the ulcer.[206-209] Treatment, however, is not curative. Acyclovir has been used for treatment since 1982, has a long track record of efficacy and safety, and has recently become available in generic formulations. New, recently approved drugs for the treatment of genital herpes include famcyclovir and valacyclovir, which offer the advantages of less frequent dosing. Local treatment is not required if systemic therapy is administered.

Suppressive Therapy

In individuals who have more than six recurrences per year or who are profoundly immunosuppressed and have recurrent disease (such as those with advanced HIV disease, transplant recipients, or patients undergoing chemotherapy) suppressive therapy is indicated. Suppressive regimens are over 90% protective in preventing recurrences.[208,210] Suppressive therapy also has a public health benefit. Studies of *dichotomous* couples (couples in which one partner is HSV-2 seropositive and the other is not) have shown that suppressive treatment of the *infected* partner, even if asymptomatic, reduces transmission of symptomatic disease by more than 90%, and a 60% reduction of asymptomatic transmission also occurs.[211] This finding has profound impact because it sets a paradigm for treatment of an infected individual—not to benefit the patient, but to benefit an exposed second party (the sexual partner).

From an epidemiologic and control perspective, the following factors are associated with increased HSV transmission:

1. Asymptomatic viral shedding: Asymptomatic viral shedding is actually implicated in more than half of the cases of new primary herpes transmission. Individuals with previous HSV-2 infection have asymptomatic shedding approximately 1–3% of the time, with an increased proportion of days that are positive in the year following the initial outbreak. From a clinical standpoint, there are no specific lesions or symptoms that are associated with asymptomatic shedding. Therefore, patients who are under the impression that if they are asymptomatic they are unlikely to shed virus can actually transmit the infection to their sexual partners.

2. Misclassification of herpes symptoms with those of other infections: Especially in women, herpes recurrences are confused with other vaginal infections, especially "yeast infections." Therefore, in situations where this is misclassified, individuals who are symptomatic due to HSV-2 infection may actually misclassify this and have sexual relations with their partners leading to increased transmission.

3. Studies in monogamous couples in which one partner is infected and the other uninfected (discordant) indicate that approximately 11% of partners will seroconvert per calendar year of exposure.[212] Studies have demonstrated that seroconversion may be less likely to occur in the face of antiviral therapy. However, studies to demonstrate this are still continuing, and even if implemented as an intervention this would be extremely expensive.

4. Prevention recommendations in the long term are difficult to implement because of the issue of asymptomatic shedding and the wide prevalence of disease. In developing countries, HSV-2 seroprevalence rates are even higher; rates of 60–80% have been reported from Thailand and Africa.[213,214]

Despite methodological challenges, condom efficacy in preventing HSV transmission has been measured. The challenges include the need to evaluate dichotomous couples, the relatively low seroconversion rate in dichotomous couples (8–11% per year), the need for periodic serological monitoring, and the reliance on self-reports for the independent variable. Nevertheless, by nesting behavioral measures into phase 3 vaccine studies for preventive HSV vaccines, condom efficacy has been shown to be over 90% for consistent users, and over 60% for inconsistent users.[215]

HSV-2 has also been conclusively implicated in HIV transmission. Prospective and retrospective studies in the United States and abroad have demonstrated that presence of HSV-2, even only serologically, is an independent predictor of increased HIV seroconversion.[216] The presence of a genital ulcer or primary infection in these cases potentiates that risk. A large meta-analysis evaluated 31 studies examining the association between HSV-2 infection and the risk for HIV acquisition, and found that HSV independently increased the risk or odds ratio between 2.9–5. Furthermore, incident HSV results in even increased risk. Studies from the Rakai prospective cohort study conducted in Uganda, which included large numbers of HIV and HSV dichotomous couples, have been able to estimate the impact of HSV on per-contact probability of HIV transmission.[217] The per-contact probability of HIV acquisition was five times greater if the susceptible partner was HSV-2 seropositive compared with partners who were HSV-2 (see Table 23-3.) seronegative. These findings, coupled with the overall consistent macroepidemiology, have prompted clinical trials of prophylactic antiherpes medication as a potential prevention intervention for HIV transmission.

Human Papillomavirus Infection

Human papillomaviruses are small DNA viruses that have the unique capacity of causing chronic infection, can cause malignant transformation, but

TABLE 23-3   Per-Contact Probability of HIV-1 Acquisition in HIV-1-Discordant Couples by HSV-2 Serology

Couple Status	Per-Contact Probability
Overall	0.0011
Susceptible HIV-1 partner, HSV-2 seropositive	0.002
Susceptible HIV-1 partner, HSV-2 seronegative	0.004 ($P = .01$)
Susceptible HIV-1 partner, HSV-2 seropositive with symptomatic GUD	0.0031
Susceptible HIV-1 partner, HSV-2 seropositive without GUD	0.0019
Susceptible HIV-1 partner, HSV-2 seronegative without GUD	0.0004 ($P = .01$)

Soure: Corey L, Wald A, Celum CA, et al. The effects of herpes simplex virus-2 on HIV-1 acquisition and transmission: a review of two overlapping epidemics. J Acquir Immune Defic Syndr. 2004;35(5):435–445.

also cannot be cultured in vitro, making diagnosis of subclinical infection difficult.[218-222]

There are over 100 subtypes of HPV. The HPV types that most commonly infect the genital tract are HPV-6, -11, -16, and -18. HPV-6 and HPV-11 have been termed low-risk types, as they are seldom associated with malignancy and instead occur on external surfaces of the vulva, anus, and vagina. In contrast, HPV-16, along with HPV-18, -31, -45, and others, are associated with invasive cervical and other epithelial cancers and are thus classified as high-risk types.

The vast majority of HPV infections are asymptomatic. A fraction develops cytological changes that progress to cervical malignancy (Figure 23-5). The genital HPV are transmitted sexually and have been identified in skin as well as genital secretions. The incubation period is not well defined, although most authorities estimate that it is approximately 3 months, with a reported range of 3 weeks to 8 months.[223,224] A small proportion of patients infected with genital subtypes 6 and 11 will develop *condyloma acuminata*, or genital warts.[222,225] These lesions are fleshy, nonvascular warts that are caused by proliferation of the keratinized epithelium and may occur anywhere on the external genitalia. In women, cervical warts are occasionally observed; in men, besides the external warts, lesions may be present inside the urethra.

HPV is sexually transmitted. HPV infection is not systemic, and transmission is thought to occur through mechanical abrasion of an infected epithelial surface with an uninfected epithelium. HPV DNA can be detected in vulvar, vaginal, cervical, oral, and anal samples in women, and penile shaft, glans, foreskin, scrotum, oral, and anal samples in men; however, most cases of HPV are clinically asymptomatic.

Estimates indicate that approximately 1% of the sexually active population in the United States have clinically apparent genital warts, and in STD clinic populations the percentage is much higher.[226] Studies that use colposcopic or cytological examination as the basis for diagnosis yield higher prevalence estimates. Estimates of infection range from 20% to above 90% depending on the specific populations studied, with college students,[227] adolescents,[228] and commercial sex workers demonstrating the highest rates. These prevalence data therefore strongly suggest that in many cases, HPV infection may also spontaneously resolve, as prevalence decreases with age.

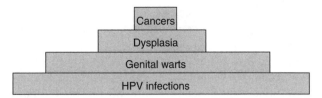

FIGURE 23-5   Human papillomavirus (HPV) pyramid.

Trend data collected by the CDC suggest that the incidence has increased over the past 30 years.

However, genital warts and cervical dysplasia represent only a small proportion of persons with infection (Figure 23-5). Prevalence and incidence studies have found that HPV infection is extremely common, with prevalence up to 50–90% in adolescent populations, and incidence rates greater than 20% per year. The highest-risk period appears to be within the year after initiating sexual intercourse.[229,230] However, it appears that over 80% of infections spontaneously clear, typically after 3–6 months. Immunity resulting from natural infection is only type specific; therefore, repeated infections and even simultaneous infection with multiple subtypes are possible.

High-risk types of HPV have been conclusively shown to be the cause of cervical and other epithelial squamous cell cancers. The sexually transmitted epithelial cancers include cervical carcinoma, vulvar carcinoma, some oral carcinomas, penile carcinoma, and anal carcinoma. Sexually transmitted HPV-associated anal and oral carcinomas are seen predominantly in homosexual men and are associated with HIV infection.[218,221]

In cervical cancer, HPV infection of the transition zone may cause a number of changes leading to malignant transformation. The hallmark of HPV infection is koilocytosis, a ballooning of the nuclear portion of the cervical epithelial cells. Left unchecked, this may lead to cervical atypia, early cervical malignant dysplasia, or frank malignant transformation. In most cases involving an immunocompetent host, the latency period from development of HPV infection to development of early cervical cancer is often 5–10 years. Advanced cervical cancer cases often take more than 20 years to develop. There are no parallel lesions in men.

The strength of association between high-risk (HR)–HPV infection and invasive cervical cancer is unprecedented in cancer epidemiology, with odds ratios exceeding 45 in most cases. Development of cancer occurs only with *persistent* infection and has a latency period of years. However, this association must be considered in the context of the high prevalence of transient HPV infection among sexually active women and the frequent resolution of HPV-associated lesions. It can therefore be concluded that HR-HPV infection is a necessary but insufficient cause of invasive cervical cancer. Besides infection with HR-HPV, the other factors influencing risk for progression to invasive cervical cancer are less well defined. Cigarette smoking has been consistently found to increase risk.[230–233] In addition, long-term use of oral contraceptives (longer than 5 years), coinfection with other sexually transmitted diseases (e.g., *Chlamydia trachomatis* or herpes simplex virus),[234–236] host immune defects such as coinfection with HIV, and inflammation have been found to increase the risk for HPV-associated cervical cancer, although these observations are generally less consistent than those demonstrated for smoking.

There is thus a continuum of HPV infection that includes asymptomatic HPV infection, development of genital warts, development of malignancies. The continuum may have discontinuities in many patients. For example, it is not uncommon for patients to develop cervical cancer who have never developed any signs of genital warts. Similarly, most patients with genital warts do not progress to develop cervical cancer.

Treatment

Treatment for condylomata (genital warts) is based on tissue-destructive therapy.[237] Genital warts are a proliferative epithelial process that is caused by HPV stimulation. In most cases, the proliferative epithelial is benign. However, therapy for genital warts is mostly cosmetic. An eradication of HPV-containing tissue is impossible because grossly and histologically appearing tissues may be infected with HPV and cannot be detected unless specifically probed for by DNA analysis. Therefore, the treatment of genital wart lesions due to HPV by traditional destructive methods such as liquid nitrogen or surgery leads to substantial recurrence rates because HPV infection is often present in the histologically normal surgical margins.

Clinical Screening for High-Risk HPV—The Pap Smear Approach

Because of the long latency period and the slow, local progression of squamous cell cervical cancer, screening for the disease is an effective prevention measure. Development of advanced cervical cancer should be considered to be a sentinel event and cause one to evaluate the cancer prevention program. For most persons, Pap smear screening is recommended every 3 years.[238] These programs have been found to be extremely effective in reducing the population-based morbidity and mortality from cervical cancer, but are expensive interventions and require access to highly trained cytotechnologists.[239–242] In HIV-infected women, screening is recommended every 6 months because of the more aggressive disease seen in these patients. If cervical abnormalities are found, then further evaluation may include colposcopy and possibly biopsy. The presence of external genital warts alone is not an indication for colposcopy.

The Pap smear approach has been traditionally oriented toward identification of HPV-adverse outcomes (i.e., cervical malignancy). In 2001, specific HPV testing was approved.[243] These tests detect a pool of high-risk HPV subtypes (i.e., those associated with development of cervical cancer). There is consensus that these tests are appropriate for use in two major circumstances. The first is in the low-grade Pap smear abnormality (for example, atypical cells of undetermined significance [ASCUS]), in which case the presence or absence of a diagnostic HPV test can help determine whether the woman needs further workup (i.e., colposcopy), or can be defined as having an inflammatory, low-risk Pap smear. A positive HPV test in this setting would result in assignment to the colposcopy intervention, whereas a negative HPV test would result in being assigned to the normal follow-up arm.[244-246] The second area of HPV testing is useful in defining women over the age of 30, who are monogamous, and who have negative HPV tests.[247] In these settings, women can be assigned to a much more infrequent Pap smear screening algorithm.

One of the most promising developments in HPV has been the development of the HPV vaccine.[248] The major approach for the HPV vaccine was initiated with HPV-16; other subtypes are currently being evaluated. The technical approach was innovative in that it utilized artificially prepared viruslike particles (VLPs) as the viral antigen in an appropriate adjuvant. In studies of over 2000 women, the vaccine was demonstrated to have an efficacy of over 99%; in fact, when both HPV as well as cytological outcomes were used, efficacy was extremely high. We anticipate the vaccine will be available for general use in 2006. One of the more intriguing aspects of the vaccine is a policy question: which population would be most appropriate to vaccinate? This is a global STD vaccine issue but one which would be precipitated by development of the HPV vaccine. Consensus among STD experts is that this vaccine should be utilized universally for women (and potentially men as well) who are 11–12 years old (i.e., before they initiate sexual activity). From a policy standpoint this presents challenges in convincing parents/guardians that STD vaccination is appropriate for this population. Qualitative work performed by Zimet in Indianapolis actually found that there was a dichotomy between population groups in that African-American inner-city mothers tended to approve STD vaccination much more readily than suburban non-African-American mothers.[249]

Primary prevention of transmission by condom use appears to be of limited effectiveness,[250] likely because of the broad range of epithelial targets for infection in men and women, absence of detectable symptoms to identify an infected partner, and inconsistent condom use (e.g., lack of use during abrasive foreplay). However, evaluation of condom effectiveness in preventing HPV transmission is complicated by the difficulty in obtaining a reliable diagnosis of HPV infection in men to confirm exposure and in accurately ascertaining proper condom use.

A sexually active couple implementing HPV prevention presents a number of important logistical and technical challenges. First, the infection in the male is not well characterized. Penile cancer is caused by HPV but in the United States and other developed countries occurs at very low frequency. Asymptomatic infection in the male is common, and no clinical evidence exists to support routine screening either using acetic acid techniques or other tissue-based techniques for diagnosis of HPV infection in men. Therefore, we are left with recommendations for consistent condom use, which may not be a practical option in couples who are monogamous and in a stable relationship. One of the major problems necessary for HPV management is partner management. There are no adequate interventions for evaluating the partner.

Vaginal Infections

When evaluating individuals with vaginal infections or vaginal discharge, it is imperative to differentiate primary vaginal infections from cervical infections presenting as vaginitis.[251,252] Clinically, women often present with nonspecific symptoms of vaginal discharge or low abdominal pain; this needs to be differentiated from vaginal disease, cervical disease, or both. Gonococcal and chlamydial infections are the most common cause of cervical disease. Vaginitis has a number of causes including trichomonas, bacterial vaginosis, and candidiasis. Because candida is not a sexually transmitted infection and has very few long-term health effects, this will not be considered here.

Trichomonas

Trichomonas infection occurs in approximately 3 million women annually.[252] The causative agent, *Trichomonas vaginalis*, is a flagellated protozoan. Signs and symptoms include a watery vaginal discharge, punctate hemorrhagic lesions on the cervix, and occasionally a frank cervicitis occurring in response to the vaginal infection. Symptoms are exacerbated during the menses because the organism can ingest hemoglobin and replication is increased during that time. Trichomonas syndromes in men have not been systematically described until recently because clinical practice was (and still is) to presumptively treat all male contacts of women with trichomoniasis.[253] Trichomoniasis does not produce systemic disease in the host.

Diagnosis

Wet mount is the most inexpensive and widely used method for diagnosis. However, culture or newer DNA-based methods may be as much as 50% more sensitive, especially in women with asymptomatic infection or in men.[254,255] The development of new testing techniques has resulted also in alternative sampling strategies. Traditional approaches to STD diagnosis in women necessitate a direct speculum examination, necessary to visualize the vaginal mucosa, cervix, and for sampling of the fornix. The availability of nucleic acid-based diagnostic technology for gonorrhea and chlamydia diagnosis prompted speculation that a speculum examination was not necessary and that a swab of the distal vaginal provided adequate specimen material. Studies by Schwebke in an Alabama STD clinic and Blake in a Baltimore adolescent clinic used culture techniques and demonstrated sensitivity of 85–90% compared to speculum examination.[256,257]

Treatment for trichomoniasis is metronidazole, 2 grams as a single dose, and is also considered safe in pregnancy.[258] Metronidazole resistance is occasionally reported.[259]

Epidemiology

Despite the availability of better diagnostic tests, basic understanding of the epidemiology of trichomoniasis has not changed greatly. From an epidemiological standpoint, trichomoniasis has characteristics of both an incident and prevalent disease; because of the large number of asymptomatic infections, determination of incidence is difficult. The CDC bases trend estimates on physician office visits but note the unreliability of these figures.[4] Nevertheless, large population-based studies of prenatal clinic attendees and STD clinic attendees have continued to find high rates of trichomonas infection

(10–15%) even when only the relatively insensitive traditional methods of diagnosis are used.[260] In contrast, infection was seen only in 2–3% of an unselected college student population.[261] Trichomonas has been associated with a number of complications, including premature rupture of membranes and potential facilitation of HIV infection.[262,263]

In men, studies from different locales have confirmed the role of trichomonas in urethritis. The prevalence of trichomonas (asymptomatic and symptomatic) in Seattle STD clinic attendees was 11%;[264] in East African truck drivers, 6.0%;[265] and in a San Francisco–area STD clinic the prevalence was 12%.[266]

For many years, trichomonas was considered to be a nuisance. Although it causes symptoms that may even occasionally be disabling, it does not cause upper tract disease nor does it cause systemic disease. In an immunocompromised host, the organism load of trichomonas may be higher (such as in HIV-infected women), but no systemic disease occurs.

However, recent studies have demonstrated that in pregnancy, it can be a contributing factor to premature rupture of membranes and consequent perinatal morbidity and mortality. The Vaginal Infections in Pregnancy Study (VIPS) evaluated 13,816 pregnant women.[267] Trichomoniasis was found in 3% of women and was associated with other clinical findings of vaginal infection, such as increased pH, vaginal discharge, and cervical friability. This demonstrated the difficulty of independently assessing trichomonas as a risk factor apart from bacterial vaginosis and chlamydia. Trichomonas was also an independent risk factor for premature rupture of membranes (PROM) in women who had intercourse more than once per week during pregnancy.

Trichomoniasis has also been associated with the development of pelvic inflammatory disease. The exact etiologic mechanism is unclear, but this finding is epidemiologically important because in many STD clinic settings the prevalence of trichomoniasis in women with chlamydia or gonococcal infection can approach 25%.[268]

Relationship to HIV Infection

Exudative STD infection, such as gonorrhea and chlamydia, have been conclusively linked to enhanced transmission of HIV. In a prospective study conducted in prostitutes in Zaire, trichomonas was found to be highly prevalent, but the association with HIV seroconversion was not statistically significant (odds ratio 1.9; 95% CI, 0.9–4.1).[269] However, because of the high coinfection rates with other STDs, it is very difficult in these studies to separate out trichomonas as an independent risk.

Bacterial Vaginosis

Bacterial vaginosis (BV) is a disorder that occurs as a result of ecological disturbances among the vaginal flora.[251,270–272] The normal vaginal flora overwhelmingly consists of lactobacilli. As a result, the vaginal host environment is acidic with a pH less than 4.5. In bacterial vaginosis, alteration of the microflora occurs with the population of lactobacilli replaced by gram-negative rods and anaerobes. As a result, the pH increases above

4.5, often to 7 or higher, and clinical manifestations include development of vaginal odor, discharge, and the microscopic appearance of clue cells, which are epithelial cells with numerous anaerobes bound to the surface creating a "ground glass" appearance. A fishy odor is often present due to the production of amine compounds by the anaerobic bacteria. Bacterial vaginosis most frequently presents as secondary to another infectious, metabolic, or iatrogenic event.

Diagnosis of BV is made on either evaluation of a vaginal smear gram stain demonstrating the characteristic alteration of the vaginal flora, or by using clinical criteria. The clinical criteria are three of the following: homogenous vaginal discharge, pH above 4.5, presence of an amine odor, and presence of clue cells. Treatment of BV uses antimicrobials effective against anaerobes, such as metronidazole or clindamycin, which then results in reestablishment of the normal vaginal microflora. Recurrences are common.

BV occurs most commonly as a secondary disorder and can be caused by infection, douching, or antibiotics (Figure 23-6). The most common causes of secondary BVs include:

- Alteration of vaginal microflora as a result of cervical infection and subsequent inflammation. In many of these cases, resolution of the primary cervical infection may result in resolution of the bacterial vaginosis.
- Alteration of vaginal microflora as a result of antibiotic use. Tetracyclines and other commonly used broad-spectrum antibiotics are especially implicated in these disorders.
- Direct instillation into the vagina of microbicides and douches.[273-275] Douching is particularly associated with development of BV. Therefore, clinical recommendations include specific recommendations not to douche.

A population of patients has primary bacterial vaginosis, meaning BV without any identifiable cause. These patients do resolve with treatment; however, BV recurs frequently in this class of patients.

The epidemiologic issues with BV are further complicated by the fact that BV occurs more frequently in sexually active women. However, correlative infectious conditions in the male host have never been demonstrated. Sexual transmission of BV has also been demonstrated to occur in lesbian patients. Treatment of bacterial vaginosis is fairly straightforward and involves specific antibiotic therapy against the anaerobic component of the BV pathogenic flora, allowing replacement with the normal lactobacilli.

BV has also been demonstrated to be a risk factor for premature rupture of membranes and premature delivery.[276-281] A large, multicenter study found that in a population of over 10,000 women, the prevalence of BV was 16%. The adjusted odds ratio of BV and delivery of a preterm, low-birth-weight infant was 1.4. A follow-up study conducted by the same group found that treatment of BV in pregnancy reduced the BV-associated preterm risk by one half to two thirds. BV was also demonstrated to be more common in black women for reasons that are not completely clear. The adjusted odds ratios for blacks compared to whites was 2.9 for bacterial vaginosis.[281] These were controlled for maternal parity, age, education, insurance status, marital status, smoking, age at first intercourse, and number of male partners in the past

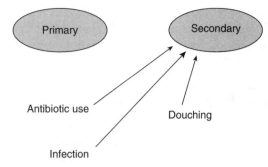

FIGURE 23-6   Bacterial vaginosis.

year. BV has also been associated with an increased incidence of postsurgical infections, including increased PID incidence after first trimester abortion and cellulitis after hysterectomy.[282] In addition, BV has recently been demonstrated to be a risk factor for HIV infection in women.[283,384] This may be a result of specific cultural practices such as dry sexual intercourse. However, further work is required in this area to conclusively define the issue.

Control of Sexually Transmitted Diseases as an HIV Prevention Intervention

Epidemiological Relationships

Sexual HIV transmission is facilitated by the same risk behaviors as those associated with the traditional STDs: multiple sexual partners, sex with prostitutes, and drug-using sexual partners.[285-287] Despite these behavioral confounders, the link between STDs and HIV infection has been conclusively demonstrated. Some examples have already been summarized. There are multiple factors that contribute to this biological relationship including the following:

1. Facilitate STD access to the vascular portal of entry.
2. Recruitment of target cells. STDs such as syphilis and chlamydia induce a lymphocytic response. Theoretically, recruitment of an increased number of CD4 target lymphocytes into an area that is exposed to HIV could facilitate infection. STDs also increase HIV receptors.
3. Potentiation of HIV replication. Studies have demonstrated that HIV replication is potentiated by presence of herpes simplex virus (viral transactivation). Recent human challenge studies of gonorrhea in HIV-infected men demonstrated that gonococcal infection increases HIV shedding by 2 logs (100-fold increase).[288] These studies suggest that the presence of other STDs may increase the inoculum size beyond the threshold required for infectivity.
4. Sexual transmission of HIV is associated with increased viral load in the infected partner. In particular, acute HIV infection is associated with viral loads in the range of 10^5–10^6, but it is paradoxically seronegative because not enough time has elapsed for seroconversion.[289] A

large study in North Carolina public clinics used HIV DNA detection of pooled specimens to identify acute HIV seroconverters; 43% of HIV transmission was estimated to occur during primary infection.[290]

Use of Epidemiologic Models to Guide Control Efforts

Epidemiologic models for STD control are based on the May-Anderson model of microparasites.[291-294] STDs form a unique subset because exposure risk is not random but determined by exposure to new sexual partners. These sexual partner characteristics, or "mixing," become critically important. These models are based on the reproductive rate equation $R_0 = BCD$, where B equals the transmission coefficient, C equals the turnover of partners, and D equals the duration of infection. As long as the reproductive rate remains above 1, the number of cases is expected to increase. Conversely, control efforts are directed toward decreasing either one or all of the constituent terms of the reproductive rate equation to drive the reproductive rate below 1.

Interventions specifically designed to decrease the transmission efficiency (B) include the use of barrier methods of contraception, use of microbicides, and recommended use of condoms. Although most interventions reduce the transmission efficiency, public health epidemiologists need to be aware that occasionally unanticipated effects may occur. For example, vaginal microbicides have been well documented to reduce the transmission efficiency of gonococcal and chlamydial infection; however, there is an increasing body of data to suggest that vaginal microbicides may actually increase HIV transmission. Therefore, in a population with high HIV exposure potential, vaginal microbicides may not be appropriate. Similarly, hormonal contraceptives may also increase the potential for HIV transmission among women who are exposed. STDs similarly increased the transmission efficiency of HIV in most settings.

Partner turnover (C) includes components that are related to the number of different partners that one is exposed to, thereby increasing the statistical risk of STD exposure, as well as the number of exposures with each partner (or dose). This actually encompasses a complex term. From a simplistic standpoint, the most effective intervention is to reduce this term to 0, which would negate the entire reproductive rate equation. This is the abstention model, which is impractical in most circumstances. Nevertheless, by reducing the number of partner exposures through risk intervention, risk reduction, education, and counseling, the reproductive rate equation can be substantially affected. Particularly effective use of this has been demonstrated recently in Thailand where reduction of high-risk exposures among Thai Army recruits both in terms of reducing partner exposures and increasing condom rates resulted in decreased STD incidence and HIV seroconversion. From a qualitative standpoint, one criticism of this model has been that the quality of partners may be just as important as the quantity of partners. For example, commercial sex workers may be particularly high risk in most settings for disease transmission and therefore qualitative factors need to be attached.

Reducing the duration of infection (D) can also decrease the reproductive rate. Reducing the duration of infection is a practical option for diseases that are curable. This essentially does not include the chronic viral diseases such as HIV, herpes simplex, and HPV. One could argue that antiviral medications, which reduce the viral load burden and shedding, actually impact transmission efficiency (*B*). Interventions that reduce the duration of infection, remove individuals from the infected pool, and reduce exposure opportunities for the population include population-based screening programs, development of effective treatment guidelines based on population base data, and partner notification. All of theses are driven by the goal to remove asymptomatic infected individuals from the population pool.

One of the most important interventions in STDs has been partner management. This has been particularly challenging, especially in environments where partners are not accessible. This can be particularly difficult in areas where commercial sex workers or gay men with anonymous sex partners are operative. Another challenge, especially in the management of gonorrhea and chlamydia infections, has been in accessing partners, especially in areas where there is poor resource availability. For example, a variety of studies has demonstrated that interventions are much more effective than traditional self-referred partner management strategies; however, resources are difficult to access. Two approaches have been utilized. One approach has included provision of partner therapy. Under this approach, an individual partner receives therapy that he or she would then give to his or her partner at home. This approach has been utilized in a number of cities but faces regulatory challenges. The regulatory challenges include liability issues (for example, the practitioner is providing therapy for an individual who is technically not the practitioner's patient); reimbursement issues, especially when both partners are not part of the same health plan; and regulatory issues from pharmacy and medical boards. Nevertheless, these barriers have been overcome in a variety of states. The most important study in addressing partner management issues was conducted by Golden.[295,296] He demonstrated that provision of partner therapy either through patient-delivered therapy or through a network of referral pharmacies substantially reduced gonorrhea reinfection in the index patients. These data, although fairly conclusive, represent an enormous investment of resources, which may not be applicable to most areas.

Prevention Issues Specific to Women

Women are at higher risk for HIV and STD transmission for both biological and behavioral factors. During unprotected intercourse, women are potentially exposed to a higher inoculum through ejaculation than their male partner. Changes in the vaginal and cervical mucosa through inflammation or hormonally induced changes can increase the tissue's friability. Hormonal contraceptives have been epidemiologically associated with increased risk of HIV transmission, which coincidentally causes a major policy dilemma in developing countries where overpopulation and the HIV epidemic coexist.

Nevertheless, women are at significant risk. In many sexual relationships, women may not be able to refuse sexual relations or require their male partner to use a condom because of either economic circumstances or fear of physical and/or emotional abuse. For example, commercial sex workers may be at an economic disadvantage if the client's preference is for unprotected intercourse. These issues have intensified the need to develop female-controlled disease-prevention methods. Female condoms are available but are not widely used. Effective vaginal microbicides still await development.

Interventions to Reduce the Risk of Sexual Exposure Through Promoting Condom Use

Condom Efficacy

Promoting condom use has been one of the central tenets of the HIV and STD risk-reduction strategy both in the United States and abroad. Large programs have developed to ensure the timely distribution of large numbers of condoms, and instructions for condom use have been part of the national STD guidelines since 1989. Condoms are effective when used correctly and consistently. Studies of HIV-discordant heterosexual couples have conclusively demonstrated that consistent use in controlled settings results in an approximately 7-fold decrease in HIV seroconversions.[297,298] Condoms are also effective in reducing the risk of sexually transmitted diseases, which attains an increasing importance as the relationships of STDs as cofactors continue to be elucidated.[299-302]

Studies of condom use have focused on understanding the determinants and issues related to their use, especially considering the low consistent use rate indicated by the national surveys. Increased condom use is influenced by the appreciation of a perceived benefit (i.e., STD/HIV prevention), peer group social norms, and sex education with specific instruction in condom use. One challenge to maintain continued use is the need to continually reinforce the perceived benefit. The result of a successful prevention is that no adverse event occurs, in contrast to other interventions or commercial marketing strategies where self-reinforcement of continued behavior is easier. As with other sex education programs, promoting condom use has not been found to increase sexual activity in adolescents or to result in earlier sexual debut.[303,304] Effective condom promotion requires integration of public health and social marketing efforts. Probably the most intensive and successful effort has been implemented in Thailand, where the "100% Condom" program has been implemented since 1991 and includes intensive advertising, an infrastructure to purchase and distribute condoms, and linkages in promoting condoms with stakeholders including the Army, provincial and municipal governments, and commercial sex workers.[305] Recent large-scale reductions in HIV seroincidence in Thailand have been in part attributed to this program. The Thai program provides a useful model on the development of an effective condom promotion and sexual risk-reduction campaign. The program includes open discussion of HIV prevention and condom promotion, mass-media campaigns, and the active participation of a large variety of stakeholders including the military, government, medical community, and even the brothels. In other words, this effective program's major accomplishment was to change the social norms across a broad spectrum of society to encourage condom use.

Core Groups and Targeting

Besides the mathematical approaches, designing control strategies also requires assessing the impact or sociogeographic effects. STDs predominantly affect specific demographic subgroups. Within the broad population strata, STDs are often concentrated in areas where poverty and other limitations on health care access exist. This has resulted in development of the "core group" concept.[306-310] The core groups are population subgroups that are disproportionately affected by STDs and which often act as the endemic reservoir of disease within a community. These may be either sociologically or geographically defined. For example, in developing countries, the predominant core groups are long-distance truck drivers and commercial sex workers, whereas in the United States, there is often a direct link to drug use.

In the United States and Western Europe, core groups are often defined geographically as being residents of defined core areas that typically are socioeconomically depressed. In the urban environment, core areas in the United States have been well documented for gonorrhea, syphilis, and HIV.[311-313] Within a core area, disease incidence may be 20–30 times that of surrounding areas. For example, in Baltimore we have identified discrete core areas where the reported gonorrhea rate in 1994 for persons aged 15–39 years was 6821/100,000 for men and 4341/100,000 for women, and areas where primary and secondary syphilis incidence had similar disproportionately high rates (Figure 23-7). The geographic core concept appears to be most relevant to incident STDs such as gonorrhea, syphilis, and chancroid, and is probably not as relevant in the chronic viral STDs. At present, chlamydia has the characteristics of a chronic infection with diffuse population-based prevalence patterns. However, with the institution of control programs, this will probably change.

The transmission efficiency of gonorrhea and syphilis through unprotected sexual exposure has been empirically estimated to be 30–50% per exposure, and treatment effectively breaks the transmission chain. Therefore, under most circumstances, introduction of gonorrhea into a community free of infection should not result in a sustained epidemic. Community-based models of STD transmission therefore postulate that core areas or epidemiologically defined core groups are critical to maintaining high rates of gonorrhea.[306] In these models, cores are characterized by a high transmission density, an empirical function that is dependent on characteristics of the sexual network. In contrast to many other infectious diseases, STD transmission is dependent on behavior—sexual intercourse. STD transmission is therefore limited to sexual networks, meaning the interrelated sexual connections of a defined social group.

Analyses of sexual networks provide a rational basis for defining transmissibility to susceptible sexual partners.[314] A sexual network is the interrelated sexual connections of a defined social group. In a dense sexual network, there are multiple pathways between sexual partners, leading to multiple sources for disease exposure.[315,316] These core group ideas have facilitated two branches of research activity in STD intervention approaches that may have profound implications for STD control.

Social Networks

Traditional STD intervention approaches have used partner notification as a major tool in control programs. As discussed earlier, for diseases such as gonorrhea—where the incubation period is short—or diseases with prolonged latency periods (asymptomatic infection) that is efficiently transmitted, such as chlamydia, partner notification may not work. In contrast, syphilis has been traditionally controlled with partner notification using the rationale of the "critical period." As a control tool, however, partner notification has never been fully and formally evaluated. In settings where partners are not named, such as in drug-related prostitution, the process fails. New approaches have utilized understanding the social network, meaning the individuals who are associated with the syphilis patient in a variety of everyday activities, and not limited to the sex partners. These approaches appear to be successful in identifying additional infected persons.

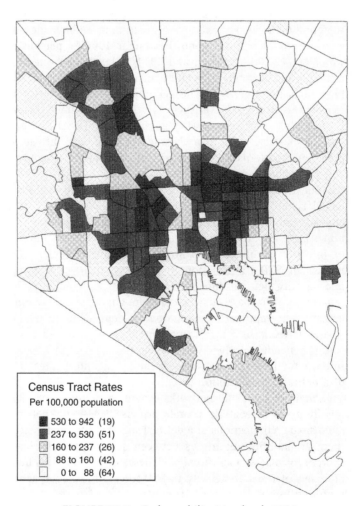

Census Tract Rates

Per 100,000 population

- 530 to 942 (19)
- 237 to 530 (51)
- 160 to 237 (26)
- 88 to 160 (42)
- 0 to 88 (64)

FIGURE 23-7   Early syphilis, Maryland, 1996.

Geographically Directed Screening

STDs, especially syphilis and gonorrhea, are associated with a host of adverse socioeconomic indicators. In the United States, these are often correlated with residential housing patterns. In highly impacted areas, STD rates, evaluated by census tract, may be an order of magnitude higher than that of surrounding areas. For example, gonorrhea rates in adolescents in the inner-city areas of Baltimore, Maryland, Washington, DC, Miami, Florida, and similar settings may be as high as 10,000–15,000/100,000 (Figure 23-8 and 23-9). In these densely populated highly impacted areas, geographically directed screening interventions represent a potential control option.

Conclusions

- STDs have major health impacts, including direct medical costs, indirect medical costs, and facilitation of HIV infection.
- STDs are predominantly asymptomatic.
- Traditional intervention strategies for STDs have been oriented toward these four goals:
  - *Reducing potential for exposure through modifying risky behavior patterns and primary STD prevention*

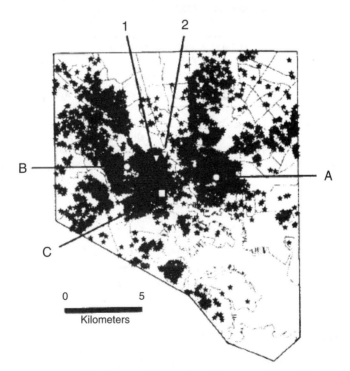

FIGURE 23-8 Dot map of reported gonorrhea for cases with valid residential addresses (*n* = 6,831), Baltimore City, Maryland, 1994. The Baltimore City Health Department sexually transmitted disease (STD) program operates two STD clinics located within high incidence areas (A & B). Point C represents the geographic centroid of the city. Point 1 represents the mean vector of private sector cases from the geographic centroid; point 2 represents the mean vector of public sector cases (see text). The scalar distance between point 1 and point 2 is 299 m.

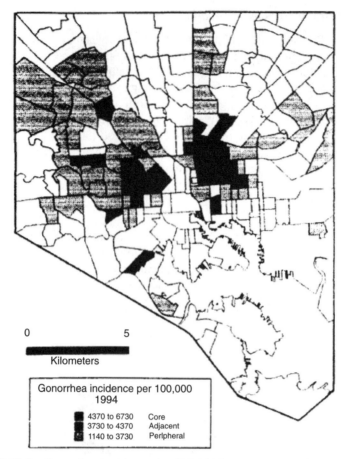

FIGURE 23-9   Gonorrhea incidence per 100,000 by census tract, for census tracts with >30 cases (1990 census), Baltimore City, Maryland, 1994. Definitions of core, adjacent, and peripheral areas are given in the text. Note that when rates are calculated, disease density is highest in the inner-city core areas.

- *Reducing of the infected pool of individuals through screening programs*
- *Providing treatment based on regimens that are known to be effective*
- *Treatment of infected partners through contact notification*

References

1. Weinstock H, Berman S, Cates W Jr. Sexually transmitted diseases among American youth: incidence and prevalence estimates, 2000. *Perspect Sex Reprod Health.* 2004;36:6–10.
2. Eng TR, Butler WT. *The Hidden Epidemic.* Washington, DC: National Academies Press; 1997.
3. Royce RA, Sena A, Cates W Jr, Cohen MS. Sexual transmission of HIV. *N Engl J Med.* 1997;336:1072–1078.

4. Centers for Disease Control and Prevention. *Sexually Transmitted Disease Surveillance, 2001.* Atlanta, Ga: US Department of Health and Human Services; 2002.

5. Day S, Ward H, Ison C, Bell G, Weber J. Sexual networks: the integration of social and genetic data. *Soc Sci Med.* 1998;47: 1981–1992.

6. Ghani AC, Swinton J, Garnett GP. The role of sexual partnership networks in the epidemiology of gonorrhea. *Sex Transm Dis.* 1997;24:45–56.

7. Potterat JJ, Rothenberg RB, Muth SQ. Network structural dynamics and infectious disease propagation. *Int J STD AIDS.* 1999;10: 182–185.

8. Upchurch DM, Levy-Storms L, Sucoff CA, Aneshensel CS. Gender and ethnic differences in the timing of first sexual intercourse. *Fam Plann Perspect.* 1998;30:121–127.

9. Hofferth SL, Kahn JR, Baldwin W. Premarital sexual activity among U.S. teenage women over the past three decades. *Fam Plann Perspect.* 1987;19:46–53.

10. Manhart LE, Aral SO, Holmes KK, Foxman B. Sex partner concurrency: measurement, prevalence, and correlates among urban 18–39-year-olds. *Sex Transm Dis.* 2002;29:133–143.

11. Ellen JM, Kohn RP, Bolan GA, Shiboski S, Krieger N. Socioeconomic differences in sexually transmitted disease rates among black and white adolescents, San Francisco, 1990 to 1992. *Am J Public Health.* 1995;85:1546–1548.

12. Hawkes S, Hart GJ, Bletsoe E, Shergold C, Johnson AM. Risk behaviour and STD acquisition in genitourinary clinic attenders who have travelled. *Genitourin Med.* 1995;71:351–354.

13. Bonell C, Imrie J. Behavioural interventions to prevent HIV infection: rapid evolution, increasing rigour, moderate success. *Br Med Bull.* 2001;58:155–170.

14. Darrow WW. Health education and promotion for STD prevention: lessons for the next millennium. *Genitourin Med.* 1997;73:88–94.

15. Ruiz M, Gable AR, Kaplan EH, Stoto MA, Fineberg HV, Trussell J, eds. *No Time to Lose—Getting More from HIV Prevention.* Washington, DC: National Academies Press; 2001.

16. Grunbaum JA, Kann L, Kinchen S, et al. Youth risk behavior surveillance-United States, 2003. *MMWR.* 2004;53:1–96.

17. Aral SO. The social context of syphilis persistence in the southeastern United States. *Sex Transm Dis.* 1996;23:9–15.

18. Moses S, Manji F, Bradley JE, Nagelkerke NJ, Malisa MA, Plummer FA. Impact of user fees on attendance at a referral centre for sexually transmitted diseases in Kenya. *Lancet.* 1992;340:463–466.

19. Tichonova L, Borisenko K, Ward H, Meheus A, Gromyko A, Renton A. Epidemics of syphilis in the Russian Federation: trends, origins, and priorities for control. *Lancet.* 1997;350:210–213.

20. Moses S, Muia E, Bradley JE, et al. Sexual behaviour in Kenya: implications for sexually transmitted disease transmission and control. *Soc Sci Med.* 1994;39:1649–1656.

21. Gangakhedkar RR, Bentley ME, Divekar AD, et al. Spread of HIV infection in married monogamous women in India. *JAMA.* 1997;278:2090–2092.

22. Edlin BR, Irwin KL, Faruque S, et al. Intersecting epidemics-crack cocaine use and HIV infection among inner-city young adults.

Multicenter Crack Cocaine and HIV Infection Study Team. *N Engl J Med.* 1994;331:1422–1427.

23. Zenilman JM. Ethnicity and sexually transmitted diseases. *Curr Opin Infect Dis (London).* 1998;11:47–52.
24. Kahn RH, Heffelfinger JD, Berman SM. Syphilis outbreaks among men who have sex with men: a public health trend of concern. *Sex Transm Dis.* 2002;29:285–287.
25. Nicoll A, Hamers FF. Are trends in HIV, gonorrhoea, and syphilis worsening in western Europe? *BMJ.* 2002;324:1324–1327.
26. Centers for Disease Control and Prevention. Trends in primary and secondary syphilis and HIV infections in men who have sex with men–San Francisco and Los Angeles, California, 1998–2002. *MMWR.* 2004;53:575–578.
27. Centers for Disease Control and Prevention. Unrecognized HIV infection, risk behaviors, and perceptions of risk among young black men who have sex with men–six U.S. cities, 1994–1998. *MMWR.* 2002;51:733–736.
28. Johnson WD, Hedges LV, Ramirez G, et al. HIV prevention research for men who have sex with men: a systematic review and meta-analysis. *J Acquir Immune Defic Syndr.* 2002;30(suppl 1):S118–129.
29. Semaan S, Kay L, Strouse D, et al. A profile of U.S.-based trials of behavioral and social interventions for HIV risk reduction. *J Acquir Immune Defic Syndr.* 2002;30(suppl 1):S30–50.
30. Beyrer C, Razak MH, Jittiwutikarn J, et al. Methamphetamine users in northern Thailand: changing demographics and risks for HIV and STD among treatment-seeking substance abusers. *Int J STD AIDS.* 2004;15:697–704.
31. Fernandez MI, Bowen GS, Varga LM, et al. High rates of club drug use and risky sexual practices among Hispanic men who have sex with men in Miami, Florida. *Subst Use Misuse.* 2005;40:1347–1362.
32. Morin SF, Steward WT, Charlebois ED, et al. Predicting HIV transmission risk among HIV-infected men who have sex with men: findings from the Healthy Living Project. *J Acquir Immune Defic Syndr.* 2005;40:226–235.
33. Semaan S, Des J, Sogolow E, et al. A meta-analysis of the effect of HIV prevention interventions on the sex behaviors of drug users in the United States. *J Acquir Immune Defic Syndr.* 2002;30(suppl 1): S73–S93.
34. Des J, Semaan S. HIV prevention research: cumulative knowledge or accumulating studies? An introduction to the HIV/AIDS prevention research synthesis project supplement. *J Acquir Immune Defic Syndr.* 2002;30(suppl 1):S1–S7.
35. Zenilman JM. Behavioral interventions–rationale, measurement, and effectiveness. *Infect Dis Clin North Am.* 2005;19:541–562.
36. Prochaska JO, DiClemente CC, Norcross JC. In search of how people change. Applications to addictive behaviors. *Am Psychol.* 1992;47:1102–1114.
37. Malotte CK, Jarvis B, Fishbein M, et al. Stage of change versus an integrated psychosocial theory as a basis for developing effective behaviour change interventions. The Project RESPECT Study Group. *AIDS Care.* 2000;12:357–364.
38. Kamb ML, Fishbein M, Douglas JM Jr, et al. Efficacy of risk-reduction counseling to prevent human immunodeficiency virus and sexually

transmitted diseases: a randomized controlled trial. Project RESPECT Study Group. *JAMA*. 1998;280:1161-1167.

39. Celentano DD, Bond KC, Lyles CM, et al. Preventive intervention to reduce sexually transmitted infections: a field trial in the Royal Thai Army. *Arch Intern Med*. 2000;160:535-540.

40. Nelson KE, Celentano DD, Eiumtrakol S, et al. Changes in sexual behavior and a decline in HIV infection among young men in Thailand. *N Engl J Med*. 1996;335:297-303.

41. Rojanapithayakorn W, Hanenberg R. The 100% condom program in Thailand. *AIDS*. 1996;10:1-7.

42. Erbelding EJ, Stanton D, Quinn TC, Rompalo A. Behavioral and biologic evidence of persistent high-risk behavior in an HIV primary care population. *AIDS*. 2000;14:297-301.

43. Erbelding EJ, Hummel B, Hogan T, Zenilman J. High rates of depressive symptoms in STD clinic patients. *Sex Transm Dis*. 2001;28:281-284.

44. Hutton HE, Lyketsos CG, Zenilman JM, Thompson RE, Erbelding EJ. Depression and HIV risk behaviors among patients in a sexually transmitted disease clinic. *Am J Psychiatry*. 2004;161:912-914.

45. Hinds MW, Gale JL. Male urethritis in King County, Washington, 1974-75: II. Diagnosis and treatment. *Am J Public Health*. 1978;68:26-30.

46. Turner CF, Rogers SM, Miller HG, et al. Untreated gonococcal and chlamydial infection in a probability sample of adults. *JAMA*. 2002;287:726-733.

47. Rogers SM, Miller HG, Miller WC, Zenilman JM, Turner CF. NAAT-identified and self-reported gonorrhea and chlamydial infections: different at-risk population subgroups? *Sex Transm Dis*. 2002;29: 588-596.

48. Hook EWI, Zenilman JM. Gonorrhea. In: Gorbach S, Bartlett JG, Blacklow N, eds. *Infectious Disease*. Philadelphia, Pa: WB Saunders; 1998:969-974.

49. Handsfield HH, Lipman TO, Harnisch JP, Tronca E, Holmes KK. Asymptomatic gonorrhea in men. Diagnosis, natural course, prevalence and significance. *N Engl J Med*. 1974;290:117-123.

50. Lebedeff DA, Hochman EB. Rectal gonorrhea in men: diagnosis and treatment. *Ann Intern Med*. 1980;92:463-466.

51. Centers for Disease Control and Prevention. Declining rates of rectal and pharyngeal gonorrhea among males–New York City. *MMWR*. 1984;33:295-297.

52. Centers for Disease Control and Prevention. Increases in unsafe sex and rectal gonorrhea among men who have sex with men–San Francisco, California, 1994-1997. *JAMA*. 1999;281:696-697.

53. McCormack WM, Nowroozi K, Alpert S, et al. Acute pelvic inflammatory disease: characteristics of patients with gonococcal and nongonococcal infection and evaluation of their response to treatment with aqueous procaine penicillin G and spectinomycin hydrochloride. *Sex Transm Dis*. 1977;4:125-131.

54. Bowie WR, Jones H. Acute pelvic inflammatory disease in outpatients: association with *Chlamydia trachomatis* and *Neisseria gonorrhoeae*. *Ann Intern Med*. 1981;95:685-688.

55. Centers for Disease Control and Prevention. Pelvic inflammatory disease: guidelines for prevention and management. *MMWR*. 1991;40(RR-5):1-25.

56. Westrom L. Effect of acute pelvic inflammatory disease on fertility. *Am J Obstet Gynecol.* 1975;121:707–713.

57. Svensson L, Mardh PA, Westrom L. Infertility after acute salpingitis with special reference to *Chlamydia trachomatis. Fertil Steril.* 1983;40:322–329.

58. Lepine LA, Hillis SD, Marchbanks PA, Joesoef MR, Peterson HB, Westrom L. Severity of pelvic inflammatory disease as a predictor of the probability of live birth. *Am J Obstet Gynecol.* 1998;178:977–981.

59. WHO Task Force on the Prevention and Management of Infertility. Tubal infertility: serologic relationship to past chlamydial and gonococcal infection. World Health Organization Task Force on the Prevention and Management of Infertility. *Sex Transm Dis.* 1995;22:71–77.

60. Washington AE, Katz P. Cost of and payment source for pelvic inflammatory disease. Trends and projections, 1983 through 2000. *JAMA.* 1991;266:2565–2569.

61. Hutt DM, Judson FN. Epidemiology and treatment of oropharyngeal gonorrhea. *Ann Intern Med.* 1986;104:655–658.

62. Koss PG. Disseminated gonococcal infection. The tenosynovitis-dermatitis and suppurative arthritis syndromes. *Cleve Clin Q.* 1985;52:161–173.

63. Rice PA, Goldenberg DL. Clinical manifestations of disseminated infection caused by *Neisseria gonorrhoeae* are linked to differences in bactericidal reactivity of infecting strains. *Ann Intern Med.* 1981;95:175–178.

64. Brown WM Jr, Cowper HH, Hodgman JE. Gonococcal ophthalmia among newborn infants at Los Angeles County General Hospital, 1957–63. *Public Health Rep.* 1966;81:926–928.

65. Laga M, Plummer FA, Piot P, et al. Prophylaxis of gonococcal and chlamydial ophthalmia neonatorum. A comparison of silver nitrate and tetracycline. *N Engl J Med.* 1988;318:653–657.

66. Gaydos CA, Crotchfelt KA, Shah N, et al. Evaluation of dry and wet transported intravaginal swabs in detection of *Chlamydia trachomatis* and *Neisseria gonorrhoeae* infections in female soldiers by PCR. *J Clin Microbiol.* 2002;40:758–761.

67. Gaydos CA. Nucleic acid amplification tests for gonorrhea and chlamydia: practice and applications. *Infect Dis Clin North Am.* 2005;19:367–386, ix.

68. Moran JS, Levine WC. Drugs of choice for the treatment of uncomplicated gonococcal infections. *Clin Infect Dis.* 1995;20(suppl 1):S47–S65.

69. Workowski KA, Berman SM. CDC sexually transmitted diseases treatment guidelines. *Clin Infect Dis.* 2002;35(suppl 2):S135–S137.

70. CDC. *Sexually Transmitted Diseases Treatment Guidelines 2002.* Atlanta, Ga: Centers for Disease Control and Prevention; 2002.

71. Lyss SB, Kamb ML, Peterman TA, et al. *Chlamydia trachomatis* among patients infected with and treated for *Neisseria gonorrhoeae* in sexually transmitted disease clinics in the United States. *Ann Intern Med.* 2003;139:178–185.

72. WHO Task Force on the Prevention and Management of Infertility. Tubal infertility: serologic relationship to past chlamydial and gonococcal infection. World Health Organization Task Force on

the Prevention and Management of Infertility. *Sex Transm Dis.* 1995;22:71–77.

73. Ghanem KG, Giles JA, Zenilman JM. Fluoroquinolone-resistant *Neisseria gonorrhoeae*: the inevitable epidemic. *Infect Dis Clin North Am.* 2005;19:351–365.

74. Jaffe HW, Biddle JW, Johnson SR, Wiesner PJ. Infections due to penicillinase-producing *Neisseria gonorrhoeae* in the United States: 1976–1980. *J Infect Dis.* 1981;144:191–197.

75. Faruki H, Kohmescher RN, McKinney WP, Sparling PF. A community-based outbreak of infection with penicillin-resistant *Neisseria gonorrhoeae* not producing penicillinase (chromosomally mediated resistance). *N Engl J Med.* 1985;313:607–611.

76. Knapp JS, Zenilman JM, Biddle JW, et al. Frequency and distribution in the United States of strains of *Neisseria gonorrhoeae* with plasmid-mediated, high-level resistance to tetracycline. *J Infect Dis.* 1987;155:819–822.

77. Zenilman JM. Update on quinolone resistance in *Neisseria gonorrhoeae*. *Curr Infect Dis Rep.* 2002;4:144–147.

78. Ghanem KG, Giles JA, Zenilman JM. Fluoroquinolone-resistant *Neisseria gonorrhoeae*: the inevitable epidemic. *Infect Dis Clin North Am.* 2005;19:351–365.

79. Moran JS, Levine WC. Drugs of choice for the treatment of uncomplicated gonococcal infections. *Clin Infect Dis.* 1995;20(suppl 1): S47–S65.

80. Schwarcz SK, Zenilman JM, Schnell D, et al. National surveillance of antimicrobial resistance in *Neisseria gonorrhoeae*. The Gonococcal Isolate Surveillance Project. *JAMA.* 1990;264:1413–1417.

81. Centers for Disease Control and Prevention. Increases in fluoroquinolone-resistant *Neisseria gonorrhoeae* among men who have sex with men–United States, 2003, and revised recommendations for gonorrhea treatment, 2004. *MMWR.* 2004;53:335–338.

82. Tapsall JW. Monitoring antimicrobial resistance for public health action. *Commun Dis Intell.* 2003;27(suppl):S70–S74.

83. Yong D, Kim TS, Choi JR, et al. Epidemiological characteristics and molecular basis of fluoroquinolone-resistant *Neisseria gonorrhoeae* strains isolated in Korea and nearby countries. *J Antimicrob Chemother.* 2004.

84. Guinan ME, Biddle J, Thornsberry C, Reynolds G, Zaidi A, Wiesner P. The National Gonorrhea Therapy Monitoring Study: I. Review of treatment results and of in-vitro antibiotic susceptibility, 1972–1978. *Sex Transm Dis.* 1979;6(suppl 2):93–102.

85. Mehta SD, Erbelding EJ, Zenilman JM, Rompalo AM. Gonorrhoea reinfection in heterosexual STD clinic attendees: longitudinal analysis of risks for first reinfection. *Sex Transm Infect.* 2003;79:124–128.

86. Webster LA, Greenspan JR, Nakashima AK, Johnson RE. An evaluation of surveillance for *Chlamydia trachomatis* infections in the United States, 1987–1991. *MMWR.* 1993;42:21–27.

87. Miller WC, Zenilman JM. Epidemiology of chlamydial infection, gonorrhea, and trichomoniasis in the United States–2005. *Infect Dis Clin North Am.* 2005;19:281–296.

88. Stamm WE, Koutsky LA, Benedetti JK, Jourden JL, Brunham RC, Holmes KK. *Chlamydia trachomatis* urethral infections in men. Prevalence, risk factors, and clinical manifestations. *Ann Intern Med.* 1984;100:47–51.

89. Hooton TM, Barnes RC. Sexually transmitted diseases. Urethritis in men. *Infect Dis Clin North Am.* 1987;1:165–178.

90. Stamm WE, Hicks CB, Martin DH, et al. Azithromycin for empirical treatment of the nongonococcal urethritis syndrome in men. A randomized double-blind study. *JAMA.* 1995;274:545–549.

91. Taylor-Robinson D. The history of nongonococcal urethritis. Thomas Parran Award Lecture. *Sex Transm Dis.* 1996;23:86–91.

92. LaMontagne DS, Fine DN, Marrazzo JM. *Chlamydia trachomatis* infection in asymptomatic men. *Am J Prev Med.* 2003;24:36–42.

93. Johnson BA, Poses RM, Fortner CA, Meier FA, Dalton HP. Derivation and validation of a clinical diagnostic model for chlamydial cervical infection in university women. *JAMA.* 1990;264:3161–3165.

94. Martin DH, Mroczkowski TF, Dalu ZA, et al. A controlled trial of a single dose of azithromycin for the treatment of chlamydial urethritis and cervicitis. The Azithromycin for Chlamydial Infections Study Group. *N Engl J Med.* 1992;327:921–925.

95. Marrazzo JM. Mucopurulent cervicitis: no longer ignored, but still misunderstood. *Infect Dis Clin North Am.* 2005;19:333–349, viii.

96. Platt R, Rice PA, McCormack WM. Risk of acquiring gonorrhea and prevalence of abnormal adnexal findings among women recently exposed to gonorrhea. *JAMA.* 1983;250:3205–3209.

97. McCormack WM, Rosner B, McComb DE, Evrard JR, Zinner SH. Infection with *Chlamydia trachomatis* in female college students. *Am J Epidemiol.* 1985;121:107–115.

98. Jacobson DL, Peralta L, Farmer M, Graham NM, Gaydos C, Zenilman J. Relationship of hormonal contraception and cervical ectopy as measured by computerized planimetry to chlamydial infection in adolescents. *Sex Transm Dis.* 2000;27:313–319.

99. Cates W Jr, Wasserheit JN. Genital chlamydial infections: epidemiology and reproductive sequelae. *Am J Obstet Gynecol.* 1991;164(6 Pt 2):1771–1781.

100. Rompalo AM, Stamm WE. Anorectal and enteric infections in homosexual men. *West J Med.* 1985;142:647–652.

101. Rompalo AM, Price CB, Roberts PL, Stamm WE. Potential value of rectal-screening cultures for *Chlamydia trachomatis* in homosexual men. *J Infect Dis.* 1986;153:888–892.

102. Quinn TC, Goodell SE, Mkrtichian E, et al. *Chlamydia trachomatis* proctitis. *N Engl J Med.* 1981;305:195–200.

103. Bauwens JE, Orlander H, Gomez MP, et al. Epidemic lymphogranuloma venereum during epidemics of crack cocaine use and HIV infection in the Bahamas. *Sex Transm Dis.* 2002;29:253–259.

104. Mabey D, Peeling RW. Lymphogranuloma venereum. *Sex Transm Infect.* 2002;78:90–92.

105. Centers for Disease Control and Prevention. Lymphogranuloma venereum among men who have sex with men—Netherlands, 2003–2004. *MMWR.* 2004;53:985–988.

106. Hillis SD, Wasserheit JN. Screening for chlamydia—a key to the prevention of pelvic inflammatory disease. *N Engl J Med.* 1996;334:1399–1401.

107. Marrazzo JM, Celum CL, Hillis SD, Fine D, DeLisle S, Handsfield HH. Performance and cost-effectiveness of selective screening criteria for *Chlamydia trachomatis* infection in women. Implications for a national chlamydia control strategy. *Sex Transm Dis.* 1997;24:131–141.

108. Rosenbaum S. Negotiating the new health system: purchasing publicly accountable managed care. *Am J Prev Med.* 1998;14(3 suppl):67–71.

109. Miller WC, Zenilman JM. Epidemiology of chlamydial infection, gonorrhea, and trichomoniasis in the United States–2005. *Infect Dis Clin North Am.* 2005;19:281–296.

110. Jaschek G, Gaydos CA, Welsh LE, Quinn TC. Direct detection of *Chlamydia trachomatis* in urine specimens from symptomatic and asymptomatic men by using a rapid polymerase chain reaction assay. *J Clin Microbiol.* 1993;31:1209–1212.

111. Gaydos CA. Nucleic acid amplification tests for gonorrhea and chlamydia: practice and applications. *Infect Dis Clin North Am.* 2005;19:367–386, ix.

112. Gaydos CA, Quinn TC. Urine nucleic acid amplification tests for the diagnosis of sexually transmitted infections in clinical practice. *Curr Opin Infect Dis.* 2005;18:55–66.

113. Addiss DG, Vaughn ML, Ludka D, Pfister J, Davis JP. Decreased prevalence of *Chlamydia trachomatis* infection associated with a selective screening program in family planning clinics in Wisconsin. *Sex Transm Dis.* 1993;20:28–35.

114. Genc M, Mardh A. A cost-effectiveness analysis of screening and treatment for *Chlamydia trachomatis* infection in asymptomatic women. *Ann Intern Med.* 1996;124(1 Pt 1):1–7.

115. Scholes D, Stergachis A, Heidrich FE, Andrilla H, Holmes KK, Stamm WE. Prevention of pelvic inflammatory disease by screening for cervical chlamydial infection. *N Engl J Med.* 1996;334:1362–1366.

116. Miller WC, Ford CA, Morris M, et al. Prevalence of chlamydial and gonococcal infections among young adults in the United States. *JAMA.* 2004;291:2229–2236.

117. Turner CF, Rogers SM, Miller HG, et al. Untreated gonococcal and chlamydial infection in a probability sample of adults. *JAMA.* 2002;287:726–733.

118. Cates W Jr, Rolfs RT Jr, Aral SO. Sexually transmitted diseases, pelvic inflammatory disease, and infertility: an epidemiologic update. *Epidemiol Rev.* 1990;12:199–220.

119. McCormack WM. Pelvic inflammatory disease. *N Engl J Med.* 1994;330:115–119.

120. Eschenbach DA, Buchanan TM, Pollock HM, et al. Polymicrobial etiology of acute pelvic inflammatory disease. *N Engl J Med.* 1975;293:166–171.

121. Eckert LO, Hawes SE, Wolner-Hanssen P, et al. Prevalence and correlates of antibody to chlamydial heat shock protein in women attending sexually transmitted disease clinics and women with confirmed pelvic inflammatory disease. *J Infect Dis.* 1997;175:1453–1458.

122. Wasserheit JN, Bell TA, Kiviat NB, et al. Microbial causes of proven pelvic inflammatory disease and efficacy of clindamycin and tobramycin. *Ann Intern Med.* 1986;104:187–193.

123. Wasserheit JN. Pelvic inflammatory disease and infertility. *Md Med J.* 1987;36:58–63.

124. Cohen CR, Brunham RC. Pathogenesis of chlamydia-induced pelvic inflammatory disease. *Sex Transm Infect.* 1999;75:21–24.

125. Westrom L. Effect of acute pelvic inflammatory disease on fertility. *Am J Obstet Gynecol.* 1975;121:707–713.

126. Westrom L. Incidence, prevalence, and trends of acute pelvic inflammatory disease and its consequences in industrialized countries. *Am J Obstet Gynecol.* 1980;138(7 Pt 2):880–892.

127. Svensson L, Mardh PA, Westrom L. Infertility after acute salpingitis with special reference to *Chlamydia trachomatis. Fertil Steril.* 1983;40:322–329.

128. Westrom L, Joesoef R, Reynolds G, Hagdu A, Thompson SE. Pelvic inflammatory disease and fertility. A cohort study of 1,844 women with laparoscopically verified disease and 657 control women with normal laparoscopic results. *Sex Transm Dis.* 1992;19: 185–192.

129. Lepine LA, Hillis SD, Marchbanks PA, Joesoef MR, Peterson HB, Westrom L. Severity of pelvic inflammatory disease as a predictor of the probability of live birth. *Am J Obstet Gynecol.* 1998;178: 977–981.

130. Clark KL, Howell MR, Li Y, et al. Hospitalization rates in female US Army recruits associated with a screening program for *Chlamydia trachomatis. Sex Transm Dis.* 2002;29:1–5.

131. Ross J. Pelvic inflammatory disease. *Clin Evid.* 2003;9:1770–1775.

132. Hu D, Hook EW III, Goldie SJ. Screening for *Chlamydia trachomatis* in women 15 to 29 years of age: a cost-effectiveness analysis. *Ann Intern Med.* 2004;141:501–513.

133. Franzini L, Marks E, Cromwell PF, et al. Projected economic costs due to health consequences of teenagers' loss of confidentiality in obtaining reproductive health care services in Texas. *Arch Pediatr Adolesc Med.* 2004;158:1140–1146.

134. Rolfs RT, Galaid EI, Zaidi AA. Pelvic inflammatory disease: trends in hospitalizations and office visits, 1979 through 1988. *Am J Obstet Gynecol.* 1992;166:983–990.

135. Lee NC, Rubin GL, Borucki R. The intrauterine device and pelvic inflammatory disease revisited: new results from the Women's Health Study. *Obstet Gynecol.* 1988;72:1–6.

136. Wolner-Hanssen P, Eschenbach DA, Paavonen J, et al. Association between vaginal douching and acute pelvic inflammatory disease. *JAMA.* 1990;263:1936–1941.

137. Centers for Disease Control and Prevention. Pelvic inflammatory disease: guidelines for prevention and management. *MMWR.* 1991;40(RR-5):1–25.

138. Washington AE, Aral SO, Wolner-Hanssen P, Grimes DA, Holmes KK. Assessing risk for pelvic inflammatory disease and its sequelae. *JAMA.* 1991;266:2581–2586.

139. Scholes D, Stergachis A, Ichikawa LE, Heidrich FE, Holmes KK, Stamm WE. Vaginal douching as a risk factor for cervical *Chlamydia trachomatis* infection. *Obstet Gynecol.* 1998;91:993–997.

140. Korn AP, Hessol NA, Padian NS, et al. Risk factors for plasma cell endometritis among women with cervical *Neisseria gonorrhoeae,* cervical *Chlamydia trachomatis,* or bacterial vaginosis. *Am J Obstet Gynecol.* 1998;178:987–990.

141. Nelson DB, Ness RB, Peipert JF, et al. Factors predicting upper genital tract inflammation among women with lower genital tract infection. *J Womens Health.* 1998;7:1033–1040.

142. Sellors J, Mahony J, Goldsmith C, et al. The accuracy of clinical findings and laparoscopy in pelvic inflammatory disease. *Am J Obstet Gynecol.* 1991;164(1 Pt 1):113–120.

143. Kahn JG, Walker CK, Washington AE, Landers DV, Sweet RL. Diagnosing pelvic inflammatory disease. A comprehensive analysis and considerations for developing a new model. *JAMA*. 1991;266: 2594–2604.

144. Beigi RH, Wiesenfeld HC. Pelvic inflammatory disease: new diagnostic criteria and treatment. *Obstet Gynecol Clin North Am*. 2003;30: 777–793.

145. Ledger WJ. Effectiveness of inpatient and outpatient treatment strategies for women with pelvic inflammatory disease. *Am J Obstet Gynecol*. 2003;188:598–600.

146. Scholes D, Stergachis A, Heidrich FE, Andrilla H, Holmes KK, Stamm WE. Prevention of pelvic inflammatory disease by screening for cervical chlamydial infection. *N Engl J Med*. 1996;334:1362–1366.

147. Hook EW III, Marra CM. Acquired syphilis in adults. *N Engl J Med*. 1992;326:1060–1069.

148. Centers for Disease Control and Prevention. Primary and secondary syphilis among men who have sex with men—New York City, 2001. *MMWR*. 2002;51:853–856.

149. Centers for Disease Control and Prevention. Primary and secondary syphilis—United States, 2000–2001. *MMWR*. 2002;51:971–973.

150. Centers for Disease Control and Prevention. Primary and secondary syphilis—United States, 2002. *MMWR*. 2003;52:1117–1120.

151. Rolfs RT, Nakashima AK. Epidemiology of primary and secondary syphilis in the United States, 1981 through 1989. *JAMA*. 1990;264:1432–1437.

152. St Louis ME, Wasserheit JN. Elimination of syphilis in the United States. *Science*. 1998;281:353–354.

153. Hook EW III. Elimination of syphilis transmission in the United States: historic perspectives and practical considerations. *Trans Am Clin Climatol Assoc*. 1999;110:195–203.

154. Gayle HD, Counts GW. Syphilis elimination: a unique time in history. *J Am Med Womens Assoc*. 2001;56:2–3.

155. Lukehart SA, Hook EW III, Baker-Zander SA, Collier AC, Critchlow CW, Handsfield HH. Invasion of the central nervous system by *Treponema pallidum*: implications for diagnosis and treatment. *Ann Intern Med*. 1988;109:855–862.

156. Centers for Disease Control and Prevention. Tertiary syphilis deaths—South Florida. *MMWR*. 1987;36:488–491.

157. Johns DR, Tierney M, Felsenstein D. Ateration in the natural history of neurosyphilis by human immunodeficiency virus infective. *N Engl J Med*. 1987;316:1569–1572.

158. Rompalo AM, Lawlor J, Seaman P, Quinn TC, Zenilman JM, Hook EW III. Modification of syphilitic genital ulcer manifestations by coexistent HIV infection. *Sex Transm Dis*. 2001;28:448–454.

159. Larsen SA, Steiner BM, Rudolph AH. Laboratory diagnosis and interpretation of tests for syphilis. *Clin Microbiol Rev*. 1995;8:1–21.

160. Quinn TC, Glasser D, Cannon RO, et al. Human immunodeficiency virus infection among patients attending clinics for sexually transmitted diseases. *N Engl J Med*. 1988;318:197–203.

161. Hook EW, III. Syphilis and HIV infection. *J Infect Dis*. 1989;160:530–534.

162. Rolfs RT, Joesoef MR, Hendershot EF, et al. A randomized trial of enhanced therapy for early syphilis in patients with and without

human immunodeficiency virus infection. The Syphilis and HIV Study Group. *N Engl J Med.* 1997;337:307–314.

163. Coles FB, Hipp SS, Silberstein GS, Chen JH. Congenital syphilis surveillance in upstate New York, 1989–1992: implications for prevention and clinical management. *J Infect Dis.* 1995;171:732–735.

164. Centers for Disease Control and Prevention. Congenital syphilis—United States, 1998. *MMWR.* 1999;48:757–761.

165. Wicher V, Wicher K. Pathogenesis of maternal-fetal syphilis revisited. *Clin Infect Dis.* 2001;33:354–363.

166. Frau LM, Alexander ER. Public health implications of sexually transmitted diseases in pediatric practice. *Pediatr Infect Dis.* 1985;4:453–467.

167. Centers for Disease Control and Prevention. Congenital syphilis—United States, 2000. *MMWR.* 2001;50:573–577.

168. Centers for Disease Control and Prevention. Congenital syphilis—United States, 2002. *MMWR.* 2004;53:716–719.

169. Lukehart SA, Godornes C, Molini BJ, et al. Macrolide resistance in *Treponema pallidum* in the United States and Ireland. *N Engl J Med.* 2004;351:154–158.

170. Andrus JK, Fleming DW, Harger DR, et al. Partner notification: can it control epidemic syphilis? *Ann Intern Med.* 1990;112:539–543.

171. Klausner JD, Wolf W, Fischer-Ponce L, Zolt I, Katz MH. Tracing a syphilis outbreak through cyberspace. *JAMA.* 2000;284:447–449.

172. Poulton M, Dean GL, Williams DI, Carter P, Iversen A, Fisher M. Surfing with spirochaetes: an ongoing syphilis outbreak in Brighton. *Sex Transm Infect.* 2001;77:319–321.

173. Edlin BR, Irwin KL, Faruque S, et al. Intersecting epidemics—crack cocaine use and HIV infection among inner-city young adults. Multicenter Crack Cocaine and HIV Infection Study Team. *N Engl J Med.* 1994;331:1422–1427.

174. Grassly NC, Fraser C, Garnett GP. Host immunity and synchronized epidemics of syphilis across the United States. *Nature.* 2005;433:417–421.

175. Mertz KJ, Trees D, Levine WC, et al. Etiology of genital ulcers and prevalence of human immunodeficiency virus coinfection in 10 US cities. The Genital Ulcer Disease Surveillance Group. *J Infect Dis.* 1998;178:1795–1798.

176. Mertz KJ, Weiss JB, Webb RM, et al. An investigation of genital ulcers in Jackson, Mississippi, with use of a multiplex polymerase chain reaction assay: high prevalence of chancroid and human immunodeficiency virus infection. *J Infect Dis.* 1998;178:1060–1066.

177. Risbud A, Chan-Tack K, Gadkari D, et al. The etiology of genital ulcer disease by multiplex polymerase chain reaction and relationship to HIV infection among patients attending sexually transmitted disease clinics in Pune, India [see comments]. *Sex Transm Dis.* 1999;26:55–62.

178. Behets FM, Andriamiadana J, Randrianasolo D, et al. Chancroid, primary syphilis, genital herpes, and lymphogranuloma venereum in Antananarivo, Madagascar. *J Infect Dis.* 1999;180:1382–1385.

179. Behets FM, Brathwaite AR, Hylton-Kong T, et al. Genital ulcers: etiology, clinical diagnosis, and associated human immunodeficiency

virus infection in Kingston, Jamaica. *Clin Infect Dis.* 1999;28: 1086–1090.

180. Patterson K, Olsen B, Thomas C, Norn D, Tam M, Elkins C. Development of a rapid immunodiagnostic test for *Haemophilus ducreyi. J Clin Microbiol.* 2002;40:3694–3702.

181. Ronald AR, Plummer FA. Chancroid and granuloma inguinale. *Clin Lab Med.* 1989;9:535–543.

182. Malonza IM, Tyndall MW, Ndinya-Achola JO, et al. A randomized, double-blind, placebo-controlled trial of single-dose ciprofloxacin versus erythromycin for the treatment of chancroid in Nairobi, Kenya. *J Infect Dis.* 1999;180:1886–1893.

183. Ronald AR, Plummer FA. Chancroid and *Haemophilus ducreyi. Ann Intern Med.* 1985;102:705–707.

184. Greenblatt RM, Lukehart SA, Plummer FA, et al. Genital ulceration as a risk factor for human immunodeficiency virus infection. *AIDS.* 1988;2:47–50.

185. Ronald AR, Plummer FA. Chancroid and granuloma inguinale. *Clin Lab Med.* 1989;9:535–543.

186. Plummer FA, Simonsen JN, Cameron DW, et al. Cofactors in male-female sexual transmission of human immunodeficiency virus type 1. *J Infect Dis.* 1991;163:233–239.

187. Schmid GP. Treatment of chancroid, 1997. *Clin Infect Dis.* 1999;28(suppl 1):S14–S20.

188. Corey L, Spear PG. Infections with herpes simplex viruses. *N Engl J Med.* 1986;314:749–757.

189. Fleming DT, McQuillan GM, Johnson RE, et al. Herpes simplex virus type 2 in the United States, 1976 to 1994. *N Engl J Med.* 1997;337:1105–1111.

190. Gottlieb SL, Douglas JM Jr, Foster M, et al. Incidence of herpes simplex virus type 2 infection in 5 sexually transmitted disease (STD) clinics and the effect of HIV/STD risk-reduction counseling. *J Infect Dis.* 2004;190:1059–1067.

191. Xu F, Schillinger JA, Sternberg MR, et al. Seroprevalence and coinfection with herpes simplex virus type 1 and type 2 in the United States, 1988–1994. *J Infect Dis.* 2002;185:1019–1024.

192. Mertz GJ, Coombs RW, Ashley R, et al. Transmission of genital herpes in couples with one symptomatic and one asymptomatic partner: a prospective study. *J Infect Dis.* 1988;157:1169–1177.

193. Mertz GJ. Epidemiology of genital herpes infections. *Infect Dis Clin North Am.* 1993;7:825–839.

194. Corey L, Holmes KK. Genital herpes simplex virus infections: current concepts in diagnosis, therapy, and prevention. *Ann Intern Med.* 1983;98:973–983.

195. Wald A, Zeh J, Selke S, Ashley RL, Corey L. Virologic characteristics of subclinical and symptomatic genital herpes infections. *N Engl J Med.* 1995;333:770–775.

196. Wald A, Zeh J, Selke S, et al. Reactivation of genital herpes simplex virus type 2 infection in asymptomatic seropositive persons. *N Engl J Med.* 2000;342:844–850.

197. Lafferty WE, Coombs RW, Benedetti J, Critchlow C, Corey L. Recurrences after oral and genital herpes simplex virus infection. Influence of site of infection and viral type. *N Engl J Med.* 1987;316:1444–1449.

198. Sucato G, Wald A, Wakabayashi E, Vieira J, Corey L. Evidence of latency and reactivation of both herpes simplex virus (HSV)-1 and HSV-2 in the genital region. *J Infect Dis.* 1998;177:1069–1072.
199. Wald A, Huang ML, Carrell D, Selke S, Corey L. Polymerase chain reaction for detection of herpes simplex virus (HSV) DNA on mucosal surfaces: comparison with HSV isolation in cell culture. *J Infect Dis.* 2003;188:1345–1351.
200. Krone MR, Wald A, Tabet SR, Paradise M, Corey L, Celum CL. Herpes simplex virus type 2 shedding in human immunodeficiency virus-negative men who have sex with men: frequency, patterns, and risk factors. *Clin Infect Dis.* 2000;30:261–267.
201. Augenbraun M, Feldman J, Chirgwin K, et al. Increased genital shedding of herpes simplex virus type 2 in HIV-seropositive women. *Ann Intern Med.* 1995;123:845–847.
202. Wald A, Ashley-Morrow R. Serological testing for herpes simplex virus (HSV)-1 and HSV-2 infection. *Clin Infect Dis.* 2002;35(suppl 2): S173–S182.
203. Brown ZA, Selke S, Zeh J, et al. The acquisition of herpes simplex virus during pregnancy. *N Engl J Med.* 1997;337:509–515.
204. Brown ZA, Wald A, Morrow RA, Selke S, Zeh J, Corey L. Effect of serologic status and cesarean delivery on transmission rates of herpes simplex virus from mother to infant. *JAMA.* 2003;289:203–209.
205. Brown ZA, Selke S, Zeh J, et al. The acquisition of herpes simplex virus during pregnancy. *N Engl J Med.* 1997;337:509–515.
206. Whitley RJ, Gnann JW Jr. Acyclovir: a decade later. *N Engl J Med.* 1992;327:782–789.
207. Rooney JF, Straus SE, Mannix ML, et al. Oral acyclovir to suppress frequently recurrent herpes labialis. A double-blind, placebo-controlled trial. *Ann Intern Med.* 1993;118:268–272.
208. Mertz GJ, Loveless MO, Levin MJ, et al. Oral famciclovir for suppression of recurrent genital herpes simplex virus infection in women. A multicenter, double-blind, placebo-controlled trial. Collaborative Famciclovir Genital Herpes Research Group. *Arch Intern Med.* 1997;157:343–349.
209. Leone PA, Trottier S, Miller JM. Valacyclovir for episodic treatment of genital herpes: a shorter 3-day treatment course compared with 5-day treatment. *Clin Infect Dis.* 2002;34:958–962.
210. Rooney JF, Straus SE, Mannix ML, et al. Oral acyclovir to suppress frequently recurrent herpes labialis. A double-blind, placebo-controlled trial. *Ann Intern Med.* 1993;118:268–272.
211. Corey L, Wald A, Patel R, et al. Once-daily valacyclovir to reduce the risk of transmission of genital herpes. *N Engl J Med.* 2004;350: 11–20.
212. Langenberg AG, Corey L, Ashley RL, Leong WP, Straus SE. A prospective study of new infections with herpes simplex virus type 1 and type 2. Chiron HSV Vaccine Study Group. *N Engl J Med.* 1999;341:1432–1438.
213. Nelson KE, Eiumtrakul S, Celentano D, et al. The association of herpes simplex virus type 2 (HSV-2), *Haemophilus ducreyi*, and syphilis with HIV infection in young men in northern Thailand. *J Acquir Immune Defic Syndr Hum Retrovirol.* 1997;16:293–300.
214. Emonyi IW, Gray RH, Zenilman J, et al. Sero-prevalence of Herpes simplex virus type 2 (HSV-2) in Rakai district, Uganda. *East Afr Med J.* 2000;77:428–430.

215. Wald A, Langenberg AG, Link K, et al. Effect of condoms on reducing the transmission of herpes simplex virus type 2 from men to women. *JAMA*. 2001;285:3100–3106.

216. Wald A, Corey L. How does herpes simplex virus type 2 influence human immunodeficiency virus infection and pathogenesis? *J Infect Dis*. 2003;187:1509–1512.

217. Serwadda D, Gray RH, Sewankambo NK, et al. Human immunodeficiency virus acquisition associated with genital ulcer disease and herpes simplex virus type 2 infection: a nested case-control study in Rakai, Uganda. *J Infect Dis*. 2003;188:1492–1497.

218. Bosch FX, Lorincz A, Munoz N, Meijer CJ, Shah KV. The causal relation between human papillomavirus and cervical cancer. *J Clin Pathol*. 2002;55:244–265.

219. Gravitt PE, Jamshidi R. Diagnosis and management of oncogenic cervical human papillomavirus infection. *Infect Dis Clin North Am*. 2005;19:439–458.

220. Koutsky LA, Galloway DA, Holmes KK. Epidemiology of genital human papillomavirus infection. *Epidemiol Rev*. 1988;10:122–163.

221. Munoz N, Bosch FX, de Sanjose S, et al. Epidemiologic classification of human papillomavirus types associated with cervical cancer. *N Engl J Med*. 2003;348:518–527.

222. Koutsky L. Epidemiology of genital human papillomavirus infection. *Am J Med*. 1997;102:3–8.

223. Moscicki AB, Hills N, Shiboski S, et al. Risks for incident human papillomavirus infection and low-grade squamous intraepithelial lesion development in young females. *JAMA*. 2001;285:2995–3002.

224. Moscicki AB, Shiboski S, Hills NK, et al. Regression of low-grade squamous intra-epithelial lesions in young women. *Lancet*. 2004;364:1678–1683.

225. Beutner KR, Reitano MV, Richwald GA, Wiley DJ. External genital warts: report of the American Medical Association Consensus Conference. AMA Expert Panel on External Genital Warts. *Clin Infect Dis*. 1998;27:796–806.

226. Kiviat NB, Koutsky LA, Paavonen JA, et al. Prevalence of genital papillomavirus infection among women attending a college student health clinic or a sexually transmitted disease clinic. *J Infect Dis*. 1989;159:293–302.

227. Bauer HM, Ting Y, Greer CE, et al. Genital human papillomavirus infection in female university students as determined by a PCR-based method. *JAMA*. 1991;265:472–477.

228. Jacobson DL, Womack SD, Peralta L, et al. Concordance of human papillomavirus in the cervix and urine among inner city adolescents. *Pediatr Infect Dis J*. 2000;19:722–728.

229. Moscicki AB. Human papillomavirus infection in adolescents. *Pediatr Clin North Am*. 1999;46:783–807.

230. Moscicki AB, Hills N, Shiboski S, et al. Risks for incident human papillomavirus infection and low-grade squamous intraepithelial lesion development in young females. *JAMA*. 2001;285:2995–3002.

231. Daling JR, Sherman KJ, Hislop TG, et al. Cigarette smoking and the risk of anogenital cancer. *Am J Epidemiol*. 1992;135:180–189.

232. Harris TG, Kulasingam SL, Kiviat NB, et al. Cigarette smoking, oncogenic human papillomavirus, Ki-67 antigen, and cervical intraepithelial neoplasia. *Am J Epidemiol*. 2004;159:834–842.

233. Thomas DB, Ray RM, Koetsawang A, et al. Human papillomaviruses and cervical cancer in Bangkok. I. Risk factors for invasive cervical carcinomas with human papillomavirus types 16 and 18 DNA. *Am J Epidemiol.* 2001;153:723–731.

234. Anttila T, Saikku P, Koskela P, et al. Serotypes of *Chlamydia trachomatis* and risk for development of cervical squamous cell carcinoma. *JAMA.* 2001;285:47–51.

235. Koutsky LA, Holmes KK, Critchlow CW, et al. A cohort study of the risk of cervical intraepithelial neoplasia grade 2 or 3 in relation to papillomavirus infection. *N Engl J Med.* 1992;327:1272–1278.

236. Smith JS, Herrero R, Bosetti C, et al. Herpes simplex virus-2 as a human papillomavirus cofactor in the etiology of invasive cervical cancer. *J Natl Cancer Inst.* 2002;94:1604–1613.

237. CDC. *Sexually transmitted diseases treatment guidelines 2002.* Atlanta, Ga: Centers for Disease Control and Prevention. *MMWR.* 2002;51 (RR-6):1–78.

238. Duncan ID. Guidelines for clinical practice and programme management. 1997. Sheffield, NHSCSP Cervical Screening Programme. MHSCSP Publication Number 8.

239. Lorincz AT, Reid R, Jenson AB, Greenberg MD, Lancaster W, Kurman RJ. Human papillomavirus infection of the cervix: relative risk associations of 15 common anogenital types. *Obstet Gynecol.* 1992;79:328–337.

240. Wright TC Jr, Denny L, Kuhn L, Pollack A, Lorincz A. HPV DNA testing of self-collected vaginal samples compared with cytologic screening to detect cervical cancer. *JAMA.* 2000;283:81–86.

241. Schiffman M, Herrero R, Hildesheim A, et al. HPV DNA testing in cervical cancer screening: results from women in a high-risk province of Costa Rica. *JAMA.* 2000;283:87–93.

242. Darwin LH, Cullen AP, Arthur PM, et al. Comparison of digene hybrid capture 2 and conventional culture for detection of *Chlamydia trachomatis* and *Neisseria gonorrhoeae* in cervical specimens. *J Clin Microbiol.* 2002;40:641–644.

243. Kulasingam SL, Hughes JP, Kiviat NB, et al. Evaluation of human papillomavirus testing in primary screening for cervical abnormalities: comparison of sensitivity, specificity, and frequency of referral. *JAMA.* 2002;288:1749–1757.

244. Cox JT. Evaluating the role of HPV testing for women with equivocal Papanicolaou test findings. *JAMA.* 1999;281:1645–1647.

245. Sherman ME, Schiffman M, Cox JT. Effects of age and human papilloma viral load on colposcopy triage: data from the randomized Atypical Squamous Cells of Undetermined Significance/Low-Grade Squamous Intraepithelial Lesion Triage Study (ALTS). *J Natl Cancer Inst.* 2002;94:102–107.

246. Cox JT. The clinician's view: role of human papillomavirus testing in the American Society for Colposcopy and Cervical Pathology Guidelines for the management of abnormal cervical cytology and cervical cancer precursors. *Arch Pathol Lab Med.* 2003;127:950–958.

247. Goldie SJ, Kim JJ, Wright TC. Cost-effectiveness of human papillomavirus DNA testing for cervical cancer screening in women aged 30 years or more. *Obstet Gynecol.* 2004;103:619–631.

248. Koutsky LA, Ault KA, Wheeler CM, et al. A controlled trial of a human papillomavirus type 16 vaccine. *N Engl J Med.* 2002;347:1645–1651.

249. Mays RM, Sturm LA, Zimet GD. Parental perspectives on vaccinating children against sexually transmitted infections. *Soc Sci Med.* 2004;58:1405–1413.

250. Manhart LE, Koutsky LA. Do condoms prevent genital HPV infection, external genital warts, or cervical neoplasia? A meta-analysis. *Sex Transm Dis.* 2002;29:725–735.

251. Sobel JD. Vaginitis. *N Engl J Med.* 1997;337:1896–1903.

252. Wendel KA. Trichomoniasis: what's new? *Curr Infect Dis Rep.* 2003;5:129–134.

253. Krieger JN, Jenny C, Verdon M, et al. Clinical manifestations of trichomoniasis in men. *Ann Intern Med.* 1993;118:844–849.

254. Wendel KA, Erbelding EJ, Gaydos CA, Rompalo AM. *Trichomonas vaginalis* polymerase chain reaction compared with standard diagnostic and therapeutic protocols for detection and treatment of vaginal trichomoniasis. *Clin Infect Dis.* 2002;35:576–580.

255. Wendel KA, Rompalo AM, Erbelding EJ, Chang TH, Alderete JF. Double-stranded RNA viral infection of *Trichomonas vaginalis* infecting patients attending a sexually transmitted diseases clinic. *J Infect Dis.* 2002;186:558–561.

256. Schwebke JR, Hook EW III. High rates of *Trichomonas vaginalis* among men attending a sexually transmitted diseases clinic: implications for screening and urethritis management. *J Infect Dis.* 2003;188:465–468.

257. Blake DR, Duggan A, Quinn T, Zenilman J, Joffe A. Evaluation of vaginal infections in adolescent women: can it be done without a speculum? *Pediatrics.* 1998;102(4 Pt 1):939–944.

258. Spence MR, Harwell TS, Davies MC, Smith JL. The minimum single oral metronidazole dose for treating trichomoniasis: a randomized, blinded study. *Obstet Gynecol.* 1997;89(5 Pt 1):699–703.

259. Lossick JG, Muller M, Gorrell TE. In vitro drug susceptibility and doses of metronidazole required for cure in cases of refractory vaginal trichomoniasis. *J Infect Dis.* 1986;153:948–955.

260. Cotch MF, Pastorek JG, Nugent RP, Yerg DE, Martin DH, Eschenbach DA. Demographic and behavioral predictors of *Trichomonas vaginalis* infection among pregnant women. The Vaginal Infections and Prematurity Study Group. *Obstet Gynecol.* 1991;78:1087–1092.

261. McCormack WM, Evrard JR, Laughlin CF, et al. Sexually transmitted conditions among women college students. *Am J Obstet Gynecol.* 1981;139:130–133.

262. Cotch MF, Pastorek JG, Nugent RP, et al. *Trichomonas vaginalis* associated with low birth weight and preterm delivery. The Vaginal Infections and Prematurity Study Group. *Sex Transm Dis.* 1997;24:353–360.

263. Moodley P, Wilkinson D, Connolly C, Moodley J, Sturm AW. *Trichomonas vaginalis* is associated with pelvic inflammatory disease in women infected with human immunodeficiency virus. *Clin Infect Dis.* 2002;34:519–522.

264. Krieger JN, Jenny C, Verdon M, et al. Clinical manifestations of trichomoniasis in men. *Ann Intern Med.* 1993;118:844–849.

265. Jackson DJ, Rakwar JP, Chohan B, et al. Urethral infection in a workplace population of East African men: evaluation of strategies for screening and management. *J Infect Dis.* 1997;175:833–838.

266. Borchardt KA, al Haraci S, Maida N. Prevalence of *Trichomonas vaginalis* in a male sexually transmitted disease clinic population by

interview, wet mount microscopy, and the InPouch TV test. *Genitourin Med.* 1995;71:405–406.

267. Pastorek JG, Cotch MF, Martin DH, Eschenbach DA. Clinical and microbiological correlates of vaginal trichomoniasis during pregnancy. The Vaginal Infections and Prematurity Study Group. *Clin Infect Dis.* 1996;23:1075–1080.

268. Paisarntantiwong R, Brockmann S, Clarke L, Landesman S, Feldman J, Minkoff H. The relationship of vaginal trichomoniasis and pelvic inflammatory disease among women colonized with *Chlamydia trachomatis. Sex Transm Dis.* 1995;22:344–347.

269. Laga M, Manoka A, Kivuvu M, et al. Non-ulcerative sexually transmitted diseases as risk factors for HIV-1 transmission in women: results from a cohort study. *AIDS.* 1993;7:95–102.

270. Spiegel CA. Bacterial vaginosis. *Clin Microbiol Rev.* 1991;4:485–502.

271. Cook RL, Redondo-Lopez V, Schmitt C, Meriwether C, Sobel JD. Clinical, microbiological, and biochemical factors in recurrent bacterial vaginosis. *J Clin Microbiol.* 1992;30:870–877.

272. Sobel JD. Bacterial vaginosis—an ecologic mystery. *Ann Intern Med.* 1989;111:551–553.

273. Schwebke JR, Richey CM, Weiss HL. Correlation of behaviors with microbiological changes in vaginal flora. *J Infect Dis.* 1999;180:1632–1636.

274. Morris M, Nicoll A, Simms I, Wilson J, Catchpole M. Bacterial vaginosis: a public health review. *BJOG.* 2001;108:439–450.

275. Holzman C, Leventhal JM, Qiu H, Jones NM, Wang J. Factors linked to bacterial vaginosis in nonpregnant women. *Am J Public Health.* 2001;91:1664–1670.

276. Kurki T, Sivonen A, Renkonen OV, Savia E, Ylikorkala O. Bacterial vaginosis in early pregnancy and pregnancy outcome. *Obstet Gynecol.* 1992;80:173–177.

277. Eschenbach DA. Bacterial vaginosis and anaerobes in obstetric-gynecologic infection. *Clin Infect Dis.* 1993;16(suppl 4):S282–S287.

278. Hauth JC, Goldenberg RL, Andrews WW, DuBard MB, Copper RL. Reduced incidence of preterm delivery with metronidazole and erythromycin in women with bacterial vaginosis. *N Engl J Med.* 1995;333:1732–1736.

279. Hillier SL, Nugent RP, Eschenbach DA, et al. Association between bacterial vaginosis and preterm delivery of a low-birth-weight infant. The Vaginal Infections and Prematurity Study Group. *N Engl J Med.* 1995;333:1737–1742.

280. Meis PJ, Goldenberg RL, Mercer B, et al. The preterm prediction study: significance of vaginal infections. National Institute of Child Health and Human Development Maternal-Fetal Medicine Units Network. *Am J Obstet Gynecol.* 1995;173:1231–1235.

281. Royce RA, Jackson TP, Thorp JM Jr, et al. Race/ethnicity, vaginal flora patterns, and pH during pregnancy. *Sex Transm Dis.* 1999;26:96–102.

282. Larsson PG, Platz-Christensen JJ, Thejls H, Forsum U, Pahlson C. Incidence of pelvic inflammatory disease after first-trimester legal abortion in women with bacterial vaginosis after treatment with metronidazole: a double-blind, randomized study. *Am J Obstet Gynecol.* 1992;166(1 Pt 1):100–103.

283. Sewankambo N, Gray RH, Wawer MJ, et al. HIV-1 infection associated with abnormal vaginal flora morphology and bacterial vaginosis [see

comments] [published erratum appears in *Lancet*. 1997;350:1036]. *Lancet*. 1997;350:546–550.

284. Taha TE, Gray RH, Kumwenda NI, et al. HIV infection and disturbances of vaginal flora during pregnancy. *J Acquir Immune Defic Syndr Hum Retrovirol*. 1999;20:52–59.

285. Fleming DT, Wasserheit JN. From epidemiological synergy to public health policy and practice: the contribution of other sexually transmitted diseases to sexual transmission of HIV infection. *Sex Transm Infect*. 1999;75:3–17.

286. Wasserheit JN. Epidemiological synergy. Interrelationships between human immunodeficiency virus infection and other sexually transmitted diseases. *Sex Transm Dis*. 1992;19:61–77.

287. Royce RA, Sena A, Cates W Jr, Cohen MS. Sexual transmission of HIV. *N Engl J Med*. 1997;336:1072–1078.

288. Moss GB, Overbaugh J, Welch M, et al. Human immunodeficiency virus DNA in urethral secretions in men: association with gonococcal urethritis and CD4 cell depletion. *J Infect Dis*. 1995;172:1469–1474.

289. Pilcher CD, Tien HC, Eron JJ Jr, et al. Brief but efficient: acute HIV infection and the sexual transmission of HIV. *J Infect Dis*. 2004;189:1785–1792.

290. Pilcher CD, Fiscus SA, Nguyen TQ, et al. Detection of acute infections during HIV testing in North Carolina. *N Engl J Med*. 2005;352: 1873–1883.

291. Garnett GP, Anderson RM. Sexually transmitted diseases and sexual behavior: insights from mathematical models. *J Infect Dis*. 1996;174(suppl 2):S150–S161.

292. Pequegnat W, Fishbein M, Celentano D, et al. NIMH/APPC workgroup on behavioral and biological outcomes in HIV/STD prevention studies: a position statement. *Sex Transm Dis*. 2000;27:127–132.

293. Woolhouse ME, Dye C, Etard JF, et al. Heterogeneities in the transmission of infectious agents: implications for the design of control programs. *Proc Natl Acad Sci U S A*. 1997;94:338–342.

294. Brunham RC, Plummer FA. A general model of sexually transmitted disease epidemiology and its implications for control. *Med Clin North Am*. 1990;74:1339–1352.

295. Golden MR, Manhart LE. Innovative approaches to the prevention and control of bacterial sexually transmitted infections. *Infect Dis Clin North Am*. 2005;19:513–540.

296. Golden MR, Whittington WL, Handsfield HH, et al. Effect of expedited treatment of sex partners on recurrent or persistent gonorrhea or chlamydial infection. *N Engl J Med*. 2005;352:676–685.

297. Padian NS, O'Brien TR, Chang Y, Glass S, Francis DP. Prevention of heterosexual transmission of human immunodeficiency virus through couple counseling. *J Acquir Immune Defic Syndr*. 1993;6:1043–1048.

298. de V, I. A longitudinal study of human immunodeficiency virus transmission by heterosexual partners. European Study Group on Heterosexual Transmission of HIV. *N Engl J Med*. 1994;331:341–346.

299. *Workshop Summary: Scientific Evidence on Condom Effectiveness for STD Prevention. 2003*. National Institutes of Health; 2001.

300. Holmes KK, Levine R, Weaver M. Effectiveness of condoms in preventing sexually transmitted infections. *Bull WHO*. 2004;82:454–461.

301. Wingood GM, DiClemente RJ, Mikhail I, et al. A randomized controlled trial to REDUCE HIV transmission risk behaviors and sexually

transmitted diseases among women living with HIV: the WiLLOW Program. *J Acquir Immune Defic Syndr.* 2004;37:S58–S67.

302. Warner L, Newman DR, Austin HD, et al. Condom effectiveness for reducing transmission of gonorrhea and chlamydia: the importance of assessing partner infection status. *Am J Epidemiol.* 2004;159: 242–251.

303. Kirby D, Short L, Collins J, et al. School-based programs to reduce sexual risk behaviors: a review of effectiveness. *Public Health Rep.* 1994;109:339–360.

304. Sellers DE, McGraw SA, McKinlay JB. Does the promotion and distribution of condoms increase teen sexual activity? Evidence from an HIV prevention program for Latino youth. *Am J Public Health.* 1994;84:1952–1959.

305. Rojanapithayakorn W, Hanenberg R. The 100% condom program in Thailand. *AIDS.* 1996;10:1–7.

306. Rothenberg RB, Potterat JJ. Temporal and social aspects of gonorrhea transmission: the force of infectivity. *Sex Transm Dis.* 1988;15:88–92.

307. Woodhouse DE, Rothenberg RB, Potterat JJ, et al. Mapping a social network of heterosexuals at high risk for HIV infection. *AIDS.* 1994;8:1331–1336.

308. Rothenberg RB, Potterat JJ, Woodhouse DE. Personal risk taking and the spread of disease: beyond core groups. *J Infect Dis.* 1996;174(suppl 2):S144–S149.

309. Rothenberg RB, Sterk C, Toomey KE, et al. Using social network and ethnographic tools to evaluate syphilis transmission. *Sex Transm Dis.* 1998;25:154–160.

310. Rothenberg RB, Long DM, Sterk CE, et al. The Atlanta Urban Networks Study: a blueprint for endemic transmission. *AIDS.* 2000;14: 2191–2200.

311. Bernstein KT, Curriero FC, Jennings JM, Olthoff G, Erbelding EJ, Zenilman J. Defining core gonorrhea transmission utilizing spatial data. *Am J Epidemiol.* 2004;160:51–58.

312. Becker KM, Glass GE, Brathwaite W, Zenilman JM. Geographic epidemiology of gonorrhea in Baltimore, Maryland, using a geographic information system. *Am J Epidemiol.* 1998;147:709–716.

313. Zenilman JM, Ellish N, Fresia A, Glass G. The geography of sexual partnerships in Baltimore: applications of core theory dynamics using a geographic information system. *Sex Transm Dis.* 1999;26:75–81.

314. Rothenberg R, Narramore J. The relevance of social network concepts to sexually transmitted disease control. *Sex Transm Dis.* 1996;23: 24–29.

315. Klovdahl AS, Potterat JJ, Woodhouse DE, Muth JB, Muth SQ, Darrow WW. Social networks and infectious disease: the Colorado Springs Study. *Soc Sci Med.* 1994;38:79–88.

316. Rothenberg RB, Potterat JJ, Woodhouse DE, Muth SQ, Darrow WW, Klovdahl AS. Social network dynamics and HIV transmission. *AIDS.* 1998;12:1529–1536.

VECTOR-BORNE AND PARASITE DISEASES

CHAPTER TWENTY-FOUR

EMERGING VECTOR-BORNE INFECTIONS

Kenrad E. Nelson

Introduction

In the last two decades several vector-borne infections have emerged as major causes of human morbidity and mortality. A dramatic recent example is the spread of West Nile virus (WNV) into the Western Hemisphere from endemic foci in the Middle East, Africa, and eastern Europe. However, it should be noted that the recent epidemic activity of WNV has also increased and expanded, even in the areas where the virus previously was endemic.

Other examples of the spread of vector-borne infections include the emergence of all four serotypes of dengue virus in the Caribbean and Central and South America, the expansion of the geographic foci of Japanese encephalitis virus to western India and Pakistan, and the emergence of yellow fever in West Africa.[1-3]

The incidence of Lyme disease in the United States and tick-borne encephalitis virus in eastern and central Europe and Russia has increased in the last decade. Malaria remains a major cause of infectious morbidity and mortality in sub-Saharan Africa and other tropical countries in Asia, the Middle East, and South America.

Although the emergence of each of these vector-borne infections is linked to unique changes in human activity and the environment, several cross-cutting factors facilitate the emergence of infectious diseases. These include the following:

- The increased ease and frequency of global travel allows infected persons to efficiently spread an infection to a new area.
- Rapid urbanization in the major cities of the tropics have created slums where the density of human populations is extreme.
- The profusion of nonbiodegradable containers (i.e., mostly plastic) has created breeding sites for many mosquitoes, especially *Aedes aegypti*, in proximity to large human populations.

- The public health infrastructure has deteriorated, and vector-control programs have been abandoned, due in part to the pressures to "privatize" the economies of developing countries.

In addition to these proximate causes for the emergence of arthropod-borne viruses, several other factors may have played a role in their emergence in the past or could become more important in the future. These factors include the following:

- Building of large dams and water projects that provide breeding sites for mosquito vectors
- Deforestation and changes in land use associated with expansion of human habitation
- Introduction of new virus-amplifying hosts or efficient vectors into new areas (e.g., introduction of *Aedes albopictus* into the Americas)

Also, climatic changes (global warming) could amplify endemic transmission by expanding mosquito breeding sites to new temperate areas and potentially decreasing the extrinsic incubation period of the virus in the mosquito.[4]

Arthropod-Borne Virus Infections

Arboviruses are important causes of encephalitis and hemorrhagic fever in many parts of the world. Only specific species of mosquitoes or ticks that are present in specific ecologic systems can transmit these viruses. Because they depend on transmission by the arthropod host, these diseases are seasonal in temperate climates yet year-round in tropical climates. The virus must replicate in the vector and travel from the mosquitoes' stomach to their salivary glands before transmission can occur. The interval between infection of the vector when blood is ingested from a viremic host until the virus appears in the salivary gland of the arthropod is referred to as the extrinsic incubation period. This period is shorter at higher temperature, but averages 6–10 days for most arboviral infections.

Arboviruses are classified into four families: Togaviridae, Flaviviridae, Bunyaviridae, and Reoviridae. The vectors, animal reservoir, and geographic distribution of some important representatives of these four viral families are shown in Table 24-1. The viruses generally are not cytopathic to the infected mosquitoes. However, some arboviruses are neurotropic in the mosquito, as well as in humans. This is especially true for Japanese encephalitis (JE) virus and may increase transmission by enhancing biting of CO_2-emitting targets, such as humans and other animals, by JE-infected mosquitoes.

The transmission of these viruses may occur throughout the year in tropical areas but increases during the rainy seasons. However, in temperate climates, infections only occur during the warmer months. The mechanism of survival of arboviruses over the winter in cold temperatures is of considerable epidemiologic interest. Although it is possible that a female mosquito could hibernate after a blood meal and reemerge the following season, this is believed to be uncommon. Generally, only nulliparous mosquitoes hibernate. Nevertheless, hibernating mosquitoes infected with West Nile virus have been found in storm sewers during the winter in the New York area.[5] The virus

TABLE 24-1 Arboviruses That Cause Encephalitis

Family Genus Complex Virus Species	Vector	Animal Reservoir	Geographical Location	Importance in Encephalitis[a]
Togaviridae[b]				
Alphavirus[b]				
Eastern encephalitis	Mosquitoes (Culiseta, Aedes)	Birds	Eastern and gulf coasts of US, Caribbean, and South America	++
Western encephalitis	Mosquitoes (Culex)	Birds	Widespread; but disease in western US and Canada	++
Venezuelan equine encephalitis	Mosquitoes (Aedes, Culex, Mansonia, etc.)	Horses and small mammals	South and Central America, Florida, and southwest US	+
Flaviviridae[c]				
St. Louis complex				
St. Louis	Mosquitoes (Culex)	Birds	Widespread in US	+++
Japanese	Mosquitoes (Culex)	Birds	Japan, China, Southeast Asia, and India	++++
Murray Valley	Mosquitoes (Culex)	Birds	Australia and New Guinea	++
West Nile	Mosquitoes (Culex)	Birds	Africa, Middle East, and southern Europe	++
Liheus	Mosquitoes (Psorphora)	Birds	South and Central America	+
Rocio	Mosquitoes (?)	Birds	Brazil	++
Tick-borne complex				
Far Eastern tick-borne encephalitis[d]	Ticks (Ixodes)	Small mammals and birds	Siberia	+++
Central European tick-borne encephalitis	Ticks (Ixodes)	Small mammals and birds	Central Europe	+++
Kyasanur Forest	Ticks (Haemophysalis)	Small mammals and birds	India	++
Louping III	Ticks (Ixodes)	Small mammals and birds	North England, Scotland, and Ireland	+
Powassan	Ticks (Ixodes)	Small mammals and birds	Canada and northern US	+
Negishi	Ticks (?)	Small mammals and birds	Japan	+

continued

TABLE 24-1   continued

Family Genus Complex Virus Species[e]	Vector	Animal Reservoir	Geographical Location	Importance in Encephalitis[a]
Bunyaviridae[e]				
Bunyavirus				
California group				
California encephalitis	Mosquitoes (*Aedes*)	Small mammals	Western US	+
La Crosse	Mosquitoes (*Aedes*)	Squirrels, chipmunks	Midwestern and eastern US	+++
Jamestown Canyon	Mosquitoes (*Culiseta*)	White-tailed deer	US and Alaska	+
Cache Valley	Mosquitoes (*Culiseta*)	Livestock and large mammals	North and South America	+
Snowshoe hare	Mosquitoes (*Culiseta*)	Snowshoe hare	Canada, Alaska, northern US, and Russia	+
Tahnya	Mosquitoes (*Aedes, Culiseta*)	Small mammals	Central Europe	+
Inkoo	Mosquitoes (?)	Reindeer, moose	Finland and Russia	+
Phlebovirus				
Rift Valley	Mosquitoes (*Culex, Aedes*)	Sheep, cattle, camels	East Africa	+
Reoviridae				
Coltivirus				
Colorado tick fever	Ticks (*Dermacentor*)	Small mammals	Rocky Mountain area	+

[a] ++++, over 10,000 cases/year; +++, common outbreaks of >100 cases/year; ++, irregular outbreaks; +, rare occurrences.
[b] Formerly group A arboviruses.
[c] Formerly group B arboviruses.
[d] Formerly Russian spring–summer encephalitis.
[e] Several other Bunyaviridae (Arbia and Toseana viruses of genus *Phlebotivirus*; Erve virus of genus *Nairovirus*), Reoviridae (Lipovnik and Tribec viruses of genus *Orbivirus*; Eyach of genus *Coltivirus*), and single tick-borne members of Bunyaviridae (Bhanjavirus) and Orthomyxoviridae (Thogotovirus) have been tentatively associated with CNS disease in Europe, Asia, and Africa (Dobler, 1996).

Source: Johnson, R. Viral Infections of the Central Nervous System, 2nd Edition, © 1998, Lippincott Williams and Wilkins.

could also be reintroduced by migrating birds. In southern areas in the United States, virus-infected mosquitoes have been found year-round.[6] Another mechanism for wintering over is the vertical transmission of the viral genome to the eggs of an infected female mosquito. This has been shown to occur for most of the viruses in the *Bunyavirus* and *Phlebovirus* groups. Also, there is experimental evidence of vertical transmission of several flaviviruses, as well as sexual transmission of these viruses from male to female mosquitoes.[7,8] Ticks do survive for several years and can spread infection during subsequent seasons after they are infected (see Chapter 25).

Flaviviruses

The Flaviviridae family contains about 68 single-stranded RNA viruses, most of which, but not all, are transmitted by arthropods. Several flaviviruses have been especially prominent among the important emerging human infections in the past decade or two. West Nile virus has spread dramatically in the Western Hemisphere, dengue in the Caribbean and Central and South America, and Japanese encephalitis virus in Asia.[9]

Dengue and Other Mosquito-Borne Infections

Although dengue has been known as a human disease for over 200 years, in the last 20 years, dengue fever, dengue hemorrhagic fever (DHF), and dengue shock syndrome (DSS) have emerged as the most important arthropod-borne viral disease of humans worldwide.[10] It is estimated that up to 100 million cases of dengue fever occur annually globally. Approximately 250,000 cases of DHF are officially reported each year, but the actual number probably is several times higher. The syndrome of DHF/DSS was first reported as an epidemic disease in the Philippines in 1954, and it gradually spread to other areas in Southeast Asia.[11] This more severe form of dengue carries a mortality of 5% to 15% and is believed to be related most often to an infection with a second dengue serotype in a person previously infected with another dengue virus.[12] The second dengue virus infection is believed to lead to vascular damage by immune mechanisms—associated with the formation of immune complexes—and the binding to FC receptors on vascular endothelial cells in a previously sensitized host. The vascular leakage from the damaged vessels can cause hemorrhage and fluid accumulation leading to DHF or DSS.

Immune enhancement was suggested as the cause of DHF in the 1997 dengue 2 outbreak in Cuba.[13] The country had been free of dengue since the outbreak of dengue 1 infection in 1981. Overall, it was estimated that 5208 cases of dengue fever and 205 cases of DHF occurred. In sharp contrast to outbreaks in Asia, nearly all dengue fever and DHF cases in this outbreak occurred in adults; all except three of the DHF cases were in adults who had been infected with dengue 1 in 1981 and experienced a secondary dengue infection in 1997.[14,15] Another outbreak of dengue in Rayong, Thailand, in 1980 found that all cases of DHF had a secondary immune response, indicating they had had a prior dengue infection.[16]

In contrast, another outbreak of dengue 2 infection occurred in Peru in 1993 in a population that had previously been infected with other dengue genotypes; however, no cases of DHF occurred.[17] This outbreak supports the second major hypothesis concerning the cause of DHF/DSS, namely, that the virulence of the dengue strain is a critical factor in the pathogenesis of DHF and more severe dengue infections. This hypothesis has been put forward by Rosen and colleagues, who have reported DHF in patients during a primary dengue infection.[18-20] The pathogenesis of DHF/DSS is not completely understood, but various data favor both immune enhancement from a secondary infection and high virulence of some dengue viruses and the combination of these factors to be related to severe life-threatening dengue infections, meaning DHF and DSS.[21]

Factors Favoring Dengue Emergence

Several factors have promoted the emergence of dengue and its spread to new geographic areas. Increases in the use and disposal of nonbiodegradable containers and their storage in peridomestic locations have provided more breeding places for the mosquito vector *Aedes aegypti* in proximity to humans. A program to eradicate *A. aegypti* from the Americas was initiated by the Pan American Health Organization (PAHO) in 1947 to control yellow fever, which is also spread by the same mosquito. Efforts were successful in a number of countries. By 1972, *A. aegypti* had been eliminated from 19 countries in the Americas, representing 73% of the area originally infected (Figure 24-1). However, the campaign gradually lost steam, and funding was withdrawn.[22] This occurred in part due to the identification of a jungle cycle of yellow fever and the recognition that, even with the elimination of

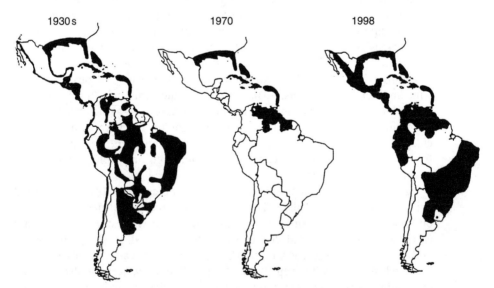

FIGURE 24-1 *A. aegypti* distribution in the Americas during the 1930s and in 1970 and 1998.
Source: Gubler D. Dengue and dengue hemorrhagic fever. Clin Microbiol Rev. 1998 Jul;11(3):480–96.

A. aegypti from urban areas, a focus of yellow fever would persist. Hence, the disease was no longer felt to be eradicable. Within about 10 years, *A. aegypti* had reestablished itself in virtually all of South and Central America (Figure 24-2). In 1981, a severe epidemic of dengue type 2 infection, with the first cases of DHF/DSS in the Western Hemisphere, occurred in Cuba.[23] In 1986, an explosive outbreak of dengue type 1, involving over 1 million cases, occurred in Rio de Janeiro. Subsequently, dengue epidemics have occurred in Paraguay, Bolivia, Peru, Ecuador, Colombia, and Venezuela. Recently, dengue outbreaks have been reported for the first time in Argentina.[24] All of the four dengue serotypes are currently endemic in Latin America. Their continued importance was evident when a large epidemic of dengue type 2 virus, with cases of DHF, occurred in Cuba in 1997.[25-27]

Reports of dengue in Africa were unusual in the 1960s and 1970s or prior to that time. In the mid-1980s, however, dengue appeared along the coast of Kenya, then in the Ivory Coast and Burkina Faso. Dengue has spread to other African countries in recent years. Also, in Asia dengue has spread westward into India, Pakistan, and the Middle East in the last decade (Figure 24-3).

Another factor that has raised considerable concern about the potential for further spread of mosquito-borne viruses in the Americas was the introduction of *Aedes albopictus* into Houston in used truck tires imported from Southeast Asia for recapping in 1985.[28] These spare tires collected rainwater and were excellent breeding sites for these mosquitoes, which could transmit dengue and yellow fever, as well as other arthropod viruses, such as eastern equine encephalitis. *Aedes albopictus* mosquitoes have also been introduced into Brazil in a similar manner; these effective vector mosquitoes are now widely distributed in 19 states of the United States (Figure 24-4). Each year, over 100 cases of dengue are reported in persons in the United States who have acquired their infections in the endemic areas of Asia, Latin America,

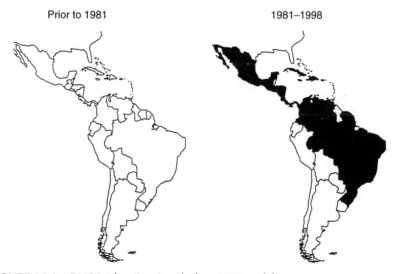

Prior to 1981   1981–1998

FIGURE 24-2   DHF in the Americas before 1981 and from 1981 to 1998. *Source:* Gubler D. Dengue and dengue hemorrhagic fever. Clin Microbiol Rev. 1998 Jul;11(3):480–96.

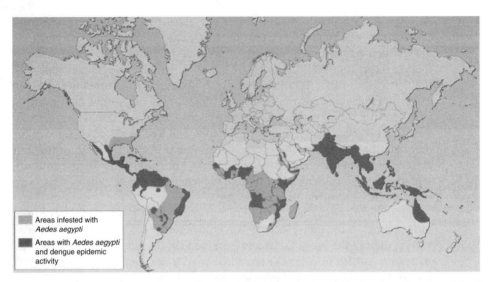

FIGURE 24-3 Dengue: its current distribution, and countries with *A. aegypti* and at risk of introduction.
Source: Mackenzie, J. et al. Emerging flaviviruses: the spread and resurgence of Japanese encephalitis, West Nile and dengue viruses. Nat Med. 2004 Dec;10(12 Suppl):S98–109.

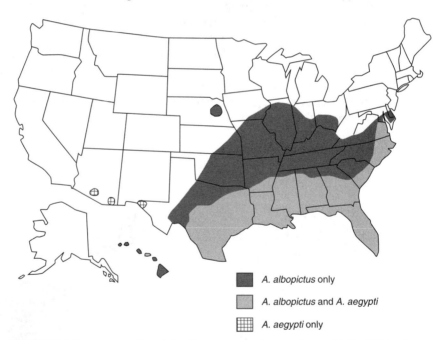

FIGURE 24-4 *A. aegypti* and *A. albopictus* distribution in the United States in 1998.
Source: Gubler D. Dengue and dengue hemorrhagic fever. Clin Microbiol Rev. 1998 Jul;11(3):480–96.

or Africa.[29] It is quite possible that these viremic individuals might eventually provide a sufficient reservoir to reestablish dengue as an endemic disease in the southern United States, with either *A. aegypti* or *A. albopictus* as the vector.

Control and Prevention of Dengue

The prevention of dengue in areas where the disease is endemic is directed at avoiding contact with an infected *A. aegypti* or *A. albopictus* vector. Dengue epidemics tend to be geographically localized where *A. aegypti* and infected humans reside. An infected mosquito remains infected for its entire life and may bite repeatedly, so it can be a highly effective vector. Because these mosquitoes are both around homes (peridomestic) and in homes, and may bite at any time, especially during the daytime, prevention is difficult. The most effective means of prevention involves destroying sites where larvae develop, such as water-filled containers in and around the house, and using strategies to prevent larval development when water-filled containers are present. Outdoor spraying to kill adult mosquitoes is much less effective than attacking the larval breeding sites, since adult *A. aegypti* may be indoors when the spraying is done.[30]

Considerable control of dengue came about as a result of the yellow fever eradication campaign which centered on elimination of *A. aegypti* by reducing larval breeding sites.[31] The campaign encouraged the removal of trash that could hold water and draining or covering other water sources. Unfortunately, this highly effective, but labor-intensive effort, was abandoned in many tropical developing countries when it was recognized that yellow fever could not be eradicated. Household screens, air-conditioning, and other methods to seal the living area from mosquitoes are also effective in preventing dengue.

A recent report describes a coordinated program to control dengue in several communities in Vietnam.[32] This program involved support from the central government (vertical) plus local community action (horizontal approach). It included destroying larval breeding sites where possible and the use of predacious copepods of the genus *Mesocyclops* as a biological agent to control *A. aegypti* larval development in water-filled containers. The program has eliminated dengue from the target area for the past two years.

Several researchers have been working for over a decade on developing a dengue vaccine.[33-35] One problem in developing an effective vaccine to prevent dengue is that the vaccine needs to be equally effective against all four serotypes and protection needs to last until dengue is no longer endemic in an area. If either of these criteria are not met, there is concern that vaccinees could be placed at increased risk of DHF or DSS when the protective immunity wanes. This theoretical risk is based upon the hypothesis that DHF/DSS occurs because of enhancing antibodies when the level of protective antibodies wanes over time.

West Nile Virus in North America

West Nile virus (WNV) is a flavivirus that was first isolated in 1937 from the blood of a febrile patient in the West Nile district of northern Uganda.[36] Subsequently, in the 1950s the virus was recognized as a cause of severe meningoencephalitis in the elderly. Equine disease due to WNV was reported in the 1960s in Egypt and France.[37] Outbreaks of WNV infection were reported in Israel, France, Russia, South Africa, and Romania in the 1970s.[38,39] Studies of these outbreaks found that birds were the reservoir and amplifying host, that infections were transmitted by mosquitoes, and that horses, birds, and humans were susceptible.[40] During 1994–2000 many outbreaks of WNV occurred in North America, Europe, and the Middle East as the geographic area for endemic WNV expanded.[40] The virus is now recognized to have an extensive distribution in Africa, the Middle East, eastern Europe, the former Soviet Union, South Asia, and in Australia, where it is known as Kunjin virus (Figure 24-5).[40] West Nile virus is antigenically related to Japanese encephalitis virus, St. Louis encephalitis virus, and Murray Valley fever virus. However, unlike the other members of the Japanese encephalitis serogroup, WNV can be divided into two lineages. Lineage 1 viruses are more pathogenic for humans, whereas lineage 2 viruses cause only mild human disease or no symptoms. Lineage 1 viruses have circulated recently in Romania (1996), Tunisia (1997), and Russia (1999) and are now epidemic in the United States and Canada.

Probably the best recent example of the introduction and rapid emergence of a human mosquito-borne viral infection from one geographic region to another is the emergence and spread of West Nile virus in North America after its introduction in the summer of 1999 into the borough of Queens, New York.[41] Subsequent genetic work has shown that the genetic structure of the North American WNV isolates and those from Israel were virtually identical.[42]

The original outbreak was recognized and reported by an infectious diseases physician, who cared for six patients with encephalitis in August 1999.[41] He suspected an outbreak of viral encephalitis based upon the patients' similar clinical presentation. Initial serological investigation of the cases detected IgM antibodies to viruses in the St. Louis encephalitis group of flaviviruses. In fact, initially the outbreak was thought to be due to St. Louis encephalitis

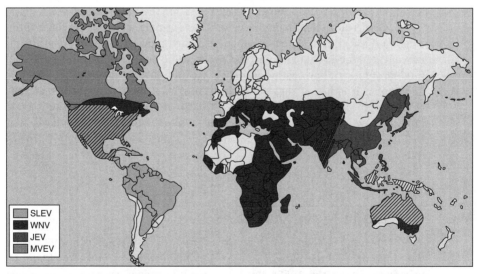

FIGURE 24-5 The global distribution and spread of the major Japanese encephalitis serological group members.
Source: Mackenzie, J. et al. Emerging flaviviruses: the spread and resurgence of Japanese encephalitis, West Nile and dengue viruses. Nat Med. 2004 Dec;10(12 Suppl):S98–109.

(SLE) virus, since SLE had been endemic in North America, although it had never been reported from New York. Subsequently 62 cases of meningoencephalitis with eight deaths were reported in the New York area in 1999.

Another unusual feature of this epidemic was the deaths of several bird species at the Bronx zoo in September 1999. Deaths occurred in a cormorant, two Chilean flamingoes, and an Asian pheasant. But in addition to the deaths of birds in the zoo, the 1999 outbreak and subsequent outbreaks of WNV were accompanied by extensive mortality among wild birds, especially crows and other corvid species. The extensive bird mortality associated with WNV infection has differentiated this virus from other arbovirus epidemics. In the 2002 WNV epidemic 124,854 dead birds were reported to state and local health departments, 31,514 were tested for WNV, and 15,745 (50%) were positive. West Nile virus has been isolated from 138 species of birds in the United States.[43] In fact, bird mortality has been a sensitive method of epidemiologic surveillance of the geographic extension of WNV activity in each of the annual epidemics since 1999.[44,45] Bird mortality has generally preceded cases of WNV infection in humans and has been used for sentinel surveillance of WNV activity (Figure 24-6). In addition, in common with several other North American arboviruses, WNV infection is commonly fatal for horses. The impact of WNV emergence in other species is an evolving story. The near elimination of corvid species from areas of the United States will alter the distribution of many other bird species. Ornithologists are actively working to determine susceptibility to WNV and minimize morbidity and mortality among endangered birds, such as the whooping crane.

After the localized epidemic in New York in the summer and fall of 1999, seasonal epidemics spread to other areas of the United States in subsequent years. In 2001, 64 cases of WNV meningoencephalitis were reported, but the cases were in 38 counties in 10 states in the eastern United States (Figure 24-7). In 2002 a major epidemic of WNV occurred and 4156 cases and 284 deaths were reported. The human cases in 2002 were concentrated in several midwestern (i.e., Michigan, Illinois, and Ohio) and southern states (i.e., Louisiana, Texas, and Mississippi).[46] In the summer and fall of 2003 another large epidemic occurred that was especially severe in several western states, including Nebraska, Colorado, North and South Dakota, and New Mexico (Figure 24-8).[47] Overall, 9862 symptomatic human WNV infections and 264 deaths were reported in 2003 (Table 24-2). In 2004 the epidemic centered in Arizona and California, and 2470 cases and 88 deaths were reported.[48] It is somewhat curious that although WNV has spread to Central America and the Caribbean, encephalitis is less frequent there than in North America.

Population surveys following epidemics of WNV have allowed the spectrum of clinical diseases associated with WNV to be better understood. It is now believed that only 1 infected person in 150 will develop frank encephalitis, whereas 20% will develop fever, headache, or milder symptoms, and 80% of infected persons will remain asymptomatic. Similar to outbreaks of St. Louis encephalitis in the United States, older persons and those who are immunosuppressed are at much greater risk of neurological disease. Extrapolation from the number of reported meningoencephalitis cases suggests that approximately 400,000–500,000 human infections actually occurred in the United States in 2003. Serosurveys of human populations in an area that has recently experienced an epidemic of WNV often detect antibodies in about

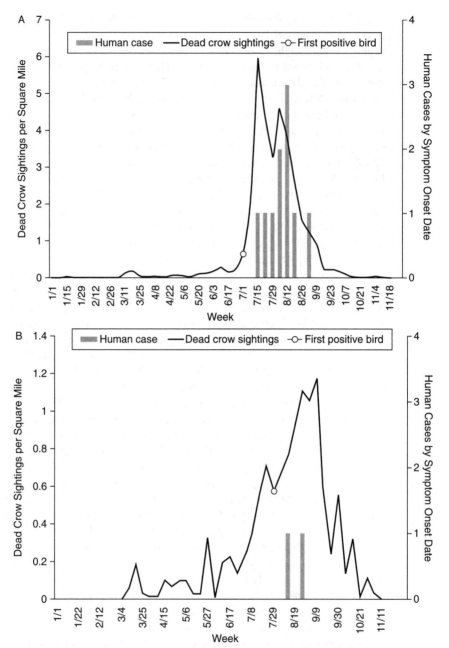

FIGURE 24-6 a, b, c, & d   Dead crow density (number of dead crow sightings per square mile) compared with number of human cases, by week. A. Staten Island, axis scale for weekly dead crow density 0 to 7; B. Brooklyn, axis scale for weekly dead crow density 0 to 1.4; C. Queens, axis scale for weekly dead crow density 0 to 0.7; D. Manhattan, axis scale for weekly dead crow density 0 to 1.4. *Source:* Edison, M. et al. Dead crow densities and human cases of West Nile virus, New York State, 2000. Emerg Infect Dis. 2001 Jul–Aug;7(4):662–4.

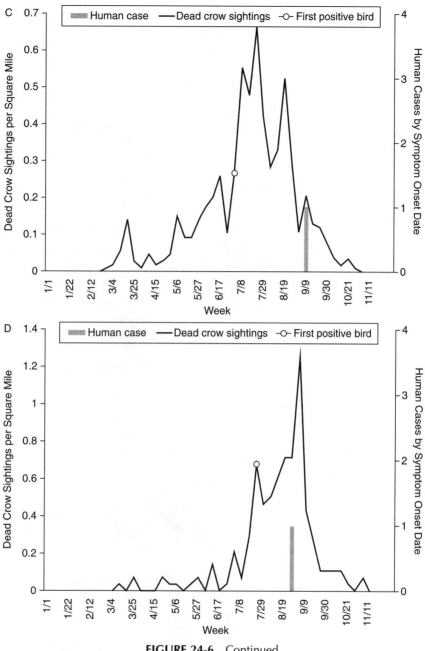

FIGURE 24-6 Continued

5% of the population.[49] These data indicate that despite the occurrence of large epidemics annually in the past six years in the United States, human immunity (i.e., herd immunity) is not likely to be a significant factor in the occurrence or absence of subsequent epidemics. However, the density of infected birds that can maintain high levels of viremia and abundant and suitable vector mosquitoes are probably critical.

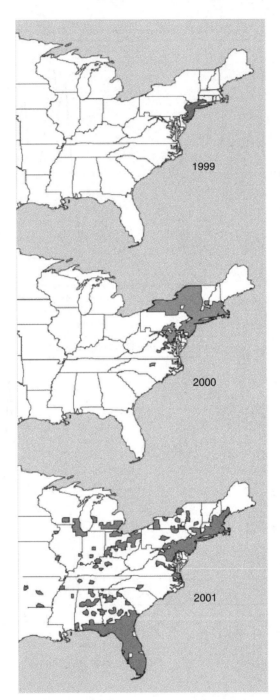

FIGURE 24-7 US counties reporting WN virus–infected birds in 1999, 2000, and 2001. Data are from the ArboNET surveillance system, Arbovirus Diseases Branch, Division of Vector-Borne Infectious Diseases, National Center for Infectious Diseases, CDC.
Source: Campbell, G. et al. West Nile Virus. *Lancet Infectious Diseases.* 2002. Vol. 2, pp. 519–529, with permission from Elsevier.

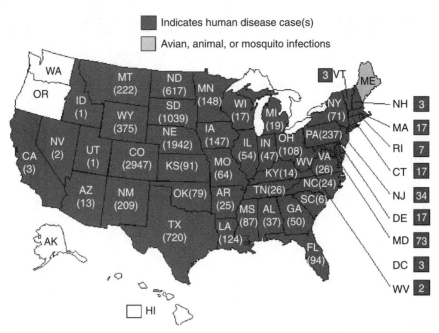

FIGURE 24-8 West Nile virus disease 2003 human cases, by clinical syndrome. *Source:* Data from the Centers for Disease Control and Prevention.

Another unique feature of the recent WNV epidemics in North America has been the broad range of mosquito species from which the virus has been isolated. In the first 4 years of the recurring epidemics, WNV has been isolated from 43 different species of mosquitoes plus several tick species (Table 24-3). The virus is primarily transmitted by *Culex* species mosquitoes. These mosquitoes are capable of hibernating during the winter and maintaining a pool of virus for the following season.[50] During the first few epidemic years in the eastern United States *Culex pipiens* mosquitoes were believed to be the main vector transmitting the virus among birds. Transmission from birds to humans may have involved not only *C. pipiens* but other culicine mosquitoes, such as *C. restuans* and *C. quinquefasciatus*. However, when the epidemic moved to the Midwest and the West, *C. tarsalis* became a major vector. *C. tarsalis* is known to be a more avid human biter than *C. pipiens* and is more difficult to eradicate from its breeding sites. During the westward movement of the epidemic center in recent years, WNV activity continued in the areas that were previously epidemic, albeit at a lower level. Because of the continued activity in many areas of the United States, the broad range of mosquito vectors, and recurring summer/fall epidemics for the past 6 years, most experts believe that yearly seasonal epidemics will continue to occur, similar to the yearly epidemics of the related virus Japanese encephalitis (JE) in many countries of southeast Asia.

St. Louis encephalitis (SLE) virus is another human flavivirus that has been endemic in the United States for the past 60 years. However, in contrast to JE and WNV, SLE tends to occur as a rare endemic infection with occasional large-scale epidemics, often separated by several years or even decades.

TABLE 24-2   2003 West Nile Virus Activity in the United States

State	Neuroinvasive disease	Fever	Unspecified	Total Human Cases Reported to CDC	Deaths
Alabama	25	10	2	37	3
Arizona	7	2	4	13	1
Arkansas	23	2	0	25	0
California	2	1	0	3	0
Colorado	621	2326	0	2947	63
Connecticut	12	5	0	17	0
Delaware	12	4	1	17	2
District of Columbia	3	0	0	3	0
Florida	61	33	0	94	6
Georgia	27	21	2	50	4
Idaho	0	1	0	1	0
Illinois	30	24	0	54	1
Indiana	15	31	1	47	4
Iowa	81	65	1	147	6
Kansas	89	0	2	91	4
Kentucky	11	1	2	14	1
Louisiana	101	23	0	124	8
Maryland	49	23	1	73	8
Massachusetts	12	5	0	17	1
Michigan	14	4	1	19	2
Minnesota	48	100	0	148	4
Mississippi	34	38	15	87	1
Missouri	39	25	0	64	8
Montana	75	135	12	222	4
Nebraska	194	1741	7	1942	29
Nevada	2	0	0	2	0
New Hampshire	2	0	1	3	0
New Jersey	21	9	4	34	3
New Mexico	74	135	0	209	4
New York	57	12	2	71	11
North Carolina	16	8	0	24	2
North Dakota	94	523	0	617	5
Ohio	84	24	0	108	8
Oklahoma	56	23	0	79	0
Pennsylvania	145	90	2	237	8

continued

TABLE 24-2   continued

State	Neuroinvasive disease	Fever	Unspecified	Total Human Cases Reported to CDC	Deaths
Rhode Island	5	2	0	7	1
South Carolina	3	3	0	6	0
South Dakota	151	869	19	1039	14
Tennessee	21	5	0	26	1
Texas	431	289	0	720	37
Utah	0	1	0	1	0
Vermont	0	3	0	3	0
Virginia	19	1	6	26	1
West Virginia	1	1	0	2	0
Wisconsin	7	2	8	17	0
Wyoming	92	210	73	375	9
Total	**2866**	**6830**	**166**	**9862**	**264**

Source: Data from the Centers for Disease Control and Prevention.

Other (nonmosquito) Routes of WNV Transmission

Another unique feature of WNV infection has been the identification of the importance of nonmosquito transmission of the virus. This possibility was first recognized when an organ donor acquired WNV after several transfusions and subsequently donated several organs, which transmitted WNV to four transplant recipients (Figure 24-9).[51] Subsequently, in 2002, surveillance of symptomatic WNV-infected patients detected 23 persons in whom the virus had been transmitted by transfusion from one of 16 viremic blood donors.[52] This was likely a significant underestimate of the risk of transfusion transmission of WNV, as only symptomatic recipients for whom the donor could be traced and shown to have been viremic when the donation occurred were detected and counted. Transmission of WNV by breast-feeding, transplacentally, and by occupational exposure has also been reported. Biggerstaff and Petersen have estimated the risk of transmission of WNV through blood transfusion during the epidemic period in various geographic areas of the United States in 2002, prior to donor screening. They estimated the risks of WNV transmission by transfusion to be 1.46–12.33 per 10,000 donations for selected high incidence areas during the 2002 epidemic.[53] These rates fluctuated markedly over time as the local epidemic peaked and waned (Figure 24-10).

The US Food and Drug Administration and the American Association of Blood Banks encouraged the pharmaceutical industry to develop screening tests for WNV nucleic acids (NAT) by July 1, 2003, the start of the next

TABLE 24-3   Species of Mosquito Positive for WNV by Year

1999	2002	2003
Aedes vexans	*Ae. aegypti*	*Ae. aegypti*
Culex pipiens	*Ae. albopictus*	*Ae. albopictus*
Cx. restuans	*Ae. vexans*	*Ae. cinereus*
2000	*An. atropos*	*Ae. vexans*
Ae. vexans	*An. barberi*	*An. atropos*
Anopheles punctipennis	*An. crucians/bradleyi*	*An. barberi*
Cx. pipiens pipiens	*An. punctipennis*	*An. crucians/bradleyi*
Culiseta melanura	*An. quadrimaculatus*	*An. punctipennis*
Ochlerotatus cantator	*An. walkeri*	*An. quadrimaculatus*
Oc. japonicus	*Cq. perturbans*	*An. walkeri*
Oc. triseriatus	*Cx. erraticus*	*Cq. perturbans*
Psorophora ferox	*Cx. nigripalpus*	*Cx. erraticus*
2001	*Cx. pipiens*	*Cx. nigripalpus*
Ae. albopictus	*Cx. quinquefasciatus*	*Cx. pipiens*
Ae. cinereus	*Cx. restuans*	*Cx. quinquefasciatus*
Ae. vexans	*Cx. salinarius*	*Cx. restuans*
An. punctipennis	*Cx. tarsalis*	*Cx. salinarius*
An. quadrimaculatus	*Cx. territans*	*Cx. tarsalis*
Coquillettidia perturbans	*Cs. inornata*	*Cx. territans*
Cx. nigripalpus	*Cs. melanura*	*Cs. inornata*
Cx. pipiens	*Deinocerites cancer*	*Cs. melanura*
Cx. quinquefasciatus	*Oc. atropalpus*	*Deinocerites cancer*
Cx. restuans	*Oc. atlanticus/tormentor*	*Oc. atropalpus*
Cx. salinarius	*Oc. canadensis*	*Oc. atlanticus/tormentor*
Cs. melanura	*Oc. cantator*	*Oc. canadensis*
Oc. canadensis	*Oc. japonicus*	*Oc. cantator*
Oc. cantator	*Oc. sollicitans*	*Oc. dorsalis*
Oc. japonicus	*Oc. taeniorhynchus*	*Oc. infirmatus*
Oc. sollicitans	*Oc. triseriatus*	*Oc. fitchii*
Oc. trivattatus	*Oc. trivattatus*	*Oc. japonicus*
Orthopodomyia signifera	*Or. signifera*	*Oc. provocans*
Ps. columbiae	*Ps. ciliata*	*Oc. sollicitans*
Uranotaenia sapphirina	*Ps. columbiae*	*Oc. sticticus*
	Ps. ferox	*Oc. stimulans*
	Ur. sapphirina	*Oc. taeniorhynchus*
		Oc. triseriatus
		Oc. trivattatus
		Or. signifera
		Ps. ciliata
		Ps. columbiae
		Ps. ferox
		Ps. howardii

Source: Granwehr, B. et al. West Nile virus: where are we now. *Lancet Infectious Diseases.* 2004. Vol. 4. 547–56, with permission from Elsevier.

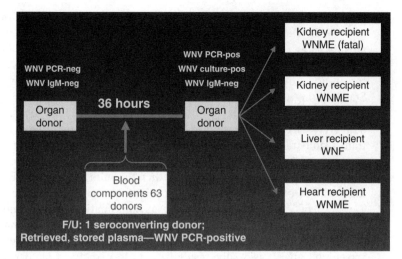

FIGURE 24-9 WN virus infection in organ donor and four organ recipients, August 2002.
Source: Data from the Centers for Disease Control and Prevention.

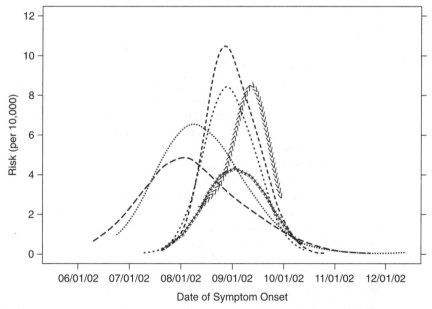

FIGURE 24-10 Estimated transfusion-associated WNV transfusion risk curves for each state. (............) Illinois; (----) Louisiana; (- - -) Michigan; (............) Mississippi; (*) Nebraska: (>)
Source: Biggerstaff, B. et al. Transfusion. 2003. Vol. 43. p. 1007, by permission of Blackwell Publishing.

WNV transmission season. A strategy to screen all blood donors with a NAT assay was felt to be feasible, since similar nucleic acid–based assays were already being used to screen donors for HIV and hepatitis C virus. Fortunately, the effort proved to be successful when two manufacturers developed NAT screening assays that were used for screening all blood donors in the United States during the 2003 WNV transmission season.

Among 6.0 million donors screened during June–December 2003, 818 WNV NAT-positive donors were detected and deferred.[54] Another six transfusion-transmitted WNV infections occurred when the screening NAT assays were false negative because the level of viremia in the donor was below the limit of detection using either the minipool NAT screening assay for testing 6 or 16 donor samples in a pool or individual donor screening.[54] The level of WNV RNA in generally asymptomatic viremic donors is often modest to quite low (i.e., <50–2000 copies/mL) compared to that found in donors infected with HIV or HCV. The use of minipool samples for donor screening can occasionally result in a false-negative test. Because of this problem many blood banks switch from minipool screening to individual donor screening during the height of WNV transmission. The decision to switch from minipool to individual screens is based on increases in the rates of NAT-positive donations at a blood collection facility.[55]

Clearly, the implementation of screening blood donors during the WNV transmission season in the United States has been very cost effective. It is likely that donor screening has prevented at least 1500 cases of WNV transmission to transfusion recipients. Because transfusion recipients are often immunocompromised or elderly, the clinical consequences of a transfusion-acquired WNV infection is much more serious in this population than in generally healthy persons who acquire the disease by mosquito bite. For example, all four of the recipients of organ transplants from the 2002 case were symptomatic, three had meningoencephalitis, and one died.

The surveillance of blood donors for WNV infection has provided extremely important clinical and epidemiological data. First, because donors are usually asymptomatic, their NAT prevalence has allowed a better estimate of the extent and geographic localization of the epidemic than data limited to clinical reports of meningoencephalitis cases. Second, quantitation of WNV RNA has provided a better understanding of the natural history of WNV infection in humans.

A model based on screening of blood donors has been developed by Busch, who estimated that the level of virus increases after infection from a mosquito bite. In the first day or so after infection the level of WNV RNA may be below the limit of detectability using an individual donation NAT assay. Then for a day or so the level of RNA can be detected only by individual donor NAT screening. For the next 3–5 days the level of RNA increases so it is detectable by minipool NAT screening, using pools of 10–16 donors developed for the commercial assays. Then the level of RNA declines and IgM and then IgG antibodies appear. Overall, it is about 7–10 days after an infectious mosquito bite that antibodies appear. No cases of transfusion transmission of virus from donors after WNV antibodies appeared have been reported. However, more data are needed on whether IgM antibodies renders' a NAT-positive donor noninfectious. Another unusual feature of WNV infection is that IgM antibodies commonly persist for a long time, up to 500 days or more. So it is not possible to interpret the presence of IgM antibodies to WNV as indicative of a recent infection.

Remaining Questions

Many questions remain about the unusual introduction and spread of WNV throughout North America. First, how was the virus introduced from its endemic focus in the Middle East? This answer will never be known for certain, but there are several possibilities. The virus could have been transported from Israel to New York aboard a plane by an infected mosquito(s), bird(s), or less likely a human. Infected birds could have migrated across the Atlantic. It has been documented that birds can cross the Atlantic aided by the wind. Or birds could have been transported by ship or have been imported illegally as a part of the trade in exotic pets. It is unlikely that an infected traveler could have started the epidemic in North America, as the levels of virus in humans usually is not sufficient for them to act as a reservoir. Intentional introduction or bioterrorism has been postulated by some but seems very unlikely.

The next question is why WNV spread so extensively in North America. The answer to this question is also uncertain. However, it should be noted that severe epidemics of WNV and expansion of the areas of endemnicity in Europe, the Middle East, and Africa have also occurred in recent years. In addition, other flaviviruses, especially dengue, Japanese encephalitis virus, and yellow fever virus have emerged and expanded their geographic range in the past decade. The westward spread of WNV has probably resulted from migrating infected birds. The future of WNV epidemiology in North America will be of great interest. Many experts believe that annual summer/fall epidemics of WNV will continue to occur, as has happened with Japanese encephalitis virus infections in Asia since they were introduced 50 or so years ago. Clearly, there is need for better surveillance, more effective mosquito control, and the development of a protective vaccine or antiviral treatment to control WNV in North America, Europe, and the Middle East in the years to come.

Japanese Encephalitis Virus

Japanese encephalitis virus (JE) is a mosquito-borne flavivirus that is endemic in eastern, southern, and Southeast Asia, Papua New Guinea, and the Torres Strait of northern Australia (Figure 24-5). It is the most important infection causing childhood neurological disease in Asia. Each year 35,000–50,000 cases of encephalitis due to JE and 10,000 deaths are reported. However, it is likely that cases may be underreported from some endemic areas. Although about 25–30% of cases of JE are fatal and 50% of survivors develop permanent neurological sequelae, most JE infections are asymptomatic; the ratio of symptomatic to asymptomatic infections ranges from 1:250 to 1:1000.[56]

The incubation period of JE is 5–15 days. Clinical disease can vary from a nonspecific febrile illness to severe meningoencephalitis with ensuing coma and seizures or aseptic meningitis with flaccid paralysis.[56] Most clinical cases occur in infants and children in the endemic areas, although adults, including travelers to rural areas, can become infected. In the rural areas that are endemic for JE, most older children and adults are immune because of subclinical infections during childhood.

Epidemiology of JE Viruses

Epidemics of JE were recognized as early as 1871 in Japan and were common in Japan, Korea, and China in the first half of the 1900s.[57] However, widespread use of the inactivated JE vaccine in Korea, Japan, and Taiwan after 1965 has reduced the number of human cases substantially. Nevertheless, the enzootic cycle of JE continues to infect wild birds and pigs in these countries. During the last several decades JE has spread widely in Asia from the originally recognized foci in Japan, Korea, and China. Although occasional cases of encephalitis had been noted in Thailand, epidemic JE was not a recognized health problem in Southeast Asia until 1969 when an epidemic of 685 cases were reported in the Chiang Mai valley in northern Thailand.[58] Subsequently, yearly outbreaks involving thousands of cases and hundreds of deaths occurred in northern Thailand. The disease continued to spread throughout Asia and is now endemic in Indonesia, the Philippines, Northern Australia, and South Asia, including Sri Lanka, most of India, and Nepal (Figure 24-5).

JE virus was first isolated from the brain of a human case in 1935 and from *Culex tritaeniorhynchus* mosquitoes in 1938. These mosquitoes breed in irrigated rice fields and other stationary water sources throughout Asia. It was subsequently established that the JE cycle in nature included transmission of the virus to aquatic birds, such as herons, egrets, and ducks. The virus titer is amplified by infection of pigs and can then be spread by mosquitoes to humans (Figure 24-11). Because of the large populations of people living in the endemic areas of rural Asia and the serious sequelae of JE, it is one of the most important emerging infections in humans.

Japanese encephalitis is largely a rural disease in Asia with *Culex tritaeniorhynchus* mosquitoes breeding in rice fields and pigs providing the major source of blood meals. There are seasonal epidemiologic patterns of JE infection. In tropical areas the virus is circulating in most months, but there is an increase in infections during times of rice field irrigation and the rainy season. In temperate areas the disease is more common in the summer and absent during the cold months in the winter. The expansion of rice cultivation and pig husbandry in rural areas of Asia in response to the tremendous population growth and need for food in the last century are important factors leading to the increased numbers of JE infections in humans and the expansion of the areas of endemicity.

Control of JE disease has largely rested on routine immunization of infants and children with an inactivated mouse-brain-derived vaccine that was originally developed in Korea. Studies of this vaccine among children in Thailand found the vaccine to be quite efficacious.[59] Several countries including Korea, Japan, China, Taiwan, and Thailand have introduced JE vaccine into the routine childhood immunization schedule, and this has reduced the number of cases substantially. However, large populations in rural South Asia remain susceptible.

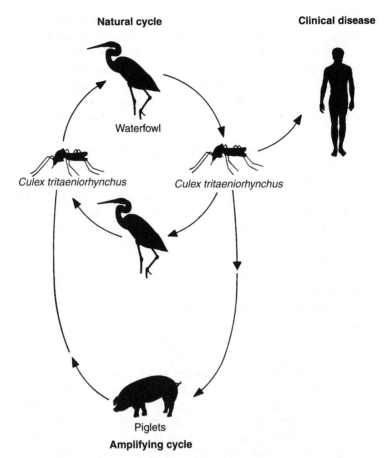

Natural cycle   **Clinical disease**

Waterfowl

Culex tritaeniorhynchus   *Culex tritaeniorhynchus*

Piglets

Amplifying cycle

FIGURE 24-11 The cycle of Japanese encephalitis virus. The natural cycle is between water birds and mosquitos, predominantly *Culex tritaeniorhynchus.* Amplification occurs in piglets and juvenile water buffalo, but older buffalo are blocking hosts. Humans are dead-end hosts.
Source: Johnson, R. Viral Infections of the Central Nervous System, 2nd Edition, © 1998, Lippincott Williams and Wilkins.

Yellow Fever

Yellow fever is the prototype member of the Flaviviridae family. Infection with yellow fever virus results in a severe systemic illness characterized by hemorrhage; hepatic, renal, and myocardial injury; and very high mortality, ranging from 20–60% or higher. The inapparent to clinical illness ratio of yellow fever infections is about 7 : 1. The disease occurs in several phases with an incubation period of 3–6 days after a bite from an infected mosquito. The acute phase is characterized by sudden onset of fever, headache, myalgia, nausea, and vomiting and lasts for about 3 days. This is followed by a toxic phase with jaundice, hematemesis, melena, coma, and death in 25–50% of the cases who progress to this stage.

Historical records indicate that yellow fever epidemics appeared in the New World in Yucatan, Cuba, and the Caribbean area in the middle of the

1600s, probably introduced into the America's by the slave trade from Africa. During the 1700s major epidemics occurred throughout North America, with high mortality.[60] The disease initially was widely believed to be transmitted as a "miasma" from sewage and rotting material, until the hypothesis of Dr. Carlos Finley of Cuba in 1881 and the subsequent experiments of Walter Reed and his group on human volunteers in Cuba demonstrated that the agent was a filterable virus that was transmitted by the bite of infected *Aedes aegypti* mosquitoes.[61,62]

In the 1920s and 1930s researchers in the United States, England, and France worked on developing a protective vaccine for yellow fever. Theiler and Smith at the Rockefeller Foundation developed a live vaccine, the 17D strain, which had been attenuated by serial passage in cell cultures and embryonated chicken eggs.[63] The 17D strain vaccine was tested in over 1 million persons in Brazil and found to be highly effective.[63] Subsequently, the French mouse-brain-derived yellow fever vaccine and the 17D vaccine were widely used in areas of previous epidemic disease. By the late 1940s, control of yellow fever had been achieved at a population level in francophone Africa.

With the knowledge that the disease was spread to humans by the bite of *A. aegypti* mosquitoes, comprehensive public health programs were implemented to control the disease by elimination of the vector. Early success in the control of yellow fever epidemics by eliminating sites for *A. aegypti* larval development were led by Gorgas and colleagues in Cuba and the Panama Canal zone. Prior to the leadership of Gorgas, efforts to build the canal had to be abandoned because over 55,000 workers had died from yellow fever or malaria.[64] Subsequently, Soper spearheaded control programs in Brazil and other neighboring countries in South America.[65] However, these successful programs to control urban yellow fever were periodically interrupted by reintroduction of yellow fever from the jungle. It was discovered in the 1930s in Rio de Janeiro that there are two yellow fever transmission cycles in nature. One, the urban cycle, involves transmission from a viremic human to another susceptible person by *A. aegypti*. The jungle cycle involves transmission of the virus among nonhuman primates by different mosquitoes. In South America the enzootic cycle involves monkeys and diurnally active tree-hole breeding mosquitoes, such as the *Haemagogus* species. In Africa *A. africanus* is an important vector of jungle yellow fever.

Brazil developed an active program to control yellow fever by eliminating the *A. aegypti* vector from key urban centers into the 1920s. This program was quite successful, but occasionally *A. aegypti* was reintroduced in the country from neighboring countries. In 1947 Brazil proposed to the Pan American Health Organization that a plan of regional elimination of *A. aegypti* from the Americas be undertaken. The other countries of Latin America signed on to this effort and in the subsequent years *A. aegypti* was reduced or eliminated from many areas in the region. However, periodically small outbreaks of yellow fever occurred due to reintroduction of the virus from the jungle areas.

Based in part on the inability to control the jungle cycle of yellow fever transmission and an assessment of the cost-effectiveness of the *Aedes aegypti* eradication effort, the program was abandoned in the 1970s. At this time *A. aegypti* mosquitoes were limited to islands in the Caribbean, the Southeastern

United States, and a few areas in northern South America (Figure 24-1). However, in the following two decades, *A. aegypti* became reestablished throughout South and Central America and the Caribbean (Figure 24-1).

Since the 1980s, yellow fever has reemerged across Africa and in South America.[65-67] In the period from 1987 to 1995 a total of 18,735 yellow fever cases and 4522 deaths were reported to the World Health Organization. This is the largest number of cases reported since reporting began in 1948. Because many of the cases occur in rural areas or in children in areas where diagnostic facilities are unavailable, it is likely that the number of cases actually is 10–500 times greater than the number reported. The WHO estimates that 200,000 cases occur every year.[65] Almost all of the cases are in sub-Saharan Africa, especially West Africa (Figure 24-12). The disease has never been reported from Asia, despite the abundance of *A. aegypti* vectors and widespread dengue epidemics. The last epidemic in the United States occurred in New Orleans in 1905 when 5000 cases and 1000 deaths occurred.[61]

In Africa both jungle and urban transmission cycles occur. Thirty-three African countries in a band from 15° north to 10° south of the equator are at risk (Figure 24-12). However, Nigeria has had the most cases in the past decade; several other West African countries have had urban epidemics.

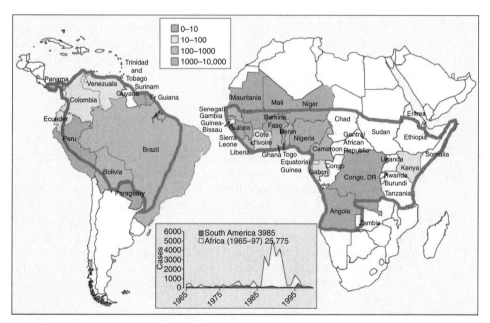

FIGURE 24-12   Yellow fever endemic regions (outlined in gray), based on serological surveys, field studies, and previous reports of human disease. The range of number of cases of yellow fever officially reported to the World Health Organization, 1990–1999, is shown by country. White indicates that no cases were reported. Inset: incidence of yellow fever in South America and Africa over the past 35 years, and the marked increase during the late 1980s–mid-1990s. Regions of the world outside the yellow fever endemic zone infested with *A. aegypti* and thus receptive to the introduction and spread of the disease include coastal areas of South America, Central America, the Caribbean, the southern USA, South Africa, India, Southeast Asia, Australia (Queensland), southern China, Taiwan, and the Pacific islands.
Source: Monath, T. Yellow Fever: an update. *Lancet Infectious Diseases.* 2001. Vol. 1. pp. 11–20, with permission from Elsevier.

Yellow fever had not been reported from east Africa for 50 years until 1992 when an outbreak of jungle type yellow fever occurred in Kenya. This outbreak was controlled with a large-scale immunization campaign.

In South America, the jungle transmission cycle predominates. Outbreaks have been reported from Bolivia, Brazil, Ecuador, and Peru during the last decade. Cases are often seen among forest workers who have not been immunized. One small outbreak of urban yellow fever was reported from Santa Cruz, Bolivia, in 1998, which was the first urban-type outbreak in South America since 1954.[68]

Experts are very concerned that the reemergence of urban-type epidemics of yellow fever in the Western Hemisphere is a real possibility.[65-67] The factors that might promote reemergence are the wide distribution of *A. aegypti* throughout the region; ease and frequency of travel from yellow fever endemic areas, which could place a viremic person in an area conducive to transmission; and the generally low levels of immunity of the population from vaccine or natural infection.

In addition to vector control, vaccination is an important tool in yellow fever control. A cost-benefit analysis of the introduction of yellow fever vaccine into the Expanded Programme on Immunization (EPI) has been done.[69] Routine use of the 17D yellow fever vaccine for infants above 6 months of age and children would be more effective in preventing deaths than the current strategy of using the vaccine only during epidemics. The vaccine cannot be used in infants under 6 months because of a higher risk of adverse reactions, such as encephalitis in young infants. It is otherwise quite safe and highly effective, however.

Tick-Borne Encephalitis Virus

Tick-borne encephalitis (TBE) virus is a member of the Flaviviridae family. The TBE viruses can be differentiated into a western and far eastern subtype using monoclonal antibodies, specific peptides, or by genetic sequencing.

Human disease due to infection with the TBE viruses has been known since the 1930s. Seasonal outbreaks of meningitis due to the western subtype of TBE were described among populations in Europe, especially Austria in 1931.[70] A survey in 1958 found that 56% of all virus diseases of the central nervous system in Austria were due to TBE.[71] The far eastern subtype of TBE is more virulent, often leading to severe encephalitis with higher mortality than the western subtype.[72]

Ticks are the vectors and reservoir hosts of TBE in nature. Several species of ticks have been found to be infected, but *Ixodes ricinus*, the common castor bean tick, is the major vector of the western TBE subtype and *Ixodes persulcatus* of the far eastern TBE subtype.[72]

These ticks parasitize many species of mammals, reptiles, and birds in addition to humans. Small mammals tend to have higher levels of viremia, sufficient to infect ticks. During the viremic stage, milk from goats, cows, and sheep may be infectious and a source of infection to humans if they consume raw milk from these animals. Infection by the oral route has been reported from Slovakia after consumption of nonpasteurized cheese from infected animals.[73] Inactivated vaccines have been prepared against both the western and far eastern subtypes of TBE virus.[72] These vaccines are quite immunogenic and effective in preventing infection in humans at risk of disease caused by TBE viruses.[72,74,75]

Other Mosquito-Borne Encephalitis Viruses in North America

La Crosse Virus

The next most frequent cause of arboviral encephalitis in the United States is that caused by infection with the La Crosse virus. In 1960, the La Crosse virus, a member of the California family of bunyaviruses, was first isolated from a child with fatal encephalitis in Wisconsin.[76] Since that time the La Crosse virus has been identified in states throughout the midwestern and eastern United States (Figure 24-13).

Since 1964 when La Crosse encephalitis was first reported, cases have been reported every year; a mean of 75 cases per year were reported between 1964 and 2000. In 2000 a total of 114 cases were reported from 14 states (Figure 24-14). The natural cycle of La Crosse virus involves transmission between *Ochlerotatus triseriatus* mosquitoes and small mammals, especially chipmunks and tree squirrels (Figure 24-15). This mosquito has a limited flight range and lives in tree holes in wooded areas. Persons living in suburban areas with trees on or near their property are at highest risk of infection. A prevention strategy is to fill tree holes with concrete, tar, or other filler to eliminate breeding areas for vector mosquitoes and to dispose of used containers that could serve as artificial tree holes.

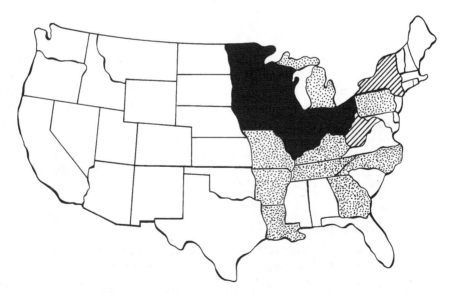

FIGURE 24-13   The geographic range of California encephalitis due to the La Crosse strain of the virus. The states that reported more than 100 cases between 1964 and 1991 are heavily shaded, the lined states reported 50 to 99 cases, the stippled states reported 5 to 49 cases, and the clear states reported 4 or fewer cases.
Source: Johnson, R. Viral Infections of the Central Nervous System, 2nd Edition, © 1998, Lippincott Williams and Wilkins.

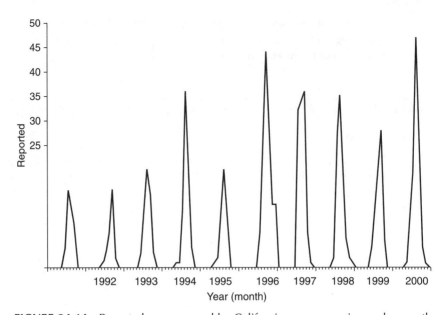

FIGURE 24-14   Reported cases caused by California serogroup viruses, by month of onset—United States, 1991–2000.
Source: MMWR Summary of Notifiable Diseases, United States, 2000, Centers for Disease Control and Prevention.

La Crosse virus and other related viruses can be maintained in nature by transovarial transmission by an infected female mosquito. Virus survival over winter by transovarial transmission has allowed some arboviruses in the *Bunyavirus* genus to become endemic in far northern latitudes. For example, the Snowshoe hare virus lives in subarctic areas that have very short summers in which mosquitoes can hatch and develop. Unless the eggs were infected when they hatched, it might not be possible for mosquitoes to acquire infection from Snowshoe hares at a rate sufficient to maintain the endemic cycle from year to year.

St. Louis Encephalitis Virus (SLE)

St. Louis encephalitis virus has become a frequent cause of arboviral encephalitis in the United States since it was originally identified in the 1940s. For the next several decades SLE was the most frequent cause of epidemics of viral encephalitis during the summer in the United States. Large epidemics of SLE encephalitis have occurred in Florida and Texas. An epidemic of over 2000 cases of encephalitis with 171 deaths occurred in 1975 in the United States; persons from 31 states became ill during this epidemic but the incidence was highest in the Midwest, especially Illinois.[76] Encephalitis cases due to SLE were reported from as far north as Canada during this outbreak.

Natural cycle   **Clinical disease**

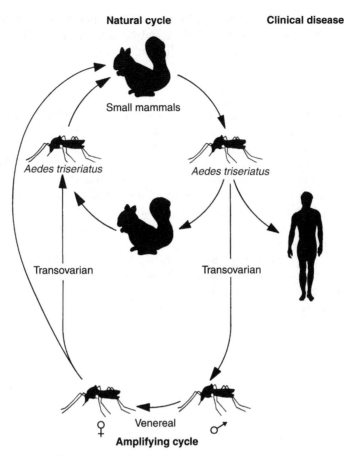

Small mammals

Aedes triseriatus   *Aedes triseriatus*

Transovarian   Transovarian

♀   Venereal   ♂
Amplifying cycle

FIGURE 24-15   The cycle of La Crosse encephalitis virus. The inapparent cycle of the La Crosse virus is between *Aedes triseriatus*, a woodland mosquito, and chipmunks and tree squirrels. The virus is maintained over winters by transovarian transmission and is amplified by venereal transmission between the infected male nonbiting mosquito and the uninfected female, which can in turn transmit either by biting or by transovarian transmission to the next generation. Humans are the only known hosts to develop clinical disease and are dead-end hosts for the virus. *Source:* Johnson, R. Viral Infections of the Central Nervous System, 2nd Edition, © 1998, Lippincott Williams and Wilkins.

This virus can be transmitted in different cycles in different locations. In the western United States SLE is spread from the reservoir in passerine birds, such as the house sparrow, by *Culex tarsalis* mosquitoes. This cycle is similar to that for western encephalitis transmission in rural areas of the western United States. In the Midwest, SLE is spread by other culicine mosquitoes, especially *Culex pipiens*. In Florida, a rural cycle involves transmission by *Culex nigrapalpus*. The epidemic activity of urban SLE is greatest in drought years, where dirty water collects due to poor drainage. However, rural SLE tends to occur more frequently in years with heavy rainfall.[77]

The inapparent to apparent infection ratio is 60–100 : 1. However, clinical encephalitis occurs more frequently in the elderly, similar to West Nile virus encephalitis. Urban epidemics tend to occur more frequently in lower socioeconomic areas.

Apart from years in which major urban epidemics occur, SLE encephalitis is only sporadic. Between 1964 and 2000 a mean of 121 cases (median 26 cases) were reported annually (Figure 24-16).

Western Encephalitis Virus (WE)

Western encephalitis virus causes sporadic cases of encephalitis in the rural areas of the western United States (Figure 24-17). This virus has been called western equine encephalitis virus because it often causes clinical encephalitis and death in horses as well as humans. The incidence of WE encephalitis increases with heavy rainfall. The virus is transmitted from the reservoir in birds to humans and horses by *Culex tarsalis*. The inapparent to apparent infection ratios are 25–50 : 1 in children and 1000 : 1 or more in adults. Most cases of clinical encephalitis from WE infection occur in children younger than 2 years of age.[78]

The most recent epidemic of western encephalitis occurred in Colorado in 1987. The reasons for the absence of epidemic transmission since then is not known. During 1964–2000 an average of 17 cases (median of 3 cases) were reported per year in the United States.

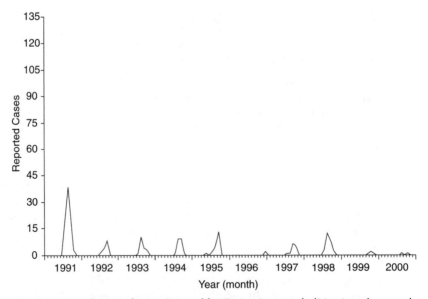

FIGURE 24-16   Reported cases caused by St. Louis encephalitis virus, by month of onset—United States, 1991–2000.
Source: MMWR Summary of Notifiable Diseases, United States, 2000, Centers for Disease Control and Prevention.

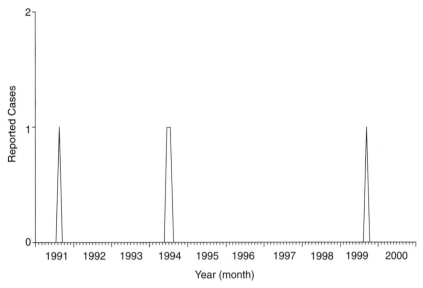

FIGURE 24-17 Reported cases caused by western equine encephalitis virus, by month of onset—United States, 1991–2000.
Source: MMWR Summary of Notifiable Diseases, United States, 2000, Centers for Disease Control and Prevention.

Eastern Encephalitis Virus

Eastern encephalitis virus is found in the eastern half of the United States, especially in the freshwater marshes along the shores of the Atlantic and Gulf coast. Human infections are rare because the natural cycle occurs in remote areas and the mosquito vector, *Culiseta melanura*, does not feed on humans. However, when human infection occurs it results in severe encephalitis with high mortality (i.e., over 20%). The inapparent to clinical infection rates are 2:1 to 8:1 in children and 4:1 to 50:1 in adults. During 1964–2000 an average of five human cases were reported each year in the United States (Figure 24-18).

Venezuelan Encephalitis

Venezuelan encephalitis (VE) is localized in the United States to Southern Florida, especially the Everglades, and south Texas. Infections caused by VE are also endemic in Central and South America. The virus can be spread by both *Aedes* and *Culex* genera mosquitoes. Major epidemics have been reported from South America and typically involve horses, which can serve as the reservoir of the virus. As with several other arboviruses, human infections are more severe in children.

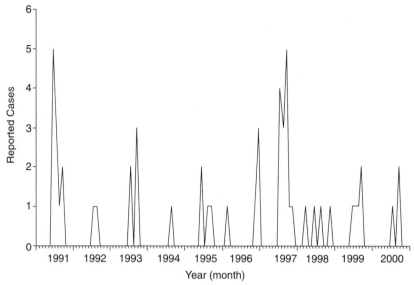

FIGURE 24-18   Reported cases caused by eastern equine encephalitis virus, by month of onset—United States, 1991–2000.
Source: MMWR Summary of Notifiable Diseases, United States, 2000, Centers for Disease Control and Prevention.

Other Tick-Borne Infections

Other tick-borne infections that are endemic in the United States have been described in recent years, and these diseases may have increased in frequency as well. However, the data on temporal trends of their incidence is less clear because the only reportable tick-borne infections in the United States are Rocky Mountain spotted fever (RMSF) and Lyme disease. The number of reported patients with RMSF increased from about 200 to 400 cases in the 1950s and 1960s to over 1000 cases in the late 1970s and 1980s. Increased opportunities for human exposure to the vectors, primarily the Rocky Mountain wood tick (*Dermocenter andersonii*) in the western United States and the American dog tick (*Dermocenter variabilis*) in the eastern United States, occurred because of the expansion of suburban housing into wooded, tick-infested areas and the increased opportunities for exposure associated with recreational activities. Currently RMSF is more common in the eastern United States.

Two forms of human ehrlichiosis, human monocytic ehrlichiosis (HME) caused by infection with *Ehrlichia chaffeeinsis* and human granulocytic ehrlichiosis (HGE) caused by infection with *Ehrlichia ewingii*, have also been recognized with increased frequency in the past few years. HME is transmitted by the dog tick and HGE by the deer tick.

Another tick-borne disease, babesiosis, an infection of red blood cells with *Babesia microti*, can be transmitted to humans by tick bites in the endemic areas in the coastal northeastern United States. It is not unusual for a patient to be seen who has both Lyme disease and ehrlichiosis after exposure to tick habitats in an endemic area. It seems likely that these other tick-borne diseases have increased in frequency similar to increases documented with Lyme disease. However, without surveillance, the documentation of this increased incidence has been difficult to interpret.

A tick-borne encephalitis virus was isolated from the brain of child who died from encephalitis after receiving a tick bite while on a vacation near Powassan, Ontario, Canada.[79] The Powassan virus, a member of the flavivirus group of viruses, occasionally causes encephalitis in Canada and the northern areas of the United States.

Lyme Disease

Lyme disease was first recognized by Steere and colleagues in 1975 following the identification of a group of children living in Old Lyme, Connecticut, who were diagnosed with juvenile rheumatoid arthritis.

In the 50 years since the recognition of Lyme disease, the number of reported cases has increased progressively, and the geographic areas of endemicity of the disease have expanded to include the coastal northeastern and mid-Atlantic states, several states in the Midwest (especially Minnesota, Wisconsin, and Michigan), and coastal California (see Chapter 25).

Colorado Tick Fever Virus

Colorado tick fever virus is transmitted by the tick *Dermacentor andersoni* in the Rocky Mountain area, where the tick is endemic. Typically the disease occurs among hikers in rural areas in the western United States during May through July. The symptoms include a febrile illness and macular papular rash occurring 3–6 days after a tick bite. Recovery without sequelae is the rule, but occasionally severe, even fatal, disease has been reported.

Human African Trypanosomiasis

Human African trypanosomiasis increased explosively in the early1900s during the era of European colonization. Massive epidemics occurred involving large areas in sub-Saharan Africa.[80] However, this led to a concerted public health effort to control the disease using vector control and treatment of human infections. By the early 1960s the disease was nearly eradicated. However, the disease has reemerged in the last 3 decades and is now a serious health problem in Africa (Figure 24-19).[80-83]

African sleeping sickness is caused by two subspecies of *Trypanosoma brucei*, an extracellular protozoan parasite. *T. brucei gambiense* is focally distributed in West and central Africa and is transmitted by riverine species of the tsetse fly (*Glossina* species). *T. brucei rhodesiense* is distributed in eastern and southern Africa and is transmitted by savannah species of the tsetse fly. The two species of trypanosomes are morphologically indistinguishable. However, the epidemiology and clinical illness in humans infected with the

No. of cases

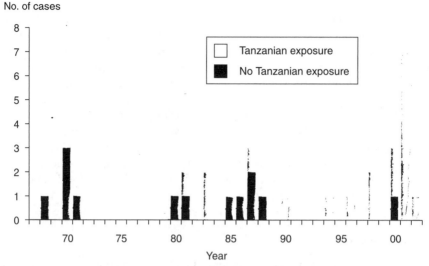

FIGURE 24-19 Imported *T. brucei rhodesiense* trypanosomiasis in the United States by year, 1967 to 2002.
Source: Emerging Infections, eds. Scheld, Murray, and Hughes. ASM Press. © 2004.

two parasites differ. *T. brucei rhodesiense* is a zoonotic parasite that infects a variety of domestic and wild animals, especially cattle, which serve as the reservoir. In contrast, *T. brucei gambiense* has a human reservoir. The tsetse fly vector of *T. brucei gambiense* inhabits humid and dark areas of vegetation along streams. Human activities, such as washing, fishing, or collecting firewood, bring humans into contact with the habitat of the tsetse fly vector.[84]

Thirty-two human infections with *T. brucei rhodesiense* have been reported to CDC in the last 35 years among visitors to game preserves in Africa.[83] Nearly all of the imported cases since 1990 were acquired in Tanzania (Figure 24-20).

Infection with either subspecies of trypanosoma leads to encephalitis; however, infection with *T. brucei rhodesiense* is usually more acute. The encephalitis is usually fatal if not treated. Therapy is usually successful with melarsopol, an organic arsenic, compared to treatment with suramin, eflornithine, or nifurtimox. However, drug toxicity during treatment is common.

Control of transmission is dependent on elimination of the vector and treatment of human infections.

Sleeping sickness emerged in Africa as a major health problem in the 1990s, fueled by wars, social disruption, and a shortage of drugs to treat the disease. However, lobbying by Medecins Sans Frontieres for improved access of developing countries to essential medicines and funding by the Gates Foundation resulted in an agreement by Aventis to provide eflornithine free of charge and also to support control activities.[81] As a result the number of cases of sleeping sickness have decreased from an estimated 450,000 in 1997 to 50,000 currently. If the current level of support can be maintained, experts at WHO now believe human African trypanosomiasis could be eliminated as a public health problem.[85]

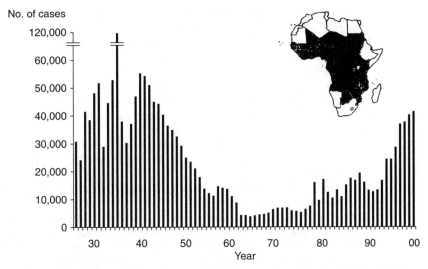

FIGURE 24-20 Reported incidence of African trypanosomiasis, 1926 to 2000. Data are from the WHO.
Source: Emerging Infections, eds. Scheld, Murray, and Hughes. ASM Press. © 2004.

Rift Valley Fever

Rift Valley fever is a phlebovirus that has been recognized for many years as a cause of disease in domestic ruminants and man in African countries south of the Sahara. In 1978, a major epidemic of RVF occurred in Egypt. This was followed by an outbreak in 1987 in Senegal after the opening of a new dam. The 1997 epidemic of RVF associated with the increased rainfall accompanying El Niño weather conditions has already been discussed.

References

1. MacKenzie JS, Gubler DJ, Petersen LR. Emerging flaviviruses: the spread and resurgence of Japanese encephalitis, West Nile and dengue viruses. *Nat Med.* 2004;10:S98–S109.
2. Solomon T. Flavivirus encephalitis. *N Engl J Med.* 2004;351:370–378.
3. Weaver SC, Barrett AD. Transmission cycles, host range, evolution and emergence of arboviral disease. *Nat Rev Microbiol.* 2004;2: 789–801.
4. Patz JA, Epstein PR, Burke TA, Balbus JM. Global climate change and emerging infectious diseases. *JAMA.* 1996;275:217–223.
5. Nasci RS, Savage HM, White DJ, et al. West Nile virus in overwintering *Culex* mosquitoes, New York City, 2000. *Emerg Infect Dis.* 2001;7: 742–744.
6. Tesh RB, Parsons R, Siirin M, et al. Year-round West Nile virus activity, Gulf Coast region, Texas and Louisiana. *Emerg Infect Dis.* 2004;10:1649–1652.
7. Rosen L, Shroyer DA, Tesh RB, Freier JE, Lien JC. Transovarial transmission of dengue viruses by mosquitoes: *Aedes albopictus* and *Aedes aegypti. Am J Trop Med Hyg.* 1983;32:1108–1119.

8. Rosen L. Sexual transmission of dengue viruses by *Aedes albopictus*. *Am J Trop Med Hyg*. 1987;37:398–402.

9. MacKenzie JS, Gubler DJ, Petersen LR. Emerging flaviviruses: the spread and resurgence of Japanese encephalitis, West Nile and dengue viruses. *Nat Med*. 2004;10:S98–S109.

10. Gubler DJ, Clark GG. Dengue/dengue hemorrhagic fever: the emergence of a global health problem. *Emerg Infect Dis*. 1995;1:55–57.

11. Halstead SB. Dengue haemorrhagic fever—a public health problem and a field for research. *Bull WHO*. 1980;58:1–21.

12. Halstead SB. Observations related to pathogensis of dengue hemorrhagic fever. VI. Hypotheses and discussion. *Yale J Biol Med*. 1970;42: 350–362.

13. Vaughn DW. Invited commentary: dengue lessons from Cuba. *Am J Epidemiol*. 2000;152:800–803.

14. Guzman MG, Kouri G, Valdes L, et al. Epidemiologic studies on dengue in Santiago de Cuba, 1997. *Am J Epidemiol*. 2000;152:793–799.

15. Kouri G, Guzman MG, Valdes L, et al. Reemergence of dengue in Cuba: a 1997 epidemic in Santiago de Cuba. *Emerg Infect Dis*. 1998;4:89–92.

16. Sangkawibha N, Rojanasuphot S, Ahandrik S, et al. Risk factors in dengue shock syndrome: a prospective epidemiologic study in Rayong, Thailand. I. The 1980 outbreak. *Am J Epidemiol*. 1984;120:653–669.

17. Watts DM, Porter KR, Putvatana P, et al. Failure of secondary infection with American genotype dengue 2 to cause dengue haemorrhagic fever. *Lancet*. 1999;354:1431–1434.

18. Barnes WJ, Rosen L. Fatal hemorrhagic disease and shock associated with primary dengue infection on a Pacific island. *Am J Trop Med Hyg*. 1974;23:495–506.

19. Rosen L. The Emperor's New Clothes revisited, or reflections on the pathogenesis of dengue hemorrhagic fever. *Am J Trop Med Hyg*. 1977;26:337–343.

20. Rosen L. The pathogenesis of dengue haemorrhagic fever. A critical appraisal of current hypotheses. *S Afr Med J*. 1986;(suppl):40–42.

21. Vaughn DW, Green S, Kalayanarooj S, et al. Dengue viremia titer, antibody response pattern, and virus serotype correlate with disease severity. *J Infect Dis*. 2000;181:2–9.

22. Gubler DJ. Dengue and dengue hemorrhagic fever. *Clin Microbiol Rev*. 1998;11:480–496.

23. Guzman MG, Kouri GP, Bravo J, et al. Dengue haemorrhagic fever in Cuba. I. Serological confirmation of clinical diagnosis. *Trans R Soc Trop Med Hyg*. 1984;78:235–238.

24. Gubler DJ. Dengue and dengue hemorrhagic fever. *Clin Microbiol Rev*. 1998;11:480–496.

25. Guzman MG, Kouri G, Valdes L, et al. Epidemiologic studies on dengue in Santiago de Cuba, 1997. *Am J Epidemiol*. 2000;152:793–799.

26. Kouri G, Guzman MG, Valdes L, et al. Reemergence of dengue in Cuba: a 1997 epidemic in Santiago de Cuba. *Emerg Infect Dis*. 1998;4:89–92.

27. Vaughn DW. Invited commentary: Dengue lessons from Cuba. *Am J Epidemiol*. 2000;152:800–803.

28. Craven RB, Eliason DA, Francy DB, et al. Importation of *Aedes albopictus* and other exotic mosquito species into the United States in used tires from Asia. *J Am Mosq Control Assoc*. 1988;4:138–142.

29. Rigau-Perez JG, Gubler DJ, Vorndam AV, Clark GG. Dengue surveillance—United States, 1986–1992. *MMWR CDC Surveill Summ*. 1994;43:7–19.

30. Gubler DJ. *Aedes aegypti* and *Aedes aegypti*-borne disease control in the 1990s: top down or bottom up. Charles Franklin Craig Lecture. *Am J Trop Med Hyg.* 1989;40:571–578.

31. Gubler DJ. Dengue and dengue hemorrhagic fever. *Clin Microbiol Rev.* 1998;11:480–496.

32. Kay B, Vu SN. New strategy against *Aedes aegypti* in Vietnam. *Lancet.* 2005;365:613–617.

33. Guirakhoo F, Weltzin R, Chambers TJ, et al. Recombinant chimeric yellow fever-dengue type 2 virus is immunogenic and protective in nonhuman primates. *J Virol.* 2000;74:5477–5485.

34. Kinney RM, Huang CY. Development of new vaccines against dengue fever and Japanese encephalitis. *Intervirology.* 2001;44: 176–197.

35. Vaughn DW, Hoke CH Jr, Yoksan S, et al. Testing of a dengue 2 live-attenuated vaccine (strain 16681 PDK 53) in ten American volunteers. *Vaccine.* 1996;14:329–336.

36. Smithburn KC, Hughes TP, Burke AW, Paul JU. A neotropic virus isolated from the blood of a native of Uganda. *Am J Tropic Med Hyg.* 1940;20:471–492.

37. Hurlbut HS, Rizk F, Taylor RM, Work TH. A study of the ecology of West Nile virus in Egypt. *Am J Trop Med Hyg.* 1956;5:579–620.

38. McIntosh BM, Jupp PG, Dos Santos I, Meenehan GM. Epidemics of West Nile and Sindbis viruses in South Africa with *Culex univittaatus Theobald* as vector. *Lancet Infect Dis.* 1976;72:295–300.

39. Work TH, Hurlbut HS, Taylor RM. Indigenous wild birds of the Nile Delta as potential West Nile virus circulating reservoirs. *Am J Trop Med Hyg.* 1955;4:872–888.

40. Murgue B, Murri S, Triki H, Deubel V, Zeller HG. West Nile in the Mediterranean basin: 1950–2000. *Ann N Y Acad Sci.* 2001;951: 117–126.

41. Nash D, Mostashari F, Fine A, et al. The outbreak of West Nile virus infection in the New York City area in 1999. *N Engl J Med.* 2001;344:1807–1814.

42. Lanciotti RS, Roehrig JT, Deubel V, et al. Origin of the West Nile virus responsible for an outbreak of encephalitis in the northeastern United States. *Science.* 1999;286:2333–2337.

43. Marfin AA, Petersen LR, Eidson M, et al. Widespread West Nile virus activity, eastern United States, 2000. *Emerg Infect Dis.* 2001;7: 730–735.

44. Eidson M, Komar N, Sorhage F, et al. Crow deaths as a sentinel surveillance system for West Nile virus in the northeastern United States, 1999. *Emerg Infect Dis.* 2001;7:615–620.

45. Kulasekera VL, Kramer L, Nasci RS, et al. West Nile virus infection in mosquitoes, birds, horses, and humans, Staten Island, New York, 2000. *Emerg Infect Dis.* 2001;7:722–725.

46. Campbell GL, Marfin AA, Lanciotti RS, Gubler DJ. West Nile virus. *Lancet Infect Dis.* 2002;2:519–529.

47. Granwehr BP, Lillibridge KM, Higgs S, et al. West Nile virus: where are we now? *Lancet Infect Dis.* 2004;4:547–556.

48. Centers for Disease Control. Arbonet Database. 2005. Available at http://www.cdc.gov

49. Mostashari F, Bunning ML, Kitsutani PT, et al. Epidemic West Nile encephalitis, New York, 1999: results of a household-based seroepidemiological survey. *Lancet.* 2001;358:261–264.

50. Nasci RS, Savage HM, White DJ, et al. West Nile virus in overwintering *Culex* mosquitoes, New York City, 2000. *Emerg Infect Dis.* 2001;7: 742–744.

51. Iwamoto M, Jernigan DB, Guasch A, et al. Transmission of West Nile virus from an organ donor to four transplant recipients. *N Engl J Med.* 2003;348:2196–2203.

52. Pealer LN, Marfin AA, Petersen LR, et al. Transmission of West Nile virus through blood transfusion in the United States in 2002. *N Engl J Med.* 2003;349:1236–1245.

53. Biggerstaff BJ, Petersen LR. Estimated risk of transmission of the West Nile virus through blood transfusion in the US, 2002. *Transfusion.* 2003;43:1007–1017.

54. Centers for Disease Control. Update: West Nile virus screening of blood donations and transfusion-associated transmission–United States, 2003. *MMWR.* 53;282–284.

55. Custer B, Tomasulo PA, Murphy EL, et al. Triggers for switching from minipool testing by nucleic acid technology to individual-donation nucleic acid testing for West Nile virus: analysis of 2003 data to inform 2004 decision making. *Transfusion.* 2004;44:1547–1554.

56. Solomon T, Vaughn DW. Pathogenesis and clinical features of Japanese encephalitis and West Nile virus infections. *Curr Top Microbiol Immunol.* 2002;267:171–194.

57. Mackenzie JS, Gubler DJ, Petersen LR. Emerging flaviviruses: the spread and resurgence of Japanese encephalitis, West Nile and dengue viruses. *Nat Med.* 2004;10:S98–S109.

58. Grossman RA, Edelman R, Willhight M, Pantuwatana S, Udomsakdi S. Study of Japanese encephalitis virus in Chiangmai Valley, Thailand. 3. Human seroepidemiology and inapparent infections. *Am J Epidemiol.* 1973;98:133–149.

59. Hoke CH, Nisalak A, Sangawhipa N, et al. Protection against Japanese encephalitis by inactivated vaccines. *N Engl J Med.* 1988;319:608–614.

60. Monath TP. Yellow fever. In: Plotkin S, Orenstein W, eds. *Vaccines.* Philadelphia, Pa: Saunders Publishing Co; 1999.

61. Bres PL. A century of progress in combating yellow fever. *Bull WHO.* 1986;64:775–786.

62. Carter HR. *Yellow Fever: An Epidemiological and Historical Study of Its Place of Origin.* Baltimore, Md: Williams & Wilkins; 1931.

63. Monath TP. Yellow fever: Victor, Victoria? Conqueror, conquest? Epidemics and research in the last forty years and prospects for the future. *Am J Trop Med Hyg.* 1991;45:1–43.

64. Soper FL. The 1964 status of *Aedes aegypti* eradication and yellow fever in the Americas. *Am J Trop Med Hyg.* 1965;14:887–891.

65. Robertson SE, Hull BP, Tomori O, Bele O, LeDuc JW, Esteves K. Yellow fever: a decade of reemergence. *JAMA.* 1996;276:1157–1162.

66. Monath TP. Yellow fever: an update. *Lancet Infect Dis.* 2001;1:11–20.

67. Tomori O. Yellow fever: the recurring plague. *Crit Rev Clin Lab Sci.* 2004;41:391–427.

68. Van der SP, Gianella A, Pirard M, et al. Urbanisation of yellow fever in Santa Cruz, Bolivia. *Lancet.* 1999;353:1558–1562.

69. Monath TP, Nasidi A. Should yellow fever vaccine be included in the expanded program of immunization in Africa? A cost-effectiveness analysis for Nigeria. *Am J Trop Med Hyg.* 1993;48:274–299.

70. Schneider K. Uber epidemische meningitis serosa. *Wien Klin Wochenschr.* 1931;44:350–352.

71. Kausler J, Kraus P, Moritsch H. Klinische and Virologisch-serologische. *Wein Klin Wochenschr.* 1958;70:634–637.

72. Barrett PN, Dorner F, Plotkin SA. Tick-borne encephalitis vaccine. In: Plotkin SA, Orenstein WA, eds. *Vaccines.* 3rd ed. Elsevier, Inc. Philadelphia: Pa; 1999:767–780.

73. Gresikova M, Sekeyova M, Stupalova S, Necas S. Sheep milk-borne epidemic of tick-borne encephalitis in Slovakia. *Intervirology.* 1975;5:57–61.

74. Klockmann U, Krivanec K, Stephenson JR, Hilfenhaus J. Protection against European isolates of tick-borne encephalitis virus after vaccination with a new tick-borne encephalitis vaccine. *Vaccine.* 1991;9:210–212.

75. Kunz C, Heinz FX, Hofmann H. Immunogenicity and reactogenicity of a highly purified vaccine against tick-borne encephalitis. *J Med Virol.* 1980;6:103–109.

76. Creech WB. St. Louis encephalitis in the United States, 1975. *J Infect Dis.* 1977;135:1014–1016.

77. Shope RE. Arbovirus-related encephalitis. *Yale J Biol Med.* 1980;53: 93–99.

78. Earnest MP, Goolishian HA, Calverley JR, Hayes RO, Hill HR. Neurologic, intellectual, and psychologic sequelae following western encephalitis. A follow-up study of 35 cases. *Neurology.* 1971;21: 969–974.

79. Mclean DM, Donohue WL. Powassan virus: isolation of virus from a fatal case of encephalitis. *Can Med Assoc J.* 1959;80: 708–711.

80. Ekwanzala M, Pepin J, Khonde S, Molisho H, Bruneel H, DeWais P. In the heart of darkness: sleeping sickness in Zaire. *Lancet.* 1996;348:1427–1430.

81. Barrett MP. The fall and rise of sleeping sickness. *Lancet.* 1999;353:1113–1114.

82. Fevre EM, Picozzi K, Fyfe J, et al. A burgeoning epidemic of sleeping sickness in Uganda. *Lancet.* 2005;366:745–747.

83. Moore AC. Human Africa trypanosomiasis: a reemerging public health threat. In: Scheld WM, Murray BE, Hughes JH, eds. *Emerging Infections.* Washington, DC: ASM Press; 2004:143–157.

84. Barrett MP, Borahmore RJS, Stich A, et al. The trypanosomiases. *Lancet.* 2003;362:1469–1480.

85. Anomymous. Human African trypanosomiases (sleeping sickness): epidemiological update. *Wkly Epidemiol Res.* 2006;81:71–80.

LYME DISEASE

Diane E. Griffin

Historical Introduction

In 1975 a concerned mother from Old Lyme, Connecticut (Figure 25-1), reported to the Connecticut State Health Department that 12 children in her small town of 5000 residents had an illness that had been diagnosed as juvenile rheumatoid arthritis. At approximately the same time a mother from nearby East Haddam told physicians at the Yale Rheumatology Clinic in New Haven that there was an epidemic of arthritis occurring in her family and neighbors. In response to this information, investigators established a system of surveillance in the communities east of the Connecticut River to identify all cases of "Lyme arthritis" in order to try and determine the cause of this new disease, suspected to be of infectious etiology. Fifty-one individuals (39 children and 12 adults) with similar symptoms of arthritis were identified. Seventeen of the 39 children lived on just four country roads, and on those roads 10% of children had the illness. Many families had more than one affected member.[1]

The disease these individuals described began with the sudden onset of pain and swelling in a knee or other large joint. The first attack of arthritis lasted about a week, but many individuals had recurrent attacks usually involving large joints with a similar distribution to that of initial attacks. More than half of those interviewed reported other flulike symptoms suggestive of an infectious disease, such as headache, chills, fever, and malaise. In addition, 13 patients said that approximately a month before the arthritis, they had noticed a red skin papule and that this lesion had developed into a large annular lesion with red margins and central clearing that continued to expand. This unique skin lesion was usually on an extremity, not painful, lasted 2–3 weeks and was consistent with a previously described disease, erythema migrans (EM). EM was recognized primarily in Europe and had been associated with bites of the sheep tick *Ixodes ricinus*, but had not been

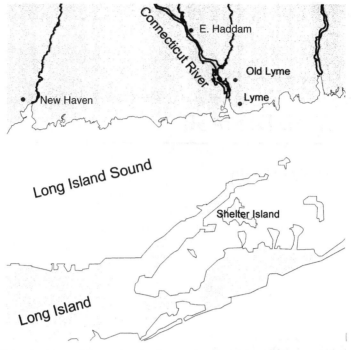

FIGURE 25-1 Map of the region in the northeastern part of the United States where Lyme disease was first recognized, where the epidemiology of the disease was defined and where *Borrelia burgdorferi* was first isolated from *Ixodes scapularis* ticks.

associated with subsequent arthritis.[2] One patient remembered having been bitten by a tick at the site where the lesion developed. These early data suggested that the disease often had manifestations other than, or in addition to, arthritis; that it was probably due to an infectious agent; and that it was likely to be arthropod-borne and potentially related to a previously described disease in Europe.[1]

Clinical Picture and Biological Information

The Vector

Cases of Lyme disease occurred primarily in the summer (Figure 25-2) indicating that the disease was seasonal and consistent with the possibility suggested by one of the original patients that it was tick-borne. Therefore, in the summers of 1976 and 1977 ticks and patients in the areas around the Connecticut River were studied.[3-5] A surveillance system was established using health care providers in the area around Old Lyme, Connecticut, including both sides of the river. To enhance surveillance, introductory lectures were conducted at three southern Connecticut hospitals and specialists in dermatology, rheumatology, pediatrics, and internal medicine were contacted. The broad scope of the surveillance program was intended to reduce bias in the

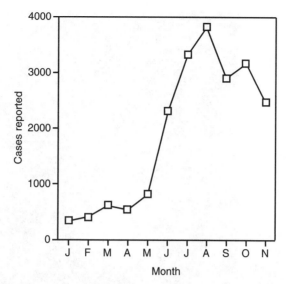

FIGURE 25-2   Seasonal incidence of erythema chronicum migrans. *Source:* Data from the Centers for Disease Control and Prevention.

collection of cases. A case was defined as a recent episode of EM or a diagnosis of Lyme arthritis. Forty-three new cases of Lyme disease were identified, mostly on the east side of the Connecticut River where the incidence was 2.8 cases/1000 residents compared to 0.1 cases/1000 residents on the west side of the river, a difference of almost 30-fold. Nine of these 43 individuals (21%) remembered a tick bite at the site of the initial skin lesion within the 3 previous weeks. One individual had saved the tick, and it was identified as the deer tick *Ixodes scapularis* (Figure 25-3). For each case, two control participants were chosen from neighbors who lived within 150 feet of the case. In addition to matching on local environmental conditions, cases and controls were matched by age and sex. Epidemiologic investigation (Table 25-1) revealed that the patients with Lyme disease had more cats and farm animals and had more often noted ticks on their pets and themselves than their neighbors without disease.[4]

Analysis of the ticks collected showed that *Ixodes scapularis* (occasionally referred to as *I. dammini*) was much more abundant on the east than on the west side of the river. Immature *I. scapularis* were 13 times more abundant on white-footed mice (*Peromyscus leucopus*), and adult *I. scapularis* were 16 times more abundant on white-tailed deer (*Odocoileus virginianus*) in communities on the east side than the west side of the river (Table 25-2). Although no pathogen was isolated from the ticks or the people with Lyme disease, these data provided strong epidemiologic evidence for a tick-transmitted agent as the cause of Lyme disease.[5]

Extensive searches for the etiologic agent of Lyme disease using a wide variety of culture techniques were unsuccessful. However, the agent was identified in the summer of 1981 when Willy Burgdorfer, a medical entomologist specializing in the study of ticks as vectors of infectious agents, was analyzing ticks from various parts of Long Island, New York. As part of his studies he noted the presence of spirochetes in the midguts of most *Ixodes*

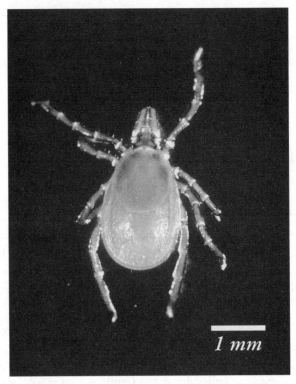

FIGURE 25-3   Adult female *Ixodes scapularis* tick collected in Maryland (photograph by Steven Dumler, Johns Hopkins University School of Medicine).

TABLE 25-1   Risk Factors for Contracting Lyme Disease: Comparison of Patients with Their Neighbors, Connecticut, 1977

Risk Factor	Cases (%)	Neighbors (%)	Statistical Significance (*P* value)
Male	53	44	ns
Rural environment	47	45	ns
Activities in woods	77	61	ns
Farm animals	26	11	<.05
Pets	86	81	ns
Cats	63	39	<.01
Ticks on pets	70	27	<.0001
Tick bites	44	25	<.05
Mosquito bites	72	70	ns

Note: ns, no significance.
Source: Steer, Broderick, and Malawista, Erythema Chronicum Migrans and Lyme Arthritis, *American Journal of Epidemiology*, 1978, Vol 108, p. 317, by permission of the Oxford University Press.

TABLE 25-2   Numbers and Types of Ticks Collected from Various Sources East and West of the Connecticut River, 1977

Source	West			East		
	Number	*Ixodes*	*Dermacentor*	**Number**	*Ixodes*	*Dermacentor*
Humans	21	8	37	27	33	20
Dogs	26	2	78	16	27	96
Cats	10	12	17	4	3	5
White-footed mice	143	29	26	197	498	143
Other mammals	10	3	15	9	9	77
Dragging	0	0	0	1	8	43
Totals	210	54	173	254	578	384

Source: Wallis, Kloter, and Main, Erythema Chronicum Migrans and Lyme Arthritis, American Journal of Epidemiology, Vol. 108, p. 325, © 1978, by permission of the Oxford University Press.

ticks collected on Shelter Island, which is located directly across Long Island Sound from the mouth of the Connecticut River (Figure 25-1). In an indirect immunofluorescent assay these spirochetes were stained by sera from patients with Lyme disease, but not by sera from individuals without a history of Lyme disease,[6] suggesting an etiologic link to the disease. In retrospect, organisms morphologically characteristic of spirochetes had been associated with EM in Europe in 1948,[7] but had not become accepted as the EM infectious agent. Subsequently, the Lyme disease spirochete was isolated from the blood and tissues of patients with Lyme disease[8,9] and was identified as a new species of borrelia, *Borrelia burgdorferi*.[10]

    I. scapularis, like most hard ticks, has a complicated life cycle that requires 2 years to complete and includes progression through the stages of egg, 6-legged larvae, 8-legged immature nymph, and the 8-legged reproductively mature adult tick (Figure 25-4). At each stage a blood meal is required for morphogenesis and progression to the next stage. Adult ticks lay eggs in the early spring that hatch to become larvae. *Ixodes,* as do all tick species, walk to the end of grasses and tree leaves where they "quest," front legs waving in the air, until a suitable host brushes past them. Ticks do not fly, hop, drop, or jump to their next meal. The larvae feed once and then rest for the remainder of the year. The following spring nymphs emerge and feed once. The white-footed mouse is a primary host for immature *I. scapularis* and develops persistent infection with *B. burgdorferi*,[11] but other mammals, reptiles, and birds, variably susceptible to persistent infection with *B. burgdorferi*, are also fed upon by *I. scapularis* ticks. Both nymphs and adults will feed on humans and can transmit Lyme disease.[12] After the nymph feeds, the adult emerges and feeds once in the summer/fall. Usually, adults feed on large mammals such as domestic pets, humans, and deer. Adults mate preferably on white-tailed deer. The male tick dies, while the female overwinters and lays eggs the following spring.

    Interstage and vertical transmission of *B. burgdorferi* is rare (<0.1%) so eggs are not commonly infected.[13] The larvae may acquire the spirochete at the first feeding. The chance of the first host being positive is dependent on the host being exposed and susceptible to *B. burgdorferi* infection. Exposure is dependent on being previously bitten by an infected tick. The white-footed mouse, for example, has as many as 10 litters of pups each year. As vertical transmission is rare, mice infected in the previous year will not pass their infection on to the next generation. Nymphal ticks, which emerge in the spring, are responsible for transmitting *B. burgdorferi* to the next generation of mice. If nymphal forms of the tick emerge and feed before the larvae hatch, as is the case in the northern United States, host populations have a higher prevalence than in the southern United States where larvae may hatch and feed before the nymphs. This order of feeding combined with feeding on *B. burgdorferi*–incompetent hosts in the southeast United States explains the high prevalence of *B. burgdorferi* in *Ixodes* ticks from the northeastern United States (50%) as compared to southeastern United States (1%).[13]

The distribution of *I. scapularis* is probably determined by the need for high humidity and availability of host species, particularly deer.[14] Populations of this tick are abundant in the United States in the northeast and upper Midwest.[14] Related ticks, *I. pacificus* (the western black-legged tick), *I. ricinus* (the sheep tick), and *I. persulcatus*, are the primary vectors for Lyme disease along the Pacific Coast of the United States, in Europe, and in Asia.[13-15] The enzootic cycles of *B. burgdorferi* on the Pacific coast and in the southeastern United States are maintained primarily between reservoir rodents and species of *Ixodes* ticks (e.g., *I. spinipalpis*, *I. affinis*, *I. minor*) that rarely bite humans.[16] The immature forms of bridge vector ticks that do bite humans (e.g., *I. scapularis*, *I. pacificus*) have a variety of suitable hosts and prefer to feed on lizards, which are not susceptible to *B. burgdorferi*,[17] rather than rodents, resulting in a low penetrance of *B. burgdorferi* in these regions.[13]

The Infectious Agent

Borrelia are motile, helical, gram-negative spirochetal bacteria that are maintained in zoonotic cycles involving a variety of wild mammals and birds as reservoirs. By definition, reservoir species are hosts that are commonly infected with an organism and remain infectious for the vector for prolonged periods of time.[11,18] For *B. burgdorferi* this is determined largely by ability of the host complement system to inactivate the spirochetes.[17,19,20] *B. burgdorferi* has been isolated from the blood of white-footed mice, which are abundant, highly susceptible to persistent infection, a preferred host of *I. scapularis* at early stages of the life cycle (Figure 25-4), and do not become resistant to repeated tick feeding.[11,16,21] Vector competence describes the inherent ability of an arthropod to become infected with the organism and subsequently to transmit the infectious agent to a new vertebrate host. Larval ticks acquire *B. burgdorferi* when they feed on infected mice, persistent infection is established in the tick, and all subsequent stages of the vector remain infected unless borrelia in the midgut are inactivated through subsequent feeding on an incompetent host.[18,19,22] Infected nymphal ticks then transmit *B. burgdorferi* to uninfected mice. All the data indicate that mice are the most important reservoir species for maintaining the invertebrate cycle of infection. Deer, although important for the tick life cycle, have blood that can inactivate borrelia and are dead-end hosts.[14,19]

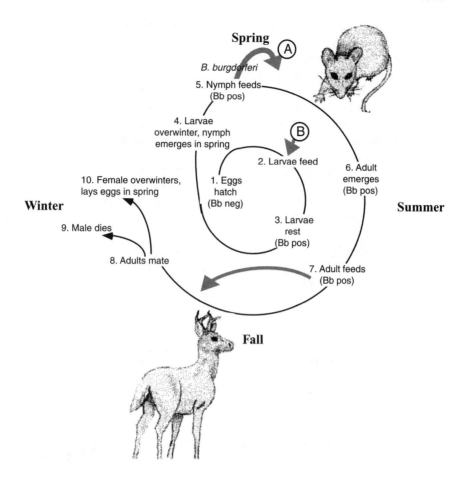

FIGURE 25-4 Life cycle of *Ixodes scapularis* indicating principal seasonal activity and hosts. The tick must overwinter twice and take 3 blood meals on two different vertebrate hosts. (A) Nymphs feed and infect white footed mice with Borrelia burgdorferi (Bb) in spring. (B) Larvae hatch and feed on the nymphally infected mice. Larvae then rest for the remainder of year. In the spring, the cycle repeats when (A) infected larvae emerge as nymphal ticks to feed and infect subsequent generations of white footed mice. Bb prevalence is lower if the larvae emerge first and feed on uninfected mice. The remainder of the tick's life cycle does not impact on Bb prevalence as the adults feed and mate once on large mammals, white tailed deer or humans.
Source: Copyright © 1999, Carolyn Masters Williams.

The genome of *B. burgdorferi* is small (~1.5 megabases) and consists of an unusual linear chromosome and 21 linear and circular plasmids that encode a remarkably large number of lipoproteins.[23] The structure includes an inner membrane, an outer membrane, and periplasmic flagella. The primary outer surface lipoproteins (Osps) vary antigenically between strains and can undergo phase shifts as an important means of organism adaptation to growth in vertebrate and invertebrate hosts.[24,25] OspA, which has multiple distinct antigenic variants, and OspB are encoded on a bicistronic operon and expressed on the surface of spirochetes within the midgut of unfed ticks. OspA and OspB bind borrelia to the tick midgut and are essential for *B. burgdorferi* colonization and survival within the tick.[26-28] When infected nymphs take a blood meal, the borrelia cease expression of OspA, thus releasing them from the gut, and begin to express OspC (Figure 25-5). This switch is induced in part by the increase in temperature and decrease in pH in the tick midgut associated with taking a blood meal.[28-30]

Infected ticks have several hundred *B. burgdorferi* in the gut lumen. When a blood meal is taken the organisms begin to proliferate and increase their numbers more than a hundred-fold. This expanded, OspC-expressing population of borrelia cross the midgut epithelium into the hemolymph and then enter the salivary glands. OspC facilitates salivary gland invasion, and it takes approximately 60 hours after tick attachment for sufficient numbers of organisms to be present in salivary glands for infection of a new host. OspC is the primary surface antigen expressed by *B. burgdorferi* in vertebrate hosts, and specific OspCs are associated with infection of different vertebrate hosts.[25,28,31-33]

Other lipoproteins expressed by *B. burgdorferi* that are important during tick feeding and host infection are proteins that bind complement regulatory factors in host plasma. Borrelia are susceptible to immobilization and lysis through the alternative complement pathway.[17] Resistance to complement-

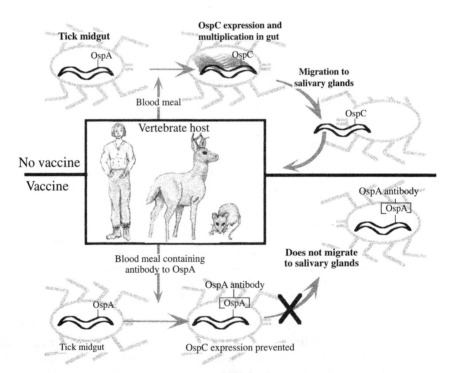

FIGURE 25-5 Schematic diagram of the changes in the expression of Osp proteins by *B. burgdorferi* (Bb) in infected ticks after taking a blood meal from an unvaccinated individual and an individual previously vaccinated against OspA. When the blood meal contains no OspA antibody *B. burgdorferi* is induced to express OspC, multiply, and spread to the salivary gland of the tick, which allows transmission to the host on which the tick is feeding. When the blood meal contains OspA, antibody to *B. burgdorferi* expression of OspC is inhibited, and neither multiplication nor spread to the salivary glands occurs.
Source: Copyright © 1999, Carolyn Masters Williams.

dependent lysis depends on the ability of borrelia to bind factor H and/or factor H-like proteins in the blood meal through complement regulatory-acquiring surface proteins (CRASPs). Complement regulatory factors in host plasma control the alternative pathway of complement activation at the level of C3b and prevent lysis by complement bound to a surface.[17] CRASPs confer complement resistance to the pathogen. This circumvention of innate immunity allows persistent infection in the vertebrate host, an important determinant of a reservoir host, and prevents lysis in the tick gut, an important determinant of vector infection and subsequent transmission. For borrelia, expression of functional CRASPs correlates directly with serum resistance. Factor H and factor H-like binding proteins are absent in serum-sensitive *B. garinii* strains. CRASPs belong to two different families of outer surface membrane lipoproteins, the polymorphic OspE/F-related proteins (Erps)(e.g., CRASP-3) and a unique lipoprotein (CRASP-1).[34,35]

Eleven genospecies of *B. burgdorferi sensu lato* (*s.l.*) are now recognized of which three, *B. burgdorferi sensu stricto* (*s.s.*), *B. afzelii*, and *B. garinii*, are associated with human disease. Each of these genospecies has different reservoir hosts and is associated with different clinical manifestations of infection.[36,37] An important determinant of vertebrate host and tick infection is susceptibility of the borrelia genospecies to complement-dependent lysis.[19] For instance, serum from lizards and deer can lyse *B. burgdorferi s.s.* and *B. afzelii*, while serum from mice and humans does not. On the other hand, *B. garinii* is lysed by serum from mice, but not by serum from birds, the reservoir host for this genospecies.[20]

The Disease

Clinical Manifestations

Early Disease

B. burgdorferi is introduced into the skin of a susceptible host by the saliva from an infected tick, and the earliest manifestation of infection is usually a slowly expanding skin lesion that appears within days to weeks at the site of the bite (Figure 25-6). The lesion starts as a red macule or papule. The later appearance of the lesion, which may become very large, is characteristic of an EM lesion with an erythematous border and a clearing center. The lesion is usually warm, but not particularly painful or pruritic. *B. burgdorferi* can be isolated from this lesion.[8,37] This stage of Lyme disease is often accompanied by flulike symptoms including fever, chills, malaise, stiff neck, and headache,[15] and *B. burgdorferi* can often be isolated from the blood.[8,9,38] Even without treatment these early signs and symptoms generally resolve within 3–4 weeks.

Secondary Disease

The secondary disseminated phase of the disease usually occurs within 1 to 6 months after exposure and may manifest in more generalized EM lesions, myocarditis, or neurological disease.[15,39] Dissemination to form multiple secondary annular skin lesions is usually accompanied by more intense systemic manifestations with severe lethargy, encephalopathy, myalgias, generalized

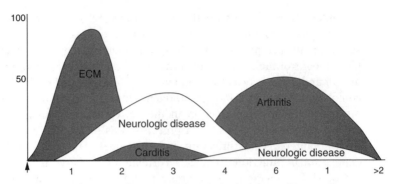

FIGURE 25-6 Schematic drawing of the clinical phases of Lyme disease indicating the approximate percentage of infected individuals that will develop the various manifestations of infection if left untreated. ECM, erythema chronicum migrans.
Source: Copyright © Diane E Griffin.

lymphadenopathy, and splenomegaly. A second type of skin eruption, lymphocytoma or lymphadenosis benigna cutis, may also be seen, particularly in Europe. This condition consists of a solitary red or violaceous lesion most commonly located on the ear lobe in children or on the nipple in adults. It may be accompanied by regional lymphadenopathy as well as other manifestations of Lyme disease.[40] Carditis occurs in approximately 5% of untreated infected individuals and presents with palpitations associated with atrioventricular conduction abnormalities and occasionally S-T segment and T-wave changes on the electrocardiogram. These signs and symptoms usually resolve within 6 weeks. *B. burgdorferi* frequently invades the central nervous system (CNS),[41] and neurological complications occur in approximately 15% of untreated patients. These complications include meningitis, meningoencephalitis, cranial nerve palsies, and radiculitis.[42] Systemic symptoms may be present, but skin lesions and lymphadenopathy have usually resolved. Approximately half of the patients with meningitis have some symptoms of encephalitis such as depressed consciousness, impaired concentration, seizures, ataxia, or behavioral abnormalities. The most characteristic neurological abnormalities are cranial and peripheral neuropathies, most commonly Bell's palsy.[42-44]

Late Disease

The later stages of Lyme disease occur months to years after infection. The most common manifestation is arthritis that may be monoarticular or oligoarticular and occurs in approximately 60% of untreated patients. Large joints, particularly the knees, are most frequently affected, but occasionally there is involvement of small joints as well. The arthritic attacks last weeks to months and can be recurrent over years.[45] *B. burgdorferi* can often be detected in synovial fluid aspirated from affected joints.[46] Chronic arthritis develops in a subset of patients with a genetic susceptibility to this complication and probably has an autoimmune component.[47] OspA cellular and humoral responses are seen in patients with Lyme arthritis resistant to treatment.[48] This complication occurs preferentially in individuals with HLA-DR4 and DR2,[47] and it has been proposed that this may be due to molecular mimicry of T-cell epitopes of OspA and human-leukocyte-function-associated antigen 1 (hLFA-1). Lyme arthritis may be the result of an autoimmune process where hLFA-1 is attacked by the patient's immune response to the OspA antigen.[15]

Late Lyme disease can also have a characteristic skin eruption, acrodermatitis chronica atrophicans, which is most commonly seen in elderly European women infected with *B. afzelii*. This chronic skin disease begins insidiously on the distal portions of the extremities with redness and swelling followed by atrophy and ultimately by loss of fingers and toes. The skin disease is associated with persistent infection and is often accompanied by joint deformities or polyneuropathy.[44] Neurological manifestations of late Lyme disease are less well defined but include chronic progressive leukoencephalitis, which may resemble multiple sclerosis and is seen most often in Europe associated with *B. garinii* infection, generalized encephalopathy, and generalized polyneuropathy.[44] These illnesses may begin many years after the primary infection and are often difficult to diagnose.[15,49]

Diagnosis

The diagnosis of Lyme disease during the early phases of the disease is based primarily on the characteristic clinical presentation. The history of tick exposure is often helpful, although because of the small size of the tick, the bite may not be recognized by the patient. Therefore, the season of the year and a history of living or vacationing in a known endemic area are also important information. The EM rash is characteristic and usually sufficient for the diagnosis of primary disease.[40] The clinical presentation of secondary disease, especially the combination of meningitis and cranial or peripheral neuropathy, should suggest Lyme disease as the leading diagnosis.[43] Culturing the organism provides a definitive diagnosis, but is positive only early in disease or in patients with acrodermatitis.[15] Borrelia DNA can be detected by PCR in synovial fluid, cerebrospinal fluid (CSF), and blood with varying levels of success.[50-52] PCR can also be used to identify the genospecies of *B. burgdorferi s.l.* causing the infection.[53]

Antibody to *B. burgdorferi* appears only weeks after infection, and even borrelia-specific IgM is often not present early in disease. IgG antibody to the organism, as measured by enzyme immunoassay or immunoblot, is usually but not always present at the time of development of carditis, neurologic disease, or disseminated skin lesions. In neurologic disease antibody may also be present in CSF. Enzyme immunoassays using recombinant or peptide antigens are more specific than those using whole cell sonicates of *B. burgdorferi* and may detect antibody earlier.[54] Currently, a two-tier approach that combines enzyme immunoassay with a confirming immunoblot is recommended for serologic diagnosis.[55]

Epidemiologic research on Lyme disease is complicated by the lack of a definitive laboratory test. In the absence of a reliable test for *B. burgdorferi*, it is difficult to determine either those with a recent infection or those with a history of infection. Epidemiologists must rely on clinical symptoms to define cases of Lyme disease. Unfortunately, the most characteristic symptom, the EM rash, does not appear in all patients.

Other Diseases

In addition to those symptoms and conditions associated with Lyme disease, others have suggested a wide range of conditions that they feel may be associated with infection with *B. burgdorferi*. Although there is no scientific data to support the claims, chronic fatigue syndrome, dyslexia, and other degenerative, inflammatory, and neuropsychiatric conditions have been linked to Lyme disease. Epidemiologic research studies designed to examine the risk of disease for populations are not able to supply answers to individuals who want to know the cause of their symptoms. Several characteristics of Lyme disease encouraged these speculative claims: it is an emerging disease, symptoms of Lyme-associated disease can occur long after the initial infection, lack of definitive tests complicates epidemiologic studies, and the high prevalence of the disease in endemic areas ensures that there are persons with both a diagnosis of Lyme disease and another condition. Only continued epidemiologic investigation coupled with improvements in diagnosis will ensure that these questions are satisfactorily answered.

Treatment

The generally accepted treatment for early Lyme disease is orally administered tetracycline, usually in the form of doxycycline in adults, or amoxicillin in pregnant women, lactating women, and young children.[15,56] Treatment is usually for 14–21 days, but 10 days may be sufficient for EM.[57] Cefuroxime axetil can be used as alternative therapy in patients allergic to tetracycline or penicillin. Treatment both shortens the course of EM and greatly reduces the later manifestations of arthritis, carditis, and neurological disease.[15,58] Patients with minor cardiac (e.g., first-degree atrioventricular block) or neurologic (e.g., Bell's palsy) involvement without other significant symptoms can be treated with the same regimen used for early disease. Those with more severe cardiac or neurologic disease or with arthritis are often treated with intravenous antibiotics, usually ceftriaxone for 14–28 days.[15,56] Symptoms of pain or fatigue that persist after treatment, sometimes called "chronic Lyme disease" or "post-Lyme disease," do not benefit from repeated or prolonged antibiotic treatment.[15] Chronic arthritis that is unresponsive to antibiotic therapy is associated with an immune response to OspA and probably is autoimmune in nature.[48,59,60]

Epidemiology

Lyme disease is endemic in several areas of the United States, eastern and central Europe, and Russia.[61] Although Lyme disease was first recognized in 1975, *B. burgdorferi* is not new to the United States or Europe. In retrospect, at least one case of Lyme disease occurred on Cape Cod in 1962,[62] and in 1970 the case of a Wisconsin physician who developed EM at the site of a tick bite was reported.[63] Museum ticks collected in Europe in 1884 and on Long Island in the 1940s were positive when examined by polymerase chain reaction (PCR) for *B. burgdorferi* DNA,[64,65] and it is likely that the organism has been present in these locations for many centuries.[66] However, cases of Lyme borreliosis are increasing in both America (Figure 25-7) and Europe.[67,68]

The incidence of Lyme disease, and seropositivity as evidence of prior infection, varies dramatically between geographic regions, and this undoubtedly correlates with the prevalence of *Ixodes* ticks that feed on humans, the proportion of these ticks that is infected, and the opportunity for human exposure to infected ticks.[69,70] The factors regulating disease prevalence vary with the geographic site and the genospecies of the pathogen. Several possible reasons for emergence have been examined. There is little evidence that climate change in the form of increasing temperatures is an important factor.[71] However, ticks require a moist environment, and precipitation in the spring affects tick abundance probably by increasing nymph survival.[72,73]

United States

Areas of the United States with frequent transmission of *B. burgdorferi* to humans are in the northeast and upper Midwest. However, a zoonotic cycle is maintained in many other parts of the United States, and cases of Lyme disease are seen by physicians in many regions because of occasional transmission and summertime vacation travel to areas of high risk (Figure 25-7). Essentially all cases of Lyme disease in the United States are due to infection with *B. burgdorferi s.s.*,[74] although regional genetic heterogeneity exists within this group.[75] The ratio of apparent-to-inapparent infections is 1:1.[62] The age distribution is bimodal with peaks in children from 5 to 14 years (9.9 cases/100,000 population/year) and adults 50 to 59 years (9.2 cases/100,000

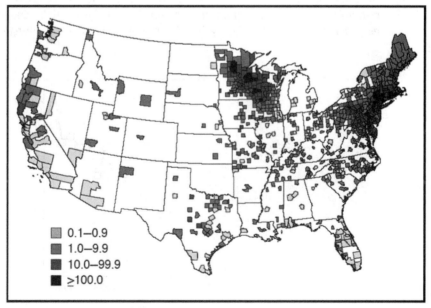

* Per 100,000 population.

FIGURE 25-7   Map of United States with Lyme disease by county for 2002. United States
Source: Lyme Disease—United States, 2001–2002. *MMWR.* 2004;53:365–369.

population/year).[68] Males and females are approximately equally affected (53% male).[68]

The vector for human infection in the northeast, southeast, and Midwest is *I. scapularis*, and the vector along the Pacific coast is *I. pacificus*. Transmission occurs primarily in the spring and early summer when ticks are most abundant and active. Disease follows a few weeks later (Figure 25-2). In some areas virtually 100% of the ixodid ticks are infected with the Lyme disease borrelia. The incidence of Lyme disease has been steadily increasing since its recognition in 1975 (Figure 25-8), and the zones of relatively high incidence are expanding. Lyme disease is currently the most common arthropod-borne disease in the United States.

The numbers of cases fluctuate from year to year. In the northeast this is likely to be linked to the fluctuating abundance of white-footed mice, a primary host for *I. scapularis* and the primary reservoir of *B. burgdorferi*. An important food source for mice is acorns that are naturally produced in increased abundance every 2–5 years. Another food source for mice are the pupae of gypsy moths. Recent experimental studies have shown that in oak forests in the eastern United States defoliation by gypsy moths and the risk of Lyme disease are determined by local interactions between acorn abundance and the numbers of white-footed mice, moths, deer, and ticks.[76] Moth increases are caused by reductions in mouse density that occur when there are no acorns because moth pupae are more likely to survive. An increase in acorns increases the numbers of mice and the densities of *I. scapularis*, predicting increased numbers of cases of Lyme disease.

On the Pacific coast and in the Southeast the transmission cycle for *B. burgdorferi* is different than it is on the Atlantic coast. In California and Oregon dusky-footed woodrats rather than white-footed mice are the primary reservoir hosts, and *I. spinipalpis*, a non-human-biting tick, maintains *B. burgdorferi* in the enzootic cycle. The primary vector of *B. burgdorferi* to

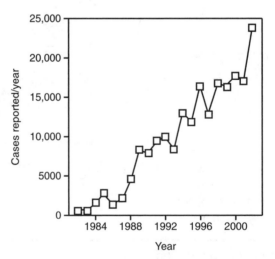

FIGURE 25-8   Numbers of cases of Lyme disease in the United States from 1982 to 2002.
Source: Based on data published by the Centers for Disease Control and Prevention.

humans is *I. pacificus*. This tick feeds on a wide variety of hosts, so only 1–2% of these ticks become infected.[77] In the Southeast cotton rats, eastern woodrats, and cotton mice are reservoir hosts, and *I. minor* and *I. affinis* are important enzootic vectors that rarely feed on humans.[16] The primary vector of *B. burgdorferi* to humans is *I. scapularis*, as in the Northeast, but many fewer are infected.

Europe and Asia

The EM skin lesion was first described in Sweden in 1909.[2] The distribution of the disease in Europe correlates with the distribution of *I. ricinus*, the transmitting vector and extends from north and central Europe into eastern Europe and Russia.[61,78] *I. persulcatus* is the most important vector in Asian Russia, China, and Japan.[36] Strains of borrelia causing infection in Europe are much more varied than in the United States and include all three genospecies of *B. burgdorferi s.l.*: *B. burgdorferi s.s.*, *B. garinii*, and *B. afzelii*,[36,55] while in Asia, *B. garinii* and *B. afzelii* are most common. The major reservoir hosts for *B. afzelii* are *Apodemus* mice and *Clethrionomys* voles, and *B. garinii* is maintained predominantly in a bird-tick cycle.[36]

In studies performed in southern Sweden, where 10–30% of ticks are infected, the highest rates of EM were found to be among children 4–9 years old and adults 60–74 years old. There was no difference in the incidence between males and females. In children, tick bites were more often about the head and neck than in adults, and bites in these regions increased the risk of neuroborreliosis.[79]

Exposure/Risk Factors

Because Lyme disease is transmitted by ticks, it is not surprising that living, working, or vacationing in a woodsy, rural environment increases risk.[69] The probability of contracting Lyme disease after a tick bite in an area of endemic disease ranges from 0.012 to 0.05.[80] Once exposed to an infected tick the likelihood of transmission of *B. burgdorferi* depends on how long the tick is attached. In mice, transmission of infection requires attachment for at least 36 hours and is most efficient between 48 and 72 hours.[81,82] In humans, the incidence of Lyme disease is significantly higher (20% vs 1.1%) if the duration of attachment is greater than 72 hours.[83] This need for prolonged attachment is explained by the time required for the borrelia in the tick midgut to multiply, shift from expressing OspA to OspC, and migrate to the tick salivary glands in sufficient numbers for transmission (Figure 25-5).

Control Measures

Prevention of a vector-borne zoonotic disease such as Lyme disease in humans can take the form of controlling the reservoir host species (mice), controlling the host species required for maintenance of the vector (deer), controlling the vector (ticks), preventing human exposure to the vector, or prophylaxis or immunization of humans against infection.[84] Essentially all of these approaches have been or are being explored as mechanisms to prevent Lyme disease in the United States.

Control of reservoir species is difficult. *Peromyscus* populations fluctuate with food supply,[76] but abundance of food in woodlands is not really amenable to human control measures. Furthermore, the diversity of hosts for the immature forms of the tick make elimination of these hosts unfeasible. The availability of diverse hosts of varying ability to serve as reservoirs will decrease the likelihood of tick infection and prevalence of disease in a community.[85]

Deer are an important host as they are the preferred site for mating. Deer populations have burgeoned in many regions and are associated with increased *I. scapularis* populations.[86] Several studies have shown that decreasing or eliminating deer populations decreases the abundance of infected ticks after several years.[87,88]

Strategies for directly reducing the tick populations have been successful in limited areas. One approach has used acaricides delivered to white-footed mice in cotton balls or bait boxes that are scattered over a wooded area. This has resulted in up to 95% reduction of *I. scapularis* populations in treated areas.[89] Another approach has been to trap and vaccinate mice with OspA to prevent infection. This approach decreased tick infection 19–23%.[90] A long-term effect on infected *I. scapularis* populations using either of these approaches would require a sustained effort that would be expensive and impractical for large areas.

Preventing exposure to the vector is inexpensive and universally applicable. Wearing light clothing so ticks are visible, avoiding grass and shrubbery where questing ticks are likely to be waiting, applying insecticide, and limiting access to skin surfaces by wearing a long-sleeved shirt and long pants tucked into socks all decrease the likelihood of tick bite. Daily "tick checks" can result in removal of ticks before the 36–48-hour period of attachment needed to transmit *B. burgdorferi*. These preventive measures are reasonable when the risk of exposure to ticks is only during certain activities. However, residents of rural areas, or those with wooded areas near their homes, are potentially exposed to ticks every day. In areas of the country where infection rates in ticks are also high, such as the northeastern United States from Maryland to Maine, people may be at risk of Lyme disease whenever they are outside. With summertime temperatures exceeding 80°F, long-sleeved shirts and long pants are not a realistic solution. In the spring, when the nymphal forms of the tick are active, daily "tick checks" are also difficult as the nymphal tick is light colored and minute. Overall, educational campaigns to decrease tick exposure have not had a demonstrable impact on the incidence of tick bites or Lyme disease.[91]

Antibiotic prophylaxis after exposure to ticks has been studied by several investigators and is generally not recommended. An analysis of cost-effectiveness concluded that empiric treatment for anyone with a tick bite is indicated if the probability of infection is >0.036. By this formula prophylaxis is not recommended in any region where the prevalence of infected ticks is less than 10%.[80] A trial of antimicrobial prophylaxis (amoxicillin for 10 days) concluded that even in highly endemic areas the risk of infection is so low that numbers of adverse reactions to antimicrobial treatment were equivalent to the cases prevented.[92] Another study showed that a single dose of doxycycline within 72 hours of exposure prevented EM, but side effects occurred in six individuals for every case of Lyme disease prevented.[84]

Vaccine

A vaccine based on the OspA protein, the Osp expressed by *B. burgdorferi* in the infected unfed tick, has been licensed in the United States. OspA immunization effectively protects mice and humans from *B. burgdorferi* infection (Table 25-3).[93-95] Antibody to OspA in the blood meal blocks borrelia development in the infected tick and the subsequent transmission of *B. burgdorferi* from the vector to the host (Figure 25-2).[29] Thus, the OspA vaccine is a transmission-blocking Lyme disease vaccine.

Two different recombinant OspA vaccines were developed and tested.[94,95] The first[94] showed a 49% vaccine efficacy in the first year (95% confidence interval [CI], 15–69%) after two immunizations and a 76% vaccine efficacy in the second year (95% CI, 58–86%) after three immunizations for preventing definite Lyme disease. The measured vaccine efficacy for preventing asymptomatic Lyme disease was 83% in the first year and 100% in the second year. Antibody levels correlated with protection. Cases of Lyme disease among vaccine recipients were found to have lower antibody titers than those subjects who did not contract Lyme disease during the follow-up period. This vaccine was licensed for use in the United States in 1998.

TABLE 25-3 Measured Vaccine Efficacy in Two Trials of OspA Recombinant Protein Vaccine

Study and Year	Vaccine Group No. Subjects (cases)	Placebo Group No. Subjects (cases)	Measured Vaccine Efficacy (95% CI*)
End of year one			
Sigal et al.[71]			
–Two injections	5156 (12)	5149 (37)	68 (37–85)
Steere et al.[70]			
–Two injections, definite Lyme	5469 (22)	5467 (43)	49 (15–69)
–Two injections, asymptomatic Lyme	5469 (2)	5467 (13)	83 (32–97)
Second year of study			
Sigal et al.[71]			
–Two injections	1379 (2)	1411 (5)	0 (0–60)
–Three injections	3745 (2)	3770 (26)	92 (69–97)
Steere et al.[70]			
–Three injections, definite Lyme	5469 (16)	5467 (66)	76 (58–86)
–Three injections, asymptomatic Lyme	5469 (0)	5467 (15)	100 (26–100)

*CI, confidence interval.

For the second vaccine[95] the measured vaccine efficacy was 68% (95% CI, 36% to 85%) for definite cases in the first year of the study and 92% (95% CI, 69% to 97%) for those receiving three injections in the second year of the study. Interestingly, this study measured zero vaccine efficacy in the second year for participants who did not receive the booster shot, although the large confidence interval indicates that there may have been an effect of the vaccine that the study was unable to measure.

Both studies reported mild to moderate side effects in the vaccine recipients, including flulike symptoms of chills, fever, and myalgias, but no severe or persistent consequences of vaccination. However, subsequent experience raised questions of the role of the immune response to OspA in chronic Lyme arthritis. To address these concerns, the manufacturer established an active surveillance system to monitor adverse events for recipients of the Lyme vaccine. This enhanced system would be expected to collect better information regarding adverse outcomes than the passive reporting system used for most licensed vaccines. The vaccine chapter has additional discussion of adverse event monitoring. However, acceptance of the vaccine by the public and by physicians was limited. The vaccine was withdrawn from the market in 2002. Reasons for limited acceptance included low risk of Lyme disease in most parts of the country, need for frequent booster injections, and relatively high cost compared to antibiotic treatment of early infection.[66,96]

Second-generation vaccines are under development. Recombinant OspA has been engineered to eliminate the potentially autoreactive T-cell epitope.[97] Antibody to OspC is borreliacidal and correlates with recovery from infection.[98] Passive transfer of OspC antibody to chronically infected immunodeficient mice leads to clearance of *B. burgdorferi* and immunization with an OspC DNA vaccine induces protective responses in mice.[99] Additional protective antigens have been identified.[100] It is possible that new vaccines will employ multiple *B. burgdorferi* immunogens.

Conclusion

Lyme disease is an example of a zoonotic vector-borne disease. Its recent "emergence" as a cause of human disease is a product of human exposure to an existing natural transmission cycle. Analyses of museum specimens have shown that the spirochete has infected ixodid ticks for decades and does not represent a new disease. The factors that have contributed to its emergence are instead changes in the host, vector, and environment relationship. The environmental movement of the last 20 years has brought about increased attention to preservation of natural areas and increased occupation of suburban, semirural housing. Deer populations have burgeoned since they were almost eliminated from the United States at the turn of the century. As deer are fringe woodland dwellers, they have adapted well to the suburban environment. The availability of deer, as the preferred mating host, has in turn allowed for an increase in the number of ticks. Humans intrude on the sylvan cycle of Lyme disease when they camp, hike, and otherwise enjoy the woodland areas around them. The epidemiologic questions surrounding the late complications of Lyme disease are difficult to answer. It is difficult to determine which diseases are truly associated with *B. burgdorferi* as the length of time between infection and disease makes causation difficult to prove.

Referencs

1. Steere AC, Malawista SE, Snydman DR. Lyme arthritis: an epidemic of oligoarticular arthritis in children and adults in three Connecticut communities. *Arthritis Rheum.* 1977;29:7-17.
2. Afzelius A. Erythema chronicum migrans. *Acta Dermatol Venereol.* 1921;2:120-125.
3. Steere AC, Malawista SE, Hardin JA, Ruddy S, Askenase PW, Andiman WA. Erythema chronicum migrans and Lyme arthritis: the enlarging clinical spectrum. *Ann Int Med.* 1977;86:685-698.
4. Steere AC, Broderick TF, Malawista SE. Erythema chronicum migrans and Lyme arthritis: epidemiologic evidence for a tick vector. *Am J Epidemiol.* 1978;108:312-321.
5. Wallis RC, Brown SE, Kloter KO, Main AJ. Erythema chronicum migrans and Lyme arthritis: field study of ticks. *Am J Epidemiol.* 1978;108:322-327.
6. Burgdorfer W, Barbour AG, Hayes SF, Benach JL, Grunwaldt E, Davis JP. Lyme disease—a tick borne spirochetosis? *Science.* 1982;216: 1317-1319.
7. Lennhoff C. Spirochaetes in aetiologically obscure diseases. *Acta Dermatol Venereol.* 1948;28:295-324.
8. Steere AC, Grodzicki RL, Kornblatt AN, et al. The spirochetal etiology of Lyme disease. *N Engl J Med.* 1983;308:733-740.
9. Benach JL, Bosler EM, Hanrahan JP, et al. Spirochetes isolated from the blood of two patients with Lyme disease. *N Engl J Med.* 1983;308: 740-742.
10. Johnson RC, Schmid GP, Hyde FW, Steigerwalt AG, Brenner DJ. *Borrelia burgdorferi* sp. nov: etiologic agent of Lyme disease. *Int J System Bacteriol.* 1984;34:496-497.
11. Bunikis J, Tsao J, Luke CJ, Luna MG, Fish D, Barbour AG. *Borrelia burgdorferi* infection in a natural population of *Peromyscus leucopus* mice: a longitudinal study in an area where Lyme borreliosis is highly endemic. *J Infect Dis.* 2004;189:1515-1523.
12. Schulze TL, Bowen GS, Lakat MF, Parkin WE, Shisler JK. The role of adult *Ixodes dammini* (Acari: Ixodidae) in the transmission of Lyme disease in New Jersey, USA. *J Med Entomol.* 1985;22:88-93.
13. Barbour AG, Fish D. The biological and social phenomenon of Lyme disease. *Science.* 1993;260:1610-1616.
14. Lane RS, Piesman J, Burgdorfer W. Lyme borreliosis. *Annu Rev Entomol.* 1991;36:587-609.
15. Steere AC. Lyme disease. *N Engl J Med.* 2001;345:115-125.
16. Oliver JH Jr, Lin T, Gao L, et al. An enzootic transmission cycle of Lyme borreliosis spirochetes in the southeastern United States. *Proc Natl Acad Sci USA.* 2003;100:11642-11645.
17. Kuo MM, Lane RS, Giclas PC. A comparative study of mammalian and reptilian alternative pathway of complement-mediated killing of the Lyme disease spirochete (*Borrelia burgdorferi*). *J Parasitol.* 2000;86:1223-1228.

18. Telford SR III, Mather TN, Moore SI, Wilson ML, Spielman A. Incompetence of deer as reservoirs of the Lyme disease spirochete. *Am J Trop Med Hyg.* 1988;39:105–109.
19. Kurtenbach K, De Michelis S, Etti S, et al. Host association of *Borrelia burgdorferi* sensu lato—the key role of host complement. *Trends Microbiol.* 2002;10:74–79.
20. Kurtenbach K, Sewell HS, Ogden NH, Randolph SE, Nuttall PA. Serum complement sensitivity as a key factor in Lyme disease ecology. *Infect Immunol.* 1998;66:1248–1251.
21. Bosler EM, Coleman JL, Benach JL, Massay DA. Natural distribution of the *Ixodes dammini* spirochete. *Science.* 1993;220:321–322.
22. Matuschka FR, Heiler M, Eiffert H, Fischer P, Lotter H, Spielman A. Diversionary role of hoofed game in the transmission of Lyme disease spirochetes. *Am J Trop Med Hyg.* 1993;48:693–699.
23. Fraser CM, Casjens S, Huang WM, et al. Genomic sequence of a Lyme disease spirochaete, *Borrelia burgdorferi. Nature.* 1997;390:580–586.
24. Anguita J, Hedrick MN, Fikrig E. Adaptation of *Borrelia burgdorferi* in the tick and the mammalian host. *FEMS Microbiol Rev.* 2003;27:493–504.
25. Templeton TJ. Borrelia outer membrane surface proteins and transmission through the tick. *J Exp Med.* 2004;199:603–606.
26. Fikrig E, Pal U, Chen M, Anderson JF, Flavell RA. OspB antibody prevents *Borrelia burgdorferi* colonization of *Ixodes scapularis. Infect Immunol.* 2004;72:1755–1759.
27. Yang XF, Pal U, Alani SM, Fikrig E, Norgard MV. Essential role for OspA/B in the life cycle of the Lyme disease spirochete. *J Exp Med.* 2004;199:641–648.
28. deSilva AM, Fikrig E. Arthropod- and host-specific gene expression by *Borrelia burgdorferi. J Clin Invest.* 1996;99:377–379.
29. de Silva AM, Telford SR, Brunet LR, Barthold SW, Fikrig E. *Borrelia burgdorferi* OspA is an arthropod-specific transmission-blocking Lyme disease vaccine. *J Exp Med.* 1996;183:271–275.
30. Schwan TG, Piesman J, Golde WT, Dolan MC, Rosa PA. Induction of an outer surface protein on *Borrelia burgdorferi* during tick feeding. *Proc Natl Acad Sci USA.* 1995;92:2909–2913.
31. Brisson D, Dykhuizen DE. OspC diversity in *Borrelia burgdorferi*: different hosts are different niches. *Genetics.* 2004;168:713–722.
32. Pal U, Yang X, Chen M, et al. OspC facilitates *Borrelia burgdorferi* invasion of *Ixodes scapularis* salivary glands. *J Clin Invest.* 2004;113:220–230.
33. Grimm D, Tilly K, Byram R, et al. Outer-surface protein C of the Lyme disease spirochete: a protein induced in ticks for infection of mammals. *Proc Natl Acad Sci USA.* 2004;101:3142–3147.
34. Hellwage J, Meri T, Heikkila T, et al. The complement regulator factor H binds to the surface protein OspE of *Borrelia burgdorferi. J Biol Chem.* 2001;276:8427–8435.
35. Kraiczy P, Hellwage J, Skerka C, et al. Complement resistance of *Borrelia burgdorferi* correlates with the expression of BbCRASP-1, a novel linear plasmid-encoded surface protein that interacts with human factor H and FHL-1 and is unrelated to Erp proteins. *J Biol Chem.* 2004;279:2421–2429.
36. Wang G, van Dam AP, Schwartz I, Dankert J. Molecular typing of *Borrelia burgdorferi sensu lato*: taxonomic, epidemiological, and clinical implications. *Clin Microbiol Rev.* 1999;12:633–653.

37. Logar M, Ruzic-Sabljic E, Maraspin V, et al. Comparison of erythema migrans caused by *Borrelia afzelii* and *Borrelia garinii. Infection.* 2004;32:15-19.
38. Wormser GP, Liveris D, Nowakowski J, et al. Association of specific subtypes of *Borrelia burgdorferi* with hematogenous dissemination in early Lyme disease. *J Infect Dis.* 1999;180:720-725.
39. Steere AC, Bartenhagen NH, Craft JE. The early clinical manifestations of Lyme disease. *Ann Int Med.* 1983;99:76-82.
40. Mullegger RR. Dermatological manifestations of Lyme borreliosis. *Eur J Dermatol.* 2004;14:296-309.
41. Luft BJ, Steinman CR, Neimark HC, et al. Invasion of the central nervous system by *Borrelia burgdorferi* in acute disseminated infection. *JAMA.* 1992;267:1364-1367.
42. Reik L, Steere AC, Bartenhagen NH, Shope RE, Malawista SE. Neurologic abnormalities of Lyme disease. *Medicine.* 1979;58:281-294.
43. Pachner AR, Steere AC. The triad of neurologic manifestations of Lyme disease: meningitis, cranial neuritis and radiculoneuritis. *Neurology.* 1985;35:47-53.
44. Oschmann P, Dorndorf W, Hornig C, Schafer C, Wellensiek HJ, Pflughaupt KW. Stages and syndromes of neuroborreliosis. *J Neurol.* 1998;245:262-272.
45. Steere AC, Gibofsky A, Patarroyo ME, Winchester RJ, Hardin JA, Malawista SE. Chronic Lyme arthritis: clinical and immunogenetic differentiation from rheumatoid arthritis. *Ann Int Med.* 1979;90:896-901.
46. Russell AS, Percy JS, Grace M. The relationship of autoantibodies to depression of cell-mediated immunity in infectious mononucleosis. *Clin Exp Immunol.* 1975;20:65-71.
47. Steere AC, Dwyer E, Winchester R. Association of chronic Lyme arthritis with HLA-DR4 and HLA-DR2 alleles. *N Engl J Med.* 1990;323:219-223.
48. Kalish RA, Leong JM, Steere AC. Association of treatment-resistant chronic Lyme arthritis with HLA-DR4 and antibody reactivity to OspA and OspB of *Borrelia burgdorferi. Infect Immunol.* 1993;61:2774-2779.
49. Logigian EL, Kaplan RF, Steere AC. Chronic neurologic manifestations of Lyme disease. *N Engl J Med.* 1990;323:1438-1444.
50. Nocton JJ, Bloom BJ, Rutledge BJ, et al. Detection of *Borrelia burgdorferi* DNA by polymerase chain reaction in cerebrospinal fluid in Lyme neuroborreliosis. *J Infect Dis.* 1996;174:623-627.
51. Nocton JJ, Dressler F, Rutledge BJ, Rys PN, Persing DH, Steere AC. Detection of *Borrelia burgdorferi* DNA by polymerase chain reaction in synovial fluid from patients with Lyme arthritis. *N Engl J Med.* 1994;330:229-234.
52. Wallach FR, Forni AL, Hariprashad J, et al. Circulating *Borrelia burgdorferi* in patients with acute Lyme disease: results of blood cultures and serum DNA analysis. *J Infect Dis.* 1993;168:1541-1543.
53. Chmielewski T, Fiett J, Gniadkowski M, Tylewska-Wierzbanowska S. Improvement in the laboratory recognition of Lyme borreliosis with the combination of culture and PCR methods. *Mol Diagn.* 2003;7:155-162.
54. Bacon RM, Biggerstaff BJ, Schriefer ME, et al. Serodiagnosis of Lyme disease by kinetic enzyme-linked immunosorbent assay using recombinant VlsE1 or peptide antigens of *Borrelia burgdorferi*

compared with 2-tiered testing using whole-cell lysates. *J Infect Dis.* 2003;187:1187–1199.

55. Wilske B. Diagnosis of Lyme borreliosis in Europe. *Vector Borne Zoonotic Dis.* 2003;3:215–227.

56. Wormser GP, Nadelman RB, Dattwyler RJ, et al. Practice guidelines for the treatment of Lyme disease. The Infectious Diseases Society of America. *Clin Infect Dis.* 2000;31(suppl 1):1–14.

57. Wormser GP, Ramanathan R, Nowakowski, J, et al. Duration of antibiotic therapy for early Lyme disease. A randomized, double-blind, placebo-controlled trial. *Ann Intern Med.* 2003;138:697–704.

58. Nowakowski J, Nadelman RB, Sell R, et al. Long-term follow-up of patients with culture-confirmed Lyme disease. *Am J Med.* 2003;115:91–96.

59. Chen J, Field JA, Glickstein L, Molloy PJ, Huber BT, Steere AC. Association of antibiotic treatment-resistant Lyme arthritis with T cell responses to dominant epitopes of outer surface protein A of *Borrelia burgdorferi. Arthritis Rheum.* 1999;42:1813–1822.

60. Gross DM, Forsthuber T, Tary-Lehmann M, et al. Identification of LFA-1 as a candidate autoantigen in treatment-resistant Lyme arthritis. *Science.* 1998;281:703–706.

61. Schmid GP. The global distribution of Lyme disease. *Rev Infect Dis.* 1985;7:41–50.

62. Steere AC, Taylor E, Wilson ML, Levine JF, Spielman A. Longitudinal assessment of the clinical and epidemiological features of Lyme disease in a defined population. *J Infect Dis.* 1986;154:295–300.

63. Scrimenti RJ. Erythema chronicum migrans. *Arch Derm.* 1970;102:104–109.

64. Persing DH, Telford SM, Rys PN, et al. Detection of *Borrelia burgdorferi* DNA in museum specimens of *Ixodes dammini* ticks. *Science.* 1990;249:1420–1423.

65. Matuschka FR, Ohlenbusch A, Eiffert H, Richter D, Spielman A. Characteristics of Lyme disease spirochetes in archived European ticks. *J Infect Dis.* 1996;174:424–426.

66. Steere AC, Coburn J, Glickstein L. The emergence of Lyme disease. *J Clin Invest.* 2004;113:1093–1101.

67. Kampen H, Rotzel DC, Kurtenbach K, Maier WA, Seitz HM. Substantial rise in the prevalence of Lyme borreliosis spirochetes in a region of western Germany over a 10-year period. *Appl Environ Microbiol.* 2004;70:1576–1582.

68. Centers for Disease Control and Prevention. Lyme Disease–United States, 2001–2002. *MMWR.* 2004;53:365–369.

69. Gustafson R, Svenungsson B, Gardulf A, Stiernstedt G, Forsgren M. Prevalence of tick-borne encephalitis and Lyme borreliosis in a defined Swedish population. *Scand J Infect Dis.* 1990;22:297–306.

70. Daniels TJ, Boccia TM, Varde S, et al. Geographic risk for Lyme disease and human granulocytic ehrlichiosis in southern New York state. *Appl Environ Microbiol.* 1998;64:4663–4669.

71. Randolph SE. Evidence that climate change has caused "emergence" of tick-borne diseases in Europe? *Int J Med Microbiol.* 2004;293(suppl 37):5–15.

72. McCabe GJ, Bunnell JE. Precipitation and the occurrence of Lyme disease in the northeastern United States. *Vector Borne Zoonotic Dis.* 2004;4:143–148.

73. Subak S. Effects of climate on variability in Lyme disease incidence in the northeastern United States. *Am J Epidemiol.* 2003;157:531–538.
74. Wilske B, Preac-Mursic V, Gobel UB, et al. An OspA serotyping system for *Borrelia burgdorferi* based on reactivity with monoclonal antibodies and OspA sequence analysis. *J Clin Microbiol.* 1993;31:340–350.
75. Bunikis J, Garpmo U, Tsao J, Berglund J, Fish D, Barbour AG. Sequence typing reveals extensive strain diversity of the Lyme borreliosis agents *Borrelia burgdorferi* in North America and *Borrelia afzelii* in Europe. *Microbiology.* 2004;150:1741–1755.
76. Jones CG, Ostfeld RS, Richard MP, Schauber EM, Wolff JO. Chain reactions linking acorns to gypsy moth outbreaks and Lyme disease risk. *Science.* 1998;279:1023–1026.
77. Brown RN, Lane RS. Lyme disease in California: a novel enzootic transmission cycle of *Borrelia burgdorferi. Science.* 1992;256:1439–1442.
78. Dekonenko EJ, Steere AC, Berardi VP, Kravchuk LN. Lyme borreliosis in the Soviet Union: a cooperative US-USSR report. *J Infect Dis.* 1988;158:748–753.
79. Berglund J, Eitrem R, Ornstein K, et al. An epidemiologic study of Lyme disease in southern Sweden. *N Engl J Med.* 1995;333:1319–1324.
80. Magid D, Schwartz B, Craft J, Schwartz JS. Prevention of Lyme disease after tick bites: a cost-effective analysis. *N Engl J Med.* 1992;327:534–541.
81. Piesman J. Dynamics of *Borrelia burgdorferi* transmission by nymphal *Ixodes dammini* ticks. *J Infect Dis.* 1993;167:1082–1085.
82. des Vignes F, Piesman J, Heffernan R, Schulze TL, Stafford KC III, Fish D. Effect of tick removal on transmission of *Borrelia burgdorferi* and *Ehrlichia phagocytophila* by *Ixodes scapularis* nymphs. *J Infect Dis.* 2001;183:773–778.
83. Sood SK, Salzman MB, Johnson BJB, et al. Duration of tick attachment as a predictor of the risk of Lyme disease in an area in which Lyme disease is endemic. *J Infect Dis.* 1997;175:996–999.
84. Hayes EB, Piesman J. How can we prevent Lyme disease? *N Engl J Med.* 2003;348:2424–2430.
85. LoGiudice K, Ostfeld RS, Schmidt KA, Keesing F. The ecology of infectious disease: effects of host diversity and community composition on Lyme disease risk. *Proc Natl Acad Sci USA.* 2003;100:567–571.
86. Rand PW, Lubelczyk C, Lavigne GR, et al. Deer density and the abundance of *Ixodes scapularis* (Acari: Ixodidae). *J Med Entomol.* 2003;40:179–184.
87. Stafford KC III, Denicola AJ, Kilpatrick HJ. Reduced abundance of *Ixodes scapularis* (Acari: Ixodidae) and the tick parasitoid *Ixodiphagus hookeri* (Hymenoptera: Encyrtidae) with reduction of white-tailed deer. *J Med Entomol.* 2003;40:642–652.
88. Rand PW, Lubelczyk C, Holman MS, Lacombe EH, Smith RP Jr. Abundance of *Ixodes scapularis* (Acari: Ixodidae) after the complete removal of deer from an isolated offshore island, endemic for Lyme Disease. *J Med Entomol.* 2004;41:779–784.
89. Dolan MC, Maupin GO, Schneider BS, et al. Control of immature *Ixodes scapularis* (Acari: Ixodidae) on rodent reservoirs of *Borrelia burgdorferi* in a residential community of southeastern Connecticut. *J Med Entomol.* 2004;41:1043–1054.

90. Tsao JI, Wootton JT, Bunikis J, Luna MG, Fish D, Barbour AG. An ecological approach to preventing human infection: vaccinating wild mouse reservoirs intervenes in the Lyme disease cycle. *Proc Natl Acad Sci USA*. 2004;101(52):18159–18164.

91. Malouin R, Winch P, Leontsini E, et al. Longitudinal evaluation of an educational intervention for preventing tick bites in an area with endemic Lyme disease in Baltimore County, Maryland. *Am J Epidemiol*. 2003;157:1039–1051.

92. Shapiro ED, Gerber MA, Holabird NB, et al. A controlled trial of antimicrobial prophylaxis for Lyme disease after deer-tick bites. *N Engl J Med*. 1992;327:1769–1773.

93. Fikrig E, Barthold SW, Kantor FS, Flavell RA. Protection of mice against the Lyme disease agent by immunizing with recombinant OspA. *Science*. 1990;250:553–556.

94. Steere AC, Sikand VK, Meurice F, et al. Vaccination against Lyme disease with recombinant *Borrelia burgdorferi* outer-surface lipoprotein A with adjuvant. Lyme disease vaccine study group. *N Engl J Med*. 1998;339:209–215.

95. Sigal LH, Zahradnik JM, Lavin P, et al. A vaccine consisting of recombinant *Borrelia burgdorferi* outer-surface protein A to prevent Lyme disease. Recombinant outer-surface protein A Lyme disease vaccine study consortium. *N Engl J Med*. 1998;339:216–222.

96. Hanson MS, Edelman R. Progress and controversy surrounding vaccines against Lyme disease. *Expert Rev Vaccines*. 2003;2:683–703.

97. Willett TA, Meyer AL, Brown EL, Huber BT. An effective second-generation outer surface protein A-derived Lyme vaccine that eliminates a potentially autoreactive T cell epitope. *Proc Natl Acad Sci USA*. 2004;101:1303–1308.

98. Jobe DA, Lovrich SD, Schell RF, Callister SM. C-terminal region of outer surface protein C binds borreliacidal antibodies in sera from patients with Lyme disease. *Clin Diagn Lab Immunol*. 2003;10:573–578.

99. Scheiblhofer S, Weiss R, Durnberger H, et al. A DNA vaccine encoding the outer surface protein C from *Borrelia burgdorferi* is able to induce protective immune responses. *Microbes Infect*. 2003;5:939–946.

100. Wallich R, Jahraus O, Stehle T, et al. Artificial-infection protocols allow immunodetection of novel *Borrelia burgdorferi* antigens suitable as vaccine candidates against Lyme disease. *Eur J Immunol*. 2003;33:708–719.

THE EPIDEMIOLOGY AND CONTROL OF MALARIA

Richard H. Morrow and William J. Moss

Background, History, and Public Health Importance

History of Malaria Control

Vertebrates, mosquitoes, and malaria have been interacting and evolving together for tens of thousands of years. Humans have been afflicted with malaria as long as there have been humans; documentation of what is certainly malaria dates back to 2700 BCE in China, and malaria is featured in the writings of Homer, Plato, Aristotle, Chaucer, Pepys, and Shakespeare.[1] It has been over 100 years since the discovery that malaria was caused by a protozoan parasite that infected red blood cells and was transmitted by mosquitoes from human to human. In 1902, Ronald Ross was awarded the Nobel Prize in medicine for his work on malaria and its transmission cycle. Over the following several decades, major scientific advances were made in understanding the parasite, its cycles within anopheline mosquitoes, and its pathogenesis in humans.

The Greeks had known the relation of fever to swamps and low-lying water since the sixth century BCE. Advances in controlling mosquito breeding through drainage and environmental control were of key importance in the development of the Panama Canal and continued to be the major approach to malaria control until after World War II. During World War II, two major biochemical/pharmaceutical advances in unrelated fields revolutionized malaria control and its treatment: dichlorodiphenyltrichloroethane (DDT) as an insecticide was found to be highly effective against anopheline vectors; and chloroquine replaced quinine as the principal antimalarial drug.

With these new tools, plans for the reduction and control of malaria were envisioned, but beyond that the exciting prospect of total eradication of this horrendous disease began to be discussed. The fundamental notion involved the complete elimination of all parasites of all human malaria species, principally by stopping the transmission by the vector from one human to the next. Residual spraying of DDT on the walls of households was the principal weapon to be employed and, in nearly all early trials, proved to be remarkably effective in killing those mosquitoes that had just enjoyed a blood meal from a sleeping household resident. The availability of chloroquine, rapidly and uniformly curative with a wide margin of safety and very low cost, to treat anyone who might be infected provided an additional tool.

Following World War II, the newly formed World Health Organization (WHO) formulated a plan for worldwide malaria eradication at the 8th World Health Assembly in 1955. It was estimated that eradication using DDT residual spraying could be accomplished at a cost of less than 25 cents per person per year; the total cost for the first 5 years would be half a billion US dollars.[2]

Plans were put into action in many areas of the world, and truly dramatic success was achieved in some regions. By 1958, the most inspirational, ambitious, complex, and costly health campaign ever undertaken was well under way.[3] Early campaign efforts in many countries in Europe, Asia, and Latin America were enormously successful. Indeed, in Malta the anopheline vector was completely eliminated.[4] However, as time passed, there seemed to be little effect in many continental tropical countries of Asia and South America. In Africa, where malaria was by far of greatest importance, virtually nothing was even attempted. Unfortunately, with the great emphasis on logistics and organizational activities, there seemed a comparable deemphasis on scientific research. Over a period extending for 20 years, virtually no innovative research on malaria was undertaken—the general opinion frequently and loudly expressed was that "We know what has to be done; let us get on with it!" An entire generation of malaria researchers was lost.

Even by the mid-1960s, it was clear that eradication would fail. The complex logistical and operational needs were too much for the weak infrastructures in most tropical countries; moreover, basic biological developments emerged including anopheline resistance to insecticides and parasite resistance to antimalarials.[5,6] The malaria eradication campaign came to be viewed as a major failure. In the wisdom of hindsight, the failure was a result of scientific arrogance and lack of foresight. In truth, however, large numbers of lives were saved in many countries, and major economic activities were spurred. Further, a major revolution in ideas about malaria control was fostered; gradually, it became clear that peaceful coexistence between humans and malaria parasites would have to be worked out.

Today, major advances have taken place in understanding the molecular biology of the malaria parasite, parasite and vector genomics and proteomics, vector control methods, development of antimalarial drugs, understanding the immunological responses to malaria infection and vaccine development, and a variety of innovative strategies for malaria control. Yet, despite these advances, a resurgence of severe malaria and an increased number of deaths, particularly in Africa, have taken place. Perhaps the term "resurgence" is not entirely apt in Africa since malaria was never under any sort of control there. Indeed, most African health officials did not rank malaria as a priority because malaria was considered an inevitable and accepted part of life for the infants and children of the rural poor and because the basic biological factors of transmission were so intractable. Other serious problems, more amenable to control, were given priority. By the 1980s, when primary health care programs aimed at diarrheal and respiratory diseases and diseases controllable through immunizations became increasingly effective in many African countries, the HIV/AIDS epidemic was rampant and fully occupied the attention of most health ministries, international agencies, and donor communities. Only quite recently has malaria been viewed as a genuine priority in Africa. Roll Back Malaria (RBM) was launched in 1998 by the World Health Organization, UNICEF, United Nations Development Programme, and the World Bank to provide a coordinated international approach to fighting malaria. The Roll Back Malaria Partnership is a global initiative made up of more than 90 partners whose goal is to halve the burden of malaria by 2010. The five years since its launch have been devoted to coordinating efforts of the many stakeholders; working toward an in-depth understanding of the ecology, biology, and epidemiology of malaria, particularly in Africa; developing comprehensive and cohesive planning; and raising funds and political support. It is hoped that in the next five years, 2006 to 2011, these plans will finally lead to action. Other important efforts to reduce malaria morbidity and mortality include the Multilateral Initiative on Malaria (MIM), the Malaria Vaccine Initiative, and the Global Fund to Fight AIDS, Tuberculosis, and Malaria.

Public Health Importance

The impact of malaria in human populations varies greatly in different parts of the world; wherever there is *Plasmodium falciparum,* there will be dire consequences. Figure 26-1 shows a map of the malaria distribution according to the level of endemicity. Although *Plasmodium vivax* malaria is a major cause of morbidity in parts of China, Southeast Asia, and Latin America, the overwhelming problems of malaria as a life-threatening disease are in those countries with *P. falciparum* malaria, especially in Africa. Most of this discussion will focus on issues related to tropical Africa, where malaria is of greatest importance and where approaches to control have had the least success.

The public health significance of a disease depends upon its incidence and resulting disability and mortality. These measures are particularly useful when the disease's distribution is known according to basic descriptive epidemiological variables, including person (age, sex, and other demographic variables such as occupation, education, socioeconomic group), place (urban and rural, or particular ecological zones), and time (including seasonal or other cyclical variation or secular trends).

Generally, the incidence of a disease is usefully expressed in terms of episodes per time period and of persons affected per time period. In many places where malaria is hypoendemic or mesoendemic, the incidence of malaria has meaning and can be expressed as number of episodes per thousand persons per year or as the number of persons having episodes per thousand persons per year. In holoendemic areas, however, with an entomological inoculation rate (EIR) ranging from dozens to hundreds of infectious bites per person per year, everyone is infected all the time and is reinfected every few days. The very idea of incidence, or indeed prevalence, has little meaning. The health status of an individual in these situations results from a balance between

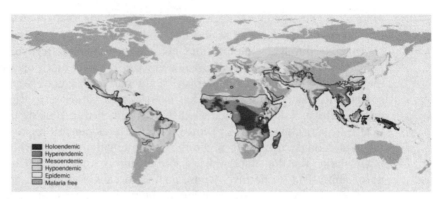

FIGURE 26-1   The Lysenko map of global malaria endemicity. Endemicity
as used by Lysenko is defined by the parasite rate in the 2–10-year cohort
(hypoendemic < 0.1; mesoendemic 0.1 – 0.5; hyperendemic 0.51 – 0.75;
holoendemic > 0.75, using the parasite rate in the 1-year-old age group). The
black line represents the 2002 limit of malaria risk. Note that the 'epidemic' class
is restricted to temperate regions in this map and is used differently today.
Source: Hay, S.I., et al., *The global distribution and population at risk of
malaria: past, present, and future.* Lancet Infect Dis, 2004. 4: pp. 327–336, with
permission from Elsevier.

the parasite and host immunity. Clearance of parasites from the host occurs
with reasonable certainty only when an individual is given an effective antimalarial drug; reinfection and, thus, "a new incident" case occurs as soon as
the level of the antimalarial drug drops below the effective therapeutic level
and recently injected sporozoites develop into blood-stage parasites.

The figure that from one to two million children die of malaria every
year has remained the quoted estimate since first put forth by the WHO in
the early 1950s.[7,8] Recently, estimates have varied more widely, ranging
from a low of 856,000 total global deaths to 1.5 to 2.7 million,[9,10] with 90%
occurring in Africa. In the 2004 World Health Report, a total of 1,272,000
malaria deaths were estimated globally, of which 1,136,000 were in Africa.
Whatever the estimate, the reality in Africa is that malaria is a major cause
of mortality in infants and children and of disability in adults. An indirect
indicator of the importance of malaria mortality is the frequency of sickle-cell
trait (AS) in tropical Africa (ranging from 16–29% AS hemoglobin in adults).
To account for this frequency, the historical case fatality rate in West Africa
attributed to malaria must be on the order of 15–20% of all children born
with AS hemoglobin (see the section on host response).[11]

Recently, composite measures of disease burden in populations have
been developed that combine the effects of disability and of mortality into a
single indicator of healthy life lost that can be used to compare the relative
importance of one disease with another.[12,13] For example, in Ghana, malaria
was the leading cause of loss of healthy life and accounted for nearly 10%
of discounted years of healthy life lost.[12,14] Although HIV/AIDS recently has
taken the lead with a total of 84,458,000 disability adjusted life years (DALYs)
lost globally, with 63,963,000 lost in Africa, deaths in Africa from malaria
have continued to increase each year; in the 2004 World Health Report,
malaria accounted for 46,486,000 DALYs lost globally of which 40,855,000
were in Africa.

The Biology of Malaria Parasites and Anopheline Vectors

Malaria Parasites and Their Life Cycle

Four species of protozoan parasites of the genus *Plasmodium* infect humans: *P. falciparum*, *P. vivax*, *P. ovale*, and *P. malariae* (Table 26-1). Although *P. vivax* is the most widespread form of malaria infection in the world, *P. falciparum* causes the most severe disease and is responsible, by far, for most deaths and serious morbidity due to malaria.

The complex life cycle of the malaria parasite is given in Figure 26-2. The parasite undergoes multiple transformations within the mosquito and human host; at least a dozen separate steps have been defined. The parasite is transmitted to humans as the sporozoite form in the saliva of an infected female anopheline mosquito taking a blood meal. Sporozoites enter the venous blood system from the subcutaneous tissues through the capillary bed, and within minutes those that avoid the defending reticuloendothelial (RE) system invade liver cells. Over the next 5 to 15 days, each sporozoite nucleus replicates thousands of times to develop into a hepatic schizont within the liver cells. When released from the swollen liver cells, each schizont splits into tens of thousands of daughter parasites called merozoites. Merozoites attach to specific erythrocyte surface receptors (Duffy blood group antigen for *P. vivax*, glycophorins for *P. falciparum*)[15] and penetrate into the erythrocyte. Each intraerythrocytic merozoite differentiates into a trophozoite that ingests human hemoglobin, enlarges, and divides, into 6 to 24 intraerythrocytic merozoites forming a schizont. The red cell swells and bursts, releasing the next batch of approximately 20 merozoites, which then attach and penetrate new erythrocytes to begin this cycle again. Along with the liberation of merozoites, the resultant hemolysis and release of "pyrogens" from infected red cells and the host's response to these toxins correspond with clinical paroxysms of fever and chills; when synchronous, the simultaneous release from many red cells account for the periodicity of these symptoms in some patients. This second stage of asexual division takes about 48 hours for *P. falciparum*, *P. vivax*, and *P. ovale*, or 72 hours for *P. malariae*.[4] A single *P. falciparum* merozoite potentially can lead to 10 billion new parasites through these recurrent cycles.[1]

After a number of cycles within red cells, some merozoites differentiate into sexual forms called gametocytes—macrogametocytes (female) and microgametocytes (male)—that are then available to be ingested by an anopheline mosquito during its next blood meal. Factors related to gametogenesis include

TABLE 26-1   Malaria Parasites of Humans

Species	Intra-RBC Schizont Period	Type of RBC	Relapse (hypnozyte)	Global Distribution
P. vivax	48 hours	Reticulocytes	Yes	Everywhere except Africa
P. ovale	48 hours	Reticulocytes	Yes	Africa
P. malariae	72 hours	Older RBCs	No	Everywhere
P. falciparum	48 hours (±)	All	No	Tropical regions

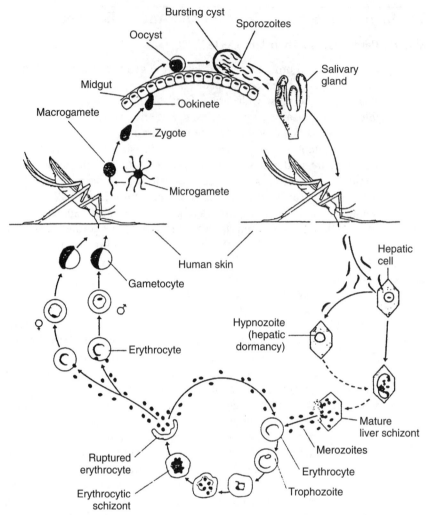

FIGURE 26-2 Life cycle of the malaria parasite.
Source: Nussenzweig V. Progress toward a malaria vaccine. Hosp Pract (Off Ed).
1990 Sep 15;25(9):25–52, 55–7.

the species of parasite, length of infection or number of intraerythrocytic cycles, density of parasitemia, drug treatment, and age or immune status of the infected individuals.

Sporogonic Development

Once in the mosquito, the red cells are digested, freeing the gametocytes, which then begin sexual reproduction leading to sporogonic development. The male and female gametes fuse, providing for genetic recombination, to form a zygote. Over the next 12 to 14 hours, the zygote elongates and forms an ookinete, which in turn penetrates the wall of the mosquito's stomach and becomes an oocyst. During the next several days, the oocyst enlarges, forming more than 10,000 sporozoites. After the oocyst ruptures into the coelomic cavity of the mosquito, the sporozoites migrate to the salivary glands, ready to be injected back into the human host to complete their life cycle. Once infected with malaria, a female anopheline remains infected for life and can transmit sporozoites with each blood meal.[4,16]

The phases of parasite development, from ingestion of gametocytes to when sporozoites in the salivary glands are poised for reinoculation into the human host, comprise the extrinsic cycle or sporogonic phase, which generally takes 7–12 days. The time required depends upon the species of parasite and the ambient temperature. For example, under optimal conditions with the temperature at 30 °C, *P. falciparum* requires 9 days; but at 20 °C it takes 23 days—a difference of 14 days for a temperature differential of 10 °C.[1,4] With an average life span for most anophelines of less than 3 weeks, the ambient temperature is critical to transmission.

During sporogonic development, each female-male pair of gametocytes potentially can produce over 10,000 sporozoites for inoculation. Because dozens to thousands of gametocytes can be ingested with one blood meal, the potential exists for millions of sporozoites to be injected with one bite. Perhaps related to damage to the mosquito from such heavy loads or insufficient nutrients/metabolites available to support these levels of parasitemia, such high inocula counts are not observed. Limited studies of naturally infected mosquitoes have found sporozoite loads (the number of sporozoites in the salivary glands of an anopheline) to range from 10 to over 100,000.[17,18]

In vitro studies using experimentally infected mosquitoes have shown most infected mosquitoes transmit fewer than 25 sporozoites per bite, but about 5% can transmit hundreds.[10] Epidemiological studies comparing sporozoite rates (the proportion of anopheline females with sporozoites in their salivary glands) with infant infection have demonstrated that less than 20% of sporozoite inoculations result in infection.[19] However, great variation in the ratio of infant conversions rate (ICR), the rate at which infants acquire malaria, to the entomological inoculation rate (EIR), roughly the number of infectious bites per person, has been found between places,[20] seasons,[21] and for evaluation of vector control.[22] In general, far lower numbers of sporozoites are delivered than are found in the salivary glands; yet, some bites do transmit high numbers of infective sporozoites, and although speculative, high inocula may lead to more severe disease.

Biological Differences Among Malaria Species

There are important species-specific differences in this generic life cycle. With *P. vivax* and *P. ovale*, some sporozoites entering hepatic cells do not immediately proceed to tissue schizogony, but become hypnozoites and lie dormant for months to years.[23] Later, these hypnozoites can differentiate into hepatic schizonts, leading to the cycle of erythrocytic schizogony and consequent relapse of symptoms. This biologic capability accounts for the relapses characteristic of *P. vivax* and *P. ovale* and the need for specific drug treatment targeted to the hypnozoite stage (primaquine). Different strains of *P. vivax* from diverse areas of the world are known to have characteristic relapse patterns. In general, following acute infection with either *P. vivax* or *P. ovale*, patients are at risk for up to 3 to 4 years of having a relapse. There is no diagnostic test available to determine whether or not individuals have hepatic hypnozoites.

P. falciparum and *P. malariae* do not produce hypnozoites and do not relapse following effective treatment, but untreated or inadequately treated infections may cause persistent low-grade parasitemia leading to recrudescent clinical disease.[24] In summary, the term "relapse" refers to renewed infection from survival of the parasite in hepatic cells as hypnozoites, whereas "recrudescence" refers to renewed infection from surviving erythrocytic forms.

The different species of human malaria parasites have affinities for particular types of erythrocytes. *P. vivax* and *P. ovale* parasites only invade the young reticulocytes; thus, the density of peripheral parasitemia in these infections rarely exceeds 3%. *P. malariae* is limited to older red cells. However, *P. falciparum* infects erythrocytes of all ages, and for this reason is able to produce high-density parasitemias with serious morbidity and high mortality.[4,16]

There also are important differences in gametocyte production among species. After infection with *P. vivax*, infective gametocytes appear in the peripheral blood almost as soon as the asexual blood-stage forms. Gametocytes are usually present when vivax malaria is first diagnosed and before antimalarial treatment has been started. *P. vivax* can be transmitted prior to symptomatic disease, and its gametocytes will not have been exposed to drug pressure that would select for drug-resistant mutants; therefore, drug-sensitive parasites are not at a disadvantage in competition with the drug-resistant strains. In contrast, following infection with *P. falciparum*, gametocytes appear only after several intraerythrocytic cycles, first appearing at least 10 days after onset of clinical symptoms. Early treatment of *P. falciparum* with an effective drug will kill blood-stage schizonts, preventing gametocytes from developing and blocking transmission. However, gametocytes that do develop will be derived from malaria parasites that survived drug treatment and may carry drug resistance genes. This strongly assists the selection and spread of drug-resistant parasites. The difference in timing of gametocyte emergence may be a major factor accounting for the much higher rate of drug resistance in *P. falciparum* as compared to *P. vivax*.[25]

Aspects of the Molecular Biology of the Malaria Parasite

Understanding the molecular biology of malaria parasites has been greatly advanced by the publication of the genome sequence of *P. falciparum* in 2002.[26] Genome sequencing of *P. vivax* is expected to be completed in 2006. Functional and comparative genomics and proteomics of the malaria parasite during different stages of its life cycle will lead to improved understanding of plasmodium biology and pathogenesis, and it is hoped to the identification of new drug and vaccine targets.

The genome of *P. falciparum* consists of 14 chromosomes containing over 5000 predicted genes. Several aspects of the molecular biology of *P. falciparum* are relevant to the epidemiology and control of malaria. A large proportion of identified genes is involved in immune evasion and host-parasite interactions. *P. falciparum* contains three families of highly variable genes, the most important of which is the *var* gene family, comprising 59 genes encoding for the *P. falciparum* erythrocyte membrane protein 1

(PfEMP1). Transcriptional switching between different *var* genes allows the parasite to evade immune responses directed against PfEMP1. These genes may also be modified by the exchange of material between chromosome ends, where these genes are located. PfEMP1 is located on the surface of infected red blood cells and mediates adherence to endothelial cells. One *var* gene encodes a protein that mediates adherence to chondroitin sulfate A in the placenta and is responsible for the severe disease observed in pregnant women. Thus, this gene family encodes for an important virulence factor responsible for the sequestration of infected red blood cells in various organs of the infected human.[26,27]

Genome sequencing of *P. falciparum* has led to the identification of metabolic pathways unique to plasmodia and not found in humans. These pathways are ideal targets for novel antimalarial drugs. For example, enzymes involved in fatty acid synthesis or protein degradation in food vacuoles may be ideal drug targets. Identification of potential antigens for vaccine development may also result from careful study of the *P. falciparum* genome, particularly the identification of conserved sequences expressed on cell surfaces during different stages of parasite development.[28] However, as the scientists responsible for the genome sequencing of *P. falciparum* wrote, "genome sequences alone provide little relief to those suffering from malaria," and much work needs to be done to convert this knowledge into effective control strategies.[26]

Although the malaria genome project focused on a single clone of *P. falciparum*, great genetic diversity is found among parasites from different geographical regions. In an early genetic analysis of dozens of *P. falciparum* isolates from three continents, all isolates were different from one another.[29] Improved understanding of the genetic differences between strains will provide insights into transmission, pathogenesis, and drug resistance.

Anopheline Mosquitoes and Their Life Cycle

Malaria is only transmitted by the genus *Anopheles* mosquitoes. Yet, over 70 species of *Anopheles* are known to be capable of transmitting malaria to humans, with only about 40 considered important vectors. The female anopheline requires protein derived from host blood for egg production; therefore, only the female is the vector for malaria. There is great variation among different species in host feeding preference, biting, and resting behavior, and in selection of larval habitat for laying the eggs. Some anophelines are opportunistic feeders on a variety of vertebrates (zoophilic), whereas others are very particular and take blood meals only from humans (anthropophilic). Some feed only indoors (endophagic), whereas others may occasionally or exclusively feed outdoors (exophagic). Whether they rest indoors (endophilic) or outdoors (exophilic) after feeding is critical in understanding transmission and effective approaches to control. Nearly all anophelines prefer clean water in which to breed, but some have very specific preferences for the aquatic environment in which to lay their eggs. For example, *Anopheles stephensi* breed in tin cans and in confined water systems, whereas *Anopheles gambiae*, the most important malaria vector in Africa, prefers small, open, sunlit pools. Knowledge of this variation is critical for effective vector control.

The mosquito goes through four stages of growth during its life cycle, from egg to larva to pupa and to adult. Shortly after emerging as an adult (eclosion) and before the first blood meal, adult anopheline females mate. They usually mate only once and store the sperm, laying a total of 200–1000 eggs in 3 to 12 batches over their lifetime.[4] A fresh blood meal is required for development of each egg batch. After hatching, an anopheline larva feeds at the water's surface and develops over 5–15 days before pupation. Within 2–3 days an adult mosquito emerges from the pupal case. The entire cycle requires a total of 7–20 days, depending upon the anopheline species and the environmental conditions. Under favorable conditions of high humidity and moderate temperatures, female anophelines can survive at least one month, time enough for the parasite to go through the sporogonic cycle of 7 to 12 days needed to develop sporozoites in the salivary glands for injection with the next blood meal. Thereafter, the mosquito is capable of transmission with each subsequent human blood meal, often taken every 2 to 3 days for the remainder of its life. Therefore, the longevity of the anopheline mosquito and host selection are critically important in determining the efficiency of transmission (see section on vectorial capacity, below).

Mosquitoes are able to seek out their host in response to a combination of chemical and physical stimuli, including carbon dioxide, body odors, warmth, and movement. Most anophelines feed at night, but some species may feed in late afternoon or early morning. During feeding, the mosquito injects salivary fluid containing enzymes into the subcutaneous tissue. These enzymes diffuse through the surrounding tissue and increase blood flow, facilitating both the blood meal and the transfer of sporozoites to the capillary bed. Anophelines generally feed on people sleeping indoors. Some species, however, bite outdoors, especially those that are forest dwellers, such as *Anopheles dirus*. After feeding, the engorged female seeks a resting place on a nearby wall or in a secluded spot outdoors. Some species alter their behavior in the presence of DDT or other insecticides, becoming irritated and flying outside to seek refuge. Engorged mosquitoes usually rest for 24–36 hours to digest the blood meal before they search for an oviposition site.

The identification of potential vectors and those that are actually involved in malaria transmission is often the starting point for investigation. Measurement of the entomological inoculation rate (EIR), as described in the section below, for each of the potential vectors is important for determining the relative contribution of each species to transmission as well as for determining the intensity of transmission in the area. The global distribution of malaria and the principal vectors have been mapped and catalogued by Haworth.[30] However, there is enormous spatial and temporal variation in vector species. Furthermore, ecological change induced by human activities such as urbanization, deforestation, and irrigation modify mosquito habitat and vector distribution. In addition, a major obstacle to species identification is the existence of species complexes, in which genetically distinct sibling groups are morphologically indistinguishable. Sibling species may vary in their potential as vectors due to differences in susceptibility to parasitic infection, resistance to insecticides, breeding habitat, geographic distribution, host preference, or biting and resting habits. For example, the *A. gambiae* complex consists of seven species, including two of the most important vectors in sub-Saharan

Africa: *A. gambiae* and *A. arabiensis*. In contrast to *A. gambiae*, *A. arabiensis* often feeds on cattle, rests outdoors, and is tolerant of low humidity. Another member of this species complex, *A. quadriannulatus*, feeds only on animals and is not a vector of human malaria. Even within *A. gambiae*, there is genetic heterogeneity with geographic and seasonal variations. Further advances in understanding the ecological, vector, host, and parasite factors should translate into improved approaches to control.

Simultaneous with the publication of the genome sequence of *P. falciparum*, a first draft of the genome sequence of *A. gambiae* was published in 2002.[31] Identification of polymorphisms within the *A. gambiae* genome will aid in the detection of insecticide resistance (e.g., detoxifying enzymes), genetic factors responsible for transmission efficiency of malaria parasites, and gene flow within mosquito populations. Genetic studies should also lead to a better understanding of the determinants of anopheline behaviors, including mechanisms by which the mosquito identifies human hosts, as well as metabolic targets for insecticide development. In addition, components of the mosquito's innate immune system have been identified that allow for a better understanding of the coevolution of parasite and vector, and potential reasons for different transmission efficiencies.[32]

Vectorial Capacity and Entomological Inoculation Rate

Understanding the dynamics of transmission is fundamental to understanding how best to reduce transmission through vector control measures. The entomological inoculation rate (EIR) and vectorial capacity (VC) are two basic indices of malaria transmission. These measures are closely related, but it is important to know how they are derived and how they are used. Both are applied to a defined ecological zone or geographical area, and both vary greatly in place and time.[20,22,33] The EIR is the number of infected bites that each person receives per night and is calculated by multiplying the human landing rate (HLR) by the sporozoite rate (SR). The HLR, previously termed the "human biting rate," is obtained by capturing all mosquitoes that land on a person, the "bait," during the night and is expressed as the number of mosquitoes landing (bites) per person per night. The SR is determined by microscopic examination of dissected salivary glands to detect sporozoites in these captured mosquitoes, expressed as the ratio of infected anophelines to the total collected. More recently, serologic and molecular techniques have been developed to measure the SR, including rapid dipstick methods that are easily used under field conditions to detect circumsporozoite proteins.[34] Even with these advances, measuring the HLR and the SR is difficult, tedious, and costly. As indicated above, only a fraction (perhaps 20%) of the sporozoites inoculated are infectious. The EIR provides a direct measure of malaria transmission and the risk of human exposure to the bites of infected mosquitoes.

In contrast, the VC measures the rate of *potentially* infective contact, meaning the potential for malaria transmission, and is based solely on key vector parameters in a particular area. In theory, it is independent of whether or not there are humans actually present. (To obtain variable *a* in the VC formula below, of course, requires that there are humans that have been bitten.) The VC is the number of potentially infective contacts an individual human could acquire in that particular area, through the vector population, per unit of time.[22,35] The formula for its calculation is:

$$VC = ma^2p^n/-\log p.$$

where m is the density of vectors in relation to humans (obtained by standardized sampling methods to give the number of female anophelines caught in a collection per person per night); a is the human biting habit (the proportion of blood meals taken from humans to the total number of blood meals taken from any animal) so that a person is bitten by ma vectors in 1 day; p is the daily survival probability of the vector; and n is the extrinsic incubation (or sporogonic) period of the vector measured in days so that a fraction p^n of the vectors survive the extrinsic cycle (incubation period). They still have an expectation of life of $1/-\log p$ (the expectation of life is assumed to be independent of age): each of the surviving vectors bites a persons per day. In principle, the VC can predict the extent to which anopheline populations must be reduced in order to reduce transmission.

It is important to understand the nonlinear relation among these variables.[36] In Figure 26-3, the prevalence of parasitemia in the human population is charted against the average annual VC.[37] Note that at low levels of VC small increases result in a rapid rise in parasitemia prevalence rate; thereafter, a long plateau is reached, where large changes in the VC do not change the level of parasitemia. This is the situation in most of tropical Africa. In these areas, reduction of several 100- or even a 1000-fold in the VC will not change the prevalence of malaria (although it may change the frequency and nature of severe malaria). For these reasons, malaria control for holoendemic areas, as in much of tropical Africa, must involve a "peaceful" coexistence rather than elimination of malaria.

Geographical Areas According to Intensity of Transmission

Traditionally, geographical patterns of transmission have been classified into four broad categories according to the intensity of transmission and based upon the percentage of children aged 2–9 with enlarged spleens and malaria parasites as follows[38,39]:

1. *Holoendemic:* Areas of intense transmission with continuing high EIRs where virtually everyone is infected with malaria parasites all the time. In older children and adults, detection of parasites may be very difficult because of high levels of immunity, but sufficient searching will generally reveal the presence of parasites. Classification on the basis of children under age 10: spleen and parasitemia rates of over 75%.
2. *Hyperendemic:* Regions with regular, often seasonal transmission but where the immunity in some of the population does not confer protection at all times. Classification as above: spleen and parasite rate in children under age 10 from 50% to 75%.
3. *Mesoendemic:* Areas that have malaria transmission fairly regularly but at much lower levels. The danger in these areas is occasional epidemics involving those with little immunity and resulting in fairly

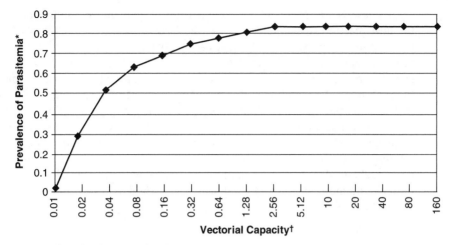

FIGURE 26-3   Prevalence of parasitemia related to vectorial capacity.
Source: Data from Garki Project Molineaux and Gramiccia, WHO, Geneva, 1980, p. 281.

high morbidity and mortality. In these areas, children less than 10 years will have spleen and parasitemia rates ranging from 10% to 50%.

4. *Hypoendemic:* Areas with limited malaria transmission and where the population will have little or no immunity. Spleen and parasitemia rates in children less than 10 years will be less than 10%. These areas, too, can sometimes have severe malaria epidemics involving all age groups.

Further classification schemes have been devised in efforts to simplify the complex epidemiological factors of malaria and to better target strategies for malaria control. An expert group was brought together by WHO in 1990 to define a set of eight major malaria paradigms intended to categorize typical transmission settings; such efforts were made to facilitate discussion and more efficient planning of control efforts.[8,40] These included malaria of the Africa savannah, forest malaria, malaria associated with irrigated agriculture, highland fringe malaria, desert fringe and oasis malaria, urban malaria, and plains and seashore malaria. Yet these, too, were oversimplifications and in general have not replaced the need to gather the detailed epidemiological and entomological data as described above.

Pathogenesis in Individual Humans

Infection and Disease

The distinction between infection and disease is particularly important in malaria. Infection with the malaria parasite does not necessarily result in disease, especially in highly endemic areas. In these regions, children may have parasitemia prevalence rates of 50% or more and yet few will have symptoms.

Disease is the result of the combination of parasite multiplication and the host reaction to the parasite. The classic description of periodic shaking chills, severe fever, and drenching sweats every two or three days can be seen in nonimmune adults infected with *P. vivax* (every other day) or *P. malariae* (every third day). The symptoms in these cases result from the host response to synchronous lysis and release of pyrogens from infected red cells. However, with falciparum malaria, clinical manifestations, particularly in children, range from asymptomatic parasitemia to severe overwhelming disease and rapid death. Children may present with drowsiness, coma, convulsions, or simply listlessness and fever with nonspecific symptoms. Abdominal cramping, cough, headaches, muscle pains, and varying levels of mental disorientation are common. Severe and complicated malaria due to falciparum malaria is a medical emergency.

Host Response

Malaria, on a population basis, is the most intense stimulator of the human immune system known. Many immunologic defense systems are activated in response to malaria infections, including the reticuloendothelial system with enhanced phagocytosis in the spleen, lymph nodes, and liver to remove infected RBCs, an intense production of antibodies—indeed humans can develop several grams per liter of immunoglobulin directed against malaria—and a range of cellular immune responses and cytokine cascades. Some of these responses are protective; others contribute to pathology (and often to both). For example, proinflammatory cytokines, severe metabolic acidosis, as well as the classical sequestration of infected RBCs that cause cerebral anoxia all may contribute to the pathogenesis of cerebral malaria; yet at the same time, the proinflammatory response and acidosis evidently account for why some patients survive without neurological complications.[41]

The host response to malaria can go wrong in several ways. For example, the pathogenesis of "big spleen disease" (tropical splenomegaly) is caused by an excessive and inappropriate host response to malaria. Tropical splenomegaly is fairly common among relatively nonimmune populations who, because they move to a malarious area or experience a change in climate, are exposed to more intense transmission. The disease starts in childhood, progressing through adolescence to young adulthood with severe anemia, high levels of IgM and antimalarial antibodies, a decrease in platelets, and a huge spleen. Malaria parasites rarely are detectable. If untreated, tropical splenomegaly is often fatal, usually from a secondary infection. Two lines of evidence indicate this is directly the result of an abnormal reaction to malaria: (1) those with sickle trait (hemoglobin SA) do not develop big spleen disease,[42-44] and (2) individuals with tropical splenomegaly who take long-term antimalarial prophylaxis have gradual reduction in spleen size and anemia, and return to normal health over many months.

Malaria parasites have evolved complex mechanisms to evade host immune responses and establish persistent or repeated infections. Understanding the basis of effective immune responses that either prevent infection or reduce disease severity is important for vaccine development. Protective immunity following natural infection takes many years to develop. However, no immunodominant response has been identified, and an effective immune response likely is the sum of cellular and humoral responses to multiple parasite antigens. Antibodies to the circumsporozoite protein can prevent the binding of sporozoites to liver cells. Cellular immune responses, specifically interferon-γ secreting T cells, are important in killing infected liver cells. Antibodies play a role in killing parasitized red blood cells and can protect from sporozoite challenge, although cell-mediated immunity contributes to blood-stage protection as well. Antibodies to erythrocytic stages may act through monocytes in a process called antibody-dependent cellular inhibition (ADCI).[45] The great antigenic variability of *P. falciparum*, as described above, is in large part responsible for the ability of the parasite to evade effective host immune responses, although other mechanisms of immune evasion have been hypothesized (e.g., induction of the immune-modulating cytokine interleukin-10).

Human Genetic Factors

As humans, mosquitoes, and malaria parasites have evolved, many human genetic characteristics that provide partial protection against malaria have emerged. These genetic polymorphisms mostly involve the red blood cell, and include structural variants in the β globin chain of hemoglobin such as sickle-cell trait (hemoglobin S) and hemoglobins C (West Africa) and E (Southeast Asia); altered α and β globin chain production leading to the α and β thalassemias (Mediterranean anemia); erythrocyte enzyme deficiencies including glucose-6-phosphate dehydrogenase (G6PD); red cell cytoskeletal abnormalities such as ovalocytosis; and changes in the red cell membrane such as the absence of the Duffy blood group factor (West Africa).[46–48] The mechanism that provides protection seems clear for sickle-cell trait—when red cells are invaded, they sickle and are preferentially removed by the RE system thus reducing parasite density levels[49]—but mechanisms have not been fully elucidated for other genetic polymorphisms. In addition to genetic changes involving hemoglobin, red cell membrane proteins, or red cell metabolism, polymorphisms in human immune response genes may also affect infection and disease. For example, HLA-B*53 was associated with protection from severe malaria in West Africa. Polymorphisms in cytokine genes or their promoters have also been associated with disease susceptibility and severity, although recent studies suggest this association is complex and requires examination of broader haplotype structure.[50]

Many polymorphisms exact a heavy burden on the homozygous individual, such as hemoglobin SS or sickle cell disease. To account for the frequency of sickle-cell trait (AS) in tropical Africa (ranging from 16–29% AS hemoglobin in adults), the historical case fatality rate that must be attributed to malaria is in the order of 10–20% of all children born with AA hemoglobin genotype.[11] If 28% of the adult population has sickle trait, then the S gene allele frequency in the adult gene pool would be half of 28%. With application of the Hardy-Weinberg law, the selection coefficient for the AA genotype would then be $0.14/(1.00 - 0.14) = 0.1628$. The ratio of AS genotype individuals to AA for survivorship to adulthood would be $1/(1.00 - 0.1628) = 1.194$, which is equivalent to nearly a 20% excess death rate for those with AA before adulthood. Since the only advantage of AS over AA is that from severe malaria, the case fatality rate due to malaria in those with

AA hemoglobin is 19.4%. The sharp age-specific rise in prevalence of sickle trait in West Africa from 20–24% in newborns to 26–29% in adults indicates that infants born without the "protective" sickle-cell trait died before adulthood. This differential survival can be expressed as the ratio of proportion of AS in adults/by that in newborns to the proportion of AA in adults/by that in newborns. In the Garki study area with very high malaria transmission and sickle-trait rates, adults were 28.96% AS and 70.2% AA (0.84% were other including those with AC and SC hemoglobin), whereas newborns were 23.6% AS and 73.78% AA (2.62% were other including 2.1% SS and 0.5% AC) giving 3.86/2.99 = 1.29. This is equivalent to a 29% case fatality rate in the AA because of malaria.[22]

Undernutrition and Micronutrient Deficiencies

Malaria is prevalent in regions where childhood malnutrition is common, and nutritional deficiencies interact with malaria infection in complex ways. Protein-energy malnutrition (PEM) applies to a group of related disorders that include marasmus, kwashiorkor, and intermediate states of marasmus-kwashiorkor. Marasmus (starvation) involves inadequate intake of protein and calories and is characterized by emaciation, whereas kwashiorkor (taken from the Ga language of Ghana and means "the sickness of the weaning" and first used by Cicely Williams in 1935[51]) refers to inadequate protein intake but with reasonable caloric (energy) intake. Edema is characteristic of kwashiorkor but is absent in marasmus. All forms of PEM impair the functioning of all bodily systems; in particular, both the cellular and humoral immune systems are weakened. Early observational studies suggested that undernourished children suffered lower morbidity and mortality than adequately nourished children.[52-54] These early reports often involved selected groups or were conducted during famine, and refeeding severely malnourished children may worsen apparent disease severity. However, more recent studies have not confirmed this association; pooled analyses of two cohort studies that examined the relationship between underweight and the severity of malaria found that malnourished children were more likely to die from malaria than adequately nourished children.[55] In any case, malaria chemoprophylaxis should be provided to famine victims or any malnourished child in malarious areas when treating PEM.

Iron deficiency is the most common micronutrient deficiency and is associated with defects in immune responses and a number of poor health outcomes. However, early observations suggested that infants with iron deficiency had less severe malaria than children without iron deficiency, and that providing iron supplementation may increase disease severity.[52,56] These observations were confirmed in a meta-analysis of iron supplementation given to children in malarious areas. Pooled analyses indicated a small but significant increase in parasitemia, and a small but not significant increase was reported in splenomegaly and clinical attack rates in those given iron.[57] However, the risk of severe anemia was reduced by 50%. The authors found no reports of increases in severe malaria and concluded that the value of iron supplementation outweighed the minor intensification of malaria parasitemia.

Vitamin A is essential for the proper functioning of the immune system in response to malaria. In contrast to the effects of iron, a trial of vitamin A supplementation in preschool children in Papua New Guinea found that vitamin A reduces clinical episodes of malaria, splenic enlargement, and parasite density, particularly in children 1 to 3 years of age.[58] However, vitamin A may not affect severe malaria or mortality. Extrapolating from this single trial, the fraction of malaria morbidity attributable to vitamin A deficiency was estimated to be 20% worldwide.[55]

Zinc is another micronutrient that is essential for both cell-mediated and humoral immunity. In randomized trials in Papua New Guinea and the Gambia, the effects of zinc supplementation on malaria morbidity and mortality were investigated.[59,60] The fraction of malaria morbidity attributable to zinc deficiency was estimated to be 20% worldwide, very similar to that for vitamin A.[55] However, in Papua New Guinea zinc supplementation reduced malaria-attributable clinic attendance by 38% and had its greatest effect on attacks having high-density parasitemia. In the Gambia, the effect of zinc supplementation was less pronounced, but the treatment group had fewer clinic visits for malaria than did the placebo group.

Improving the nutritional status of children, particularly supplementation with vitamin A and zinc, may significantly reduce malaria morbidity and mortality.

The Diversity of Falciparum Malaria Disease

As notions of eradication, with its focus on parasites and vectors, faded, more research was undertaken to define and understand the clinical and epidemiological features of malaria. Advances have been made in differentiating distinctive forms of severe falciparum malaria and in understanding underlying pathogenic factors, for example, inoculum size, differing strains of falciparum, differing immunologic responses, and various cofactors. This in turn contributed to an appreciation of distinctive epidemiological features of different forms of clinical disease. A synthesis of new information from thorough clinical studies in diverse ecological settings has led to new ideas about malaria disease and new approaches to control that focus on reducing death and enhancing immune defenses rather than reducing transmission as an end in itself. Such an approach requires an understanding of the relation of disease manifestations to intensity and constancy of transmission due to ecological factors, genetic characteristics of the parasite, and genetic and acquired immune mechanisms in humans.

The first important clinical distinction to be made is between severe and nonsevere disease caused by *P. falciparum*.[61] Severe malaria in children in holoendemic areas behaves as a different disease from nonsevere malaria. Although there may be value in differentiating various forms of nonsevere falciparum, this chapter will focus on the distinctive features of the various forms of severe malaria, particularly those of cerebral malaria and of severe anemia with and without respiratory distress.[62-64]

Severe Malaria

Disease caused by *P. falciparum* is a major cause of death in children wherever there is a high intensity of infection. Results from community-based intervention studies indicate that malaria may account for nearly half of the mortality rate of children younger than 5 years in holoendemic areas.[65,66] In hospitals throughout tropical Africa, a very large proportion of under-5 admissions and deaths is due to malaria. However, this is a small proportion of malaria cases and deaths in the community; in tropical Africa more than 80% of under-5 deaths occur at home. The pattern of disease as seen in hospitals is determined by access and health-seeking behavior as well as by the nature of the disease and, thus, may not provide a good guide to the pattern of disease in the community.

In holoendemic areas, severe disease in children does not progress from mild or moderate illness; it strikes abruptly without warning. Mothers are frequently unable to get their infants and young children to a health center in time to provide treatment before the child dies, even when facilities with trained health workers are readily available. If they do manage to reach a hospital, many die within 24 hours of admission despite treatment efforts.[67-69] Antimalarial prophylaxis was compared to clinic-based treatment in a clinical trial in the Gambia. This trial found that children less than 5 years old had much lower mortality if they were from a family randomized to receive regular prophylaxis versus those who depended upon the use of well-staffed, nearby primary health care facility.[70]

Rapid progression to severe disease is not characteristic in areas with less intense transmission. In Southern Asia, malaria typically slowly progresses in severity over several days in both children and in adults and does so in both major types of severe disease that occur there: cerebral malaria, which has a median time of five days from onset to cerebral symptoms, and multiple organ dysfunction syndrome (MODS), which is somewhat slower in development and has a median time of eight days.[71] Early effective treatment before the onset of the severe phase is the key to reducing mortality in these circumstances, an option difficult to achieve with the fulminant African form. Although these slowly progressive types are also seen in Africa, they are distinctly less common in holoendemic areas than the rapid severe forms in children.

Clinical Patterns

The starting point for understanding the pathogenesis of severe malaria is a clear description of the clinical course of the disease. There are now a number of systematic clinical studies describing the presenting symptoms and clinical characteristics of children under age 5 years admitted to hospitals in Africa with severe malaria from areas ranging from relatively low moderate to highly intensive transmission. These include studies from Kilifi, Kenya, with moderate seasonal transmission with EIR of up to several dozen annually[62,67]; Ifakara, Tanzania, with intense, year-round transmission and annual estimated ERI of over 300[72]; Malawi with intense perennial transmission, EIR of 300; the Gambia with moderate seasonal transmission, EIR of 60–120[73]; Dakar, Senegal, with low-intensity seasonal transmission, EIR of 10–80[74];

Tamale, Ghana, with intense seasonal transmission, EIR of 300[75]; and Burkina Faso with low-intensity seasonal transmission in the urban areas with an EIR of less than 10 and intense seasonal transmission in the rural areas with an EIR of over 300.[76]

All studies used the WHO definition of severe malaria of 1990 and/or as modified in 2000 that was based on the 10 clinical manifestations (coma, severe anemia, respiratory distress, hypoglycemia, circulatory collapse, renal failure, spontaneous bleeding, repeated convulsions, acidosis, and hemoglobinuria) and five additional conditions (impaired consciousness, jaundice, prostration, hyperpyrexia, and hyperparasitemia).[63,77] The revised 2000 WHO criteria provided a simplified tool for rapid and sensitive diagnosis of severe malaria with less dependence upon laboratory tests often not available outside of major hospital facilities. However, as compared to the 1990 criteria, it was somewhat less specific.[74,75]

Keeping in mind that those hospitalized with malaria are a small and selected fraction of those with severe malaria in the community, review of these studies provided useful generalizations regarding the relation of intensity of transmission with the clinical presentation and course of disease. Most children presenting with severe malaria could be placed in one of three distinctive syndromes that emerged from review of these studies: two syndromes that are readily delineated clinically when the child is first seen—those with neurological deficit (about 20% of admissions with about 15% mortality) and those with respiratory distress (about 14% of admissions also with about 15% mortality), plus a third life-threatening syndrome, not so readily apparent clinically when first seen, of severe anemia (about 18% of admissions with about 5% mortality). The roles of both hypoglycemia and metabolic acidosis in the pathogenesis of severe disease are clearly central. Hypoglycemia, difficult to diagnose on clinical grounds alone, had a prevalence equivalent to that of respiratory distress and an even higher mortality (about 22%). Hypoglycemia associated with cerebral malaria certainly contributed to the death of those classified as unarousable coma and probably those with acidosis.[62]

Cerebral Malaria

The classical histopathological picture of cerebral malaria is intense sequestration of infected cells in the cerebral microvasculature,[78] and clinically is associated with case-fatality ratios ranging from 10% to 50%.[8,79] Cerebral malaria is heterogeneous and includes four overlapping syndromes fulfilling the WHO definition of cerebral malaria with different pathogenic mechanisms: (1) prolonged postictal state, characterized as deep sleep, headache, confusion, and muscle soreness; (2) covert status epilepticus, characterized by continual seizures; (3) severe metabolic derangement (particularly with hypoglycemia and metabolic acidosis); and (4) children with a primary neurological syndrome. Commonly more than one of these situations coexists. A child may be acidotic, have hypoglycemia, and be in status epilepticus; recognition and proper management of all three in addition to treatment of the malaria are critical.[80,81] These distinctions are important for appropriate therapy, of course, but careful delineation also may help in defining underlying pathogenic factors.

Hypoglycemia is especially common in severe pediatric malaria wherever it occurs. In Thailand 23%[82] and in Malawi 33%[83] of pediatric patients admitted for severe malaria had hypoglycemia; the outlook was grim for these patients. In the Malawi study, 37% with hypoglycemia died and 26% were discharged with brain damage—many times higher than those diagnosed as cerebral malaria but with normal blood sugar levels. The combination of hypoglycemia with lactic acidosis as described below is particularly devastating.

In Kilifi, survivors of those with cerebral malaria had a much higher rate of both epilepsy (11.5%) and of cognitive impairment (24%) than did the survivors of other forms of severe malaria (2.2% and 9.2%, respectively) (personal communication, Kevin Marsh, 2003).

Respiratory Distress

Pulmonary edema, often seen with acute respiratory distress syndrome (ARDS), is included in the WHO criteria for severe malaria and has long been recognized as a serious, frequently fatal complication of malaria in nonimmune adults.[63] Respiratory distress per se did not appear in the original WHO criteria, but it is a valuable defining characteristic because with minimum training the clinical signs can be applied with good interobserver consistency. The clinical signs of hyperventilation, driven by efforts to reduce CO_2, are highly sensitive and specific for the diagnosis of respiratory distress.[84]

Cardiac failure, coexistent pneumonia, direct sequestration of malaria parasites in the lungs, and increased central drive to respiration in association with cerebral malaria all contribute to respiratory distress, but the main factor is metabolic acidosis largely due to lactate production caused by reduced oxygen to the tissues. In addition, several factors increase lactic acidemia: the metabolic processes of the malaria parasite itself; reduced hepatic blood flow[68] leading to reduced lactate clearance; and high levels of cytokines that directly impair cellular metabolism and increase lactate production.

Severe Anemia

The third major clinical manifestation of severe malaria is severe anemia; it, too, has a complex pathogenesis and varies considerably geographically, partly due to the extent of interaction with PEM, marasmus, and iron deficiency. It tends to be the predominant form in areas of the most intense transmission and is common in the youngest age groups. In northern Ghana with an EIR of over 300 per year, severe anemia was the predominant form and associated with young age, malnutrition, and hyperlactatemia, but not with hyperparasitemia.[75] In Tanzania, malaria was a more important cause of anemia than malnutrition, whereas in Burkina Faso, it was the other way around.

Different manifestations of severe malaria arise from interaction of a limited number of pathogenic processes: metabolic acidosis, red cell destruction, toxin-mediated activation of cytokine cascades, and infected cell sequestration in tissue microvascular beds. All lead to reduced tissue oxygenation as a unifying process in the pathogenesis of these major clinical syndromes of severe malaria.[80] Other severe but less common causes of malarial mortality include renal failure, pulmonary edema with acute respiratory distress syndrome, and disseminated intravascular coagulopathy (DIC).

Factors such as malnutrition, anemia, dehydration, and HIV, in addition to the clinical signs and symptoms of severe malaria as given by the WHO definitions, may greatly influence both appropriate treatment and expected outcome. In contrast to traditional teaching, malnourished children were at increased risk of death from malaria. They were more likely to be hypoglycemic and more likely to develop respiratory distress than the better nourished. Also those who were dehydrated were at a disadvantage. Preexisting anemia from any cause was an additional risk factor beyond that resulting from the malaria in several studies. In addition, HIV coinfection has profound consequences as discussed below.

Epidemiological Features of Severe Malaria

Though it now seems useful to consider three main severe malaria syndromes as discussed above, most descriptions of severe malaria in African children have focused on differentiating those with severe anemia from those with cerebral and neurological involvement.[63,66,68,85] Clear epidemiological differences parallel these distinctive clinical forms of severe malaria. As the intensity of transmission increases from one geographic area to another, the proportion of the population having severe malaria as compared to nonsevere shifts increasingly to younger age groups. Similarly, with increasing transmission intensity, the proportion with asymptomatic malaria compared to those with symptoms is shifted to younger ages in the nonsevere malaria group. Thus, in the areas with the most intense transmission, severe malaria and death are restricted largely to children younger than 5 years, and most clinical disease is seen in those under age 10.[61]

Within any endemic area, the pattern of severe morbidity varies with age; severe anemia predominates in younger children with a median age of 15 to 24 months whereas coma is more common in older children with a median age of 36 to 48 months. Between endemic areas with different levels of transmission intensity, there may be a marked difference in the age distributions of children with severe malaria and in the relative importance of different clinical syndromes. For example, severe malaria usually presents as severe anemia and occurs at a younger age in Ifakara where transmission is intense with an inoculation rate over 100 infectious bites per year per person, as compared to Kilifi with moderate transmission where the inoculation rate is less than 10, and children with severe disease more commonly present with cerebral symptoms at an older age. Despite these differences, the overall incidence of severe disease in a cohort is about the same.[61,86,87] An additional factor that apparently affects the nature of severe malaria in a population is the constancy of transmission. An area of intense perennial transmission had a higher incidence of severe anemia; whereas in an area with intense seasonal transmission there was a higher rate of cerebral malaria.[62,64]

Previous evidence that indicated there was space-time clustering of severe malaria has recently been strengthened in the Kilifi area through the use of a geographical information system and more sophisticated statistical analyses.[88,89] The same analyses were carried out for child deaths due to all causes, but no space-time clustering was found. The interpretation is that severe malaria occurs in localized microepidemics, but whether the space-time clustering of severe malaria is different from that which may occur with nonsevere malaria will be exceedingly difficult to discern as most episodes of nonsevere malaria are not reported in any consistent fashion. Certainly there are marked local variations in transmission intensity in holoendemic areas, but whether these variations are related to the space-time clustering of severe malaria remains to be explored.

In areas of intense transmission, the prevalence and density of both asexual and gametocyte stages of *P. falciparum* reach a peak in early childhood and decline thereafter. Density of parasitemia drops off before prevalence, and density of gametocytes declines before that of asexual stages. The density of asexual parasites at which symptoms appear increases in early life and declines thereafter. This indicates a separate immune response to toxic products of red cell rupture from that against the response to the parasites themselves. The antitoxic immunity builds rapidly with early infections but declines thereafter as effective immune responses to the parasites themselves slowly develop and thus directly reduce toxic products.[61,90]

Many questions remain about super infection, defined as infection concurrent with an already existing infection, common in holoendemic malaria areas with an EIR of dozens to hundreds each year. An important epidemiological point is that the incidence of malarial disease, whether mild or severe, is limited to the period of transmission in areas of holoendemic seasonal malaria. Interpretation of this is that disease onset must require a recent inoculation.[66,91] In some way, the newly inoculated parasite must differ from those parasites already present in that particular child. Quantitatively there are more parasites already in the blood than will be released from the liver cells derived from the new batch of sporozoites. During the low-transmission season, each child continues with the same parasite type and remains without symptoms, but during the high-transmission season parasite isolates are quite diverse, and there is rapid shifting of types within each child. Those that become symptomatic do so only with a new parasite type. Only some of the new types are associated with symptoms, but these types vary from child to child.[91]

There is some evidence that those with severe malaria have received no more inocula than those with nonsevere malaria,[92] but much work remains to be done to relate number of sporozoites injected by individual inoculum to clinical disease. Reports on the effectiveness of insecticide-impregnated bed nets indicate that the impact on mortality, or on severe malaria, is greater than the impact on nonsevere malaria; likewise, there is a greater reduction in clinical disease than in prevalence of asymptomatic parasitemia.[93]

In most child deaths in tropical Africa malaria is a contributing factor even though death may be attributed to another cause such as diarrhea or pneumonia. When malaria is controlled in holoendemic areas, a major reduction in overall child mortality occurs, though previously much may have been attributed to other causes.[11]

Malaria in Pregnancy

Women infected with malaria while pregnant are at much greater risk of serious consequences than women who are not pregnant (or than men);

host defense mechanisms apparently are much dampened during and for several weeks postpartum with reductions in both cell-mediated and humoral responses.[94-97]

In all areas endemic for malaria, pregnant women are more likely to be bitten by malaria vectors.[98] This increased risk of bites has been hypothesized to be related to the higher metabolic rate of pregnancy that increases body temperature and CO_2 release, both of which are attractants for mosquitoes. However, in a study of risk behaviors, it was also noted that pregnant women were more exposed to mosquitoes when they left the home to urinate at night. Pregnant women are also at higher risk of infection with malaria of all types and are more likely to develop severe, complicated malaria and die than the nonpregnant women. Adverse outcomes of their pregnancies are also higher, due to active malarial infection of the placenta.[99]

The maternal mortality ratio (MMR) for women infected with malaria ranges from 100 to over 1000 per 100,000,[100,101] and relative risks for maternal mortality for women with malaria as compared to those without range upward from two-fold. The MMR is as high in low-transmission areas as it is in high-transmission areas, but the nature of the complications and those at greatest risk are different. In low-transmission areas, pregnant women across the spectrum of parity die from severe, complicated malaria, particularly with cerebral symptoms, hypoglycemia, and acute respiratory distress syndrome. MMRs of up to 1000 per 100,000 live births are reported during malaria epidemics in low-transmission areas. In areas of high transmission, the risk of severe disease and death is mainly among women in their first pregnancy (over 1000 per 100,000 MMR) even though they had acquired a high level of immunity prior to their pregnancy; mortality is mainly related to severe anemia.

The prevalence of parasitemia is highest during the second trimester regardless of the transmission intensity. In low-transmission areas, women with malaria virtually always have symptoms and generally have parasitemia regardless of parity. In contrast, in high-transmission areas, pregnant women often have asymptomatic parasitemia; it is only primigravidae that have symptoms and a high risk of complications.[102]

Malaria infection during pregnancy commonly leads to infection of the placenta.[103,104] The effects of both present and past placental infection together with the often-intense host responses contribute to the high fetal losses due to malaria. There is often a discrepancy in parasitemia between the placenta and the peripheral blood especially in high-transmission areas where there may be an intense placental parasitemia but few if any parasites found in the peripheral blood. Although not fully understood, the reasons seem related to the distinctive placental and uterine immunological and biochemical responses and associated immunological memory. Local uterine and placental responses apparently are least effective in first pregnancies, but increase with "renewed parasite acquaintance" in subsequent pregnancies.[105] In high-transmission areas, women, when they become pregnant for the first time, lose their high levels of malaria immunity; yet somehow they regain much of it after the first pregnancy and virtually fully after their second, presumably through a uterine immunological memory mechanism. Much work is going on at the molecular level concerning adherence and binding of infected RBCs and the cascade of cytokines and other factors in the placenta, but a full understanding of these complex interactions is some way off.

Pregnant women with malaria have a higher rate of low weight births and of stillbirths than those without malaria. The proportion of low-birth-weight (LBW) infants is elevated in both low-transmission and high-transmission areas, but the reasons for the low weight may be different: preterm delivery (PTD) is common in low-transmission areas especially in association with acute febrile episodes caused by malaria in the third trimester; whereas in high-transmission areas there is fetal growth retardation (FGR) associated with chronic placental inflammatory damage. In addition, maternal malaria leads to a higher perinatal and infant mortality rate in keeping with the high rate of low-birth-weight infants.[99] In areas of moderate transmission such as Kilifi, women with malaria of all parities have a substantially higher risk of low birth weight and severe anemia. The risk of low birth weight is particularly high in children whose mothers had either chronic or past placental malaria and severe anemia.[106]

Steketee et al reviewed studies performed between 1985 and 2000 and summarized the malaria population attributable risk (PAR) that accounts for both the prevalence of the risk factors in the population and the magnitude of the associated risk for anemia, LBW, and infant mortality (IM).[107] Consequences from anemia and HIV infection in these studies were also considered. Population attributable risks were substantial: malaria was associated with anemia (PAR range 3–15%), overall LBW (8–14%), PTD (8–36%), FGR (13–70%), and IM (3–8%). Human immunodeficiency virus was associated with anemia (PAR range 12–14%), LBW (11–38%), and direct transmission in 20–40% of newborns, with direct mortality consequences. Maternal anemia was associated with LBW (PAR range 7–18%), and fetal anemia was associated with increased IM (PAR not available). They estimate that each year 75,000 to 200,000 infant deaths are associated with malaria infection in pregnancy.

With viral and some bacterial infections, it is infection in the first trimester that leads to anomalies and excess fetal death, but there are virtually no reports concerning the possible effects of malaria in the first trimester of pregnancy. It is clear that reduction or prevention of infection in the second and third trimesters greatly reduces the adverse consequences of malaria both for the mother and for the fetus—though not to the levels common in nonmalarious areas. Now, with the potential for protection from malaria throughout pregnancy by use of bed nets, it may be possible to eliminate or reduce the possible consequences of first-trimester malaria.

In Africa especially, MMR has actually increased in the last decade in concert with the emergence of drug-resistant falciparum and the HIV epidemic. HIV has profound effects on infant and maternal morbidity and mortality and increases susceptibility to maternal malaria.[99] HIV impairs the ability of pregnant women to control parasitemia and shifts the usual gravidity-specific pattern of malaria burden from the primigravidae to all pregnant women.[108] Where severe anemia from malaria requires blood transfusion, the dangers of HIV and hepatitis B virus transmission are added risks to the consequences of malaria.

Malaria and HIV

Early investigations concluded that there were no significant interactions between HIV and malaria coinfection, with the exception of malaria in HIV-infected pregnant women as discussed above. Subsequently, HIV-infected Ugandan adults were observed to have twice as many episodes of symptomatic parasitemia than HIV-uninfected adults, and the parasite density and clinical signs and symptoms were correlated with the degree of immunosuppression.[109] In Malawi, plasma HIV-1 RNA levels in adults were almost twice as high during periods of malaria parasitemia that resolved within a few weeks after antimalarial treatment,[110] suggesting malaria may enhance HIV disease progression and aid HIV transmission. Few studies have investigated malaria in HIV-infected children, the age group at greatest risk of morbidity and mortality caused by malaria. Although not definitive, these studies suggest malaria may be more severe and less responsive to therapy in HIV-infected children and, further, that malaria may adversely affect HIV disease progression.

Human Activities and the Epidemiology of Malaria

Human activities, particularly at the population level, but also at the individual behavioral level, strongly influence the epidemiological pattern of malaria and the efforts to control it. Agricultural development, population movement, and urbanization are important determinants of the pattern of malaria transmission. All control measures involve the interplay of broad social, cultural, and economic factors.

Malaria has long been linked to farming practices. In sub-Saharan Africa, the clearing of forest for crop production has led to increased breeding of *A. gambiae*, the most efficient vector of human malaria, which prefers sunlit open pools of standing water to the full shade of tropical forest. The formation of small towns, dams, and irrigation schemes arising in concert with agricultural development in much of Africa has concentrated populations of humans and vectors in relatively confined areas near water supplies. Additionally, agricultural use of pesticides has been a major factor in the development and spread of insecticide-resistant vectors. Thus, the very efforts to promote economic development and improve human conditions have increased the intensity of malaria transmission.

Population movements throughout Africa have contributed toward an increased intensity of malaria transmission. Traditionally, in many parts of Africa seasonal migration has been a part of life with people moving from their village settlements to rural farms during the early months of the wet season when cultivation, planting, and weeding are carried out. Often intensity of transmission is much higher in these areas than in their settled home villages where water supplies are controlled. In a similar way, many pastoral Africans are exposed to higher transmission as they move their livestock between highland and lowland pastures with the seasons.

Other reasons for population movement are related to population expansion with movement into previously unoccupied and more marginally productive areas. The living and working conditions in these areas often result in greater exposure to malaria vectors. Africa has been especially afflicted with drought, famine, war, and political upheavals resulting in mass population displacement and refugee movements, all of which are frequently associated with increased malaria transmission. These groups frequently are poorly served by government health and malaria control programs and have less access to antimalarials and other aspects of health care. Disasters and conflicts, so prominent in Africa for decades, greatly contribute to the transmission of malaria and inhibition of antimalaria control efforts.

Malaria in Complex Emergencies

Approximately one third of malaria deaths in sub-Saharan Africa occur in countries affected by complex emergencies. Factors facilitating malaria mortality in complex emergencies include migration of nonimmune people to hyperendemic areas, overcrowding, interruption of vector-control programs, and inadequate access to health care.[111] Multiple interventions, including provision of shelter, vector control, case management, and surveillance, are required for malaria control in complex emergencies. Insecticide-treated plastic sheeting may be an effective means of vector control in complex emergencies and has the potential to reduce the vectoral capacity.[112]

Urban Migration

In contrast to the types of population movement described above, the major secular migrations to urban areas throughout Africa generally have little influence on malaria transmission. Although malaria in Africa is principally a rural rather than an urban disease, some anopheline species have come to be well adapted to city life. For example, *A. arabiensis* has become a transmitter of malaria in many cities of Nigeria.[8] Generally, this vector is restricted to semiurban slum areas rather than the highly concentrated populations in urban centers.

Social Class

Although malaria can infect and cause severe disease in anybody, it is principally a disease of the poor and uninformed. Loss of healthy life due to malaria is much higher in poor rural areas of Africa than in the better-developed urban areas. Some notion of the difference in impact on different social groups can be seen in the studies by Oduntan in Nigeria,[113] who found that the sickle-trait rate among elite school children in Ibadan was under 20%, whereas in rural children not attending school, the AS rate was 26.3%. To account for this marked differential, the mortality rate due to malaria among those with AA hemoglobin in the poor must be many times greater than that in the elite who would have had better nutrition and access to health services. If one assumes that at birth the distributions of AA, AS, and SS genotypes were the same, and further that none of the elite with AA died by school age, then 29.9% of those with AA in the nonelite would have died from malaria. However, with the strong tendency for social classes to intermarry, it is likely that the distributions would not have been the same and that at least some of this marked differential could be attributed to lower malaria mortality and less benefit from AS in the last generation or two among the elite. The interplay between environmental factors (malaria) and genetics (hemoglobin genotypes) ensures that the sickle-trait rate will continue to be reduced among the better off in whom the balanced polymorphism from selective protection for sickle-trait no longer holds. The dramatic differential in mortality from malaria by social class provides clear evidence that malaria control efforts should contribute to improved equity of health status.

Health-Seeking Behavior

Individual and community behavior are important factors influencing the population effects discussed above and are crucial in determining the success of malaria control. In Africa, there is great diversity in cultures and community structures. Understanding and acting in accord with the prevailing belief systems are essential; otherwise, these beliefs may serve as barriers to adoption of effective interventions. Health-seeking behavior, key for obtaining timely treatment, depends upon understanding the need for treatment; thus, people's perceptions of malaria and its causes are very important. Even in communities that have an appreciation of the importance of malaria and need to obtain appropriate treatment, the symptoms of cerebral malaria may be misunderstood because it produces convulsions and confusion. People frequently do not recognize these as signs for urgent treatment for malaria; indeed, such symptoms often are attributed to belief of supernatural causes, not something that modern medicine can affect, and the advice of traditional healers is often sought.[114,115]

As detailed in the section on antimalaria interventions, virtually all approaches to control require a good understanding of what factors contribute to malaria and the active participation of the community, families, and individuals for effective control.

Diagnosis and Treatment

A definitive diagnosis of malaria is made by demonstration of parasites in red blood cells. The standard technique is microscopic examination of a Giemsa-stained thick and thin smear of blood on glass microscope slides. This technique will likely remain the gold standard. The thick smear is the more sensitive method for the detection of parasites. With thin films, skilled technicians can determine not only the species of malaria, but also can obtain reliable estimates of the number of parasites (parasite density). The ability to detect parasites depends on the number of fields examined and the experience of the technician viewing the slide.

Although this approach continues as standard, there are problems of practical implementation and interpretation. At the practical level, Giemsa-stained blood smears examined with standard light microscopes have been used for 70 years in every area in the world. Yet the work is tedious and requires continuous concentration; delays in viewing smears can result in delayed treatment; maintenance of the microscope and staining materials requires rigorous control; and training technicians and supervising their activities require discipline difficult to maintain. Quality control methods are essential, and approaches to maintain good morale among the technicians are critical.

The problems of interpretation of blood smears are two-fold. First, peripheral smears may be falsely negative before red blood cells are infected and later during schizongony when infected red blood cells are sequestered in the capillary beds. Second, the peripheral smear may be "falsely" positive in the sense that the presence of parasites in a blood smear from a febrile patient in an endemic area does not necessarily mean that the symptoms are due to malaria. Most school-aged children in holoendemic areas will have malaria parasites in the blood all the time. Thus, there is no specific approach to diagnosing clinical disease in this situation. In highly endemic areas, patients are treated on the basis of clinical symptoms alone. Usually a clinician, quite appropriately and in accordance with the Integrated Management of Childhood Illness (IMCI) guidelines, will give antimalarials to any child with fever. Such an approach may be necessary to provide early treatment to young children with severe malaria, but also can result in overdiagnosis, the misuse of antimalarials, and the inappropriate treatment of other causes of fever.

Many efforts have been expended to develop rapid methods of diagnosis that do not involve such demanding discipline and technical skills. A variety of immunochromatographic assays have been developed that detect a variety of malaria antigens, including histidine-rich protein 2 (HRP2) and lactate dehydrogenase (LDH).[116] These rapid diagnostic tests have been designed for use as dipsticks and are easy to use in health centers without equipment and with minimal training. Trials of a dipstick assay based upon antigen capture of HRP2 antigen (ParaSight-F test) showed high sensitivity and specificity with moderate parasite densities but reduced sensitivity at lower parasite densities.[117] The use of simple, inexpensive, and rapid diagnostic tests for malaria may be of increasing importance as countries in Africa shift from the use of low-cost antimalarials (chloroquine and sulphadoxine/pyrimethamine) to more expensive drugs (artemisinin-based combination therapy) in the face of widespread drug resistance.

Although not appropriate for the diagnosis of malaria in endemic areas, the use of polymerase chain reaction (PCR)–based assays can provide high sensitivity in persons with low-level parasitemia. These molecular diagnostic tools can distinguish infections with multiple *Plasmodia* species and can provide quantitative measures using real-time PCR that may prove useful in following responses to treatment.[118] PCR-based genotyping is valuable in the analysis of malaria parasites in drug efficacy trials by distinguishing recrudescences from new reinfections. Molecular epidemiology also assists in analyzing parasite populations during and after vaccine trials and changes in parasite populations resulting from vector control or environmental alterations.[119]

Treatment

The history of drug treatment of malaria goes back hundreds of years. In the early 1600s, Jesuit missionaries brought back to Europe cinchona bark used by Peruvian healers against fevers for generations. In 1820, the active ingredient was identified as the alkaloid quinine,[1,4] the first highly active drug against a specific infection known to man that continues as an important therapeutic agent for drug-resistant falciparum malaria. In China, extracts of the plant *Artemisia annua* (wormwood) have been in use for centuries; recently a family of highly effective antimalarials, the artemisinins, has been derived from this plant and is coming into widespread use especially in combination with other antimalarials for drug-resistant malaria.

At the time of the Second World War, several compounds were found to be highly effective against malaria, including chloroquine, primaquine, and sulfadoxine-pyrimethamine. Chloroquine was synthesized in the late 1930s in Germany. During the war, the Allies captured some chloroquine and found it to be highly effective against malaria.[1,8] Chloroquine is rapidly absorbed after oral administration and is active against the asexual stages of all human species except for strains of *P. falciparum* that have become resistant. Chloroquine interferes with the degradation of haem, allowing the accumulation of toxic metabolic products that kill the parasite within the red blood cell. In appropriate doses, it is well tolerated even when taken for long periods, and it is safe for young children and pregnant women. The only important side effect is intense pruritis reported uniquely but frequently by black Africans. Because of low toxicity, low cost, and effectiveness, chloroquine was the drug of choice to treat malaria for decades following World War II. Only after parasite resistance to chloroquine was demonstrated (see below) were serious efforts focused on developing alternative antimalarials.

Primaquine was developed by the US Army during World War II. It is the only drug effective against sporozoites and the hepatic forms, and it can be used to prevent infection in the liver (referred to as a "causal" prophylaxis) and to eliminate the hypnozoite stages of *P. vivax* and *P. ovale* that lead to relapse (antirelapse treatment).[120,121] It is also effective in eliminating gametocytes and theoretically could play a role in reducing transmission and preventing the spread of drug-resistant strains. Primaquine causes hemolysis in persons with glucose-6-phosphate dehydrogenase (G6PD) deficiency, common in those of African and Mediterranean descent.

Sulfadoxine-pyrimethamine (Fansidar, SP), originally developed and promoted for its efficacy against chloroquine-resistant *P. falciparum*, has been widely used for treatment to replace chloroquine in areas of drug resistance. Both compounds inhibit enzymes in the folic acid synthesis pathway. Because it is single-dose therapy and inexpensive, SP is widely used in Africa to treat malaria, is the preferred antimalarial for pregnant women, and can be used for intermittent prophylactic treatment of young children. Adverse reactions, some which are severe—including Stevens-Johnson syndrome—have been reported when used for prophylaxis.

Chloroquine and sulfadoxine-pyrimethamine have been the most commonly used drugs to treat malaria in Africa, but widespread drug resistance has significantly reduced their effectiveness. Although several other antimalarial drugs are available and have been used alone or in combination, no widely used, new antimalarials have been developed in decades.

Mefloquine, a synthetic compound structurally related to quinine and quinidine, was developed for its activity against chloroquine-resistant *P. falciparum* by the US Army in the late 1960s. Mefloquine has an unusually long half-life and is used for chemoprophylaxis and for treatment in combination with artesunate in Thailand. However, resistance to mefloquine has emerged in Southeast Asia. Frequent reports of adverse mental reactions have led to reduction in its use.

Artemisinin and related compounds (e.g., artesunate, arthemether), the active agent of the Chinese herbal medicine, are metabolized to the active form, dihydroartemisinin, and act by inhibiting a calcium-pumping enzyme *P. falciparum* ATP6. These drugs quickly clear blood-stage parasites and gametocytes and provide a rapid clinical response. Importantly, resistance to artemisinins has not been observed yet. When used alone, however, recrudescence is common, and so these drugs are usually combined with other antimalarials.

The most significant change in the treatment of malaria has not been the introduction of novel antimalarials but the use of older drugs in combination. Because of rapid and widespread emergence of resistant parasites in Southeast Asia, combination therapy, particularly of artesunate and mefloquine, has been used there for many years. In sub-Saharan Africa combination therapy has been introduced much more recently. Not only is combination therapy more effective in regions where resistance to chloroquine and sulfadoxine-pyrimethamine is widespread, but also combination therapy can improve compliance by shortening the duration of therapy. Importantly, combination therapy can decrease the risk of resistant mutations arising during therapy, similar to the principles guiding combination therapy for HIV-1 infection and tuberculosis. Many combinations of antimalarials have been used. Some combinations do not include an artemisinin, such as clindamycin/quinine, chlorproguanil/dapsone, and atovaquone/proguanil. However, the most widely used combinations include an artemsinin, referred to as artemisinin-based combination therapy (ACT). Examples include artemether/lumefantrine (available as a fixed-dose formulation), artesunate/amodiaquine, and artesunate/mefloquine. The major disadvantage of ACT is the high cost of artemisinin derivatives.

Drug Resistance

The emergence and spread of drug-resistant malaria, particularly of chloroquine- and sulfadoxine-pyrimethamine-resistant *P. falciparum*, are of major public health importance and likely responsible for the doubling of child mortality attributable to malaria in parts of Africa.[122] These once highly effective, affordable, and safe drugs are no longer useful in many malaria endemic regions, forcing countries to switch to more expensive artemisinin-based combination therapies. Resistance to more recently introduced antimalarials, such as mefloquine and atovaquone, developed quickly, and many experts believe it is only a matter of time before resistance develops to artemisinins. The emergence of drug resistance to the artemisinins may be delayed because of their short half-life and ability to reduce gametocyte carriage. Antimalarial drug resistance is largely a problem with *P. falciparum* infection, although chloroquine-resistant *P. vivax* is prevalent in Papua New Guinea and Irian Jaya. Clinically relevant drug resistance in *P. malariae* and *P. ovale* has not been documented.[123]

Many factors contribute to the emergence and spread antimalarial drug resistance, including pharmacologic properties of the drug, host immunity, parasite genetics, and transmission characteristics. For example, use of anti-malarials with a prolonged half-life (such as sulfadoxine-pyrimethamine), poor compliance, or inappropriate use can expose parasites to subtherapeutic drug levels, thus increasing the risk of emergence of drug-resistant parasites. An effective host immune response can clear drug-resistant parasites that escape being killed, making the transmission of drug resistance more likely in immunologically naive hosts.[123]

Antimalarial drug resistance can be assessed in several ways, including evaluation of therapeutic responses in vivo, measurement of parasite growth ex vivo, and identification of genetic mutations associated with resistance. However, there is great need for a rapid, simple, and inexpensive field test to detect antimalarial drug resistance. The traditional method of in vivo resistance testing was developed by the WHO.[120,121] Infected patients are given an antimalarial drug according to an established regime, and parasite counts are performed at the start of therapy, at 24 hours, at 7 days, and at 28 days after the start of treatment. If parasites are not detectable at the end of 7 days (and still not detectable at 28 days), the malaria parasites are considered sensitive to the drug. If there is clearance of parasites at 7 days, but recrudescence 8 or more days after the start of treatment, the parasites are stage RI resistant. If there is reduction in parasitemia but not complete clearance at 7 days, the parasites are considered stage RII resistant. If there is no evidence of response, the parasites are considered to be fully resistant, RIII.

In the absence of molecular epidemiologic tools, however, distinguishing recrudescence from reinfection is not possible. To overcome this limitation in regions of intense transmission, WHO introduced a modified protocol based on clinical response rather than parasitemia. Adequate clinical response is distinguished from early and late treatment failure. A limitation in interpreting in vivo testing is that persons with immunity will improve even if the parasites are moderately resistant to the drug.

In vitro testing of *P. falciparum* drug resistance relies on short-term culture of malaria parasites. Blood from a parasitemic individual is prepared for culture and incubated with increasing concentrations of an antimalarial drug. Several assay end points have been developed to measure parasite growth in the presence of different drug concentrations, including schizont maturation, radioisotope incorporation, and detection of the parasite enzyme LDH or HRP2.[124] The advantages of in vitro resistance testing are that these assays are independent of individual variation in drug levels and immune responses.

In vivo and in vitro test systems provide two complementary approaches to determine drug resistance of malaria parasites and are used to monitor the distribution and levels of drug resistance in particular geographic areas. This monitoring provides a basis for judging effective antimalarials for use in the area, but afford little basis for certainty in any particular individual. Particularly for severe malaria in children, which strikes with great speed, neither of these test systems is useful for making immediate decisions about what treatment should be provided for the individual patient.

Genetic polymorphisms are associated with drug resistance and are best characterized for chloroquine and sulfadoxine-pyrimethamine resistance. Chloroquine resistance is associated with mutations in the *pfcrt* gene that codes for a membrane transporter protein that allows the parasite to excrete chloroquine so that intracellular concentrations do not reach toxic levels.[125] One particular mutation, the substitution of threonine for lysine in codon 76 (Th76), is highly associated with chloroquine resistance. More is known about the mutations that decrease the binding affinity of *P. falciparum* enzymes to sulfadoxine-pyrimethamine. At least five different point mutations in the gene encoding the enzyme dihydropteroate synthetase (*dhps*) confer resistance to sulfadoxine. Resistance to pyrimethamine is caused by specific point mutations in the gene encoding dihydrofolate reductase (*dhfr*). Accumulation of three or four mutations confers high-level resistance to pyrimethamine. Mutations in the *pfmdr1* gene is associated with resistance to mefloquine, chloroquine, and other antimalarials.[126]

Although not feasible for case management, identification of these polymorphisms in clinical isolates is a useful but expensive tool for monitoring drug resistance in populations. However, the identification of specific mutations does not always correlate with in vivo drug resistance. For example, the presence of the Th76 mutation in the *pfcrt* gene predicted only one third of treatment failures, although the absence of this mutation was highly predictive of chloroquine susceptibility.[127] Drug resistance and parasite fitness are likely conferred by multiple mutations, all of which have not yet been identified.

Epidemiology of Drug Resistance in Malaria

Chloroquine resistance in *P. falciparum* was first reported in the late 1950s in South America in areas between Venezuela and Colombia and in Southeast Asia along the Thai-Cambodian and Thai-Burma borders.[128-131] Although it was nearly 20 years later that resistance was first demonstrated in Africa,[132] chloroquine-resistant malaria is now widespread in Africa. Only in Central America and the Caribbean has chloroquine resistance not yet been documented. Along the Thai-Cambodian border, *P. falciparum* was first noted to be resistant to sulfadoxine-pyrimethamine in the mid-1960s, with more widespread resistance reported in the late 1970s after the drug was introduced into the malaria control program. In Africa, resistance to sulfadoxine-pyrimethamine was first noted in the late 1980s, with high-level resistance and treatment failures most common in East Africa. Mefloquine resistance also was first observed near the Thai-Cambodian border in the late 1980s. Clinically significant resistance to mefloquine, however, is rare in Africa.

The origins and mechanisms of spread of drug-resistant strains of *P. falciparum* are of great public health importance. Chloroquine resistance is conferred by a complex set of genetic mutations, making multiple independent origins unlikely. Resistance to chloroquine appears to have originated only four times, and to have spread from Asia to Africa.[133,134] Because of the less complex nature of resistance to sulfadoxine-pyrimethamine, and the ease in which resistance mutations can be induced in the laboratory, resistance to sulfadoxine-pyrimethamine was thought to have multiple, independent origins. However, genotyping of microsatellite markers flanking the *dhfr* gene suggests that high-level resistance to sulfadoxine-pyrimethamine (i.e., triple or quadruple mutant *dhfr* alleles) originated in Southeast Asia and subsequently spread to Africa.[135]

Of considerable debate is whether drug resistance evolves faster in areas of high or low malaria transmission.[136,137] This question has important public health implications, as interventions to reduce transmission could affect rates of drug resistance. Lower transmission was hypothesized to increase rates of drug resistance by enhancing parasite inbreeding, thus lowering the rate of genetic recombination and increasing the probability that drug resistance mutations would spread in the parasite population. Inbreeding is more frequent when transmission rates are lower as infection with multiple different strains is less likely. The frequent emergence of resistance along the Thai-Cambodian border supports the hypothesis that lower transmission facilitates the emergence of drug resistance. However, the true situation is more complex than this simple analysis suggests.[136,138] Reduced transmission in Zimbabwe through residual insecticide spraying of households was associated with suppressed levels of drug resistance, suggesting that malaria control measures that reduce transmission will not increase drug resistance.[139]

Vaccines Against Malaria

Prospects for a successful vaccine against malaria have been considered bright for several decades; unfortunately, they have remained prospects and to date no vaccine has been sufficiently effective to warrant widespread use. However, progress has been made. Vaccine development has largely focused on *P. falciparum*, although efforts have been made to develop vaccines against *P. vivax*. The overwhelming evidence that humans develop protective immune responses against *P. falciparum* when repeatedly exposed to infection indicates that development of an effective vaccine should be possible. By the age of 6 years, most children in holoendemic regions have acquired substantial immunity. These children are protected from severe and fatal malaria, even though they may have parasitemia and occasional bouts of fever. The population will have paid a high price for this protection, however, since under-5 mortality from malaria is very high. Early studies by Ian McGregor et al. demonstrated that serum from immune adults in the Gambia could be used to treat young children with malaria in East Africa.[140] In the early 1970s, David Clyde and others demonstrated that injection of sporozoites derived from irradiated *P. falciparum*-infected mosquitoes provided protective immunity against challenge.[141,142] However, the immunologic basis of protection induced by natural infection or irradiated sporozoites is not completely understood.

In addition to the empirical evidence for an effective acquired immune response, important advances have taken place in sequencing the genomes of *P. falciparum*, the *Anopheles gambiae* vector, and the human host, with hopes that genomics and proteomics will spur novel vaccine development. In addition, progress has been made in understanding the immunology and pathogenesis of malaria, and advances have been made in vaccinology. Subunit vaccines composed of synthetic peptides or recombinant proteins, newer vaccine strategies (e.g., prime-boost and the targeting of dendritic cells), and novel adjuvants and protein conjugates give hope that the formidable impediments to malaria vaccine development will be overcome.

Several high-risk groups would greatly benefit from a malaria vaccine that decreases morbidity and mortality, including young children and primagravida women in endemic areas. In addition, immunologically naive travelers to malaria endemic regions would benefit from a vaccine that prevents infection. These different risk groups necessitate different types of vaccine. The different stages of the malaria parasite outlined in Figure 26-2 provide potential targets for immunization. Vaccine development has focused largely upon three parasite stages: (1) preerythrocytic sporozoite and hepatic forms to prevent infection; (2) asexual erythrocytic forms to reduce morbidity and mortality; and (3) sexual forms within the mosquito to prevent transmission. By the end of 2004, over 90 malaria vaccine candidates were in various stages of development, with over 40 in clinical trials in humans.

Much effort has gone into development of sporozoite vaccines because immunity was induced by immunization with irradiated sporozoites,[141,143] even though there is little evidence of effective natural immunity to sporozoites. A single sporozoite that evades the immune response could potentially generate thousands of merozoites capable of infecting red blood cells. Efforts to develop a preerythrocytic vaccine have focused largely on targeting the circumsporozoite (CS) protein, a major component of the sporozoite surface. One of the more promising CS vaccines, RTS,S/AS02A, consists of recombinantly expressed *P. falciparum* CS peptides fused to a portion of the hepatitis B virus surface antigen and administered with an adjuvant (AS02A). In a much publicized clinical trial, both the first clinical episode of malaria and episodes of severe malaria were reduced in Mozambican children for 6 months following vaccination.[144] However, protective efficacy for the first clinical episode of malaria was only 30%, and antibody titers decayed rapidly. In addition to this subunit vaccine, other vaccine constructs targeting the preerythrocytic stages include using viral vectors or plasmid DNA to express recombinant CS, thrombospondin-related adhesion protein (TRAP), or liver-stage antigen (LSA). Other approaches include pursuit of a radiation-attenuated sporozoite vaccine and vaccines based on genetically modified sporozoites.[145,146]

Vaccines against asexual blood stages of *P. falciparum* would seem a promising approach, as passive transfer of immunity has been shown with antimerozoite immunoglobulin.[140] However, as described above, the *P. falciparum* genome contains a number of highly polymorphic gene families, most importantly the *var* genes encoding the surface protein PfEMP1 that allows successive waves of parasites to express new variant surface antigens. Thus, antibodies directed against these variable surface proteins are unlikely to remain effective for long. There appears to be, however, a limited number of conserved surface antigens against which protective immunity can be established.[147] Children surviving malaria eventually mobilize a sufficiently diverse set of antibodies that provide protection against severe disease. In holoendemic Africa, where the entomological inoculation rate may be hundreds a year, protective immunity takes place over several years, representing thousands of inoculated parasites. The hope is to develop a vaccine that can induce similar levels of immunity in weeks or months, and by age 6 months rather than 6 years. A synthetic peptide vaccine SPf66, directed at blood-stage parasites, was promising in early trials in South America and Tanzania but later was found to have little efficacy in other trials in Africa.[148] Most current vaccine candidates against blood-stage parasites are directed toward merozoite surface proteins (e.g., MSP-1) or apical membrane antigens (AMA).

Finally, substantial work has been done on vaccines directed against gametocytes that block parasite development within the mosquito, termed "transmission blocking" vaccines. These vaccines represent an interesting approach in that the vaccine would not protect the vaccinated individual but would reduce transmission from those who are infected, analogous to the use of residual insecticides in households. Preclinical studies have demonstrated that antibodies against sexual-stage antigens expressed by *P. vivax* and *P. falciparum* can prevent the development of infectious sporozoites in the mosquito salivary gland. Actual interruption of malaria transmission in communities, however, would require sustained high levels of vaccine coverage.[149] The potential usefulness of this kind of vaccine is discussed below.

Approaches to Control

The complexity of the malaria transmission cycle provides a wide variety of opportunities to stop or slow transmission of parasites. Historically, though based on the flawed theory of miasma that disease was caused by "evil winds," the major public health approach to malaria was the establishment of communities away from low-lying swamps to reduce vector contact.[8]

Approaches to malaria control include a variety of strategies directed against the vector and parasite. Detailed knowledge of the ecological and epidemiological circumstances, and of the human economic, cultural, and social situation, is as vital for determining how best to intervene as are the specifics of the vector, parasite, and intervention tool itself. Control strategies that may be of particular value in Africa and new tools to support them are outlined in Table 26-2.

Vector Control Methods

The array of vector control methods is based upon attacking the mosquito in various stages of its life cycle: control of breeding sites to reduce vector density by drainage and waterway engineering and application of specific larvacides and biological agents; the use of mosquito netting, screens, and repellents for personal protection from bites; aerosol distribution of insecticides to reduce adult mosquito densities; killing adult mosquitoes after they have taken a blood meal by use of residual insecticides within households; and the development of insecticide-impregnated bed nets and curtains that kill or reduce those adults seeking a blood meal.

Breeding Site and Larva Control

After the discovery of the role of mosquito vectors, efforts were directed toward elimination or reduction of vector breeding sites by swamp drainage and environmental control, including water source diversion, water management with flushing and sluicing, covering of wells, clearing vegetation, and reforestation. DDT, other insecticides, and larvacides were additional breeding site control methods, particularly in urban settings. In addition to these

TABLE 26-2 Control Strategies for Malaria in Africa

What can be done now:
- General infrastructure/institution improvement
- Role of vector control with
  - Environmental improvements to reduce breeding
  - Impregnated bed nets
  - Personal protection
- Household use of antimalarials for those under 5 years of age
- Intermittent preventive treatment for infants and pregnant women
  - Monitoring for antimalarial resistance
- Strengthened nutrition programs
- Improved immunization coverage especially in remote areas in anticipation of effective vaccines

New tools:
- Vaccine development, especially asexual phase
- Drug development and acceleration of those in the pipeline
- Understanding of the molecular biology of the parasite
- Understanding of the sporogonic cycle to aid in reengineering of the anopheline
- Improved entomological field methods for better understanding of microepidemiological variation
- Understanding mechanisms of drug resistance and factors that contribute to its spread
- Better diagnostic tests that rapidly and inexpensively indicate drug resistance

engineering and insecticide approaches, various biological methods including larva predators, such as larvivarous fish and bacteria such as *B. thuriagensis* that produce specific antilarval toxins, are selectively used. Approaches to vector control through reduction of breeding sites continue to play a major role in malaria control strategies.

Adult Vector Control

The use of DDT for household residual spraying had great impact on malaria control in many areas of the world, and its initial successes served as the rationale for the eradication efforts in the 1950s and 1960s. The conceptual foundation for eradication through use of residual insecticides was based upon anopheline resting behavior after a blood meal as discussed in previous sections of this chapter: the success of this approach depends upon the biting and resting behavior of the mosquito and upon the willingness of the human population to have their households sprayed. The effect is upon the mosquito that has already bitten an infected human in the household and rests nearby after engorgement. No protection is provided to those in the treated household itself. Instead, the protection is to those in other households whom these mosquitoes would have bitten for their next blood meal. The dilemma is that to reduce transmission, almost all households in the neighborhood must be sprayed. The higher the intensity of transmission, the more difficult it is to achieve a sufficient level of coverage. Success with residual household spraying was achieved in large areas of Europe, Asia, and Latin America, but in areas with EIRs of dozens per year as in much of tropical Africa, control by residual spraying alone was not possible.

But where residual spaying was successful, a different obstacle to its use arose: anopheline resistance to DDT became widespread. Although other insecticides were substituted, they were generally difficult to formulate for residual spraying and were much more expensive and toxic to humans and other mammals. Unfortunately, DDT was also an excellent agricultural insecticide, and its widespread use in agriculture has been implicated as the cause of anopheline resistance. Residual spraying of DDT for malaria control required a minute amount of pesticide that was not used outside and did not disperse into the environment as it was absorbed by the wall material. Because of this, it is felt that antimalaria use of DDT was not a factor in the development of anopheline resistance nor in the devastation of bird populations by DDT thinning of egg shells. The ecological effects of agricultural use led to major restrictions and, in many countries, complete banning of DDT for any use. As production dropped, the cost of DDT increased. Sadly enough, these restrictions, and economic realities, affected antimalarial residual spraying programs, curtailing an effective public health tool.

Notwithstanding these problems, the use of household residual insecticides, even DDT in some countries, continues as an important vector control measure in many countries.

Insecticide-Impregnated Treated Bed Nets

In the last 10 years increasing experience with insecticide-treated impregnated bed nets (ITNs), including four large-scale randomized, controlled trials in different areas of Africa,[150-153] has demonstrated that their use leads to reductions in transmission, clinical disease, and overall childhood mortality. Although not all studies have demonstrated such positive benefits,[154] there seemed sufficient evidence for the Roll Back Malaria global partnership to recommend ITNs as a key method for reducing the burden of malaria in high-transmission areas of Africa. At the Abuja Summit in 2000, representatives from 44 African countries agreed to a goal of providing ITNs for 60% of those at risk of malaria, especially pregnant women and children under 5 years of age.[155]

Despite this strong support for concerted action, there remained serious issues to be resolved. None of the trials had been conducted in an area of intense year-round transmission, and scrutiny of the completed trials showed a trend toward decreasing efficacy with increasing intensity of transmission. Additional concerns were raised about the feasibility of such a level of coverage and its sustainability. Surveys from 29 African countries conducted between 1998 and 2001 found that an average of only 2% of under-5 children were sleeping under an ITN. For these reasons, a large-scale, randomized controlled trial was carried out in an area of intense perennial transmission in western Kenya with special focus on a multidisciplinary approach to community sustainability and equitable distribution of benefits.[156] This work in western Kenya confirmed the value of ITNs in reducing all-cause postneonatal mortality, maternal mortality, stillbirths and prematurity, and all-cause hospital admissions in a cost-effective manner. Under the conditions of this study, it was possible to achieve the high level of community cooperation with ITNs needed for effectiveness. The three key determinants of effectiveness were coverage (proportion of households with ITNs), adherence (the proportion of individuals properly deploying ITNs each night), and net treatment care (the proportion of nets properly treated with insecticide). These three determinants should serve as the foundation for implementation of national ITN programs, and efforts should continue to improve the intervention tools (the net, the insecticide, and methods for durable treatment and retreatment) and their deployment.[157]

Personal and Household Protection

Repellants of various types, protective clothing, screening, bed nets, and other forms of personal protection against the bite of mosquitoes are all of importance and widely recommended, but aside from educational campaigns and exhortations this approach has never been viewed as a major component in malaria control programs.

Treatment Strategies

Passive Case Finding and Treatment

In tropical Africa, the principal approach of antimalaria programs has been through the use of antimalarial drugs in passive case finding and treatment of those who present to clinics or pharmacies with symptoms of malaria.[158] Health workers in Africa are taught about the major symptoms of malaria and the need to treat it promptly with an appropriate antimalarial drug. Treatment of malaria in childhood is accorded a prominent place in the Integrated Management of Childhood Illnesses (IMCI).[159] This important provider-oriented, facility-based approach focuses upon assessment and treatment of the major causes of child mortality.

Unfortunately, severe malaria kills children so rapidly in most of Africa that often mothers cannot get their children to facility-based treatment in time. An effective case treatment strategy for reducing under-5 mortality must include community mobilization and education for families, particularly for the mother or caretaker, to understand the urgency to obtain treatment of their sick child. The range of IMCI activities extends beyond the health facility to include critical family and community aspects, but so far there has been little impact in reducing under-5 mortality from malaria.

Home Treatment

A relatively untried strategy for timely provision of antimalarials is to teach mothers to recognize symptoms of malaria in their children and to treat immediately at home. If mothers could be taught to recognize and promptly treat their children, and if they had an appropriate antimalarial supply immediately at hand, it seems reasonable to expect that many children could be saved in high-transmission areas that are dying under current health care conditions.

This approach was tested in a randomized trial in Tigray, Ethiopia. Village-based mother coordinators (MCs) received training and supervision to teach neighboring mothers to recognize symptoms of malaria in their children and to promptly administer the antimalarial. Overall under-5 mortality was reduced by 40% at very low cost.[160]

Home treatment of children by their mothers had not been seriously considered as a viable approach by most malaria experts because of concerns that "illiterate women" would misuse, sell, or waste the drugs; that they would not know when or at what dose to give it; and that indiscriminant use of antimalarials would lead to increased drug resistance. But this study gave dramatic evidence to the contrary, demonstrating the high degree of effectiveness of home treatment by mothers in the circumstances in Tigray.

The special circumstances in Tigray included the following: the presence of chloroquine-sensitive falciparum malaria; a disciplined and coherent population related to the rigors imposed by 20 years of conflict; and lack of alternative employment opportunities for the MCs. Resistance to chloroquine in high-transmission areas is now virtually universal; the combination antimalarial drugs required are more expensive and have a higher rate of adverse reactions. But the rationale for home treatment by mothers (or caretakers) remains valid as do the requirements for teaching mothers to recognize malaria, to administer the correct dose, and to assure a home-based supply of antimalarial drug. These requirements may well be met in other ways than through the MC approach that worked so well in Tigray. Depending upon local circumstances, the teaching of mothers and supplying of antimalarials could involve women's groups, NGOs, and various information, education, and communication (IEC) programs. Training private drug vendors about appropriate drugs and dosages for malaria treatment may be a useful supplement, but the primary need is to empower mothers to treat their children at home.

Prophylaxis

Prophylaxis with antimalarials has been the standard procedure for travelers and short-term residents of endemic areas. It has also been an effective approach for selected "captive" populations, such as plantation workers or miners. From the public health viewpoint, prophylaxis has also been shown to be highly beneficial in pregnancy, both for the pregnant woman and for the fetus, especially for first and second pregnancies.[105] This strategy now has been replaced by intermittent preventive (full) treatment (IPT) that involves administration of a full-treatment course each month during antenatal care.

The role of prophylaxis for infants and young children is still not clear. In pilot studies in the Gambia, prophylaxis was more effective than use of nearby primary health care facilities for treatment of children. The reason was that the rapid course of severe malaria did not give time for mothers to procure treatment.[93] There have been two major concerns about antimalarial prophylaxis: it might suppress development of an immune response, and it might favor development of drug resistance, but there is little firm evidence for either. Even in tightly run prophylaxis programs, little retardation in development of immunological defenses has been observed. Mathematical modeling could help to determine the proportion of the parasite population in a human population that would be affected by prophylaxis of under-2-year-olds and provide some indication of likelihood of enhancing resistance. The optimal age for reducing or stopping prophylaxis in children has not been established, but certainly before age 5 would seem reasonable for most areas. In many respects, household treatment of possible malaria symptoms as discussed above would be equivalent, would not inhibit host defense mechanisms, would require less antimalarial distribution, and would provide for a natural stopping age for use of antimalarials.

Intermittent Preventive Treatment

An alternative strategy to prevent malaria in young children is the use of intermittent preventive treatment. This strategy differs from chemoprophylaxis in that infants and children receive periodic treatment doses of antimalarials, rather than continuous prophylactic regimens. Intermittent treatment can be offered at the time of routine childhood immunization, a strategy referred to as intermittent preventive treatment in infants (IPTi). Two large trials of intermittent preventive treatment have been conducted in Tanzania. In the first, children were randomly assigned to receive sulphadoxine-pyrimethamine or placebo at 2, 3, and 9 months of age along with routine vaccinations.[161] During the first year of life, the protective efficacy against clinical malaria was 59%, and severe anemia was reduced in half. In the second trial, amodiaquine was administered three times over 6 months to infants in the first year of life.[162] The protective efficacy against malaria fevers was 65% and 67% for anemia. The logic would suggest that IPT need not be limited to infancy, but rather that IPT be given to every child under age 5 when seen for any other reason. No evidence exists that IPTi interferes with the immune responses to childhood vaccines, although this requires further study.[163] As with chemoprophylaxis, intermittent preventive treatment potentially could affect drug resistance rates and the development of protective immunity. Furthermore, the low childhood vaccination coverage rates in parts of sub-Saharan Africa need to be increased to maximize the impact of IPTi.[164]

A major threat to any strategy using antimalarials is that of parasite resistance. The monitoring of parasite sensitivity to drugs must be a component of all strategies that involve antimalarials. As discussed above in the section on treatment of malaria, no antimalarial drug should be used alone. But the use of combination therapy does increase both the cost and risk of adverse reactions.

Strategies for Vaccine Use

Even after development of one or several vaccines, the most appropriate vaccine and its use will depend upon the epidemiological situation. A sporozoite vaccine is designed to prevent infection. A potential danger, however, is that if any sporozoite bypasses host defenses and invades a liver cell, a full-blown malaria episode could follow. An antisporozoite vaccine is likely to have a limited duration of protection and to have limited, if any, natural boosting. Thus, it could be useful for visitors to endemic areas, but would not be as effective for those living in endemic areas.

An asexual stage vaccine, however, would mimic natural immunity, and could be targeted to children and pregnant women in holoendemic areas. Natural infection could provide the booster effect. In such a situation, it could be counterproductive to reduce transmission as the transmission would be the method for vaccine boosting.

The use of vaccines directed against the sexual, gamete forms (the "transmission blocking" vaccine) is more problematic: it might be useful as an additional control component in areas of relatively unstable malaria where other control measures are in place. It might be a particularly useful supplement to reduce the spread of drug-resistant parasites. Mathematical modeling could help in working through circumstances in which this type of vaccine would be advantageous. It could only be used where malaria control efforts were focused on reduction or elimination of transmission; it would be counterproductive to use with an asexual, blood-form vaccine that depends upon the booster effect of natural immunity to maintain an effective level of immunity.

Although this section has discussed approaches to control that are separately focused on vector control, antimalarial treatment, or use of vaccines, most malaria control programs need to use a combination of antimalarial measures tailored to fit the epidemiological and ecological circumstances.

The Future

Doing Better with What We Have

The first priority for reducing the continuing, appallingly high mortality from malaria in Africa is to improve the use of currently available tools. To do so requires strengthened planning based upon detailed epidemiological data combined with improved management and operational research capacity of the health system, particularly that of primary health care and its support systems at the local community and district levels. It also requires basic human development improvements including strengthened infrastructural and institutional support for enhanced employment opportunities, strengthened women's groups, better access to microcredit, augmented community and family education, and better communication and transport systems. These general development improvements are needed because the strategies as elaborated above to achieve effective malaria control require understanding and concerted action at the household and community levels. The fundamental institutional and profound structural reconstruction required to achieve these basic changes is only recently being enacted in a handful of African countries. The sectorwide action programs (SWAPs) in which all donors contribute to a common "basket" for which host country decision makers are responsible should assist in these changes when undertaken by countries with a sufficient technical and political competence to effectively use and account for the funding.[165] Globally, the need for improved equity to generate the capacity for all countries and locales to make decisions for themselves not only must be recognized, but the wealthy nations (and their voters) must be convinced that it is in their long-term interest.

Operational research to support better planning and management, largely country and even locale specific, is needed with special attention to quality management and support supervision to enhance health worker performance. In particular, if the antimalaria strategies discussed above are to be effective, more work must be devoted to the following:

- Approaches to training of trainers for distribution and use of anti-malarials by mothers in the household to treat their children.
- Community-based programs for distribution, use, and continuing retreatment of insecticide-treated bed nets.
- Increased monitoring for drug resistance.
- Support for communities to work through their own approaches to control malaria, including reduction of vector habitats, especially in areas with marginal or highly variable transmission.
- Continued improvement in immunization coverage, particularly to the underserved populations in anticipation of an effective antimalarial vaccine.
- Add antimalarial distribution at every immunization and at every clinic visit of under-fives.

New Tools at Last

Certainly, better intervention tools are needed. Research on nearly all aspects of control measures against parasites and vectors as outlined above should be valuable, but until quite recently, very little had been done. The most important reason was that global research agencies had put paltry sums to this effort. With the publication of *Investing in Health Research and Development* in 1996 that gave some sense of priority for global health research,[166] and the initiation of Roll Back Malaria in 1998, there has been a renewal of interest in malaria research. With the MIM, the Malaria Vaccine Initiative, the Global Fund against AIDS, Malaria, and Tuberculosis, and further support from the Gates Foundation, there is now a much stronger international effort focused on malaria research.

Basic research priorities include the following:

- Development of asexual phase vaccines, especially now that health infrastructures in many African countries are sufficiently developed to deliver childhood vaccines to at least 75% of their population. Many consider this the first priority.
- Continued efforts for drug development.
- Continued work to understand the molecular biology of the parasite, especially the metabolic pathways contributing to virulence that might be amenable to rational drug development.
- Further work on the much neglected sporogonic cycle, which may aid in efforts to reengineer anophelines as discussed below.
- Continued development of mathematical modeling done in direct concert with field investigations may facilitate a deeper understanding

of the critical quantitative relationships involved in transmission control.

- Improved entomological field methods for better understanding of microepidemiological variation and for local anopheline control efforts.
- Better understanding of the mechanisms underlying drug resistance and factors contributing to its spread will likely require a combined understanding of genetics, entomology, and epidemiology.
- Simple, inexpensive, rapid, and robust diagnostic tests that can provide for quantification of parasite density and that can indicate drug sensitivity (or resistance).
- Reengineering anophelines so they do not adequately support the parasite through completion of the sporogonic cycle.

Regarding the last point, progress has been made in developing the techniques to genetically modify mosquitoes, including the germline transformation of mosquitoes and the development of transgenic mosquitoes that express antiparasitic genes in their midgut.[167,168] However, much remains to be learned about how best to introduce genetically modified mosquitoes into communities and how anopheline population genetics will be altered. In addition, numerous ethical and political issues remain unresolved regarding the release of genetically modified insects. In the long run, reservations remain about the likely success of this approach. Species such as the *A. gambiae* complex have so effectively evolved through the centuries in concert with human *Plasmodia* species, and have demonstrated such enormous capacity to rapidly adapt to a wide variety of changing conditions, that successfully displacing them is a major challenge.

Reduction of the continuing high mortality and morbidity from malaria in Africa will require both better use of current control measures (necessitating better epidemiological and ecological information for better planning); better management of control programs; increased direct involvement of families and communities; accelerated research toward vaccines, drugs, and vector control approaches; and fundamental understanding of the biology of parasite, vector, and human host as outlined above. Table 26-2 outlines control strategies for Africa.

References

1. Bruce-Chwatt LJ. History of malaria from prehistory to eradication. In: Wernsdorfer WH, McGregor I, eds. *Malaria: Principles and Practice of Malariology*. Edinburgh: Churchill Livingstone; 1988:1–69.
2. International Development Advisory Board. *Malaria Eradication: Report and Recommendations of the International Development Advisory Board*. International Development Advisory Board; 1956.
3. World Health Organization Expert Committee on Malaria. WHO Technical Report Series No. 357. Geneva, Switzerland: WHO; 1967.
4. Russell PF, West LS, Maxwell RD, MacDonald G. *Practical Malariology*. 2nd ed. Oxford University Press; 1963.
5. World Health Organization. *Re-examination of the Global Strategy of Malaria Eradication*. WHO Official Records No. 176. Geneva, Switzerland: World Health Organization; 1969.

6. Krishna S. Malaria. *BMJ.* 1997;315:730–732.

7. World Health Organization. *Malaria Eradication from the Ninth Plenary Meeting.* Geneva, Switzerland: World Health Organization; 1955.

8. Oaks SC Jr, Mitchell VS, Pearson GW, Carpenter CJ, eds. *Malaria: Obstacles and Opportunities.* Washington, DC: National Academies Press; 1991.

9. Murray CJL, Lopez AD, eds. *Global Comparative Assessments in the Health Sector.* Geneva, Switzerland: World Health Organization; 1994.

10. Beier JC. Malaria parasite development in mosquitoes. *Ann Rev Entomol.* 1998;43:519–543.

11. Morrow RH. The application of a quantitative approach to the assessment of the relative importance of vector and soil-transmitted diseases in Ghana. *Social Science Med.* 1984;19:1039–1049.

12. Ghana Health Assessment Project Team. A quantitative method of assessing the health impact of different diseases in less developed countries. *Int J Epidemiol.* 1981;10:73–80.

13. Jamison DT, et al, eds. *Investing in Health. World Development Report, 1993.* New York, NY: The World Bank, Oxford University Press; 1993.

14. Hyder AA, Rotlant G, Morrow RH. Measuring the burden of disease: healthy life years. *Am J Public Health.* 1998;88:196–202.

15. Miller LH, Mason SJ, Clyde DF, et al. The resistance factor to *Plasmodium vivax* in blacks: the Duffy blood-group genotype, Fy-Fy. *N Engl J Med.* 1976;295:302.

16. Garnham PCC. *Malaria Parasites and Other Hemosporidia.* Oxford, UK: Blackwell Scientific Publications; 1966.

17. Beier JC, Onyango K, Ramadhan M, et al. Quantitation of malaria sporozoites in the salivary glands of wild Afrotropical *Anopheles. Med. Vet. Entomol.* 1991;5:63–70.

18. Pringle G. A quantitative study of naturally acquired malaria infections in *Anopheles gambiae* of East Africa. *Trans Roy Soc Trop Med Hyg.* 1966;60:626–632.

19. Pull JH, Grab B. A simple epidemiological model for evaluating the malaria inoculation rate and the risk of infection in infants. Vol 51. World Health Organization Geneva, Switzerland; 1974;51(5):507–516.

20. MacDonald G. *The Epidemiology and Control of Malaria.* London, UK: Oxford University Press; 1957.

21. Beadle C, McElroy PD, Oster CN. Impact of transmission intensity and age on *Plasmodium falciparum* density and asociated fever implications for malaria vaccine trial design. *J Infect Dis.* 1955;172:1047–1054.

22. Molineaux L, Gramiccia G. *The Garki Project: Research on the Epidemiology and Control of Malaria in the Sudan Savanna of West Africa.* Geneva, Switzerland: World Health Organization; 1980.

23. Krotoski WA, Collins WE, Bray RS, et al. Demonstration of hypnozoites in sporozoite-transmitted *Plasmodium vivax* infection. *Am J Trop Med Hyg.* 1982;31:1291–1293.

24. Schwartz IK. Prevention of malaria. *Infect Dis Clin North Am: Health Issues Int Travelers.* 1992;6:313–331.

25. Mendis N, Sina BJ, Marchesini P, Carter R. The neglected burden of *Plasmodium vivax* malaria. *Am J Trop Med Hyg.* 2001;64:S97–S106.

26. Gardner MJ, Hall N, Fung E, White O, et al. Genome sequence of the human malaria parasite Plasmodium falciparum. *Nature.* 2002;419(6906):498–511.

27. Rowe JA, et al. *J Infect Dis.* 2002;185:1207–1211.
28. Hoffman SL, Subramanian GM, Collins FH, Venter JC. Plasmodium, human and Anopheles genomics and malaria. *Nature.* 2002;415: 702–709.
29. Creasey A, Fenton G, Walker A, et al. Genetic diversity of *Plasmodium falciparum* shows geographic variation. *Am J Trop Med Hyg.* 1990;42:403.
30. Haworth J. The global distribution of malaria and the present control effort. In: Wernsdorfer WH, McGregor I, eds. *Principles and Practice of Malariology.* Edinburgh, UK: Churchill Livingstone; 1988.
31. Holt RA, Subramanian GM, Halpern A, Sutton GG, et al.: The genome sequence of the malaria mosquito *Anopheles gambiae. Science.* 2002; 298:129–149.
32. Christophides GK, Vlachou D, Kafatos FC. Comparative and functional genomics of the innate immune system in the malaria vector Anopheles gambiae. *Immunol Rev.* 2004;198:127–148.
33. MacDonald G. The measurement of malaria transmission. *Proc Roy Soc Med.* 1955;48:295–301.
34. Appawu MA, et al. Detection of malaria sporozoties by standard ELISA and VecTestTM dipstick assay in field-collected anopheline mosquitoes from a malaria endemic site in Ghana. *Trop Med Int Health.* 2003;8:1012–1017.
35. Garrett-Jones C. The human blood index of malaria vectors in relation to epidemiological assessment. *Bull WHO.* 1964;30:241–261.
36. Dye C, Lines JD, Curtis CF. A test of the malaria strain theory. *Parisitol Today.* 1996;12:88–89.
37. Dietz K, Molineaux L, Thomas A. A malaria model tested in African savanna. *Bull WHO.* 1974;50:347–357.
38. Metselaar D, van Thiel PM. Classification of malaria. *Trop Geogr Med.* 1959;11:157–161.
39. Molineaux L. The epidemiology of human malaria as an explanation of its distribution including some implications for its control. In: Wernsdorfer WH, McGregor I, eds. *Malaria: Principles and Practices of Malariology.* Edinburgh, UK: Chruchill Livingstone; 1988: 913–998.
40. Najera JA. Malaria and the work of the WHO. *Bull WHO.* 1989;67: 229–243.
41. Miller LH, Baruch DI, Marsh K, Doumbo OK. The pathogenic basis of malaria. *Nature.* 2002;415:673–679.
42. Bryceson AD, Fleming AF, Edington GM. Splenomegaly in northern Nigeria. *Acta Tropica.* 1976;33:185.
43. Fleming AF, Allan NC, Stenhous NS. Splenomegaly and sickle cell trait. *Lancet.* 1968;2:574–575.
44. Hamilton PJS, Morrow RH, Ziegler JL, et al. Absence of sickle-cell trait in patients with tropical splenomegaly syndrome. *Lancet.* 1969; 2:109.
45. Drulhe P, Perignon JL. Mechanisms of defense against *Plasmodium falciparum* asexual blood stages in humans. *Immunology Letters.* 1994;41:115–120.
46. Fleming AF, Storey J, Molineaux L, Iroko EA, Attai EDE. Abnormal haemoglobins in the Sudan Savana of Nigeria. *Ann Trop Med Parasitol.* 1979;73:161–172.
47. Weatherall DJ. Common genetic disorders of the red cell and the 'malaria' hypothesis. *Ann Trop Med Parasitol.* 1987;81:539–548.

48. Miller LH. Impact of malaria on genetic polymorphism and genetic diseases in Africans and African-Americans. *Proc Natl Acad Sciences.* 1994;91:2415–2419.
49. Luzatto L, Nwachuku-Jarret ES, Reddy S. Increased sickling of parasitised erythrocytes as mechanism of resistance against malaria in the sickle-cell trait. *Lancet.* 1970;1:319–321.
50. Ackerman HC, Ribas G, Jallow M, et al. Complex haplotypic structure of the central MHC region flanking TNF in a West African population. *Genes and Immun.* 2003;4:476–486.
51. Williams CD. Kwashiorkor: a nutritional disease of children associated with a maize diet. *Lancet.* 1935;229:1151–1152.
52. Gilles HM. The development of malarial infection in breast-fed Gambian infants. *Ann Trop Med Parasitol.* 1957;51:58–72.
53. Edington GM. Pathology of malaria in West Africa. *British Medical Journal.* 1967;1:715–718.
54. Hendrickse RG. Interactions of nutrition and infection: experience in Nigeria. In: Wolstenholme GEW, O'Connor M, eds. *Nutrition and Infection. Ciba Foundation Study Group 31.* London, UK: J & A Churchill; 1967:98–111.
55. Caulfield LE, Richard SA, Black RE. Undernutrition as an underlying cause of malaria morbidity and mortality in children less than five years old. *Am J Trop Med Hyg.* 2004;71(suppl 2):55–63.
56. Smith AW, Hendrikse RG, Harrison C, Hayes RJ, Greenwood BM. The effects on malaria of treatment of iron-deficiency anaemia with oral iron in Gambian children. *Ann Trop Paediatr.* 1989;9:17–23.
57. Shankar AH, Stoltzfus RJ. A meta-analysis of controlled trials of iron supplementation to infants and children in malarious areas. 1998.
58. Shankar A, Genton B, Semba RD, et al. Vitamin A supplementation reduces morbidity due to *P. falciparum:* a randomized trial in preschool children in Papua New Guinea. 1998.
59. Shankar AH, Genton B, Baisor M, et al. The influence of zinc supplementation on morbidity due to *Plasmodium falciparum:* a randomized trial in preschool children in Papua New Guinea. *Am J Trop Med Hyg.* 2000;62:663–669.
60. Bates CJ, Evans PH, Dardenne M, et al. A trial of zinc-supplementation in young rural Gambian children. *Br J Nutr.* 1993;69:243–255.
61. Molineaux L. *Plasmodium falciparum* malaria: some epidemiological implications of parasite and host diversity. *Ann Trop Med Parasitol.* 1996;90:379–393.
62. Marsh K, English M, Crawley J, Peshu N. The pathogenesis of severe malaria in African children. *Ann Trop Med Parasitol.* 1996;90(4):396–402.
63. Warrell DA, Molyneux ME, Beales PF. Severe and complicated malaria. *Trans Roy Soc Trop Med Hyg.* 1990;84(suppl 2):1–65.
64. Slutsker L, Taylor TE, Wirima JJ, Steketee RW. In hospital morbidity and mortality due to malaria-associated severe anaemia in two areas of Malawi with different patterns of malaria infection. *Trans Roy Soc Trop Med Hyg.* 1994;88:548–551.
65. Alonso PL, Lindsay SW, Armstrong JRM, et al. The effect of insecticide-treated bed nets on mortality of Gambian children. *Lancet.* 1991;337:1499–1502.
66. Greenwood B, Marsh K, Snow R. Why do some African children develop severe malaria. *Parasitol Today.* 1991;7:277–281.

67. Marsh K, Forster D, Waruiru C, et al. Indicators of life-threatening malaria in African children. *N Engl J Med*. 1995;322:1399–1404.
68. Molyneux ME, Taylor TE, Wirima JJ, Borgstein A. Clinical features and prognostic indicators in pediatric cerebral malaria: a study of 131 comatose malarian children. *Quart J Med*. 1989;71:441–459.
69. Brewster DR, Kwiatkowski D, White NJ. Neurological sequelae of cerebral malaria in children. *Lancet*. 1990;336:1039–1043.
70. Greenwood BM, Greenwood AM, Bradley AK, et al. Comparison of two strategies for control of malaria within a primary health care programme in The Gambia. *Lancet*. 1988;1:1121–1127.
71. Alles HK, Mendis KN, Carter R. Malaria mortality rates in South Asia and in Africa: implications for malaria control. *Parasitol Today*. 1998;14:369–375.
72. Schellenberg D, Menendez C, Kahigwa E, et al. African children with malaria in an area of intense *Plasmodium falciparum* transmission: features on admission to the hospital and risk factors for death. *Am J Trop Med Hyg*. 1999;61:431–438.
73. Waller D, Krishna S, Crawley J, et al. Clinical features and outcome of severe malaria in Gambian children. *Clin Infect Dis*. 1995;21:577–587.
74. Imbert P, Gerardin P, Rogier C, et al. Severe falciparum malaria in children: a comparative study of 1990 and 2000 WHO criteria for clinical presentation, prognosis and intensive care in Dakar, Senegal. *Trans R Soc Trop Med Hyg*. 2002;96:278–281.
75. Mockenhaupt FP, Ehrhardt S, Burkhardt J, et al. Manifestation and outcome of severe malaria in children in northern Ghana. *Am J Trop Med Hyg*. 2004;71:167–172.
76. Modiano D, Sirima BS, Sawadogo A, Sanou I, Konaté A, Pagnoni F. Severe malaria in Burkina Faso: influence of age and transmission level on clinical presentation. *Am J Trop Med Hyg*. 1998;59:539–542.
77. WHO. Severe falciparum malaria. *Trans R Soc Med Hyg*. 2000;94(suppl 1):S1–S90.
78. McPherson GG, Warrell MJ, White NJ, Looareesuwan S, Warrell DA. Human cerebral malaria: a quantitative ultrastructural analysis of parasitized erythrocyte sequestration. *Amer J Path*. 1985;119:385–401.
79. Warrell D, Looareesuwan S, Warrell MJ, et al. Dexamethasone proves deleterious in cerebral malaria. *N Engl J Med*. 1982;306:313–319.
80. Marsh K, Snow RW. Host-parasite interaction and morbidity in malaria endemic areas. *Philos Trans R Soc Lond B Biol Sci*. 1997;352:1385–1394.
81. Waruiru CM, Newton CR, Forster D, et al. Epileptic seizures and malaria in Kenyan children. *Trans Roy Soc Trop Med Hyg*. 1996;90:152–155.
82. White NJ, Warrell DA, Chanthavanich P, et al. Severe hypoglycemia and hyperinsulinemia in falciparum malaria. *N Engl J Med*. 1983;309:61–66.
83. Taylor TE, Molyneux ME, Wirima JJ, Fletcher KA, Morris K. Blood glucose levels in Malawian children before and during the administration of intravenous quinine for severe falciparum malaria. *N Engl J Med*. 1988;319:1040–1047.
84. English M, Waruiru C, Amukoye E, et al. Deep breathing reflects acidosis and is associated with poor prognosis in children with severe malaria and respiratory distress. *J Trop Med Hyg*. 1996;55:521–524.
85. Marsh K. Malaria—a neglected disease? *Parasitology*. 1992;104(suppl):s53–s69.

86. Snow RW, De Azevedo IB, Lowe BS, et al. Severe childhood malaria in two areas of markedly different falciparum transmission in East Africa. *Acta Tropica.* 1994;57:289–300.
87. Snow RW, Marsh K. Will reducing *Plasmodium falciparum* transmission alter malaria mortality among African children? *Parasitol Today.* 1995;11:188–190.
88. Snow RW, Armstrong-Schellenbert JR, Peshu N, et al. Periodicity and space-time clustering of severe childhood malaria on the coast of Kenya. *Trans Roy Soc Trop Med Hyg.* 1993;87:386–390.
89. Armstrong Schellenberg JRM, Newell JN, Snow RW, et al. An analysis of the geographic distribution of severe malaria in children in the Kilifi District, Kenya. *Int J Epidemiol.* 1998;27:323–329.
90. Smith T, Genton B, Baea K, et al. Relationships between *Plasmodium falciparum* infection and morbidity in a highly endemic area. *Parasitology.* 1994;109:539–549.
91. Lines J, Armstrong JRM. For a few parasites more: inoculum size, vector control and strain-specific immunity to malaria. *Parasitol Today.* 1992;8:381.
92. Adiamah JH, Koram KA, Thomson MC, Lindsay SW, Todd SW, Greenwood BM. Entomological risk factors for severe malaria in a peri-urban area of The Gambia. *Ann Trop Med Parasitol.* 1993;87:491–500.
93. Alonso PL, Lindsay SW, Armstrong Schellenberg JR, et al. A malaria control trial using insecticide-treated bed nets and targeted chemoprophylaxis in a rural area of The Gambia, West Africa. 6. The impact of the interventions on mortality and morbidity from malaria. *Trans Roy Soc Trop Med Hyg.* 1993;87(suppl 2):37–44.
94. Rasheed FN, Bolmer JN, Dunn DT, Menendez C, et al. Suppressed peripheral and placental blood lymphoproliferative responses in first pregnancies: relevance to malaria. *Am J Trop Med Hyg.* 1993;48:154–160.
95. Brabin BJ, Rogerson SJ. *The Epidemiology and Outcomes of Maternal Malaria.* Taylor and Francis; 2001.
96. Brabin BJ. The risks and severity of malaria in pregnant women. *TDR/Applied Field Research in Malaria Reports, No. 1.* Geneva, Switzerland: World Health Organization; 1991.
97. Diagne N, Rogier C, Sokhna CS, Tall A, et al. Increased susceptibility to malaria during the early postpartum period. *N Engl J Med.* 2000;343:598–603.
98. Lindsay S, Ansell J, Selman C, Cox V, et al. Effect of pregnancy on exposure to malaria mosquitoes. *Lancet.* 2000;355:1972.
99. Nosten F, Rogerson SJ, Beeson JG, McGready R, Mutabingwa TK, Brabin B. Malaria in pregnancy and the endemicity spectrum: what can we learn? *Trends Parasitol.* 2004;20:425–432.
100. Menendez C, Fleming AF, Atfonso PL, et al. Malaria-related anaemia. *Parasitol Today.* 2000;16:469–476.
101. Shulman CE, et al. Malaria as a cause of severe anaemia in pregnancy. *Lancet.* 2002;360:494.
102. Brabin BJ. An analysis of malaria in pregnancy in Africa. *Bull WHO.* 1983;61:1005–1016.
103. Bulmer JN, Rasheed FN, Morrison L, et al. Placental malaria. I. Pathological classification. *Histopathology.* 1993;22:211–218.
104. Rogerson SJ, Pollina E, Getachew A, et al. Placental monocyte infiltrates in response to *Plasmodium falciparum* malaria infection and

their association with adverse pregnancy outcomes. *Am J Trop Med Hyg.* 2003;68:115–119.

105. McGregor IA. Epidemiology, malaria and pregnancy. *Am J Trop Med Hyg.* 1984;33:517–525.

106. Shulman CE, Marshall T, Dorman EK, et al. Malaria in pregnancy: adverse effects on haemoglobin levels and birthweight in primigravidae and multigravidae. *Trop Med Int Health.* 2001;6: 28–35.

107. Steketee RW, Nahlen BL, Parise ME, Menendez C. The burden of malaria in pregnancy in malaria-endemic areas. *Am J Trop Med Hyg.* 2001;64:28–35.

108. Kuile FO, Parise ME, Verhoeff FH, et al. The burden of co-infection with human immunodeficiency virus type 1 and malaria in pregnant women in sub-Saharan Africa. *Am J Trop Med Hyg.* 2004;71(2 suppl): 41–54.

109. Whitworth J, Morgan D, Quigley M, et al. Effect of HIV-1 and increasing immunosuppression on malaria parasitaemia and clinical episodes in adults in rural Uganda: a cohort study. *Lancet.* 2000;356:1051–1056.

110. Kublin JG, Patnaik P, Jere CS, et al. Effect of *Plasmodium falciparum* malaria on concentration of HIV-1-RNA in the blood of adults in rural Malawi: a prospective cohort study. *Lancet.* 2005;365:233–240.

111. Connolly MA, Gayer M, Ryan MJ, Salama P, Spiegel P, Heymann DL. Communicable diseases in complex emergencies: impact and challenges. *Lancet.* 2004;364:1974–1983.

112. Graham K, Mohammad N, Rehman H, et al. Insecticide-treated plastic tarpaulins for control of malaria vectors in refugee camps. *Med Vet Entomol.* 2002;16:404–408.

113. Oduntan SO. The health of Nigerian children of school age (6–15 years). *Ann Trop Med Parasitol.* 1974;68:129–143.

114. Winch PJ, Makemba AM, Kamazima SR, et al. Local terminology for febrile illnesses in Bagamoyo district, Tanzania and site impact on the design of a community-based malaria control programme. *Soc Sci Med.* 1996;42:1057–1067.

115. Tarimo DS, Lwihula GK, Minjas JNa, Bygbjerg IC. Mothers' perception and knowledge on childhood malaria in holoendemic Kibaha district, Tanzania: implications for malaria control and the IMCI strategy. *Trop Med Int Health.* 2000;5:179–184.

116. Murray CK, Bell D, Gasser RA, Wongsrichanalai C. Rapid diagnostic testing for malaria. *Trop Med Int Health.* 2003;8:875–883.

117. Moody A. Rapid diagnostic tests for malaria parasites. *Clin Microbiol Rev.* 2002;15:66–78.

118. de Monbrison F, Angei C, Staal A, Kaiser K, Picot S. Simultaneous identification of the four human *Plasmodium* species and quantification of *Plasmodium* DNA load in human blood by real-time polymerase chain reaction. *Trans R Soc Trop Med Hyg.* 2003;97: 387–390.

119. Snounou G, Beck H-P. The use of PCR genotyping in the assessment of recrudescence or reinfection after antimalarial drug treatment. *Parasitol Today.* 1998;14:462–467.

120. Wernsdorfer WH. Epidemiology and drug resistance in malaria. *Acta Tropica.* 1994;56:143–156.

121. Bruce-Chwatt LJ, Black RH, Canfield CJ, Clyde DF, Peters W, Wernsdorfer WH. Chemotherapy of malaria. *WHO Monograph*

Series no. 27. 2nd rev. edn. ed. Geneva, Switzerland: World Health Organization; 1986.

122. White NJ. Antimalarial drug resistance. *J Clin Invest.* 2004;113: 1084–1092.

123. Wongsrichanalai C, Wernsdorfer WH, Meshnick SR. Epidemiology of drug-resistant malaria. *Lancet Infect Dis.* 2002;2: 209–218.

124. Noedl H, Wongsrichanalai C, Wernsdorfer WH. Malaria drug-sensitivity testing: new assays, new perspectives. *Trends Parasitol.* 2003;19: 175–181.

125. Krogstad DJ, Herwaldt BL. Chemopro-phylaxis and treatment of malaria. *N Engl J Med.* 1988;319:1538.

126. Reed MB, Saliba KJ, Caruana SR, Kirk K, Cowman AF. Pgh1 modulates sensitivity and resistance to multiple antimalarials in *Plasmodium falciparum. Nature.* 2000;403:906–909.

127. Djimde A, Doumbo OK, Cortese JF, et al. A molecular marker for chloroquine-resistant falciparum malaria. *N Engl J Med.* 2001;344:299–302.

128. Thaithong S, Beale GH, Fenton B, et al. Clonal diversity in a single isolate of the malaria parasite *Plasmodium falciparum. Trans Roy Soc Trop Med Hyg.* 1984;78:242–245.

129. Maberti S. Desarollo de resistencia a la pirimetamima. Presentacion de 15 casos estudiados en Trujillo. *Med Trop Paras Med.* 1960;3: 239–259.

130. Harinasuta T, Migasen S, Boonag D. UNESCO 1st Regional Symposium on Scientific Knowledge of Tropical Parasites. November 5–9, 1962. University of Singapore.

131. Krogstad DJ. Malaria as a reemerging disease. *Epidemiol Rev.* 1996;18:77–79.

132. Campbell CC, Collins WE, Chin W, Teutsch SM, Moss DM. Chloroquine-resistant *Plasmodium falciparum* from East Africa. *Lancet.* 1979;2:1151–1154.

133. Wootton JC, Feng X, Ferdig MT, et al. Genetic diversity and chloroquine selective sweeps in *Plasmodium falciparum. Nature.* 2002;418:320–323.

134. Wellems TE, Plowe CV. Chloroquine-resistant malaria. *J Infect Dis.* 2001;184:770–776.

135. Roper C, Pearce R, Nair S, Sharp B, Nosten F, Anderson T. Intercontinental spread of pyrimethamine-resistant malaria. *Science.* 2004;305:1124.

136. Hastings IM. Malaria control and the evolution of drug resistance: an intriguing link. *Trends Parasitol.* 2003;2:70–73.

137. Mharakurwa S. *Plasmodium falciparum* transmission rate and selection for drug resistance: a vexed association or a key to successful control? *Int J Parasitol.* 2004;34:1483–1487.

138. Dye C, Williams BG. Multigenic drug resistance among inbred malaria parasites. *Proc R Soc Lond B Biol Sci.* 1997;264:61–67.

139. Mharakurwa S, Mutambu SL, Mudyiradima R, Chimbadzwa T, Chandiwana SK, Day KP. Association of house spraying with suppressed levels of drug resistance in Zimbabwe. *Malar J.* 2004; 3:35.

140. McGregor IA, Carington SP, Cohen S. Treatment of East African *P. falciparum* malaria with West African human gammaglobulin. *Trans Roy Soc Trop Med Hyg.* 1963;57:170–175.

141. Clyde DF, McCarthy VC, Miller RM, Woodward WE. Immunization of man against falciparum and vivax malaria by use of attenuated sporozoites. *Am J Trop Med Hyg.* 1975;24:397–401.

142. Clyde DF, Most H, McCarthy VC, Vanderberg JP. Immunization of man against sporozoite-induced falciparum malaria. *Am J Med Sci.* 1973;266:169–177.

143. Nussenzweig R, Vanderberg J, Most H, Orton C. Protective immunity induced by the injection of X-irradiated sporosoites of *Plasmodium berghei. Nature.* 1967;216:160–162.

144. Alonso PL, Sacarlal J, Aponte JJ, et al. Efficacy of the RTS,S/AS02A vaccine against *Plasmodium falciparum* infection and disease in young African children: randomised controlled trial. *Lancet.* 2004;364:1411–1420.

145. Luke TC, Hoffman SL. Rationale and plans for developing a non-replicating, metabolically active, radiation-attenuated *Plasmodium falciparum* sporozoite vaccine. *J Exp Biol.* 2003;206:3803–3808.

146. Mueller AK, Labaied M, Kappe SH, Matuschewski K. Genetically modified *Plasmodium* parasites as a protective experimental malaria vaccine. *Nature.* 2005;433:164–167.

147. Gratepanche S, Gamain B, Smith JD, Robinson BA, Saul A, Miller LH. Induction of crossreactive antibodies against the *Plasmodium falciparum* variant protein. *Proc Natl Acad Sci.* 2003;100:13007–13012.

148. Graves P, Gelband H. Vaccines for preventing malaria. *Cochrane Database Syst Rev.* 2000;(2):CD000129.

149. Ballou WR, Arevalo-Herrera M, Carucci D, et al. Update on the clinical development of candidate malaria vaccines. *Am J Trop Med Hyg.* 2004;71(suppl 2):239–247.

150. Binka F, Kubaje A, Adjuik M, et al. Impact of permethrin impregnated bednets on child mortality in Kassena-Nankana district, Ghana: a randomized controlled trial. *Trop Med Int Health.* 1996;1:147–154.

151. Habluetzel A, Diallo DA, Esposito F, et al. Do insecticide-treated curtains reduce all-cause child mortality in Burkina Faso? *Trop Med Int Health.* 1997;2:855–862.

152. Nevill C, Some E, Mung'ala V, et al. Insecticide-treated bednets reduce mortality and severe morbidity from malaria among children on the Kenyan coast. *Trop Med Int Health.* 1996;1:139–146.

153. D'Alessandro U, Olaleye BO, McGuire W, et al. Mortality and morbidity from malaria in Gambian children after introduction of an impregnated bed-net programme. *Lancet.* 1995;345:479–483.

154. D'Alessandro U, Olaleye B, Langerock P, et al. The Gambian National Impregnated Bed Net Programme: evaluation of effectiveness by means of case-control studies. *Trans Roy Soc Trop Med Hyg.* 1997;91:638–642.

155. Roll Back Malaria Cabinet Project. The African Summit on Roll Back Malaria, Abuja, Nigeria. 2000.

156. Nahlen BL, Clark JP, Alnwick D. Insecticide-treated bed nets. *Am J Trop Med Hyg.* 2003;68(suppl 4):1–2.

157. Hawley WA, Ter Kuile FO, Steketee RS, et al. Implications of the western Kenya permethrin-treated bed net study for policy, program implementation, and future research. *Am J Trop Med Hyg.* 2003;68(suppl 4):168–173.

158. Buck AA, ed. *Proceeding of the Conference on Malaria in Africa: Practical Considerations on Malaria Vaccines and Clinical Trials.* Washington, DC: American Institute of Biological Sciences; 1986.

159. Gove S. Integrated management of childhood illness by outpatient health workers: technical basis and overview. For the WHO Working Group on Guidelines for Integrated Management of the Sick Child. *Bull WHO.* 1997:7–24.

160. Kidane G, Morrow RH. Teaching mothers to provide home treatment of malaria in Tigray, Ethiopia: a randomized trial. *Lancet.* 2000;356: 550–555.

161. Schellenberg D, Menendez C, Kahigwa E, et al. Intermittent treatment for malaria and anaemia control at time of routine vaccinations in Tanzanian infants: a randomised, placebo-controlled trial. *Lancet.* 2001:1471–1477.

162. Massaga JJ, Kitua AY, Lemnge MM, et al. Effect of intermittent treatment with amodiaquine on anaemia and malarial fevers in infants in Tanzania: a randomised placebo-controlled trial. *Lancet.* 2003;361:1853–1860.

163. Rosen JB, Breman JG. Malaria intermittent preventive treatment in infants, chemoprophylaxis, and childhood vaccinations. *Lancet.* 2004;363:1386–1388.

164. Kruger C. Malaria intermittent preventive treatment and EPI coverage. *Lancet.* 2004;363:2000–2001.

165. Cassels A. *A Guide to Sector-Wide Approaches for Health Development.* Geneva, Switzerland: World Health Organization; 1997.

166. Ad Hoc Committee on Health Research Relating to Future Intervention Options. *Investing in Health Research and Development.* Geneva, Switzerland: World Health Organization; 1996.

167. Ito J, Ghosh A, Moreira LA, Wimmer EA, M J-L. Transgenic anopheline mosquites impaired in transmission of a malaria parasite. *Nature.* 2002;417:452–455.

168. Riehle MA, Srinivasan P, Moreira CK, Jacobs-Lorena M. Toward genetic manipulation of wild mosquito populations to combat malaria: advances and challenges. *J Exp Biol.* 2003;206:3809–3816.

CHAPTER TWENTY-SEVEN

EPIDEMIOLOGY OF HELMINTH INFECTIONS

Clive Shiff

Introduction

Parasitism is a way of life. Over evolutionary time the niche by which one species depends on another for subsistence has been elaborated in countless ways. Not only have parasitic species developed a means to adapt to existence in the gut, tissues, and within the cells of their hosts, these species also have evolved mechanisms to distribute their progeny so that they can readily find and be taken up by a new host. Parasites have adopted a variety of forms, some of which may appear grotesque. They have evolved stratagems to evade the immune defenses of their hosts, and they have coevolved with their hosts to the extent that they adapt to the behavior patterns of normal life and exploit these to enable them to migrate to other sources of hosts. All of these factors influence in some way the epidemiology of parasitic infections.

Transmission and acquisition of parasites by any naive host involve three factors: a source of infection or reservoir must be present from which the parental generation of the parasite radiates, a means of transmission must exist by which the parasite gains access to the host, and a susceptible host must be available. As these factors bear directly on the severity of parasitic infections and their importance in the communities of humans, they must be considered in any study on the epidemiology, health impact, and control of the infections. Parasites have evolved numerous strategies to be successful within their various hosts, but transmission essentially involves two types of cycle. The first is the *direct cycle* where transmission is from person to person, usually through fecal waste in the environment. The second is the *indirect cycle,* which involves additional hosts or vectors that actively transfer the parasite from one host to another.

To demonstrate the complexity of this process, one example of each cycle will be discussed in detail. The direct cycle will be explained through consideration of the life cycle and epidemiology of hookworms. The indirect cycle will consider the complex epidemiology of schistosomes. The hookworms

1139

affecting humans belong to two species of nematode parasites, which produce similar infections, but because they are difficult to differentiate clinically and epidemiologically they usually are considered together. Transmission of these parasites depends on fecal contamination of the environment, absence of acceptable latrines, and a bare foot lifestyle. The schistosome parasite is a blood-dwelling trematode that has a complex life cycle involving living in freshwater molluscs as well as the blood stream of its definitive host. The parasite has coevolved in tandem with its aquatic and human hosts, producing a well-balanced association. However, the recent settling of human populations, with their need for water and their changing agricultural activities, as well as the burgeoning expansion of these human populations, has increased the transmission of the parasite and, thus, has produced severe and debilitating infections. Therefore, overt disease caused by these parasites often results when the ecological balances, to which the various populations have been adapted, have become unstable or have broken down, resulting in increasingly severe levels of infection.

Hookworm Parasites of Humans

Hookworms belong to the phylum Nematoda. Nematodes are tubular animals, diecious, with a definite body cavity in which the various organs are suspended. The gut is tubular, commencing in a complex oral region where the mouth and pharynx may have cutting teeth or plates, and the pharynx may be adapted for sucking and ingesting food. The body is covered with an outer cuticle, which is a complex structure consisting of several layers and which serves as a protective cover for the worms. The parasites are equipped only with longitudinal muscles, which accounts for the sinuous movements characteristic of the group. In parasitic nematodes the female is usually larger and packed with large ovaries and uterus. The males may exhibit complex external copulatory structures, which are characteristic of some species and which are used in identification. Eggs, which are usually characteristic for each species, are laid in large numbers; they may be embryonated or contain developing larvae. Usually the larval development takes several days and a first-stage larva (L1) emerges. This stage is able to ingest food and will proceed through two molts to reach the L3 stage, which in hookworms is infective; at this point larvae can no longer ingest food. The infective L3 larva (called the *filariform* stage) is able to attach to and penetrate the skin of the next host by using proteolytic enzymes secreted in the apical area of the worm. Altogether, four larval molts occur before the adult develops, and it is always the third-stage larva that is infectious.

Life Cycle

Two species of hookworm are known to infect humans: *Ancylostoma duodenale* and *Necator americanus*. The life cycles of these two parasites are similar and, thus, will be discussed together (Figure 27-1). Embryonated eggs are passed in the feces of an infected person. In a suitable environment, one that is shady or dark, moist, and warm (22°C to 32°C), the eggs will hatch within 24 to 48 hours, releasing first-stage larvae. These are not infective; they can

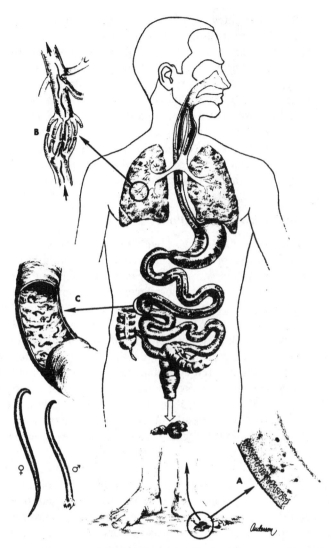

FIGURE 27-1 Life cycle of the hookworm. Filariform larvae in the soil penetrate the skin (A), are carried via the circulation to the lungs where they break out of the capillary bed into the alveolar spaces (B), then are swept up the bronchial tree, are swallowed, and become adult worms in the small intestine (C).
Source: Reprinted with permission from Beck & Davis, *Medical Parasitology*, 3rd edition, p. 150, © 1981, W.B. Saunders Company.

ingest food, and will soon molt into second-stage larvae after about 3 days. A second molt occurs after about 6 days, and the resulting third-stage larva is infectious—at the filariform stage. These larvae are unable to feed; however, under ideal conditions, they can survive and remain infectious for several weeks. Larvae invade by penetrating the skin between the toes or through the feet or ankles. However, they can also be transmitted through eating or handling unwashed, contaminated vegetables. Evidence also suggests that *A. duodenale* can be transmitted to suckling infants through milk. The filariform larvae secrete proteolytic enzymes that facilitate the penetration through the skin; they then enter the blood circulation and usually molt once more as they pass through the lungs. From the alveolar spaces, the larvae are coughed up in sputum, are swallowed, and thus gain entry to the human gut. The worms then reach the intestine where, as adults, they mate. They adhere to and lacerate the intestinal mucosa with their strong oral plates or teeth. They pump blood into the gut by means of the powerful muscular pharynx, and can continue to flush their gut with a stream of blood from the intestinal vessels they have penetrated. Thus, apart from consuming blood as a source of food, the parasites also cause considerable amounts of blood to be lost and voided in the feces of the host. Egg production commences 4 to 8 weeks after the initial infection, and the worms can live approximately 3 years.

Epidemiology of Hookworm Infections

Hookworm infection is a worldwide problem that is most prevalent in warm, humid areas or environments. It is commonly found in the tropics, although it is also common in warm, wet areas of the temperate zones; it is frequently associated with anemia in the affected populations.

Vulnerable populations are children, pregnant or lactating women, or women who menstruate heavily. The prevalence of geohelminth infections is age related, possibly because of immunological factors or specific activities or behavior patterns related to age. The prevalence of hookworm is found to be lower among children aged under 5 years, and it gradually increases with age; by age 8 years, a marked increase in prevalence occurs, which diminishes in later life. A clustering of infections is seen in certain children: evidence shows that heavily or lightly infected children have a statistical predisposition to acquire similar infection intensities following deworming procedures if patterns of exposure have not changed.

The highest prevalence of hookworm infection is found in males, teenagers, and young adults, which may be related to occupational hazards. For example, tending crops such as in rice paddies where one must stand in the fields for many hours increases the exposure to hookworm and the likelihood of becoming infected. Other risk factors are associated with the extent of outdoor defecation, presence of defecation fields, and the type of soil, which should be loose and hold moisture well, thus providing a refuge for the infective larvae. Poor standard of living and sanitation are the major determinants of hookworm prevalence. Infection is usually higher in rural areas than in urban areas, and higher in people low on the socioeconomic scale. In parts of Europe and North America where hookworm was previously common, the infections have been all but eradicated because of improved access to effective sanitation and improved living conditions, including the wearing of shoes. Figure 27-2 shows a photograph of *Ancylostoma duodenale*.

Control Measures

No prophylactic drugs are available for hookworm infections, although iron therapy is useful in preventing serious nutritional depletion, especially in women and children. Mebendazole is often used to treat both hookworm and other geohelminth infections. Mass chemotherapy is effective in reducing the prevalence of all geohelminths, but the effects are short lived if no

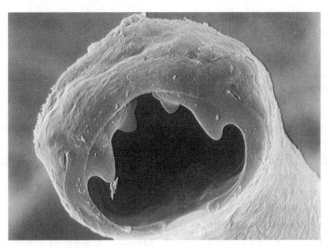

FIGURE 27-2   Photograph of *Ancylostoma duodenale*.
Source: Courtesy of Dr. G. Schad.

improvements are made in sanitation and health education. Considerable lack of knowledge exists about the transmission of intestinal parasites in many parts of the world. A study of mothers in urban slums in Sri Lanka demonstrated that 42% of mothers thought that parasites were acquired through eating sweets, 25% thought that they were transmitted through other children, and 25% did not know. None were aware of the relationship between contamination of soil with feces and transmission of the worms.[1] Kendall et al also mention that some societies consider worms to be normal symbiotes of the gut, which when mistreated (e.g., during a period of starvation or low food intake) can cause illness such as diarrhea.[2]

One of the best protective measures an individual can take is wearing adequate footwear. This reduces the risk of infection, especially if worn in latrines, in the vicinity of human habitation, and during agricultural work. The appropriate use and maintenance of latrines also makes a difference. Hookworm eggs and larvae do not survive more than 1 or 2 months in soil, even under ideal conditions. Use of latrines helps reduce contamination of soil with the parasite, and, therefore, this use also reduces transmission. Additionally, reducing the use of night soil as a fertilizer helps prevent the contamination of vegetables with parasites. Measures that can be used to prevent the transmission of all geohelminths include cleaning up stools of infants too young to use latrines; personal hygiene and care in preparing food, especially vegetables; the use of adequate footwear; and public education in elementary sanitation. During the past decade there has been an international initiative to reduce the global burden of geohelminths by attacking the reservoir of infection that mainly exists in children living in endemic areas. This is being done by mass treatment operations directed at school-age children.[3] If sustained it will likely have a significant impact on the prevalence of a wide range of parasites,[4,5] although the long-term effects of such interventions may have unforeseen effects, as there is some evidence that children infected with geohelminth parasites may have reduced risk of atopy.[6] Are there implications that the immune responses that protect against parasites have an unforeseen advantage to people that we might lose when we reach such Utopian conditions?

Schistosome Parasites in Humans

Three important species of schistosomes infect humans, with an additional two that occur in restricted areas. *Schistosoma haematobium* occurs primarily in Africa with extensions in the Middle East and western Asia. This species lives in the vesicular veins and capillaries of the bladder mucosa and causes the condition known as urinary schistosomiasis (bilharzia). *Schistosoma mansoni* occurs primarily in Africa, but also in the northern parts of South America (Brazil) and the Caribbean. Adults of this species normally live in the capillaries that drain the mesenteries; also sometimes found in the liver sinuses, they can produce the condition known as intestinal schistosomiasis (also known as intestinal bilharzia). *Schistosoma japonicum* occurs mainly in China and parts of Southeast Asia, particularly in the Philippines. This species, which occupies the same region of the body as *S. mansoni*, is a more virulent form of the parasite, and it frequently produces severe sequelae. The other species are *S. meekongi*, which is related to *S. japonicum,* found in Vietnam and adjoining territories, and *S. intercalatum*, which is related to *S. haematobium,* found in Cameroon and parts of West Africa. Because of their reliance on freshwater snails as aquatic intermediate hosts, the entire distribution of these parasites is associated with water resources in which the appropriate snail species are found.

Life Cycle

Adult schistosomes differ from typical trematode worms in their narrow, elongate shape and separate sexes. The male is the larger of the two, approximately 1.0 to 1.5 cm in length, with a cylindrical body folded to form a ventral gynecophoric canal in which the longer, slender female is embraced for most of the time. Both worms have two suckers, an oral sucker surrounding the mouth and a ventral sucker or acetabulum. The mouth leads into a blind gut that bifurcates along most of the length of the body. In the female, this is dark with hematin derived from the digestion of blood cells. The number of testes in the male, the length of the uterus in the female, and the shape of the eggs are distinctive to the species.

Eggs are deposited in the fine capillaries of the organ where the worms are living. In vesicular schistosomiasis, this is the bladder; in the intestinal form, this is the intestinal mucosa. The eggs break through into the lumen of the bladder or gut, usually with a small amount of bleeding, and are passed to the exterior in the urine or feces. Many eggs do not break through the mucosa and remain in the tissue or are flushed into the liver where they form a nidus for granulomata to develop. In severe infections, these granulomata damage the affected organ. In some cases of ectopic egg deposition, severe long-term paraplegia can occur when the base of the spinal cord is involved. There is a considerable amount of inflammation associated with the eggs while they are occluded in tissue. With *S. haematobium* this can be associated with onset of bladder cancer in adults.

If schistosome eggs are deposited in freshwater, or in a place where they can be soon washed into the water, the cycle continues. The eggs hatch and a free-living, ciliated form, the miracidium, emerges. These miracidia use a number of environmental cues to seek out appropriate intermediate host snails. Miracidia move quite rapidly and can cover great distances in their search for snails. In some recent studies in Egypt, *S. mansoni* miracidia were shown commonly to infect snails 5 to 6 m distant, and some infected snails more than 20 m distant. The association is specific, and so only the correct species of mollusk will sustain the infection. The miracidia do not ingest food and so have an infective life limited to approximately 5 to 6 hours. During this time, they must find the appropriate snail. The miracidium attaches to the snail and secreting proteolytic enzymes penetrate into the tissues of the snail. The parasite then commences a process of asexual development. The miracidium enlarges into a mother sporocyst, a saclike organism that later buds off additional daughter sporocysts from layers of germinal epithelium. These daughter sporocysts migrate to the digestive gland of the snail where they grow and finally produce copious numbers of the next larval stage, the cercaria.

Cercariae emerge from infected snails in response to sunlight after a prepatent period of about 30 days, although this could be much longer in cool weather. Cercariae normally emerge around midmorning, and continue emerging from the snails throughout the day, although by afternoon the numbers soon decline. The cercariae are furcocercous (Figure 27-3) and move by vibrating the forked tail. Their main movement is up and down, vertical rather than horizontal, and their target is the skin of a nearby human being. They respond to appropriate skin lipids that stimulate the process of penetration, a process that must occur within 6 to 12 hours after emergence, as cercariae, too, have no means to ingest nutrients. When they commence penetration, cercariae secrete proteolytic enzymes, bore through the skin of the victim, then shed the tail, and, by contortions, penetrate into the subdermis, invade the lymphatic system, and move via the circulatory system to the lungs. In the lungs, the developing form, known as the schistosomulum, remains for a few days before continuing in the circulatory system to the liver. In the liver, the schistosomula mature into adult worms and move to the end organ system in pairs.

Epidemiology of Schistosomiasis

Reservoir of the Parasite Population

Of the various important species of schistosome that affect human populations, *S. haematobium* and *S. mansoni* are primarily anthropophilic. The reservoir is almost entirely confined to humans, although occasional episodes of transmission have been ascribed to other primates. With *S. intercalatum*, the picture is unclear; however, with *S. japonicum* and related species, the parasites are found in a wide range of animals as well as the human population. The source of the reservoir fundamentally affects the epidemiology of schistosomiasis and will have an impact on attempts to control the disease.

As with most other parasitic infections, schistosomes are overdispersed or aggregated in the human population. That is, many hosts harbor few

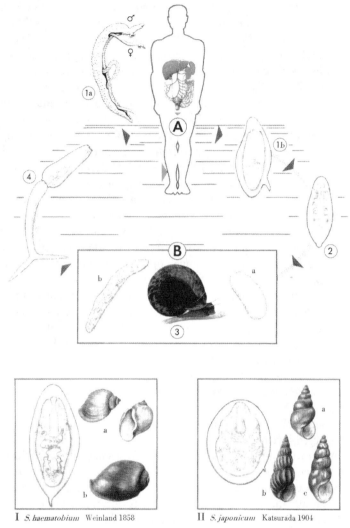

FIGURE 27-3 Illustration of the schistosomes, miracidia, and cercariae life cycles.
Source: G. Pierkarski, *Medical Parasitology*, translation of *Medizinische Parasitologie in Tafeln*, 3, Aulage, © 1987, Springer-Verlag New York, Inc.

parasites, whereas a few hosts harbor many parasites with the distribution fitting the negative binomial. This aggregated distribution has been ascribed to numerous factors: the degree of individual susceptibility, patterns of exposure to transmission foci, age difference in susceptibility, and the development of acquired resistance to further infection. Each of these factors should be considered in the epidemiology of schistosomiasis.

Age Prevalence of Schistosomiasis

Examination of the prevalence of *Schistosoma* infection in any population living in an endemic region will show a typical distribution (Figure 27-4). The proportion of infected persons increases with age to a peak in childhood

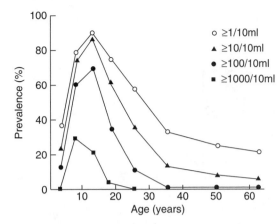

FIGURE 27-4 Prevalence and distribution of *Schistosome haematobium* egg output in relation to age in a Gambian community.
Source: H.A. Wilkens et al, The Significance of Proteinuria and Haematuria in Schistosoma Haematobium Infection, *Transactions of the Royal Society of Tropical Medicine and Hygiene*, Vol. 73, p. 75, © 1979, Royal Society of Tropical Medicine and Hygiene.

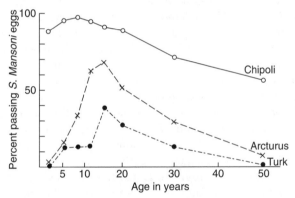

FIGURE 27-5 Prevalence of *Schistosome haematobium* infections in relation to age in three communities of Zimbabwe.
Source: V. de V. Clarke, The Influence of Acquired Resistance in the Epidemiology of Bilharziases, *Central African Journal of Medicine*, Vol. 12, No. 6, Supplement, p. 9, © 1966, Central African Journal of Medicine.

and adolescence. After the early 20s, age prevalence declines, and in adult life it remains about one third as high as at the peak until old age when it declines further. The peak seen in these age prevalence curves is a factor of the endemicity or transmission rate (incidence) of infection, as can be seen in Figures 27-5 and 27-6, which show the pattern of infection in three regions of Zimbabwe wherein a high, medium, or low level of transmission occurs. These data clearly show how prevalence in the community is age specific and that it is strongly influenced by the transmission rate, which itself is a function of the amount of surface water in the area and the extent of human contact with the water.

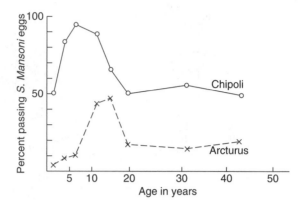

FIGURE 27-6 Prevalence of *Schistosome haematobium* infections in relation to
age in two communities of Zimbabwe.
Source: V. de V. Clarke, The Influence of Acquired Resistance in the
Epidemiology of Bilharziases, *Central African Journal of Medicine*, Vol. 12, No. 6,
Supplement, p. 9, © 1966, Central African Journal of Medicine.

Schistosomes are long-lived parasites. Estimations based on die-off of
infections under conditions where snail control operations were carried out
suggest a mean life of 5 to 6 years; in numerous instances, however, parasites
have been found to live several decades. The decline in the level of infection
seen in adults living in endemic areas may be related to acquired resistance
induced by the current infection. This is a condition known as premunition,
or acquisition of immunity in people subjected to infection by this parasite.
Certainly, antibodies are produced by people, even those who no longer show
evidence of infection by passage of parasite eggs in the excreta. Furthermore,
treatment of the infection does not appear to annul this protection, and the
rate of acquisition of new infections among recently treated people, although
high in children, declines abruptly in older children and adults (Figure 27-
7). Recently, it has been suggested that the onset of puberty and the sexual
maturation of the human host affect the ability of the parasite to survive
invasion of the adult host. Numerous studies on human behavior and water
contact have failed to show that this decline in prevalence in adults is a function of decreased water contact with age. However, when naive adults become
infected with schistosomes, acute sequelae develop rapidly, which suggests
that sexual maturity plays little role in acquisition of infection.

Compiling of age prevalence curves of schistosome infection is necessary
to determine the public health impact of the disease. Overall figures taken
from a community as a whole might mask the severe impact the disease has
on children. Furthermore, one must have some indication about the intensity
(severity) of the infection. This can be obtained by estimating the intensity of
infection or the associated worm burden. Actually, it is not possible to get an
approximation of the number of worms infecting a patient; however, if the
number of eggs passed in urine or feces is counted and expressed as a rate
per 10 mL urine or gram of feces, then it is possible to predict where and in
whom the most serious pathology may develop. Also, these estimates provide
a good indication of the extent of the reservoir for the next generation of
parasites. Egg burden in relation to age is clearly shown in Figure 27-7. In

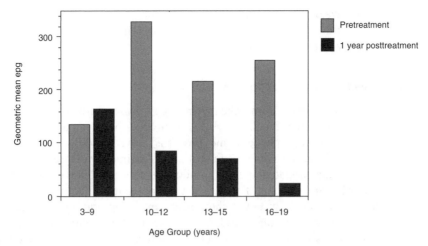

FIGURE 27-7 Geometric mean intensities of reinfection by age, one year after treatment of children in a high-transmission area (Mbugua et al in preparation). *Source:* Reprinted with permission from Butterworth et al, Immunity and Morbidity in Human Schistosomiasis, in *New Strategies in Parasitology*, K.P.W.J. McAdam, ed., p. 201, © W.B. Saunders Company.

an intensive study in Zimbabwe, Clarke translated this feature into a parameter he called the "infection potential."[7] He showed that in high endemic areas, between 82% to 92% of *S. haematobium* eggs passed in a community were from children aged less than 12 years. The pattern with *S. mansoni* was similar, although in areas of lower prevalence, the egg load appeared to be more evenly distributed in the population. Studies in the Philippines and China indicated that age-related egg passage does not follow changes in prevalence as consistently as in *S. haematobium*.[8]

Transmission and the Role of the Intermediate Host

Knowing about the distribution of the intermediate host snails is a key to understanding the epidemiology of schistosomiasis. In all instances, the snails involved are freshwater gastropod mollusks; they are entirely aquatic, although they can survive dry periods in small number within mud refuges. They belong to the family Planorbidae and the genera *Biomphalaria* (which transmit *S. mansoni*) and *Bulinus* (which transmits *S. haematobium*). In the *S. japonicum* cycle, the snails are prosobranchs, which have an operculum to close the main aperture of the snail; thus, they are amphibious and can survive periods of dryness and spend part of their life out of water. These snails are pioneering species with rapid rates of reproduction, and they can reach huge numbers when conditions are ideal. They are detritus feeders and, hence, in their environment are seldom restricted by shortages of food. Although certain predacious animals consume snails, under natural conditions the predators have little impact on the snail populations. Snails are cold-blooded and reproduce more rapidly in summer than in winter. They lay eggs in small batches on plant surfaces, stones, or other objects, even plastic sheets floating in the water. Each snail can produce several hundred eggs a week. These eggs will hatch in about 7 days, and the emerging snails will mature in about 6 weeks. Snails surviving dry periods can repopulate ponds within a short time.

Factors Affecting Snail Infection Rates

Miracidia emerge from schistosome eggs passed into water, and they will detect and infect snails nearby. The process of development in the snails is temperature dependent and proceeds more rapidly in warmer weather. In Zimbabwe, it has been shown that the rising temperatures of spring will shorten the prepatent period, producing a heavy load of cercariae in the water in early summer. Patterns of snail population fluctuation and presence of infected snails in Egypt show peaks in spring and again in autumn. The intense heat of summer and the cold in winter negatively affect the snail populations as well as the number of infected snails. These factors produce a seasonal pattern to the risk of infection in endemic areas.[9]

The Susceptible Human

Transmission of schistosomes requires contact of a susceptible host with cercariae-infested water. Such contact with water can involve ritual ablution, domestic chores, agricultural activities, gardening, or fishing, or even recreation and bathing. Occasionally an infection will occur from casual contact with water, even if the host is unaware of the contact. In most endemic areas, however, water contact is regular and systematic and part of a daily routine of life that entails a sustained exposure to the water and the risk of acquiring an infection when cercariae are present. It may be assumed that the longer the duration of contact, the heavier will be the worm burden, but this is not always the case because as people get older, the likelihood of reinfection diminishes, as discussed. The actual incidence of infection in a community is difficult to assess because in an endemic area a large proportion of the people will be infected, and it is hard to assess acquisition of new infections. It is possible to treat a cohort of people and reexamine them after a period of time to assess the number of reacquired cases. However, because a strong immune response militates against reinfection, measurement of incidence in this way can only be done in young children who are still susceptible to reinfection. Recently, it has been shown that a circulating antigen can be detected in active cases, and this may make further epidemiologic studies easier to carry out.[10]

Schistosomiasis in the Community

Schistosome parasites have evolved a well-adapted association with their human hosts. This association has probably developed over evolutionary time, particularly because of a nomadic lifestyle. However, with the more recent development of agriculture and settling of the human population in village communities, infection severity has increased, and the ill effects of the disease have become more noticeable. Where new dams have been constructed, where population movements have occurred bringing naive hosts into contact with the parasite, and where conditions have led to expansions of snail populations, the cycle of transmission has been exacerbated and the people have acquired disease. Thus, the public health problem of schistosomiasis is a product of perturbed ecological processes, and control of the disease needs to focus on reducing the increased contact between host, snail, and parasite. To do this, a careful consideration of all aspects of the complex life cycle and its various components must figure high in the development of control strategies.[11]

Review of Other Geohelminths

Worm Infections with Direct Life Cycles

A life cycle is considered direct when no intermediate host is involved and transmission is directly from one human host to another. The following species are transmitted directly, and they provide examples of direct cycles: *Strongyloides stercoralis*, *Trichuris trichiura*, *Ascaris lumbricoides*, and *Enterobius vermicularis*. Life cycles and brief notes on the epidemiology are discussed.

Strongyloidiasis

The life cycle of *Strongyloides stercoralis* is similar to that of hookworm with some important modifications. Both a free-living cycle and a parasitic cycle exist. In the free-living cycle, larvae are passed in the feces of infected people. In the presence of waterlogged soil and abundant feces, the larvae mature into *rhabditiform* males and females. These are a nonparasitic, noninfective form. With ideal conditions, the adults mate and produce several cycles of free-living worms; however, as food declines or the habitat desiccates, a filariform generation will develop, leading to a third stage—filariform larvae—which will remain on the fecal mass and penetrate through the skin of anyone contacting the larvae. The larvae circulate through the pulmonary alveolae, are coughed up, and migrate to the pharynx and finally to the intestine. They penetrate the mucosa in the duodenum and upper jejunum, molt twice, and become mature females in about 2 weeks. There are no parasitic males, so reproduction is parthenogenetic at this stage. The female is a delicate filariform worm 2 to 3 mm in length and 30 to 40 microns in width. Females produce an indeterminate number of embryonated eggs daily; these usually hatch in the mucosa, and the larvae escape in the feces. Autoinfection can occur if the emerging first-stage larvae molt twice internally and develop into the third filariform stage. These may reinvade the mucosa and proceed to reestablish a secondary infection. In immunocompromised hosts, this represents a severe stage of the infection.

With the advent of human immunodeficiency virus (HIV) infection and in cases of decreasing immunocompetence particularly associated with old age, cancer, or in patients receiving immunosuppressive drugs, strongyloidiasis has become increasingly important. In such people, dormant or new infections can disseminate and spread throughout the body. The infection is sporadic, particularly in communities where sanitation facilities are inadequate or defective.

Several species of *Strongyloides* occur in animals and the infection is known to be a zoonosis with reservoir populations in a variety of animals. This makes the infection difficult to control with chemotherapy alone. The best approach is treatment of positive cases together with emphasis on general use of latrines.

Trichuriasis (Human Whip Worm Infection)

Adults of *Trichuris trichiura* live attached to the wall of the cecum, and humans are the only source of infection. The adult worms have a large fleshy body and are attenuated in the anterior two thirds of the length, giving the picture of a whip. The mouth, at the distal end of the whip, is provided with a stylus, and it is connected to a thin, capillary-like esophagus. This thin portion of the worm is insinuated into the mucosa of the cecum and large bowel, and it anchors the worms in place. The presence of the worms causes irritation, probably as a result of the feeding process, which seems to involve tissue lysis by the parasite. The female is 35 to 50 mm in length with the male slightly smaller. Eggs are produced in situ and passed in the feces. These are characteristically barrel shaped and robust and are laid unembryonated. Development of the larvae takes about 3 weeks after which the eggs are infective. Eggs are not resistant to desiccation or bright sunlight. Transmission is most efficient in warm, humid, moist conditions, and infection results from swallowing infective eggs. In areas of high endemicity, small children seem most vulnerable, and they can develop heavy infections, which may be caused by geophagy. *Trichuris* does not respond well to treatment, probably because its favored habitat is the lower bowel, a site difficult to reach with active drugs.

Ascariasis

Ascariasis is caused by *Ascaris lumbricoides*, the large round worm of humans. This is one of the world's most ubiquitous parasites, and it has been recognized since ancient times. The adults, which are free living in the intestine, are very large; the female is 20 to 35 cm in length and 3 to 6 mm in diameter, and the male is slightly smaller. The severity of infection depends on the number of worms a patient carries; however, the worms produce prodigious amounts of eggs on a continuous basis—approximately 200,000 eggs per female can be passed in a daily stool. The eggs may be either fertile or infertile. Fertile eggs are encased in a thick shell consisting of three layers. The eggshell is remarkably stable and resistant to desiccation. It also prevents toxic substances from reaching the developing embryo. Thus, the eggs of *A. lumbricoides* can survive the rigors of sewage treatment and remain infective for many months, even years under ideal conditions.

The eggs produced are unembryonated and as such are not infective. A period of development and two molts take place in the egg prior to it becoming infective. This takes place by ingestion, either in fecally contaminated food or in water, or even inhaled through dust. The larvae emerge in the intestine and immediately penetrate the gut epithelium and circulate through the blood system to the lungs where they may remain for 9 to 15 days. They are then coughed up and swallowed and finally return to the gut. In 8 to 10 weeks, worms are mature; if males and females are present, the females will start to produce fertile eggs.

Pinworm

Pinworm is caused by *Enterobius vermicularis*, a cosmopolitan parasite more common in temperate climates than in warmer areas, when less frequent bathing and infrequent washing of underclothes occurs. The worms are small nematodes, the male being somewhat smaller (2 to 5 mm in length and not more that 0.2 mm wide) than the female (2 to 13 mm long and up to 0.5 mm in diameter). The worms live in the cecum, appendix, and adjacent areas of the ascending colon. They occupy the mucous layer between the mucosa and the fecal matter. The gravid female becomes distended and is packed with eggs. At this time, it migrates down the colon and out the anus. Normally, the eggs are deposited at one time, after which the female disintegrates. Eggs are not commonly laid in the bowel, although they are sometimes found in the feces. Usually, eggs are smeared over the perianal region and can best be seen and identified by the "Scotch tape" test. For this test, a 6-cm length of clear Scotch tape is placed over the anal area, pressed against the skin, and removed. The tape is then placed on a glass microscopic slide, with the tacky side to the glass. Eggs adhering to the adhesive can be seen by observing the glass slide under a low-power microscope.

The eggs are elongate-ovoidal, distinctly compressed laterally, and flattened on one side; they measure 50 to 60 by 20 to 30 microns. The shell is relatively thick and colorless. The eggs embryonate and become infective a few hours after being laid. They are robust and resistant to disinfectants and drying and may remain viable for up to 2 weeks. Eggs that are swallowed hatch when they reach the intestine, and the development to adult usually takes about 1 month.

The epidemiology is associated with contact between individuals usually living together or people who handle soiled clothing, particularly night clothes. Frequently, this occurs within families. Eggs are transferred from hand to mouth, particularly following scratching the perianal area after females have emerged and laid eggs, through inhalation of dust particles in bedrooms where an infected person may sleep, or similar person-to-person contact. Transmission is efficient and can lead to very severe infestations.

Control is a matter of treatment and prevention. As the eggs are resistant to disinfection, it is best to consider any contaminated area as infective for up to 2 weeks after treatment of any cases, and to maintain a high level of cleanliness and hygiene to prevent the cycle from restarting.

Examples of Worms with Indirect Cycles (Including a Vector-borne Stage)

The parasites with indirect cycles belong to a group (or superfamily) of nematode worms called the Filarioidea. They live in the tissues or body cavity of a mammalian host and are transmitted by the bite of an arthropod vector. The females produce microfilariae, which are unique in that they are less differentiated than the first-stage larvae of other nematodes. Highly motile and threadlike, they exist in the blood or subcutaneously in the mammalian host. The microfilariae in blood exhibit diurnal periodicity and are usually present in the peripheral circulation synchronized with the biting behavior of the insect vector. When taken up by an arthropod vector, they migrate through the gut wall into the hemocoel and then into the thoracic muscles of the insect. They proceed through two stages of development, finally reaching the third-stage larva (L3), which is infective and which invades a new mammalian host during the next blood meal. Seldom are more than two or three L3 forms found in one mosquito.

Bancroftian Filariasis (Elephantiasis)

Elephantiasis is a condition caused by one of two parasites, *Wuchereria bancrofti*, which is widespread in most tropical areas, and *Brugia malayi*, which is an important human parasite in Southeast Asia and the Pacific Islands. In most of their distribution, both species exhibit nocturnal periodicity, and microfilariae are in the peripheral circulation only at night.

The adults of these two species are threadlike and long; males are approximately 40 mm in length, whereas the females are approximately 100 mm in length. They are normally found coiled in lymph nodes in the inguinal region, although they can also occur in axillary nodes. Infiltration of plasma cells, macrophages, and eosinophils around the infected nodes occurs and eventually results in inflammation and swelling. In time the nodes become blocked and proximal lymphatic vessels become stenotic and obstructed, which leads to lymphedema and thickening of the subcutaneous tissue and eventually to elephantiasis. Approximately 8 to 12 months after an active infection is established, the worms become sexually mature and microfilariae appear in the blood and circulate in the peripheral blood according to the diurnal periodicity described above. It appears from experimental work with animal models that the microfilariae can live as long as 200 days.

The epidemiology is very much associated with the local distribution of mosquito vectors. However, as several genera of mosquito can transmit microfilariae, the endemic areas are extensive. Peridomestic breeding places for culicine mosquitoes are becoming increasingly important, particularly in urban areas. Infection occurs in young people; however, because the vectors carry small numbers of infective parasites, it normally takes many years before noticeable sequelae of the infection occur.

Control of the disease depends on reducing the number of breeding sites of the vectors, particularly those in close proximity to houses. In areas where sewage treatment is inadequate and wastewater is allowed to stand in pools, and where effluent from domestic water usage occurs, mosquito populations abound and present serious problems. Control by various methods, such as vector control, reduction of potential mosquito breeding sites, the use of insect repellents, and extensive chemotherapy needs to be implemented. It has recently been shown that use of the drug ivermectin will reduce considerably the level of microfilaraemia and, in this way, restrict the reservoir of infection. A combination of these various approaches will likely be successful in reducing the prevalence of both these parasites.[12]

Onchocerca volvulus

Onchocerca volvulus is associated with the condition known as river blindness. The adults live in subcutaneous nodules where they lie in tangled masses of male and female worms. They reproduce by producing unsheathed micro-filariae, which migrate through the skin intradermally. These forms are not found in the blood, but they frequently occur in the vitreous humor of the eye. The microfilariae are ingested during the process of feeding by blackflies (*Simulium* species), which breed in well-oxygenated, fast-flowing water, and are pests to people living near streams and rivers.

The microfilariae pass through two molts in the blackfly, and after about 6 to 8 days exist as L3 forms in the thoracic muscles of the fly; finally they migrate to the mouth parts of the fly. At the next blood meal, the larvae leave the fly and penetrate the wound caused during the feed. Once in the skin of a new host, the larvae migrate to various parts of the body, penetrate through the subcutaneous tissue, molt further, and finally mature into adults. The prepatent period in humans is 3 to 15 months. The parasites reside in nodules, which may be in the deep fascia or in subcutaneous tissue. They are frequently palpable and can be removed surgically. The onchocercal nodules usually cause no symptoms, although they can be somewhat deforming. The main problems from the infection come from the long-lived microfilariae in the skin and eye. In chronic infections, a progressive loss of subcutaneous connective tissue occurs and the skin becomes loose and depigmented. Dermatitis and infiltration by lymphocytes can occur, adding to the irritation and disfigurement of the host.

Severe ocular pathology is frequently associated with savannah oncho-cerciasis transmitted by blackflies of the *Simulium damnosum* species group. Transmission in the forest environment can be intense, and the prevalence of infection is high; however, blinding onchocerciasis is seen less frequently in people exposed to the forest dwelling species of blackflies.

The distribution of onchocerciasis is extensive in West and Central Africa and stretches into East Africa as far south as Malawi. It also exists in the Arabian peninsula, Yemen, Central America, and the northern part of South America. However, in the Americas, although ocular infiltration and damage occurs, little blindness is associated with the infection. To under-stand the epidemiology of onchocerciasis, it is important to know something about the vector. The blackfly belongs to the genus *Simulium*. Members of this genus, who are voracious blood feeders, are cosmopolitan in distribu-tion. Both males and females take blood, and they are worrisome nuisance pests associated with strong flowing water. Not all *Simulium* species carry *Onchocerca*. In Africa, the vectors belong to the *S. damnosum* complex and *S. neavei* group, whereas in South America, several anthropophilic species transmit the parasite.

The flies lay their eggs in water, preferably on rocks or emergent vegeta-tion washed with fast-flowing, usually well-oxygenated water. The larval and pupal forms of the insect live on firm substrates immersed in the water where they feed on plankton and suspended particles. The adult flies do not normally venture far from their breeding sites, hence transmission of this parasite is associated with rivers. In parts of Africa, prior to the major control efforts of the Onchocerciasis Control Programme, villages near rivers and the associated lands were abandoned by peasant farmers who feared the infection.

Control of the disease has been based on a two-front attack using both chemical control of the vector and treatment of the infection among humans. Because of their restricted breeding habits, blackflies can be controlled by treating the rivers with specially formulated insecticides. The insecticide is adsorbed on clay particles suspended in the fast-flowing water and is selectively toxic to filter-feeding insects. This has been done for the past 20 years in a large part of West Africa, and it has been successful in reducing both the blackfly population and the transmission of *O. volvulus*. More recently, a drug (ivermectin), which eliminates the microfilariae from the skin of infected people for up to a year, has been used to augment the vector control efforts. Together, this work has reduced morbidity and blindness in a large section of the West African population. Because the drug does not kill adult worms, treatment has to be repeated every 12 months; however, methods to overcome this drawback are being developed and some hope exists that the infection will decline in importance as a public health problem.[13]

References

1. De Silva NR, Chan MS, Bundy DA. Morbidity and mortality due to ascariasis: re-estimation and sensitivity analysis of global numbers at risk. *Trop Med Int Health*. 1997;2:519–528.
2. Kendall C, Foote D, Martorell R. Ethnomedicine and rehydration therapy: a case study of ethnomedical investigation and program planning. *Soc Sci Med*. 1984;19:253–260.
3. Booker S, Whawell S, Kabatereine NB, et al. Evaluating the epidemiological impact of national control programmes for helminths. *Trends Parasitol*. 2004;20:537–545.
4. Mani TR, Rajendran R, Muniranthanum A, et al. Efficacy of co-administration of albendazole and diethylcarbamazine against geohelminthiases. A study from South India. *Trop Med Int Health*. 2002;7:541–548.
5. De Rochars MB, Direny AN, Roberts JM, et al. Community-wide reduction in prevalence and intensity of intestinal helminths as a collateral benefit of lymphatic filariasis elimination programs. *Am J Trop Med Hyg*. 2004;71:466–470.
6. Cooper PJ, Chico ME, Rodrigues LC, et al. Reduced risk of atopy among school age children infected with geohelminth parasites in a rural area of the tropics. *J Allergy Clin Immunol*. 2003;111:995–1000.
7. Clarke V de V. The influence of acquired resistance in the epidemiology of bilharziasis. *Cent Afr J Med*. 1966;12(suppl 6):1–30.
8. Jordan P, Webbe G. Epidemiology. In: Jordan P, Webbe G, Sturrock RW, eds. *Human Schistosomiasis*. Oxford, UK: CAB International; 1993: 87–158.
9. Shiff CJ, Coutts WCC, Yiannakis C, et al. Seasonal patterns in the transmission of *Schistosoma haematobium* in Rhodesia. *Trans R Soc Trop Med Hyg*. 1974;73:375–380.
10. Ndhlovu P, Cadman H, Gunderson H, et al. Circulating anodic antigen levels in a Zimbabwe rural community endemic for *Schistosoma haematobium* using the magnetic beads antigen-capture enzyme linked immunoassay. *Am J Trop Med Hyg*. 1996;54:637–642.
11. Gryseels B. Human resistance to schistosome infections. *Parasitol Today*. 1994;10:380–384.
12. Nicholas L, Plichart C, Nguyen LN, Moulia-Pelat JP. Reduction of *Wucheraria bancrofti* adult worm circulating antigen after annual

treatments of dethylcarbamazine combined with ivermectin in French Polynesia. *J Infect Dis.* 1997;175:489–492.

13. Molyneux DH, Davies JB. Onchocerciasis control: moving towards the millennium. *Parasitol Today.* 1997;13:418–425.

INDEX

page numbers followed by *t, f, b, or e* denote tables, figures, boxes, or exhibits respectively

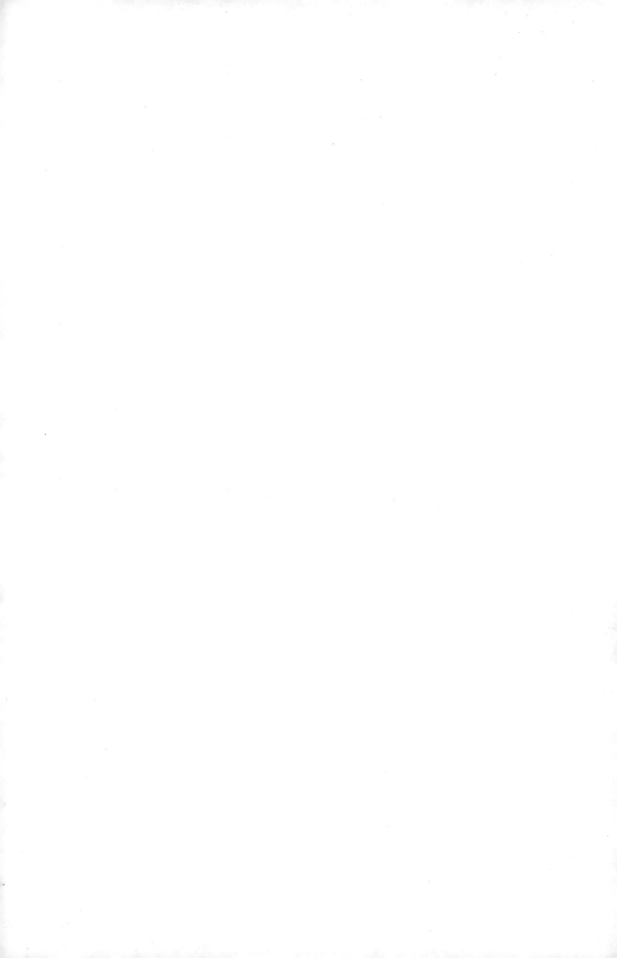